Scientific Foundations
of
Dentistry

Edited by

BERTRAM COHEN

D.D.S.(Rand), M.S.D.(Northwestern), F.D.S.R.C.S. Eng.,
F.D.S.R.C.S. Edin., F.F.D.R.C.S. Irel., F.R.C.Path.

*Nuffield Professor, Director of Department of Dental Science,
Royal College of Surgeons of England*

and

IVOR R. H. KRAMER

M.D.S.(London), F.D.S.R.C.S. Eng., F.F.D.R.C.S. Irel., F.R.C.Path.

*Professor of Oral Pathology, University of London.
Dean and Director of Studies and Head of Department
of Pathology, Institute of Dental Surgery, University of London;
Head of Department of Pathology, Eastman Dental Hospital*

LONDON
WILLIAM HEINEMANN MEDICAL BOOKS LTD

first published 1976

© William Heinemann Medical Books Limited 1976

ISBN 0 433 06185 5

Text set in 10/11 pt. Monotype Times Roman, printed by letterpress,
and bound in Great Britain at The Pitman Press, Bath

PREFACE

The idea that the Scientific Foundations of Dentistry could be presented between the covers of a single volume is not one that originated in the minds of the editors. It was our publishers, encouraged by the success of other books in this series (of which 'Surgery' was the first and of which 'Dentistry' will be the seventh), who persuaded us that the attempt should be made.

The book is intended primarily for dental graduates studying for higher qualifications; since the area it covers is so extensive we hope that in many parts it will also be of assistance to dental teachers. It seeks to provide the reader with a comprehensive background to fundamentals essential to many different aspects of dental learning. The separate chapters, written by a selection of authorities in particular fields, are in no sense intended as reviews of literature, but rather as expositions of the views of the individual authors.

It has been a difficult task to delineate the subject matter appropriate to the title of this book. Strictly speaking there is no part of biological science that does not provide a basis for dental application but, even more than that, there is much within the different branches of dentistry that is founded upon such basic sciences as chemistry and physics. To some extent, therefore, the choice of subject matter is a reflection of editorial interests, and there may well be omissions that detract from the value of this book to some with specialized needs. We have, for instance, omitted entirely the subject of dental materials—not because we do not recognize the importance of this subject to dentistry but merely because its inclusion would call for so substantial an increase in the size of this book. Nevertheless, it is our hope that the range covered is wide enough to present, within this single volume, much of the material that postgraduate students would otherwise have to sift from many different books and periodicals.

We felt that, in a book involving many authors, it would be neither desirable nor practicable to impose complete uniformity of style. Thus, the character and method of presentation of each contributor is preserved, just as it would be if the contributors had been taking part in a symposium or a lecture course. Some degree of overlap between chapters is always a problem when several authors are involved. Our policy has been to allow repetition where it is necessary to the development of an author's argument, rather than inflict upon the reader constant cross-reference between chapters.

One of the most difficult decisions of editorial policy concerned the inclusion of references to the literature. We agreed with our publishers that lengthy bibliographies were inappropriate to a work of this nature. We sought from our authors a succinct account of the scientific foundations of their subjects and, because we believed that the authors chosen were authorities, we specifically requested that they should not provide detailed accounts of the views of those who had built up this knowledge. We felt particularly that no references should be included for the purpose of authenticating statements made, nor should they be incorporated for the purpose of according recognition or acknowledging priority. Most of our authors found that this restriction ran counter to their scruples—and possibly to habits ingrained in scientific writing.

If in any instance omission of references should give offence, the authors are exonerated, for ours is the responsibility. We recognize the need, and the desirability, for both authentication and acknowledgement. In this instance, however, we believe that comprehensive bibliographies would add enormously to the size of the book, and that this is not a text designed to be consulted as a source for references. We also believe that there are many readers who would be daunted rather than assisted by lengthy lists of additional reading.

Authors were therefore asked to provide only the minimum of references, and the only ones to be included should either be particularly recent, or reviews which cover essential material that could not be included within the compass of a single chapter, or articles indispensable to the reader.

Two distinguished contributors to this book, Sir Wilfred Fish and Professor W. J. Hamilton, did not live to see it in its final form. We are indebted to Dr. D. V. Hamilton for the proof reading of his father's chapter.

Colleagues to whom we are indebted are too numerous to mention by name, but we have been particularly helped by Dr. J. E. Eastoe and Mr. M. B. Edwards. We are grateful to Mrs. Carol Sheward, Mrs. Geraldine Forsythe and Miss Carole Meadows for bearing the considerable burden of secretarial assistance.

We owe our thanks to Mr. Richard Emery of Messrs. Heinemann for his patient help in bringing this enterprise to fruition during a period in which publishers have been beset by more than their usual share of problems and, while on this topic, we also express our thanks for their forebearance to those of our authors who delivered their typescripts on time and have had to wait unduly long to see the end result.

B.C.
I.R.H.K.

CONTENTS

vii

SECTION X

SALIVARY GLANDS

SECTION XI

BONE

SECTION XII

THE MUSCLES OF MASTICATION AND THE TEMPOROMANDIBULAR JOINT

SECTION XIII

SOME SPECIAL CONSIDERATIONS

LIST OF CONTRIBUTORS

O. F. ALVARES, D.D.S., M.S., Ph.D.
Visiting Associate Professor of Oral Biology, School of Dentistry, University of Washington, U.S.A.

D. J. ANDERSON, B.D.S., M.Sc., Ph.D.
Professor of Oral Biology, University of Bristol.

D. J. BECK, M.S., D.D.S., F.R.A.C.D.S.
Professor of Preventive and Social Dentistry, University of Otago Dental School, Dunedin, New Zealand.

D. C. BERRY, M.D.S., Ph.D.
Professor of Dental Surgery, University of Bristol.

ROSEMARY BIGGS, B.Sc., Ph.D., M.D., M.R.C.P., M.A.
Director, Oxford Haemophilia Centre, Churchill Hospital; Lecturer in Haematology, Oxford University.

H. J. J. BLACKWOOD, M.D., F.F.D., F.R.C.Path.
Professor of Oral Anatomy, Vice-Dean of the Royal Dental Hospital of London School of Dental Surgery, University of London.

W. H. BOWEN, B.D.S., D.Sc., Ph.D., F.F.D., F.D.S.
Chief, Caries Research and Prevention Programme, National Institute for Dental Research, Bethesda, Md., U.S.A.

A. BOYDE, Ph.D., B.D.S., L.D.S.R.C.S.
Reader in Dental Anatomy at University College, London.

ORLA M. BROWNE, L.R.C.P., L.R.C.S., D.Ch.
Lecturer and Research Fellow, Department of Pathology, Royal College of Surgeons in Ireland.

R. A. CAWSON, M.D., M.R.C.Path., B.D.S., F.D.S.
Professor of Oral Medicine and Pathology, Guy's Hospital Medical School, London.

D. M. CHISHOLM, B.D.S., Ph.D.
Lecturer in Oral Medicine and Pathology, Department of Oral Medicine and Pathology, University of Glasgow.

B. COHEN, D.D.S., M.S.D., F.D.S.R.C.S., F.F.D., F.R.C.Path.
Nuffield Professor, Director of Department of Dental Science, Royal College of Surgeons of England.

M. F. COLE, Ph.D., B.D.S.
Florence Mills Research Fellow, Royal College of Surgeons of England.

P. CRITCHLEY, B.Sc., Ph.D.
Manager of Skin Group; formerly Manager of Dental Biochemistry and Dental Therapeutic Group, Unilever Research Labs., Isleworth, Middx., England.

E. M. DARMADY, M.A., M.D., F.R.C.P., F.R.C.Path.
Emeritus Clinical Professor of Pathology, University of Southampton; formerly, Senior Pathologist of Portsmouth and Isle of Wight Area Pathological Service.

G. N. DAVIES, D.D.S., F.D.S.R.C.S., F.A.C.D., F.R.A.C.D.S.
Professor of Social and Preventive Dentistry, University of Queensland, Brisbane, Australia.

C. DAWES, B.Sc., B.D.S., Ph.D.
Professor of Oral Biology, Faculty of Dentistry, University of Manitoba, Winnipeg, Canada.

R. DUCKWORTH, M.D., B.D.S., F.D.S.R.C.S., F.R.C. Path.
Professor of Oral Medicine in the University of London, at the London Hospital Medical College.

J. E. EASTOE, D.Sc., Ph.D., A.R.C.S.
Research Fellow in the Department of Dental Science, Royal College of Surgeons of England.

M. B. EDWARDS, B.D.S., F.D.S.R.C.S.
Research Fellow in Oral Pathology, Department of Dental Science, Royal College of Surgeons of England.

D. H. ENLOW, Ph.D.
Professor and Chairman, Department of Anatomy, School of Medicine, West Virginia University, Morgantown, West Virginia, U.S.A.

J. M. FACCINI, Ph.D., M.B., B.S., B.D.S.
Reader in Pathology of Oral Diseases, University College Hospital Medical School, London.

SIR WILFRED FISH, M.D., Ch.B., D.D.Sc., D.Sc., F.R.C.S., F.D.S.R.C.S.
Formerly Hon. Director, Department of Dental Science, Royal College of Surgeons of England.

J. R. GARRETT, B.Sc., Ph.D., M.B., B.S., M.R.C.Path., L.D.S.R.C.S.
Professor of Oral Pathology and Head of Department of Oral Pathology and Oral Medicine, The Dental School, King's College Hospital Medical School, London.

S. J. GERSON, D.D.S., M.S., Ph.D.
Professor of Oral Pathology, University of Illinois College of Dentistry, Chicago, U.S.A.

L. E. GLYNN, Ph.D., F.R.C.P., F.R.C.Path.
Director, Mathilda and Terence Kennedy Institute of Rheumatology, London; Deputy Director, M.R.C. Rheumatism Unit, Canadian Red Cross Memorial Hospital, Taplow, England.

W. J. HAMILTON, M.D., D.Sc., F.R.C.S., F.R.C.O.G., F.R.S.E.
Professor Emeritus of Anatomy, University of London; formerly Regius Professor of Anatomy, University of Glasgow.

P. D. J. HOLLAND, F.R.C.P., F.R.C.Path.
Professor of Pathology, Royal College of Surgeons in Ireland, Senior Consultant Pathologist, St. Lawrence's Hospital, Dublin.

M. S. ISRAEL, M.B., M.R.C.P., M.R.C.Path., D.C.P.
Senior Lecturer in Pathology, Institute of Basic Medical Sciences, Royal College of Surgeons of England.

G. N. JENKINS, M.Sc., Ph.D.
Professor of Oral Physiology, Dental School, University of Newcastle-upon-Tyne.

R. B. JOHNS, Ph.D., L.D.S.R.C.S.
Senior Lecturer, Department of Conservative Dental Surgery, Guy's Hospital, London.

T. LEHNER, M.D., M.B., B.S., B.D.S., F.D.S.R.C.S., M.R.C.Path.
Professor of Oral Immunology, University of London; Head of Department of Oral Immunology and Microbiology; Honorary Consultant Pathologist, Guy's Hospital, London.

R. B. LUCAS, M.D., F.R.C.P., F.R.C.Path., F.D.S.
Professor of Oral Pathology, University of London; Pathologist, Royal Dental Hospital of London.

R. G. MACFARLANE, C.B.E., F.R.S., M.A., F.R.C.P.
Emeritus Professor of Clinical Pathology, Oxford University; Oxford Haemophilia Centre, Churchill Hospital, Headington, Oxford.

D. K. MASON, B.D.S., M.D., F.D.S.R.C.S., M.R.C.Path.
Professor of Oral Medicine, Department of Oral Medicine and Pathology, University of Glasgow.

R. M. H. McMINN, M.D., Ph.D.
Sir William Collins Professor of Human and Comparative Anatomy, Royal College of Surgeons of England; Professor of Anatomy, Institute of Basic Medical Sciences, University of London.

A. H. MELCHER, M.D.S., H.D.D., Ph.D.
Professor of Dentistry and Director, Medical Research Council Group in Periodontal Physiology, University of Toronto, Canada.

JULIA MEYER, Ph.D.
Professor of Oral Pathology, University of Illinois College of Dentistry, Chicago, U.S.A.

A. E. W. MILES, D.Sc., L.R.C.P., M.R.C.S., F.D.S.
Professor of Oral Pathology, London Hospital Medical College, University of London; Hon. Curator, Odontological Museum, Royal College of Surgeons of England.

J. R. E. MILLS, D.D.S., M.Sc., F.D.S., D.Orth.
Professor of Orthodontics, Institute of Dental Surgery, University of London.

F. F. NALLY, F.D.S.R.C.S.(Eng.), F.F.D., L.R.C.P., L.R.C.S.
Senior Lecturer, Institute of Dental Surgery, University of London; Hon. Consultant, Eastman Dental Hospital, London.

J. P. PAYNE, M.B., F.F.A.R.C.S., D.A.
Professor and Director of Research, Department of Anaesthetics, Royal College of Surgeons of England; Consultant Anaesthetist, St. Peter's Hospitals, London.

J. J. PINDBORG, D.D.S., Dr.Odont., Odont.Dr.h.c., F.D.S.R.C.S., F.R.C.Path.
Professor of Oral Pathology, Royal Dental College, Copenhagen; Head, Dental Department, University Hospital, Copenhagen, Denmark.

D. E. POSWILLO, D.Sc., D.D.S., F.D.S.R.C.S., F.R.A.C.D.S., F.I.Biol., M.R.C.Path.
Professor of Teratology, Department of Dental Science, Royal College of Surgeons of England; Consultant Oral Surgeon, Queen Victoria Hospital, East Grinstead; Hon. Tutor, Guy's Hospital, London.

J. J. PRITCHARD, M.A., D.M., F.R.C.S.
Professor of Anatomy, The Queen's University, Belfast.

FELICITY REYNOLDS, M.D., F.F.A.R.C.S.
Lecturer, Department of Pharmacology, St. Thomas's Hospital Medical School, London.

A. R. SANDERSON, B.Sc., Ph.D.
Assistant Director of Research, Blond Laboratories, McIndoe Research Unit, Queen Victoria Hospital, East Grinstead, England.

H. E. SCHROEDER, Dr. Med. Dent.
Professor and Chairman, Department of Oral Structural Biology, Dental Institute, University of Zurich, Switzerland.

M. SHEAR, D.Sc.(Dent.), M.D.S., M.R.C.Path., H.Dip.Dent.
Professor of Oral Pathology, University of the Witwatersrand, Johannesburg, South Africa.

E. J. SHILLITOE, B.D.S., L.D.S.R.C.S.
Research Assistant, Department of Oral Immunology and Microbiology, Guy's Hospital, London.

L. M. SILVERSTONE, D.D.Sc., Ph.D., B.Ch.D.
Senior Lecturer in Child Dental Health, The London Hospital Medical College; Consultant Dental Surgeon, The London Hospital.

G. H. SLOANE-STANLEY, M.A., D.Phil., M.I.Biol.
Senior Lecturer in Biochemistry, Institute of Basic Medical Sciences, Royal College of Surgeons of England and University of London.

C. J. SMITH, B.D.S., Ph.D., M.R.C.Path., L.D.S.R.C.S.
Professor of Oral Pathology, University of Sheffield.

H. SMITH, Ph.D., D.Sc., F.R.C.Path.
Professor of Microbiology, University of Birmingham; formerly, Deputy Chief Scientific Officer, Microbiological Research Establishment, Porton, England.

J. A. SOFAER, B.D.S., Ph.D.
Lecturer in Genetics as it relates to Dentistry, University of Edinburgh School of Dental Surgery and Department of Human Genetics, Edinburgh, Scotland.

R. W. STANFORD, M.A., F.I.P., F.A.I.P., F.R.A.C.R.
Head of Department of Medical Physics, Royal Perth Hospital, Perth, W. Australia; Visiting Lecturer, University of Western Australia.

N. B. B. SYMONS, M.Sc., B.D.S., F.F.D., F.D.S.R.C.S.
Professor of Oral Anatomy, University of Dundee.

D. TARIN, B.Sc., D.M.
Senior Registrar in Neuropathology, General Infirmary, Leeds.

PAMELA J. TARIN, B.Sc., B.M., B.Ch.
Lecturer in Anatomy, Medical School, Leeds.

J. W. THOMPSON, M.B., B.S., Ph.D.
Professor of Pharmacology, University of Newcastle-upon-Tyne; Hon. Consultant in Pharmacology to the Newcastle University Hospitals.

P. A. TOLLER, F.D.S.R.C.S.
Consultant Oral Surgeon, Canadian Red Cross Memorial Hospital, Taplow, and Mount Vernon Hospital, Northwood, England.

C. H. TONGE, T.D., D.D.Sc., M.B., B.S., B.D.S., F.D.S.R.C.S.
Professor of Oral Anatomy and Postgraduate Sub-dean of the Dental School, University of Newcastle-upon-Tyne.

J. L. Turk, M.D., D.Sc., M.R.C.P., F.R.C.Path.
Sir William Collins Professor of Human and Comparative Pathology, Royal College of Surgeons of England; Institute of Basic Medical Sciences, University of London.

J. G. Walton, B.D.S.
Senior Lecturer in Operative Dental Surgery, Lecturer in Dental Pharmacology, University of Newcastle-upon-Tyne; Hon. Consultant, Newcastle-upon-Tyne Dental Hospital.

Lyal Watson, F.R.A.C.P., M.R.C.P.
Consultant Physician, University College Hospital, London.

J. G. Whitwam, M.B., Ch.B., Ph.D., M.R.C.P., F.F.A.R.C.S.
Reader in Clinical Anaesthesia, Royal Postgraduate Medical School; Hon. Consultant Anaesthetist, Hammersmith Hospital, London.

B. D. Wyke, M.B., M.D., B.S.
Head of the Neurological Laboratory, Royal College of Surgeons of England; Senior Lecturer in Applied Physiology, Institute of Basic Medical Sciences, University of London.

R. Yemm, B.D.S., B.Sc., Ph.D.
Lecturer in Dental Surgery and Physiology, University of Bristol, England.

ACKNOWLEDGMENTS

The Editors and Contributors wish to thank owners of copyright for permission to reproduce illustrations and other material. In most instances this has been mentioned in the appropriate legends.

In addition, acknowledgment is made to Messrs. Butterworths of London for kindly permitting reproduction of part of Chapter 16 which the author first published in "Operative Surgery". In Chapter 43 acknowledgment is due to the Editors of the Journal of Physiology for permission to reproduce figure 3; Academic Press, Inc., for the use of figure 7 (McCann, 1968); Microfilms International Marketing Corporation and the Editor of Archives of Oral Biology for permission to use figure 8 and Pergamon Press and the Editor of Archives of Oral Biology for permission to publish figure 9.

In Chapter 28 Mr. P. A. C. Baigrie, Mr. R. Smith, and Mr. W. Smith assisted in the preparation of illustrations. In Chapter 42, the diagrams were drawn by Mrs. S. Kemplay, Miss A. Kidd prepared the material for figures 6 and 11, and the photomicrographs were done by Mr. K. J. Davies.

Finally acknowledgment is made in Chapter 11 to Mr. Keith Wood, A.I.S.T. for graphic work; in Chapter 24 to Mr. J. D. Langdon of the London Hospital for information about clinical trials and Messrs. Astra Chemicals and Messrs. Wigglesworth for information; and in Chapter 59 for the assistance of Dr. J. T. Scales of the Royal National Orthopaedic Hospital and the Institute of Orthopaedics.

SECTION I

GROWTH AND DEVELOPMENT

1. THE INFLUENCE OF HEREDITY

J. A. SOFAER

TERMS AND DEFINITIONS

Variation

When observing an organism, or when studying its development, it is important to realize that every character and every developmental process is subject to some degree of variation. No attribute, whether anatomical or physiological, normal or pathological, has an identical manifestation in all individuals, and there is no single rigid path of growth and development that is common to all members of a species. All characters therefore show some differences of nature or degree between individuals, and these differences are due partly to the inheritance of different genes and partly to chance and differences in the environment to which individuals have been subjected.

The first step in investigating the influence of heredity on growth and development is to observe the ways in which individuals differ with respect to any character of interest, and to study the patterns of variation of the character within families and within and between populations. A variety of analytical methods can then be applied to estimate the extent to which differences between individuals are due to genetic differences rather than to the influence of different non-genetic factors. Once something is known about the genetic contribution to the observed variation, established hereditary variants can be used to draw conclusions about developmental processes and their genetic control.

Differences occur not only between populations and between individuals but also, within individuals, between tissues or regions of the body. These differences begin to appear early in development when cells or groups of cells start to differentiate along a variety of developmental pathways. The basis for this differentiation seems to be that only particular genes have been "switched on" in particular cells, the majority of genes remaining inactive for most of the time. In certain circumstances it may be possible to compare gene activity in different tissues, and this can be a powerful way in which to study the effects of heredity on development.

Another kind of within-individual difference is that which occurs between paired structures on the two sides of the body. As hereditary potential and the general environment are expected to influence both sides of the same individual equally, asymmetry can be assumed to indicate lack of ability of a developing organ to buffer itself against chance developmental fluctuations and variation in its own local environment within the developing individual. The symmetry of bilateral structures is therefore an estimator of developmental stability, which, like any other character, is affected by both hereditary and environmental influences.

In addition to studying the variation of each character of interest separately, it may be useful to consider how two or more characters vary together. In the case of a syndrome of abnormalities produced by a single gene it is fair to assume that all characters showing some sign of abnormality are associated during development. When two characters that are correlated appear to be affected by several genes, it may be possible to estimate the degree to which their observed patterns of variation are due to common genetic influences and thereby draw conclusions about their developmental relationships.

Genes and Chromosomes

The variation observed among living things is composed of hereditary and environmental components. Heredity supplies the potential and the environment dictates the manner and degree to which this potential is expressed. The determinants of hereditary potential are the genes, each gene being an item of stored information that can be used to produce or control the production of a particular substance. The products of gene activity are ultimately partly responsible for all the physiological and anatomical properties of the individual. The fundamental property of the gene itself is its capacity for self-replication. The information contained in it can therefore be passed from one cell generation to the next, and from a parent to its offspring. However, since genes cannot be observed directly, the existence of any gene can only be inferred from a study of variation in the character or characters it helps to produce.

The term **gene** is sometimes too general, and it may be more appropriate to talk of a **locus,** which is the site on a chromosome occupied by a gene, or an **allele,** which is one of a number of alternative forms that a gene may take. For example, at the MN blood group locus in man there may be either an "M-substance" producing allele or an "N-substance" producing allele. Allelic differences like this form the basis of the genetic component of variation, and, conversely, it is the possession of common alleles, derived from a common ancestor, that is responsible for the resemblance between relatives.

The nucleus of each human somatic cell normally contains 23 pairs of chromosomes. One member of each pair is derived from each parent so that each pair comprises a maternal and a paternal chromosome. One of the 23 pairs is a pair of **sex chromosomes** and the other 22 pairs are called **autosomes.** Each gamete contains only one member of each chromosome pair. At fertilization one gamete from each parent unite to form a single-celled **zygote** that subsequently develops into a new individual. As the zygote receives one chromosome of each pair from each parent, it is able to start its development with the full somatic complement.

The two members of each pair of autosomes are potentially identical in that the same loci are normally present in the same sequence in both. The only differences are allele differences that may be present at all, any or none of the loci. Each pair of autosomes is normally completely different from each of the others so that there are only two autosomal loci of each kind in each individual. Therefore, no matter how many alleles are available for a particular autosomal locus, no more than two will normally be present in each individual. If both alleles at a given locus are identical the individual is said to be **homozygous** at that locus for that allele, and if the alleles are different the individual is said to be **heterozygous.**

The sex chromosomes differ from the autosomes in that there are two alternative forms. One is the **X-chromosome,** which can be regarded as comparable to an autosome, and the other is the **Y-chromosome.** Loci carried by the X-chromosome are said to be **X-linked** or **sex-linked,** but no corresponding Y-linked loci have been demonstrated. The Y-chromosome can therefore be regarded as relatively inert. All viable individuals possess at least one X-chromosome, sex being dependent on whether the other member of the pair is another X-chromosome (which confers femaleness) or a Y-chromosome (which confers maleness). Females can therefore be either homozygous or heterozygous for all X-linked genes, but as males possess only one allele at each X-linked locus they can be neither. Males are consequently said to be **hemizygous** at all X-linked loci.

If an individual is homozygous (or hemizygous) at a given locus for any allele, then the observed effect is that of this allele alone. When an individual is heterozygous, and there are therefore two different alleles at the same locus, the outcome is dependent on the relationship between the alleles. If the two alleles are symbolized by A_1 and A_2, and in heterozygotes the observed effect is entirely that of A_2, then A_2 is completely **dominant** over A_1, and A_1 is completely **recessive** to A_2. All levels of dominance can occur from complete dominance of one allele over its partner to a situation of no dominance where each allele is expressed unaffected by the other.

Alleles are not absolutely stable entities. Although they are usually transmitted unaltered from generation to generation through the process of self-replication, rare events occur to cause changes within them. These events are called **mutations,** the new allele is a **mutant allele,** and individuals who show the effect of the mutant allele are known as **mutants.** The chromosomes themselves are also not entirely stable, and aberrations of the chromosomal complement, some of them associated with physical or mental abnormalities, may occur at low frequencies in all populations.

Genotype and Phenotype

The genetic constitution of an individual is known as his **genotype.** Genotype may refer to a specified locus or loci, or to all loci in general. An individual's **phenotype** is the final observed product of a combination of genetic and environmental influences. Phenotype may be used to refer to a specified character, or to the observable properties of the individual in general.

Different types of character can be thought of as being different distances from the fundamental level of gene activity. The further a character is removed from this fundamental genetic level, the greater the likelihood that its variation is dependent on allele differences at more than one locus, and also on environmental fluctuations. Enzymes, for example, are substances that are almost direct products of gene action, and in most cases it has been shown that the molecular structure of a single enzyme is dependent on a single gene. This means that variation in the structure, and consequently the function, of a particular enzyme is usually due to allele differences at a single locus. Morphological characters, on the other hand, are furthest from the fundamental genetic level and are the end results of a vast complexity of interacting developmental processes controlled by many genes and sensitive to external influences.

Since ontogeny has a basically diverging nature, the earlier an event occurs the more widespread its effects are likely to be. Each gene therefore probably affects many morphological characters, the breadth of its influence depending on the developmental stage at which it becomes active. It has in fact been observed that detectable single allele substitutions usually produce syndromes of morphological effects. Different aspects of such a syndrome may at first appear unrelated, but connections between them can often be established by probing back into their developmental relationships (Grüneberg, 1963).

TYPES OF VARIATION

Discrete Variation

Characters that show discrete variation exist in two or more qualitatively different forms. It is therefore not possible to compare individuals by their measurements on a simple common scale. The best examples of discrete variables are found among biochemical or immunological characters such as blood groups. Here individuals are either of one blood type or another and there is no continuum of intermediates. Characters that exist in two forms only, such as sex, are examples of **dimorphisms**; and characters that exist in more than two forms, such as ABO blood type, are examples of **polymorphisms.** Variation within a population implies that not all individuals are of the same type. Variation between populations implies that the frequencies of the different forms in one population are different from those in another.

Discrete variation is often due to allele differences at a single locus. This can be demonstrated by studying the pattern of distribution of the character's different forms within families. The investigator compares the pattern with the theoretical expectations associated with different modes of genetic control, and by a process of elimination arrives at the most likely genetic hypothesis to explain the observations.

Continuous (Quantitative or Metric) Variation

Continuous variables, such as height, weight, tooth size and eruption time, are characters that can be measured against a continuous scale. In any range on any scale of

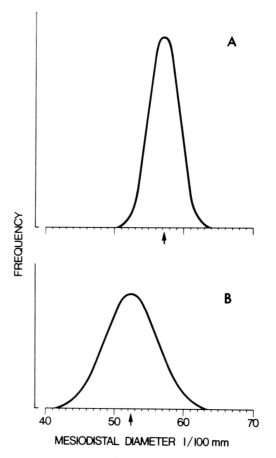

FIG. 2. Normal distributions corresponding to the data in Fig. 1. The means (indicated by arrows) of groups A and B are respectively 57.2 and 52.4, and the variances are 4.5 and 12.3.

measurement there is theoretically an infinite number of possible values, but for practical purposes it is usual to measure in terms of a chosen size of subdivision. For example, the mesiodistal diameter of mouse lower third molars can be measured to the nearest 1/100 mm. Variation within a population can then be expressed by the number of individuals that fall within each subdivision, and populations can be compared by the way in which individuals are distributed over all subdivisions of the scale (fig. 1).

The general form of each distribution in fig. 1 approximates to the most commonly encountered type of distribution, the **normal** distribution, the "ideal" shape of which is described by the normal curve. The position of such a distribution on the scale and the variation within it can be expressed in precise statistical terms as the mean and variance, and differences between populations can be established by a comparison of means and variances. The "ideal" distributions of the data in fig. 1 are shown as corresponding normal curves in fig. 2. The horizontal axis is still a scale of tooth diameter, but the vertical axis now measures the frequency with which teeth of a particular size occur in each group.

Continuous variables usually have a **multifactorial** basis; that is, several genes and environmental influences, each with a relatively small effect, contribute to an individual's

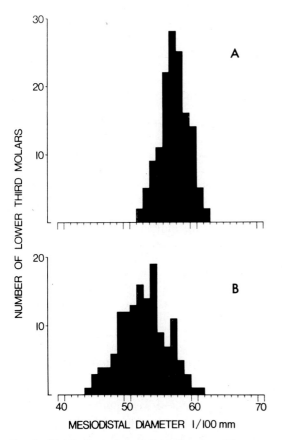

FIG. 1. Distributions of mesiodistal diameter of lower third molars in two genetically different groups of mice, A and B. The two groups differ with respect to both position and spread on the scale.

position on the continuous scale. Investigating the genetic control of continuous variables is then a problem of estimating the proportion of the observed variation due to genetic differences between individuals, and the proportion due to differences of environment. More specifically, it is a question of partitioning the observed or phenotypic variance, V_P, into its genetic and environmental components.

The total genetic variance is itself made up of a number of components, the most important being the **additive genetic variance,** V_A, which is the main cause of resemblance between relatives. The proportion of the phenotypic variance taken up by the additive genetic component is known as the **heritability,** and is symbolized by h^2. Thus: $h^2 = V_A/V_P$. Heritability is an expression of the reliance that can be placed on an individual's phenotype as an indication of the phenotype of his relatives. It is therefore useful when attempting to predict a course of development in a growing child, or the likelihood of his developing a disease for which there is a heritable predisposition.

The estimation of heritability depends on an analysis of resemblance between relatives. Consider a character that has no genetic component of variation. Phenotypic differences between individuals then have nothing to do with genetic differences and are due entirely to chance or environmental factors. Provided all individuals are exposed to the same environment, a group of related individuals is just as random a sample of the population as a group of unrelated individuals, as far as the character is concerned. Suppose, now, that the character does have some additive genetic component of variation. Related individuals, with more alleles in common than unrelated individuals, are expected to be more alike. The phenotypic variance of a group of related individuals is then lower than that of a random sample of the population, and these variances can be used to estimate the heritability of the character.

A common way of expressing the degree of resemblance between relatives is by a regression of offspring mean on **midparent value** (the mean of measurements of the character in the two parents of each family). If the two parental phenotypes are p_1 and p_2, the midparent value, $\bar{P}$, is then: $\bar{P} = (p_1 + p_2)/2$. Consider that $h^2 = 1$. All phenotypic variation is then due to additive genetic effects, and the phenotype of an individual is an exact indication of his genotype. Since each individual receives, on average, half his genetic information from one parent and half from the other, the mean of offspring, $\bar{O}$, is on average equal to: $\bar{O} = (p_1/2) + (p_2/2)$. Therefore $\bar{O}$ tends to equal $\bar{P}$, and if $\bar{O}$ is plotted against $\bar{P}$ for several different families the results average out as a straight line with a slope of 1. Thus, when $h^2 = 1$, the regression of offspring on midparent value, $b_{\bar{O}\bar{P}} = 1$; so that $h^2 = b_{\bar{O}\bar{P}}$. When $h^2 = 0$, and assuming that there is no environmental reason why offspring should be like their parents, each offspring is equivalent to a randomly selected individual from the general population, and the offspring means of all families vary around the mean of the general population. The results of plotting $\bar{O}$ against $\bar{P}$ then average-out as a straight line with zero slope. Thus, when $h^2 = 0$, $b_{\bar{O}\bar{P}} = 0$; so that in this case also $h^2 = b_{\bar{O}\bar{P}}$ (fig. 3). The equality of h^2 and $b_{\bar{O}\bar{P}}$ can in fact be shown to apply for all values of h^2.

Further details of these and other methods of estimating the heritability of continuous variables are given in Falconer (1964).

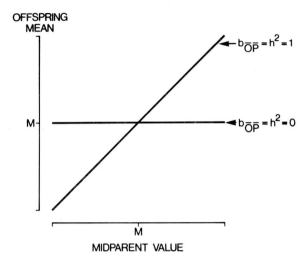

Fig. 3. The regression of offspring mean on midparent value. The two lines indicate the average relationships between parents and offspring for the two extremes of heritability. M is the mean value of the character in the population.

Quasi-continuous Variation

Characters that are either present or absent, but when present vary continuously, are known as quasi-continuous variables. The accepted model of quasi-continuous variation is based on the assumption that there is an underlying scale of continuous variation of some attribute (the result of a combination of all the genetic and environmental factors involved) that is immediately related to the development of the character. The character is absent in individuals who occupy a position on the scale below a critical **threshold** value, and present in those who occupy a position above it. The more the level on the underlying scale exceeds the threshold the more intense is the expression of the character. A quasi-continuous character can therefore be regarded as a continuous variable whose expression has a "visible" and a "non-visible" range.

In a population of individuals, some of whom show a quasi-continuous character and others of whom do not, the distribution on the underlying continuous scale is divided by the threshold. The shape of the whole distribution is therefore not disclosed, and unless there is reason to think otherwise it may be useful to assume it is normal. It is then possible, by consulting standard statistical tables of the normal distribution, to establish x, the distance of the threshold from the mean of the distribution in terms of σ, the distribution's standard deviation. The only information required is the proportion of the population, q, that falls above the threshold (fig. 4).

A simple comparison between populations can be made of means arrived at in this way, but such a comparison suffers from the possibly over-simplified assumption that the variances of all populations are the same. In order to compare variances as well as to make a more accurate comparison of means, the variable concerned must be capable of being scored in three categories rather than two: non-affected, minimally affected, and moderately to maximally affected. In such a situation there are therefore two thresholds, and variances and means can be expressed in terms of what is assumed to be a constant interval between the two thresholds.

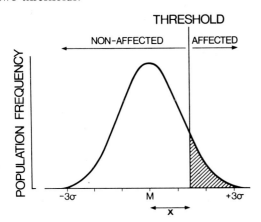

FIG. 4. The model of quasi-continuous variation. Only those individuals who fall above the threshold can be measured but the distribution on the underlying continuous scale is assumed to be normal. The distance, x, of the threshold from the mean, M, in terms of the standard deviation, σ, can be derived from tables given the proportion of affected individuals, q (hatched area as a proportion of the total area under the curve).

Figure 5 illustrates how such comparisons can be made. Applying proportions of each population to tables, as already described, q_{A1} will give x_{A1}, the distance of threshold 1 from the mean of distribution A; and q_{A2} will give x_{A2}, the distance of threshold 2 from the mean of distribution A. Both these distances are in terms of σ_A, the standard deviation of distribution A. A similar procedure can be adopted for distribution B. Thus the interval between the two thresholds, t, is equal to:

$$t = (x_{A2} - x_{A1})\sigma_A = (x_{B2} - x_{B1})\sigma_B$$

If for the sake of simplicity the distance between the two thresholds, t, is defined as unity, or one *threshold unit*, then the standard deviations of the two populations are equal to:

$$\sigma_A = 1/(x_{A2} - x_{A1}) \text{ threshold units,}$$

$$\sigma_B = 1/(x_{B2} - x_{B1}) \text{ threshold units,}$$

and the variances follow as $\sigma_A{}^2$ and $\sigma_B{}^2$. It follows also that the mean of distribution A:

$$M_A = -x_{A1}\sigma_A \text{ threshold units from threshold 1,}$$

and the mean of distribution B:

$$M_B = -x_{B1}\sigma_B \text{ threshold units from threshold 1.}$$

Greater detail of this kind of analysis is given in Falconer (1964, 1965).

Certain features of quasi-continuous variation are illustrated by a dental morphological variant in the mouse, a supernumerary cusp that has been found to occur at high frequency on the lower first molars of the Tuck No. 1

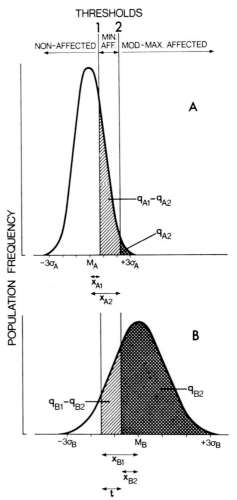

FIG. 5. Quasi-continuous variation with two thresholds. Values of x can be derived from tables given the appropriate proportion, q; and variances and means can be compared in terms of the threshold interval, t.

strain (fig. 6). Individual mice can be regarded as either non-affected (normal) or affected (variant), and affected animals can be classified according to four levels of expression of the cusp. Crosses of Tuck animals with other strains have resulted in groups of progeny with different frequencies of the cusp. Each group was genetically different from the others, and the different frequencies presumably reflect different mean levels of underlying genetic potential for cusp formation. These groups make it possible to test whether the relationship between the frequency of affected animals and the observed mean score of affected animals (observed MSA) conforms with what would be expected of normal distributions occupying different positions on the underlying continuous scale. The higher the frequency of affected individuals, the more severely they should be affected on average.

Just as it is possible to locate the mean of an entire distribution relative to the threshold, it is also possible to determine from tables the position of the mean of only those individuals who fall above the threshold. This, then, is the theoretical position of the mean of affected individuals (expected MSA) based on the frequency of affected animals in each group. Expected MSA values were calculated for six groups of mice, making allowance for differences of variance by using the two-threshold model described above.

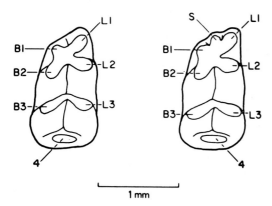

FIG. 6. Diagrams of occlusal surfaces of normal (left) and Tuck (right) lower left first molars. Both teeth have three buccal and three lingual cusps, B1–3 and L1–3, and a single distal cusp, 4. The Tuck tooth has an additional cusp, S. Reproduced with the permission of Pergamon Press Ltd. from Sofaer (1969a).

Figure 7 shows the relationship between observed and expected MSA values. There is a high correlation ($r = 0.98$), and the regression ($b = 0.86$) is not significantly different from 1. The mean levels of expression of the cusp in groups

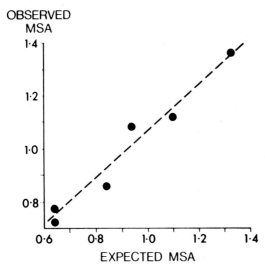

FIG. 7. The relationship between observed and expected MSA values for 6 groups of mice produced by crossing Tuck animals with different strains. Redrawn from Sofaer (1969a).

showing different frequencies of affected individuals therefore conform with what would be expected on the basis of the model of quasi-continuous variation.

As with continuous variables, the expression of a quasi-continuous character is usually dependent on a combination of many genes and environmental factors. It is therefore appropriate to be able to estimate the heritability, and, as with continuous variables, this is done by studying the

resemblance between relatives. Consider the case of cleft lip with or without a cleft of the palate, CL(P). The assumption is that for each individual a combination of genetic and environmental influences determines the level of disposition to develop the malformation. An individual whose level falls below the threshold is normal, whereas one whose level falls above it is affected.

If CL(P) has no hereditary basis and is produced entirely by chance or environmental factors, then, provided all individuals are exposed to the same environment, a group of relatives of CL(P) individuals is equivalent to a random sample of the population with an incidence of the malformation approximating to that of the general population itself. On the other hand, if CL(P) is under some degree of genetic control the frequency of this abnormality among relatives of CL(P) cases should be higher than among the general population. Thus, assuming that there is no environmental reason why relatives should tend to be alike, d, the distance between the mean of a group of relatives of CL(P) individuals and the mean of the general population, is a measure of the degree to which CL(P) is a heritable condition. This is simply the difference between x_g and x_r derived from applying the proportions q_g and q_r to tables as described above (fig. 8). It should be pointed out here

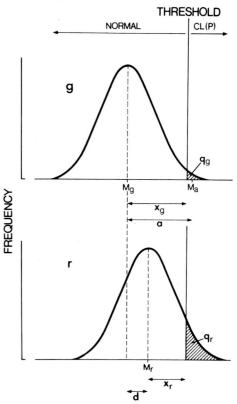

FIG. 8. Heritability estimation for a quasi-continuous character, CL(P). Distributions of the general population, **g**, and of a group of relatives of affected individuals, **r**, are shown. The values of x_g and a, and x_r, are derived from tables given the proportions q_g and q_r. The distance d, relative to a and the degree of relationship of the relatives used, provides the estimate of heritability.

that, as this is a single-threshold situation, it must be assumed that the variances of the general population and the group of relatives are the same.

The difference d has however to be considered in relation to a, the distance of the mean of affected individuals in the general population from the general population mean; and also to r, the degree of relationship of the relatives being used. The distance a is the maximum value that d can assume, and this can only occur if $h^2 = 1$ and if the relatives are monozygotic twins (genetically identical with their originally identified CL(P) cases, with $r = 1$). If the relatives used are first-degree (full sibs, parents or children), second-degree (aunts, uncles, nieces or nephews) or third-degree relatives (first cousins) then $r = \frac{1}{2}$, $\frac{1}{4}$ and $\frac{1}{8}$ respectively, as these relatives have on average $\frac{1}{2}$, $\frac{1}{4}$ and $\frac{1}{8}$ of their genes in common with their originally identified CL(P) cases. The maximum values of d when using first-, second- and third-degree relatives are accordingly $a/2$, $a/4$ and $a/8$, and these can only occur if $h^2 = 1$. The actual value of the heritability is simply the difference d expressed as a proportion of its maximum possible value. Thus: $h^2 = d/ar$ (Falconer, 1965).

Estimates of heritability for familial CL(P) from first-, second- and third-degree relatives by this method are respectively 0·83, 0·78 and 0·81 (Ross and Johnston, 1972). These values suggest that the differences between familial CL(P) cases and normal individuals could be largely due to the inheritance of different genes.

GENETIC VARIATION AND DEVELOPMENT

Normal Variation

The differences that are observed between "normal" individuals are often referred to as constituting **normal variation**. These differences may be due to allelic differences at single loci, as in the case of blood-group variants, and are then likely to be discrete differences; or they may have a multifactorial basis, as appears to apply to most dental characteristics, in which case variation is usually continuous or quasi-continuous. Investigating the genetic basis of normal variation in dental characteristics therefore depends largely on estimating the relative contributions of inherited and environmental differences to the observed differences between individuals. This is done by studying the degree of resemblance between relatives, which is often expressed as a heritability estimate for the character concerned. Since heritability is the ratio of the additive genetic variance to the total phenotypic variance, alteration of either the environmental or the genetic component will affect its value. This applies equally to any other expression of resemblance between relatives. Comparison of the resemblance between relatives for similar structures in the same population, such as neighbouring teeth, may therefore provide some information about the relative stability of the local environment around each developing structure within the developing individual as a whole.

Estimates of resemblance between relatives with respect to tooth size in man show that within each morphological class (incisors, premolars and molars) relatives tend to be most alike with respect to the teeth that develop early, and

least alike with respect to those that develop late. That is, environmental variation contributes proportionally more to the observed differences between individuals in the later-developing teeth of each class (fig. 9, Table 1). Since, as is widely recognized, later-developing teeth show greater phenotypic variability, it follows that environmental variation also contributes more in absolute terms to the observed size differences between individuals in the later-developing teeth of each class. The point of interest here is what this pattern of hereditary *versus* environmental influence suggests about the way in which teeth develop. A possible interpretation is as follows. The early tooth of each class is the first to develop in its own region of the jaw and is therefore not initially in competition with any closely adjacent tooth germs. The later-developing tooth, on the other hand, must compete with already established tooth germs from the start, making do with what remains of any nutritional requirements that are necessary for growth. Consequently, variation in the supply of these requirements, within certain limits, is likely to affect the later rather than the earlier developing tooth of each class.

Abnormal Variation

The term **abnormal variation** is usually used to refer to gross differences from the population norm, many of which are due to single genes with major phenotypic effects, or to aberrations of whole chromosomes or parts of chromosomes. A study of the effect of a single gene on development generally consists of working back from the adult phenotype through to earlier and earlier stages, comparing normal and mutant individuals until there is no discernible difference between them. In doing this, it may be possible to formulate a hypothesis about the developmental basis of the mutant phenotype. It may even be possible to associate the observed abnormalities with a fundamental biochemical difference between normal and mutant individuals. On the other hand, a chromosomal aberration involves many loci, so there is unlikely to be a simple genetic cause for an associated syndrome of abnormalities. Investigation of a chromosomal aberration at the biochemical and even developmental level is therefore a more complex problem than the study of single genes.

Examples of single genes with major phenotypic effects in the mouse are the X-linked gene *tabby*, and two autosomal recessive genes, *crinkled* and *downless*. Each produces the same syndrome of abnormalities of hair, teeth and certain exocrine glands; all structures formed by the downgrowth of an epithelium into the underlying mesenchyme. These genes therefore presumably affect in some fundamental way the interaction that is known to occur between epithelium and mesenchyme during the formation of such structures, and, since the phenotypes they produce appear to be indistinguishable, their activities must be closely related during development.

Dental manifestations of the mutants include reduced size of the teeth and a characteristic mutant molar morphology (fig. 10), the rare occurrence of a supernumerary tooth just anterior to the first molar, and, very rarely, a composite tooth, apparently composed of incompletely

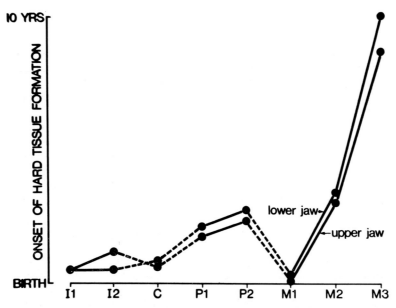

FIG. 9. The pattern of developmental timing (data from Orban, 1957) for incisors (I1 and I2), canine (C), premolars (P1 and P2) and molars (M1, M2 and M3). Solid lines connect points for teeth of the same class, and broken lines connect points for adjacent teeth of different classes.

TABLE 1

THE RESEMBLANCE BETWEEN RELATIVES WITH RESPECT TO MESIODISTAL TOOTH DIAMETER. THE DATA OF LUNDSTRÖM ARE RATIOS OF "HEREDITY/ NON-HEREDITY" DERIVED FROM A COMPARISON OF IDENTICAL AND FRATERNAL TWINS; THOSE OF BOWDEN AND GOOSE ARE THE COMBINED CORRELATIONS FOR ALL PAIRS OF FIRST-DEGREE RELATIVES; AND THOSE OF SOFAER, BAILIT AND MACLEAN ARE CORRELATIONS BETWEEN FIRST-DEGREE RELATIVES

		Upper Jaw						
		I1	I2	P1	P2	M1	M2	M3
Lundström (1948)	Identical-twin pairs	91	90	62	53	—	—	—
	Fraternal-twin pairs	94	98	73	60	—	—	—
	Heredity / Non-heredity	3·9	2·8	5·1	2·8	—	—	—
Combined from Bowden and Goose (1969)	Pairs of first-degree relatives	308	284	—	—	—	—	—
	Correl. coeff.	0·49	0·38	—	—	—	—	—
Sofaer, Bailit and MacLean (1971)	Pairs of first-degree relatives	224	229	216	194	243	152	63
	Correl. coeff.	0·47	0·42	0·51	0·44	0·51	0·30	0·33
		Lower Jaw						
		I1	I2	P1	P2	M1	M2	M3
Lundström (1948)	Identical-twin pairs	93	95	80	62	—	—	—
	Fraternal-twin pairs	91	94	85	67	—	—	—
	Heredity / Non-heredity	3·3	3·5	3·6	2·5	—	—	—
Sofaer, Bailit and MacLean (1971)	Pairs of first-degree relatives	214	222	209	193	233	167	62
	Correl. coeff.	0·22	0·30	0·53	0·25	0·26	0·31	0·18

separate first molar and supernumerary elements. Embryological study has shown that the most fundamental mutant characteristic observed is a partial suppression of growth and differentiation of dental epithelium during a particular phase of development. The reduced size of the teeth and

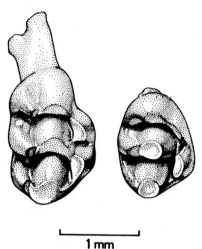

1 mm

FIG. 10. Occlusal views of normal (left) and tabby (right) upper right first molars. Reproduced with the permission of Professor H. Grüneberg and The Company of Biologists Ltd. from Grüneberg (1965).

the mutant molar morphology seem to be due directly to the suppression of growth without an associated comparable delay in the onset of calcification, since the morphology of fully formed mutant molars corresponds in most respects to the morphology of an earlier stage of development in normal animals. The supernumerary tooth was found to arise independently from a normal extension of dental

recently been released from the effects of the suppressive influence (fig. 11c). Since the supernumerary tooth arises independently, the composite teeth observed in adult animals are likely to be the result of fusion of the supernumerary and first molar germs. Thus, a complex pattern of dental abnormalities appears to result from a basically simple genetically controlled defect of epithelial function. This defect could be either intrinsic to the epithelium itself or secondary to an abnormality in the related mesenchyme.

These mutant mice do not provide the only example of an inherited association between fused and supernumerary teeth. Such an association can occur in the incisor region of dogs, and has led to the proposal of a mechanism whereby fusion might take place. It has been suggested that rapid growth of adjacent tooth germs can result in stripping of the external enamel epithelium from the dental lamina separating adjacent teeth, allowing the internal enamel epithelium of neighbouring germs freedom to come into contact and fuse. A further example is provided by the rice rat, a rodent native to the southern United States. In this case a supernumerary tooth sometimes develops posterior to the three molars of the normal series, and fusion may involve the first two molars, or all three molars of the normal series. Breeding records provide some evidence that the condition is caused by a single recessive gene. A section of a developing composite tooth composed of first, second and third molar elements is shown in fig. 12. It illustrates the bizarre result of fusion, the anterior end of the composite tooth germ showing an advanced state of histodifferentiation but the posterior end barely having progressed beyond undifferentiated internal enamel epithelium.

The reason for the association between supernumerary and fused teeth is not entirely clear, but may simply be related to the amount of space available to the developing tooth germs. Crowding of adjacent germs at a critical stage

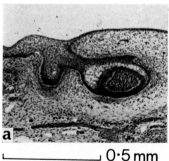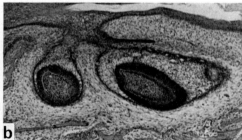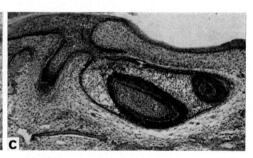

FIG. 11(a). Tabby heterozygote lower first molar at 17 days of gestation showing a large bud of dental lamina anteriorly.
(b) Tabby heterozygote lower first molar at 19 days of gestation with a small supernumerary germ anteriorly.
(c) Lower first molar from the opposite side of the same animal as in (b) showing a laminal downgrowth that has failed to form a supernumerary tooth germ. (Anterior to the left.) Reproduced with the permission of the Company of Biologists Ltd. from Sofaer (1969b).

lamina anterior to the point of origin of the first molar, apparently as a response to small size of the first molar at the end of the suppression phase (fig. 11a and b). However, an overgrowth of dental lamina elicited at this stage does not necessarily progress to form a supernumerary tooth. Regression of the laminal downgrowth may occur, possibly as a result of competition with a first molar germ that has

of development may predispose to epithelial stripping and subsequent fusion, and crowding may result from the presence of an additional tooth germ. Conversely, fusion, since it usually results in a smaller volume of developing tooth material than normal, may allow the lamina to proliferate further and form a supernumerary tooth. On the other hand, it could be that the basis of the association lies in the lamina itself, and that there is some inherited quality of the dental lamina predisposing to epithelial stripping and laminal hyperactivity.

In man, a relatively commonly occurring inherited abnormality is the absence of one or both upper lateral incisors. There is some evidence that the abnormality is due to a single gene, but the situation is not sufficiently clear cut to regard this as proved. In any event, it is certain that the condition

operate with lip furrow epithelium, and even with epidermis from the plantar surface of the foot, to form teeth; whereas the enamel organ becomes a stratified keratinizing epithelium when confronted with plantar surface dermis. The specificity for continued dental development therefore seems to reside in the dental papilla rather than the enamel organ at this stage (Kollar, 1972).

Direct evidence of differential gene action in the different

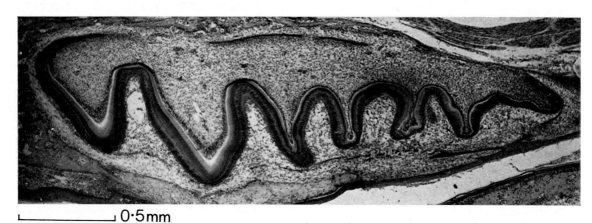

FIG. 12. Rice rat fused upper molar at one day after birth composed of first, second and third molar elements. (Anterior to the left.) Reproduced with the permission of The Company of Biologists Ltd. from Sofaer and Shaw (1971).

is largely genetic in origin, the most informative kind of case perhaps being one in which an upper lateral incisor is absent on one side and present and of normal size on the other. In such a case, the two central incisors developed under different conditions, one having adjacent tooth germs on both sides, and the other having an adjacent germ on one side only. Unilateral absence therefore provides a simple situation in which to study the effect of local competition between tooth germs during development. In a sample of over 13,000 school-children from Hawaii unilateral absence, with a normal lateral on the other side, was observed in 77 cases. Measurements of the widths of the central incisors showed that the centrals tended to be larger on the side where the lateral was missing than on the side where the lateral was present and of normal size. This hereditary variant has thus revealed an association between local competition during development and final tooth-size.

Within-Individual Differences

(a) Tissue and Regional Specificities

Differences may occur within individuals between tissues or regions of the body in terms of their developmental potencies. These potencies appear to be under the control of different sets of genes that have become activated in the different tissues. Variation in developmental potency is illustrated by studies of epidermis-dermis interaction that have involved separation of epidermis and dermis and the recombination of epidermis and dermis from different sources, allowing continued growth in culture. The results of such recombination procedures indicate that dental papillae from early tooth germs of mouse embryos are able to co-

tissues may be forthcoming if a suitable mutant affecting the system is available. Instead of making reciprocal recombinations between epidermis and dermis from different regions it is then possible to make combinations of normal epidermis with mutant dermis, and *vice versa*. In the case of *downless* mice, the dental abnormalities of which

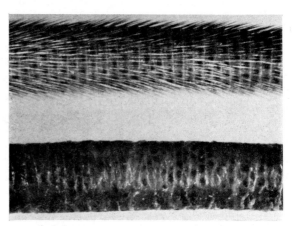

FIG. 13. Segments of normal (above) and downless homozygote (below) adult tails.

have already been mentioned, a simple difference between normal and mutant animals caused by the abnormality of epidermis-dermis interaction presents itself in the tail. The tails of normal mice are covered with hair whereas those of the mutants are bald (fig. 13). This results from suppression of formation of hair follicles in mutant tails, and could be due to a failure in either the epidermal or dermal component of the system. Recombinations between epidermis and dermis from embryonic tails of *downless* homozygotes (phenotypically mutant) and *downless* heterozygotes (phenotypically normal) have been made at a stage well before the first signs of tail hair follicle formation in normal mice. After further development in culture, recombinations containing *downless* heterozygote epidermis and *downless* homozygote dermis produced hair follicles, whereas those containing *downless* homozygote epidermis and heterozygote dermis did not. Phenotypically normal epidermis was therefore required for follicle initiation, and mutant dermis did not prevent initiation from taking place. The mutant defect therefore appears to be restricted to the epidermis. Thus it seems reasonable to suppose that all the abnormalities shown by *downless* mice are due to a primary epithelial defect resulting from the presence of the mutant gene.

An example of regional rather than tissue specificity is the difference of morphology shown by different teeth along the length of the jaw. These differences have been explained in terms of **developmental fields** that may be related to gradients of evocating substances along the length of the developing tooth row. It is assumed that all prospective tooth germs have identical **prepatterns,** that is to say each is competent to form a complete set of morphological components in a prescribed relationship; but that the presence and relative size of each component depends on the level of the appropriate gradient at the position in which a tooth germ finds itself. Both prepatterns and gradients are presumably under genetic control, so that a study of variation in morphological fields may help to indicate how they are established during development.

(b) Asymmetry

The difference between sides within individuals with respect to a bilaterally represented character is of considerable interest in the study of development. As already noted, the level of asymmetry can be taken as a measure of developmental instability. Numerous studies using experimental animals have shown that normal phenotypes are relatively stable, or, put another way, normal development is narrowly canalized. On the other hand, if a major genetic or environmental influence acts to produce an abnormal phenotype, the abnormal phenotype is frequently much more variable. Abnormal development is therefore usually poorly canalized, and is accordingly associated with a relatively high level of asymmetry. In the case of an inherited malformation it is of interest to know whether the instability of development is restricted to the areas of the body primarily affected by the abnormality, or whether poor canalization is a general feature of development of affected individuals.

Two measures of developmental instability have been made in individuals suffering from familial CL(P) (cleft lip with or without cleft palate). As seen above, this condition has a high heritability, indicating that differences between CL(P) and normal individuals are largely due to the inheritance of different genes. The first measure of instability was the asymmetry of the lower first molar teeth. Although part of the same developmental complex as that affected by the malformation, these teeth are remote from the site of the cleft. The second measure was the asymmetry of the *atd* angle, a feature of the dermatoglyphic pattern of the palm of the hand. The *atd* angle is clearly far removed in developmental terms from the lip, alveolus and palate. Both the lower first molar and the *atd* angle showed greater asymmetry in familial CL(P) cases than in a control group, suggesting that developmental instability is not restricted to the area immediately related to the cleft. The interpretation of this finding was that there is a system of normal genes that buffers development against environmental fluctuations, that replacement of these normal genes by deleterious alleles lowers developmental stability, and that when buffering becomes too low to compensate for adverse environmental influences a major malformation in a particularly sensitive region may occur.

Animal experiments have shown, too, that developmental stability is reduced not only by major genetic or environmental influences but also through **inbreeding.** That is, as a result of a population becoming progressively more homozygous over all loci by the mating of closely related individuals, the phenotype becomes more unstable. Rapid progress towards a high level of homozygosity in laboratory animals is achieved by successive generations of brother-sister mating. In human populations lower levels of inbreeding may result from cousin marriages, or may occur in small isolated communities where potential mates are likely to be related. Instability may follow for two reasons. Firstly, homozygosity allows the expression of deleterious recessive alleles whose effects are masked by normal dominant counterparts in heterozygotes; and secondly, homozygosity provides the developing organism with a poorer choice of genes with which to deal with fluctuations of the developmental process. In keeping with the experimental findings is the association with inbreeding of an increased variance of tooth size and a suggestion of increased dental asymmetry in man.

By comparing different populations, it may be possible to learn more about the relative contributions of the genetic and environmental sources of instability. Four populations subject to different environmental conditions have been studied with this in mind. These were: natives of Tristan da Cunha, two distinct groups from the Solomon Islands (Kwaio and Nasioi), and Boston school-children. Dental asymmetry was found to be greatest in the population subject to the greatest environmental stress (Tristanites), as assessed by a consideration of climate, housing, diet and disease experience; and progressively lower in those subject to lower levels of environmental stress (Kwaio—Nasioi—Boston school-children). The measure of asymmetry used was the intraclass correlation between the mesiodistal diameters of antimeric teeth, and for all but one of the populations (Boston school-children) correlations for several pairs of teeth could be combined into a mean z score for each individual. The frequency distributions of individual z scores of males are shown for the other three populations in fig. 14. A lower z score means lower correlation between sides and therefore greater asymmetry. There is clearly a definite separation between the populations.

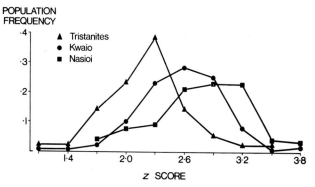

FIG. 14. Frequency distributions of individual z scores expressing dental asymmetry in three populations. Redrawn from Bailit, Workman, Niswander and MacLean (1970).

Correlated Characters

Correlation between characters in adult individuals may be the result either of common genetic control or of common environmental influence, or a combination of both. Associations between various dental characteristics have been discussed in the past; for example, third molar agenesis appears to be related to agenesis of other teeth and to retarded development. However, although plausible explanations may be advanced as to the basis of any association, it is not possible to determine the underlying nature of the observed correlation unless family data are available. Through an analysis of the resemblance between relatives, comparable to that by which heritabilities are estimated, a **genetic correlation** between characters can be calculated (Falconer, 1964). This is an expression of the degree to which characters are associated because they are influenced by the same genes. A high genetic correlation indicates a high degree of common genetic control, whereas a low genetic correlation implies that the characters vary together largely because of common environmental influences during development.

REFERENCES

Bailit, H. L., Workman, P. L., Niswander, J. D. and MacLean, C. J. (1970), "Dental Asymmetry as an Indicator of Genetic and Environmental Conditions in Human Populations." *Hum. Biol.*, **42**, 626.

Bowden, D. E. J. and Goose, D. H. (1969), "Inheritance of Tooth Size in Liverpool Families," *J. med. Genetics*, **6**, 55.

Falconer, D. S. (1964), *Introduction to Quantitative Genetics*. Edinburgh: Oliver and Boyd.

Falconer, D. S. (1965), "The Inheritance of Liability to Certain Diseases, Estimated from the Incidence Among Relatives," *Annals Hum. Genetics*, **29**, 51.

Grüneberg, H. (1963), *The Pathology of Development*. Oxford: Blackwell.

Grüneberg, H. (1965), "Genes and Genotypes Affecting the Teeth of the Mouse," *J. Embryology and Experimental Morphology*, **14**, 137.

Kollar, E. J. (1972), "Histogenetic Aspects of Dermal-Epidermal Interactions," in *Developmental Aspects of Oral Biology* (Slavkin and Bavetta, Eds.). New York and London: Academic Press.

Lundström, A. (1948), *Tooth Size and Occlusion in Twins*. Basle and New York: S. Karger.

Orban, B. J. (1957), *Oral Histology and Embryology*, 4th edition. St. Louis: The C. V. Mosby Company.

Ross, R. B. and Johnston, M. C. (1972), *Cleft Lip and Palate*, Chap. 3. Baltimore: The Williams and Wilkins Company.

Sofaer, J. A. (1969a), "The Genetics and Expression of a Dental Morphological Variant in the Mouse," *Arch. oral Biol.*, **14**, 1213.

Sofaer, J. A. (1969b), Aspects of the Tabby-Crinkled-Downless Syndrome. I. The Development of Tabby Teeth. II. Observations on the Reaction to Changes of Genetic Background. *J. Embryology and Experimental Morphology*, **22**, 181 and 207.

Sofaer, J. A., Bailit, H. L. and MacLean, C. J. (1971), "A Developmental Basis for Differential Tooth Reduction During Hominid Evolution," *Evolution*, **25**, 509.

Sofaer, J. A. and Shaw, J. H. (1971), The Genetics and Development of Fused and Supernumerary Molars in the Rice Rat. *J. Embryology and Experimental Morphology*, **26**, 99.

2. PRENATAL GROWTH AND DEVELOPMENT

W. J. HAMILTON

Branchial arches

Development of the face

Nasal cavity

Floor of the mouth
   Tongue

Lips, cheeks and gingiva

Salivary glands

Pharyngeal grooves and pouches and their derivatives
   The first pharyngeal endodermal pouch
   The second pharyngeal endodermal pouch

   The third pharyngeal endodermal pouch
   The fourth pharyngeal endodermal pouch
   Thyroid gland

The cervical sinus and cervical vesicles
   Cervical cysts and fistulae of developmental origin

Neural crest

INTRODUCTION

An understanding of the development of the face, nose, mouth, palate, air sinuses and pharynx requires a knowledge of the formation and the fate of the primitive foregut.

This, in turn, presupposes a grasp of the arrangement of the original yolk sac vesicle and an appreciation of the folding of the embryonic head.

At about the 12th day of human development, the embryo itself consists of two apposed layers of cells—embryonic ectoderm and embryonic endoderm. The embryonic ectoderm forms the "roof" of the primary yolk sac (fig. 1). The next phase of development consists in the formation of a third layer, the intra-embryonic mesoderm, which arises from the primitive streak and lies between the embryonic ectoderm and endoderm throughout the whole of the length of the embryonic disc except at the site of the prochordal plate and the cloacal region, at the very rostral and caudal portions of the embryo, where only the two layers exist.

As the embryonic disc elongates, it becomes oval and then pear-shaped. At the same time it develops head and tail folds and bulges slightly upwards into the amniotic cavity. With the formation of the head fold, the cranial portion of the yolk-sac cavity is enclosed within the embryo and appears as a tube-like endodermal diverticulum dorsal to the portion of the embryo forming the pericardial cavity and the septum transversum (diaphragm). This diverticulum is the foregut (fig. 2). It is situated in a median position, the notochord being at first embedded in its roof and separating it from the hindbrain. The blind cranial extremity of the foregut diverticulum lies in part immediately adjacent to the surface ectoderm of the stomatodaeum. The stomatodaeum is a depression which occurs with further extension of the head fold. It is bounded above by the projecting forebrain, laterally by the maxillary processes, and laterally and caudally by the mandibular processes and by the pericardial swelling (figs. 3 and 4). The junction of the ectodermal stomatodaeum and the endodermal cranial portion of the foregut is the buccopharyngeal membrane (fig. 2).

Immediately in front of the buccopharyngeal membrane (fig. 2) an ectodermal diverticulum, Rathke's pouch, arises from the stomatodaeal roof and grows towards the ventral aspect of the forebrain (prosencephalon). In embryos of about 26 days, the buccopharyngeal membrane ruptures and continuity is established between the foregut and the ectodermal stomatodaeum (figs. 4 and 6). Soon all traces of the membrane disappear and the line of junction between ectoderm and endoderm is no longer identifiable (fig. 8). Consequently, in the description of the developmental history of the mouth region and its derivatives, both endodermal and ectodermal epithelia must be considered.

The paraxial mesoderm of each side of the notochordal process is present as thickened longitudinal masses which become subdivided into somites (fig. 6). With the possible exception of the somites for the eye muscles, no somites are found in the mesoderm cranial to the notochord, nor is there an intermediate cell mass. The diffuse, unsegmented mesoderm does exist, however, as far forward as the rostral extremity of the embryonic disc. It is this mesoderm (branchial) which condenses cranially as the forerunner of the branchial arch components (fig. 11) and also surrounds the more caudal derivatives of the foregut proper.

The foregut can now be subdivided into cranial and caudal portions. The former, flanked by the branchial mesoderm, gives origin to the endodermal part of the mouth, to the greater part of the pharynx, and to the endodermal epithelium of the respiratory system. The ectodermal part of the mouth cavity and the nasal cavities, with the disappearance of the buccopharyngeal membrane, becomes continuous with the cranial part of the foregut and will be described with it. In this chapter, the fate of the caudal portion of the foregut will not be discussed.

BRANCHIAL ARCHES

In the head region, a series of elevations, formed from the unsplit branchial mesoderm, the branchial arches, develops lateral to the stomatodaeum and to the embryonic pharynx (figs. 3–7). These surface elevations, or arches, are separated from each other by grooves. Each arch gradually extends ventrally and comes to merge with its fellow of the opposite side. In this way, five or six bars, pharyngeal, branchial, or visceral arches are formed.

In each of these mesodermal condensations, a cartilaginous bar and branchial musculature differentiate (fig. 8). The musculature of each arch is supplied by a branchial (special visceral) efferent nerve and the related endoderm by branchial efferent fibres from the nerve (post-trematic) of the immediately succeeding arch (fig. 9). Each arch has also associated with it, for at least part of the embryonic life, a branchial (pharyngeal) or aortic arch artery which passes from the aortic sac to the corresponding dorsal aorta. Between the successive arches the foregut endoderm extends laterally in the form of endodermal pharyngeal grooves which soon become pouch-like and come into contact with similar, but shallower, ectodermal grooves (figs. 3, 8, and 10). In lower vertebrates, the ectodermal grooves become continuous with the corresponding endodermal pouches by the rupture of the intervening branchial membrane, and thus the definitive gill clefts are established. In terrestrial vertebrates, however, such rupture never normally occurs, as a thin layer of mesoderm becomes interposed between the ectoderm and endoderm, and the endodermal pouches become modified to form structures as diverse as the middle-ear cavity and the parathyroid and thymus glands.

In vertebrates with functional gill-clefts, the sensory component of each branchial nerve is distributed to the cranial and caudal surface of the corresponding cleft. The fibres to the cranial surface form the pre-trematic branch of the branchial nerve and those to the caudal surface form the post-trematic branch. The motor component of each branchial nerve is included in the post-trematic branch. It follows from this arrangement that two cranial nerves are represented in each arch—the post-trematic branch of the branchial nerve corresponding to that arch and the pre-trematic branch of the immediately succeeding arch.

The first, or mandibular arch, is interposed between the mouth and the first ectodermal groove. The major portion, or mandibular process, of this arch forms the lower jaw, and an extension, the maxillary process, from its dorsal end, cranial to the stomatodaeum, contributes to the upper jaw. The second pharyngeal arch is often called the hyoid arch.

In the 14-somite stage (15th day), the head region, which is now becoming established, shows certain marked features

—the maxillary and mandibular processes bounding the stomatodaeum, and the hyoid arch can now be identified. Between the mandibular process and the hyoid arch the depression of the first pharyngeal (branchial) ectodermal groove is seen and, caudal to the hyoid arch, the second pharyngeal ectodermal groove is evident. A thickening of the ectoderm dorsal to the second pharyngeal groove marks the position of the otic placode. Ventral to the pharyngeal arches is the pericardial elevation.

In the 20-somite embryo (26th day), the buccopharyngeal membrane is in the process of rupturing to establish communication between the ectodermal stomatodaeum and the endodermal foregut. The third pharyngeal arch is now appearing and the otic placode of earlier stages has now become the otic depression.

After the rupture of the buccopharyngeal membrane, the roof of the primitive buccal cavity is lined by stomatodaeal ectoderm and foregut endoderm; the junctional area is indicated by the attachment of Rathke's pouch. A thin layer of mesoderm in the anterior part separates the ectodermal roof from the forebrain. In the middle line, more caudally, the notochord is interposed between the endoderm and the nervous system.

DEVELOPMENT OF THE FACE

In late somite embryos (25–28 somites), the optic vesicle projects from the forebrain and can be seen through the overlying ectoderm. The otic depression has separated from the surface ectoderm to form the otic vesicle.

Above the margin of the stomatodaeal orifice, the nasal placodes appear as convex thickenings of the surface ectoderm (fig. 5). Growth changes in the forebrain and the proliferation and differentiation of the surrounding mesoderm accompanying the formation of the medial and lateral nasal folds, or processes, cause the nasal placodes to become depressed to form the olfactory pits (fig. 12). Soon the openings of these pits come to lie on the stomatodaeal margin where they are bounded by the medial and lateral nasal folds (figs. 12 and 13). The elevation produced by the forebrain and the proliferation of mesoderm round the olfactory pits is the fronto-nasal process. Current embryological opinion regards the elevation, or "processes", of the developing facial region as in the nature of surface swellings produced by proliferations of the underlying mesoderm. The furrows between the elevations become smoothed out in subsequent development as growth and fusion of the mesodermal centres proceeds beneath the ectoderm. "Under the circumstances no ectoderm requires absorption; it is simply flattened out in adaptation to the changed surface" (Streeter, 1948). Nevertheless, for descriptive purposes, it is convenient to retain the term maxillary, mandibular and fronto-nasal processes.

With further growth of the nasal folds each olfactory, or nasal, pit becomes deeper, forming a nasal sac (fig. 14). Each sac then extends dorsocaudally above the level of the corresponding medial and lateral nasal folds. The apposed epithelial surfaces of these folds fuse, in the floor of the nasal sac, to form a longitudinal epithelial septum (Epithelmaeuer, of Hochstetter, 1944; the nasal fin, of Streeter, 1948). Anteriorly, mesoderm soon extends across this line of epithelial fusion. This mesodermal junction is immediately behind the original nasal pit, the opening into which can now be called the anterior naris. The mesodermal fusion itself can be considered to result in the establishment of the primordium of the primitive palate which then separates the nasal sac from the mouth cavity. Posteriorly, however, the epithelial nasal fin becomes stretched and thinned, forming a temporary bucconasal membrane (fig. 14) behind the primitive palate. In embryos of 12–14 mm. CR length (38–40 days) the bucconasal membranes rupture and continuity is established on each side between the corresponding nasal sac and the roof of the mouth. The regions of continuity are the primitive posterior nares, and they lie behind and above the primitive palate.

Meanwhile, the epithelium of each maxillary process fuses with the corresponding lateral nasal process. Mesodermal continuity between the two processes is soon established and further medial extension of the maxillary mesoderm results in its intermingling with that of the fronto-nasal process (figs. 15, 16 and 17). The medial extension of the maxillary mesoderm is considered by some embryologists to reach the midline in the lower part of the fronto-nasal process, where it fuses with the corresponding mesoderm from the opposite side. With this interpretation, the upper lip is considered to originate chiefly from the two maxillary processes. Many embryologists, however, believe the mesoderm of the central part of the upper lip to be of fronto-nasal origin (see Vermeiz-Keers, 1972 for review).

NASAL CAVITY

As a result of the forward growth of the maxillary processes and the establishment of the fronto-nasal process, the buccal cavity becomes highly vaulted (figs. 14 and 17). The sacs, now called the primitive nasal cavities, have become much more extensive, but remain separated, however, by a deep portion of the fronto-nasal process which progressively becomes relatively thinner to form the primitive nasal septum. This septum gradually extends backwards and downwards as a distinct midline elevation with a free edge, the upper part of which reaches as far as the attachment of Rathke's pouch (figs. 16 and 17). The septum forms a marked projection between the two nasal cavities. Later cartilage and bone will appear in the mesoderm of this septum.

While the nasal septum is developing, each mass of maxillary mesoderm gives origin to a vertically directed extension—the palatal process (figs. 14, 15 and 16). This process extends medially as a free edge below and behind the primitive posterior nares on a level with the primitive palate. The tongue, which is developing from the floor of the mouth, lies below the primitive palate in front while, more posteriorly, it projects upward, for a time, between the maxillary palatal processes and the developing nasal cavity. At first, the posterior parts of these processes are directed vertically downwards on each side of the tongue. As the tongue descends in the developing mouth cavity in fetuses of about 20 mm. CR length (45–50 days), the palatal processes take up a horizontal position. With further growth, the free edges of the maxillary palatal processes fuse, first with the posterior margin of the primitive palate, and then progressively, from before backward, with each other in the middle line and eventually with the lower free edge of the nasal septum (figs. 16 and 17). The posterior part of the soft palate and the uvula are formed by subepithelial merging of mesenchymal tissues which proliferate from the posterior edge of each palatal maxillary process. These developmental changes result in the subdivision of the stomatodaeum and olfactory pits into an upper pair of nasal fossae and a lower cavity, the definitive mouth (fig. 18). The changes obviously constitute the embryological basis for the separation of the respiratory and alimentary systems in the facial region; the former now bypasses the mouth and each system is enabled to perform its own specific function. During the changes the tongue is gradually excluded from the nasal cavities by the progressive fusion, from before backwards, of the maxillary palatal processes with the primitive palate and with each other. This fusion also results in a gradual posterior migration of the posterior nares so that they come to lie on each side of the posterior free edge of the adult nasal septum. Pourtois (1972) using mice and rat embryos, has shown that a wedge-like projection develops from the caudal segment of each palatal shelf between the tongue and the roof of the stomatodaeum. He suggests that it may be the primordium of the horizontal part of the palatine bone.

In later development, there are extensions of membranous ossification from the pre-maxillae into the primitive palate, and from the maxillae and palatine bones into the maxillary palatal processes. The posterior portions of the latter, however, do not become ossified; they extend beyond the nasal septum and fuse to form the soft palate and uvula (fig. 20). A small opening, the naso-palatine canal, persists for a time in the middle line between the primitive palate and the maxillary palatal processes. Eventually epithelial fusion obliterates the naso-palatine canal. Its position is represented throughout the life, however, in the hard palate by a foramen known as the incisive canal.

While these changes are progressing, a number of elevations appear on the lateral wall of each nasal cavity; these will develop into the **superior, middle** and **inferior conchae** (fig. 20). The olfactory placodes are now represented by olfactory epithelium situated in the roof and adjacent parts of the walls of each nasal cavity (fig. 21). Neuroblasts in the olfactory epithelium differentiate into nerve cells. These cells give origin to the olfactory nerve fibres which grow into the olfactory bulbs of the cerebral hemispheres (fig. 14). The **paranasal** sinuses appear in late fetal and early postnatal life as small diverticula of the lateral nasal wall which, in childhood, come gradually to invade the substance of the maxilla, the ethmoid, the frontal and the sphenoid bones. The maxillary sinuses are the first to appear and are followed before birth by the sphenoidal sinuses. The other sinuses are represented at full term merely by dimples in the nasal wall. After formation of the epithelial **nasolacrimal duct,** approximately in the line of fusion of the superficial surfaces of the maxillary and fronto-nasal processes, the lower end of this duct grows actively and comes to terminate in the lateral wall of the nasal cavity below the inferior concha (fig. 20).

FLOOR OF MOUTH

In an embryo of 4–5 mm. CR length (30th to 32nd day), the floor of the mouth has the appearance seen in fig. 9. The ventral portions of the endodermal pharyngeal grooves. and the arches between them, extend towards the middle line. The first and second arches of each side meet their fellow in the middle line where the medial ends of the first arches produce a small pair of swellings. A small median eminence, the **tuberculum impar,** soon appears between and caudal to these mandibular swellings while the second arches appear to be directly continuous across the midline. Owing to the development of another, more caudal, median swelling, the **hypobranchial eminence,** the third and fourth arches, in surface relief, do not reach the middle line. The succeeding arches are not yet well established and, indeed, the fifth soon disappears. Immediately caudal to the hypobranchial eminence the **tracheobranchial groove** can be seen, bounded laterally by the sixth arch rudiments. A narrow portion of the foregut, the primitive oesophagus, lies caudal to the tracheal groove and is flanked by the **pericardioperitoneal canals** (pleural cavities) (fig. 9).

At this time the endoderm can no longer be distinguished from the stomatodaeal ectoderm and there is probably a considerable amount of intermingling of the two epithelia. The boundary line, however, is behind that part of the epithelium of the mandibular process which gives origin to the teeth since the enamel organs of the latter are of ectodermal origin as is the epithelium lining the cheek and the parotid gland derived from it. The boundary in the adult can be indicated by approximately a line between the gingiva and the attachment of the tongue to the floor of the mouth. As the lip lies external to the teeth of the lower jaw its epithelium is also ectodermal. From the undulating endodermal floor of the primitive buccal cavity and the associated mesoderm the **tongue,** the **epiglottis** and the **submandibular** and **sublingual salivary glands** are derived.

Tongue

The tongue initially consists of:

(a) an anterior portion which arises from the tuberculum impar and the adjacent regions of both mandibular arches; and

(b) a posterior, paired, portion which arises from the ventro-medial ends of the second (hyoid) arches; later these paired portions fuse, in front of the hypobranchial eminence, to form a single swelling, sometimes known as the copula, to which the third arch mesoderm later contributes.

The anterior part of the tongue first appears as the tuberculum impar (fig. 9), but soon elevations of the ventro-medial portions of the first (mandibular) arches arise on each side of this tubercle and by their growth merge with it and with each other. From the resulting single eminence the anterior two-thirds of the adult tongue arises. Its position can be identified however, in later stages of development, owing to the fact that the thyroid gland takes origin as an endodermal downgrowth, the site of origin of which is marked by the **foramen caecum,** immediately caudal to the tubercle. As the mandibular arches form the anterior two-thirds of the tongue the epithelial nerve supply is from the mandibular division (post-trematic first arch nerve) of the trigeminal nerve and from the chorda tympani (sometimes regarded as a pre-trematic) branch of the facial (second arch) nerve. The posterior one-third of the tongue has a more complicated developmental origin, in that it appears to be developed by a subepithelial overgrowth of the third arch mesoderm, together with its nerve supply, over the second arch mesoderm, which is consequently separated from the surface of the adult tongue. The third arch meso-derm fuses with the first arch mesoderm, thus obliterating the ventral portions of the first and second pharyngeal endodermal grooves. The epithelial nerve supply of this part of the tongue, therefore, is the third arch nerve (glosso-pharyngeal). The extreme posterior part of the tongue, which lies immediately in front of the hypobranchial eminence, receives its epithelial supply from the fourth arch nerve (superior laryngeal branch of the vagus).

It will be seen that the greater part of the mesoderm under-lying the epithelium of the tongue is derived from the ventro-medial extremities of the first and third pharyngeal arches. The line representing the junction of the two portions is indicated in the epithelium by the **sulcus terminalis,** but this is not an absolute boundary since glossopharyngeal nerve fibres cross it to supply taste buds which develop in the region immediately anterior to the sulcus. The branchial mesoderm underlying the epithelium forms the general con-nective tissue of the tongue. In the human embryo, it is possible that the musculature of the tongue arises *in situ*: but from the morphology of the hypoglossal nerve and comparative embryology, it is reasonable to assume that the striated lingual musculature is really derived from a ventral migration of three or more **occipital myotomes**. The tongue, therefore, results from the developmental inter-locking of pharyngeal endoderm, branchial mesoderm and occipital myotomes, and its nerve supply from diverse sources (Vth, VIIth, IXth, Xth and XIIth cranial nerves) is thus explained.

The lingual epithelium is at first a single layer of cuboidal cells. The layer soon becomes two or three cells thick. At about the 25 mm. stage (50 days) the epithelium of the dorsum and tip becomes stratified and the **papillae** make their appearance; of the latter the **vallate** and **foliate** are the first, and are found in close relation with terminal branches of the glossopharyngeal nerve which may induce their development. The fungiform papillae appear rather later under the influence of the chorda tympani branch of the facial nerve. All of these papillae soon develop taste buds. The filiform papillae arise in fetuses of about 45 mm.

LIPS, CHEEKS AND GINGIVA

The lower lip is formed from the free edge of the mandib-ular process by the separation of its superficial portion from the remainder by an arched groove, the **labio-gingival sulcus.** Internal to, and parallel with, this groove another deeper groove, the **linguo-gingival sulcus,** separates the mandibular portion of the developing tongue from the remainder of the mandibular process. The portion of the mandibular process between the lower lip externally and the tongue internally forms the primitive gingiva and, eventually, the tooth-bearing area. The upper lip is formed in its lateral parts from the maxillary processes in a manner similar to that described for the formation of the lower lip from the mandibular process. Its median portion, related to the lower end of the fronto-nasal process, is formed by the lower part of this process and, as indicated earlier, it is generally considered that the whole of the central portion of the upper lip is developed from the lower portion of the fronto-nasal process. It has, however, been suggested that medial extensions of the two maxillary processes pass super-ficial to the lower end of the fronto-nasal process which, therefore, contributes only to the deep aspect of the median part of the upper lip. The **philtrum** of the upper lip appears to be formed by the heaping up of maxillary mesoderm on either side of the middle line. It is absent in cases of bilateral hare-lip.

The musculature of both upper and lower lips is derived from hyoid arch mesoderm which migrates early from its site of origin in the second branchial arch into the tissue of the developing face. It is therefore supplied by the VIIth cranial nerve which is the nerve of the hyoid arch.

SALIVARY GLANDS

The salivary glands arise as solid outgrowths of the buccal epithelium (fig. 19). The submandibular gland makes its appearance in embryos of about 15 mm. CR length (32 days) as a ridge-like antero-posterior epithelial thickening, probably endodermal, in the floor of the mouth between the tongue and developing gingivae. The ridge is gradually separated from the buccal epithelium, the process starting posteriorly, so that eventually it is attached only at its anterior extremity. It is then an epithelial cord in the substance of the mesoderm of the floor of the mouth. A little later the parotid gland arises as an epithelial prolifer-ation, probably ectodermal, on the deep aspect of the cheek immediately posterior to the angle of the mouth. The pri-mordium of the greater sublingual gland then appears immediately lateral to the submandibular gland. Finally, the primordia of the lesser sublingual glands, 5–14 in num-ber, arise in the linguo-gingival sulcus. The submandibular and parotid glands do not arise in the position where the openings of the ducts are found in the adult, for closure of gutter-like grooves of the buccal epithelium causes elonga-tion of the ducts in an anterior direction. The elongation of the submandibular duct results in the inclusion within it of the duct orifice of the greater sublingual gland so that the two glands share a common opening. The lesser sublingual glands are later surrounded by a common connective tissue sheath and so appear in the adult as a single gland with multiple orifices.

In the third month of intra-uterine life the distal extremi-ties of the epithelial cords of the salivary glands branch repeatedly. The solid primordia develop lumina and, by the sixth month, are completely canalized. The definitive histological appearances of serous secretory activity are found only after birth, but mucin is secreted much earlier.

PHARYNGEAL GROOVES AND POUCHES AND THEIR DERIVATIVES

The lateral walls and floor of the cranial part of the early foregut become much altered by the development of the pharyngeal pouches in this region. These pouches first appear as grooves which extend ventrally across, or towards, the middle line (figs. 9 and 11). A comparative study of the developmental history of the pharynx shows that, in Man and other terrestrial vertebrates, these grooves have marked resemblances, in their early stages, to the endodermal part of the gill region of aquatic vertebrates. In their later development, however, they become greatly modified to give origin to a number of diverse structures. These include the tympanic (middle ear) cavity, the **parathyroid glands** and the **thymus**. The **thyroid gland** arises from the mid-pharyngeal floor and is conveniently considered with the derivatives of the pouches.

While these modifications are occurring in the pharyngeal grooves and pouches, correlated changes take place in the ectodermal clefts. These changes result in the eventual disappearance of all the ectodermal clefts, except a restricted portion of the first which becomes the external auditory meatus, and are a necessary prelude to the formation of a smooth contour to the neck. The structures found in the wall of the pharynx are shown in fig. 9.

The First Pharyngeal Endodermal Pouch

This lies between the first (maxillo-mandibular) and the second (hyoid) arches (fig. 8) and becomes obliterated in its ventral portion by the development of the tongue, but its dorsal portion becomes pouch-like and, with the adjacent pharyngeal wall, possibly including part of the second dorsal pouch, forms the tubo-tympanic recess, which lies between the dorsal ends of the first (Meckel's) and the second (Reichert's) arch cartilages.

The Second Pharyngeal Endodermal Pouch

This lies between the second and third pharyngeal arches and is obliterated ventrally by the development of the tongue. The lateral portion persists as the second pharyngeal pouch. The dorsal portion of this pouch possibly contributes to the corresponding tubo-tympanic recess. The ventral portion of the pouch soon loses its contact with the ectoderm and is almost completely obliterated by the proliferation of its endodermal lining, only a small portion possibly persisting as a small recess, the **tonsillar fossa**.

The Third Pharyngeal Endodermal Pouch

Each third pouch becomes apparent in the pharyngeal wall at about the 10-somite stage (23rd day) and is soon in contact with the corresponding third ectodermal cleft. Growth changes result in the narrowing of the communication (**ductus pharyngobranchialis** III) between the pouch and the pharynx. Contact with the ectoderm is soon lost and the pouch grows in a ventro-medio-caudal direction. The pouch is thick-walled with a dorsocranial bulbous portion, and a caudal narrower portion. The antero-lateral wall of the bulbous portion begins to differentiate into parathyroid tissue—**parathyroid** III. The remaining part of the third pouch develops into the corresponding half of the **thymus**.

The Fourth Pharyngeal Endodermal Pouch

The fourth pouch eventually separates from the wall of the pharynx by rupture of the ductus pharyngobranchialis IV. It soon becomes solid by proliferation of the endodermal cells of its walls and its dorsal portion shows a differentiation into parathyroid tissue. This is **parathyroid** IV, or the superior parathyroid in the adult (fig. 9). The fate of the ventral and larger part of the fourth pouch has been much debated. In the earliest stages of its development the fourth pouch has situated caudal to it a transient, fifth, "ultimo-branchial" pouch. It is generally assumed that this fifth pouch disappears completely or is "taken-up" into the fourth pouch which is then termed the "caudal pharyngeal complex". The derivation of parathyroid IV from this complex is universally accepted. There is never a well-defined capsule to the fetal parathyroid glands and little connective tissue is found in them although they are vascularized early. The evidence suggests that the parathyroid glands become functionally active very early in fetal life and regulate fetal calcium metabolism.

Thyroid Gland

In early somite embryos the thyroid gland first appears as a thickening of the endoderm of the floor of the pharynx in the middle line just caudal to that portion which becomes the tuberculum impar (fig. 9). This thickening soon forms a diverticulum which, in early post-somite embryos, is a small bi-lobed, flask-like structure attached to the buccal cavity by a narrow stalk, the **thyroglossal duct.** In subsequent development the duct elongates and forms a solid cord and the bi-lobed nature of its terminal glandular swelling becomes more marked. During the 7th week, the thyroid reaches its definitive location anterior to the first six tracheal cartilages. The thyroid loses its attachment to the pharynx when the thyroglossal duct and the pharyngo-branchial duct become obliterated during the 6th to 8th weeks. The hormones of the thyroid gland are probably first produced in the 5th month.

THE CERVICAL SINUS AND THE CERVICAL VESICLES

As was stated earlier, profound changes occur in the ectodermal clefts behind the first one (which persists, at least in part, as the external auditory meatus). These changes result in their disappearance and in the establishment of a smooth contour to the developing neck. During these alterations, which occur in embryos of between 5 and 15 mm. CR length, the so-called "cervical sinus" which is the depression found between the second arch (hyoid) elevation and the region of the developing upper thoracic wall, disappears. In the course of disappearance of the cervical sinus, two small ectodermal cysts are separated from the surface ectoderm and come to lie in the depths of the developing neck. These are the cervical vesicles and they represent the epithelium of the ectodermal placodes associated with the early stages of development of the IXth and Xth cranial nerves. One of them, which has its origin from the second ectodermal cleft, and can be named cervical vesicle II, and which is closely related to the glosso-pharyngeal nerve, is transient and normally disappears by the time of "closure" of the cervical sinus. The other cervical vesicle (IV) has its origin from the epithelium of the fourth ectodermal cleft. It is larger and persists longer than vesicle II. It has intimate relations with the vagus nerve and may indeed contribute cells to its ganglion inferius. Normally, however, cervical vesicle IV has disappeared completely by the 25 mm. stage.

Cervical Cysts and Fistulae of Developmental Origin

Abnormalities arising from persistence in whole or in part of the ectodermal branchial clefts or the endodermal pharyngeal pouches are not uncommon. Four types of abnormality are described; cysts, external sinuses, internal sinuses and complete fistulae. These are usually lined by stratified epithelium but internal sinuses and complete fistulae may in part possess a columnar ciliated lining. Cysts are usually unilateral; fistulae, however, are bilateral in about 30 per cent of cases. The external sinuses and complete fistulae usually open to the surface at some point along the anterior border of the sternomastoid muscle. Internally the opening of a fistula is usually situated on the anterior aspect of the posterior pillar of the fauces just behind the tonsil. Large cervical cysts may arise from a failure of obliteration of the cervical sinus; the explanation of many of the cysts, however, seems to lie in the persistence of the cervical vesicle.

NEURAL CREST

The sensory cells and fibres of the peripheral nervous system and probably most of the peripheral cells of the autonomic nervous system are derived from the neural crest. The neural crest arises as a strip of specialized ectoderm flanking each side of the neural plate and interposed between it and the somatic ectoderm. When the neural plate becomes depressed to form the neural tube, the primordium of the neural crest is found at the neurosomatic junction. The crest of each side appears as a column of isolated cells along the dorsal aspect of the neural tube. Subsequently, the neural crest cells migrate ventrolaterally and come to lie along the dorsolateral aspect of the neural tube where they form an interrupted column of cells on either side along the whole length of the nervous system from the future mesencephalic region. The neural crest tissue, craniocaudally, can be subdivided into the following primordia:

(a) trigeminal;
(b) facial and auditory;
(c) glossopharyngeal and vagal complex;
(d) occipital; and
(e) spinal.

These primordia, with the exception of the occipital which appears to retrogress, give origin to sensory cells of the cranial nerve ganglia and, by segmentation of the spinal primordium, to the chain of spinal posterior root ganglia.

It is agreed that most of the cranial and all of the spinal sensory ganglion cells arise by differentiation of neural crest cells. There has been much discussion on the additional potentialities of these cells and there is evidence, derived especially from experiments on the development of lower vertebrates, that the neural-crest cells can differentiate into the following cell types:

(a) unipolar dorsal root ganglion cells, and the equivalent cells of the sensory ganglia of the Vth, VIIth, IXth, Xth and XIth cranial nerves through the stages of bipolar neuroblasts. The central process of the T-shaped axon of a unipolar sensory neurone grows into the dorsal portion of the neural tube to form a fibre of a posterior or sensory nerve root. The peripheral process joins the ventral root or, in the cranial nerves, the corresponding motor root, to constitute a mixed spinal or cranial nerve. Eventually, such peripheral processes from the ganglion cell grow out to innervate sensory receptor organs;
(b) probably all of the persistently bipolar cells of the auditory nerve;
(c) sympathetic neuroblasts which may differentiate into either sympathetic ganglion cells or chromaffin cells;
(d) the Schwann cell sheath of all the peripheral sensory and motor nerves;
(e) on the basis of experiments on amphibian larvae, the leptomeninges (pia and arachnoid);
(f) mesenchymal cells of the head and branchial cartilage cells (see Horstadius, 1950 for a review); odontoblasts are also probably of neural crest origin; and
(g) epithelial and connective-tissue pigment cells (see Boyd, 1960 and for a recent review on the neural crest see Weston, 1970).

The role of the neural crest in odontogenesis is dealt with in Chapter 26.

REFERENCES

Boyd, J. D. (1960), "The Embryology and Comparative Anatomy of the Melanocyte," in *Progress in the Biological Sciences in Relation to Dermatology*, (Rook, Ed.). London: Cambridge University Press.
Hochstetter, F. (1944), "Über die Art und Weise, in welcher sich bei Saugerieren und beim Menschen aus der sogennanten Tiechgrube die Nasenhöhle entwickelt," *Z. Anat. EntwGesch.*, II 3, 105.
Horstadius, S. (1950), *The Neural Crest*. London: Oxford University Press.
Pourtois, M. (1972), "Developmental Aspects of Oral Biology," in *Morphogenesis of the Primary and Secondary Palate*.
Streeter, G. L. (1948), "Developmental Horizons in Human Embryos. Description of Age Groups XV, XVI, XVII and XVIII, Being the Third Issue of a Survey of the Carnegie Collection," *Contr. Embryol. Carneg. Instn.*, **32**, 133.
Vermeiz-Keers, C. (1972), Springer-Verlag, Berlin, Heidelberg, New York.
Weston, J. A. (1970), "The Migration and Differentiation of Neural Crest Cells," in *Advances in Morphogenesis*, Vol. 8, (Abercrombie, Brachet and King, Eds.). New York and London: Academic Press.

PLATE SECTION

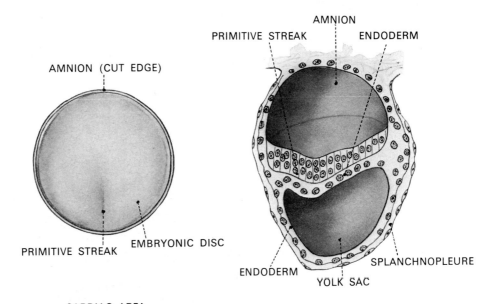

AMNION (CUT EDGE)

PRIMITIVE STREAK   EMBRYONIC DISC

PRIMITIVE STREAK   AMNION   ENDODERM

ENDODERM   SPLANCHNOPLEURE
YOLK SAC

FIG. 1. Schemes to show the development of the embryonic disc.

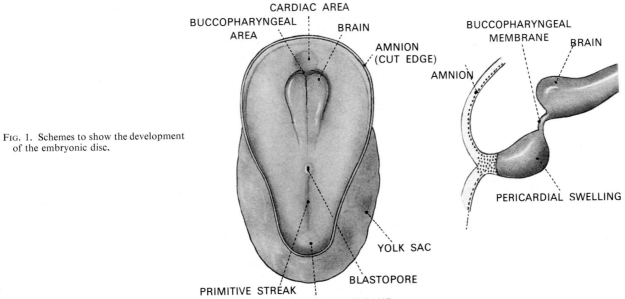

CARDIAC AREA
BUCCOPHARYNGEAL AREA   BRAIN
AMNION (CUT EDGE)

BUCCOPHARYNGEAL MEMBRANE   BRAIN
AMNION

YOLK SAC
BLASTOPORE
PRIMITIVE STREAK
CLOACAL MEMBRANE

PERICARDIAL SWELLING

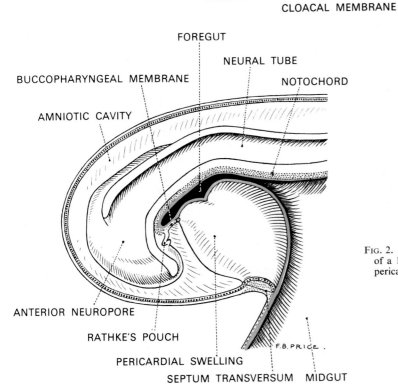

FOREGUT
NEURAL TUBE
BUCCOPHARYNGEAL MEMBRANE   NOTOCHORD
AMNIOTIC CAVITY

ANTERIOR NEUROPORE

RATHKE'S POUCH

PERICARDIAL SWELLING
SEPTUM TRANSVERSUM   MIDGUT

F.B.PRICE.

FIG. 2. A schematic drawing of a longitudinal section of the head region of a 14 somite human embryo. It shows the relationship between the pericardial swelling, the foregut and the stomatodaeum.

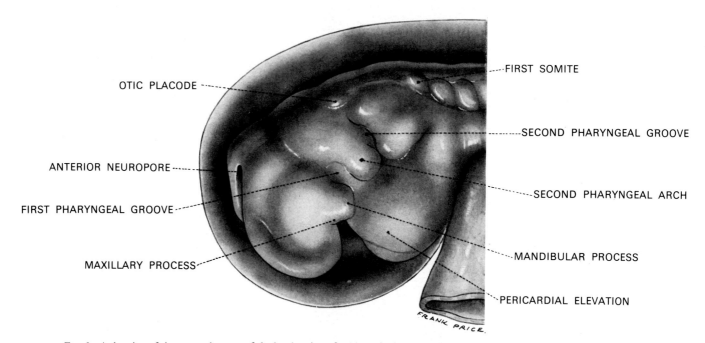

FIG. 3. A drawing of the external aspect of the head region of a 14 somite human embryo to show the developing pharyngeal region.

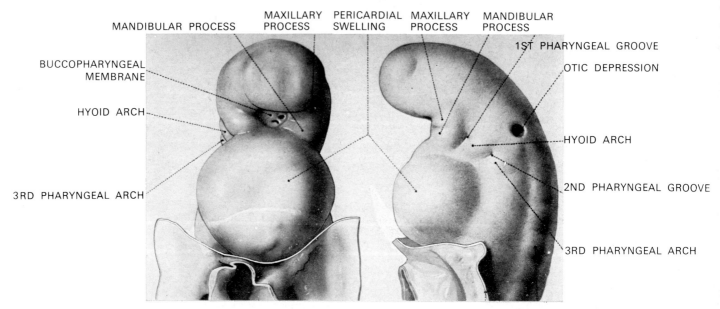

FIG. 4. A drawing of the ventral aspect of a 20 somite human embryo. It shows the breaking down of the buccopharyngeal membrane.

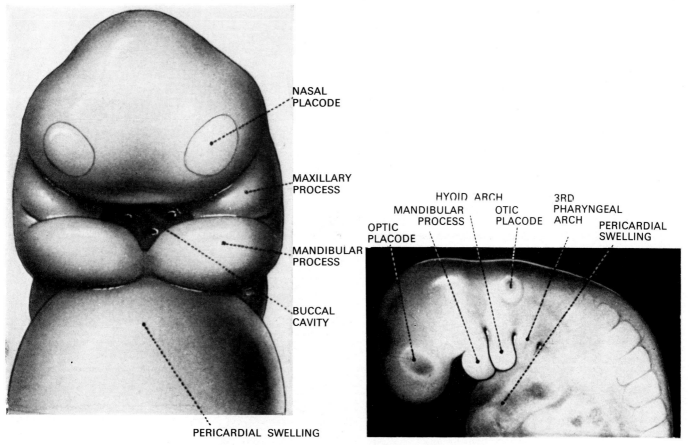

NASAL
PLACODE

MAXILLARY
PROCESS

MANDIBULAR
PROCESS

BUCCAL
CAVITY

PERICARDIAL SWELLING

FIG. 5. A drawing of the ventral aspect of the head region of a 2·5 mm. human embryo.

OPTIC
PLACODE

MANDIBULAR
PROCESS

HYOID ARCH

OTIC
PLACODE

3RD
PHARYNGEAL
ARCH

PERICARDIAL
SWELLING

FIG. 6. A photograph of the left side of the head region of a 28 somite human embryo.

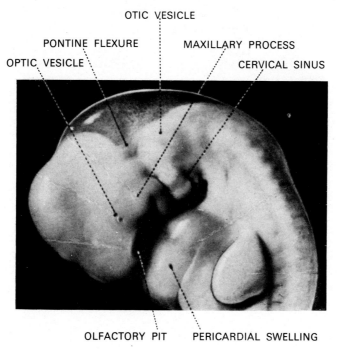

OTIC VESICLE

PONTINE FLEXURE

OPTIC VESICLE

MAXILLARY PROCESS

CERVICAL SINUS

OLFACTORY PIT   PERICARDIAL SWELLING

FIG. 7. A photograph of the left side of the head region of a 6–7 mm human embryo.

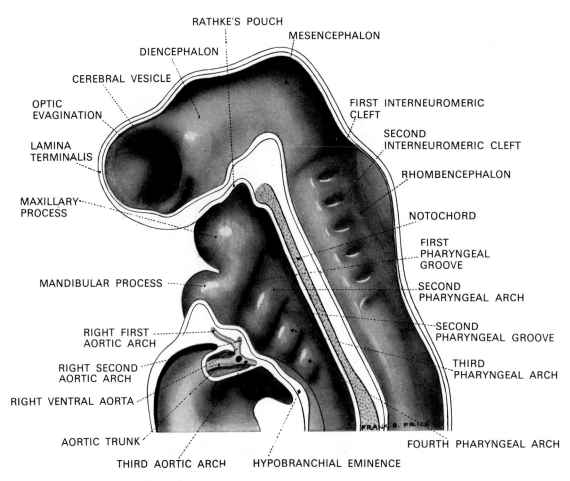

Fig. 8. A drawing of the right half of a sagittally sectioned reconstruction of the cephalic region of a 4·2 mm. human embryo (modified from His). The interrupted line A represents the approximate site of the previous attachment of the bucco-pharyngeal membrane, *i.e.*, the boundary between ectoderm and endoderm.

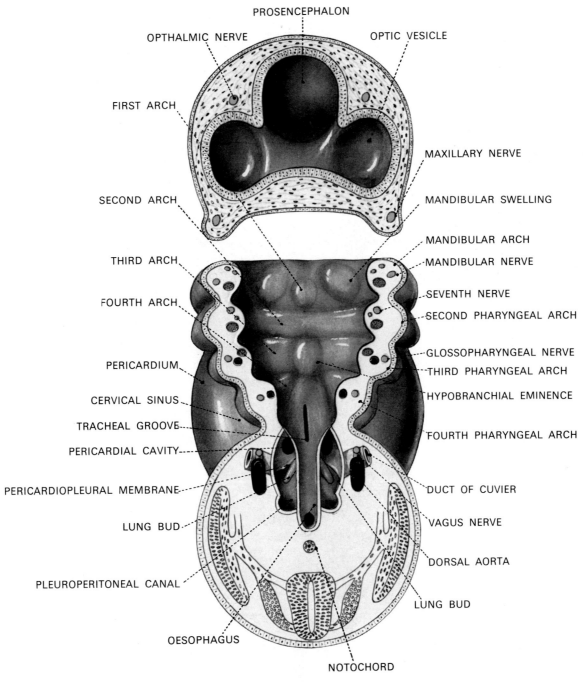

PROSENCEPHALON

OPTHALMIC NERVE

OPTIC VESICLE

FIRST ARCH

MAXILLARY NERVE

MANDIBULAR SWELLING

SECOND ARCH

MANDIBULAR ARCH

MANDIBULAR NERVE

THIRD ARCH

SEVENTH NERVE

SECOND PHARYNGEAL ARCH

FOURTH ARCH

GLOSSOPHARYNGEAL NERVE

THIRD PHARYNGEAL ARCH

PERICARDIUM

HYPOBRANCHIAL EMINENCE

CERVICAL SINUS

TRACHEAL GROOVE

FOURTH PHARYNGEAL ARCH

PERICARDIAL CAVITY

PERICARDIOPLEURAL MEMBRANE

DUCT OF CUVIER

VAGUS NERVE

LUNG BUD

DORSAL AORTA

PLEUROPERITONEAL CANAL

LUNG BUD

OESOPHAGUS

NOTOCHORD

Fig. 9. A horizontal section through a reconstruction of a 5 mm. human embryo (seen from above) to show the pharyngeal arches, the structures in the floor of the developing pharynx and the primitive pleural cavity. The rudimentary sixth pharyngeal arches bound the tracheal groove.

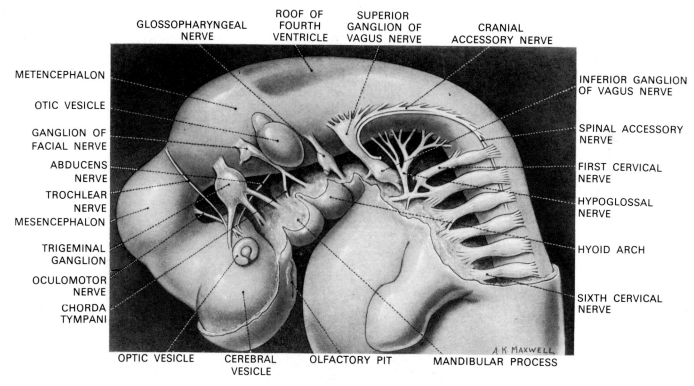

GLOSSOPHARYNGEAL NERVE

ROOF OF FOURTH VENTRICLE

SUPERIOR GANGLION OF VAGUS NERVE

CRANIAL ACCESSORY NERVE

METENCEPHALON

OTIC VESICLE

GANGLION OF FACIAL NERVE

ABDUCENS NERVE

TROCHLEAR NERVE

MESENCEPHALON

TRIGEMINAL GANGLION

OCULOMOTOR NERVE

CHORDA TYMPANI

INFERIOR GANGLION OF VAGUS NERVE

SPINAL ACCESSORY NERVE

FIRST CERVICAL NERVE

HYPOGLOSSAL NERVE

HYOID ARCH

SIXTH CERVICAL NERVE

OPTIC VESICLE

CEREBRAL VESICLE

OLFACTORY PIT

MANDIBULAR PROCESS

A.K. MAXWELL

FIG. 10. Dissection of the head region and cranial and upper spinal nerves in a 10 mm. human embryo. × *ca.* 10.

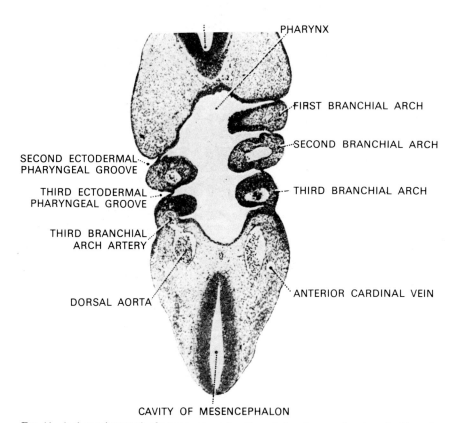

PHARYNX

FIRST BRANCHIAL ARCH

SECOND BRANCHIAL ARCH

SECOND ECTODERMAL PHARYNGEAL GROOVE

THIRD ECTODERMAL PHARYNGEAL GROOVE

THIRD BRANCHIAL ARCH

THIRD BRANCHIAL ARCH ARTERY

ANTERIOR CARDINAL VEIN

DORSAL AORTA

CAVITY OF MESENCEPHALON

FIG. 11. A photomicrograph of a transverse section through the pharyngeal region of a 28 somite human embryo to show the branchial arches and vessels. × *ca.* 70.

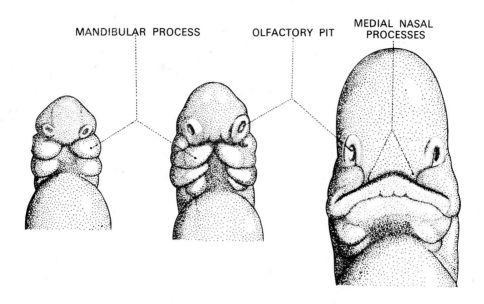

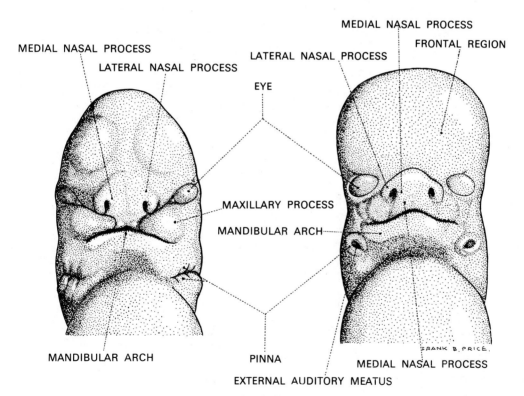

FIG. 12. Drawings of the ventral aspect of the head region of human embryos to show the development of the face at: 5·7 mm.; 6·7 mm.; 11·8 mm.; 14 mm. (Based on Streeter.)

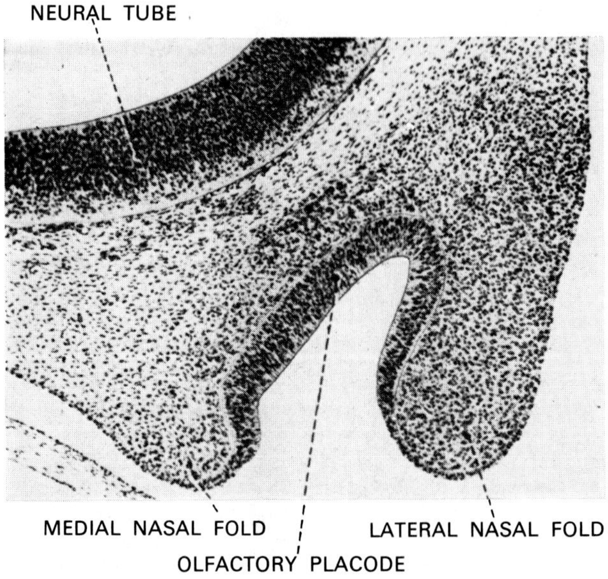

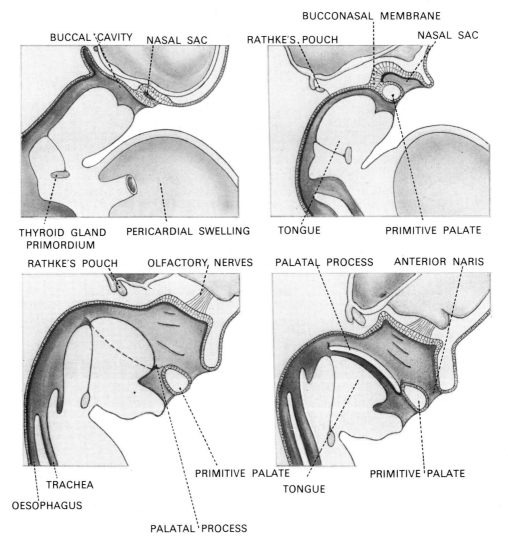

NEURAL TUBE

MEDIAL NASAL FOLD   LATERAL NASAL FOLD

OLFACTORY PLACODE

FIG. 13. Photomicrograph of a section through the developing olfactory
placode of a 10 mm. human embryo. × ca. 70.

BUCCONASAL MEMBRANE

BUCCAL CAVITY   NASAL SAC   RATHKE'S POUCH   NASAL SAC

THYROID GLAND   PERICARDIAL SWELLING   TONGUE   PRIMITIVE PALATE
PRIMORDIUM

RATHKE'S POUCH   OLFACTORY NERVES   PALATAL PROCESS   ANTERIOR NARIS

TRACHEA   PRIMITIVE PALATE   PRIMITIVE PALATE

OESOPHAGUS   TONGUE

PALATAL PROCESS

FIG. 14. Schemes of sagittal sections through the head regions to show successive stages in the development
of the buccal and nasal cavities.

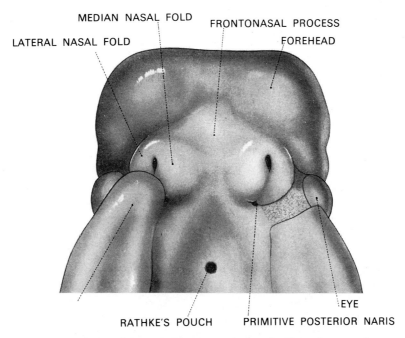

MEDIAN NASAL FOLD   FRONTONASAL PROCESS

LATERAL NASAL FOLD   FOREHEAD

EYE

RATHKE'S POUCH   PRIMITIVE POSTERIOR NARIS

FIG. 15. A drawing of the roof of the stomatodaeum of a 12 mm. human embryo to show the development of the primitive anterior and posterior nares by the approximation of the maxillary processes to the lateral and medial nasal folds. Part of the left maxillary process has been removed.

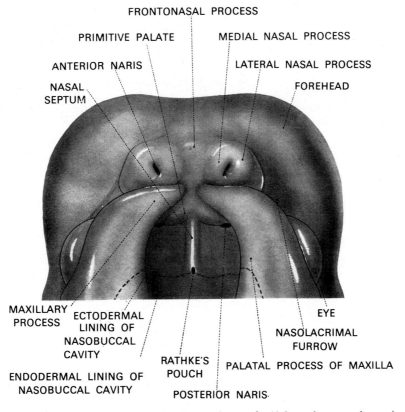

FRONTONASAL PROCESS

PRIMITIVE PALATE   MEDIAL NASAL PROCESS

ANTERIOR NARIS   LATERAL NASAL PROCESS

NASAL SEPTUM   FOREHEAD

MAXILLARY PROCESS   ECTODERMAL LINING OF NASOBUCCAL CAVITY   EYE

NASOLACRIMAL FURROW

ENDODERMAL LINING OF NASOBUCCAL CAVITY   RATHKE'S POUCH   PALATAL PROCESS OF MAXILLA

POSTERIOR NARIS

FIG. 16. A drawing of the roof of the stomatodaeum of a 13·5 mm. human embryo. A distinct palatal process from the maxillary mesoderm is now present. This will later meet its fellow of the opposite side and fuse with it and with the down-growing nasal septum. The latter is now seen as a ridge in the roof of the primitive nasal cavity portion of the stomatodaeum. The previous site of attachment of the buccopharyngeal membrane is shown by the interrupted line.

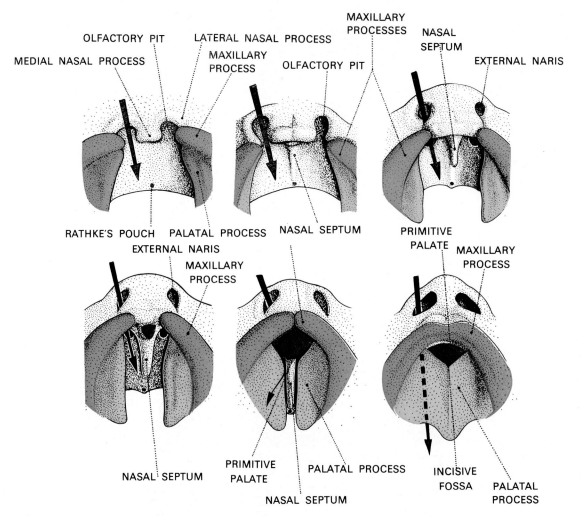

FIG. 17. Schemes to show stages in the development of the palate. The arrow passes through the anterior and posterior nares. The maxillary process is shown in blue, the medial nasal process in red and the palatal processes in yellow.

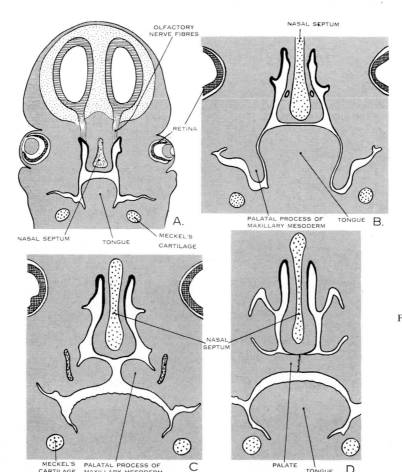

OLFACTORY
NERVE FIBRES

RETINA

NASAL SEPTUM   TONGUE   MECKEL'S
                                       CARTILAGE

A.

NASAL SEPTUM

PALATAL PROCESS OF   TONGUE
MAXILLARY MESODERM

B.

NASAL
SEPTUM

MECKEL'S   PALATAL PROCESS OF
CARTILAGE   MAXILLARY MESODERM   C

NASAL
SEPTUM

PALATE   TONGUE   D

Fig. 18. Schemes showing stages in the development of the palatal processes, palate and nasal septum.

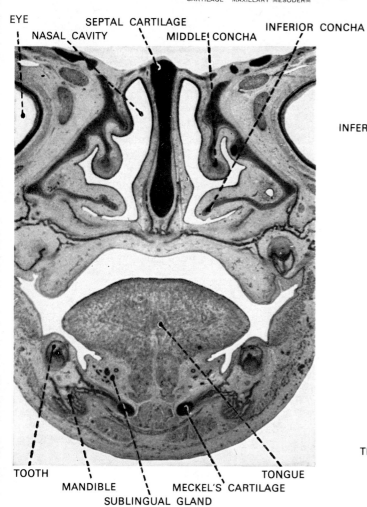

EYE   SEPTAL CARTILAGE
NASAL CAVITY   MIDDLE CONCHA   INFERIOR CONCHA

TOOTH   TONGUE
     MANDIBLE   MECKEL'S CARTILAGE
          SUBLINGUAL GLAND

Fig. 19. Photomicrograph of a section through the developing mouth and nasal cavity of an 80 mm. human fetus. × ca. 10.

Fig. 20. A sagittal section of a fetal head to show the lateral wall of the nasal cavity and the palate. The nasal septum has been removed. Maxillary ossification has extended into the anterior two-thirds of the maxillary palatal process and the palatal process of the premaxilla is extending into the primitive palate.

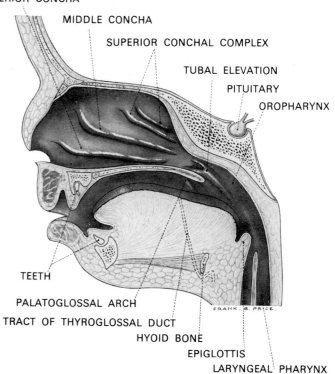

INFERIOR CONCHA

MIDDLE CONCHA

SUPERIOR CONCHAL COMPLEX

TUBAL ELEVATION
PITUITARY
OROPHARYNX

TEETH

PALATOGLOSSAL ARCH

TRACT OF THYROGLOSSAL DUCT

HYOID BONE

EPIGLOTTIS

LARYNGEAL PHARYNX

FRANK. B. PRICE.

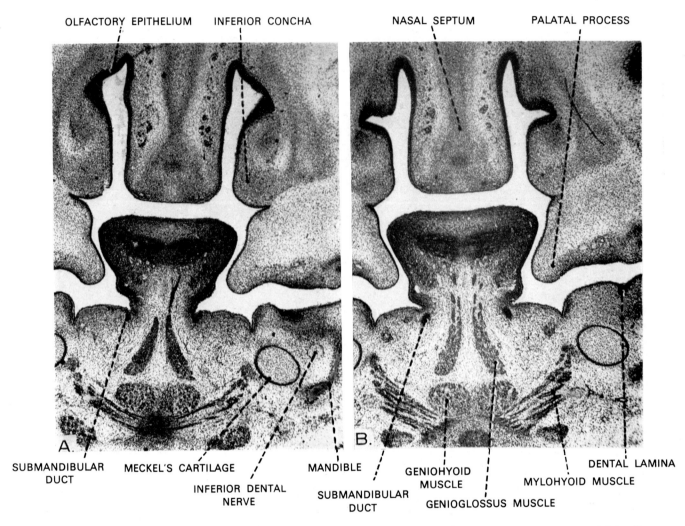

Fig. 21. Photomicrographs of sections through the developing mouth of a 20 mm. human embryo. × *ca.* 25. A is more cranial than B.

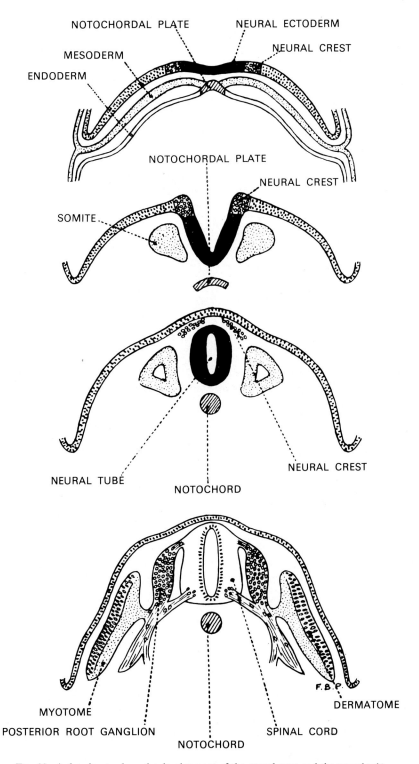

Fig. 22. A drawing to show the development of the neural crest and the neural tube.

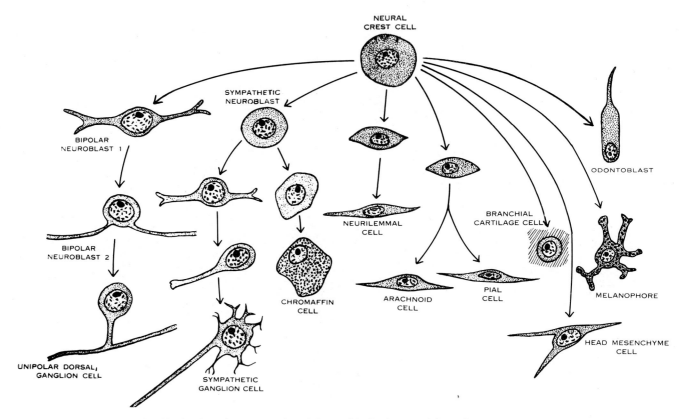

Fɪɢ. 23. A schematic representation of the possible developmental fates of a neural crest cell.

3. POSTNATAL GROWTH AND DEVELOPMENT OF THE FACE AND CRANIUM

DONALD H. ENLOW

Craniofacial morphogenesis
 Stages in craniofacial morphological development

*The morphological basis of variations in craniofacial form
 and pattern*

Intrinsic compensations

*The role of the cranial base in establishing facial form and
 pattern*

INTRODUCTION

Many different kinds of bone tissue are involved in the growth of the skull. "Haversian" bone, contrary to popular assumption, is not the predominant skeletal tissue present in the growing child. Other, much more prevalent types exist throughout the greater part of virtually all the bones in the growing face and cranium. These different kinds of bone tissue are adaptations to the rate of osseous formation in any particular part of the bone; to the amount of bone tissue being deposited in any given area of the bone; to the inward or outward direction in which that area is growing; to the presence or absence of any muscle, tendon, or tooth attachments; to the size of a given bone or bony part; and to the age of the individual. For example, the most common type of bone during the childhood period is densely vascular and has a canal system that is largely primary (non-Haversian) in nature. Bone tissues in older individuals tend to be less vascular and are also characterized by an increasing accumulation of osteons because replacement and turnover of bone due to remodelling associated with growth have ceased. The osteon is a secondary structure that is involved in the reconstruction of compact bone and functions to replace old or necrotic areas with new bone tissue. Haversian systems can also occur in some localized areas of the young skeleton, however, and in such locations function in the movement and relocation of muscle and tendon attachments on the surface of elongating bones as well as attachments on resorptive surfaces of a bone. (For a more detailed account of these basic types of bone tissues, see Enlow, 1968b.)

Deposition of bone on the periosteal side of a cortical plate, together with proportionate resorption from the endosteal surface, move the plate in an outward direction. Conversely, deposition on the inside surface together with periosteal resorption combine to produce a resultant inward (endosteal) direction of growth. Periosteal and endosteal types of bone tissues are thereby formed, respectively, and can be readily identified and distinguished microscopically. Significantly, about half or more of the cortex (compact bone) in most craniofacial elements is composed of endosteal bone tissue. How a bone can actually enlarge by a

growth process involving widespread periosteal resorption and endosteal deposition is explained in Chapter 45.

Changes in the inward and outward directions of growth occur in local areas of a bone as the whole bone continues to enlarge. This produces a stratification of endosteal and periosteal zones of bone tissue within the cortical plate, and each such zone is separated from the others by a **reversal line**. The outer surface of any bone during periods of growth is characterized by a mosaic pattern of well defined, circumscribed resorptive and depository growth fields associated with respective inward and outward directions of growth

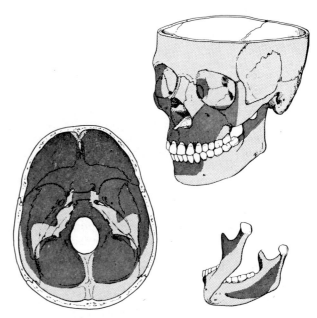

FIG. 1. The distribution of growth fields. The dark areas are resorptive fields, and the light areas are depository fields. (From Enlow and Moyers, *J. Amer. dent. Ass.*, **82**, 1971. Copyright by the American Dental Association. Reprinted by permission.)

movement (figs. 1, 4 and 5). Each area is outlined and separated from the next by a reversal line which angles down into the cortex between the endosteal and periosteal layers. The positions of reversal lines become changed on the growing surface of the bone so that, as the whole bone enlarges, the regional growth fields surrounded by these boundaries also enlarge proportionately.

It is important to understand that any given facial or cranial bone does not grow by a generalized process involving, simply, deposition of new bone on external cortical surfaces and resorption of older bone from internal surfaces. A facial bone does not grow in such a manner that already existing surfaces and contours merely expand by uniform, overall additions of new periosteal bone around the entire perimeter (fig. 2). The facial bones, also, do not simply grow "forward and downward" (figs. 9, 10 and 11). Many divergent, regional, inward and outward directions of growth take place during the whole bone's enlargement. Those particular surfaces, either periosteal or endosteal, that face toward the direction of growth receive new bone

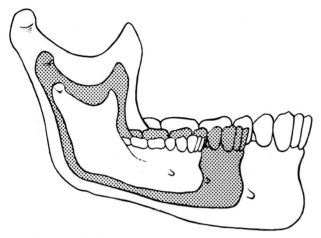

FIG. 2. This diagram illustrates a manner of enlargement that does not occur during the growth of a bone. See text for explanation.

deposits. Conversely, surfaces that point away from the regional growth direction are ordinarily resorptive. An entire cortical plate thus moves ("drifts") in a specific, regional direction, and this movement constitutes a basic part of the process of skeletal growth itself.

A process of differential growth occurs during the enlargement of any craniofacial bone. Some areas grow faster and involve more extensive deposition or resorption than other regions. Particularly active areas are sometimes indentified as growth sites ("centres"). These include the maxillary tuberosity, lingual tuberosity (the direct anatomical and morphogenic counterpart of the maxillary tuberosity), the bony alveolar ridges, the anterior and posterior margins of the ramus, sutures, condyles, and synchondroses. However, virtually all other endosteal and periosteal surfaces are also active during growth, either in deposition, resorption, or sequentially in both. While the extent of such regional activities may be less marked in some areas, their role in the overall, composite plan of growth is no less important.

Due to the differential nature of enlargement, the shape and dimensions of a bone would soon become disproportionate without complementary remodelling, which functions to sustain the bone's configuration during continued growth. Remodelling is an integral part of the growth process itself and is carried out by the same depository and resorptive activities utilized to produce the cortical movements involved in enlargement, as described above. Growth and remodelling, are effected by the same actual process.

As bone is differentially added in some parts, the relative positions of other regions in that bone necessarily become shifted. This is termed relocation and is the underlying basis for the remodelling process. For example, the mandible grows posteriorly by deposition on the posterior margin of the ramus (in conjunction with growth at the con-

dyle, as explained later). Regions once occupied by the ramus are progressively remodelled to become new additions to the corpus, which is lengthened by this remodelling conversion process (fig. 6). The complex alterations in regional morphology associated with the relocation of parts are accomplished by the same resorptive and depository growth activities that also function to enlarge the component areas. Remodelling, in brief, is the process of resizing and reshaping as any one area becomes sequentially relocated into the next during the increase in size of the bone as a whole.

Growth fields are under the developmental control of overlying soft tissues and function to enlarge the entire bone (even though some areas actually decrease in size because of regional relocations) and, at the same time, to provide relocation (remodelling) of all local areas, parts, tuberosities, fossae, crests, and so on. A single growth field can encompass different parts of several separate bones all of which take part in a common growth movement even though separated by sutures, synchondroses, or condyles. A growth field moves as each whole bone enlarges. This progressive movement in turn produces the relocation of the bony parts involved. As the coverage of the soft tissue matrix expands, the regional portions of the bones which it houses correspondingly expand.

Variations in the morphology of a bone between individual persons are produced by:

(a) basic differences in the pattern of surface resorption and deposition;
(b) the specific placement of the reversal lines that separate growth fields;
(c) the differential rates of deposition and resorption associated with particular fields; and
(d) by the timing that occurs in the growth activities among the different fields.

Two basic and separate kinds of growth movement occur during morphogenesis. One is **direct cortical growth** and is produced by deposition and resorption on contralateral sides of the cortex, as already described. This process is termed **cortical drift**. The second is a physical movement of whole bones, a process termed **displacement** (Enlow, 1968b; Moss and Salentijn, 1969). As two or more contiguous bones grow, a displacement of each bone occurs because of the increasing size of all of the bones growing in relation to each other. The pulling and pushing forces that produce displacement are believed to include the growth of bones against each other wherever intervening compression-resistant cartilage is present and, especially, movement of the bone produced by the growth expansion of enclosing soft tissues.

Growth by the process of cortical drift in any given region of a bone may be opposite in direction to that bone's displacement, or the two may complement each other in direction. Complex combinations ordinarily occur among the many parts of a bone.

A distinction between these two basic modes of growth, *i.e.* growth movement by cortical drift and growth movement by displacement, is important to an understanding of the overall, composite process of craniofacial enlargement (fig. 3). In cephalometric analyses of serial growth changes, the relative contributions of each cannot be determined for most of the individual bones unless metallic implants are used (Björk, 1947; Enlow and Moyers, 1971). Only the cumulative, summated result of both can be seen and measured. This greatly complicates, and severely limits, interpretations and analyses of growth changes in serial headfilms.

The "forward and downward" doctrine of facial growth is misleading because the overall growth process involves

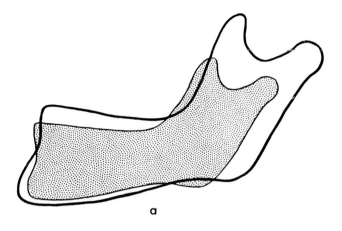

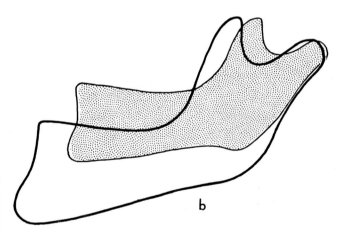

FIG. 3. Enlargement of a bone by the process of deposition and resorption is shown in (a). The simultaneous process of displacement is shown in (b).

cumulative combinations of growth changes among separate bones by the process of drift in conjunction with the displacement of all these bones in relation to one another (Enlow, 1968b; Moss et al., 1969). For the most part, the bones involved do not simply "grow" anteriorly and inferiorly. The periosteal surface on the forward part of the bony maxillary arch, for example, is actually resorptive, yet this same surface moves anteriorly. The forward direction of movement, of course, is produced by the displacement ("carry") that occurs as other parts of the nasomaxillary complex simultaneously grow in an actual posterior direction by cortical drift.

Sutures are believed to be tension-adapted growth sites not ordinarily able to accommodate direct bone-to-bone compression. As contiguous bones become separated by the force of soft tissue growth (e.g. the enlarging brain), new bone is laid down on the sutural edges within a localized field of tension. Such sutural bone growth takes place in conjunction with the remodelling growth that occurs in other parts of the bone. While the extent of such remodelling growth is minimal in the bones comprising the calvaria, it is widespread and marked in degree in the facial bones. Growth in the facial sutures does not cease at a relatively early age to be replaced by a process of "generalized surface growth", as previously believed. Growth of sutures continues so long as the whole bone continues to enlarge. The sutural membrane itself is structurally comparable with the periosteum. They are directly continuous, and their respective functional layers are equivalent (Enlow, 1968b).

Epiphyses, condyles and **synchrondroses** are believed to represent pressure-adapted growth sites, although the levels of actual compression may vary considerably among different bones. While such sites provide regional bone increases in their own particular areas, it is important to understand that they do not exert any overall growth control influence over the remainder of the bone. The mandibular condyle, for example, does not function as a "master centre" that regulates the many regional growth fields throughout the mandible as a whole (Enlow, 1968b; Moss, 1968).

The avascular nature of the cartilage, its interstitial growth process, the usual absence of a covering membrane, and the provision for endochondral bone replacement combine to make possible bone lengthening in a direction toward the compression. Free articular movement is provided at the same time wherever a synovial joint is involved. These key relationships are in contrast to the intramembranous mode of growth associated with the periosteum, sutures, and the periodontal membrane, which have a growth process that is basically tension-adapted.

The displacement movement of the bones in the upper and midfacial regions had at one time been assumed to be a compressive pushing apart of the separate bones by continued bony deposits within the various facial sutures. Because current theory, however, holds that the sutural growth mechanism is specifically tension rather than pressure adapted, this is no longer regarded as a tenable explanation. The expansion of the nasal septum was subsequently suggested as the force responsible for forward and downward midfacial displacement since it is a cartilaginous structure presumed to be capable of growth expansion within a field of compression (Scott, 1959). Although still supported by many investigators, this explanation has been questioned on the basis that actual genetic and developmental control lies within the "functional matrix" (see below) rather than the developmentally dependent tissue of the cartilage itself.

Although sutures, condyles and synchondroses are important sites of regional growth, all of the many other endosteal and periosteal surfaces throughout the remainder of the entire bone represent regional growth and remodelling sites of equal importance. The composite of all produces the overall enlargement and remodelling of the bone as a whole.

Wolff's law is a well known principle stating, in general, that the morphology of a bone becomes progressively adapted to the sum of all the changing mechanical forces exerted upon it during growth and development. When these forces attain functional equilibrium with the physical properties of the bone, growth ceases and the morphology of that bone is then in balance with the mechanical needs of its various functions While this principle is essentially

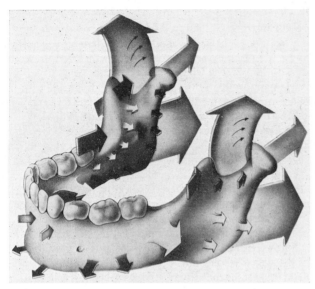

FIG. 4. The enlargement of the mandible involves inward and outward directions of growth according to the distribution of resorptive and depository fields shown in fig. 1. (From Enlow and Harris, *Amer. J. Orthodont.*, **50**, 1964).

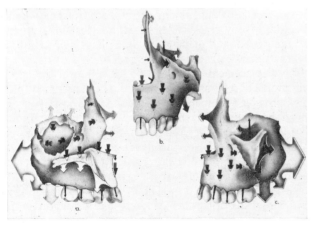

FIG. 5. The multidirectional growth of the maxilla is shown. This corresponds to the distribution of resorptive and depository growth fields illustrated in fig. 1. (From Enlow, D. H.: *The Human Face*, Harper and Row, 1968).

valid, some of the traditional tension-pressure explanations of its actual mode of operation are oversimplified or incorrect since many known growth changes do not coincide with the patterns of pressure and tension that have been presumed to produce and regulate them. Wolff's law is a descriptive account of what happens during the process of growth and its control. It does not explain how this process

is carried out. The question of growth control is one of the foremost biological problems of our time (Enlow, 1973b).

The functional matrix concept states, in general, that a bone grows in relationship with the sum of its associated soft tissues, and that the soft-tissue matrix represents the governing determinant of the skeletal growth process (Moss *et al.*, 1969). The course and the extent of bone growth are secondarily dependent upon the growth of the soft tissues. However, the bone itself and any cartilage present are involved in the operation of the functional matrix since an essential feedback exists in the bone-soft tissue interrelationship. The "functional matrix" is a meaningful title that describes morphological and morphogenetic growth relationships. The principle is not intended to represent an explanation of how the mechanisms actually operate. The

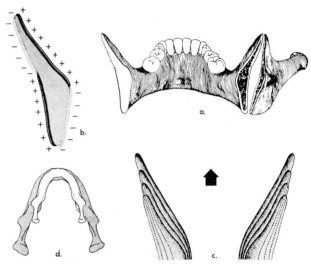

FIG. 6. Growth of the mandibular ramus. See text for explanation. (From Enlow and Harris, *Amer. J. Orthodont.*, **50**, 1964).

basic factor of local growth control is at present an incompletely understood process (the reader is referred to Enlow, 1968a, 1973b and 1973c for an evaluation of the complex factors involved in the control of facial growth).

CRANIOFACIAL MORPHOGENESIS

Figures 1, 4 and 5 show the typical distribution of depository and resorptive fields of growth in the various parts of the face and cranium. Figures 9, 10 and 11 show the growth process as visualized using two-dimensional headfilm tracings. As this sequence of diagrams is followed, the changes that occur in each region of each bone should be correlated with the resorptive and depository growth activity illustrated in figs. 1, 4 and 5. It should be possible to visualize the three-dimensional nature of the growth processes when viewing conventional headfilm tracings, including changes on those surfaces not representable because of the two-dimensional nature of the tracing.

The plan for the growth sequence shown in figs. 9, 10 and 11 is as follows. Firstly, all growth increases are made in such a way that they are "balanced". As a result, the enlarged facial composite in the last stage has the same form and pattern as the first stage without changes in proportions or facial symmetry. Such a completely balanced growth process, of course, never occurs in facial development but has been depicted in this series of diagrams so that the

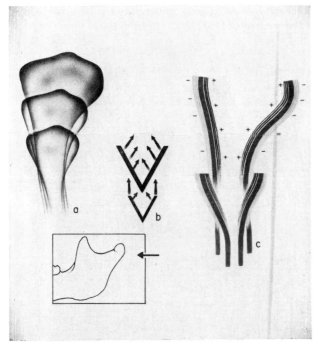

FIG. 7. Diameter of condylar neck (a) is progressively reduced from the wider dimensions of the posterior-moving condyle. Inward growth of buccal and lingual cortices (c) is accomplished by a combination of periosteal resorption (−) and endosteal deposition (+). This is an example of the "V principle" (b).

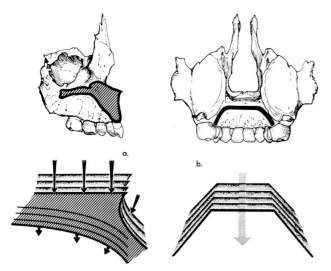

FIG. 8. Vertical growth of the palate and maxillary arch. See text for explanations. (From Enlow and Bang, *Amer. J. Orthodont.*, **51**, 1965).

developmental basis for alterations and variations in facial form can later be shown and so that the morphological basis for different facial types and malocclusions can be more effectively explained.

Secondly, the growth of each bone is described in two separate phases:

(a) resorptive and depository changes (fine arrows); and

(b) the displacement (carry) of the whole bone that accompanies these surface changes (coarse arrows).

It is essential to understand that they occur simultaneously; each of these phases must be shown and described in separate diagrams, however, in order to demonstrate their respective morphological effects.

Thirdly, the many growth events in all of the various bones and bony parts throughout the face and cranium all take place more or less at the same time but are shown individually as separate stages so that regional relationships can be explained. Each figure is cumulative and includes all growth changes of the stages that precede it.

Fourthly, the growth changes shown in the sequence of illustrations are based on the "counterpart principle" (Enlow, Kuroda and Lewis, 1971a). Growth changes in any given part of a bone must be accompanied by equivalent growth increases in certain specific parts of other bones if the same overall facial form and balance is to be retained. If disproportionate growth changes occur among these specific "parts and counterparts", however, corresponding changes in facial pattern are produced. Such relationships are the morphological and developmental basis for normal facial variations among different individuals, the facial changes associated with ageing, and those that underlie the development of malocclusions. These are described in later sections of this chapter after a "balanced" sequence of growth increases is first described.

To identify specific combinations of parts and their counterparts, the following question is asked: "If a change is observed in some given part, exactly where must corresponding, equivalent changes also be made if continuing form and balance are to remain unchanged?" In the descriptions that follow, the growth of each regional part is related directly to its particular counterpart(s) so that the fundamental plan of craniofacial enlargement can be recognized and followed. A horizontal and a vertical reference line are provided so that the direction and the extent of each change can be visualized.

The first and last stages are superimposed in the conventional manner using sella as a registration point to show the tracing overlay familiar to dentists and cephalometric investigators (figs. 9a to 11e). This illustrates the well-known "forward and downward" change in the face relative to the cranial base. However, this picture is often mistakenly presumed to demonstrate the manner of direct, actual growth in the various regional parts of each bone involved. It must be understood that this overlay represents a cumulative composite of changes that are produced, firstly, by bony resorptive and depository processes, and secondly, by the process of displacement that accompanies these changes. It is important to note that the face does now merely "grow" from the younger state to the older in the manner suggested by the overlay. Rather, all of the complex, regional, interrelated growth and remodelling processes described below are involved. The series begins arbitrarily with the maxillary arch.

Stage 1 (figs. 9a and 9b)

The actual lengthening of the bony maxillary arch is produced by continued deposition of bone in a posterior direction on the posterior-facing maxillary tuberosity. This is represented by a movement of PTM posteriorly. The

direction (Enlow, 1968b). Since the processes of backward maxillary growth and forward displacement (Stages 1 and 2) occur simultaneously, the position of PTM actually remains stable on the vertical reference line, and the PA dimension of the pharynx remains unchanged. The force that produces maxillary displacement is controversial but has been attributed to nasal septum expansion, as previously

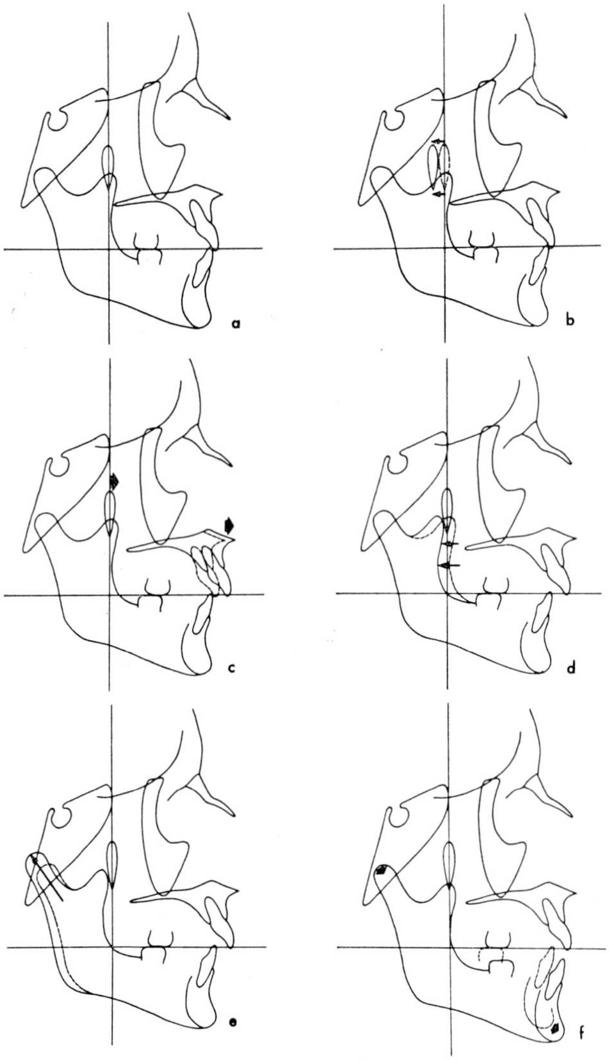

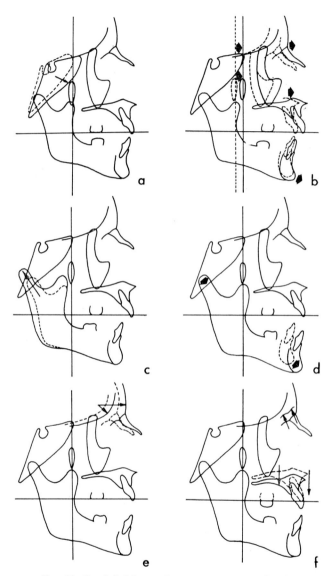

FIG. 9. Craniofacial growth sequence. See text for descriptions. (From Enlow and Moyers, *J. Amer. dent. Ass.*, **82**, 1971. Copyright by the American Dental Association. Reprinted by permission.)

FIG. 10. Craniofacial growth sequence. See text for descriptions.

maxillary sinus correspondingly expands in a like direction by resorption from the endosteal side of the bony cortex. These growth changes take place in conjunction with the separate process of maxillary displacement (next stage).

Stage 2 (fig. 9c)

As bone is added to the posterior surface of the tuberosity, the entire maxilla becomes displaced in an opposite anterior

mentioned. The entire "functional matrix" of the midface, however, is now believed to be involved (Moss and Greenberg, 1967).

Stage 3 (fig. 9d)

To retain equivalent dimensions and proper positioning of other facial parts with respect to the maxilla, the various horizontal counterparts of the maxillary arch change correspondingly and proportionately. One of these counterparts is the bony arch of the mandible. The actual bony changes are shown first, and the accompanying displacement of the mandible is then illustrated. In terms of growth and functional relationships, the mandible is not a single skeletal unit but a composite of several regional parts. The whole mandible is not a counterpart of the maxilla; only the mandibular corpus is directly related to the bony maxillary arch. The mandibular ramus is a functional counter-

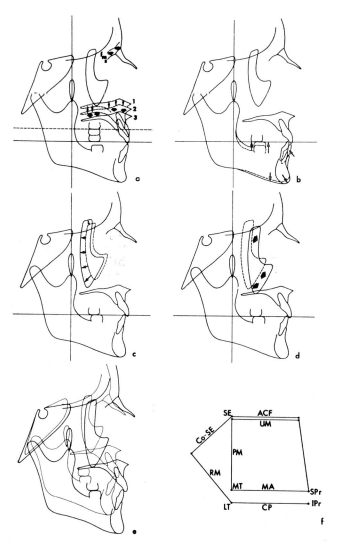

FIG. 11. Craniofacial growth sequence. See text for descriptions. Co-SE is the middle cranial fossa from condylion to the sphenoethmoidal or sphenofrontal junction; the other segments represent the anterior cranial floor (ACF), the upper maxilla (UM), the posterior nasomaxillary vertical plane (PM), maxillary tuberosity (MT), lingual (LT), ramus (RM), corpus (CP), superior prosthion (SPr), and inferior prosthion (IPr).

part of other regional components in the craniofacial composite.

Figure 9d shows the process by which the mandibular corpus lengthens. This may take place simultaneously with the elongation of the maxillary arch, or a lag may occur producing a transient imbalance between the dimensions of the arches (i.e. a Class II type of relationship in early

childhood can become materially decreased as mandibular growth eventually approximates that of the maxilla).

Just as the maxilla increases in horizontal length by actual bony growth in a backward direction, the bony mandibular arch also lengthens in a corresponding posterior direction (Björk, 1947; Enlow, 1968b). Unlike the maxillary arch, however, the mandible has an additional and functionally separate component, the ramus, that bridges the pharyngeal space to articulate with the cranial floor. The lengthening of the mandibular corpus is accomplished by a process of remodelling conversion directly from the ramus, as seen in fig. 6. The entire ramus, as a part of this process, relocates in a posterior direction by its own growth process (fig. 6). In two-dimensional tracings of serial cephalograms, this would appear to be a result, simply, of resorption from its anterior margin and deposition on the posterior margin. This is an incomplete explanation. As seen in figs. 4 and 6, which illustrate the three-dimensional growth process, it is evident that the buccal and lingual sides of the ramus are also directly involved in its posterior growth movement. The ramus is not oriented in a straight-line, posteroanterior manner; it has, rather, a propeller-like twist so that the lingual side of the coronoid process faces posteriorly. This surface is depository (it faces toward the direction of growth) and the contralateral buccal surface is resorptive, thereby producing a posterior growth movement. The lingual side of the coronoid process also faces superiorly and medially, and the same deposits of bone that result in its posterior growth are responsible for upward lengthening (fig. 6). Most of the inferior part of the ramus has an opposite combination of deposition and resorption in relation to the direction its surfaces face due to the torque of ramus configuration. As the coronoid process and the entire remainder of the ramus move posteriorly, the corpus lengthens at the same time as a result of the medial direction of growth in the anterior portion of the ramus where it joins the corpus. Note that the mandibular arch and lingual tuberosity are positioned well medially with respect to the ramus.

Stage 4 (fig. 9e)

The mandibular condyle is a regional site providing a superoposterior direction of growth for this part of the ramus. Since the articulation between the condyle and the fossa involves compression, an endochondral growth mechanism is utilized. The condyle does not, as often presumed, serve as a master centre that directly controls growth activities throughout the mandible as a whole.

It should be noted that the periosteal surfaces of some parts of the condylar neck on both the lingual and buccal sides are resorptive in nature (fig. 7). If one examines a hand-held mandible, it is apparent that the endosteal surfaces of the condylar neck in these regions actually face the posterosuperior direction of growth, and that the periosteal side is oriented inferiorly away from this direction. The combination of endosteal deposition and periosteal resorption thus moves the cortices of the neck, which are composed of endosteal bone tissue in such areas, upward and backward together with the condyle as the latter moves in a like direction. A remodelling conversion from condyle to neck is thereby involved in a continuing process of relocation of parts. The broad condyle is remodelled into the more narrow neck by this means as the condyle continues to move by its own growth process (fig. 7). As the condyle grows posteriorly, new bone is proportionately added to the posterior edge of the ramus.

In fig. 9e, the ramus has now been brought to the same horizontal dimension as Stage 1; its own PA breadth has not increased during this particular operation since the present growth phase is concerned with increasing only the length of the mandibular corpus in relationship with the horizontal elongation of the maxillary arch. Horizontal increase in the ramus dimension itself is associated with other relationships described later.

During continued growth, the ramus becomes more upright with respect to the corpus in order to accommodate the vertical lengthening of the nasomaxillary complex. This is accomplished by differential extents of deposition and resorption on the superior and inferior parts of the anterior and posterior borders of the ramus (not shown in fig. 9e since constant form is being retained). Thus, the "gonial angle" becomes progressively reduced with age.

Stage 5 (fig. 9f)

The growth and remodelling changes responsible for lengthening the mandibular corpus were described in Stages 3 and 4 above. These changes are simultaneously accompanied by the forward and downward displacement of the whole mandible. Whether the force that brings about this displacement movement is a pushing action caused by condylar growth into the glenoid fossa or a passive carry produced by the expansion of the functional matrix is currently controversial. The latter, however, is now becoming the favoured explanation.

In summary, precisely balanced growth and retention of facial pattern without change involves equal increments of:

> (a) posterior growth of the bony maxillary arch at its posterior tuberosity;
> (b) anterior displacement of the maxilla;
> (c) resorption from the anterior margin (and other areas) of the ramus;
> (d) deposition of bone on the posterior margin (and other areas) of the ramus;
> (e) condylar growth; and
> (f) forward displacement of the mandibular corpus.

In fig. 9e, it is seen that the oblique direction of condylar growth necessarily produces vertical as well as horizontal lengthening of the ramus. Complementary vertical changes in the maxilla are described in later stages.

Stage 6 (fig. 10a)

The size and configuration of the frontal lobes of the cerebrum determine the corresponding size and configuration of the anterior cranial fossa. The floor of this fossa is a structural "counterpart" of the horizontal superior part of the nasomaxillary complex. This is a significant relationship since the configuration of the frontal lobes and the floor of the anterior cranial fossa establish certain basic features of facial form, structure, topography, and appearance (Enlow

and McNamara, 1971). The size and configuration of the temporal lobes determine the corresponding size and configuration of the middle endocranial fossa the floor of which, in turn, is a horizontal counterpart of the pharynx and the ramus of the mandible. Note that the vertical reference line (termed the PM line) in the accompanying figures is a natural boundary between these various cranial and facial horizontal parts and counterparts (fig. 20 and 21). This important line passes through the sphenoethmoidal junction and sphenofrontal sutures of the cranial floor, along the anterior margin of the greater sphenoidal wings which are the anterior limits of the middle endocranial fossae, along the posterior maxillary tuberosity (PTM), and (in a "balanced" face) along the lingual tuberosity (not identifiable in lateral headfilms). The posterior margin of the lingual tuberosity is the effective dividing-point between the corpus and ramus, although the oblique nature of the ramus produces an overlap of its anterior margin and the region of the last molar.

The vertical reference line (PM line) is thus a natural morphological and morphogenic boundary that separates the anterior cranial fossa-upper nasomaxilla-maxillary arch-mandibular arch group of horizontal counterparts from the middle cranial fossa-pharynx group of horizontal counterparts. This line passes along major sites of growth, remodelling, and displacement for each of the parts involved. The PM line is a natural cephalometric plane and is certainly one of the most important with regard to the basic architecture and development of the face. It should also be noted that the PM line is approximately perpendicular to the neutral axis of vision.

In conjunction with the expansive growth of the temporal lobe, the middle endocranial fossa expands by a combination of resorption on the meningeal surface and deposition on the ectocranial side. This growth change is shown in fig. 10a. It is important to realize that the entire width of the cranial floor from condyle to condyle is involved and not merely the midventral part customarily represented in headfilm tracings. The mandibular and maxillary arches lie laterally as they relate to the cranial floor. The region of the clivus (and sella) is not directly involved, developmentally or structurally, with the cranial template that establishes basic facial form.

Stage 7 (fig. 10b)

The growth process described in the previous stage produces a forward displacement of the anterior cranial fossa, the entire nasomaxillary complex and, to a much lesser extent, the mandible. In fig. 10b, note that the vertical reference line becomes moved anteriorly to an extent corresponding with the expansion of the middle fossa and, of course, the temporal lobes of the cerebrum. This particular displacement effect is to be distinguished from the previously described anterior displacement of the maxilla produced by the functional matrix of the midface (or by the nasal septum according to older theory).

Note that the pharyngeal space and airway have now become enlarged by this growth process, and that the horizontal dimensions involved are not independently determined but are established primarily by the temporal lobes.

The growth of the middle cranial fossa also increases the

overall vertical dimensions of the cranial floor-and-mandibular ramus composite. This raises the maxillary arch and lowers the mandibular dental arch correspondingly. Equivalent vertical maxillary changes that serve to match this vertical cranial floor-ramus growth are described in later stages.

Stage 8 (fig. 10c)

The horizontal mandibular counterpart of the temporal lobe, the middle endocranial fossa, and the pharyngeal region is the ramus. The mandibular ramus bridges the pharyngeal region, extending from the temporocondylar articulation to the maxillary tuberosity, and places the mandibular corpus into occlusal relationship with the maxillary arch. To match the forward displacement of the maxilla by the expansion of the middle cranial fossa (Stage 7), the ramus correspondingly increases in equivalent dimensions to displace the mandibular arch anteriorly to the same extent (assuming "balanced" growth). The ramus grows posteriorly by the same complex process described in Stage 4. It now increases in horizontal size to the same extent as its counterpart, the middle cranial fossa.

Stage 9 (fig. 10d)

Simultaneous with the growth process described in Stage 8, the whole mandible undergoes forward and downward displacement. This places the mandibular arch in proper horizontal position relative to the maxillary arch. Note that these changes also add to the vertical dimension of the cranial base-ramus composite, however, thereby continuing to lower the mandibular occlusal plane.

Stage 10 (fig. 10e)

As the frontal lobes of the cerebrum expand, the floor of the anterior cranial fossae likewise lengthens and widens to a corresponding extent. It is noted, at the age levels used in these diagrams, that the anterior cranial fossae have already actually completed growth (the middle cranial fossae still continue to expand, however). Since the purpose of these descriptions is to explain the basis for "balanced" growth, expansion of the anterior fossae is, nevertheless, included in order to illustrate the growth process involved. The forehead and lateral walls of each fossa move anteriorly and laterally, respectively, by a combination of resorption and deposition on the appropriate surfaces of the inner and outer cortical tables. When cerebral growth ceases, growth of the inner table stops. The outer table of the forehead, however, continues to grow forward as it keeps pace with the horizontal growth of the ethmomaxillary complex. This produces a progressively enlarging frontal sinus. The inner and outer tables thus become progressively separated in conjunction with long-term upper facial expansion. The volume of the frontal sinus varies according to age, sex and ethnic group since the morphology of the ethmomaxillary region differs according to these factors.

In contrast to the bony maxillary arches, which lengthen for the most part by growth at the maxillary tuberosity, the ethmomaxillary region grows by complex combinations of sutural growth and resorption-deposition on the topographically complex bony surfaces involved. The nasal

chambers, in general, expand by resorption from the mucosal sides of the cortices and deposition on the outer sides.

Stage 11 (fig. 10f)

In preceding stages, the mandibular corpus was lowered by composite growth changes in the cranial floor and the mandibular ramus, as described in Stages, 5, 7 and 9. Simultaneously, however, the entire nasomaxillary complex and the alveolar regions of the mandibular arch also increase in their respective vertical dimensions. The vertical size of the cranial floor and ramus, together, represent a composite counterpart of the vertical dimensions of the nasomaxillary complex and the alveolar portion of the mandibular corpus. If their respective increases are balanced, facial form is retained without change (as represented by these diagrams).

The nasal side of the hard palate is resorptive and the oral side is depository (figs. 5 and 8). This combination produces a direct growth movement (relocation) of the palate inferiorly. In conjunction with this, the alveolar cortices of the maxillary arch also move downward by direct resorption and deposition on appropriate upward- and downward-facing surfaces. This results in an inferior movement of the bony arch involving successive new generations of bone tissue occupying progressively new, more inferior levels. The bony arch constantly changes in substance as it grows. Significantly, the teeth are being carried inferiorly by this process, which involves deposition and resorption of the alveolar bone lining the sockets. These same depository-resorptive changes also produce the mesial drift of teeth as well as any tipping, rotation, and distal movements that may occur during maxillomandibular growth and the establishment of occlusion. The teeth, thus, undergo vertical as well as horizontal drifting. The extent of vertical tooth drift is significant, accounting for approximately half of the total vertical distance involved in downward maxillary growth (displacement accounts for the other half, as described in Stage 12). Vertical drift is to be distinguished from the separate process of eruption, which is a vertical movement that takes place in addition to the drift of each tooth.

In figs. 1, 5 and 8, it is seen that much of the labial surface of the anterior maxillary bony arch is resorptive (the lingual side is depository). The growth movement in this part of the arch proceeds essentially straight downward. This is in contrast to the growth of a "muzzle" on the face of other primate and non-primate species where a depository type of labial cortex grows anteriorly as well as inferiorly, thereby producing more pronounced maxillary protrusion. Only in the flat, vertical face of man does the forward part of the arch have a resorptive external surface. The morphogenic basis for this is apparent in fig. 8. The surface contour of the bony arch in the incisor region is either concave or labially inclined. The portion inferior to A point necessarily requires resorption on the labial (upward-facing) sides of the cortices and deposition on the lingual (downward-facing) sides in order to achieve direct downward growth. Were the converse combination to occur in a growing child, a "muzzle" would be produced. The portion superior to A point has a depository type of labial surface since it faces inferiorly toward the direction of growth. The reversal line is precisely at *A* point.

In fig. 10f, growth at the maxillary sutures is also represented. Although changes in the tracing are represented only by the frontomaxillary suture, growth occurs at the various other sutures as well, including the ethmomaxillary, zygomaticomaxillary, ethmofrontal, nasofrontal, nasomaxillary, lacrimal, zygomaticofrontal, and the vertical palatal sutures. Sutural growth and growth by generalized periosteal and endosteal activity are not separate processes. They are regional expressions of essentially the same intramembranous growth process involved in the overall, proportionate enlargement of the entire bone and all of its surfaces.

Stage 12 (fig. 11a)

The inferior displacement of the nasomaxillary complex is represented in this stage. It is important to understand that enlargement of each bony component by bone deposition in sutures does not actually "push" the maxilla and other contiguous bones downward and away from the cranial floor. Rather, these bony parts are carried downward and, as this takes place, the bones themselves simultaneously enlarge. Thus, new bone is added on to sutural contact surfaces as each bone becomes displaced by expansive forces other than the process of bone enlargement itself. These forces, according to present theory, are the same as previously described in Stage 2, *i.e.* the functional matrix of the midface (and/or the expanding nasal septum according to older theory).

In fig. 11a, the movement of the maxillary arch and palate from level 1 to level 2 is accomplished by resorption on the nasal surface of the palate and deposition on the oral side in conjunction with the other growth and remodelling changes outlined in Stage 11. The movement from level 2 to 3 is produced by the downward displacement of the ethmomaxillary complex as a whole. These composite, cumulative movements proceed simultaneously.

Stage 13 (fig. 11b)

As the mandible is displaced inferiorly (described in previous stages), the bony alveolar ridges of the mandibular corpus grow in a superior direction at the same time. Accompanying this, the mandibular teeth move upward by vertical drift, a movement that is additional to the eruption of each tooth. This brings the upper and lower dental arches into occlusion. It should be noted that the posteroanterior positions of the teeth are now in proper (Class I) relationship as a composite result of all the previously described, balanced horizontal and vertical growth movements. Comparing fig. 11b with fig. 11a, it is apparent that the extent of upward drift by the mandibular teeth is much less than downward maxillary dental arch movement. This is due to the additional presence of the nasal chambers and their expansive changes within the maxillary complex.

The extent of vertical nasomaxillary growth equals the combined vertical increases of the cranial floor, the ramus, and the vertical adjustments of the mandibular dental arch and alveolar bone if their respective changes are all balanced. If imbalances occur, dimensional disproportions and skeletal rotations are produced which cause specific types of facial variations, as described later.

Bone deposition takes place on the inferior as well as lateral and medial surfaces of the mandibular corpus. This enlarges the corpus and thickens its cortical plates proportionately with overall mandibular enlargement. To bring the mandibular incisors into occlusal relationship with the maxillary incisors, a backward tipping of the former takes place bringing them into more upright placement behind the upper incisors. This is accomplished by resorption on the labial-facing cortical surfaces and deposition on the lingual side. The combination of posterior mandibular incisor relocation, a resorptive alveolar region on the labial side, and continued anterior growth on the underlying basal bone results in a progressively enlarging chin as the child ages. This combination is also related to the crowding of incisor teeth in both the mandible and maxilla (the incisor area of the maxillary arch also having a resorptive type of labial surface, as previously described).

Stage 14 (fig. 11c)

Just as the maxillary arch lengthens by a posterior direction of bony growth, the contiguous malar region correspondingly enlarges by a backward mode of growth. The anterior surface of the malar protuberance is resorptive. The zygomatic complex lengthens vertically at the zygofrontal suture and, laterally, by deposition on the lateral surface of the zygoma with proportionate resorption from the medial side. The zygomatic arch enlarges by continued bone deposition on its inferior side.

While not representable in a lateral headfilm tracing, the superior side of the orbital floor is of a depository nature. The opposite endosteal side of this thin cortical plate is resorptive, thereby producing an upward expansion of the underlying maxillary sinus in conjunction with sinus enlargement in all other directions except toward the nasal side (the nasal chamber is expanding in a lateral direction as well). It would appear that bone deposited on the inner side of the orbital cavity (superior side of the orbital floor) would progressively decrease its size. This is not the case. The orbital floor slopes so that it faces obliquely in an anterior as well as upward direction. Bone deposition on this surface thus functions to move this part of the orbit anteriorly as the whole orbit grows forward with temporal and frontal lobe expansion. The orbital floor does indeed rise during growth as a consequence, however, but this important growth movement functions to sustain its constant position with relation to the eyeball. Bone additions at the frontomaxillary suture accompany the significant extent of downward displacement of the whole maxilla. This downward movement would result in a disproportionate lowering of the orbital floor except that compensatory bone additions on the superior side of the floor simultaneously move it upward. The position of the orbital floor remains essentially stable, although a slight net inferior repositioning may occur as the orbital soft tissues enlarge. Thus, a differential extent of downward movement occurs between the floor of the orbit and the floor of the nasal chamber even though both are parts of the same skeletal unit.

Stage 15 (fig. 11d)

The inferior and anterior displacement of the zygomatic complex is represented by this stage, a movement that simultaneously accompanies the resorptive and depository growth changes described in Stage 14. Just as the maxilla grows backward together with displacement in an opposite forward direction, the contiguous malar region, correspondingly, follows the same growth and displacement combination. It is apparent that the cheek area could not grow in a direct forward manner simply by deposition of bone on its forward-facing surface (as one might mistakenly presume). This would alter the positional relationship between the malar protuberance and the maxillary arch; *i.e.* they would be growing in opposite directions and their positions and surface contours would become progressively divergent. In fig. 11d, the position of the zygoma has been placed in proper location with respect to the maxillary arch by the forward and downward displacement of the zygoma.

THE MORPHOLOGICAL BASIS FOR VARIATIONS IN CRANIOFACIAL FORM AND PATTERN

In order more readily to understand the complex anatomical and architectural factors that underlie the wide range of normal and abnormal variations which commonly occur in facial form, the simplified diagram in fig. 11f is used. The segments in this diagram represent key parts in the cranial and facial composite directly involved in the basic growth and remodelling changes described in the preceding section (Stages 1 to 15). The changes illustrated in these stages can be effectively repeated and demonstrated using this schematic representation. The basis for anatomical and topographical variations in facial form produced by variations in regional growth changes can thus also be demonstrated.

Each segment in the diagrammatic plan represents a specific, major site of growth, remodelling and/or displacement. This is in contrast to most conventional cephalometric planes and angles. Sella-nasion, for example, does not represent any specific site or sites of growth, and it actually bypasses the relevant centres of growth along its course. This plane, like many others commonly used in cephalometrics, begins and ends at points and passes across bones in such a way that specific areas involved in actual, key growth changes are not recognized or represented. Such planes, also, do not recognize counterpart relationships, which are fundamental to the basic geometric plan of craniofacial construction and growth.

Two basic considerations are involved in determining the nature of the geometrical and structural relationships among separate bones and their parts. The first is the overall horizontal or vertical length of a whole bony segment or the length of some particular, architecturally effective portion of that bone (such as the horizontal dimension of the ramus). The second consideration is the manner of alignment of each particular bony segment. The nature of alignment (angulation) of any given part determines the expression of that segment's actual dimension. For example, a more upright alignment of the ramus serves to increase its vertical expressed (not actual) dimension but reduces the

expression of its horizontal dimension. Any consideration of the relationships among the parts of the craniofacial composite must consider both the "actual" vertical and horizontal dimensions and the nature of alignment of each part relative to the others so that the "expressed" dimensions can be appraised.

The following descriptions are selected examples of various dimensional and alignment combinations. Many other commonly encountered patterns also occur, and these can be worked out by the reader utilizing this same basic procedure (Enlow and Moyers, 1971).

Figure 12a. In this figure, the upper horizontal segment of the nasomaxillary complex is dimensionally "long" relative to its various geometric counterparts, including the floor of the anterior cranial fossa, the palate (which is not represented in these particular schematic diagrams), the maxillary skeletal arch, and the mandibular arch. The outer cortical table of the frontal bone grows forward in company with the upper face, but the inner table remains fixed in contact with the frontal lobes which have already ceased growth. As a result, an enlarged frontal sinus and a sloping forehead are formed. A high nasal bridge is produced, and the cheek area appears recessed due to the anterior projection of the nasal region. A marked extent of forward growth by the upper nasal region relative to the palatal area results in a bent, aquiline, or "Roman" type of nose. Due to the

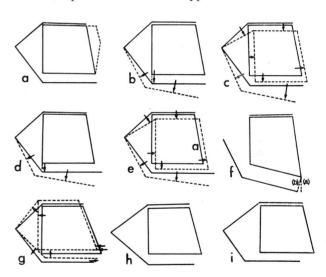

Fig. 12. Schematic craniofacial diagrams showing various combinations of the structural parts. See text for descriptions and fig. 11 for identification of the various segments.

protrusion of the upper part of the face, the profile suggests retrognathia. This does not necessarily exist, however, since the arches themselves may be in proper dimensional and positional balance.

Should the upper ethmomaxillary and anterior cranial floor relationship be in close dimensional balance, conversely, a more upright and bulbous forehead, small frontal sinus, low nasal bridge, shorter nose, and prominent-appearing cheekbones occur. These various relationships are associated with characteristic features of the face related directly to differences in the shape of the brain among ethnic groups, and they are also associated with age and sex differences (Enlow *et al.*, 1971b, 1973a).

Figure 12b. This relationship involves a nasomaxillary complex that is vertically long with respect to its structural counterpart, the vertical length of the combined ramus-middle cranial fossa. This results in a downward and backward rotation of the ramus which increases the expressed vertical length of the ramus to accommodate the long midface. Because of this, however, the expression of the horizontal ramus dimension is also changed, resulting in a decrease with respect to its horizontal structural counterpart, the middle cranial fossa. This change in ramus alignment produces a retrognathic relationship even though the upper and lower arches themselves, as well as the horizontal ramus and middle fossa "actual" dimensions, are all in dimensional balance. Due to the posterior offset of the mandibular arch, a Class II molar relationship occurs. Note also that the downward rotation of the whole mandible results in a consequent downward-inclined occlusal plane, which is a common feature in facial types having a vertically long midface.

In contrast to the above, a vertically short midface leads to a prognathic facial profile and a Class III molar relationship due to the forward and upward nature of ramus alignment.

Figure 12c. A forward-inclined alignment of the floor of the middle cranial fossa, as seen in this diagram, increases the horizontal "expressed" dimension with respect to its counterpart, the ramus, and also lowers the nasomaxillary complex relative to the condyle. The latter causes a downward and backward rotation of the ramus in order to accommodate the more inferior positioning of the maxillary arch. The result is twofold. Firstly, the nasomaxillary complex is placed in a more forward position and, secondly, the mandibular arch is placed in an opposite, posterior position. Retrognathia is the composite result, and a Class II molar relationship occurs even though all the various bony segments themselves can be in actual dimensional balance (as in the example illustrated). The expression of these dimensions, however, has been altered due to a chain of alignment responses originating with the ventral contour of the temporal lobes of the brain.

In contrast to the above, a backward-inclined alignment of the middle cranial fossa leads to mandibular protrusion, a prognathic facial profile, and a Class III molar relationship. If the mandibular corpus should also be horizontally "long" relative to the maxilla, or if the actual horizontal dimension of the ramus is long with respect to the middle cranial fossa, the mandibular protrusive effect is increased in proportion.

Figure 12h. A "short" mandibular arch relative to its geometrical counterpart, the bony maxillary arch, produces one type of a retrognathic relationship if other additional, compensatory factors are not involved. This combination in itself does not necessarily result in a severe Class II "molar relationship", however, since the posterior portions of the respective arches (the maxillary and lingual tuberosities) are in proper juxtaposition.

Figure 12i. This diagram illustrates a dimensional imbalance between the ramus of the mandible and its particular structural counterpart, which is that part of the middle cranial fossa from the apical point of the mandibular condyle (condylion) to the boundary between the middle and anterior cranial fossae*. This boundary is in direct line with the posterior margin of the maxillary tuberosity, as previously described, and lies on the vertical PM reference line in fig. 11f. The horizontal dimension of the middle cranial fossa in this example exceeds that of the ramus, and the mandibular arch is thereby placed in a retrognathic position; *i.e.* posteriorly offset with respect to the maxilla. This relationship underlies one of several combinations that produces a Class II molar relationship since the posterior end of the mandibular arch is situated behind the posterior end of the maxillary arch. Even though mandibular retrusion results, however, note that the arches themselves are dimensionally balanced in the example illustrated.

In contrast to the above, a horizontally broad ramus with respect to the middle cranial fossa produces a prognathic facial profile and a Class III molar relationship due to an anterior offset of the mandible. The respective arches, however, may be dimensionally balanced. If they are not, the extent of mandibular protrusion would be either increased or decreased depending upon which arch is dimensionally "short".

INTRINSIC COMPENSATIONS

The above examples show several regional dimensional and alignment relationships that produce characteristic types of resultant facial patterns. In any given individual person, many such combinations of relationships always exist (Enlow *et al.*, 1971b). If all or most of these regional factors contribute to a protrusion of the maxilla and/or retrusion of the mandible, a severe Class II cumulative pattern is produced. Conversely, if all or most of the regional relationships throughout the craniofacial composite contribute to mandibular protrusion, a more or less severe, cumulative Class III pattern results. In the great majority of individuals, however, mixed combinations of maxillary-protrusive and mandibular-protrusive regional relationships exist. The nature of the aggregate balance among all of them determines the final, composite facial form in any given person. In most individuals, the nature of the offsetting balance of underlying, regional Class II and Class III features results in a Class I or only a tendency toward a Class II or III pattern. Any individual having normal or a Class I type of facial pattern actually represents a mixture of maxillary and mandibular protrusive-causing characteristics throughout the craniofacial composite. In this sense, a separate "Class I" type of facial pattern, in contrast to Class II and III types, does not exist as such.

Figure 12d. In many ethnic groups, the nasomaxillary complex tends to be vertically "long" causing a downward and backward alignment of the whole mandible. In the absence of compensatory features, this would produce a retrognathic facial pattern. In many such individuals, however, the dimension of the mandibular corpus is horizontally long relative to the maxilla. The degree of compensation

---

* Both the ramus and the middle cranial fossa are obliquely oriented. However, their respective "effective" dimensions are determined by appraising the horizontal span covered by each.

may be sufficient to produce an orthognathic profile, or it may fall at some point between this and the full possible extent of retrognathia caused by the backward alignment of the ramus. Because of the offsetting, compensatory nature of this common combination, a Class I profile, a Class II molar relationship, and a Class III type of mandibular corpus exist. The presence of a downward-inclined occlusal plane caused by the mandibular rotation should be noted.

The result of a forward-inclined middle cranial fossa was previously described and illustrated in fig. 12c. A frequently observed relationship involves the development of an increased horizontal dimension of the ramus which compensates for the increased "expressed" horizontal dimension of the middle cranial fossa due to the nature of its alignment. This is common in Class I caucasoids having a dolichocephalic head form. This feature is also characteristic in blacks; the extent of horizontal ramus increase is notably marked, causing mandibular protrusion to a degree that results in anterior maxillary incisor tipping and consequent bimaxillary protrusion.

The combination seen in fig. 12e may also occur. A horizontally long mandibular corpus compensates for the forward alignment of the middle cranial fossa. Although an orthognathic profile exists, a Class II molar relationship can exist due to the ramus middle cranial fossa offset.

Figure 12f. A Class II occlusal pattern does not necessarily accompany a retrognathic profile (a) for the reason illustrated in this diagram. Because various rotational alignments are always involved in any craniofacial composite, different planes of reference show different kinds of structural relationships. Although the mandible is in a retrognathic profile position due to its downward inclination, the upper and lower arches themselves may or may not remain properly aligned in the incisor region as indicated by a perpendicular to the occlusal plane. The reference plane for occlusal alignment is separate from the reference plane for the facial profile. In this diagram, a horizontally long mandibular corpus has compensated for the backward rotation of the mandible. The upper and lower incisors are in proper relationship even though the chin is receded (b).

Figure 12g. This diagram illustrates an upward and backward alignment of the middle cranial fossa in combination with a horizontally "short" mandibular arch (relative to its counterpart, the maxillary arch). As a result, a Class II type of mandible-maxillary dimensional relationship exists in conjunction with a Class III type of molar relationship and a Class I facial profile. The nature of middle cranial fossa alignment reduces its expressed horizontal dimension relative to the ramus, thereby producing a mandibular protrusive effect. This is compensated, however, by the dimension of the mandibular corpus.

Figure 13a to 13e. This series of diagrams illustrates the basis for the development of the curve of Spee, which is a compensatory mechanism involving the development of the dental arches (Enlow *et al.*, 1971b). As previously pointed out, a vertically long midface characterizes many individuals and results in a backward and downward inclination of the whole mandible (fig. 13b). In itself, this would result in an

anterior open bite (in addition to retrognathia) should adaptive skeletal or dental compensations fail to occur. In fig. 13c, those maxillary teeth that are mesial to the last molar extrude until full-length occlusion is obtained (a process of inferior dental drift). The straight-line nature of the resultant, downward-inclined occlusal plane should be noted. The reader should also observe the overjet of the maxillary incisors caused by the backward and downward rotation of the mandible.

Figure 13d shows an extrusion of the maxillary teeth, but the anterior teeth descend only about the same extent as the posteriors; the increasing amounts needed in the canine and

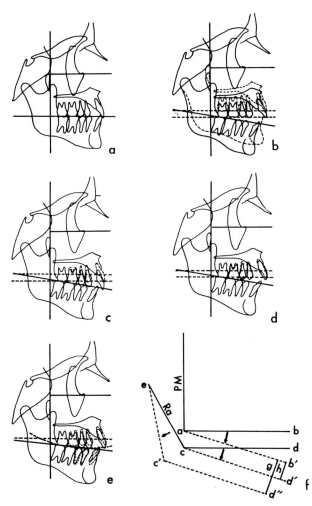

FIG. 13. The developmental basis for the curve of Spee is illustrated in figures a, b, c, d, e. Figure f shows the contrasting effects of downward rotations of the mandibular ramus and corpus. A backward and downward rotation of ramus from ec to ec' carries the corpus from cd to c'd". The corpus becomes placed posteriorly relative to the maxillary arch (g). A rotation of the maxillary and mandibular arches ab and cd to positions ab' and cd' places the mandibular arch in a more protrusive position relative to the maxillary arch (h).

incisor regions thus fall short. An anterior open bite remains, although of lesser severity than seen in fig. 13b. In this case, however, the premolars and incisors of the mandible can extrude to complete closure of the occlusion (fig. 13e). A curved occlusal plane thus results with full-length contact. The mandibular incisors have become positioned, characteristically, well above the plane of the molars and premolars. This feature is commonly encountered among long-faced individuals.

The developmental and morphological basis for the characteristic varieties of facial types seen among ethnic groups or between individuals in any given group involves different combinations of the kinds of structural relationships described in the preceding sections. Many of these facial features are based on the shape, size and topographical nature of the brain, since the size, shape and surface contours of various cerebral lobes determine the corresponding form of the cranial floor which, in turn, provides the template upon which the various parts of face develop.

Some caucasoid groups have an elongated, dolichocephalic head (and brain) form, and many individuals in these groups characteristically demonstrate a Class II tendency. Also, a much greater incidence of Class II rather than Class III malocclusions exists. The reasons are as follows. The elongated shape of the brain results in an open cranial base angle (a more forward inclination of the middle endocranial fossa). This in turn places the maxilla anteriorly and causes a downward and backward rotation of the ramus

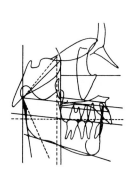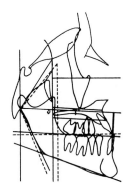

FIG. 14. The structural basis for a Cl II malocclusion (left) is contrasted with that of a Cl III. In both instances, the resultant malocclusion is caused by a summation of many mandibular retrusive and/or protrusive factors in various parts of the craniofacial composite. Each of these malocclusion types is thus a composite of many features and is not simply produced by a "short" or a "long" mandible or maxilla. In the Cl II, note the forward alignment of the middle cranial fossa (solid line rotated anteriorly with respect to the dashed "neutral" line), the backward alignment of the ramus, the horizontally short mandibular corpus, the forward placement of the maxillary complex by the middle cranial fossa, and the alignment of the mandibular corpus ("closed" gonial angle). All of these regional factors contribute to the composite basis for mandibular retrusion. In the Class III, conversely, note that each of these various relationships has an opposite, mandibular protrusive effect. A degree of compensation has been provided in both the Cl II and Cl III individuals, however, by the broad and the narrow horizontal dimensions of the ramus, respectively. From Enlow, *et al.*, *Angle Orthodont.*, **41**, 1971 (a).

due to the downward positioning of the midface. If characteristic compensatory factors (as previously discussed) are operative, these underlying maxillary-protrusive and mandibular-retrusive features are partially or completely offset, and a more or less normal (Class I) facial composite results.

If adequate compensatory features are absent, however, a Class II malocclusion occurs since the underlying Class II tendency then becomes fully expressed (fig. 14a). Other ethnic populations, including some other caucasoid and most oriental groups, have a brachycephalic head (and brain) form which produces a more upright middle cranial fossa alignment, and an opposite, Class III underlying tendency is therefore present (fig. 14b). These groups are characterized by a higher incidence of Class III than Class II mal occlusions (fig. 14b).

Figure 13f. A downward inclination of the mandibular corpus at the ramus-corpus junction (not the condyle) has a mandibular protrusive effect. A converse, upward inclination has a mandibular retrusive effect. This differs from upward and downward directions of mandibular rotation at the condyle which have opposite effects, as previously described.

Such a downward-inclined mandibular corpus often occurs in conjunction with features in other regions that have maxillary-protrusive effects. The alignment of the corpus (*i.e.* the "gonial angle") is thus a factor that can partially compensate for any underlying Class II tendency, or it can augment the tendency to make it more severe.

ROLE OF THE CRANIAL BASE IN ESTABLISHING FACIAL FORM AND PATTERN

The upright, bipedal stature of man involves a number of specialized phylogenetic interrelationships among the different areas of the body as a whole; the morphological design of the feet, vertebral column, pelvis, shoulder girdle, free arms, manipulative hands, binocular vision, unobstructed muzzleless vision of close hand-held objects, a mind to direct the hands, and a cranial base flexure that allows a vertical spine and upright posture together with forward-directed vision and jaws which are perpendicular to body stance (Enlow, 1968b). All of these features require all of the rest in order to carry out the functions of each.

The face is not structurally and developmentally independent of the floor of the cranium. The cranial floor is the template upon which the face develops, and the shape, dimensions, contours and alignment of the various parts of the cranial floor establish a number of fundamental relationships that determine, at least in part, the basic shape, dimensions, contours and the profile of the face itself (Enlow, 1973a).

The massive enlargement of the cerebrum appears to be a pacemaking factor that has led to the interrelated development of the rest of the above-mentioned human anatomical features. Regardless of its phylogenic priority, however, the morphological consequences of the shape and the size of the brain involve several clear-cut effects on facial form. First, the disproportionately large extent of cerebral growth relative to the slower, lesser growth of the midventral portion of the brain has caused a bending of the ventral side of the brain as a whole. This is the developmental basis for the flexure of the cranial base which, in turn, produces several key changes in the structure of the human face and its relationships. These are outlined below and illustrated in figs. 15 to 23 inclusive.

(1) The flexure of the cranial base, together with the massive enlargement of the frontal, temporal, parietal and occipital lobes, places the foramen magnum in a midventral position with a vertically-aligned spinal cord (compare fig. 16 with fig. 19).

(2) Cranial base flexure, as it relates to frontal lobe enlargement, produces a rotation of the eyeballs and orbits into forward-directed positions perpendicular to the spinal cord (figs. 15, 18 and 19). Thus, the eyes and the face point in the direction of general body movement. The orbital rims rotate, in conjunction with the enlarged

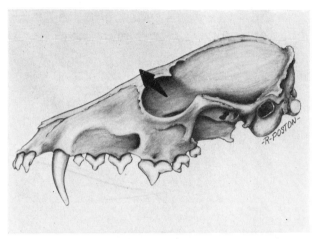

FIG. 15. In relation to the size of the frontal and temporal lobes of the cerebrum, the orbits of this carnivore point obliquely superiorly and laterally.

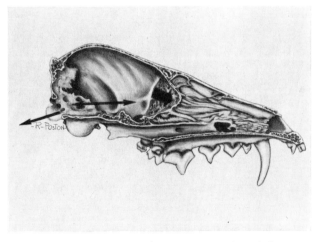

FIG. 16. In relation to the size of the cerebral hemisphere, the cranial floor is unflexed, the spinal cord is aligned horizontally, and the olfactory bulbs (cribriform plates) are obliquely vertical and lie in a perpendicular relationship with a more horizontal, elongate muzzle and snout.

frontal lobes, into a vertical plane. The frontal lobes also produce a vertical forehead which, together with the vertical rims of the orbit, shortened nose, and bimaxillary retrognathism give the face a flattened, vertical profile. The lateral expansion of the cerebrum provides the structural basis for the widened human face in comparison with other mammals.

(3) The enlarged temporal lobes, together with the

frontal lobes, are related to a rotation of the eyes toward the midline. This produces approximately parallel axes of bilateral vision pointing essentially straight forward in a binocular manner.

(4) Convergence of the eyes toward the midline, however, also reduces the relative dimension of the interorbital region, which is the root of the nasal chamber. This narrowing of the nasal bridge is accompanied by shorten-

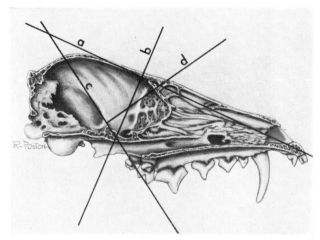

FIG. 17. The midfacial plane (a) from the edge of brain to superior prosthion is perpendicular to the plane of the cribiform plates (b). The PM line (c), which passes from the boundary between the middle and anterior cranial fossae down to the edge of the posterior maxillary tuberosity, is approximately perpendicular to the neutral orbital axis (d). See PM plane on fig. 22.

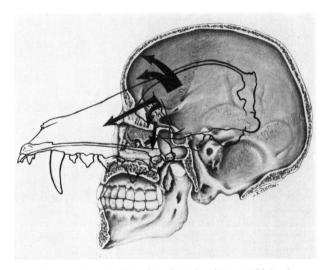

FIG. 18. The expansion of the frontal and temporal lobes is related to the vertical rotation of the orbital rims and a horizontal rotation of the cribriform plates. Note the resultant vertical alignment of the human face.

ing in the extent of snout protrusion because the architectural base of the nose is reduced as well as the physiological capacity of olfaction. A narrow nose in any species is necessarily shorter, functionally and structurally, than a broad nose.

(5) Expansion of the frontal lobes displaces the olfactory bulbs from a vertical or oblique position, as found

in non-human species, into a horizontal one. The alignment of the olfactory bulbs is a key relationship that contributes to facial position and profile. The plane of the midfacial region in any species is approximately perpendicular to the olfactory bulbs since this is the axis of olfactory nerve spread. Thus, the vertical or oblique nature of olfactory bulb alignment in non-human groups

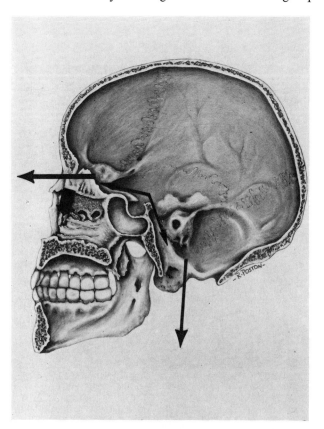

FIG. 19. The expansion of the cerebrum is associated with a flexure of the cranial floor, a vertically aligned spinal cord, a horizontal displacement of the olfactory bulbs, a vertical face, and a neutral orbital axis that is perpendicular to the spinal cord. Compare with fig. 16.

having smaller frontal lobes is related to a more horizontally aligned midface which protrudes as an elongated, horizontal or oblique snout. This occurs in conjunction with the more broad interorbital dimension (see 4 above) that provides the architectural and physiological base for a protrusive snout. In man, the olfactory bulbs are rotated into a horizontal position by frontal-lobe expansion (figs. 18 and 19) and the face thereby develops in a vertical plane perpendicular to the bulbs (i.e. the cribriform plates of the anterior cranial floor).

(6) Reduced protrusion of the snout, based on the two relationships described in (4) and (5) above, is accomplished by reduction of the bony maxillary arch. The nasal and the oral surfaces of the palate are, in effect, two sides of the same coin, and any reduction of one must necessarily be accompanied by a more or less equal reduction in the other. Two factors are involved. Firstly, the decreased relative volume of the olfactory region caused by orbital convergence toward the midline reduces the

horizontal expanse, both laterally and posteroanteriorly, of the nasal chamber and palate. Secondly, the horizontal rotation of the olfactory bulbs causes a corresponding "rotation" of the nasomaxillary complex into a vertical and more posterior placement. This carries the maxillary arch into a largely suborbital position (in contrast with other species) and is accompanied by the development of a complete orbital floor and the formation of the large suborbital (maxillary) sinuses. The configuration of the maxilla becomes rectangular rather than triangular as a consequence (fig. 23). The face of man thus lies under rather than anterior to the anterior cranial fossae. The mandibular ramus, also, has become vertically elongate to accommodate the more vertical disposition of the mid-

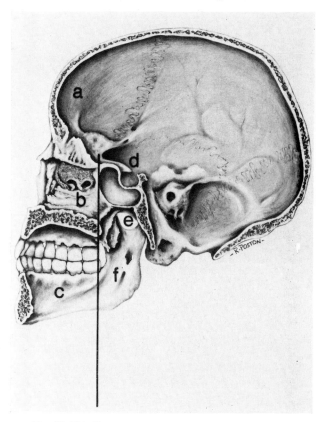

FIG. 20. This diagram illustrates the subdivisions of the face in relation to corresponding compartments of the brain. The vertical PM line is a natural anatomical and developmental boundary that separates the floor of the anterior cranial fossa (a) and its counterparts (b and c) from the floor of the middle cranial fossa (d) and its counterparts, the pharynx (e) and the ramus (f).

face, and the horizontal length of the mandibular corpus has become adapted to the length of the maxillary arch. Due to the nature of placement of the mandibular incisors lingually in relation to the maxillary incisors as a factor involved in bimaxillary reduction and the vertical alignment of the midface, a "chin" is formed (fig. 11b).

(7) The face is subdivided according to matching cranial base compartments established by the lobes of the brain. The size and the shape of these various cerebral lobes determine the corresponding boundaries of the underlying facial parts (figs. 12, 20 and 21). Thus, the

temporal lobe of each cerebrum establishes the perimeter of the middle endocranial fossa which determines the boundaries of the pharynx and is related, in turn, to the horizontal breadth of the ramus which functions to bridge the pharyngeal space. The ramus may or may not match the dimensional span of the pharynx since it is involved

the anterior boundary of the brain-midfacial profile, *i.e.* a line along the upper front edge of the brain down to superior prosthion perpendicular to the cribriform plate (fig. 22). The upper face among persons with a dolicho-

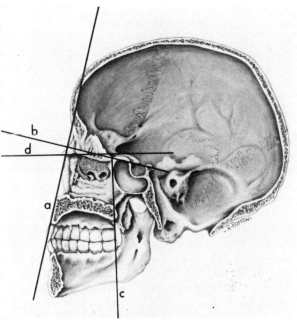

FIG. 22. The dimensions of certain facial parts are determined by corresponding dimensions of the various lobes of the brain. The alignment of these parts is determined by the alignment of the olfactory and orbital sense organs. Thus, the anterior boundary of the midface (a) and the midfacial plane are established by a line from the front edge of the frontal lobes perpendicular to the cribriform plates down to superior prosthion (b). The posterior boundary of the midface (c) is established by the posterior edge of the frontal lobes (junction of anterior and middle cranial fossae) approximately perpendicular to the neutral orbital axis (d). This is the PM plane. Compare with fig. 17.

FIG. 21. This is a headfilm tracing showing the placement of the vertical PM line, which extends from the intersection of the great wings of the sphenoid and the cranial floor down to the most inferior point of PTM. As in fig. 20, counterparts a, b, and c are separated from counterparts d, e, and f by this key line. The ramus (f) is a highly variable structure involved in craniofacial compensations. Because its horizontal breadth and the nature of its vertical alignment varies in response to disproportions in other parts of the craniofacial composite, the ramus lies at correspondingly variable positions relative to the vertical PM. From Enlow, *et al., Angle Orthodont.*, **41**, 1971a.

in maxillo-mandibular compensations (described in a previous section).

Each frontal lobe establishes the perimeter of the anterior cranial fossa and provides the template from which the underlying nasal part of the face develops. The latter, in turn, is related to the development of the palate and the maxillary arch. The placement of the mandibular arch relative to the maxilla is variable and is determined by the horizontal lengths of the frontal lobes and the midface, the vertical length of the midface (causing ramus rotations), the adaptive breadth of the ramus, and of course, the horizontal length of the mandibular corpus itself in any given individual.

(8) The breadth, horizontal and vertical lengths of the brain establish the corresponding breadth and the horizontal and vertical lengths of the face. A long, narrow configuration of the brain (dolichocephalic head form) is characterized by a narrow and a vertically long face. The anterior boundary of the frontal lobes establishes

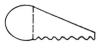

FIG. 23. These schematic diagrams depict the vertical rotation of the face in conjunction with phylogenetic frontal and temporal lobe expansion and the consequent realignment of the arches into horizontal positions. This results in a change from a triangular maxillary configuration to a rectangular one, the formation of orbital floors, and the development of large suborbital (maxillary) sinuses.

cephalic head form tends to be protrusive due to the more open nature of alignment of the anterior-to-middle cranial fossae, as described earlier. Conversely, a short, broad brain (brachycephalic) is characterized by a wide face and a vertically shorter nasomaxillary region. The face is correspondingly less protrusive due to the more upright nature of the cranial base flexure.

(9) The placement of the maxillary arch in any species, including man, is determined by the olfactory and orbital senses. The anterior and posterior boundaries of the maxillary arch are established by the horizontal dimensions of the frontal lobe (anterior cranial fossa), which is the structural "counterpart" of the maxilla (fig. 22). The placement of the anterior plane of the midface in almost all species is determined by a line from the anterior-superior edge of the brain perpendicular to the olfactory bulb. The posterior plane of the maxillary arch is determined by a line from the posterior–inferior edge of the frontal lobe (sphenofrontal suture; junction of anterior and middle cranial fossae) perpendicular to the neutral geometrical axis of the bony orbital cavity. This is the key PM line and passes along the posterior maxillary tuberosity through PTM.

(10) The alveolar ridge of the midface grows inferiorly down to the inferior-most level of the occipital lobe (in man and most other mammalian groups except some species having a highly specialized maxillary configuration). A line may thus be drawn (in the adult) from prosthion through the posterior–inferior corner of the maxillary tuberosity to the floor of the posterior cranial fossa.

BIBLIOGRAPHY

Björk, A (1947), "The Face in Profile," *Berlingska Boktrycheriet.*

Enlow, D. H. (1968a), "Wolff's Law and the Factor of Architectonic Circumstance," *Amer. J. Orthodont.*, **54**, 803.

Enlow, D. H. (1968b), *The Human Face: An Account of the Postnatal Growth and Development of the Craniofacial Skeleton.* New York: Harper and Row.

Enlow, D. H. and Moyers, R. E. (1971), "Growth and Architecture of the Face," *J. Amer. dent. Ass.*, **82**, 763.

Enlow, D. H., Kuroda, T. and Lewis, A. B. (1971a), "The Morphological and Morphogenetic Basis for Craniofacial Form and Pattern," *Angle Orthodont.*, **41**, 161.

Enlow, D. H., Kuroda, T. and Lewis, A. B. (1971b), "Intrinsic Craniofacial Compensations," *Angle Orthodont.*, **41**, 271.

Enlow, D. H. and McNamara, J. (1973a), "The Neurocranial Basis for Facial Form and Pattern," *Angle Orthodont.*, **43**, 256.

Enlow, D. H. (1973b), "Growth and the Problem of the Local Control Mechanism," *Amer. J. Anat.*, **136**, 403.

Enlow, D. H. (1973c), "Alveolar Bone," in *International Prosthodontic Workshop on Complete Denture Occlusion*, Chap. 1 (C. C. Kelsey and B. R. Lang, Eds.). The University of Michigan School of Dentistry.

Moss, M. L. and Greenberg, S. N. (1967), "Functional Analysis of the Human Maxillary Bone. I. Basal Bone," *Angle Orthodont.*, **37**, 151.

Moss, M. L. (1968), "Functional Cranial Analysis of Mammalian Mandibular Morphology," *Acta anat.*, **71**, 423.

Moss, M. L. and Salentijn, L. (1969), "The Capsular Matrix," *Amer. J. Orthodont.*, **56**, 474.

Scott, J. H. (1959), "Further Studies on the Growth of the Human Face," *Proc. roy. Soc. Med.*, **52**, 263.

4. DISTURBANCES OF PRENATAL GROWTH AND DEVELOPMENT

D. E. POSWILLO

Causal agents and mechanisms

Cleft lip

Cleft palate

Other anomalies of the craniofacial complex
First and second branchial arch anomalies

The cause, the course, and the consequence

Anomalous development of the cranio-facial complex has been described and discussed in the literature for centuries. In the past, the principal concern was with the surgical and prosthetic reconstruction of congenital defects. More recently, the problem of anomalous development has been accepted as a challenge on the biological as well as the therapeutic front. The problems of treatment have been investigated from all sides by many related disciplines; opportunity for research into fundamental causes of facial deformity has opened up new possibilities. The stage has not yet been reached where the pathogenesis of these anomalies is clear, and the causative factors understood. Nonetheless, considerable progress has been made in unravelling many of the complex factors involved in the origins of abnormal cranio-facial morphology.

In the light of present knowledge it seems probable that while the causal agents which initiate cranio-facial deformity may number hundreds, and be both genetic and/or environmental in origin, the causal mechanisms involved may be very few. Thus the identification of mechanisms of malformation may provide clues to the character of the initiating agents, and assist predictability in the screening of environmental teratogens. Such advances could have far-reaching consequences in the prevention of deformity.

It is not easy to define a mechanism of teratogenesis. This is in part due to limited knowledge of the causal mechanisms of malformation in man, and in part due to the possible overlap between initiating mechanisms and secondary mechanisms, all of which may play a part in dysmorphogenesis (fig. 1). A causal mechanism of malformation can best be defined as a derangement of the tissues, cells, or cellular components resulting from the action of a teratogenic agent and producing a deviation from the normal pattern of development. Despite a great deal of research into the effects of teratogenic agents on morphogenesis, there are as yet few established mechanisms known to pro-

attempts are made to progress from the level of morphology to levels of cytophysiology and histochemistry the problems of reconstruction of the sequence of normal development become even more complex.

In the absence of sufficient human embryonic material for the study of normal and abnormal embryogenesis considerable information may be obtained by investigation of appropriate animal models. Cranio-facial anomalies arise spontaneously in many species of animals; they may also be induced by known human teratogens in others. When a reliable animal model of malformation has been established, considerable information may be obtained on the

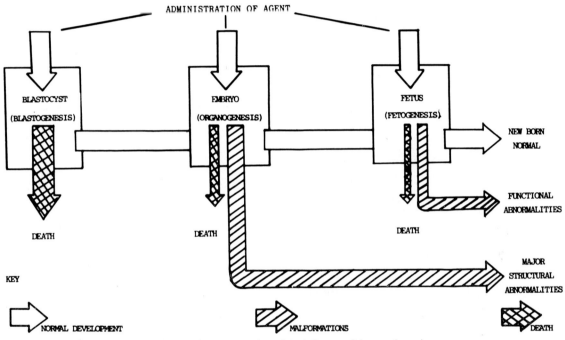

FIG. 1. Schematic representation of the influence of dysmorphogenic agents on the various stages of prenatal development.

duce cranio-facial anomalies in man. The probable mechanisms include:

(a) mutation;
(b) chromosomal aberrations;
(c) mitotic inhibition and cell death;
(d) deviations from normal nucleic acid synthesis and function;
(e) mechanical factors;
(f) embryonic haemorrhage; and
(g) viral infections.

Normal morphogenesis of the oro-facial tissues involves complex step-by-step sequences of migration of cells, and interaction between cell groups. Only by the systematic study of human embryonic specimens obtained at short intervals over the period extending from day 25 to day 45 of development can the sequential development of the face be reconstructed. Unfortunately, this volume of material has not yet become available; even if it were to, serial sampling of multiple embryos enables at best only static reconstructions of a fluid and dynamic process. When

causal mechanisms of dysmorphogenesis. In the succeeding sections of this chapter attention will be paid to the more common anomalies of the cranio-facial complex, and the clinical and experimental findings which suggest their mode of genesis.

CLEFT LIP

Cleft lip, with or without cleft palate, is a relatively common malformation (fig. 2); it occurs most frequently in the Mongoloid race and least frequently in Negroes. In Caucasians, it occurs once in 750 live births. More males than females are affected and the cleft may be complete or incomplete. When the cleft involves only one side of the lip, it is found more frequently on the left than the right. No significant relationship between maternal age and cleft lip and palate has been found. While many investigators have attempted to identify a genetic basis for cleft lip and palate, there is widespread agreement that only 20–30 per cent of all cases show a positive hereditary basis. Even in these cases there is no general agreement on how the phenotype is inherited. The polygenic inheritance hypothesis is the most useful, and it is easier to understand the contribution of environmental factors when cleft lip and palate is considered as a threshold phenomenon resulting from a variety of responses in the developing embryo.

While human embryonic specimens of cleft lip and palate are rare, spontaneous clefts of the lip and palate occur in about 10 per cent of offspring of the A/Strong mouse. These clefts show many of the features observed in the human embryo (fig. 2) and it is likely that a similar mechanism of malformation exists in the two species. Serial studies of the development of cleft lip, by comparison with normal lip

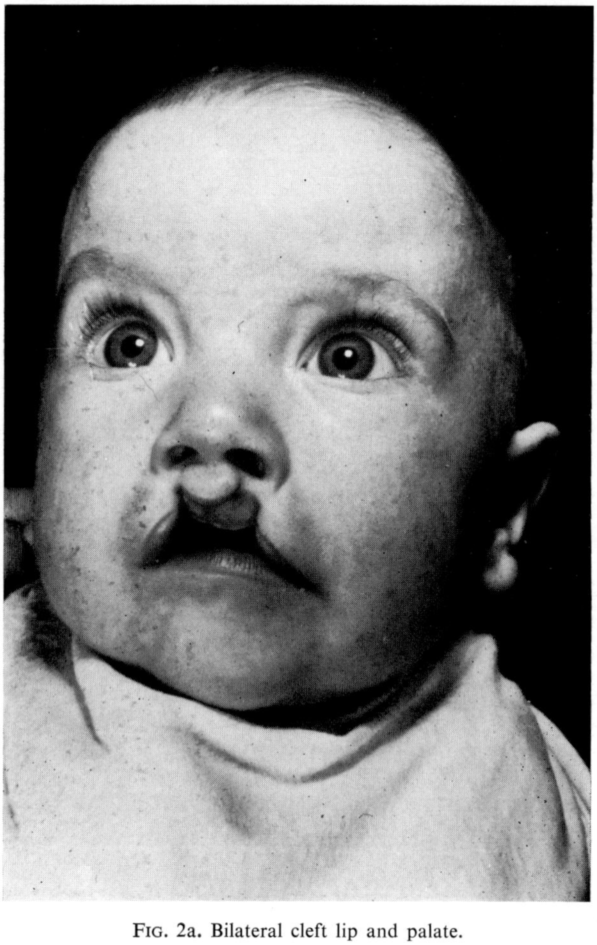

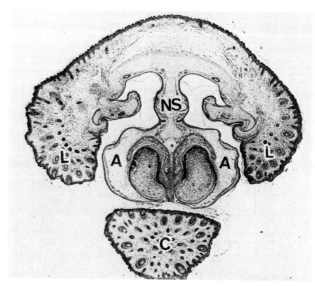

FIG. 2a. Bilateral cleft lip and palate.

morphogenesis, reveal that in the A/Strong mouse there are probably two factors involved. The first of these operates after the flow of neural crest mesenchyme has spread from the lateral nasal and maxillary prominences to the median nasal prominence, thus producing an isthmus of mesoderm in the site of the future lip and premaxilla. Indenting the isthmus from below is the nasal fin of epithelial cells which is soon to be removed by programmed cell death and resorption. The autolysis and disappearance of the epithelial fin, and the coalescence and expansion of the mesenchymal masses finally establishes the morphology of the lip and primary palate.

The critical stage of development for complete formation

of the lip comes at that period when the lateral nasal process and the median nasal process move against each other and coalesce. Animal experiments have shown that two mechanisms of maldevelopment may arise at this stage and initiate cleft lip. It has been shown that the administration of salicylates to pregnant mice prior to the stage of fusion reduces the appositional pressure of one process upon the other. The area of contact is thus insufficient for complete coalescence to take place and cleft lip may result. Where the anatomical configuration of the median nasal process

FIG. 2b. Frontal section through maxilla and mandible of A/Strong mouse with bilateral cleft lip and palate. NS—Nasal septum, L—Lip, A—Alveolus, C—Chin.

is such that the juxtaposition of the coalescing processes is angular rather than linear, i.e. in a "pointed" as opposed to a "flat" face, the predisposition to cleft lip is higher. In the A/Strong strain mouse the median nasal process is ventral to the lateral nasal process and the susceptibility to salicylate-induced cleft lip is enhanced. In the C57 B1 strain, which has a flat broad face, the resistance to induced cleft lip is high. The hypothesis that susceptibility to cleft lip may be related to the shape of the embryonic face, and consequently the adult face, was tested by measuring the facial shape in cleft and non-cleft families. The results supported the hypothesis that parents of children with cleft lip, with or without cleft palate, appear to have facial dimensions which differ from those of the general population.

The secondary mechanism by which cleft lip may arise at the time of coalescence of the facial processes is related to premature and excessive autolysis of the epithelial fin. The administration of the antimetabolite Hadacidin has been found to affect the onset of autolysis and phagocytosis of the epithelial fin and the neighbouring mesenchyme. By premature autolysis and an intensification of the normal process of programmed cell death, local mesenchyme is destroyed. The lip fusion which does take place is either materially reduced in size, with partial clefting, or so small that the processes split apart again under the influence of growth. This leads to a complete cleft which may extend into the nose and the alveolus. The median nasal process, thus freed from its lateral support, grows at a rate which increases the separation of the parts. This becomes particularly apparent in the condition of bilateral cleft lip where the premaxillary segment may protrude some distance beyond the lateral alveolar margins.

When it is appreciated that the lip and primary palate are formed by a series of morphogenetic movements and concurrent cellular phenomena, all closely interdependent in time and space, it is not difficult to envisage the "threshold" nature of the phenomenon of cleft lip. In a heterogeneous population affected by both protective and noxious agents the variations in susceptibility to malformation appear as a continuously distributed series of values. Close to the threshold will be found those individuals who fall short of gross deformity and who exhibit only microforms of cleft lip such as irregularities of the alar base and the lateral incisor tooth; at a distance beyond the threshold exist those with complete bilateral cleft of the lip and palate.

The frequent association of cleft palate with the cleft lip anomaly has been investigated by many workers. As has already been described, animal embryos susceptible to cleft lip have a large median nasal process. It has been shown that in such circumstances, at the commencement of palatal shelf closure, the tongue does not move forward between the lips as is usually the case. Instead, the tip of the tongue remains pressed against the median process and arches up into the nasal cavity between the palatal shelves. Thus movement of the shelf or shelves towards the midline is impeded. Therefore, in an embryo with cleft lip it is likely that cleft palate results because movement of the shelves from vertical to horizontal is delayed by the intervening tongue. If eventually the shelves do become horizontal it is unlikely that they will meet each other, or the nasal septum, so that fusion will fail to take place.

Although median cleft of the upper lip occurs naturally in rodents and lagomorphs, i.e. "hare-lip", this cleft is exceedingly rare in man. When it does arise it may involve either the upper or lower lip and may vary in degree from a notch in the vermilion border to a full thickness cleft. In man the incidence of median cleft is reported to be 4:1,000 of all types of cleft. True median clefts of the upper lip are occasionally found in association with other median clefts of the face, e.g. bifid nose, and with orbital hypertelorism. The pathogenesis of median cleft is unresolved. It is probable that these clefts represent persistence in the upper lip of the paired primordia of the median nasal processes which have failed to form a single globular process; developmental arrest may account for this failure to merge. In the lower lip the cleft probably results from failure of fusion of the paired mandibular processes in the midline, a developmental stage found at about 6 weeks in the normal embryo.

Oblique facial clefts are the most uncommon. The line of these clefts extends from the upper lip through or near the ala of the nose to the lower border of the eye. Again the pathogenesis is unclear. Because they are often accompanied by coloboma of the eyelid it has been suggested that the cause may be absence of a specific portion of embryonal mesoderm in the naso-optic groove. Some support has been produced for the suggestion that such clefts may arise from mechanical factors caused by the fetus swallowing the free end of a strip of amnion. When this happens the attached end remains fixed to the fetal sac and the free end stays in the fetal pharynx; the intermediate portion of this band then ulcerates obliquely through the tissues of the lip and cheek.

Transverse facial clefts of the mouth result in macrostomia. These clefts may be unilateral or bilateral, but rarely extend beyond the anterior border of the masseter muscle. True macrostomia is very rare, and should not be confused with pseudo-macrostomia which occasionally accompanies either cranio-facial or otomandibular dysostosis.

A syndrome consisting of bilateral pits of the lip in association with cleft lip and/or cleft palate has been reported frequently in the literature. There appears to be neither sex limitation nor sex linkage in this condition of variable expression. The relationship between the lip pits and facial clefts may be temporal, rather than causal. It is probable that during the early development of the lip the lateral sulci fail to merge, leading to persistent furrows which eventually shrink into blind tubes or pits.

While cleft lip, with or without cleft palate, has so far been discussed as a single developmental problem it is not always so. It has been shown that facial clefts are associated with at least one other malformation in about 8 per cent of cases. In about one-third of the multiple anomaly cases, clubfoot is associated with facial clefts. Polydactyly appears to be more commonly associated with cleft lip and palate than with either of these anomalies alone. There is a plethora of malformation syndromes, documented in detail by Gorlin (1971), in which the facial cleft is just one feature of a characteristic syndrome. A significant feature of these syndromes is that they may exhibit either cleft lip or cleft palate, or both in combination, but with one exception (Van der Woude's lip pit syndrome) separate defects of lip and palate never occur in the same subject. The relationship between facial clefts and other anomalies in these syndromes is probably temporal. Where a teratogenic influence is operating over a reasonably long period of time many developing systems come to be affected; palate closure, being near the end of the first trimester, is very likely to be affected by a long-acting dysmorphogenic process which has already left its mark on other parts.

CLEFT PALATE

Clefts of the posterior palate (fig. 3) may be classified into two principal groups. In one there are those clefts, both unilateral and bilateral, which accompany cleft lip. In the other are the solitary clefts of the secondary palate. Clinically, these two groups may easily be distinguished, and most authors agree that they are distinct entities. Differences in incidence, sex predisposition, and prevalence of associated anomalies all support this division into cleft lip and palate and isolated cleft palate.

The prevalence figures for isolated cleft palate are lower than those for cleft lip and palate, but the ratio of racial incidence is much the same. In Caucasians it occurs once in 3,000 live births; in Negroes it is 1:5,000 and in Japanese,

1:2,000. Cleft uvula is about ten times more prevalent than cleft lip and palate. An excess of females over males in the ratio of 60:40 exists in isolated cleft palate. Associated congenital anomalies occur twice as often with isolated cleft palate as with combined lip and palate clefts. Micrognathia has a very high association with isolated cleft palate

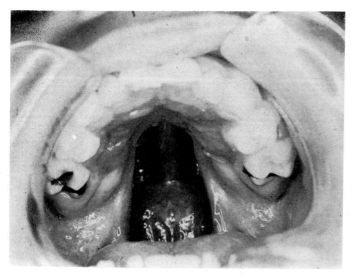

FIG. 3a. Isolated cleft of the posterior palate.

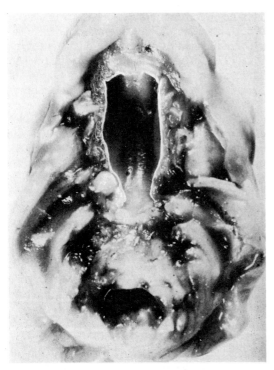

FIG. 3b. Cleft palate induced in the rat by steroids, to produce a model for the study of failure of palatal shelf closure. (Margins of palatal shelves retouched).

due in part to the simultaneous occurrence of the two anomalies in the Pierre Robin syndrome.

Normal palate fusion involves synchronized interaction between growth and convergence of the palatal processes,

tongue withdrawal and muscular activity, mandibular growth, changes in cranial base and cranial flexure, and steady increases in the width of the developing head. It can be postulated that any significant interference with these time-specific interactions could lead to incomplete fusion of the palatal shelves, both with each other and with the nasal septum. In addition, changes affecting the fusion and subsequent breakdown of the epithelial seam between the shelves could induce malformation. Shelves which merge and fuse could be later disrupted, either by abnormal mechanical pressures or by growth traction if mesodermal bridging is incomplete. Such phenomena could lead to palatal fistula, submucous clefts, or even complete rupture of the palate. One can hypothesize, therefore, that cleft palate may arise from one or more of the following causes:

(a) interference with the forces which elevate the vertical shelves into a horizontal position;
(b) excessively small palatal shelves and/or an excessively wide inter-shelf distance;
(c) tongue obstruction preventing shelf contact;
(d) failure of epithelial fusion and/or breakdown;
(e) failure of mesodermal penetration; and
(f) post-fusion rupture.

When first proposed, the existence of an intrinsic shelf force was ascribed to the presence of elastic fibres within

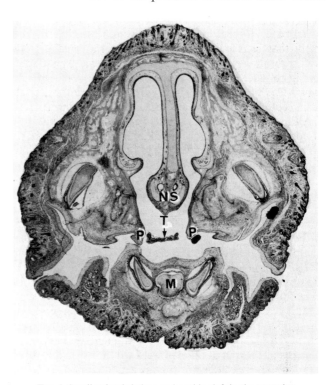

FIG. 4. Small palatal shelves and a wide cleft in the posterior palate are seen in this frontal section of a marmoset with isolated cleft palate induced by X-irradiation. The top of the tongue (T) sits between the shelf margins (P). NS—Nasal septum. M—Mandible.

the shelf mesoderm, and later elevation of the shelf was attributed to hydration of mucopolysaccharides. It seems likely that the force originates from a combination of the expanding fibrillar mesoderm and increased mitotic activity along the lower margin of the shelf, especially since increasing mitotic activity has been shown to contribute to the rise in tension of the shelf tissues. It has also been proposed that a gradual decrease in the angulation of the cranial base could provide the "internal shelf force", and work on cortisone-induced oligohydramnios further supports the hypothesis that factors which interfere with extension and elongation of the cranial base could be responsible for cleft palate. In a multi-factorial system such as palate closure it is likely that interference with the cranial base, be it

withdrawal followed by tongue pressure on the aligning shelves plays an essential role in closure of the palate. Complete tongue obstruction over a time-specific period can produce 100 per cent cleft palate in rodents, accompanied by a high proportion of moulding defects of the Pierre Robin type when induced by amniocentesis (fig. 5). (Poswillo, 1966.)

It has been shown that glucocorticoids produce oligohydramnios in mice, with postural-type defects of the palate caused by interference with angulation of the cranial base and subsequent tongue withdrawal. The role of corticosteroids in the induction of cleft palate is still not clear. Some

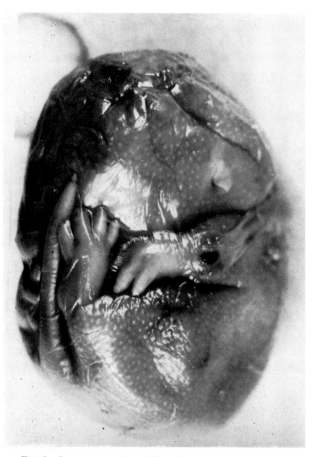

FIG. 5a. Severe postural moulding (chin-chest compression) of rat fetus (with cleft palate) induced by aminocentesis.

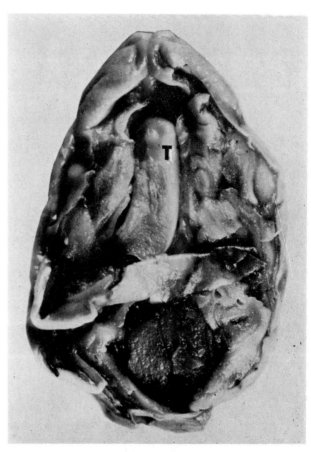

FIG. 5b. Plan view of tongue and palate (mandible removed) of fetus seen in Fig. 5a. Note that the tongue (T) remains impacted in the wide cleft in the posterior palate.

mechanical or biochemical (*i.e.* by alteration in the mucopolysaccharides) will contribute to failure of palate closure.

Small palatal shelves may also contribute to palatal clefting; X-irradiation produces reduced mitotic activity and small palatal shelves in both rodents and primates (fig. 4). Other teratogens, including glucocorticoids, have been shown to do likewise. Mesenchymal deficiency, however it may arise, will obviously affect the developing palatal shelf mechanism with consequences leading towards malformation.

The role of the tongue in palate closure is still a matter for debate. Demonstrations in rodents suggest that tongue

believe that their teratogenicity is related to their myopathic effects and the resulting redirection in tongue activity. Others, however, could not produce cleft palate in mice by the administration of muscle relaxants and suggested that the effects of the corticosteroids are more likely to be related to the induced "stress" situation. It has often been demonstrated that pregnant mice exposed to starvation, noise, cold, or transportation near the critical time for palate closure will have a high incidence of cleft palate in their offspring.

Disturbances of fusion have been held responsible for

cleft palate. *In vitro* studies suggest that an area of programmed cell death produces breakdown of the medial

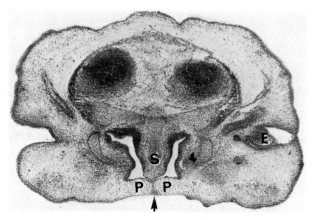

FIG. 6. The epithelial seam (arrowed) a potential site for postfusion rupture, seen in the mouse fetus soon after initial palate closure. P—Palatal process. S—Septum. E—Eye.

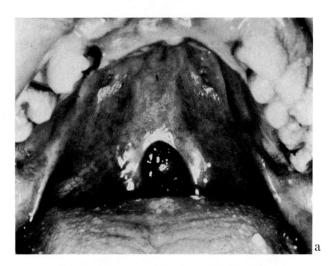

FIG. 7a. Submucous cleft palate with bifid uvula.

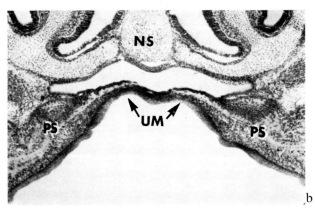

FIG. 7b. Induced submucous cleft palate in the mouse, showing tenuous soft tissue bridge of unsupported mucosa (UM), between the palatal shelves (PS). NS—Nasal septum.

edges of the palatal shelves prior to contact, and it has been suggested that altered epithelial degeneration and/or desquamation of the shelf margins may prevent epithelial

adhesion or promote early rupture of the epithelial seam (fig. 6).

Submucous cleft palate, in association with bifid uvula (fig. 7a and b) is likely to be a microform of posterior cleft palate. In animal experiments a delay in the centripetal flow of palatal shelf ossification, of increasing magnitude from before backwards, leaves an unreinforced palatal vault which is prone to rupture under growth traction or tongue pressures. The absence of bony reinforcement across the midline of the vault, combined with a deficient osseous inductive force in the midline of the palate, contributes to the failure of the velar mesenchyme to merge and elongate. Thus bifid uvula, either alone or combined with submucous cleft palate, may result from disturbances in the processes of ossification and merging which take place between the 7th and 10th weeks of human development.

OTHER ANOMALIES OF THE CRANIO-FACIAL COMPLEX

Many and diverse are the cranio-facial anomalies reported to affect structures beyond the lip and palate. Gross defects

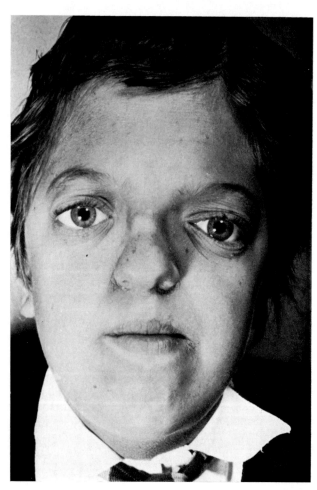

FIG. 8. Characteristic facies observed in Crouzon's syndrome.

of cranial development such as acrania, anencephaly and cranioschisis (major cranial osseous defects) are usually incompatible with life. In many instances major monstrosities such as the cyclops fetus and holoprosencephaly have many systems affected, and their survival is limited to a few hours. Of the defects of the cranium consistent with survival, the most interesting are those in which the time of closure of the sutures has been disturbed. Interference with normal closure of the sutures may result in bizarre distortions of skull shape such as are found in Apert's and

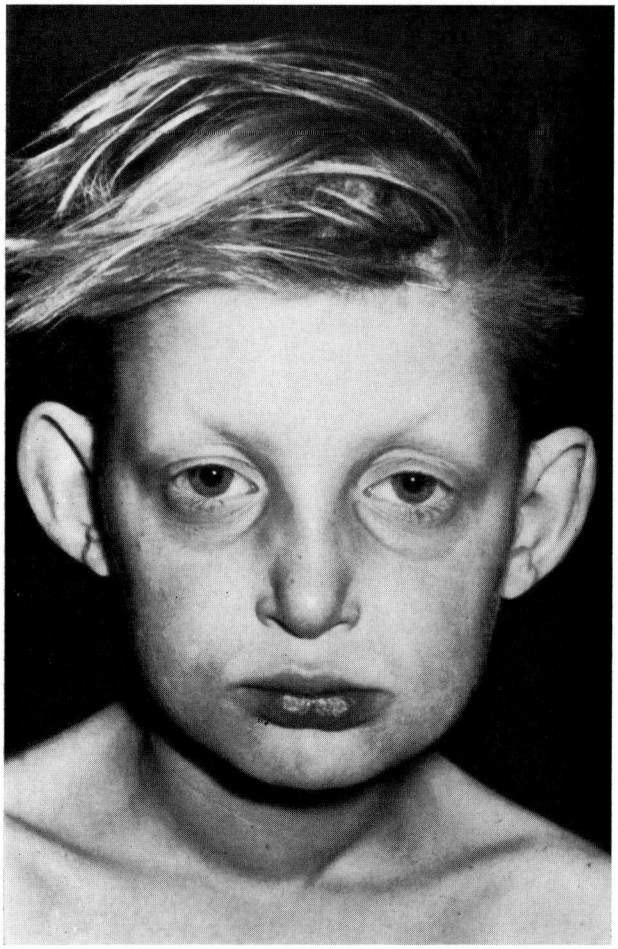

A broad high forehead, saddle nose, supravalvular stenosis and mental retardation are found associated in infants suffering from congenital cortical hyperostosis. There is evidence to suggest that excessive maternal intake of vitamin D may induce these anomalies.

Saddle nose, though rare in the congenital form, occasionally accompanies other congenital syndromes such as

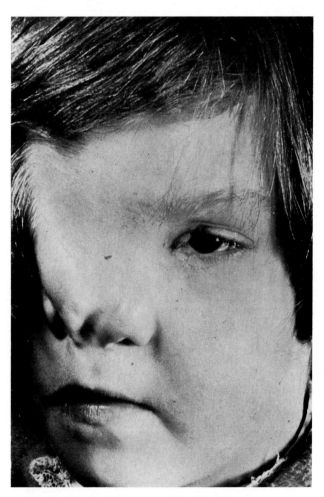

FIG. 10. Holoprosencephaly with bifid nose.

FIG. 9. Saddle nose and sparse facial hair seen in association with dental anomalies in the condition of anhidrotic ectodermal dysplasia.

Crouzon's syndromes. In both these conditions premature fusion of the coronal, sagittal and lambdoid sutures occurs. The result of early synostosis is a peaking of the vault of the skull producing such variations as oxycephaly, acrocephaly or turricephaly. These anomalies worsen as growth continues, and the development of the orbit and mid-face is severely affected (fig. 8). Recent studies suggest that the creation of an artifical pericoronal suture in the first year of life prevents the development of these cranial deformities.

Delayed mid-line ossification of the frontal and sagittal sutures, with an open anterior fontanelle, is a common occurrence in such congenital anomalies as cleido-cranial dysostosis, cretinism and Down's syndrome. The delay results in a brachycephalic skull characterized by hypertelorism, a broad forehead, and a "dish-face" maxilla.

anhidrotic ectodermal dysplasia (fig. 9) and Down's syndrome. In both instances the nasal bones may be deficient or absent.

Errors of commission, as opposed to errors of omission, are even more rare in the formation of the face. The gross anomalies of bifid nose and holoprosencephaly (fig. 10) are seen occasionally, and probably represent disorganization of the programme of cell death which shapes and reduces the triangular area of the primitive forebrain in the early stages of morphodifferentiation.

First and Second Branchial Arch Anomalies

Anomalies affecting structures derived from the first and second branchial arches have attracted the attention of both artists and clinicians from very early days in man's history.

There are beautiful carvings of heads showing both symmetrical and asymmetrical anomalies of the first and second branchial arches in the terracottas found in the remains of pre-Columbian cultures prior to 3,000 B.C.

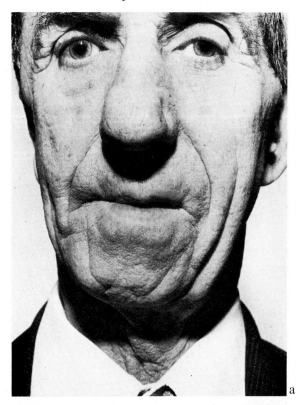

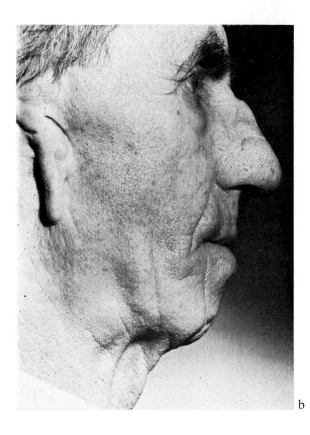

Anomalies of the first and second branchial arches have been classified into those that are usually unilateral (hemifacial microsomia and Goldenhar's syndrome) and those that are usually bilateral (mandibulo-facial dysostosis, and the Hallerman-Streif syndrome). Studies into the pathogenesis of these syndromes have shown that they can be categorized further into asymmetrical anomalies which comprise the predominantly unilateral group, and the symmetrical anomalies which are entirely bilateral in expression.

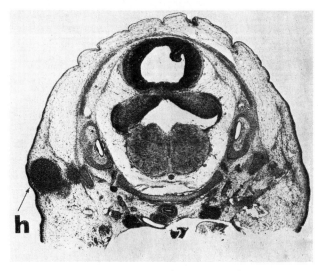

FIG. 11. Full face (a) and affected side (b) in the first and second branchial arch syndrome. The focal haematoma (h) believed to be responsible for this anomaly is seen in the frontal section (above) of an animal model in which the malformation had been induced by a folic acid antagonist.

Hemifacial microsomia (1st and 2nd arch syndrome) and Goldenhar's syndrome are characterized by asymmetrical anomalies of the pinna and middle ear, deficiencies in the malar and squamous temporal bones, and ramus of the mandible, facial paresis, and pseudomacrostomia (fig. 11). Prior to the introduction of thalidomide these anomalies occurred spontaneously, without a familial history, at the rate of 1:3,000 births. One feature of the thalidomide embryopathy was the high incidence of cases of induced otomandibular dysostosis which closely resembled hemifacial microsomia. Before thalidomide it had been proposed that the anomalies of the first and second branchial arches resulted from the absence or anomalous development of the stapedial artery about the 6th week of embryonic life. Recently, the study of animal models of both hemifacial microsomia and thalidomide otomandibular dysostosis have shown that while faulty development of the stapedial arterial stem was not the initiating factor in these disorders, a locally destructive haematoma did arise from the anastomosis of those developing vessels which initiated the stapedial arterial stem. The displacement and destruction of local mesenchyme by this expanding haematoma caused delays in differentiation of first and second branchial arch structures and the neighbouring squamous temporal bone which lead to the asymmetrical anomalies found in the first and second arch disorders. The comparability of the gross anomalies, in rodents, non-human primates, and in man provides strong evidence to support this hypothesis of a common causal mechanism of malformation.

The Treacher Collins syndrome (fig. 12), while variable in expression, is invariably symmetrical insofar as the human face is ever symmetrical. There is a family history in about 50 per cent of affected cases and the mode of transmission is autosomal dominant. In the remaining 50 per cent of cases the cause is not found. The familial incidence has been

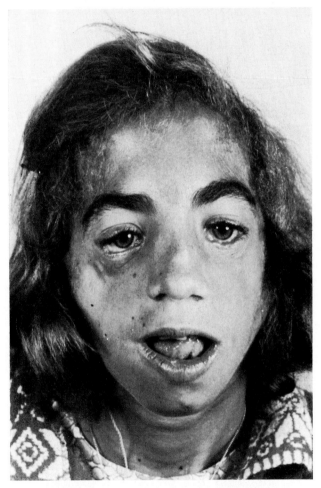

FIG. 12. Characteristic facies of Treacher Collins syndrome.

known for a long time; even in the pre-Columbian terracottas there is a collection of carvings representing a family group affected by Treacher Collins anomalies. The principal features of the condition are the antimongoloid obliquity of the palpebral fissures, notched lower eyelids with colobomata at the junction of the outer and middle thirds, hypoplasia of the malar bones and mandibular rami, concavity of the lower border of the mandible, deformity or displacement of the external ear, or anotia, and middle-ear defects. Occasionally cleft palate is also found. There are usually anomalies of the teeth, and malocclusion.

The genetically programmed nature of the disorder and the symmetry of the facial anomalies, despite the variability found between individual cases, suggested that the pathogenesis differed materially from that of the hemifacial

microsomia-like anomalies. Studies on the effect of vitamin A and cortisone on the development of the cranio-facial complex revealed that symmetrical anomalies of the facial bones were induced. The bones affected were the malars and ramus of mandible, and the palate was cleft. The anomalies resembled those seen in symmetrical malformations of the cranio-facial complex in man. Further descriptions of the effect of vitamin A on endoderm during early rat embryogenesis and the subsequent reduction in size of the sub-cephalic pocket into which the branchial arches develop (fig. 13) prompted further study of the vitamin A-cortisone dosed animal system for elucidation of the pathogenesis of Treacher Collins anomalies. It now seems that the symmetrical anomalies of the Treacher Collins syndrome may be related to disturbances in distribution of neural crest-derived mesenchyme.

Early mechanical interference with the downward and forward development of the branchial arches results from the failure of development of the customary sub-cephalic pouch. It is probable that in the syndrome found in man, this subcephalic space fails to develop because of genetically programmed interference with the extension of the cranial flexure responsible for lifting the embryonic head off the foregut; this results in mechanical compression of the expanding first branchial arch. Consequently, there is abnormal invagination of the neighbouring otic placodes into first rather than second arch territory. The migrating neural crest cells are disorganized by the aberrant forerunner of the otic structures. Neural crest cells destined to provide mesenchyme for the expansion of the malar arches and mandibular structures, lower eyelids, and palate are syphoned away, as it were, into the neighbourhood of other branchial arches and are redistributed in a haphazard fashion. Thus the normal synchrony of differentiation is disturbed, and hypoplasia of the facial bones and deficiencies of the soft tissues occur in a symmetrical fashion to produce the characteristic Treacher Collins facies.

THE CAUSE, THE COURSE, AND THE CONSEQUENCES

There exists, in normal embryogenesis of the craniofacial region, a continuum of development that requires the synchronous and appropriate interaction between cellular and inductive processes in time and space for subsequent normal development of succeeding and neighbouring parts. When developmental processes get out of step in the morphogenesis of the face, whatever the causal agent, a mechanism of malformation may be initiated that can proceed inexorably to dysmorphism.

Disturbances of morphogenesis arising from either environmental or genetic factors, or both, are, to all intents and purposes, irreversible. Some evidence exists that a degree of embryological "catchup" can take place after an embryological accident such as focal haematoma formation, or postural deformation. Changes in the DNA, RNA, and protein content of teratogen-affected tissues may be induced, but the capacity for recovery is limited. Such responses, however, in both early and late pregnancy, draw attention to the danger of attributing undue significance to

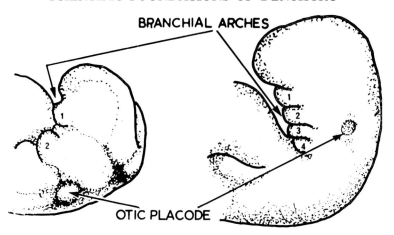

FIG. 13a. The elevation of the head off the foregut which accompanies the induction of the otic placode. This creates the subcephalic pouch into which the first and second branchial arches extend during the formation of the face.

post-natally observed changes in malformed tissues and organs as indicators of pathogenesis. The finite, observed defect represents the effects of both teratogenic insult and repair. Thus morphogenesis and development should not be regarded as rigid programmes executed in a series of

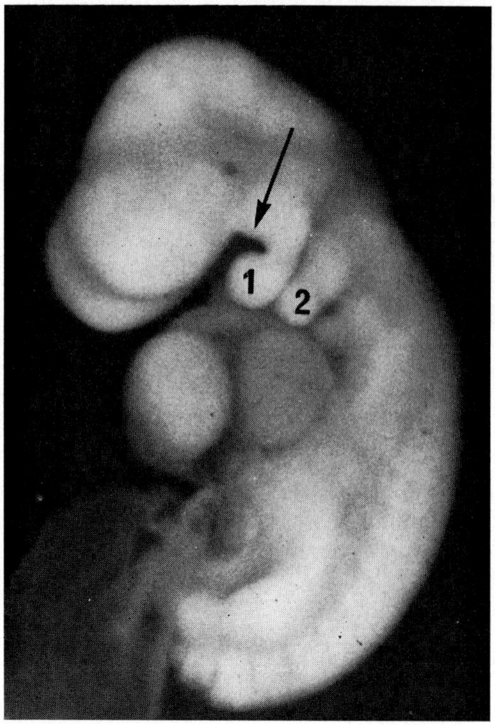

interval exists between the embryonic accident and the spontaneous shut-down of morphogenetic processes at the end of the first trimester. Notwithstanding all the provisos, the cranio-facial anomaly seen at birth has probably been modified considerably from that anomaly which existed at about the 12th week of intra-uterine life.

FIG. 13b. Normal sub-cephalic pouch (arrowed) in early embryogenesis.

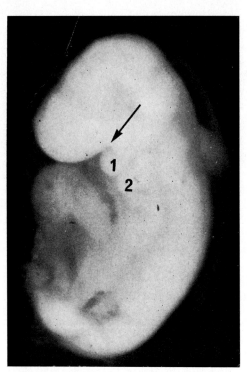

FIG. 13c. Deficient sub-cephalic space (arrowed) in animal model of the Treacher Collins syndrome.

rigorously controlled steps, but rather as continuously modulated processes.

For a substantial degree of tissue or organ "catchup" to be achieved, the appropriate inductive forces would need to be acting in sufficient degree and direction to overcome all the handicaps of delayed morphogenesis; this is unlikely to be achieved in any instance where a relatively short

In a disorganized anatomical system the patterns of growth and development are unlikely to follow normal parameters. There has been considerable speculation on the changes which take place in the bilateral cleft of lip and palate during the second and third trimesters of intra-uterine development. While it has been suggested that overgrowth of the premaxillary "snout" is caused by lack of restraint from intact oral sphincters during ante-natal growth, there has been no conclusive evidence presented to support this. It seems unlikely that, in the absence of adequate primate material, this question can be resolved directly. As long as the role of the nasal septum in the growth of the mid-face remains unresolved, the hypothetical concept of "as they are cleft, so do they grow" will remain unproven. From an examination of both normal and malformed specimens, investigators have been unconvinced of the dominant role of the nasal septum. It is believed that the maxillae, even in the presence of a palatal cleft, exercise their inherent potential for postero-superior growth in such a way that the facial bones are displaced downwards and forwards in a normal manner.

Questions concerned with the effect of pre-natal growth and development on cranio-facial anomalies have more than academic importance. Improved methods of pre-natal diagnosis of deformity, particularly of the cranio-facial regions and limbs, suggest the possibility of pre-natal surgical repair of the more accessible defects. For such procedures to be of value, in the face of the obvious hazards of operating on the fetus *in utero*, the gains would need to be considerable. It has already been demonstrated that repair of skin and mucosal wounds, carried out *in utero*, leaves little or no trace of the operative procedure when examined at birth. If the influence of pre-natal growth on deformities of the oro-facial complex is such as to increase the degree of deformity, and scar-free ante-natal repair is feasible in humans, as it is in non-human primates, then the role of reconstructive surgery in the management of cranio-facial deformity may be revised in a dramatic fashion.

It is the responsibility of the scientist to explore, with the surgeon and physician, those new and expanding horizons in the fields of cranio-facial teratology that may lead to a reduction in human anguish and suffering. The aim of the basic scientist should differ but little from that of the clinician to achieve the objective first expressed in 1597 by Gaspare Tagliacozzi, "to restore, repair, or make whole those parts of the face which Nature has forgotten or Fortune has taken away; not so much that we may delight the eye, but that we may buoy up the spirit, and help the mind of the afflicted".

REFERENCES

Gorlin, R. J. (1971), "Facial Clefting and its Syndromes in Birth Defects XI," *Orofacial Structures*, **3**, 50.
Poswillo, D. E. (1961), *The Embryology of Cleft Palate*, p. 39. University of New Zealand.
Poswillo, D. E. (1966), "Foetal Posture and Causal Mechanisms of Deformity of Palate, Jaw and Limbs," *J. dent. Res.*, **45**, 584.
Poswillo, D. E. (1973a), "The Pathogenesis of the First and Second Branchial Arch Syndrome," *Oral Surgery, Oral Medicine, Oral Pathology*, **35**, 302.
Poswillo, D. E. (1973b), "The Pathogenesis of Submucous Cleft Palate," *Proceedings of Second International Conference on Cleft Palate*, p. 182. Copenhagen.
Poswillo, D. E. (1975), "The Pathogenesis of the Treacher Collins Syndrome," *British Journal of Oral Surgery*, **13**, 1.

5. DISTURBANCES OF POSTNATAL GROWTH AND DEVELOPMENT

J. R. E. MILLS

Modifications of the genotype
   The skeletal pattern
   The soft tissues

Abnormalities of the cellular processes
   Cartilaginous growth
   The sutures
   Surface deposition of bone

INTRODUCTION

The human head has evolved over many millions of years to fulfil five functions; that is, to contain the brain, ears, eyes, nose and teeth. The first two of these functions hardly concerns us in the present context. As a primate, man is an aberrant member of a predominantly tree-living group.

For life in the trees a sense of smell is of limited value, while vision, and particularly binocular vision, is of great value. As a result the snout is reduced, while the eyes are positioned so that they look forwards rather than sideways. The remainder of the face is made up of the jaws, whose sole purpose is to carry the teeth.

The upper and lower jaws are not very closely related to each other. The mandible articulates only with the squamous part of the temporal bone. The maxilla is only connected to this glenoid fossa via sutures with the intervening sphenoid bone. Nevertheless, in most animals, and in primitive man, the growth of these bones—not only the jaws themselves but also those in the base of the skull—is so accurately synchronized that the upper and lower teeth erupt into a position of perfect occlusion, with each cusp fitting neatly into its opposing groove or fossa, with little or no post-eruptive adjustment. This synchronization of growth continues as the individual matures, so that ideal occlusion is maintained with slight and usually predictable minor changes.

The actual mechanism of this growth involves deposition and resorption of bone, with the periosteum, the sutures and the cartilaginous growth centres all playing a part; but these histological changes seem to occur in response to the needs of the master plan.

Moreover, the erupted teeth are very labile in their positions. A gentle force is sufficient to cause them to move—a fact well known to those familiar with orthodontic treatment. It follows that in a normal mouth the teeth must lie in a position of balance between the adjacent structures, so that they remain stationary. These structures are in fact the soft tissues of the lips, cheeks and tongue.

It is, perhaps, surprising that this delicately balanced system functions so well, so often. When it goes wrong it may be for one of two reasons. Firstly the master plan—the genotype—may become modified, usually as a result of genetic factors. Secondly the cellular mechanisms necessary for the fulfilment of the genotype may be abnormal. While this may appear an over-simplification, it is proposed to consider the problem in this light.

MODIFICATIONS OF THE GENOTYPE

In primitive races of mankind normal dental occlusion is the rule, and malocclusion, if present, is usually mild. With the coming of civilization it becomes more common, rising to epidemic proportions in industrialized nations in the last couple of centuries.

There would seem to be three factors involved in this process. The first lies in the literal meaning of civilization itself; a tendency for populations to change from small rural communities, breeding within their own tribe or group, to come to live in towns and cities. This was suddenly much increased with the advent of the industrial revolution, and consequent massive migration of populations. This increase in the size of the gene pool greatly increases the chance of an individual inheriting "components" of the face and jaws which do not "match". This has been demonstrated in the experimental breeding of dogs.

The second factor arises from the greatly increased survival rate. In a primitive community the majority of babies do not live long enough to have children themselves. If they did so, the population would increase dramatically as, indeed, it did in the early years of the industrial revolution in England. In nature, an increased survival rate is accompanied by an increase in variation; "survival of the fittest" comes to include some of the less fit. In modern society, we have virtually eliminated natural selection, and even the most grotesque may survive and reproduce.

The third factor is more favourable. The organism has a strong natural tendency to be viable, and will make suitable compensations to do its best with the materials which the genes have provided. To quote a crude example, we see individuals in whom the mandible seems small relative to the maxilla, and the alveolar process may be narrow in the molar region, producing a cross-bite. Nevertheless,

intercondylar width is always equal to the width between the glenoid fossae, so that the mandible can function.

This type of abnormality must therefore be considered as an extreme variation of the normal, resulting from an enlargement of the gene pool from which the individual is produced. In sterner times the individual might not have survived, or would have had greater difficulty in attracting a mate, so that the less desirable genes would have been eliminated. Unfortunately, the processes of natural selection no longer operate in civilized man. The result may be due to a disproportion of the bony skeleton, the surrounding soft tissues or—all too often—an interaction of the two.

The Skeletal Pattern

The relationship and development of the components of the face have been studied mainly by the use of standardized cephalometric lateral skull radiographs, and knowledge of these matters is therefore much greater in the two dimensions which can be seen therein—the antero-posterior and vertical—than in the third, lateral dimension. Broadbent (1947) was the first to make use of lateral radiographs for this purpose, illustrating cases where superior and inferior protrusion of the teeth was apparently due to corresponding variations in the size of the lower law. Björk (1947) analysed the skulls of a large number of 12-year-old Swedish schoolboys, and also of a similar number of 20–21-year-old conscripts to the Swedish army. From these analyses, he prepared diagrams to represent the average skulls of individuals of these ages. He then used his average figures for comparison with individuals within the two groups who showed marked departures from the normal. He found that where a discrepancy in dental arch relationship existed, this frequently was associated with a discrepancy in jaw relationship. There were, however, many different ways in which an apparently similar discrepancy could be produced. For example, a protrusion of the upper incisors, with an Angle's Class II Division 1 malocclusion, could be the result of a large maxilla or a small mandible, as one might suspect. It could, and frequently was, the result of abnormalities at more distant sites. A long anterior base of skull would carry the maxilla too far forward. A long posterior base would similarly carry the temporomandibular joint, and hence the mandible, too far posteriorly. The same result would occur if the angle between the anterior and posterior parts of the skull base, where they meet at the sella turcica (the so-called "saddle angle") were unusually high. Even this is not a complete list of the possibilities, and, indeed, Björk stated that in the cases he studied it was never possible to select a single factor as responsible for the discrepancy. Sometimes, two or more factors reinforced each other, sometimes one factor would counteract the effect of another. Björk's findings have been confirmed, with minor modifications, by other authors.

The Soft Tissues

The bones do not grow up in isolation. It has been observed that the alveolar processes grow from the earliest stages in close proximity to the muscular tissue of the lips and tongue, and that these muscles are apparently capable of actively functioning as early as the third month of intra-uterine life. Vertical development of the alveolar process and the teeth, takes place within the influence of these muscles which, both during activity and in their normal resting posture, control the labiolingual position of the teeth and, to a lesser extent, of the alveolar bones supporting them. This may worsen a malocclusion, but frequently helps to compensate for a skeletal discrepancy. For example, in cases of mandibular prognathism the lower incisors lean lingually in an effort to meet the upper incisors;

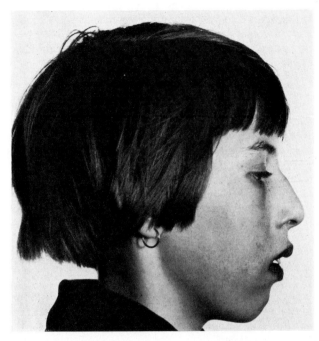

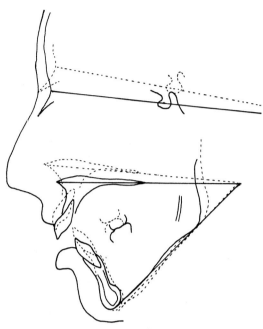

Fig. 1C.

FIG. 1. A. Profile photograph of 11 year old girl, showing unusual amount of vertical growth of upper jaw. B. Tracing of lateral skull radiograph of the same girl (solid outline), superimposed on Björk's diagram of average facial form (broken outline). C. Tracing as in B superimposed on tracing of same girl eight years later, using mandibular structures suggested by Björk (1969) as points of superimposition. D. Simulated tracing of same 11 year old girl with mandible in rest position, showing soft tissues.

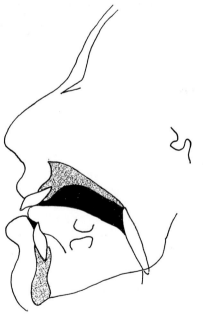

Fig. 1D.

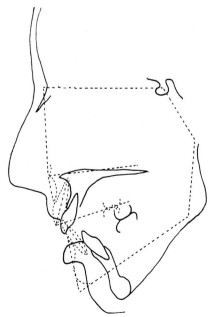

Fig. 1B.

although there is individual variation, they make, on average, an angle 10° lower with the lower border of the mandible than do those of a comparable control group.

Although scientific evidence is hard to produce, there can be little doubt that soft tissues can influence the positions of the teeth and alveolar processes. Their effect on the form of the more basal part of the bones is more problematical, although aspects of this will be considered later.

It is now proposed to illustrate these concepts with a consideration of two children who show gross skeletal discrepancies, associated with severe malocclusions.

The girl shown in fig. 1 was first seen at the age of 11 years. As will be seen from the photograph (fig. 1A), her upper incisors were protruding, and she had an anterior open bite. She had a long face, the lower part of her face being especially long, and she had a receding chin. He lips were apart at rest. In fig. 1B the tracing of a lateral skull radiograph of this girl has been superimposed on the "polygon" produced by Björk to represent the average facial shape for 12–year-old Swedish boys. There are obvious shortcomings in using the average shape of 12-year-old Swedish boys to assess an 11-year-old English girl, but the discrepancy from this source is slight compared with the discrepancy between this girl and the average. The abnormality would seem to arise from the fact that the face, and especially the lower face, has grown downwards to an excessive extent, with some posterior component, instead of the anterior growth component normally seen.

Figure 1C is a little more difficult to explain. In recent years Björk (1963, 1969, 1972) has carried out growth studies with the aid of metal implants in the skull. In particular, he has inserted a number of such implants into the mandibles of growing children. In most cases, these implants can be seen to remain in a constant relationship to each other, and it therefore seems reasonable to assume that they are remaining stationary in the bone—the alternative, that they are all migrating in the same direction at the same speed seems highly improbable. By superimposing tracings of lateral skull radiographs on the shadow of these implants, it is possible to see the effects of growth in literal terms of deposition and resorption of bone. In most cases, growth was regular, and much as would be expected. In a few cases it was very different from what might be expected. In particular, he found that when the tracings of two successive radiographs of the same individual were superimposed on the shadows of the implants in the mandible, the rest of the skull appeared to rotate relative to the mandible.

Björk (1969) went on to state that the same effect could be produced by superimposing the mandibles on certain natural structures, which his studies had shown to remain as stationary as the implants. Specifically, he mentioned the internal outline of the compact bone seen in the cross-section of the symphysis menti, the anterior point of the bony chin and the outline of the inferior dental canal below the molar teeth. Figure 1C has therefore, been constructed from the same tracing as that seen in fig. 1B, by superimposing it on these structures on the tracing of a radiograph of the same girl taken eight years later. It will be seen that the upper part of the skull appears to have rotated in a clockwise direction relative to the mandible. It is, of course, more logical and equally true to say that the mandible has rotated relative to the skull in an anticlockwise direction.

This further complicates the picture of the growth of this girl. It would now seem to show growth of the maxilla which is excessive in the vertical dimension. The growth

of the mandible is inadequate to keep pace with this, and therefore it hinges open about the condyles. This would tend to produce an anterior open bite and also a postnormal position of the tooth-bearing areas, as the mandible swings downwards and backwards. The natural tendency to compensate for abnormalities now enters the scene. The anterior teeth, failing to meet an antagonist, continued to develop towards each other, and reference to fig. 1B shows that the alveolar processes have, in fact, grown further from their respective bases than in Björk's average individual. Nevertheless, they have been unable to compensate completely, leaving her with an anterior open bite.

Figure 1D shows the same face, but with an attempt to show the mandible at rest, and with the surrounding soft tissues in place. It will be noticed first that the lips are apart at rest. This is a common clinical picture, sometimes incorrectly called "adenoid facies"—like most such individuals this girl breathed through her nose, and the adenoid tissue was apparently healthy. The upper and lower lips were inserted into their respective jaws in the usual positions, and were of normal length. Because of the skeletal discrepancies, the vertical and horizontal distances between these insertions were increased, and this made it impossible for her to hold her lips together comfortably. It is, however, essential that the anterior part of the mouth is efficiently sealed, to permit nasal respiration and to prevent drooling of saliva. In this case the anterior oral seal is produced by resting the tongue between the incisors, in contact with the lower lip. This tongue position will help to maintain the anterior open bite.

It will also be seen from fig. 1 that the lower incisors and indeed their supporting alveolus are proclined labially. This, again, is presumably a result of the soft-tissue balance, and is not uncommon in conjunction with a postnormal mandible. It is another example of natural, if inadequate compensation.

Moss, in numerous papers (see, e.g., 1968), has put forward a concept of the "functional matrix". He believes that the jaws and teeth develop, as do many structures around a matrix, and that in this case the matrix is provided by their function. He states that "there are no genes for bones". It is difficult to accept this hypothesis in full, but this principle of the "functional matrix" explains the way in which the individual compensates for inherent discrepancies. (See also Chapter 3.)

Figure 2 illustrates another extreme variant which is in some ways the opposite of the previous case. The records refer to a boy, first seen at the age of 10 years. The superimposition on Björk's diagram for 12-year-old Swedish boys shows a marked discrepancy from both this average and from the previous case. The growth of the posterior face was reasonably normal, but the anterior ends of both jaws were lacking in both anterior and vertical growth. The lack of anterior growth, not surprisingly, was associated with extreme crowding of the dentition, the only feature which he had in common with the girl. Measurement of the vertical distance from the tip of the upper incisor to the floor of the nose, and similarly from the tip of the lower incisor to the lower border of the mandible, shows these distances to be less than in the average face. The very deep overbite occurred in spite of this, and was primarily due to the very shallow facial height.

Figure 2B shows the same tracing superimposed on one of a radiograph taken seven years later, as suggested by Björk (1969). Here, again, an apparent rotation of the skull relative to the mandible is seen, but in the direction

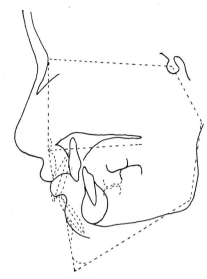

FIG. 2. Tracings of lateral skull radiographs of 10 year old boy, showing minimal vertical growth of face. A. Superimposed on Björk's average diagram of facial form (broken outline). B. Superimposed on tracing of radiograph of same boy taken seven years later, using mandibular points suggested by Björk (1969) for superimposition. C. Tracing of radiograph taken in rest position, showing soft tissues.

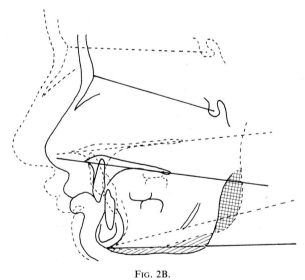

FIG. 2B.

opposite to that seen in the previous case. It is noticeable, however, that the outline of the mandible remained much the same, due to resorption of an area of bone at the lower border of the mandible, indicated by shading, and deposition in the cross-hatched area of the posterior side of the vertical ramus. The actual process of deposition and resorption again seems to have occurred as became necessary in order to produce and maintain the shape of the phenotype.

It has been found, from electromyographic studies, that muscular contraction in this type of case produces greater force than average, whereas in the type of case seen in fig. 1, where the rotation is in the opposite direction, muscular force is less than average. This, again, would seem to be an interaction between skeletal and soft tissues,

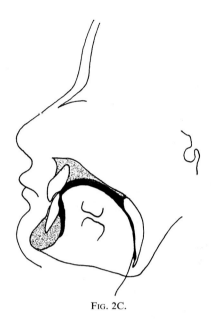

FIG. 2C.

and further investigations along these lines should add greatly to knowledge.

Figure 2C is a tracing of a radiograph taken in the rest position of the mandible, showing the surrounding soft tissues. In the true, endogenous rest position of the individual the mandible is lowered slightly by a hinge action at the temporomandibular joint, so as to produce a gap of 2–3 mm. between the molars. In the present case, the rest position was modified by displacing the mandible downwards and forwards, so as to bring the incisor teeth into a more acceptable relationship to each other, and to eliminate some of the overbite. Here again, the lips were probably normal in individual shape and size, but, because of the reduced lower facial height, their insertions were close together, causing them to appear unduly full, especially in the occlusal position (fig. 2A). This also had the effect of causing the lower lip-line to be high relative to the upper incisors. This high lip-line upset the balance between lips and tongue and caused the incisors to be retroclined lingually. In some cases, although not in this one, the lips appear hyperactive in facial expression, and this brings about further retroclination.

These two cases have been chosen as extreme examples to illustrate the ways in which the human face and jaws in industrialized communities depart from the genotype to produce appearances which at times border on the grotesque. This type of abnormality is the genetic result of the environment. The gene pool has increased due to the migration of populations, while improvements in the environment have virtually eliminated the beneficial effects of natural selection on human populations, so that all but the unfittest survive. Nevertheless, the "functional matrix" operates to "make the best of a bad job". The actual mechanisms of bone deposition and resorption are usually secondary to the need to produce a viable organism, and compensate for discrepancies, with variable success.

ABNORMALITIES OF THE CELLULAR PROCESSES

It would appear that the actual mechanics of growth are usually secondary to the genetically determined "master plan", and deposition and resorption of bone takes place as and when necessary to produce this. At times, however, these cellular mechanisms can go wrong, for a variety of reasons. Here again, the maximum possible compensation is usually seen, but even so the results are often considered as pathological.

It is not proposed to give a catalogue of the conditions where abnormal growth mechanisms are seen; these may be studied in standard text-books. It is proposed rather to describe the principles underlying these conditions, and to mention specific conditions merely as examples.

The bones of the skull grow through three mechanisms, any of which may be disturbed. They are cartilaginous growth, surface deposition of bone, and sutural growth, the last being a special type of surface growth.

Cartilaginous Growth

Growth in cartilage occurs in two main areas, the base of the skull, where the cartilage is the remnant of the cartilaginous precursor of the whole skull case, and the mandibular condyle. This latter is secondary cartilage, whose precise function in the growth of the mandible has recently been the subject of controversy. There can be little doubt that it plays an important part in mandibular growth, even if its importance has been exaggerated in the past.

Cartilaginous growth of the base of skull takes place in two synchondroses. That between the sphenoid and ethmoid bones ceases at about 7 years of age, while that between sphenoid and occipital remains patent throughout growth. Abnormalities are produced by a reduction or premature cessation of growth at these sites, producing an unusually short base of skull. The bones of the upper jaw are consequently retroposed, giving a false appearance of mandibular prognathism. A classical and extreme form of this is seen in achondroplasia and, in a less marked form, in Down's syndrome and many other, rarer, syndromes. It is not infrequently seen in individuals who are otherwise normal, as in the girl whose radiograph is shown in fig. 3. This was a healthy intelligent girl, whose facial appearance was spoilt by the short skull base and by a degree of ocular hypertelorism. It is notable, again, that the upper incisors and their alveolar processes have proclined to compensate for the skeletal discrepancy.

This shortness of the skull base is usually combined with hypertelorism. Adult man is unique in having a very narrow bridge of his nose, the eyes having come together, allowing binocular vision. It is not present in any other animal, nor in the human fetus. During development from the fetal stage, the eyes come together due to differential growth of the bone around the orbits. Hypertelorism is due to a failure of this maturation. It has been suggested that a narrow nasal bridge can only occur in animals with an extreme reduction in the snout, probably for mechanical reasons. It may be that where the anterior base of the skull is short, increased width is essential, to provide adequate strength to this part of the skull.

If the importance of the cartilage of the mandibular condyle has been exaggerated in the past, nevertheless its significance is emphasized by the abnormalities to which it

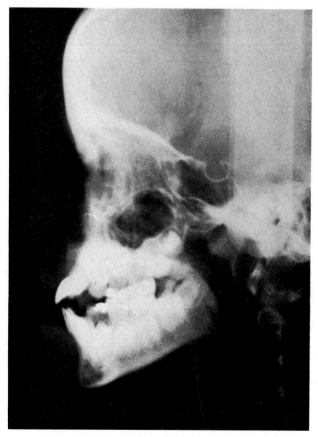

FIG. 3. Lateral skull radiograph of girl aged 12 years with unusually short anterior base of skull.

may give rise. The effect of excessive condylar growth is seen in the asymmetrical mandible which arises in unilateral condylar hyperplasia, illustrated in fig. 4. This is a case of the vertical type of hyperplasia, and the alveolar processes on the affected side have developed vertically to maintain an occlusion of the teeth on that side. Similarly, in acromegaly, although all the tissues grow excessively, the ability of the condylar cartilage to continue or recommence growth in early adult life produces a mandibular prognathism.

A reduction of condylar growth may occur spontaneously, as in condylar hypoplasia, or may be the result of trauma or infection in infancy, causing destruction of the condylar growth centre. Again there is an increased surface deposition of bone, and marked proclination of the lower teeth, in an effort to compensate for the discrepancy, but a marked mandibular micrognathia remains.

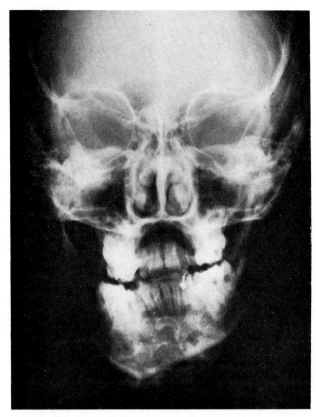

FIG. 4. Postero-anterior skull radiograph of girl aged 12 years, in rest position of mandible, showing unilateral condylar hyperplasia.

The Sutures

Growth at the sutures is a specialized form of surface deposition. Their function is well seen in the cranial vault. The developing brain, increasing in size, tends to spread the cranial bones apart, and the sutures compensate for this, keeping their margins in contact; that is, the sutures are not so much a growth mechanism as an "infilling" process, acting secondarily to the primary growth mechanism. Nevertheless, if the sutures close prematurely, the shape of the skull becomes deformed, as in oxycephaly or plagiocephaly, where growth can take place only in those sutures which remain patent.

Surface Deposition of Bone

A large part of the growth of the face and skull is brought about by surface deposition by the osteogenic layer of the periosteum, especially in the so-called membrane bones. The condition of cleidocranial dysostosis affects such bones, and rather small jaws are a feature of the condition. Since the cartilaginous growth at the condyle is unaffected, a relative prognathism is present. Again, a lack of periosteal bone may be seen, as in fig. 5, in individuals who are otherwise normal and healthy.

There are many conditions, mostly rare and usually extremely rare, which may interfere with facial growth at the

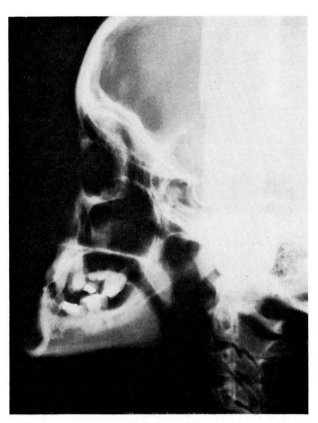

FIG. 5. Lateral skull radiograph of girl aged 16 years, showing deficiency of appositional bone growth.

cellular level. Some are the result of genetic abnormalities, and may be inherited. Others are local manifestations of generalized pathological conditions, or even of trauma or infection. In contemplating the effect of these conditions, a knowledge of the mechanism of growth is valuable. The division of abnormalities into two types, one an extreme of normal variation of the genotype, the other more truly pathological, may constitute an over-simplification, but the division is a real one.

REFERENCES

Björk, A. (1947), "The Face in Profile," *Svensk tandläk. Tidskr.*, **40,** suppl. 5B.

Björk, A. (1963), "Variations in the Growth Pattern of the Human Mandible: Longitudinal Study by the Implant Method," *J. dent. Res.*, **42,** 400.

Björk, A. (1969), "Prediction of Mandibular Growth Rotation," *Amer. J. Orthodont.*, **55,** 585.

Björk, A. and Skieller, V. (1972), "Facial Development and Tooth Eruption," *Amer. J. Orthodont.*, **62,** 339.

Broadbent, B. H. (1947), *Practical Orthodontics* (G. M. Anderson, Ed.). London: Kimpton.

Moss, M. L. (1968), "The Primacy of Functional Matrices in Orofacial Growth," *Trans. Brit. Soc. Orthodont.*, **54,** 107.

6. CELL STRUCTURE

R. M. H. McMINN

In 1665 Robert Hooke, inventor of the spirit level and later secretary of the Royal Society, published an illustration of the structure of the bark of the cork tree. He called the small compartments of which it was composed "cells", but it was almost another two centuries before it became recognized that cells were the basic components of all living matter. Credit for this is usually given to a botanist, Schleiden (1838), and a zoologist, Schwann (1839), and the

establishment of the cellular basis of pathological lesions in man and animals is usually attributed to Virchow (1858). Many remarkably prophetic (and sometimes imaginative) observations were made by the early microscopists with what would now be regarded as most primitive apparatus, but as in other scientific fields more knowledge about cell structure and function has been gathered in the last quarter of a century than in all preceding eras. In other words, this increased understanding has occurred during the lifetimes of the younger postgraduates reading this book.

Any present-day student of animal or human biology will have been made aware that use of the electron microscope (EM) has revolutionized our concept of the structure of the cell and its constituents. Among other things, it has shown how the interior of the cell is not the more or less homogeneous mass it so often appears to be under the optical microscope, but is divided into compartments, thus allowing fundamentally different chemical reactions to take place perhaps in close proximity but without interfering with one another. However, it is important to recognize that while the EM has contributed enormously to our appreciation of form, the all-important correlation with function has been possible largely because of the concomitant use of other techniques, but perhaps particularly by the use of the ultracentrifuge. By this means, different cellular components can be isolated from one another, because different kinds of components separate out at different levels of the centrifuge tube. In this way, relatively large concentrations of any one type of component can be analysed biochemically, and a correlation between form and function may be inferred or established.

At this point it should be emphasized that in many respects we do not yet understand precisely how our methods of specimen preparation for the EM affect the structural components of the cell. It is important to appreciate that what we visualize on the EM screen and later on a photographic print are the end results of the scattering of electrons, the scatter being produced by aggregations of atoms (single atoms are not sufficient). The higher the atomic number of the atoms, the greater is the scatter and the darker the image. The atoms of most biological tissues (carbon, hydrogen, oxygen, nitrogen) have very small atomic numbers and so produce little scatter, but we can increase the contrast of parts of the image by introducing heavy metals such as lead or osmium. The problem that then emerges is to know with which macromolecules of the structure we are investigating the newly introduced atoms have become bound, and to know whether this artefact is reproducible under standard conditions. With these questions answered, and with the aid of other biophysical and biochemical techniques such as histochemistry, autoradiography and X-ray diffraction, it may be possible to arrive at an accurate interpretation of structure in terms of its components parts, or at least an interpretation that leads to a testable hypothesis.

The purpose of this chapter will be to examine the various

structural components of the cell with some reference to their function, so indicating how cells may differ from one another in their form and function on the basis of their component parts. For further detailed consideration of all topics the reader is referred to the recent works on cell biology edited by Bittar (1973), Giese (1973) and Beck and Lloyd (1974). More general accounts are available in textbooks of histology and electron microscopy (*e.g.* Bloom and Fawcett, 1975; Ham, 1974; Toner and Carr, 1971; Greep and Weiss, 1973).

CELL COMPONENTS AND CYTOPLASM

The cell consists essentially of nucleus and cytoplasm, the latter bounded by the cell membrane. The cytoplasm contains various components which are often classified as organelles and inclusions. Organelles can be defined as living structural components concerned with synthetic and metabolic activities, and although perhaps varying in quantity in different physiological states they can usually be regarded as permanent features of the cell. They comprise the endoplasmic reticulum (ER), Golgi apparatus, mitochondria, lysosomes, annulate lamellae, ribosomes, fibrils, microtubules and centrioles. Because of their structure, all except the last four in this list may be termed membranous organelles. In view of their functional importance both the nucleus and the cell membrane are sometimes included among the organelles. Inclusions are accumulations of products, many of which may be only "temporary residents" of the cell—secretion granules, storage granules, pigments and crystals. It is principally the differing proportions of the various organelles and inclusions that enable cell types to be distinguished from one another, although size and shape may sometimes be characteristic also.

The cytoplasm is the part of the cell in which the various organelles and inclusions are embedded; it is bounded by the cell membrane and surrounds the nucleus. In most cells the volume of cytoplasm is several times the nuclear volume, but in some, *e.g.* small lymphocytes, the amount of cytoplasm is minimal. In preparations for optical microscopy, staining reactions such as "cytoplasmic basophilia" (p. 77) are due to organelles and not to the cytoplasm itself, which is sometimes known as hyaloplasm or cytoplasmic matrix. Different regions of the cytoplasm may exist in the sol or gel states, and there may be rapid changes from one to the other. This may play a part in the motility of free connective-tissue cells in the adult and in other cell types during embryonic development and reparative processes.

Although the cytoplasmic matrix contains large numbers of molecules, many of which are enzymes that react with other constituents, much of the activity of the cytoplasm is due to the organelles it contains, and their performance in the life of the cell is determined by information derived from the nucleus (p. 74).

BIOLOGICAL MEMBRANE STRUCTURE

Since so many parts of the cell are composed of membranes, it is appropriate before describing any further cellu-lar details to give some consideration to the general structure of biological membranes before meeting them in various cell components.

Using the currently accepted methods of tissue preparation for the EM, a typical biological membrane appears as a three-layered structure—a sandwich of two dark layers (electron-dense) enclosing a light layer (electron-lucent). This is commonly referred to as the trilaminar or unit membrane (fig. 1), and has an overall thickness of something of the order of 7·5 nm.*, each dense layer being approximately 2·0 nm. thick with the light zone about 3·5 nm. These dimensions must not be considered absolute, for there is a considerable range in the total thickness from about 5–12 nm., depending not only on the method of preparation but also on the type of cell or organelle and the physiological state of the tissue at the time of fixation. With well-preserved and well-prepared specimens, and with sections cut at right-angles to the membrane, electron micrographs at a magnification of about 70,000 and above should show this pattern, although at the more commonly used routine levels of magnification, say 5–30,000, the triple layering will not (of course) be apparent.

This basic pattern is found not only in the membrane that forms the boundary of the cell but also in the nuclear membrane and in those cytoplasmic organelles that are of a membranous nature (*i.e.* endoplasmic reticulum, Golgi apparatus, mitochondria, lysosomes and annulate lamellae —see below). This is not to say that the chemical (macromolecular) composition of the membrane in these diverse situations is identical; it is certainly not, but this does not alter the fact that the fundamental pattern is common to most if not all membranes.

Numerous biochemical and biophysical methods of examination have established that the unit (trilaminar) membrane consists mostly of protein and lipid, with a small amount of carbohydrate. The lipid is probably arranged in the form of a double (bimolecular) layer with protein on either side, the carbohydrate being combined either with some of the lipid as glycolipid or with some of the protein as glycoprotein. Thus there are basically four layers of macromolecules (protein–lipid–lipid–protein) which must react with fixatives and other processing reagents to give the three-layered ultrastructural pattern. The lipid molecules are arranged at right angles to the surface of the membrane, with their polar groups at opposite ends of the molecules and closely associated with the overlying protein. The protein with part of the lipid gives the electron-dense "bread" of the sandwich (or inner and outer leaflets of the membrane), the remainder of the lipid being the pale "filling".

From time to time there has been criticism of the above concept of membrane structure which owes its origin to the theoretical model of Danielli and Davson (1935) and which received experimental support from Robertson (1957) who introduced the term "unit membrane". Although there are many detailed problems that remain unresolved, recent

---

* International units of measurement: 1 mm. = 1,000 μm. (micrometre, formerly μ or micron); 1 μm = 1,000 nm. (nanometre, formerly mμ or mμm., millimicron). The Angstrom unit, Å., is no longer an official unit; 1 nm. = 10 Å.

critical reviews suggest that in general it is the concept or model which most widely stands up to the various tests to which it has been subjected. Possibly the most likely alternative arrangement is that the lipid is not in a continuous bimolecular layer but in the form of globules (micelles).

It is important to emphasize that the protein–lipid–protein formula refers only to the general architectural make-up of the membrane, and does not specify what lipid or what protein molecules are taking part. It must not be inferred, for example, that the proteins on the inner and outer aspects of the membrane are the same, or that those in different regions of the membrane are identical, or that they are never found anywhere but on the surface; some glycoprotein molecules, for example, are known to extend throughout the whole thickness of the membrane. The widely differing functions of membranes in different sites would make it surprising if their components did not differ. Also, the proportions of the three principal constituents (protein, lipid and carbohydrate) show considerable variation in different organelles, and even in different parts of the same organelle. For example, in the plasma membrane of the red blood cell, protein, lipid and carbohydrate are found in the percentages of 49, 43 and 8 respectively, whereas in myelin, which is a fused spiral of membrane, the proportions are 75, 20 and 5. Mitochondrial membranes have other proportions (p. 78).

CELL MEMBRANE

All cells are bounded by a cell membrane, properly known as the cytolemma or plasmolemma (correctly so spelt, not

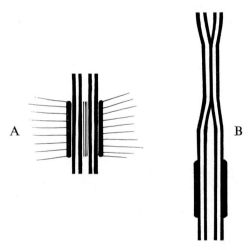

FIG. 1. A diagrammatic representation of the trilaminar appearance of the cell membrane (plasma membrane), as seen in adjacent epithelial cells with specialized regions of attachment. A: at a desmosome, where there is a condensation of cytoplasm (with fibrils) immediately adjacent to the inner leaflet of each membrane. B: above, at a tight junction, where the outer leaflets of each membrane fuse; below, at an intermediate junction, where there is a thickening of the inner leaflet of each membrane.

plasma*lemma*), and commonly called the plasma membrane, since it forms the limiting boundary between the cytoplasm of the cell and its environment. In histological

preparations, this membrane cannot be identified as a distinct entity, being in thickness much below the resolving power of the optical microscope, but in many tissues (*e.g.* epidermis, oral epithelium, the collecting tubules of the kidney) some linear demarcation between individual cells is usually observed. This represents not only the adjacent cell membranes but a certain amount of adjoining cytoplasm and intercellular material as well, all combining to give an apparently single line.

The EM reveals that the individual plasma membrane (figs. 1 and 2) has the typical unit membrane appearance (described above) and is usually about 7·5 nm. thick. In

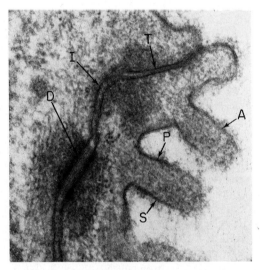

FIG. 2. Parts of two adjacent epithelial cells (from the stomach) showing several features of the plasma membrane described in the text. The trilaminar nature of the plasma membrane can just be discerned where it covers a cytoplasmic process (as at P). On other regions of the surface, the plasma membrane has not been sectioned in the correct plane for visualizing this structural detail (as at A); this is not uncommon in electron micrographs and must not be interpreted as indicating absence of the membrane. Some of the material adhering to the surface of the membrane represents the surface coat (as at S). Also shown are a tight junction (T), intermediate junction (I) and desmosome (D). × 750,000.

the most superficial layer of cells of the urinary bladder, the membrane of the free surface is thicker (about 12 nm.), due to a wider outer leaflet with unusual structural features—probably an example of a local specialization of function associated with the need for a urineproof lining—while in intestinal epithelium the microvilli (see below) are bounded by a membrane with an overall thickness of about 10 nm. In all cells the membrane forms a continuous boundary between the cytoplasm and the exterior; even where cells are fenestrated (as in some capillary endothelial sites) the gaps are of course entirely bordered by membrane. The term sarcolemma, often used to refer to the boundary of muscle cells, is a composite term that includes both the plasma membrane and the basal lamina (see below). Likewise, neurolemma includes the plasma membrane and basal lamina of the neurolemmal (Schwann) cell.

Surface Coat

Sometimes (as on the microvilli of intestinal epithelium or the surface of the superficial layer of oral epithelium) material of moderate electron density with a filamentous component can be demonstrated on the exterior of the plasma membrane, apparently adhering to the outer leaflet (fig. 2). Not all methods of preparation allow it to be observed readily, but when preserved it can be as much as 30 nm. or more thick, *i.e.* considerably more than the plasma membrane itself. It is commonly called the surface coat, or fuzzy coat, or more elegantly the glycocalyx ("sweet husk"). It has a high carbohydrate (acid mucopolysaccharide and glycoprotein) content but few details are known of its exact make-up. It is secreted by the cell to which it adheres; precursors have been identified in the Golgi apparatus, but it is not clear by what routes it reaches the cell surface. It appears to be undergoing continual renewal. It must not be confused with the basal lamina (see below) which is an entirely different structure, and on intestinal cells it is not simply secreted mucus adhering to the plasma membrane. It can be stained with colloidal thorium and the periodic acid–silver methenamine technique, and there are some reports indicating that it may be present to some extent around almost all cells. In epithelia it is only absent at the sites of tight junctions and gap junctions (p. 72). It follows closely all the contours of the plasma membrane, and can therefore be seen as an internal lining for phagocytic and pinocytic vesicles (p. 73).

The surface coat must be regarded as an additional part of the cell's permeability barrier, and it may function as an intercellular cement. Some authorities consider it and the plasma membrane to be a single complex forming the cell boundary. Whatever one defines as the real surface, the nature and configuration of the molecules at that surface play an important part in the immunological properties of the cell as well as in its permeability and other functions.

Basal Lamina

At the junctions of epithelia with connective tissue, the EM reveals a moderately electron-dense layer of material about 30–70 nm. thick (fig. 3). Commonly termed the basal lamina (see below) it possesses fine collagenous filaments embedded in a mainly carbohydrate matrix and is separated from the epithelial cells by a clear interval of about 30 nm. It forms a (usually) continuous sheet separating the epithelium from the underlying connective tissue fibres, cells and ground substance. Descemet's membrane under the (inner) endothelium of the cornea of the eye is an exceptionally thick basal lamina (5–10 μm.) and easily seen histologically. Sometimes filaments extend into the basal lamina from epithelial hemidesmosomes (p. 70), and similar strands may fan out into underlying tissue—a particularly prominent feature in oral mucosa. There is evidence, at least in some cells, that the basal lamina is a product of the epithelium, and it should not be regarded as a condensation of connective tissue ground substance containing some fine fibrils. It must be distinguished from the surface coat (described above) which lies between the plasma membrane and the basal lamina. Unlike the surface coat, the basal lamina does not contain acidic polysaccharides and it is fairly easily detached from its overlying cells experimentally (*e.g.* by microinjection between cell and lamina). From its position it must be penetrated by any substances entering or leaving the cell via the connective tissue, so that it is at least a potential barrier. However, even such large structures as migrating leucocytes seem to be able to puncture it easily, and it is probably not so obstructive as its appearance in electron micrographs would lead one to believe.

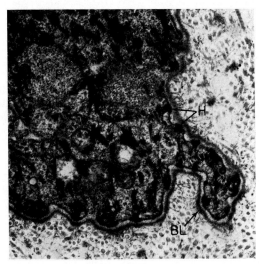

Fig. 3. The basal lamina (BL) beneath part of a basal cell of the epidermis. Also shown are a number of hemidesmosomes (H), and bundles of fibrillar material (F) in the cytoplasm. × 18,750.

A basal lamina of the type just described is also associated with cells other than epithelia. It underlies the external surface of most capillary endothelia (both vascular and lymphatic, though its presence under lymphatic endothelium is variable and there is none under the endothelium of hepatic sinusoids), and in electron micrographs of the kidney, for example, it forms a distinctive feature separating the capillary endothelium from the foot processes of the podocytes (glomerular visceral epithelial cells). Similarly in the lung, both alveolar epithelium and capillary endothelium each have their own basal laminae which, in the walls of the air sacs, fuse into a single layer separating the basal plasma membranes of these two cell types. A basal lamina completely surrounds the various kinds of muscle cell, only being absent where there are plasma membrane specializations for adhesion (p. 70). The satellite cells of skeletal muscle lie internal to the basal lamina of the parent cell, but there is no basal lamina between the adjacent interfaces of satellite and parent. A basal lamina also completely surrounds neurolemmal (Schwann) cells where it remains as an overall external sleeve without dipping down where the plasma membrane forms a mesaxon (p. 72). After crush injury to peripheral nerves, persistent basal laminae help to form the endoneural tubes that guide growing axons back to the periphery.

Terminology: Basal Lamina and Basement Membrane

It has been suggested that in non-epithelial tissues, where there is no polarization of the cell into apex and base, the term **basal** lamina is a misnomer and that **external** lamina would be more appropriate, but it remains to be seen whether this term will be adopted in future literature. This area is already beset with problems of terminology, for the basal lamina is sometimes referred to as the basement membrane. This is an old-established histological term that includes not only what we now know as the basal lamina (which is itself beyond the resolving power of the optical microscope) but also an amount of underlying connective tissue containing fine (rather than coarse) collagen fibres and ground substance. This composite structure, the basement membrane of optical microscopy, is clearly seen histologically at epithelial-connective tissue junctions and is particularly prominent in the nose and trachea. It would help to avoid confusion if the single structure described here as basal lamina could always be referred to as such (or even as external lamina), so keeping the term basement membrane for the composite structure. Those who insist on using basement membrane as a term in electron microscopy should make clear whether they are using it as a synonym for basal lamina or in its wider context.

Free Surface Specializations

Microvilli

Microvilli are nonmotile fingerlike processes (fig. 4A) consisting of a central core of cytoplasm covered by plasma

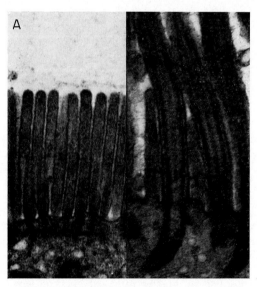

FIG. 4. A: microvilli at the surface of small intestinal epithelial cells, forming a regular array of fingerlike processes, each of which is bounded by the plasma membrane. B: cilia at the surface of a tracheal epithelial cell, photographed at the same magnification as the microvilli. If shown throughout their full length, cilia may be ten times as long as microvilli. × 30,000.

membrane of the usual trilaminar appearance, with an outer surface coat. The most striking examples of microvilli

are seen on the columnar cells of the intestine and the proximal convoluted tubules of the kidney, where they form a close-packed regular array of 2–3,000 processes on the free surface of every single cell. An individual microvillus is here about 1 μm. in height and 0·1 μm. in diameter, with a boundary plasma membrane about 10 nm. thick. Such a configuration increases the surface area of the cell by about twenty times—presumably a desirable feature where absorption is concerned. Collectively microvilli form the "brush border" (striated border) of optical microscopy. In the cytoplasmic core of intestinal microvilli there are a number of fine filamentous structures (microfilaments, perhaps as many as 50) which extend into the apical cytoplasm of the cell.

Many other cells exhibit more sparsely situated microvillous processes (sometimes called filopodia) of very variable size and shape, e.g. on the free surface of exocrine gland cells such as the serous cells of the parotid or pancreas, on the lateral surface of liver cells (hepatocytes) whose microvilli lie in the perisinusoidal space, and at the surface of macrophages where they are perhaps concerned with the motility of the cells.

Stereocilia

Closely allied to microvilli are the processes known as stereocilia, which are nothing more than exceptionally long microvilli. They have a similar structure and are seen typically in the epididymis and ductus deferens. They must not be confused with the next kind of specialization to be discussed, cilia proper.

Cilia

Cilia are motile cell processes which are entirely different in composition from microvilli and stereocilia, and are typically found on the cells of respiratory epithelium, i.e. in the lining of the nasal cavity, air sinuses, trachea and bronchial tree, and also on some cells of the uterine tube. They are larger than microvilli, up to 10 μm. long and 0·2 μm. broad (fig. 4B), and usually easily seen with the optical microscope. Their characteristic structural features are best seen in transverse section; the cytoplasmic core, bounded by plasma membrane, contains a constant number of fibrillar elements arranged as two central and nine peripheral fibrils. Each central fibril appears as a hollow circle or microtubule, while each of the peripheral fibrils has a figure-of-eight pattern (a pair of microtubules) with two small attached "arms". The nine peripheral fibrils extend into the apical cell cytoplasm and constitute the basal body of the cilium. The basal body is in fact a modified centriole (p. 81), and the cilium itself an extension or outgrowth of the centriole. In a cell that is about to develop cilia, a hundred or more centrioles (formed by duplication from an original pair) accumulate in the apical cytoplasm. The flagellum of a spermatozoon is basically an elongated cilium, with the same 9 + 2 structure.

The fibrillar or microtubular structures are composed of contractile proteins of as yet uncertain composition; in some respects they resemble the actin and myosin of muscle (but they are not identical), and they are responsible for the beating movement. However, the control mechanisms are quite unknown.

Basal Infoldings

In some epithelial cells the plasma membrane at the epithelial-connective tissue junction is not always more or less flat but may be elaborately infolded (as "basal infoldings") to receive matching projections from neighbouring cells. The result is a series of interdigitating cytoplasmic processes that fit together like cogwheels. This pattern probably reaches its highest degree of complexity in the proximal convoluted tubules of the kidney, but has also been noted in salivary-gland cells. If a surface coat is present, it will adhere to all the infoldings, but the basal lamina does not—it remains as a boundary between the epithelium and the underlying connective tissue.

specializations of certain parts of the plasma membrane that are the main factors in maintaining cells in close apposition.

Desmosomes and Hemidesmosomes

The term desmosome, properly called macula adherens (plural, maculae adherentes) refers to a button-shaped or plate-like area of two adjacent plasma membranes together with the intervening intercellular space, *i.e.* there is a half desmosome on each of the two plasma membranes (figs. 1A, 2, 5 and 6A). They are present in all epithelia, but are particularly numerous in oral epithelia and epidermis. They are too small to be identified with the optical microscope, so that knowledge of them dates only from the EM era.

At the site of a typical desmosome the intercellular space

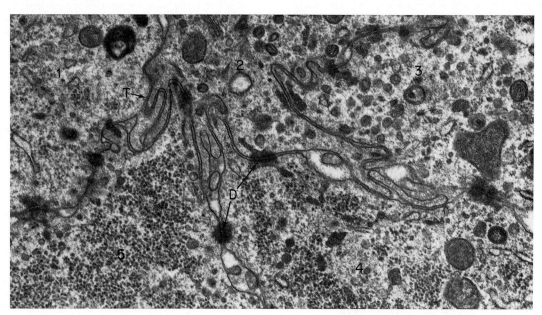

Fig. 5. Parts of five cells (numbered 1–5) of the stratum spinosum of epidermis, showing interdigitation of adjacent plasma membranes (T) and several desmosomes (D). × 24,000.

Contact Specializations

In epithelia, where the cells are arranged in single sheets or numerous layers, the plasma membranes of adjacent cells lie parallel with one another and normally separated by a remarkably constant interval of about 15–20 nm. This intercellular space is electron-lucent and is thought to contain something more than just tissue fluid; special staining techniques may reveal the surface coat (described above) which possibly acts as an intercellular cement. If there is an adhesive there, it must be relatively weak, for under some physiological and pathological conditions it seems easy for fluid to accumulate in the intercellular space and enlarge it.

The sides of adjacent epithelial cells, although normally remaining parallel with one another, are rarely straight for any distance but are frequently interdigitated with one another like pieces of an elaborate, irregular jigsaw puzzle (fig. 5). These interdigitations presumably play some part in holding cells together. However, there are important

may measure 20–25 nm. in width, and contains material that is rather more electron-dense than intercellular substance elsewhere, and which may contain a mucopolysaccharide that acts as a glue. The most striking feature of the desmosome is the very electron-dense, plate-like concentration of cytoplasm that lies immediately adjacent to the plasma membrane. Numerous fine fibrils or filaments can be observed radiating from the dense plaque into the surrounding cytoplasm, and some of the filaments can be traced to other desmosomes. Although some of the filaments may end in, and be attached in some way to, the condensation of cytoplasmic matrix, many of them form hairpin loops in the plaque, entering it at one point and leaving at another.

Observations of epithelia wherein the intercellular spaces have become dilated, together with microdissection studies, all indicate that desmosomes are regions of firm adherence. Apart from being found in all kinds of epithelia, including epithelial derivatives such as ameloblasts, they are also present as attachments between the endothelial cells of vascular and lymphatic vessels, whether capillaries or channels of larger dimensions. Although not usually found on the majority of connective tissue cell types, they do exist on odontoblasts, at least where these cells are not separated by intercellular clefts. As well as acting as attachment plaques, they are probably sites of low-resistance electrical communication between cells.

On the plasma membrane that forms the base of single-layered epithelial cells or the base of the basal layer of stratified epithelia, there are structures commonly known as hemidesmosomes. As the name implies, they resemble exactly one-half of a desmosome, consisting of a dense cytoplasmic plaque immediately adjacent to the plasma membrane, with filaments radiating into the cytoplasm (fig. 3). As there is no underlying epithelial cell, the other half of a normal desmosome is missing. Presumably they act as areas of adherence, for there is usually some evidence of attachment to the basal lamina by very fine filaments which may extend into the underlying basal lamina and connective tissue.

Intermediate Junctions

The intermediate junction (zonula adherens) is not found alone but always in association with the third type of intercellular junction, the tight junction (described below). These

At an intermediate junction there is an intercellular gap of about 20 nm. separating adjacent cell membranes which themselves show some localized thickening of their inner (cytoplasmic) leaflets (figs. 1B, 2 and 6). There is usually no evidence of any particularly dense intercellular material in this region, and no dense plaque of cytoplasm as there is at a desmosomal site, although fine fibrils that are apparently attached to the membrane radiate into the cytoplasm. But the main feature to appreciate about the intermediate junction (zonula adherens) is that it forms a continuous girdle round the cell (zonula means girdle or belt). This is its main distinguishing difference from the desmosome or macula adherens (macula means spot) which is a very localized region of attachment.

Tight Junctions

The tight junction, properly known as the zonula occludens, forms a complete girdle round the apices of columnar or cubical epithelial cells, and is found immediately above the zonula adherens. Most electron micrographs of tight junctions indicate that in these regions the intercellular space is obliterated and the adjacent plasma membranes fuse together by their outer leaflets for a distance of not more than 500 nm. (figs. 1B, 2 and 6). In the cytoplasm adjacent to the site of membrane fusion there are no dense condensations and no filamentous attachments.

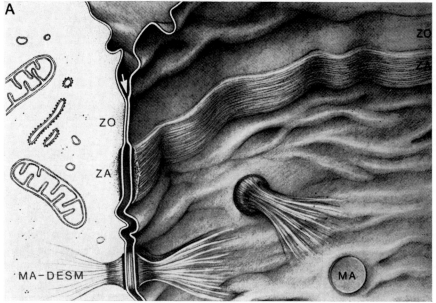
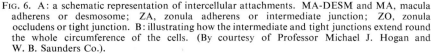
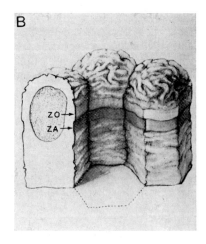

FIG. 6. A: a schematic representation of intercellular attachments. MA-DESM and MA, macula adherens or desmosome; ZA, zonula adherens or intermediate junction; ZO, zonula occludens or tight junction. B: illustrating how the intermediate and tight junctions extend round the whole circumference of the cells. (By courtesy of Professor Michael J. Hogan and W. B. Saunders Co.).

two features are found near the apices of the cells of single-layered epithelia, e.g. gastro-intestinal cells, and near the upper poles of ameloblasts and odontoblasts. The intermediate junction is always situated just below the tight junction, e.g. in an intestinal cell it is a little farther from the internal surface of the gut than the tight junction; in an odontoblast it is a little farther from the main mass of dentine.

The presence of the tight junction, which is an undoubted area of firm adhesion, means that many substances that are being absorbed (e.g. by intestinal cells or by the proximal convoluted tubules of the kidney) cannot pass through the lining epithelium between cells; they must enter the cell through its apex and either pass out through the base or, more likely, through the side of the cell into the intercellular space which can easily become dilated, except of course where the plasma membranes are held in apposition by any of the adhesive structures just described. At the sides of the apices of single-layered epithelial cells it is common for a tight junction, intermediate junction and a desmosome to be found close together; such a combination of these three elements is now known as a junctional complex, which corresponds to the "terminal bar" of pre-EM days. ("Terminal web" is the name given to the cytoplasm that extends across the cell at the level of the junctional complex. Ameloblasts have a corresponding region at the level of the tight junction and known as the basal web.) Odontoblasts and ameloblasts exhibit tight and intermediate junctions, and there may or may not be nearby desmosomes.

Apart from acting as adhesion sites, tight junctions are regions where small molecules (with molecular weights up to about 20,000) can pass from one cell to another, despite the lack of any cytoplasmic continuity.

Gap Junctions

In the last few years another type of cell contact has been described, the gap junction. It appears that in the past this has been confused with the tight junction, but there are distinct differences. Primarily, at the gap junction the adjacent plasma membranes are not fused but remain separated by a narrow gap of 2 nm. However, this is not an empty space, for there is evidence of a very regular hexagonal array of material that does in fact join the membranes together (the term gap junction is thus already a misnomer). Whereas the tight junction in epithelia is a belt-like structure completely encompassing the cell near its free border, the gap junction is plaque-like, resembling a desmosome, but there are no adjacent cytoplasmic condensations or filamentous attachments. Gap junctions have been described as attachment areas between various epithelial cells, and between visceral and cardiac muscle cells, where they apparently function not only as anchors but as sites of increased permeability and electrical conductivity. The latter is particularly important in visceral and cardiac muscle where not all the cells receive a nerve ending. They have not yet been identified in odontoblasts or ameloblasts.

The term "nexus" has been used as a synonym for gap junction, and also for the tight junction before the existence of the gap junction was recognized. Confusion will persist until these structures have been more clearly defined.

Synapses

The synapse is a specialized region of plasma membranes and adjacent cytoplasm where part of one neuron communicates with another by means of a transmitter substance.

A typical synapse is formed by a process (axon or dendrite) of one neuron and a process or cell body of another neuron (fig. 7). The afferent side of the synapse is usually in the form of an expanded end of a neuronal process, and is still often known by the old French term bouton (presynaptic bouton) or alternatively as the synaptic or presynaptic bulb, bag or ending. This nerve ending consists of cytoplasm bounded by plasma membrane but without any surrounding Schwann cell or basal lamina. The ending contains perhaps a few mitochondria and fine fibrils, but its

most characteristic features are the synaptic vesicles. These are rounded membrane-bound bodies about 20–60 nm. in diameter which lie near the extremity or "business end" of the synapse, where the cytoplasm immediately adjacent to the plasma membrane shows a desmosomal-like density. An interval about 20 nm. wide, the synaptic cleft, separates the bouton from the postsynaptic region of the neuron with which communication is being made. This region has a similar desmosomal density of cytoplasm but does not possess synaptic vesicles. This is the prime distinction between the pre- and post-synaptic parts of the communication complex, and usually enables the afferent and efferent

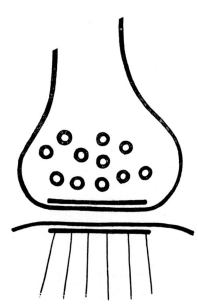

FIG. 7. A diagram of a synapse, showing presynaptic vesicles and the post-synaptic web of filaments. The unit (trilaminar) membrane is here indicated by a single line.

sides to be identified. On the postsynaptic side, fine fibrils may radiate into the cytoplasm from the dense region, and constitute the subsynaptic web—another distinguishing feature from the presynaptic bouton.

The synaptic cleft seems to contain fine filamentous material of slight electron density and unknown composition. The presynaptic vesicles are thought to contain the transmitter substances. When an action potential reaches the ending, some vesicles rapidly fuse with the plasma membrane and the transmitter is liberated into the synaptic cleft, so reaching the postsynaptic membrane. Vesicles that contain acetyl choline (at somatic and preganglionic autonomic endings) are electron-lucent, but at adrenergic endings their contents are rather dense. Synaptic transmission can be regarded as one form of neurosecretion (p. 81).

The pre- and post-synaptic membranes of the synapse bear some structural resemblance to a desmosome, and at these regions the two membranes certainly adhere to one another. When nervous tissue is homogenized and centrifuged, presynaptic bulbs with adherent post-synaptic membranes can be isolated, constituting the particles known as synaptosomes. It is from such preparations that the contents of synaptic vesicles can be analysed.

Motor Nerve Endings

Allied to synapses are the endings of efferent nerves on muscle and gland cells—another example of cell contact or communication where a transmitter substance is required.

At a motor endplate on skeletal muscle, the nerve axon (which at this level is now devoid of myelin sheath, Schwann cell and basal lamina) divides into a number of fingerlike or bulbous endings that sink into shallow depressions or furrows in the sarcolemma (consisting of both plasma membrane and basal lamina—the latter does not disappear at motor endplates as it does at synapses and other cell contacts). In the depths of the furrow there are small folds of muscle-cell plasma membrane containing basal lamina but no axonal processes. The axoplasm at the ends of the axonal processes contains mitochondria and a large number of vesicles about 45 nm. in diameter containing acetyl choline. The distance between the axolemma and the plasma membrane component of the sarcolemma is 40–60 nm. (about twice the width of a synaptic cleft).

In cardiac and smooth muscle there are unmyelinated autonomic nerves which end as nodules adjacent to the sarcolemma, forming endings that are less complicated than somatic motor endplates and which have certainly been less extensively investigated. While any one skeletal muscle cell normally receives only one endplate, many cardiac and smooth muscle cells receive no motor endings; impulse transmission occurs through the tight junctions or nexuses. Some smooth muscle cells, on the other hand, may have more than one motor ending.

Gland cells have contacts with neuronal processes but there is less information about them than about synapses and endplates. In salivary glands (see Chapter 42) there is a nerve network derived from the postganglionic fibres of the appropriate parasympathetic ganglia and making a contact with acinar cells to provide the secretomotor stimulus. The nerve terminals penetrate the basal lamina and come to lie against or between the secretory cells with an intervening synapse-like space of about 20 nm. There are vesicles in the neuronal processes but no membranous or cytoplasmic dense area.

Permeability and Transport

The plasma membrane is not simply an inert boundary for cytoplasm but is vital to the whole life of the cell as a site for the exchange of materials. It is involved in the transport of many substances that enter or leave the cytoplasm, by mechanisms known biochemically but which cannot yet be visualized microscopically. For this purpose, enzymes may be incorporated within the membrane; thus it contains ATPase which acts on the ATP that has become liberated from mitochondria and diffuses through the cytoplasm to reach the plasma membrane, providing the necessary energy for transport mechanisms. Specialized areas may have their own complement of enzymes, e.g. the membrane of the microvilli of intestinal absorptive cells contains various peptidases and disaccharidases that are involved in the digestion of protein and carbohydrate. In neurons and muscle cells the membrane is concerned with excitability and impulse conduction which depend on ionic and electrical changes.

However, there are other transport mechanisms that can be recognized at optical and EM levels. These include secretory processes (exocytosis) involving granule formation (to be described on p. 81) as well as phenomena concerned with the intake of materials—phagocytosis and pinocytosis, sometimes collectively known as endocytosis.

Phagocytosis

Macrophages and other cell types that can exhibit macrophagic activity (such as polymorphonuclear leucocytes, monocytes, Kupffer cells of liver sinusoids and microglial cells of the central nervous system) have the ability to ingest particulate matter, including bacteria and cell debris, by the process of phagocytosis. This involves contact (or nearcontact) of the particle with part of the plasma membrane (or surface coat), which invaginates to surround the ingested material and then forms a complete membranous sac or phagosome that breaks away from the surface membrane. There must be a rapid restoration of continuity at the site where the phagocytic vacuole becomes nipped off. (The fate of such phagocytic vacuoles is discussed in the section on lysosomes, below.) Any cell that is engaged in extensive phagocytic activity is therefore required to manufacture new plasma membrane to replace that which is lost to the surface boundary by continual vacuole formation.

Pinocytosis

Closely allied to phagocytosis, which deals with solid matter, is the process of pinocytosis which refers to the ingestion of fluid by vacuoles that again become pinched off from the plasma membrane (fig. 8). These fluid packages are often so small that they are detectable only with the EM, in which case the process is called micropinocytosis. A typical example is in capillary endothelium, where the small vesicles, here known as caveolae, have been shown to cross from one side of the flattened endothelial cell to the other in a time of about 1 sec., so transporting material from lumen to tissue (or from tissue to lumen) but at the same time keeping it segregated from the cytoplasm. Vesicle production again involves synthesis of more plasma membrane; but there is another problem, for when vesicles traverse the cell and fuse with the membrane on the opposite side there must be an equal amount of disappearance or degradation of the boundary on that side if a state of equilibrium is to be maintained and the wall there is not to become unduly lengthened. It is not yet clear how this occurs.

Myelin

The plasma membranes of the oligodendrocytes of the central nervous system and of the neurolemmal (Schwann) cells of peripheral nerves make a unique contribution to the nerve fibres associated with these cells, for the myelin that surrounds so many axons and dendrites consists of plasma membrane that has become wound round and round the fibres in a spiral fashion. The more heavily myelinated the nerve fibre, the more spiral turns of membrane there are surrounding it. Myelin therefore consists, at the EM level, of closely-packed membrane lamellae, which give a characteristic pattern (periodicity) of alternating light and dark bands with a spacing or repeating distance between like bands of about 12–15 nm.

In peripheral nerves that are non-myelinated, the axons simply sink into the Schwann cell and remain surrounded

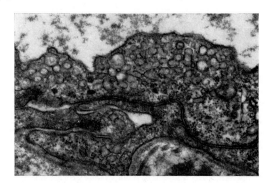

FIG. 8. Part of the lining of a small blood vessel, showing numerous pinocytic vesicles or caveolae in the endothelium. × 30,000.

by a single layer of plasma membrane (as in the earliest fetal stage of myelination) (fig. 9). In contrast to myelinated fibres, a dozen or more non-myelinated fibres may be enveloped by a single Schwann cell, but in both types of nerve the basal lamina remains as a general investment for the cell and does not follow the invaginated portions of membrane.

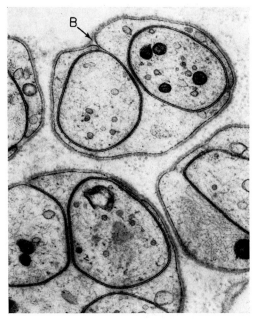

FIG. 9. Unmyelinated nerve fibres and Schwann cells. Each fibre has become surrounded by part of a Schwann cell plasma membrane, but the basal lamina external to the plasma membrane is not incorporated with the invaginating fibre and remains on the surface (as in B). × 14,250. (By courtesy of J. H. Kugler.)

NUCLEUS

In histological preparations the most obvious constituent of the average cell is its nucleus. It stains blue with haematoxylin and other basic dyes, because of its high content of nucleic acids (DNA and RNA) and is usually seen as a round or oval body about 4–10 μm. in diameter somewhere near the centre or base of the cell. Nearly all human cell types contain a single nucleus; the prominent exceptions are erythrocytes and the surface cells of stratified squamous keratinizing epithelia, which have none. Occasional cells (*e.g.* in the liver) are binucleate. Osteoclasts and some macrophages (foreign-body giant cells) may have tens or even hundreds of nuclei. The longer skeletal muscle cells probably have the most of all; they average 80 nuclei per millimetre of cell length, so that a cell with a length of 5 cm. will have about 4,000 nuclei. In skeletal muscle the nuclei are not situated in the central regions of the cells but lie characteristically immediately adjacent to the plasma membrane. The part of a neuron (nerve cell) that contains the nucleus is commonly called the cell body (or perikaryon) to distinguish this part of the cell from the remainder which is composed of processes (axons and dendrites). (The term neuron is often confusingly and erroneously used to refer to the cell body only, when in fact the term comprises both the cell body and all its processes.)

Nuclear Membrane

The nucleus is separated from the cytoplasm by the nuclear membrane (nuclear envelope). It consists of two

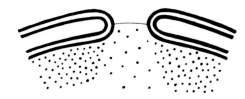

FIG. 10. A diagrammatic representation of the double nuclear membrane, enclosing the perinuclear space, and indicating the site of a nuclear pore.

membranes, each of typical trilaminar appearance and about 7–10 nm. thick, separated by a variable interval which is commonly about 30–50 nm. wide and electron-lucent—the perinuclear space (fig. 10). The two membranes are referred to as the inner and outer nuclear membranes, and they become continuous with one another at the margins of nuclear pores (figs. 10–13). These are unique features of the nuclear membrane, and in many nuclei have been shown to be arranged in a regular pattern. There may be as many as 65 pores per square micrometer of membrane surface, and they may occupy 10 per cent or so of that surface. Each is round (or perhaps octagonal) and about 40–60 nm. in diameter; the rim or margin of the pore may have a thickened appearance forming the annulus. Although acting as passages of communication between nucleus and cytoplasm, the pores are not simply gaps in the membrane, for in suitable preparations they are usually seen to be "closed" by a fine diaphragmatic structure which, in ways not yet understood, may control nucleocytoplasmic interchange. Furthermore, pores are not constant in number in any given nucleus, for they seem to vary with different physiological states.

The perinuclear space is sometimes observed to be in continuity with the cisternae of rough ER, and ribosomes may be found on the cytoplasmic surface of the outer nuclear membrane. (At the end of mitotic division, the new nuclear envelope is thought to be re-formed from ER.) The perinuclear space is another site for possible communication between the nucleus and the extranuclear world; the nuclear pores must not be considered the only such chan-

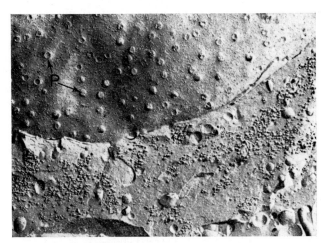

FIG. 11. A specimen prepared by the "freeze-cleave" technique showing numerous pores (as at P) in the nuclear membrane. × 14,250. (By courtesy of Professor A. S. Breathnach and the Editor of the British Journal of Dermatology).

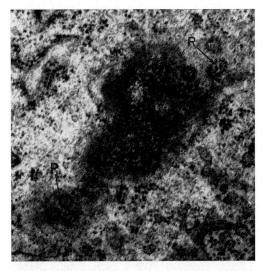

FIG. 12. A tangential section through the edge of a nucleus, showing (at P) three pores in the nuclear membrane viewed *en face*. A polysome with ribosomes arranged in spiral form is seen at R. × 30,000.

nels. Material may pass through the inner nuclear membrane into the perinuclear space and so into the ER, and *vice versa*.

Chromatin

Chromatin is a biochemical complex consisting mainly of DNA and histones (a group of proteins). DNA is the genetic material of the cell, and is localized in the chromosomes of the nucleus. In the resting (as opposed to the mitotic) nucleus, the chromosomes are not recognizable as

distinct entities, but are in the form of long threadlike structures, tangled up like an irregular ball of wool. Some parts of the threads may be coiled and stain deeply, giving a dense appearance to parts of the nucleus. This kind of chromatin is called heterochromatin, to distinguish it from

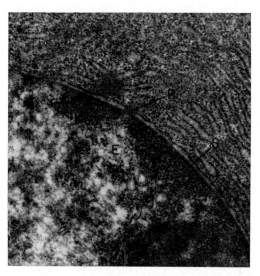

FIG. 13. Part of the nucleus of a serous secretory cell, showing areas of heterochromatin (H) and euchromatin (E), part of the nucleolus (N), a nuclear pore (P), and the double nuclear membrane with the intervening perinuclear space (S). × 30,000.

the lighter (uncoiled) areas which are said to consist of euchromatin. Thus a typical nucleus contains irregular masses of heterochromatin and euchromatin (fig. 13), representing aggregated and dispersed chromosomal material respectively. The heterochromatin often forms clumps adjacent to the plasma membrane, and if similar clumps extend towards the centre of the nucleus a "cartwheel" effect is obtained (a common feature of plasma cells). In those areas of the nucleus immediately opposite nuclear pores only euchromatin is present, so that a break in an otherwise dense mass of heterochromatin may indicate the site of a pore.

In some types of cell in the female, a particularly dense chromatic mass may be seen adhering to the inner surface of the nuclear membrane. This is the so-called sex chromatin, and is thought to represent one of the two X-chromosomes of the female which remains as a tightly coiled mass and does not disperse into a threadlike structure. It can usually be detected easily with the optical microscope in scrapings or sections of female buccal mucosa.

The DNA of the nucleus has two specific functions: it is concerned with: (1) cell division and reproduction, which involve replication of the DNA molecule (*i.e.* making an exact copy), and (2) growth and differentiation of the cell, which involve the transmission of the genetic message (that is encoded in the DNA) to RNA molecules. The term transcription refers to the synthesis of RNA on a single strand of DNA; this takes place in the nucleus. (The term translation refers to the assembly of a chain of amino acids to form a polypeptide (protein); this takes place at polysomes in the cytoplasm—see p. 80.)

In man there are 46 chromosomes (23 pairs, including the one pair of sex chromosomes) in a typical nucleus, and this total is referred to as the diploid number ($2n$). In germ cells (ova and spermatozoa) only one of each pair is present, the haploid number (n), so that if fertilization occurs the diploid state is restored. In preparation for division by mitosis, the DNA content of the nucleus doubles, so that the daughter cells will each possess a normal amount. The amount of DNA in any somatic nucleus in constant for any one species; in human nuclei it has been estimated as 6.5×10^{-6} g.

The genetic material in a cell nucleus is potentially capable of causing the cell to differentiate along any line of development; the information encoded in its DNA could theoretically result in a cell with all the characteristics of, say, a fibroblast, an odontoblast, a skeletal muscle cell and a neuron—all mixed up in one cell. In practice, only one group of features normally ensues in any one cell, because the genetic expression of all the other possible combinations has become suppressed. Most of the genetic material in a nucleus is not in fact allowed to express itself. In lower organisms such as bacteria various "operators", "regulators" and "repressors" have been described to explain how only particular parts of the genetic message are allowed to be transcribed. The whole story of this kind of genetic control in mammalian cells has yet to be worked out, but is obviously of fundamental importance in cell behaviour, both normal and pathological.

Nucleolus

The nucleolus is a densely-staining region of the nucleus that has a high content of RNA. Any one nucleus may contain several nucleoli; generally speaking, the more protein manufacture taking place in the cell, the greater the number. With the EM, the nucleolus is seen to have fibrillar and granular components—fibrils 6–8 nm. in thickness and granules 15 nm. in diameter. These appear to be the precursors of the RNA of ribosomes; the precursors leave the nucleus via the pores in the nuclear membrane, and when in the cytoplasm they combine to form true ribosomes. There is no membranous structure separating the nucleolus from the rest of the nucleus.

Not all the RNA of the nucleus is concentrated in the nucleolus; some of it is messenger RNA transcribed from the DNA of euchromatin.

ENDOPLASMIC RETICULUM

In many cells, especially those that are responsible for the secretion of protein, ER is a prominent feature. This organelle is recognized as a system of membranes which in sections appear as elongated closed sacs, tubules and vesicles of varying shapes and sizes (figs. 14–16). The spaces enclosed by the membranes are the cisternae of the ER, and when visualized in three dimensions (fig. 14) the cisternae form one continuous irregular space which is separated from the rest of the cytoplasm by the membrane of the ER. The internal space of the ER may be in continuity, at least in some functional states of the cell, with the

perinuclear space, and possibly with the cisternae of the Golgi apparatus, or even with the extracellular environment if the ER membranes join the plasma membrane. The membrane is of typical trilaminar appearance, about 7·0 nm. in thickness.

Two kinds of ER are described. One variety, known as rough or granular ER, is recognized by the presence of numerous ribosomes (see below) that are attached to the outer (cytoplasmic) surface of the membranous profiles; the other, the smooth or agranular ER, is devoid of ribosomes. In cells possessing quantities of rough ER, the protein manufactured by the ribosomes is passed into the cisternae of the ER through its membranes, so becoming segregated from the cytoplasm. These activities represent an early phase of secretion, hence any cells that are preparing protein material for export usually have large amounts of

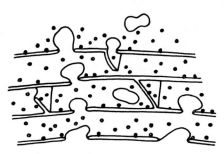

FIG. 14. A diagrammatic representation of endoplasmic reticulum, with ribosomes adhering to the outer surface of the membrane that forms the boundary of the cisternae. The unit (trilaminar) membrane is here indicated by a single line.

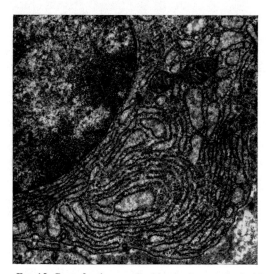

FIG. 15. Part of a plasma cell with cytoplasm packed with rough endoplasmic reticulum, mostly in the form of flattened cisternae. × 14,750.

rough ER. These include such apparently diverse cells as parotid or pancreatic exocrine cells producing enzymes, plasma cells (fig. 15) secreting antibody, fibroblasts (fig. 16) liberating tropocollagen molecules (the precursors of collagen fibrils), and osteoblasts, odontoblasts and ameloblasts preparing their specific matrices. In the epithelial cells of exocrine glands the rough ER is typically concentrated in the basal part of the cell, and in histological sections is responsible for the cytoplasmic basophilia seen with basic dyes. This kind of staining sometimes presents as small irregular areas in the cytoplasm, and in neurons under the optical microscope these received the name chromidial substance, Nissl substance or Nissl granules. All these terms are now known to indicate and refer to one and the same thing—rough ER, which itself is still sometimes called ergastoplasm.

When cells are homogenized, the rough ER breaks up and forms the rounded bodies known as microsomes—small vesicular-shaped fragments of ER membrane with

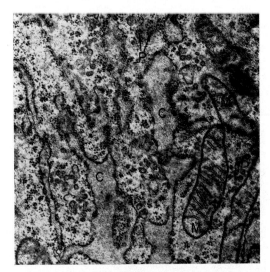

FIG. 16. Part of an active fibroblast, showing endoplasmic reticulum consisting of dilated cisternae (C). There are numerous ribosomes, attached to the outer surface of the cisternae and also lying free in the cytoplasm where they can be seen occasionally as polysomes in the form of spirals or rosettes (as at P). Mitochondria (M) are present on the right. × 30,000.

ribosomes still attached to the outer surface. Microsomes are therefore not normal cell organelles but an artefact of homogenization; they are used for analytical purposes since they can be separated from other components by ultracentrifugation.

The smooth variety of ER is functionally less well defined but more diverse. It is especially prominent in cells producing steroid hormones (adrenal cortex, endocrine cells of the testis), in sebaceous glands and in cells synthesizing glycogen (liver cells). In skeletal and cardiac muscle cells the smooth ER becomes known as the sarcoplasmic reticulum, and is part of the T-system of tubules concerned in impulse conduction.

GOLGI APPARATUS

The Golgi apparatus is a membranous system which in some respects resembles smooth ER (from which it is probably derived) in that it consists of flattened sacs and vesicles, but these are often closely stacked against one another in a somewhat curvilinear array giving a lamellated appearance (figs. 17 and 18). The Golgi membranes have

the common trilaminar form, but are usually rather thinner than plasma membrane or ER membrane, being about 6 nm. wide.

This organelle is a prominent feature in all kinds of secretory cells, for it is a region of segregation and packaging for newly synthesized products. In protein-secreting cells, the polypeptide chains manufactured by the ribosomes of the rough ER become transferred to the Golgi sacs. Sometimes there is evidence of direct continuity between the ER and the Golgi apparatus, but it is rare for this continuity to be "captured" in electron micrographs, and it seems that the common mode of transport from ER to Golgi sacs is by "transfer vesicles" which break off from the ER and pass through intervening cytoplasm to fuse with some part of the Golgi complex. In their turn, vacuoles loaded with the secretion product break off from the Golgi apparatus and pass as secretion granules towards the cell surface (fig. 18).

Apart from merely collecting and redistributing sub-

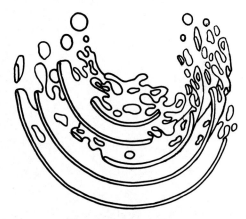

FIG. 17. A diagrammatic representation of the Golgi apparatus—a system of membranous sacs, parts of which may eventually break away as secretion granules. The unit (trilaminar) membrane is here indicated by a single line.

stances synthesized elsewhere, the Golgi apparatus itself can indulge in synthetic activity. In particular, it is the site of production of the carbohydrate fraction of the mucus molecule; the protein part from the rough ER is also here conjugated with the carbohydrate portion. In goblet cells, it has been estimated that one saccule is liberated from the Golgi stack every 2–4 min.

The Golgi apparatus is typically situated between the nucleus and the surface of the cell from which secretory products are to be discharged. Ameloblasts afford a good example of the functional locus of this organelle within the cell: before enamel matrix is laid down, the Golgi membranes and vesicles are poorly developed and lie on the stellate reticulum side of the cell, but when amelogenesis begins they increase in amount and move to the enamel-forming side. In most EM sections they usually appear as several discrete clumps in different regions of the supranuclear cytoplasm rather than as a single continuous entity. In three dimensions the whole complex can be visualized as a stack of curved saucers or basins with the hollow opening facing the surface of the cell from which secretion granules will be discharged (fig. 17). The outer surface of the complex is the "forming face" and receives the transfer vesicles, while the inner surface from which the secretion granules are derived is the "maturation face".

MITOCHONDRIA

Mitochondria are discrete membranous organelles that play a vital part in the oxidative metabolism of the cell, for they contain the citric acid cycle enzymes and the cytochromes required for the formation of ATP (see Chapter

cristae. These extend into the central part of the organelle which contains finely granular material of slight electron density—the mitochondrial matrix. The cristae may be sparse or closely packed, and usually form incomplete partitions for the matrix; it seems rare for them to stretch right across. Close inspection of the inner mitochondrial membrane and cristae at very high magnification reveals that their inner surfaces (those in contact with the matrix) are studded with large numbers of knoblike bodies, attached to the membrane by a thin short stalk. These are known as subunits or elementary particles, and are a unique feature

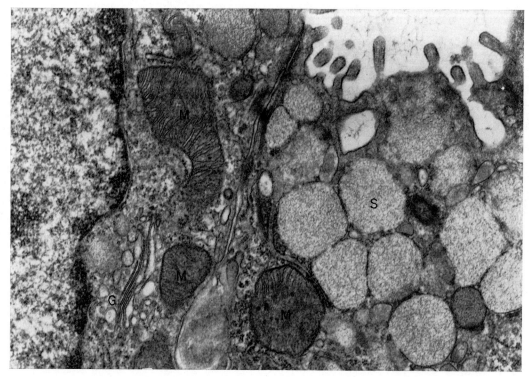

Fig. 18. Adjacent parts of two mucus-secreting cells, showing in one of them flattened sacs and vesicles of the Golgi apparatus (G), and in the other mucous granules (S) awaiting discharge from the apex. M, mitochondria. × 30,000.

7). They vary greatly in size and number; the largest can be seen with the optical microscope, but the EM is required to discern structural details. Many types of cell contain several hundred mitochondria; some liver cells (hepatocytes) and gastric parietal cells (secreting hydrochloric acid) may contain over two thousand; erythrocytes have none (their energy requirements being obtained by glycolysis).

Mitochondria (figs. 16 and 18) are often sausage-shaped but they may be more elongated and tubular, or round or oval. It is difficult to give average sizes, but they may range from 1–5 μm. or more in length and from 0·3–1·0 μm. wide. In skeletal muscle some are 10 μm. long. They consist of inner and outer membranes, both of which have a typical unit membrane appearance in EM sections and are about 6 nm. thick, separated by an interval of 8 nm. The percentages of protein and lipid in the outer membrane are 52 and 48 respectively, but in the inner the values are 76 and 24; there is very little carbohydrate in either. The outer mitochondrial membrane is smooth, but the inner one is thrown into numerous folds or corrugations known as

not found on any other unit membrane. A small number of round dense granules about 50 nm. in diameter may be scattered in the matrix.

In general, the greater the metabolic activity of the cell, the greater the number of mitochondria it possesses, or perhaps more accurately, the greater the area of the inner mitochondrial membrane and cristae. The cytochromes concerned with electron transport have been shown to be attached to the inner membrane, probably to the elementary particles, whereas the Krebs cycle enzymes are located in the matrix. In ameloblasts the matrix is particularly electron dense, but the significance of this is not known. The small dense granules of the matrix seem to be sites of cation concentration, especially calcium, but again the functional implications have not been revealed.

Mitochondria contain some DNA and RNA and are able to multiply by growth and division, but little is known about their formation de novo. How they may disappear is also a mystery, but at least some seem to be digested by lysosomes.

LYSOSOMES AND ASSOCIATED BODIES

The membranous organelles described so far were all known to the older histologists, albeit without precise knowledge of structural details, but lysosomes were only discovered in the 1950s.

They are round or oval cytoplasmic particles of up to

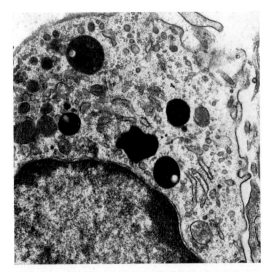

FIG. 19. Part of a monocyte, showing several lysosomes, the large dense bodies lying among other cytoplasmic constituents. The membrane bounding the lysosomes is not apparent at this magnification due to the density of their contents. × 15,000.

about 80 nm. in diameter bounded by a single trilaminar membrane, with contents that are heterogeneously dense and granular (fig. 19). They are probably derived from the Golgi apparatus, and are scattered in the cell cytoplasm. They are found in varying numbers in most cells; in liver cells, which are an abundant source, there may be 200 or more. Most of the granules in neutrophils are lysosomes. Biochemical analysis shows that they contain forty or more enzymes, mostly of a hydrolytic nature, such as acid phosphatase, cathepsin, β-glucosidase and β-glucuronidase. Lysosomes in fact act as storage organelles for these enzymes, segregating them from the rest of the cell, and in this form they are called primary lysosomes. Positive histochemical tests for these enzymes are usually taken as evidence for the presence of lysosomes, for which the EM is required for confirmation. Similarly, an organelle in an electron micrograph that is suspected of being a lysosome should strictly speaking only be identified as such if it can be shown to have an appropriate enzyme content.

Lysosomes are brought into functional activity when they unite with phagosomes (p. 73) containing material that has been ingested by the cell. The membranes of these two structures fuse and break down at their area of contact, so forming a single membrane-bound body, the secondary lysosome. The contained enzymes are then able to act upon and break down the ingested material. These biochemical reactions take place within a membrane-bound space so that there is no enzymatic degradation of the surrounding cell cytoplasm. Lysosomes have sometimes been called

"organelles of intracellular digestion". Why lysosomal enzymes do not normally digest their own surrounding membrane is, as they say, a good question that has not been precisely answered.

Secondary lysosomes may unite with additional phagosomes, but eventually their enzymatic activity ceases and they become known as residual bodies containing a variety of partially digested or indigestible debris. These may either remain in the cell or be discharged to be taken up by some other phagocyte.

Apart from dealing with material brought into the cell by phagosomes, lysosomes are also responsible for removing the cell's own damaged or unwanted organelles. They then become known as autophagic vacuoles or cytolysosomes. However the digestion of material taken up, phagocytosis, must not be considered the only function of lysosomes, for they are involved in many other activities. For example, in the thyroid the thyroglobulin stored in the colloid is absorbed into the thyroid cells where lysosomes release from it the active principles. In other endocrine organs, such as the anterior pituitary, lysosomes may remove secretion granules and so play a part in controlling the amount of hormone liberated.

A further variety of lysosome contains peroxidase, and for this reason is sometimes called a peroxisome, while yet another is distinguished by containing catalase and is known as a microbody (although this term is often used to embrace peroxisomes as well). Both are found especially in hepatocytes, renal tubule cells and macrophages; some of the lysosomes of polymorphonuclear leucocytes are peroxisomes.

ANNULATE LAMELLAE

These are among the least understood of all the organelles. Structurally they have features like those of both nuclear membrane and ER, for they consist of parallel rows or stacks of double membranes, each 7–9 nm. thick, the pairs being separated by a cisternal space 30–50 nm. in diameter. The double sheets of membrane are perforated at regular intervals (say, 150 nm.) by pores (about 75 nm. in diameter) formed by the union of the two membranes.

Annulate lamellae are typically but not exclusively found in male and female germ cells and in some tumour cells but so far their function is unknown. It is also not clear whether they are developed from nuclear membrane or ER, or whether they arise *de novo*.

RIBOSOMES

Ribosomes, the first of the non-membranous organelles in this discussion, are very small granular bodies, individually well beyond the resolving power of the optical microscope. However, aggregations of them are indicated histologically by cytoplasmic basophilia which is due to the ribosomes' own high content of protein, and to the fact that they are sites of protein synthesis.

A single ribosome is roughly shaped like a figure 8, with one part of the 8 being broader than the other. The whole article is about 25 nm. long and 15 nm. broad. In all but the higher-powered electron micrographs (say, less than ×100,000) the above shape is not apparent, and they present as very electron-dense roundish granules (figs. 14–16). They are either found scattered in the cytoplasm among the other organelles (free ribosomes), or attached to ER (attached ribosomes) forming the rough or granular type of this organelle (as described on p 76). Their precursors are present in the nucleoplasm and within the nucleolus (p. 76). Ribosomes contain about 85 per cent of the cell content of RNA.

Whether free or attached, ribosomes function not singly but in small groups or clusters of up to 50 or so, strung like beads on a strand of messenger RNA. Such a functional grouping is called a polysome or polyribosome (figs. 12 and 16), recognized in electron micrographs as a spiral or rosette-shaped arrangement of ribosomes (the RNA strand is not normally visible but has been observed when the EM is pushed to the limits of its resolving power). Amino acids are brought to the ribosomes by molecules of transfer RNA and assembled in the order dictated by the messenger RNA to form proteins. As a general rule, free ribosomes manufacture proteins for the cell's own metabolic needs, while the products of the attached variety are passed into the cisternae of the ER and destined for export from the cell.

FIBRILS

Many cells possess fibrillar or filamentous structures, sometimes apparently randomly scattered in the cytoplasm among other organelles, and sometimes in more definite patterns. They attain their highest degree of organization in striated muscle, where the filaments—collectively known as myofilaments—are arranged in the characteristic interdigitating bundles to form myofibrils which in turn lie in phase with one another in the cell cytoplasm to produce the well-known transverse striations of skeletal and cardiac muscle. The filaments here are mainly of the two proteins actin and myosin. The myosin filaments are about $1 \cdot 5 \mu m$. long and 10 nm. wide, while actin filaments (which are attached at one end to the so-called Z-line) are about the same length but only 5 nm. thick. Visceral (smooth) muscle cells do not show transverse striations, but it is important to appreciate that they do contain both actin and myosin. What is not yet known is exactly how these contractile proteins are arranged to produce shortening of the visceral muscle cell. Actin filaments lie longitudinally and are probably responsible for the finely fibrillar appearance of visceral muscle cytoplasm, but it seems that the visualization of myosin with the EM requires specialized preparative techniques that have only recently been developed.

The filaments of non-muscular cells do not present a striated pattern. Some have been shown to be composed of actin but the chemistry of others is unknown. Fibroblasts and macrophages among other cells display in suitable EM sections bundles of filaments that are often concentrated near the plasma membrane, and are probably responsible for localized areas of membrane motion, as in amoeboid or pseudopodial movement. In many epidermal and oral epithelial cells filaments may be seen converging on desmosomes (as described on p. 70), and in these stratified epithelia they are often known as tonofibrils (fig. 20). Fine filaments of unknown composition and commonly called microfibrils or microfilaments are a feature of such structures as odontoblast and ameloblast processes, intestinal microvilli (p. 69) and neurons, where they may have a role in the preservation of shape, like certain microtubules (below).

MICROTUBULES

The cytoplasmic elements known as microtubules probably play a mainly supporting role in many cells. However,

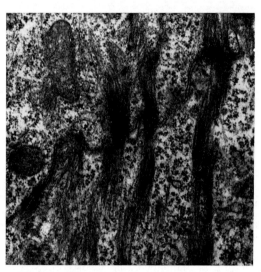

FIG. 20. Tonofibrils in epidermal cells. × 30,000.

some specialized tubular structures are concerned with movement.

The microtubules that are thought to act as an internal scaffolding are hollow unbranched cylinders of varying length (maybe several μm.) and a diameter of about 25 nm. The wall is electron-dense, not of trilaminar appearance and about 5 nm. thick, and the inside of the cylinder is electron-lucent. Probably the best examples are found in the processes of odontoblasts, and also in neuronal processes (axons and dendrites), where they are thought to assist in the preservation of shape and are often called neurotubules. They may also act as conduits for material passing along the processes (axonal flow). Microtubules are a prominent feature of the mitotic spindle formed during cell division.

Contractile forms of microtubule have already been mentioned in connection with cilia (p. 69), and another variety is found in centrioles.

CENTRIOLES

In many cells a pair of organelles, centrioles, can be found in a region of the cytoplasm known as the centrosome or cytocentrum and situated near the nucleus. In suitable sections they are detectable with the optical microscope as small dots, but the EM reveals that they are cylindrical, measuring about 0·5–2 μm. long and 0·15 μm. wide. They are usually close together and at right-angles to one another. Each centriole is composed of nine microtubular structures, each of which consists of three microtubular subunits, the one nearest the centre of the organelle having a pair of short arms. Each subunit is 25 nm. in diameter, with a wall 4·5 nm. thick which does not exhibit the trilaminar membranous appearance. The central area of the centriole is more electron-dense than the surrounding cytoplasm, but in the latter immediately adjacent to the centriole there are often small dense bodies called satellites which may provide precursor material for new centrioles.

Before mitotic division of the nucleus, the original two centrioles duplicate and a pair moves to opposite ends of the nucleus where they form the poles of the mitotic spindle. The origin of cilia from centrioles has already been described (p. 69), but much remains to be discovered about how centrioles reproduce themselves and what the controlling mechanisms are. It should be noted that while the compound microtubular structure consists of three subunits and a pair of arms, the peripheral filament of a cilium has only two subunits and a pair of arms.

SECRETION GRANULES

It has been described in earlier sections how secretory material becomes packaged by the Golgi apparatus, resulting in the formation of membrane-bound "granules" (fig. 18). The word granule has an air of solidity about it, especially when many methods of histological and EM preparation make vesicular contents appear dense, but in life secretory products are fluid and the discharged products from a cell must not be imagined as solid pill-like bodies. Secretion granules vary greatly in size in different types of cell, although any one type seems to have its own characteristic size. The main point to appreciate is that in endocrine cells they remain relatively small, say up to 300 nm. in diameter, whereas in exocrine cells they are larger, up to 1 μm. or more.

Most secretory material is liberated from cells by a process known as exocytosis, wherein the membrane that bounds the granule becomes fused with the plasma membrane, so allowing the release of the contained material. This is the mode of discharge of most secretory products, whether exocrine or endocrine, and in endocrine organs is sometimes called reverse pinocytosis. Thus, the zymogen granules of the parotid, insulin from the pancreatic islets and steroid hormones from the adrenal cortex are all liberated in this way, as are the neurotransmitter substances at synapses and motor endplates. The production of export material by neurons, whether synaptic or substances such as those derived from the hypothalamic cells associated with pituitary control, constitutes neurosecretion. The fusion of the boundary membranes of granules with the plasma membrane would lead to a great increase in the area of the plasma membrane, and there must be some way (not yet defined) by which membranous material is destroyed so that the cell surface maintains equilibrium.

The old histology terms apocrine and merocrine secretion, which dealt rather fancifully with the amount of apical-cell cytoplasm that was apparently lost, have no precise meaning in terms of what we now know about secretion at the EM level, and they should be abandoned. The sister term holocrine secretion may perhaps be retained, for here the whole cell breaks up to discharge its products and so dies; it can only be replaced by the formation of a new cell by division and differentiation of those that remain. Continuous holocrine secretion thus depends on a pattern of cell death and replacement, and in man is unique to the sebaceous glands.

Autoradiographic studies with labelled precursors (such as tritiated amino acids) have shown that in typical serous-secreting cells the time taken for synthesis of an enzyme and its discharge into the lumen of the gland is about 45 min. This period includes the time required for the precursor material to enter the cell cytoplasm, for it to be incorporated into a polypeptide chain by polysomes, segregated into cisternae of the ER, passed to the Golgi apparatus and finally to be packaged as a secretion granule whose boundary membrane fuses with the apical cell membrane. The ground substance of connective tissue is secreted by fibroblasts (e.g. in healing wounds) in a similar manner via the Golgi apparatus which is where the carbohydrate part of the mucopolysaccharide molecule is added to the protein fraction (p. 77), but it is possible that tropocollagen molecules (the precursors of collagen fibrils) are liberated from the fibroblasts after passing through the ER cisternae only. In this way the Golgi apparatus is bypassed; collagen precursors are not observed to be part of the typical secretion granules and indeed their mode of discharge from the fibroblast is not clear. Possibly because fibroblasts are not polarized, as gland cells are with a base and apex, some kind of "round-the-clock" discharge from any part of the cell surface is more appropriate for a free connective-tissue cell. However, in the processes of odontoblasts, which certainly are polarized, there are elongated granules and vesicles which have been shown to contain collagen precursors that have passed through the Golgi apparatus. Ameloblast processes contain the more typical rounded form of secretion granule.

STORAGE GRANULES, PIGMENTS AND CRYSTALS

Apart from secretion granules, which are usually destined for fairly rapid export from the cell, other granular or globular inclusions may be found such as glycogen granules or fat globules. These may be stored for varying periods ranging from perhaps a few minutes or hours in the case of glycogen in liver or muscle cells to the lipid of adipose tissue cells which may persist for months or years (although the "turnover rate" of stored material may be greater than is often supposed).

Crystals are another form of cellular inclusion, but in normal human tissue are rather uncommon. (The crystalline structures in teeth and bone are extracellular.) The best examples are in the granules of eosinophils, in the β cells (insulin-secreting) of the pancreatic islets, and in certain testicular cells.

Pigments may be mentioned as a final group of inclusions, the most obvious being melanin in the epidermis, iris and certain cells of the central nervous system. Others include breakdown product of haemoglobin, in particular haemosiderin which contains iron and is found in macrophages of the liver, spleen and bone marrow. Lipofuscin is a brownish pigment that increases in amount with age especially in liver, nerve and cardiac muscle cells, and is often a constituent of lysosomes. Carbon particles from inspired dust are taken up by pulmonary macrophages and cause varying degrees of pigmentation in the lung.

THE LIVING CELL

The examination of tissue sections with the microscope in itself reveals little of the dynamic state of the cell. We may see secretion granules or myofibrils or lysosomes, but our concept of function usually requires a combination of techniques so that dimensions of time as well as space can be brought into our formulation of what is going on. The constant coming and going of molecules through membranes, enzyme reactions that occur in fractions of a second, the formation and disruption of vesicles, mitochondria and lysosomes—all these cellular activities normally take place in a purposeful manner but under control mechanisms that are largely unknown. We have seen how much of cell life depends on membranes, and although something of their structure and function has been gleaned from biochemical and biophysical methods, their mode of formation is still not clear. Autoradiographic studies have been of immense value in helping to visualize the rate of some cellular processes, and time-lapse cinematography of cells in culture can give a vivid impression of membranous and cytoplasmic movement. The microscope in all its forms provides an interpretation of the structure of life, but to bring life into structure the viewer of cells in sections must not forget to appreciate that in order to produce a living body cells become organized into tissues, and that the static microscope picture must be mentally translated into one of continuous activity.

REFERENCES

Beck, F. and Lloyd, J. B. (Eds.) (1974), *The Cell in Medical Science*, 4 vols. London and New York: Academic Press.
Bittar, E. E. (Ed.) (1973), *Cell Biology in Medicine*. New York: John Wiley & Sons.
Bloom, W. and Fawcett, D. W. (1975), *A Textbook of Histology*, 10th edition. Philadelphia: W. B. Saunders Co.
Danielli, J. F. and Davson, H. A. (1935), "A Contribution to the Theory of Permeability of Thin Films," *J. cell. comp. Physiol.* **5**, 495.
Giese, A. C. (1973), *Cell Physiology*, 4th edition. Philadelphia: W. B. Saunders Co.
Greep, R. O. and Weiss, L. (1973), *Histology*, 3rd edition. New York: McGraw-Hill Book Co.
Ham, A. W. (1974), *Histology*, 7th edition. Philadelphia and Toronto: J. B. Lippincott Co.
Robertson, J. D. (1957), "The Cell Membrane Concept," *J. Physiol.*, **140**, 58.
Schleiden, M. J. (1838), "Beiträge zur Phytogenesis," *Archiv fur Anatomie, Physiologie und wissenschaftliche Medicin*, p. 137.
Schwann, T. (1839), *Mikroskopische Untersuchungen über die Uebereinstimmung in der Struktur und dem Wachsthum der Thiere und Pflanzen*. Berlin: G. E. Reimer.
Toner, P. G. and Carr, K. E. (1971), *Cell Structure. An Introduction to Biological Electron Microscopy*, 2nd edition. Edinburgh and London: Churchill Livingstone.
Virchow, R. (1858), *Die Cellularpathologie in ihrer Begründung auf physiologische und pathologische Gewebelehre*. Berlin: A. Hirschwald.

7. CELL CHEMISTRY

G. H. SLOANE-STANLEY

The need for metabolism
  The small molecules involved
  Cellular energy: adenosine triphosphate

The production of adenosine triphosphate
  Glucose entry and activation
  Glycolysis to pyruvate or lactate

  Acetyl-coenzyme-A formation
  The citrate cycle
  Oxidative phosphorylation
  Fatty acid and ketone body oxidation

The Use of ATP
  Some obvious functions
    Cell movement

Ion extrusion
Emergency energy stores
Cell maintenance
  Carbohydrates
    Gluconeogenesis
    Glycogen
    Proteoglycans, glycoproteins and glycolipids
  Lipids
  Proteins
    Amino-acid metabolism
    Polypeptide synthesis
    Ribonucleic acids
    Protein maturation and structure
      Chemical alterations
      The conformational effects of chemistry
      Secondary, tertiary and quaternary structures

The chemistry of cell structures

Cellular identity and the nucleus
  Deoxyribonucleic acids
  Ribonucleic acid supply
  Deoxyribonucleic acid replication
  Genes and DNA

THE NEED FOR METABOLISM

All living human cells are fundamentally very much alike; most strikingly, they use energy all the time, at a minimum average rate equivalent to heating themselves

TABLE 1

SOME SMALL IONS AND MOLECULES
OF
EXTRACELLULAR AND INTRACELLULAR FLUIDS

Substance	Approx. Concentration (mM)	
	Extracellular	Intracellular
Na$^+$	150	10
K$^+$	5	150
Ca^{2+}	2	0–1
Mg^{2+}	1	8
Cl$^-$	105	0–10
HCO$_3$$^-$	27	9
SO$_4$$^{2-}$	0·5	8
H$_2$PO$_4$$^-$ + HPO$_4$$^{2-}$	1	5–10
Glucose	4·5	1
Amino acids	4	30

through about 1°C per hour (*i.e.* 1 cal./g./hr.). They must use some for "work," ranging from the obvious perpetual activity of the heart down to the continuous slow excretion

of mucus and the endless rebuilding of bones and epithelia, and some to keep themselves warm; but they need much of this substantial power-turnover just to keep themselves alive.

The reason why cells need energy for their mere living survival seems to be that their activities change so much with time, their structures are so complex and delicate and their internal chemistry so different from that outside (Table 1), that their parts are constantly degraded and must therefore be constantly re-formed: even a cell in a museum preparation, dead, deformed and functionless, will deteriorate quite quickly if the preservative fails. Not the least of every cell's needs is to keep its working and fuel-converting parts ready for maximum output: some human cells can vary their energy-consumption at least a hundred-fold.

The energy balance of a cell can be trisected into production, use for work, and use for maintenance. Most human cells can produce energy by: the partial breakdown of **glucose** or **glycogen** to **pyruvate,** called **glycolysis,** which yields little energy but can be "self-supporting" in the absence of oxygen, when the pyruvate is eliminated as **lactate;** or, in the presence of oxygen, the complete **oxidation** of this pyruvate to carbon dioxide and water, which yields a great deal of energy; or the equally efficient oxygen-requiring combustions of **fatty acids** or of **ketone bodies** to carbon dioxide and water. Glucose, pyruvate and ketone bodies are often derived from **amino acids.**

The Small Molecules Involved

A brief outline of the chemistry of glucose, the fatty acids and the ketone bodies is shown in fig. 1. The "hexagonal" structure of glucose, shown as though seen from somewhat above one side, is that nearest to the form in which most molecules spend most of their time, although glucose's space-filling properties would probably be best represented by a picture of a small cumulus cloud. The rectangular diagram is still found in some books because it is easy to print, but antedates the discovery of actual molecular shapes and is not correct. The "open-chain" structure represents a stage through which all free glucose molecules pass (probably in a bent form) in their continual interconversion from the α- to the β-form: it also shows the **aldehyde group** which gives glucose its **reducing** power (see also **acetaldehyde** in fig. 1), because it can easily be oxidized by, i.e. take up oxygen from, some other substance such as copper oxide, which is thus **reduced** to metallic copper (Fehling's solution), while the aldehyde group becomes a **carboxylic acid group** (see **acetic acid** and fatty acids in fig. 1). The other obvious characteristic of glucose is its fringe of -OH groups, called **hydroxyls.** These are also described as **alcoholic groups** (see ethyl alcohol = **ethanol** and isopropylalcohol = isopropanol in fig. 1) and can be oxidized: that on carbon atom No. 6 (-CH$_2$-OH, called **primary**) to an aldehyde, which can in turn be oxidized to a carboxylic acid, as for ethanol → acetaldehyde → acetic acid in fig. 1, while any of the others (> CHOH, called **secondary**) can only be oxidized to **ketone groups** (> C = O, cf. isopropanol → **acetone** in fig. 1).

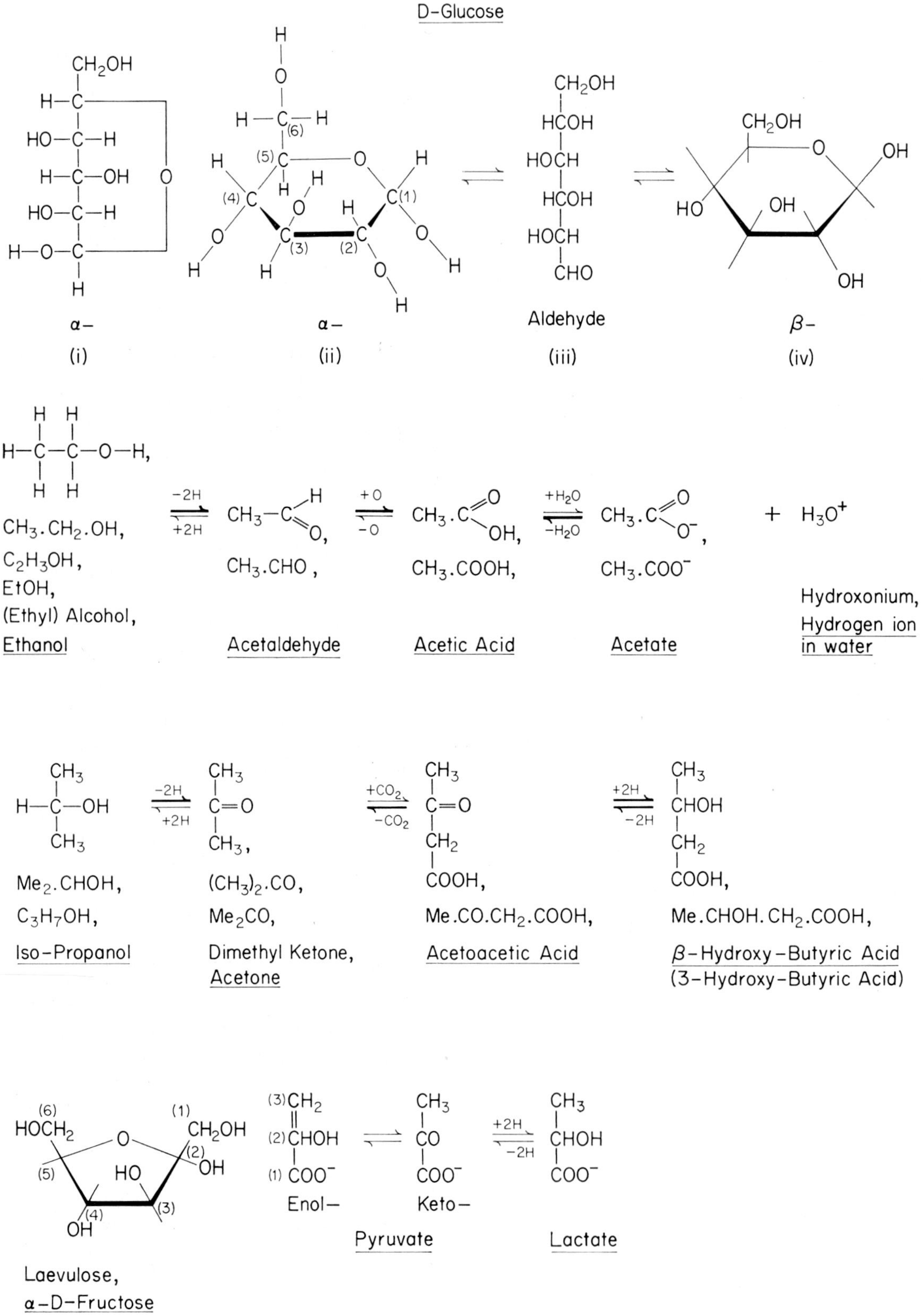

D-Glucose

CH₂OH

α–
(i)

α–
(ii)

Aldehyde
(iii)

β–
(iv)

CH₃.CH₂.OH,
C₂H₅OH,
EtOH,
(Ethyl) Alcohol,
Ethanol

CH₃.CHO,

Acetaldehyde

CH₃.COOH,

Acetic Acid

CH₃.COO⁻,

Acetate

+ H₃O⁺

Hydroxonium,
Hydrogen ion
in water

Me₂.CHOH,
C₃H₇OH,

Iso-Propanol

(CH₃)₂.CO,
Me₂CO,

Dimethyl Ketone,
Acetone

Me.CO.CH₂.COOH,

Acetoacetic Acid

Me.CHOH.CH₂.COOH,

β–Hydroxy–Butyric Acid
(3–Hydroxy–Butyric Acid)

Laevulose,
α–D–Fructose

Enol–

Keto–
Pyruvate

Lactate

Fɪɢ. 1.

Carbohydrates generally are given names ending in **-ose;** they are polyhydroxylic alcohols mostly with terminal reducing groups. Glucose, with an aldehyde group in the open chain form, is called an **aldose,** sometimes an aldo**pyranose** because of its 6-membered ring structure, while **fructose,** another reducing sugar whose open-chain structure ends in the ketonic group $-\overset{\parallel}{\underset{O}{C}}-CH_2OH$ is called

a keto**furanose** for its 5-membered ring.

The fatty acids are both chemically and metabolically related to acetic acid, and react reversibly with water in the same way (fig. 1), by **dissociation (ionization)** into positively charged hydrogen ions (**cations**) and negatively charged **carboxylate anions,** so called because they move towards the positive pole of a battery (from the Greek for "wanderer", "down" and "up" respectively); hydrogen ions in fact react much more readily with fatty carboxylates than water does with undissociated fatty acids (see below). Water itself, the main component (about 75 per cent by weight) of all our cells, ionizes very weakly on its own: $2 H_2O \rightleftharpoons H_3O^+ + OH^-$, OH^- being called the **hydroxyl ion.** In pure **neutral** water, with no extra acid (source of hydrogen ions) nor **base** (source of hydroxyl ions), the concentration of H_3O^+, which is a good measure of acidity and can be written $[H_3O^+]$, is equal to $[OH^-]$ at about 10^{-7} M, where M = **molar,** *i.e.* **moles,** Mol. (= gm. — molecular weights) per litre. The atomic weight of hydrogen being called 1 Dalton by convention, that of oxygen can be shown to be 16 Daltons, so that 1 mole (gm.-ion) of H_3O^+ weighs 19 gm. Concentrations are often, alternatively, expressed as **normalities:** 1 N means 1 gm.-**equivalent** (1 Eq.) per litre, the equivalent weight of a molecule, ion or atom being the molecular (ionic, atomic) weight divided by the valency for the reaction being considered; thus from a purely ionic viewpoint, **sulphate,** SO_4^{2-}, m.w. 96 has an e.w. of 48, while **ferric** iron, Fe^{3+}, a.w. 55·8, has an e.w. of 18·6 and **ferrous** iron, Fe^{2+}, has e.w. 27·9.

Since $[H_3O^+]$ can vary enormously under entirely practical conditions — 10^5-fold in the human body — acidity is usually expressed as the numerically more convenient quantity **pH** = $-\log_{10}[H_3O^+]$; then a neutral solution has a pH of 7, and gastric juice has pH $\leq$ 2. Most cells probably have an internal pH of about 6·8, *i.e.* are a little more acid than blood (pH 7·4); in either of these places, fatty acids in physiological concentrations are almost entirely in the anionic forms acetate, oleate and the like, since $[H_3O^+]$ is too low to re-form any significant proportion of undissociated —COOH groups.

The hydrogen ion can exist, though not in water, as a naked proton, H^+; this symbol is often used instead of the correct H_3O^+, for brevity and to simplify equations, as will be done frequently below.

The strength (tendency to dissociate) of an acid is indicated by its pK; pK = $-\log_{10}$ Ka, where

$$Ka = \frac{[H_3O^+][Anion^-]}{[Undissociated\ Acid]},$$

$[H_2O]$ being large and constant. An acid's pK is therefore the pH at which a dilute solution is half-dissociated, when $[Anion^-]$ = [Undissociated Acid], and is lower the stronger the acid; fatty acids have pKs about 5. Cells' most important mineral acid, **phosphoric,** is also relatively weak: $H_3PO_4 + H_2O \rightleftharpoons H_3O^+ + H_2PO_4^-$, pK 2·1, followed by $H_2PO_4^- + H_2O \rightleftharpoons H_3O^+ + HPO_4^{2-}$, pK 7·2, then $HPO_4^{2-} + H_2O \rightleftharpoons H_3O^+ + PO_4^{3-}$, pK 11·8. The really strong acids are always fully ionized in water (*e.g.* $HCl + H_2O \rightarrow H_3O^+ + Cl^-$), as are **salts** and **alkalis** even when solid (*e.g.* Potassium acetate, $K^+ CH_3COO^-$; sodium hydroxide = caustic soda, $Na^+ OH^-$; **choline** hydroxide, $HO.CH_2.CH_2.NMe_3^+ OH^-$).

Weak bases such as **ammonia** and **amines** (NH_3, RNH_2 primary, R_2NH secondary or **imines,** R_3N tertiary) generate hydroxyl ions by reacting with water ($NH_3 + H_2O \rightleftharpoons NH_4^+ + OH^-$) or combine directly with hydrogen ions ($RNH_2 + H^+ \rightarrow RNH_3^+$). Oxyacids (*i.e.* acids ionizing: $R-O-H \rightleftharpoons R-O^- + H^+$) can be condensed with such bases, losing water and forming **amides** such as $CH_3-\overset{\parallel}{\underset{O}{C}}-NH_2$, $CH_3.CONH_2$, **acetamide;** *N*-acetyl-galac-tosamine, chondrosamine (fig. 12, p. 96) and **phospho-creatine** (fig. 9, p. 93); but these reactions require considerable energy.

An organic molecule can also have both acidic and basic (**amino, imino**) groups at once, as in the amino-acids such as **glycine,** amino-acetic acid, $H_2N.CH_2.COOH$; they are in fact almost always fully ionized, as though $H_2N.CHR.COOH \rightarrow H_2N.CHR.COO^- + H^+ \rightarrow H_3N^+.CHR.COO^-$. The structures of the extremely important α-(2-) amino-acids ("α-", "2-" refer to the position of the NH_3^+-carrying C atom relative to the COO^- group) from which cells make proteins are given in fig. 2, which also shows the principles of the formation and structure of "an amino-acid amide of another amino-acid," *i.e.* a **peptide;** the bond between them is called a peptide bond.

The ketone bodies (fig. 1), metabolically derived from fatty and amino acids, conventionally include β-**hydroxy-butyrate** because it is made from and turned into **aceto-acetate,** some of which further decomposes to acetone and CO_2.

All acids can condense with alcohols to give **esters** such as ethyl sulphate, $C_2H_5.O.SO_3H$, or ethyl acetate, usually written $CH_3.COO.Et$ or EtOAc, where "Et" means an **ethyl** group, $-C_2H_5$ ("Me" = **methyl,** $-CH_3$) and "Ac" means an **acetyl** group, $CH_3.CO-$ ($H_3C-\overset{\parallel}{\underset{O}{C}}-$).

Oxyacids can be condensed with any other acids, to form **anhydrides,** such as **acyl** anhydrides $R.CO-O-OC.R$ (*e.g.* Acetic anhydride, Ac_2O, $Ac \sim Ac$), **pyrophosphates** $RO-PO_2^- -O-PO_2^- -OR$, $RO- \circledP \sim \circledP -OR$ ($\circledP$ = phosphate) or **acyl phosphates,** $R.CO-O-PO_3H^-$ (*e.g.* $Ac \sim \circledP$), which have strong tendencies to regain water and re-form the free acids (*e.g.* $H_2P_2O_7^{2-}$, inorganic pyrophosphate, $\circledP \sim \circledP$, "PP_i", $+ H_2O \rightarrow 2H_2PO_4^-$, inorganic ortho-phosphate, "P_i"), so that this reaction gives out energy.

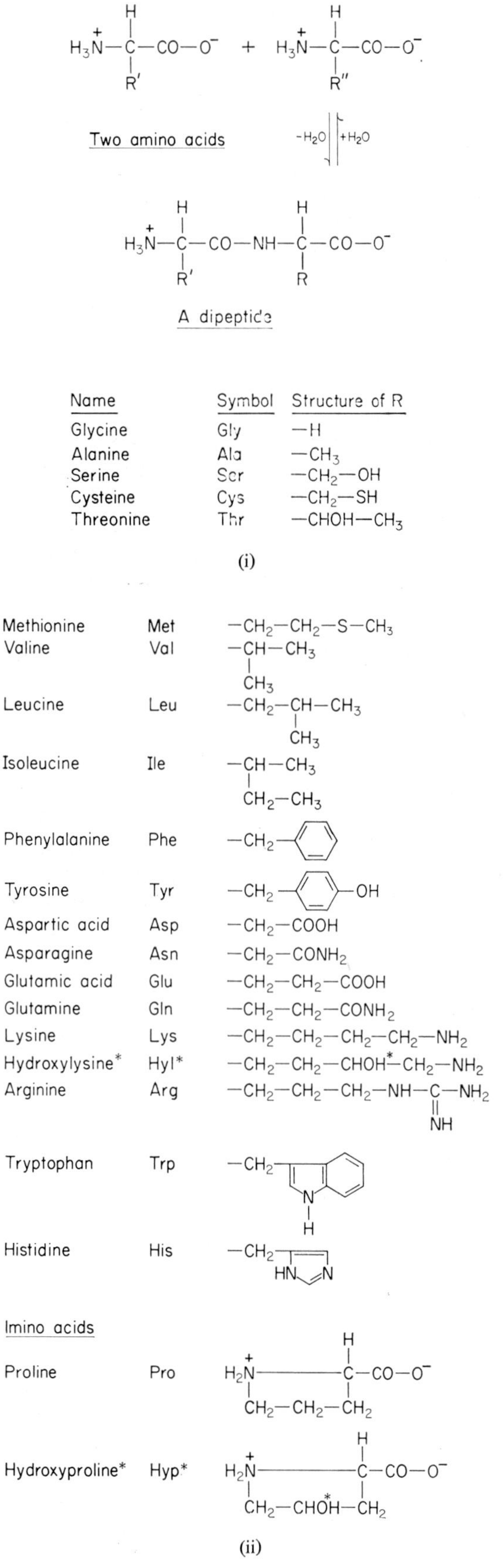

$$H_3\overset{+}{N}-\overset{\overset{\displaystyle H}{|}}{\underset{\underset{\displaystyle R'}{|}}{C}}-CO-O^- \quad + \quad H_3\overset{+}{N}-\overset{\overset{\displaystyle H}{|}}{\underset{\underset{\displaystyle R''}{|}}{C}}-CO-O^-$$

Two amino acids $-H_2O \;|\; +H_2O$

$$H_3\overset{+}{N}-\overset{\overset{\displaystyle H}{|}}{\underset{\underset{\displaystyle R'}{|}}{C}}-CO-NH-\overset{\overset{\displaystyle H}{|}}{\underset{\underset{\displaystyle R}{|}}{C}}-CO-O^-$$

A dipeptide

Name	Symbol	Structure of R
Glycine	Gly	$-H$
Alanine	Ala	$-CH_3$
Serine	Ser	$-CH_2-OH$
Cysteine	Cys	$-CH_2-SH$
Threonine	Thr	$-CHOH-CH_3$

(i)

Methionine	Met	$-CH_2-CH_2-S-CH_3$
Valine	Val	$-CH-CH_3$ with CH_3
Leucine	Leu	$-CH_2-CH-CH_3$ with CH_3
Isoleucine	Ile	$-CH-CH_3$ with CH_2-CH_3
Phenylalanine	Phe	$-CH_2-\langle ring\rangle$
Tyrosine	Tyr	$-CH_2-\langle ring\rangle-OH$
Aspartic acid	Asp	$-CH_2-COOH$
Asparagine	Asn	$-CH_2-CONH_2$
Glutamic acid	Glu	$-CH_2-CH_2-COOH$
Glutamine	Gln	$-CH_2-CH_2-CONH_2$
Lysine	Lys	$-CH_2-CH_2-CH_2-CH_2-NH_2$
Hydroxylysine*	Hyl*	$-CH_2-CH_2-CHOH^*-CH_2-NH_2$
Arginine	Arg	$-CH_2-CH_2-CH_2-NH-\underset{\underset{NH}{\|}}{C}-NH_2$
Tryptophan	Trp	$-CH_2-\langle indole ring\rangle$
Histidine	His	$-CH_2-\langle imidazole ring\rangle$

Imino acids

Proline	Pro	$H_2\overset{+}{N}-\overset{\overset{\displaystyle H}{|}}{C}-CO-O^-$ with $CH_2-CH_2-CH_2$
Hydroxyproline*	Hyp*	$H_2\overset{+}{N}-\overset{\overset{\displaystyle H}{|}}{C}-CO-O^-$ with $CH_2-CHOH^*-CH_2$

(ii)

FIG. 2. General and particular structures of amino-acids and peptides.

These compounds are therefore called "energy-rich", the readily-**hydrolysed** bonds being indicated in shortened formulae by "∼", "squiggle", the symbol of the **energy-rich bond.** There are several types, but the one most important to cells is the $\rightarrow P-O-P\leftarrow$ bond found in pyrophosphates and the higher ("meta"-) phosphates containing 3 or more phosphate groups linked anhydridically, and their esters.

Cellular Energy: Adenosine Triphosphate

The energy derived from cells' foods is indeed provided and used, for function and maintenance, mainly as one energy-rich substance called **adenosine triphosphate,** ATP (fig. 3). This is as true of bacteria, protozoa, plants and invertebrates as it of humans—even viruses can only replicate with its aid—which makes ATP the universal intracellular energy-currency *par excellence.* Its business end is a tri-meta phosphate, esterified to C-5 of the 5-carbon sugar (**pentose**) called **ribose,** which is in turn linked via its reducing group on C-1 (**glycosidically**) to the **purine**-type base **adenine.**

Cells' energy-using processes are adapted to use the pyrophosphate-bond energy of ATP without wasting much, although if hydrolysed non-enzymically ATP loses all its bond-energy as heat. The whole compound, like its analogues of which more anon, is called a **nucleotide** because it is related to **nucleic acids,** while the adenosine part (sugar + base only) is called a **nucleoside.** Figure 3 (insert) also indicates the structure of **deoxy-ATP,** dATP, an essential precursor of **deoxyribonucleic acids** (see p. 102). The first functional hydrolysis-product of ATP, from which it is most easily re-formed, is adenosine **diphosphate** (ADP, fig. 3); the further breakdown of ADP to **adenylate** (adenosine monophosphate, AMP, fig. 3) is little if at all used by cells, although it should yield about as much energy. The precise energy-yield from the hydrolysis of ATP to ADP and P_i depends on the conditions, but a useful approximation is 10 kcal./mole. The main alternative functional hydrolysis-products of the nucleoside triphosphates are combined forms of the monophosphates, and PP_i; since the latter is also energy-rich, these reactions are often truly reversible, but are usually driven to completion by the rapid hydrolysis of PP_i to 2 P_i (figs. 10, 11 and 18). All pyrophosphates, but especially nucleoside triphosphates and PP_i, bind bivalent cations like Ca^{2+} and Mg^{2+}, which of course largely discharge them; indeed Mg^{2+} is usually essential to the activities of enzymes metabolising them.

THE PRODUCTION OF ADENOSINE TRIPHOSPHATE

Glucose Entry and Activation

Although many types of human cell get most of their energy most of the time from the combustion of fatty acids or ketone-bodies and even the brain can adapt to doing so, few function at their best in the absence of glucose, which

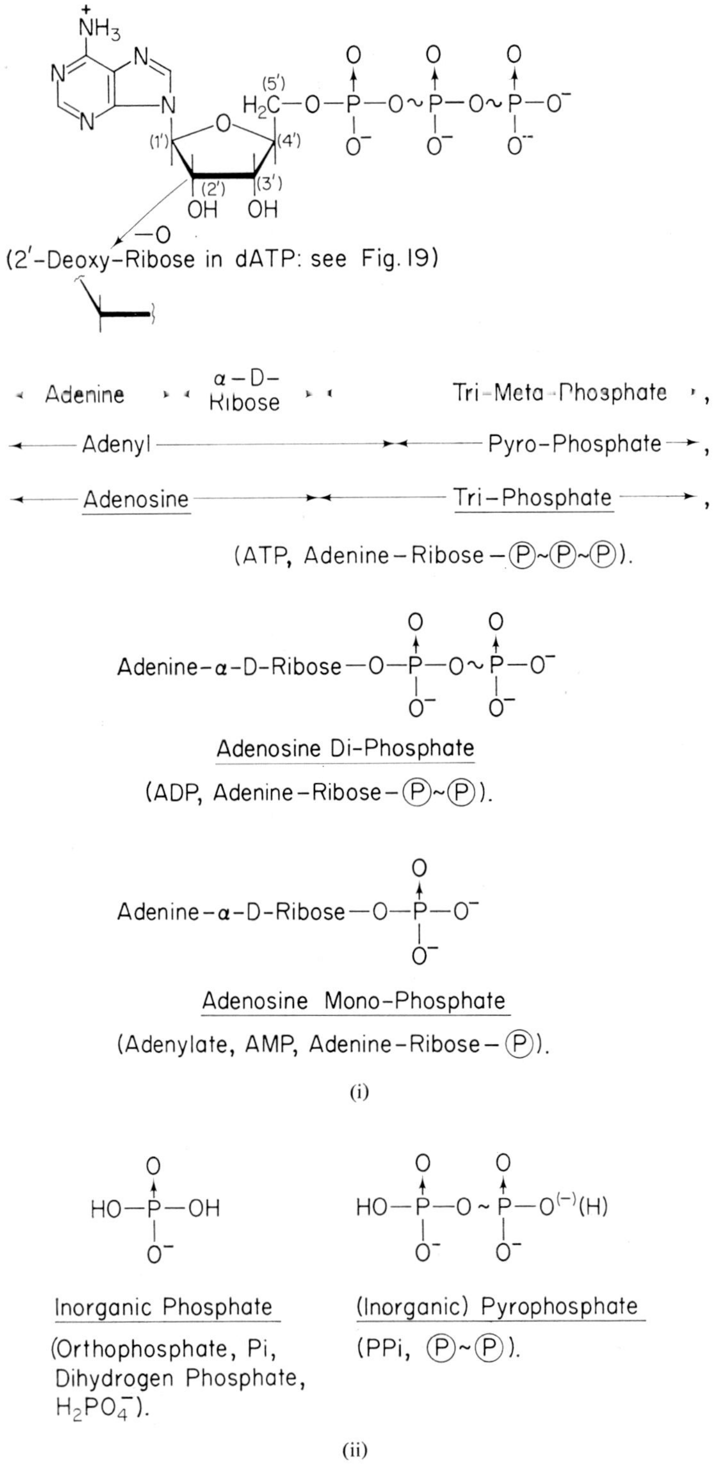

(2'-Deoxy-Ribose in dATP: see Fig. 19)

Adenine · α-D-Ribose · Tri-Meta-Phosphate ·,

Adenyl · Pyro-Phosphate →,

Adenosine · Tri-Phosphate →,

(ATP, Adenine–Ribose – (P)~(P)~(P)).

Adenine–α-D-Ribose—O—P—O~P—O⁻

Adenosine Di-Phosphate

(ADP, Adenine–Ribose – (P)~(P)).

Adenine–α-D-Ribose—O—P—O⁻

Adenosine Mono-Phosphate

(Adenylate, AMP, Adenine–Ribose – (P)).

(i)

HO—P—OH   HO—P—O ~ P—O⁽⁻⁾(H)

Inorganic Phosphate   (Inorganic) Pyrophosphate

(Orthophosphate, Pi,   (PPi, (P)~(P)).
Dihydrogen Phosphate,
$H_2PO_4^-$).

(ii)

FIG. 3. Adenosine triphosphate (ATP) and some important related phosphates.

is nutritionally essential for some of the brain's needs (and all those of erythrocytes). The general reasons for this are not yet entirely clear, but are largely to do with the fact that the terminal stages of the combustion of all three types of foodstuff are the same and depend on a constant supply of pyruvate. The absence of oxygen is of course

even more disastrous: the complete combustion of glucose via pyruvate must therefore be extremely important to cells. Paradoxically, the glycolipoprotein plasma membranes (Chapter 6; and see Table 3) of several, but not all, human cells resist the entry of glucose, except through special and mysterious portals opened only by that unique key, insulin, whose functional deficiency (diabetes mellitus) shows the importance of glucose to cellular metabolism. Once glucose has crossed the plasma membranes—a process which in most cells requires the simultaneous entry of Na^+ (see pp. 93, 97)—it is kept in by rapid conversion to substances which cannot get out.

As might be expected, the first such reaction transfers the terminal phosphate group of ATP to glucose (fig. 4), yielding the acidic ester glucose-6-phosphate (glucose-6-(P)). This can be used as an example of most other intracellular reactions, in that it does not occur if solutions of glucose and ATP are simply mixed, but absolutely requires a specific catalyst, i.e. an agent which—itself unmoved—will direct the rapid occurrence of this precise reaction between many thousands of pairs of the appropriate reactants (**substrates**) under the moderate conditions of temperature, pH, ionic strength and substrate concentration in a cell. The catalyst used is called **hexokinase** (HK), which is a protein—i.e. an enzyme—and therefore itself has complex labile molecules, and requires fairly closely defined conditions of pH (ca. 6·5), temperature (ca. 37°C.) and ionic balance (activated by Mg^{++}, inhibited by Ca^{++} and Na^+). Various substances inhibit it either by damaging the protein or interfering with one of its substrates: heavy metals react with—SH (**sulphydryl**) groups (see pp. 88, 99), Be^{2+} imitates and F^- precipitates Mg^{2+}, while 6-deoxy glucose (an artificial substance) and ADP compete with glucose and ATP respectively. Glucose-6-(P), the main product, is, however, a specific and functionally important non-competitive inhibitor.

The enzyme's name's ending, "kinase", now used generally for enzymes transferring (P) from ATP to other substances, is derived from "-ase" for "enzyme" and the Greek word for "motion", as though the inert "wagon", glucose, needs a "coupling", phosphate, before it can be moved on! HK activity is indeed the first stage in the generation of fats, proteins and other cell structures as well as energy (ATP), from glucose through glycolysis.

Glycolysis to Pyruvate or Lactate

This well-known process is so fully described in every relevant textbook that a simplified outline (fig. 4) will suffice for the discussion of its important points.

Hexose monophosphate (HMP), an equilibrium mixture of glucose-6-(P), fructose-6-(P) and **glucose-1-(P),** equally easily obtainable from glycogen, is maintained by the activities of hexose phosphate isomerase and **phosphogluco-mutase** (PGM; fig. 10).

Further progress requires the "loss" of a further unit of ~ (P), i.e. ATP, catalysed by **phosphofructokinase** (PFK); this enzyme, whose activity is increased by P_i, ADP and AMP but decreased by ATP and **citrate,** is thought to be one of the main "throttles" for the control of the rate of carbohydrate breakdown. The speed of glycolysis also depends, of course, on the thermodynamically inevitable effects, on the rates of its reversible reactions, of changes in the concentrations (more correctly, **activities,** *i.e.* "chemically effective concentrations") of their substrates and products: this "mass action control" is as absolute as that of non-enzymic reactions like the ionization of weak acids (p. 85).

The **triose phosphates** are also the source of glycerol for fat synthesis (p. 96), but more immediately important because their oxidation (**dehydrogenation**) by NAD^+ (fig. 5) is in life closely coupled to the condensation of 2 moles of P_i with 2 of ADP to give 2 moles of ATP per mole of

epithelial lesions (pellagra, stomatitis), yet NAD and NADP are essential components of every cell in the body. This tissue-specific need for a "universal" vitamin is in fact usual.

The penultimate stage, the conversion of **phospho-(enol-)pyruvate** (PEP) and ADP to pyruvate and ATP is as irreversible as the other kinase reactions, but in the opposite direction, because phospho-pyruvate seems more energy-rich than ATP. This step, catalysed by **pyruvate kinase** (PK), is another "control point"; this enzyme's activity requires a high $[K^+]$, and is inhibited by fatty acids, *i.e.* when the cell is well fed, as it is also by ATP; the latter effect is, very logically, opposed by AMP. Finally, under anaerobic conditions, the resulting pyruvate

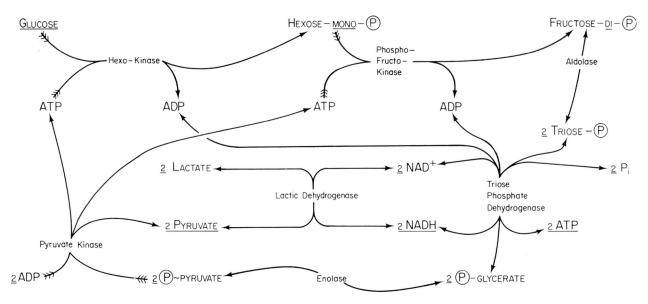

Fig. 4. Anaerobic glycolysis from glucose to lactate. Substrates in capitals, enzymes in lower-case.

starting glucose. This process (dissectable *in vitro* into at least 3 steps) is the "point of attack" of that ancient poison, arsenate, which "imitates" phosphate only too successfully in the early reactions but not the later ones; triose phosphate dehydrogenase is also particularly susceptible to poisoning by "heavy metals" (Hg^{2+}, Pb^{2+}), organic arsenicals and alkylating agents, by reason of the sensitively reactive —SH groups which must remain, uncombined, in one of the enzymes involved (*cf.* HK, p. 87); restores energy-balance to the cell; and introduces NAD (fig. 5), quantitatively the most important hydrogen-carrying **cofactor** (co-enzyme) of oxidation in cells.

NAD^+ is readily and reversibly **hydrogenated** (reduced) and dehydrogenated in the presence of appropriate enzymes and substrates (man-made reagents can be used *in vitro*), with accompanying changes in $[H^+]$ (see fig. 5). The closely-related NADP, which is in equilibrium with NAD (normally, $[NAD^+ + NADH] > [NADP^+ + NADPH]$ and $[NAD^+] \gg [NADH]$, but $[NADPH] \gg [NADP^+]$), is mainly used as NADPH for biosyntheses, particularly of fatty acids (p. 95–96).

These coenzymes are the active forms of the B-vitamin **nicotinamide;** deficiencies thereof seem to cause, mainly,

is reduced by NADH and lactate dehydrogenase; this is essential for the restoration of NAD^+ and completes anaerobic glycolysis.

The net production of only 2 moles of ATP (20 kcal.) per mole of glucose by glycolysis seems likely to be very inadequate, as we know from the effects of anoxia on most cells that it is, when compared with the total heat obtainable—686 kcal.—by burning glucose to CO_2 and water. It is, however, sufficient for erythrocytes—it is all they get—, and for skeletal muscle during temporary oxygen deficits, and for *Lactobacilli*. Normally respiring cells do much better by oxidizing the pyruvate and the NADH separately, thus breaking the glycolytic cycle, but getting much more from it.

Acetyl-Coenzyme-A Formation

All the reactions yet described are cytoplasmic, but the oxidative ones converting pyruvate to CO_2 and water, and their coupling to the generation of ATP, are carried out in the mitochondria (Chapter 6).

Pyruvate is first oxidatively decarboxylated and converted to "active acetate," **acetyl coenzyme A** (AcCoA), by a cycle of reactions involving three vitamins of real nutritional importance, viz. **thiamine** (aneurine, B1) helping to remove the CO_2, nicotinamide in NAD, and **riboflavine** (B2, more correctly **ribityl**flavine) as an intermediate hydrogen-carrier, as well as two others which the body never seems to be short of: **pantothenate** in **Coenzyme A** (CoA, CoA.SH), and **lipoate** as a hydrogen-acceptor and "active acetyl group"-carrier (fig. 6). The enzymes and cofactors catalysing the whole process can be isolated together as the **pyruvate dehydrogenase complex,** with a

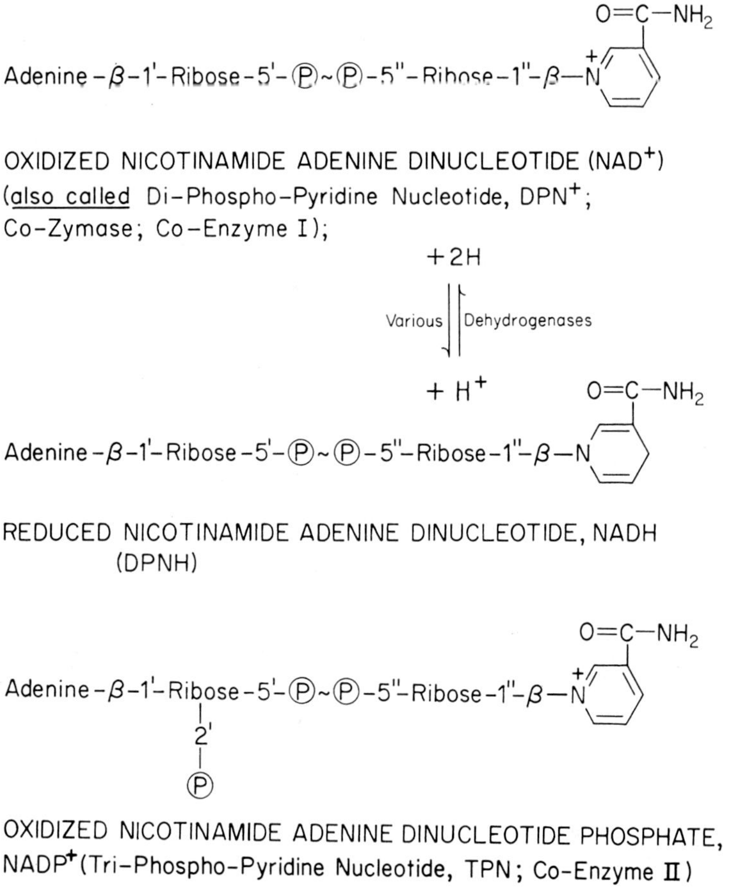

bolism; they are therefore the link between these, the cell's three main sources of energy.

The Citrate Cycle

The next stage of AcCoA metabolism is the condensation of its acetate with **oxaloacetate** to form citrate, under the influence of "condensing enzyme", **citrate synthase;** this reaction goes because AcCoA, being a **thio**-ester, CoA.S

Adenine$-\beta-1'-$Ribose$-5'-$(P)$\sim$(P)$-5''-$Ribose$-1''-\beta-$N

$O=C-NH_2$

OXIDIZED NICOTINAMIDE ADENINE DINUCLEOTIDE (NAD$^+$)
(<u>also called</u> Di-Phospho-Pyridine Nucleotide, DPN$^+$;
Co-Zymase; Co-Enzyme I);

$+2H$

Various | Dehydrogenases

$+ H^+$ $O=C-NH_2$

Adenine$-\beta-1'-$Ribose$-5'-$(P)$\sim$(P)$-5''-$Ribose$-1''-\beta-$N

REDUCED NICOTINAMIDE ADENINE DINUCLEOTIDE, NADH
(DPNH)

$O=C-NH_2$

Adenine$-\beta-1'-$Ribose$-5'-$(P)$\sim$(P)$-5''-$Ribose$-1''-\beta-$N
$|$
$2'$
$|$
(P)

OXIDIZED NICOTINAMIDE ADENINE DINUCLEOTIDE PHOSPHATE,
NADP$^+$(Tri-Phospho-Pyridine Nucleotide, TPN; Co-Enzyme II)

Fig. 5.

"molecular" weight of 10^6 Daltons. Its rate of action is functionally controlled by its inhibition by ATP (see p. 88); it can also be poisoned, via the SH groups of the lipoate, by, say, trivalent arsenicals (*cf.* triose phosphate dehydrogenase, p. 88).

Thiamine and lipoate seem to be used only here and, similarly, in **α-keto-glutarate dehydrogenase** (p. 90); but **ribitylflavine-5′-phosphate** ("flavine mononucleotide," FMN) either alone, or as here, in FAD, has functions like NAD's, although it appears in more disguises because it is always tightly bound to protein. Pantothenate, in the form of its derivative (P)-**pantetheine,** an —SH compound, seems always to function as a carrier of acyl groups, both in CoA and, combined with protein instead, in fatty acid synthesis (p. 95). Acetyl CoA and CoA are in fact equally essential to pyruvate, fat and ketone-body meta-

$\sim CO.CH_3$, is energy-rich. Thus begins the "**Citrate** (Krebs', Tricarboxylic Acid) **Cycle,**" a well-known bane to students (fig. 6); it is none the less given here in full because it is, as shown, an essential junction between carbohydrate and amino-acid metabolism, and because almost every step is a source of energy (see pp. 90–91).

Citrate synthase is probably controlled *in vivo* by its inhibitions by ATP, and (under other circumstances) by long-chain fatty acyl CoA esters, so that the energy-yielding oxidation of glucose is switched off, either when the cell is already energy-rich, or when carbohydrate is short and ketogenesis needs to be encouraged in starvation or diabetes mellitus. The Cycle is also regulated—apart from mass-action control (p. 88)—by the special influences of ADP (stimulatory) and NADH (inhibitory) on isocitrate dehydrogenase; of P_i, **succinate** and fumarate (stimulatory)

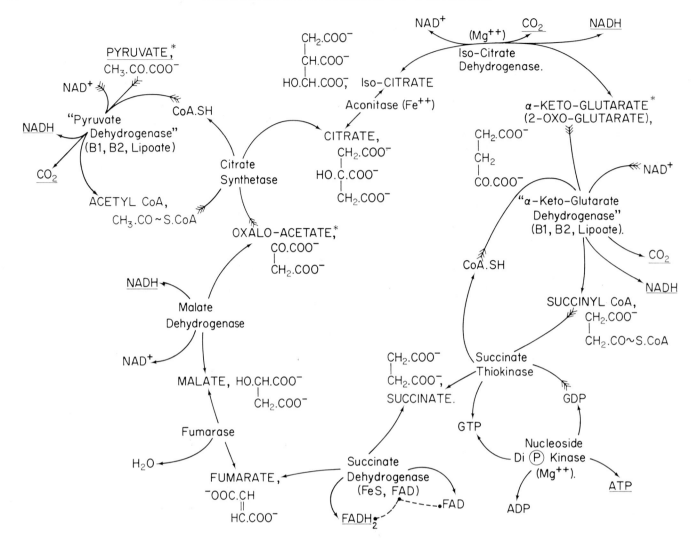

FIG. 6. The Citrate Cycle. * = substance in equilibrium with the corresponding amino-acid. ●...● = succinic dehydrogenase's FAD is its own hydrogen-carrier. Co-factors' names are in parentheses. Other conventions as Fig. 4.

and **oxaloacetate** (inhibitory) on succinic dehydrogenase; and of ATP (inhibitory) on fumarase.

Oxidative Phosphorylation

When the remnants of the glucose molecule have finally been demolished by the Citrate Cycle to CO_2, but not to water, 2 more $\sim$Ⓟs have turned up and there are 12 hydrogenated molecules awaiting their cues: the liberation and oxidation of their 24 H atoms into water is the real driving power of every respiring cell.

The reactions involved are catalysed by a rigidly organized group of enzymes and carrier-proteins in the inner mitochondrial membranes, the **electron transport system** (ETS), whereby the transfer of hydrogen from $NADH + H^+$ and $FADH_2$ to oxygen is coupled to the combination of P_i with ADP to form ATP; the organization of this system is only schematically outlined in fig. 7.

Succinic dehydrogenase and the fatty-acid-oxidizing **flavoprotein** are put on a branch to show why they yield only 2 ATP's per $FADH_2$ oxidized ("P/O ratio" = 2),

whereas the dehydrogenation of NADH has a P/O ratio of 3. The mechanisms of the **coupling factors** remain unknown, but their "locations" are as indicated.

Under aerobic conditions, each mole of glucose yields 2 moles of NADH and 2 of ATP via the Glycolytic Cycle; 2 of NADH via the conversion of pyruvate to AcCoA; and 6 of NADH, 2 of succinate dehydro enase's $FADH_2$ and 2 of ATP via the oxidation of AcCoA through the Citrate Cycle: the final yield of ATP by oxidative reactions is therefore $10 \times 3 (\leftarrow NADH) = 30, + 2 \times 2 (\leftarrow FADH_2) = 4$, total 34 moles; added to the 4 of ATP produced directly, these give the cell 38 moles of ATP per mole of glucose "burnt", *i.e.* 380 kcal. of usable energy, which represents over 55 per cent conversion and is—whatever the caloric equivalent of ATP—19 times as much as can be got by anaerobic glycolysis. It is therefore hardly surprising that most human cells must have oxygen for life.

The ETS is not only a site of action of riboflavin, but also, uniquely, for **Coenzyme Q** (ubiquinone: chemically, but not necessarily otherwise, related to vitamin K) and the **cytochromes**. The latter are reversibly-oxidizable **haem** proteins (ferrohaem containing $Fe^{2+} \rightleftharpoons$ ferrihaem containing Fe^{3+}, $+ e^{-}$, an **electron**); not to be confused with **haemoglobin** (Hb) (or **myoglobin,** Mb), which is reversibly **oxygenatable** ($Hb + O_2 \rightleftharpoons Hb.O_2$), but converted to the inactive Met Hb (or Met Mb) if its haem's Fe^{2+} is oxidized to Fe^{3+}. Although the body contains only a thousandth as much of the cytochromes as of Hb, they are evidently no less necessary for our use of oxygen.

The ETS is affected by various poisons (useful for research purposes), but is mainly controlled *in vivo* by the obligatory coupling of oxidation with phosphorylation: except perhaps in brown fat, a central heating system in babies, phosphorylation depends on oxidation, and oxidation does not occur unless there is an energy-deficit expressed as significant concentrations of ADP and P_i, NADH and/or $FADH_2$.

$CoA.SH + 7\ FAD + 7\ NAD^+ + 7\ H_2O \rightarrow 8\ CH_3.CO \sim S.CoA$, acetyl CoA, $+ 7\ FADH_2 + 7\ NADH + 7\ H^+$.

In principle, the AcCoA should be straightforwardly dealt with by the Citrate Cycle and all the resulting NADH and $FADH_2$ oxidized by the ETS, giving a correspondingly large yield of ATP, all in the mitochondria (figs. 6 and 7). This does indeed occur in many tissues, but liver cells in particular would need abnormally rapid carbohydrate breakdown to replenish oxaloacetate quickly enough for their Citrate Cycle to be able to keep up with their catabolism of fatty acids to AcCoA, which has therefore to be dealt with otherwise. The main processes used are: 2 AcCoA $\rightleftharpoons$ Acetoacetyl CoA, AcAcCoA, + CoA; then AcAcCoA + AcCoA $\rightarrow$ Hydroxymethylglutaryl CoA, HMGCoA, + CoA; HMGCoA can then be used either for the quantitatively inadequate synthesis of mevalonate and its derivatives

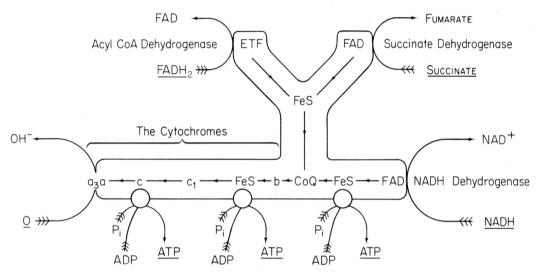

FIG. 7. The electron transport system (ETS) of mitochondria. ———→— = electrons (hydrogen equivalents) move this way. ETF = electron-transporting flavoprotein. FAD belongs to succinic dehydrogenase. FeS (ferrous sulphide) and CoQ (coenzyme Q) are co-factors of enzymes at these "points". a_3, a, c_1, b = cytochromes. Arrowed circles in bottom line = proteins coupling phosphorylation to oxidation ("coupling factors").

Fatty Acid and Ketone Body Oxidation

Cellular fat metabolism, which supplies much of the body's energy (p. 83), begins with the entry of free fatty acids, to which the plasma membrane is no barrier, or with their hydrolytic release from extracellular or intracellular fat by the appropriate lipase. These processes are no doubt helped by the next step, the ATP-driven enzymic activation of fatty acids with $CoA:R.CO.O^- + ATP + CoA.SH \rightleftharpoons R.CO \sim S.CoA + AMP + PP_i$, drawn "to the right" by: $PP_i + H_2O \rightarrow 2P_i$ (p. 85).

Long-chain acyl CoAs are then catabolized by mitochondria, after reaction with carnitine to convert them to acylcarnitines, which can cross the inner membrane and react with CoA to re-form long-chain acyl CoAs inside it. The details of the rest of the process are not given here because *in vivo*, no intermediates are found, and the individual enzymes involved are tightly bound together in a complex (with at least 3 vitamins: nicotinamide, riboflavin and pantothenate). A typical overall equation is: $CH_3.(CH_2)_{14}.CO \sim S.CoA$, **Palmityl** CoA, + 7

the **poly-isoprenoids** (see p. 96), or—most of it—for the formation of ketone bodies: $HMGCoA \rightarrow AcCoA +$ Acetoacetate, $AcAc^-$; then either $AcAc^- \rightarrow$ Acetone + CO_2, or $AcAc^- + NADH + H^+ \rightleftharpoons \beta$-Hydroxy-Butyrate, BHB^-, $+ NAD^+$. Other tissues can and do normally use ketone bodies, particularly BHB^- after dehydrogenation to $AcAc^-$, which they (but not liver) can activate: $AcAc^- + CoA + \sim ⓟ \rightarrow AcAcCoA$; then $AcAcCoA + CoA \rightleftharpoons 2\ AcCoA$, which they oxidize through the Citrate Cycle as before.

Fatty acids and ketone bodies compare well with carbohydrates in the energy derived from their oxidation. For instance, the oxidation of oleate (18 carbons, one "double bond", residue weight 281 Daltons) needs 1 ATP initially, then produces 9 AcCoA, 8 NADH and 7 $FADH_2$, whose complete oxidation through the Citrate Cycle and the ETS gives as usual 12 ATP per AcCoA, 3 per NADH and 2 per $FADH_2$, *i.e.* 145 ATP in all; or 48 ATP per 6 carbon atoms or 93 ATP per 180 Daltons, whereas glucose gives only 38 ATP per molecule (C_6, 180 Daltons). No wonder fat is such a useful energy store; these differences arise from its high proportion of hydrogen and low proportion of oxygen, which also make it both light and immiscible with water. The energy got from BHB (C_4, 103 Daltons) is closer to that from glucose: $BHB^- + NAD^+ \rightleftharpoons AcAc^- + NADH + H^+$, then $AcAc^- + 2\,CoA + \sim ℗ \rightarrow 2\,AcCoA$, then $2\,AcCoA + NADH \rightarrow 27\,ATP$ as usual, net yield 26 ATP per molecule, *i.e.* 39 per 6 carbons or 45 per 180 Daltons.

It must be remembered, however, that all these reactions are strictly aerobic: human cells get no energy from fatty acids or ketone bodies without oxygen.

THE USE OF ATP

The consumption of energy by a cell ought logically to fall into two sets of processes, those required merely to keep the cell alive and those needed for its duties to the whole organism. In practice, specialized versions of the former "maintenance" reactions are used for much of the latter "work", particularly by neurones, hepatocytes, kidney and gut cells, and even for the control and sustenance of cellular movement.

Some Obvious Functions

Cell Movement

Cellular contractions probably all use essentially the same set of chemical compounds and reactions, the **actomyosin** system; the meaning of its fine details remain obscure, but the general principles have been established with skeletal muscle. They even have some accidental resemblances to those used for cellular movements brought about by the more widespread (and primitive?) microtubules (Chapter 6).

The main ultrastructural basis of the actomyosin system is two sets of interdigitating protein fibrils, **actin** and **myosin**. Actin fibrils are long thin "pieces of string" each made of a loosely-twisted (coarse-pitched) pair of chains (polymers) of globular molecules of "G-actin", the monomers, with high affinities for ADP and Ca^{2+}. Myosin fibrils are thicker rods made up of myosin monomers, each much larger and more complex than G-actin and with one end in the body of the rod and the other projecting towards the actin.

The general arrangement and working of this machinery, crudely illustrated in fig. 8, depends absolutely on Ca^{2+} and ATP. Its thermodynamic efficiency is high, the power obtainable being at least 70 per cent of that calculated from the loss of $\sim ℗$; but in living normal muscles, no falls— even small rises—in [ATP] may happen during contraction, for reasons explained on p. 93. The precise functions of the auxiliary proteins now known to control the interaction and behaviour of actin and myosin are not yet clear enough to merit description here.

Microtubular movements, such as the beating of cilia and the separation of chromosomes by the spindle during cell division (Chapter 6), are also suspected of being based on the sliding of an ATPase-containing protein structure, in this case called **dynein,** past the far more obvious microtubules themselves, which are in turn built up of

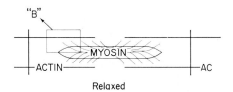

Relaxed

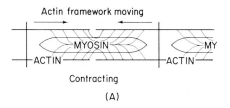

Contracting

(A)

FIG. 8A. General arrangement of the actomyosin system in skeletal muscle. $\times 200{,}000$.

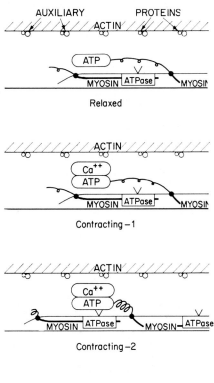

FIG. 8B. A "molecular" view of the actomyosin system at work. $\times 10^6$.

tubular arrays (looking like factory chimneys built of large rather rounded bricks) of rectangulo-globular monomers of the protein **tubulin;** chemically, however, dynein and tubulin are entirely different from myosin and actin.

Ion Extrusion

The Ca^{2+} ions needed for muscular contraction are released from the sarcoplasmic reticulum (SR; see Chapter 6) into the muscle fibre's interior, where their "resting" concentration is negligible; relaxation occurs when the stimulus (**membrane depolarization**) for their release stops, and they are reabsorbed by the SR, with the hydrolysis of 2 ATP (to ADP and P_i) per Ca^{2+}. This "calcium pump" closely resembles that found in mitochondria.

The membrane depolarization mentioned above means

Emergency Energy Stores

Besides "energy transducers", many cells also need a particularly rapid means of keeping [ATP] up during or following bursts of vigorous activity.

Of the two such reactions shown in fig. 9, the less striking "myokinase" reaction, actually found in most cells, is probably used mainly for the "recovery" of AMP.

The more specialized creatine phosphokinase (CPK) system is found particularly in muscle and nerve cells, where phosphocreatine (PC) is the main large immediate $\sim$ ⓟ store or **phosphagen,** [PC] (4–5 × [ATP]) and [CPK] being so high and judiciously located that such

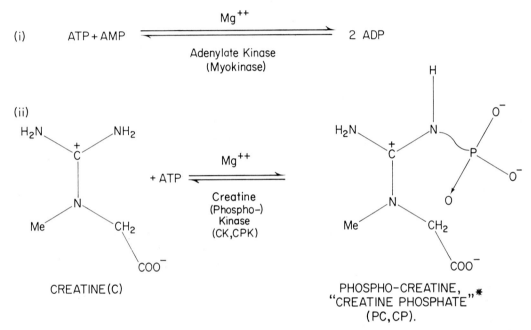

FIG. 9. The replenishment of ATP from ADP alone or from ADP and phosphocreatine. * = the name "creatine phosphate" is often used but is misleadingly wrong.

the abolition of the normal **resting potential** of most cells—particularly excitable ones—which results from the difference in $[K^+]$ (Table 1) across plasma membranes; since the latter are freely permeable to K^+, the difference has to be maintained by an opposite difference in $[Na^+]$ (Table 1). This requires continuous extrusion of Na^+, to which these membranes are not totally impermeable, and which must also enter cells during such events as passage of nerve-impulses and the entry of glucose (p. 87) and amino acids (p. 97).

Plasma membranes therefore contain a **sodium pump,** driven by the hydrolysis of ATP to ADP and P_i, and expelling $3Na^+$ per $\sim$ ⓟ; it is stimulated by Na^+ inside cells and K^+ outside, and needs Mg^{2+} for activity, so that in broken-cell preparations *in vitro*, it behaves as an "Na-K-Mg-ATPase", also now called "pump ATPase". It is particularly active in nerve, gut and kidney cells, because Na^+-extrusion is perforce an important part of their various functions; its inhibition by the "cardiac glycoside" **ouabain** is equally suggestive.

events as brief (3 secs.) sprints, or convulsions, lower only [PC] but not [ATP].

Creatine has to be made continuously (fig. 17) in order to maintain [PC], because PC breaks down slowly but irreversibly all the time to P_i and creatine's anhydride, the **creatinine** found in urine.

Cell Maintenance

Cells must not only maintain their obviously labile components, such as ATP and a high $[K^+]$, but also their "frameworks"—not entirely proteinaceous—and their food stores, while almost identical chemical reactoins are used by gland, gut, liver and plasma cells for supplying proteins, foodstuffs and other necessities to the whole body; these processes are best classified here chemically.

Carbohydrates

Gluconeogenesis. Some cells—particularly liver, kidney and gut—can resynthesize HMP from pyruvate or oxalo-acetate and therefore from amino acids, but not simply by reversing glycolysis, since the kinase reactions are irreversible (fig. 4).

The conversion of pyruvate into PEP needs an elaborate mechanism passing through oxaloacetate, involving CO_2-fixation (for which Mg^{2+}, Mn^{2+} and the "vitamin" biotin are essential), requiring activation by AcCoA, and con-

(polysaccharide) of glucose, "insoluble" and osmotically inert because of its enormous molecular weight ($> 10^6$); some aspects of its structure, formation and breakdown are shown in fig. 10. Glycogen consists of α-glucose residues, each glycosidically (see p. 86) linked to C-4 of a second and (not shown, about every twelfth unit) to C-6 of a third which results in branching of the macromolecule;

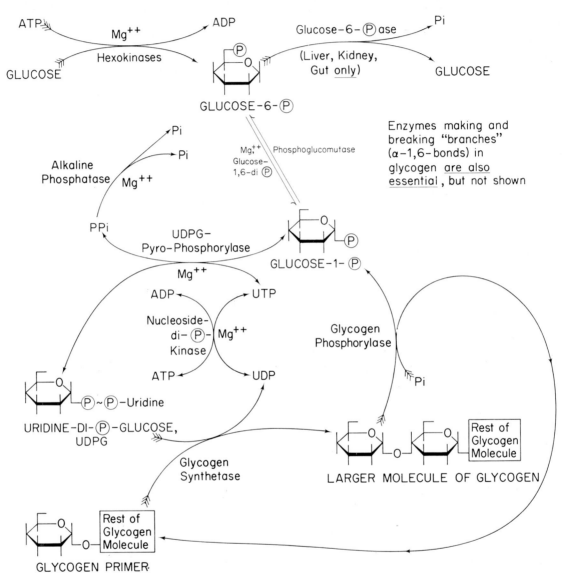

FIG. 10. Glycogen metabolism (making and breaking of α-1, 6-linked "branches" also essential, but not shown). Substrates in capitals; some parts of substrates, enzymes and co-factors given in lower-case.

suming at least 2 Eq. of $\sim$ ℗ per mole; a mere phosphatase (specific, and controlled by inhibition by AMP) suffices to hydrolyse fructose-di-℗ into P_i and HMP. The whole process thus needs at least 6 Eq. of $\sim$ ℗ per mole of HMP, which is twice as much as direct reversal would cost.

These cells, but no others, contain glucose-6-℗-ase, and can therefore split HMP to P_i and glucose.

Glycogen. Most cells, but particularly liver and skeletal muscle, store carbohydrate food as **glycogen**, a polymer

the **monosaccharide**, glucose, is thus distinguished from the **polysaccharide**, glycogen, by having an unbroken chain of carbon atoms. The **uridine triphosphate** (UTP) needed for the formation of **uridine diphosphate glucose** (UDPG), the energy-rich compound needed directly for glycogen synthesis, is an ATP-analogue with the **pyrimidine**-type base **uracil** replacing adenine.

Glycogen metabolism is very sensitive to hormonal influences, of which the most striking are on **phosphorylase** (fig. 10); the reactions leading to the activation and inactivation of this enzyme are summarized in fig. 11. The complexity of this cascade has the useful property of allowing a small quantity of hormone to release a large amount of glucose-6-Ⓟ.

These hormones also affect glycogen synthesis via the cyclic AMP system (fig. 11) but in the opposite direction, because de-phosphated **glycogen synthetase** is the active form of this enzyme; its total quantity is increased slowly by insulin and decreased by its antagonists, presumably via the cells' protein-synthesizing machinery (fig. 18).

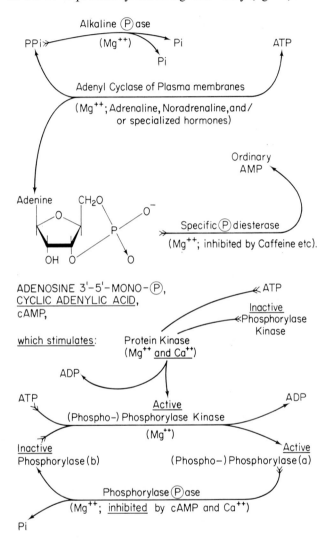

FIG. 11. The hormonal control of phosphorylase through cyclic adenylic acid. Enzymes (and co-factors) are beside arrows connecting substrates and products, which include enzymes catalysing later reactions in the cascade.

Special hormonal effects on the liver also control the supply of glucose to cells in general: **glucagon** here stimulates **adenyl cyclase** (fig. 11), while growth hormone slowly increases and insulin slowly decreases the amount of phosphorylase; **cortisol** slowly increases and insulin slowly decreases the amount of glucose-6-Ⓟase; and insulin slowly increases the amount of the liver's special **gluco-kinase,** which is specific for glucose, in high concentrations, and is not inhibited by glucose-6-Ⓟ.

The chemistry and pathology of glycogen are complicated by its "α-1,6" links, which have to be made and broken by special branching and debranching enzymes, and by the (as yet unexplained) need for some degradation by a lysosomal "acid maltase" (see Table 3). Any of these, as well as glucose-6-Ⓟase or phosphorylase, can be hereditarily deficient, yet the patients survive the resulting bizarre abnormalities of glycogen storage and glucose metabolism, often for several years and sometimes into adulthood; this suggests that glycogen is useful rather than essential.

Proteoglycans, Glycoproteins and Glycolipids. The synthesis of these complex materials, incorporating mono-, oligo- and/or polysaccharides, is of great dental importance, not only because they form parts of the cells themselves (Chapter 6; and this Chapter, Table 3), but particularly because they are essential components of the intercellular structures described in Chapters 36 and 46 and of salivary and other mucins. Here again, therefore, "work" and "maintenance" overlap. They also have considerable significance in the pathogenesis of dental caries (Chapters 31 and 34).

The two chief general chemical principles observed in the formation of these substances are that the process always begins with the attachment of monosaccharides to proteins or lipids by covalent bonds, and that further assembly is always done by the transfer of additional sugars from nucleoside-diphosphate-monosaccharides such as UDPG (cf. glycogen, fig. 10), via **dolichol-**Ⓟ carriers. All these activated precursors arise from HMP, by 3 main routes, all shown diagrammatically in simplified forms in fig. 12, except that the strongly acidic sulphate groups, found esterified or amidated to many of the proteoglycans and some glycolipids, are added after (or at a late stage in) the formation of the polysaccharide components and are supplied by 3'-phospho-adenosine-5'-phospho-sulphate (i.e. adenine-ribose-3'-Ⓟ-5'-Ⓟ ∼Ⓢ; also called "active sulphate" or PAPS).

These processes seem to occur largely in the vesicles or on the membranes of the smooth endoplasmic reticulum (SER) and/or the Golgi apparatus (Chapter 6), which carry the necessary enzymes.

Lipids

Most cells, particularly in the fetus, can make their own lipids including the fatty acids, almost entirely; but adults' peripheral tissues probably get most of their fatty acids from the gut, liver, and fat depots via the plasma.

Fatty acids are synthesized from AcCoA, but not by direct reversal of their oxidation. The process is catalysed by 2 cooperating enzyme complexes in the cytoplasm; the first uses CO_2 and ATP to carboxylate successive acetate units, and the second condenses them together and decarboxylates them, hydrogenates them with $NADPH_2$ and dehydrates them. The first complex contains biotin and Mn^{2+} (cf. gluconeogenesis, p. 94) and is stimulated by citrate (from carbohydrate) but inhibited by long-chain acyl CoA (from fat); the second contains bound Ⓟ-pantetheine (p. 89). The overall equation is:

$$8 \, \text{AcCoA} + 7 \, \text{ATP} + 14(\text{NADPH} + \text{H}^+) + \text{OH}^- \rightarrow$$
$$\text{CH}_3.(\text{CH}_2)_{14}.\text{COO}^-, \textbf{palmitate}, + 8 \, \text{CoA} + 7 \, \text{ADP} + 7 \, \text{P}_i + 14\text{NADP}^+.$$

AcCoA, which cannot get out of mitochondria, has to be supplied as citrate, which can; the formation of the necessary ATP- and Mg^{2+}-requiring **citrate lyase** is regulated by hormones.

The other main essential substrate, NADPH (fig. 5), is supplied by the cytoplasmic reduction of NADP^+ by glucose-6-Ⓟ (fig. 13); this series of reactions is also the source of **pentoses,** the central components of nucleotides.

Full blown "fats" ("neutral fat," **triglycerides),** and the complex polar lipids of membranes, have to be made by the combination of fatty acids with hydrophilic linking structures, particularly glycerol or the amino group of **sphingosine;** for adequate surface-activity, membrane lipids need additional polar groups, as shown in fig. 14 for **lecithin** and **sphingomyelin.** Their biosyntheses—only selected examples are illustrated—need activated forms of all components, *e.g.* fatty acyl CoAs (p. 91), **glycerophosphate** (⇌ triose Ⓟ, fig. 4, + NADH, catalysed by glycero Ⓟ dehydrogenase) and CDP choline, analogous to

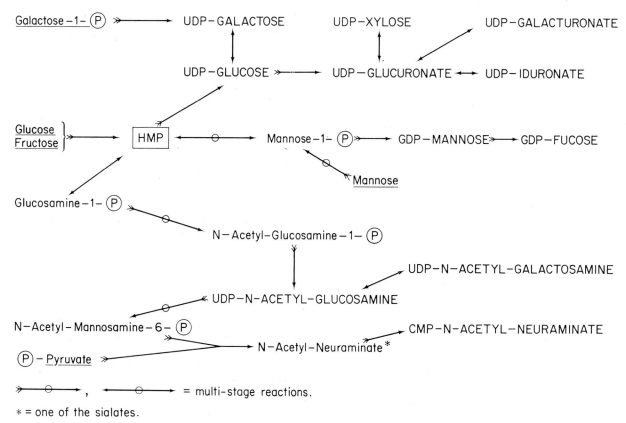

FIG. 12. Biosyntheses of the activated precursors (names in capitals) of the proteoglycans, glycoproteins and glycolipids (for structures, see Chapter 34). Enzymes and most auxiliary substrates omitted. Starting-materials underlined.

Its dehydrogenases are controlled by direct product inhibition by NADPH (cf. HK, p. 87).

Most cells also make their own polyisoprenoids (p. 91) by complex processes driven mainly by ATP and NADPH, yielding ultimately squalene (found in sebum), dicholⒹs (p. 95) and sterols (cholesterol of membranes and plasma lipoproteins; vitamin D precursors; steroid hormones; bile salts), all functionally important but small in amount and useless as fuel, because the body cannot catabolize them.

There are, however, lipid components which the body cannot make *de novo* and which are therefore "vitamins", though of uncertain significance in adult human nutrition; these are the **essential fatty acids, arachidonate** (see fig. 15) and its precursor **linoleate,** which can be converted into arachidonate, just as the body can convert palmitate into, say, stearate, oleate, nervonate and hydroxynervonate.

UDPG *etc.* (figs. 10 and 12). Although lecithin occurs in the largest quantities, several other polar lipids are qualitatively as important; they include the precisely analogous compounds of serine, **ethanolamine,** glycerol and **inositol** and its phosphates, besides sphingomyelin and the other **sphingolipids** which include the glycolipids (p. 95). An example called **cardiolipin** for historical reasons (fig. 15), but found in the ETS (fig. 7) which does not work without it, is so drawn as to illustrate both the way in which lipids are believed to be arranged in unit membranes (Chapter 6) and the structure of arachidonate (see above), of which this is one of the essential functions.

Proteins

Protein synthesis is fundamental to that of carbohydrates and lipids, because their formation and all other metabolism has to be carried out by proteins, the enzymes. A constant supply of proteins is therefore vital to a cell; it is also a complex matter, because of the large number of different proteins which a cell must have and their elaborate structures.

Amino Acid Metabolism. Cells do not obtain their enzymes and structural proteins from the plasma, even though small amounts of such "effector" proteins as

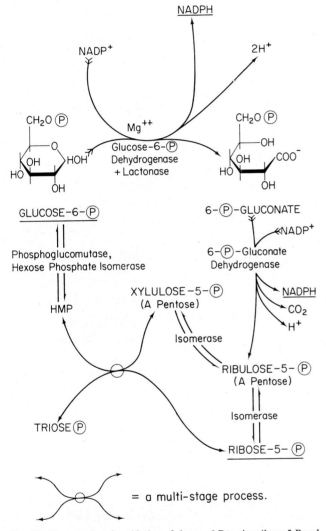

FIG. 13. The cytoplasmic oxidation of glucose-6-P to give ribose-5-P and NADPH. Also called "the HMP shunt", or the "pentose-P", "P-gluconate oxidative" or "Warburg–Dickens–Horecker" "pathway". Arrows connect substrates and products, and have enzymes and cofactors beside or within them.

hormones and bacterial exotoxins can get in, and must therefore make all their own from amino acids; a constant supply of the 20 necessary for protein synthesis, and in the right proportions, is therefore essential. The metabolism needed to ensure this being complex, and much of it confined to the liver, only a few reactions of universal significance will be described here.

All cells have mechanisms for the abstraction and concentration of amino acids from the plasma, driven by the simultaneous entry of Na^+ and its subsequent removal

by the sodium pump (p. 93). Most cells can also **decarboxylate** several amino acids and **transaminate** them with keto acids, both reactions using **pyridoxal phosphate,** a derivative of vitamin B6 (pyridoxine) as coenzyme; the examples given in fig. 16 are parts of glutamate metabolism, but amino acid decarboxylation is also the first step in the production of important amines such as dopamine and **putrescine,** the precursors of (nor)adrenaline and **spermine** (p. 102) respectively. Glutamate's unique oxido-reductive interconvertibility with α-keto-glutarate, a component of the Citrate Cycle (fig. 6), and its relationship with glutamine, our main soluble non-toxic carrier of ammonia, make it a major "metabolic crossroads" between amino acids, other nitrogen compounds and carbohydrates.

The specific metabolism of methionine (fig. 17), a nutritionally-essential amino acid, is important in all cells because of its biosynthetic ramifications; it has unique roles in protein synthesis (Table 2) and in several indispensable **methylations.** One form of "active methyl" is **S-adenosyl-methionine** (SAM, fig. 17), whose energy-rich sulphonium ($\equiv S^+$) atom allows ready transfer of its methyl group, particularly to N atoms to form, say, creatine (fig. 9), adrenaline, lecithin (fig. 14), and N-methylhistidine in actomyosin (p. 92). Figure 17 also shows some additional functions of several vitamins, particularly the anti-anaemic B_{12} (**cobalamin**) and **folate;** the latter is used by cells, as **methylene** (—CH_2—) or **methenyl** (—CH=) **tetrahydrofolate** (FH_4) in other "one-carbon" transfers, particularly in the biosyntheses of the nucleotide bases, besides its use as Me-FH_4, the other form of "active methyl".

Nucleotide synthesis is indeed very important biologically, and also clinically because it is highly susceptible to nutritional, hormonal and toxic influences; the latter can be beneficial, as in cancer chemotherapy, as well as harmful, as in carcinogenesis.

The processes involved are excessively complex, but it should be known that most cells can make their own from simple starting materials, ribose-5-phosphate (figs. 3 and 13), ammonia, aspartate, CO_2, glutamine, glycine and "one carbon", with the aid of the expected cofactors ATP, biotin, iron, K^+, methenyl- and methylene-FH_4, Mg^{2+}, NAD, NADPH and riboflavin.

Polypeptide Synthesis is doubly unique. Firstly, unlike all the other kinds of biochemical reaction yet discussed, its mechanism and substrates (fig. 2) are virtually the same in all cells of all living organisms. Secondly, the only direct controls on the biosyntheses described above are the specificities and relative Activities of the necessary enzymes and the substrates presented to them, so that the products can vary with the local conditions (*e.g.* polysaccharides and fats, pp. 95, 96), but most proteins' structures are totally determined by pre-arranged patterns, only the quantities made being variable—from zero to immense.

A crude outline of the process is given in fig. 18. The initial activation of the amino acids is more complex than that of sugars or fatty acids: each is esterified via its carboxyl group with a unique substance, its own **transfer ribonucleic acid** (tRNA), by a unique enzyme. The pattern

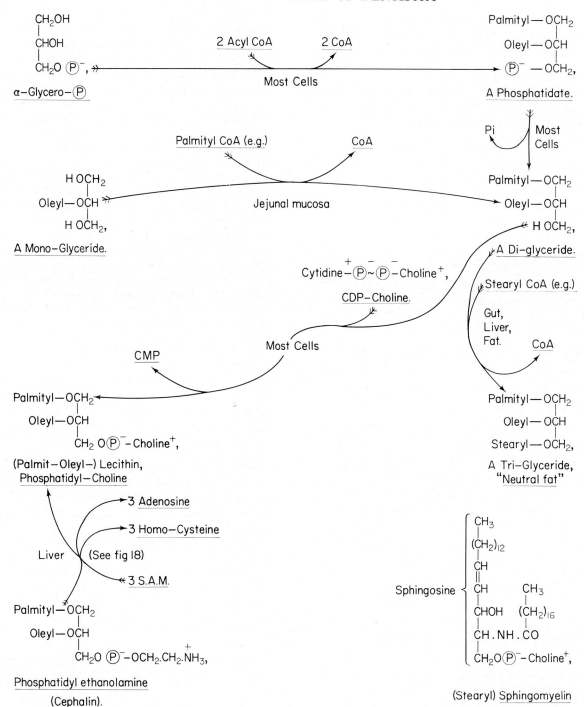

FIG. 14. The major complex lipids, and some of their biosyntheses from activated fatty acids and hydrophilic components.

used to specify the **amino-acyl tRNA's** arrangement is a long, extended, single-stranded molecule of RNA called a **messenger RNA** (mRNA).

Enzymes and energy are also needed, to initiate polypeptide synthesis, to attach each amino-acyl tRNA in turn to the mRNA, to transfer it to the end of the growing peptide chain, to form the necessary peptide bond (fig. 2) thereto, thus releasing the previous amino-acid's tRNA for re-use, and finally to release each complete polypeptide chain from the mRNA; these enzymes, and some auxiliary

proteins and RNA (rRNA, function uncertain) are packaged as **ribosomes** (Chapter 6). It will be seen that the amino acids are placed not by means of their own structures, but according to those of certain parts of their tRNAs and the mRNA, as shown in fig. 18.

This process is normally controlled by the supply of mRNA, ribosomes and tRNAs (pp. 104, 105), or of amino acids and/or ~ ℗; or by "feed-back-inhibition", as when Hb α-**globins** are not released from their polysomes until β-globins are available to combine with them. Polypeptide synthesis is also seriously deranged by various more or less specific poisons and antibiotics, as used in chemotherapy.

Ribonucleic Acids have rather simple structures, being just linear **poly-ribo-nucleotides;** their general arrangement and the structures of all their usual bases, as well as those of **poly-deoxy-ribo-nucleotides (deoxyribo-nucleic acids, DNAs)** are shown in fig. 19 (*N.B.* The nucleoside and nucleotide containing **hypoxanthine** are called **inosine** and **inosinic acid** respectively, hence the representation of

either from those amino acids having more than one tRNA each, or from their anti-codons' first bases being I, U or G, which pair imperfectly (see above). All polypeptides are indeed initiated with methionine (**N-formylated** in bacteria and a few important ETS enzymes synthesized in mito-chondria), although few mature proteins have methionine as their **N-terminal** amino acid.

Protein Maturation and Structure. The nature of mRNA ensures that every polypeptide's initial structure must be

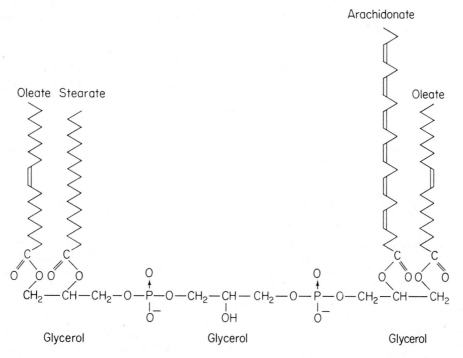

FIG. 15. A typical "cardiolipin" (diphosphatidylglycerol). An essential component of mitochondrial ETS (see Fig. 7).

hypoxanthine itself by "I" in some diagrams. Hypoxan-thine should be renamed "Inidine"!).

Figure 19 also shows how each base projecting from the RNA's **-ribose-Ⓟ-ribose-Ⓟ-** backbone goes opposite a particular complementary base, purines opposite pyrimidines, "A" opposite "U", "C" opposite "G" and *vice versa* (fig. 18), as determined both by the shapes of the bases and by **hydrogen bonding.** This phenomenon of **base pairing** not only determines the placing of amino acyl tRNA's on mRNAs, but also holds tRNAs in their "twisted clover leaf" structures (fig. 18) stabilized by the additive strengths of large numbers of the individually weak bonds involved (*cf.* DNA, p. 102). Some modified bases, including hypoxanthine, found "only" in the "ends of the loops" of tRNAs, pair weakly if at all due to their "wrong" shapes or lack of hydrogen-bonding groups; and occasionally, U can pair with G and G with C.

The complementary triplets of bases on mRNAs and tRNAs which locate amino acids (fig. 18) are called **codons** and **anticodons** respectively; Table 2 gives an approximate full list of codons, the Genetic Code. The "degenerate" codes, with variable third bases ("Y" in fig. 18), arise

purely linear; the complexity and variety of the structures of mature, functioning, proteins can only, therefore, be derived by folding, aggregation, cross-linking and/or chemical alteration of these initially simple chains of amino acid residues.

(i) *Chemical Alterations* greatly affect the folding, cross-linking and aggregation of polypeptides, and occur at an early stage in their lives, some before or soon after release from the ribosomes, but most are made in the smooth endoplasmic reticulum and Golgi apparatus (Chapter 6). They include glycosylation (p. 95); methylation (p. 97); the reversible oxidation of cysteine residues to **cystine** ($R—S—H + H—S—R' \rightleftharpoons R—S—S—R' + 2 H$), giving immediate cross-linking between different polypeptides or different parts of the same one (a process often hormonally controlled, and one which can be pathologically imitated by heavy metals, as in hexokinase—pp. 87, 88—: $R—S—H + Hg^{2+} + H—S—R' \rightarrow R—S—Hg—S—R' + 2 H^+$); the hydroxylation of proline and lysine residues in **procollagen** and **proelastin,** a reaction needing O_2, Fe^{2+}, α-ketoglutarate and ascorbic acid (vitamin C), and the oxidation of these lysine and hydroxylysine residues by a

Cu^{2+} enzyme, both reactions essential for the subsequent cross-linking and glycosylation (p. 95) needed for these polypeptides' final maturation, so that their failures in scurvy or lathyrism are responsible for the lesions occurring in these diseases; attachment of substances essential to function, such as haem in the cytochromes (p. 90) and FAD, lipoate, Ⓟ-pantetheine and biotin in the enzyme-complexes of carbohydrate and lipid metabolism (pp. 89–95); and finally, the removal of "blocking" or "molecule-shaping" peptides, as in the conversion of

TABLE 2
THE GENETIC CODE

Amino Acid	Code†	Amino Acid	Code†
"BEGIN"	**AUG**	Leucine*	CUA, C, G, U UUA, G
Alanine	GCA, C, G, U	Lysine*	AAA, G
Arginine	AGA, G, CGA, C, G, U	Methionine*	AUG
Asparagine	AAC, U	Phenylalanine*	UUC, U
Aspartate	GAC, U	Proline	CCA, C, G, U
Cysteine	UGC, U	Serine	AGC, U UCA, C, G, U
Glutamate	GAA, G	Threonine*	ACA, C, G, U
Glutamine	CAA, G	Tryptophan*	UGG
Glycine	GGA, C, G, U	Tyrosine(*)	UAC, U
Histidine	CAC, U	Valine*	GUA, C, G, U
Isoleucine*	AUA, C, U	"END"	**UAA, G** UGA

† Bases: Adenine, Cytosine, Guanine, Uracil.
Multiple codes abbreviated: *e.g.*: "AUA, C, U" means "AUA, AUC or AUU".
* Nutritionally essential. Tyrosine(*) ← Phenylalanine* *in vivo*.

pro-insulin, pro-collagen (see (iii) below) and **trypsinogen** to their final forms.

(ii) *The Conformational Effects of Chemistry* are decisive: the folding and/or aggregation of protein molecules are entirely determined by their chemical structures and the local physico-chemical conditions, without any other agency. The primary structure of a polypeptide is the order of its amino-acid residues, "native" or altered or combined with other substances; individual side-chains or attached groups may be hydrophilic like glutamine or oligosaccharides, hydrophobic like phenylalanine or cytochromes' haem, positively or negatively charged like histidine or glutamate, or chain-distorting like proline (see fig. 2). Hydrophobic side-chains tend to attract or associate with other hydrophobic substances (lipids, haemoglobins' unbound haem), and

each other, so that globular proteins physically resemble lipid micelles and may act as detergents. Electrically charged side-chains are hydrophilic, affect proteins' general ionic environments, and/or specifically attract ions such as Ca^{2+}, Zn^{2+}, Cl^- and I^-, as well as oppositely-charged groups in the same molecules; hydrophilic groups usually lie on the outsides of globular proteins. Chemically

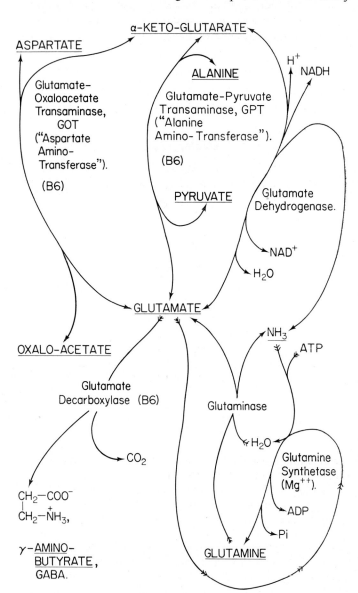

Fig. 16. Glutamate Metabolism. Substrates and products in capitals, main ones underlined; enzymes in lower-case. B6 = pyridoxal phosphate, a coenzyme.

reactive side-chains are the sites of the alterations mentioned in (i) above, independent of their physical properties; and certain residues, particularly serine, cysteine and histidine, seem particularly valuable in the active centres of enzymes, while serine is the site of the phosphorylations and dephosphorylations controlling glycogen and fat metabolism (figs. 10 and 11) and the functions of the histones (fig. 20). Certain residues, largely unidentified, must also be responsible for attachments such as that of

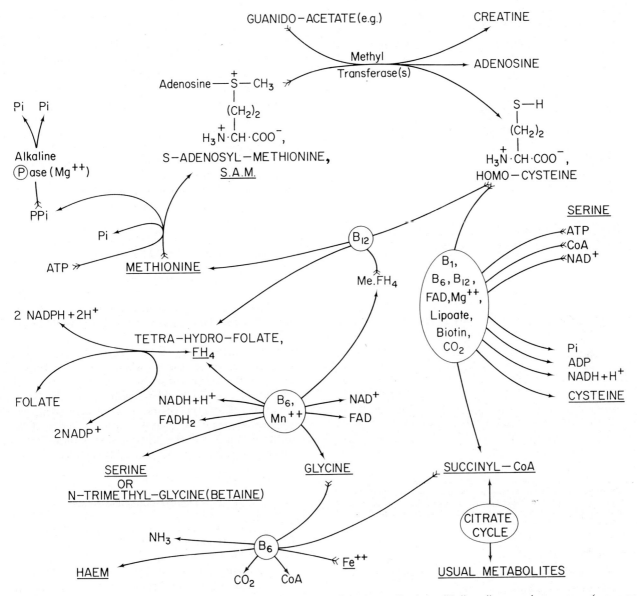

FIG. 17. Methionine metabolism, the anti-anaemia vitamins, and some of their main ramifications. "Balloons" = complex processes (names or co-factors enclosed).

citrate to PFK (p. 87) which affect enzymes' activities, often via conformational (**allosteric**) changes.

(iii) *Secondary, Tertiary and Quaternary Structures.* Polypeptide chains in general tend to have a **secondary** structure consisting of a tight right-handed spiral, the α-**helix,** but this is often broken, in particular by residues of the imino-acid proline; indeed collagen polypeptides, which are exceptionally rich in proline, give open left-handed spirals.

The **tertiary** structure of a protein is the total conformation of a single complete molecule, comprising the spirals mentioned above, bends, cross-links and co-factors. The **quaternary** structure refers to aggregation of these molecules; it may be of little apparent significance, or result in the "averaging" of the properties, or in functionally important interactions, of slightly different monomers (*e.g.* lactic dehydrogenase, p. 88; Hb, p. 97), or be

essential to the function of special mixtures of proteins (*e.g.* pyruvate dehydrogenase, p. 89).

Both are much influenced by local physico-chemical conditions such as pH, ion concentrations and the presence of lipids, as well as by the primary and secondary structures of the proteins themselves; they may be temporary and reversible (*e.g.* PFK, p.), or 87 alter definitely but reversibly during function (*e.g.* haemoglobin, cytochrome), or be rigid, permanent and irreversibly brought about by substantial chemical change. A relevant example of the last is again collagen, which matures roughly as follows: 3 (Fresh **Procollagen**) + O₂ →, enzymically as stated in (i), 3 (Procollagen-with-hydroxylated-lysine-and-proline-residues, "HO-Procollagen"); then 3 (HO-Procollagen) →, non-enzymically, (Procollagen)₃, the **Triple Helix**, a right-handed "rope"; then (Procollagen)₃ →, by enzymic proteolysis, (**Tropocollagen**)₃ + 3 (**Aggregating Peptide**), without which tropocollagen molecules cannot aggregate properly; followed by extracellular cross-linking of these new "short" "soluble" triple helices through the aldehydes

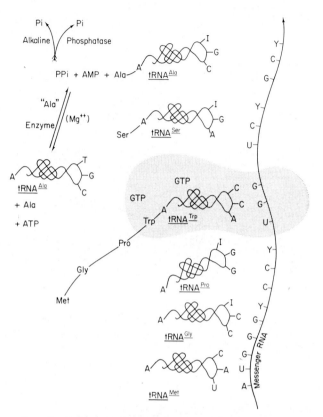

Fig. 18. Polypeptide biosynthesis and ribonucleic acids in the rough endoplasmic reticulum. Shaded area = a ribosome, moving up the mRNA; substances neither in it nor attached to it are free in the cytoplasm, and moving anticlockwise.

produced by lysine and hydroxy-lysine oxidation (see (i) above), and end to end linkage (mostly electrostatic) to form mature insoluble collagen fibres.

THE CHEMISTRY OF CELL STRUCTURES

As a prelude to discussion of the ultimate mechanism whereby a cell controls its own structure and working, the general steady-state chemical compositions of some better-known parts of cells are given in Table 3.

It must be remembered that such values could only be obtained by the analysis of centrifugally-separated collections of material from broken-cell preparations *in vitro*, and are therefore inevitably subject to several causes of uncertainty, including: impurity of the organelles analysed (*e.g.* contamination of mitochondria with lysosomes); changes due to enzymic action, interaction of one part of a cell with another, or mere instability, all of which are likely to be greater the greater the care—*i.e.* time—taken to "purify" the sample; and the mixture of cells present in every real tissue.

Cellular membranes' plentiful lipids may be nearly as

indispensable as proteins, not only structurally but also because several enzyme systems (*e.g.* pump ATPases, pp. 93, 97; the ETS, p. 90) work only in the presence of suitable lipids, either to ensure correct spatial arrangement or to provide "dry" conditions for the reactions to be catalysed. These lipids may be relatively unspecific; even cardiolipin (p. 96) can be replaced *in vitro* by other phospholipids of similar physical properties. Another function of intracellular lipids is to control membrane permeability; for instance, neither acyl CoAs (pp. 96, 91) nor NADH can enter or leave mitochondria, so that special mechanisms are needed for exchanging activated acyl groups and "hydrogen atoms" between mitochondrial and cytoplasmic enzyme systems.

CELLULAR IDENTITY AND THE NUCLEUS

Our small molecules, carbohydrates and lipids, are entirely products of our cells' vital proteins; but their production in turn depends absolutely on RNAs. Our lives therefore hang on the activities of the RNA-suppliers, our cells' nuclei.

Every nucleus has to be able to supply thousands of different RNAs, exactly when and as required, with absolute reliability, throughout its life; it must also have the power to reproduce itself with total fidelity at every cell division. These processes, like protein synthesis, need substrates, enzymes, energy, patterns and controls; the patterns used are the outstanding components of the nucleus, its deoxyribonucleic acids (DNAs).

Deoxyribonucleic Acids

The general structure of DNA is the same as that of RNA (fig. 19), except that 2'-deoxy-ribose replaces ribose, and **thymine** (5-methyl uracil, T for short) replaces uracil but has identical base-pairing properties; DNAs therefore pair readily either with RNAs (fig. 19) or with each other. When two fully complementary DNAs pair, they form the famous **Double Helix,** a "solid" right-handed screw with one large and one small groove, of rather coarse pitch (10 pairs of nucleotides per turn). This is the structure of nuclear DNA. It is very stable *in vivo*: individual human nuclei can survive without replication in almost unchanging cells like brain neurones, which are none the less very active metabolically as well as functionally, for up to 150 years. The durability of nuclear DNA may be partly due to the **supercoiling** needed to fit it into the nucleus: one average human chromosome contains about 0·14 pg. ($8·4 \times 10^{10}$ Daltons) of DNA, *i.e.* 40 mm. of Double Helix.

Nuclear DNA is usually neutralized by Mg^{2+} and quite large amounts of very simple basic proteins (almost identical in all metazoa) called **histones,** and is therefore most easily extracted as **nucleohistone** (equated to the cytologist's chromatin); but in rapidly-dividing cells, histones may be partly replaced by the polyamines spermine and spermidine (pp. 97, 105) or neutralized by the nuclear **non-histone proteins.**

TABLE 3

APPROXIMATE CHEMICAL COMPOSITION OF AN AVERAGE MAMMALIAN[1] CELL

Whole Cells contain about 75% of water, 20% of protein, 5% of lipids, 1% of nucleic acid and innumerable metabolic intermediates, including 1% of glycogen and (concn., very approximate, mM.): glucose 1, fatty acids 2, lactate 1, pyruvate 0·1, ketone bodies 0·2; total CoA 0·1, total carnitine 1; HMP 1, FDP 0·02, triose $\circledP$ 0·1, $\circledP$-glycerates 0·1, PEP 0·1; citrate 0·5, α-ketoglutarate 0·2, malate 0·3, oxaloacetate 0·01; NAD$^+$ 0·5, NADH 0·1, NADP$^+$ 0·005, NADPH 0·1; ATP 4, ADP 0·5, AMP 0·1, P_i 5, PP_i 0·003, PC 5, C 5; glycero $\circledP$ 0·1, pentose $\circledP$ 2; Glu + Gln 7·5, Asp + Asn 1, Gly 3, Ala 4, Ser + Thr 3, Cys 2, glutathione 5, NH_3 1, taurine 50.

Organelle	% of Cell's Dry Weight	Protein	Lipids Phospho-[2]	Lipids Other[3]	Combined Sugars[5]	RNA	DNA	Characteristic Enzymic Functions[10]
Plasma membrane[6]	2	50	30 L > K ≥ Spm > PS ≥ PI ≥ Ly	15[4]	4	1	0	Na$^+$-pump ATPase; adenyl cyclase; 5′-nucleotidase; leucine aminopeptidase; items of phospholipid metabolism.
Cytosol	50	95	4 L > K ≈ PA > PI, Spm, PS		1	1	0	Glycolysis and the "pentose shunt"; fatty acid synthesis; PEP-carboxykinase; transamination; amino-acyl-tRNA-forming particles; haem synthesis; carbonic anhydrase; cAMP diesterase.
Endoplasmic reticulum[6] — Rough (including ribosomes)	10	60	15 L > K > PI ≈ Spm	—	—	25	0	POLYPEPTIDE SYNTHESIS.
	(3)	(55)	—	—	—	(45)	0	
Endoplasmic reticulum[6] — Smooth	7·5	65	30 L > K > Spm > PI ≈ PS	2	0·3	2	0	Glucose-6-$\circledP$ase, Cytochrome P450 and b5 systems, hydroxylation, fatty acid desaturation; alkaline $\circledP$ase (PP$_i$-ase); lipid assembly; polyisoprenoid synthesis; fatty acid activation; aryl esterase.
Golgi apparatus[9]	2	55	25 L ≫ K > PI > Spm > PS > Ly	20[7]	—	—	—	Glycosylation of proteins and lipids; phospholipases; UDP-ase; ADP-ase.
Lysosomes	1	60	30 L > K ≥ Spm > PS ≥ PI ≥ Ly	4	4			Hydrolases with acid pH-optima: $\circledP$-ase, maltase, proteases, RNAse, DNAse, uronidases, sialidases, sulphatases, glycosidases, lipidases, lysozyme.
Peroxisomes	2	90(?)						Oxidases; catalase.
Glycogen particles	1	30			70			Phosphorylase; glycogen synthetase.
Mitochondria — Outer membranes	1	55	40 L > K > Spm ≈ PI	1	3	—	—	Fatty acid elongation; mono-amine oxidase.
Mitochondria — Inter-membrane spaces	2	90(?)						Nucleoside-di-$\circledP$-kinase; adenylate kinase.
Mitochondria — Inner membranes	9	75	20 L > K > CL > PI > Spm	1	1·5	0·5	0·05	Pyruvate dehydrogenase system; α-ketoglutarate and succinate dehydrogenases; the Electron Transport System; β-hydroxybutyrate dehydrogenase; CoA-carnitine acyl transferase; specific "translocases".
Mitochondria — Matrices[8]	8	90(?)				0·5	0·05	The Citrate Cycle[11]; fatty acid oxidation; glutamate dehydrogenase; pyruvate carboxylase.
Nucleus — Membrane	1	70	20 L > K ≫ PS ≈ PI ≈ Spm	2	3	4	1	Related to Smooth ER's, including glucose-6-$\circledP$ase and Mg^{2+}-activated ATPase.
Nucleus — Nucleoplasm	1	75				16	6	DNA-dependent DNA-polymerase; some glycolysis.
Nucleus — Chromatin	6	60	3 L > K ≫ Spm ≥ PS ≥ PI	1		2	30	DNA-dependent RNA-polymerase; ATPase; special methylases.
Nucleus — Nucleoli[8]	2	80				10	5	

— Low, uncertain, perhaps nil. Blank spaces: NO DATA.
[1] Majority of original data from rat liver.
[2] L = Lecithin (phosphatidylcholine), K = Kephalin (cephalin, phosphatidylethanolamine; often rich in pg); PS = phosphatidylserine, PI = phosphyl inositol, CL = cardiolipin, PA = phosphatidic acid, Spm = sphingomyelin, pg = plasmalogens (1-alkenylethers), Ly = lysophosphatides (monoglyceride- phosphatides).
[3] Mainly cholesterol, its esters, and some glycerides; glycolipids (cerebrosides, sulphatides and gangliosides) less frequent.
[4] Including 3% glycolipids.
[5] Neutral, amino and (in plasma membrane) sialates; as proteoglycans *and/or* glycolipids except in glycogen.
[6] Included in "microsomes".
[7] Including 1% glycolipids.
[8] Solids ≥ 50%.
[9] Resembles both plasma membrane and SER.
[10] Any enzyme may occur secondarily elsewhere. In particular: those of glycolysis or the "pentose shunt" may be partially bound to mitochondria or the ER, under the influence of substrates, products and salts; while alkaline $\circledP$ase and cAMP diesterase may alternatively be found in the plasma membrane.
[11] Except α-ketoglutarate and succinate dehydrogenases.

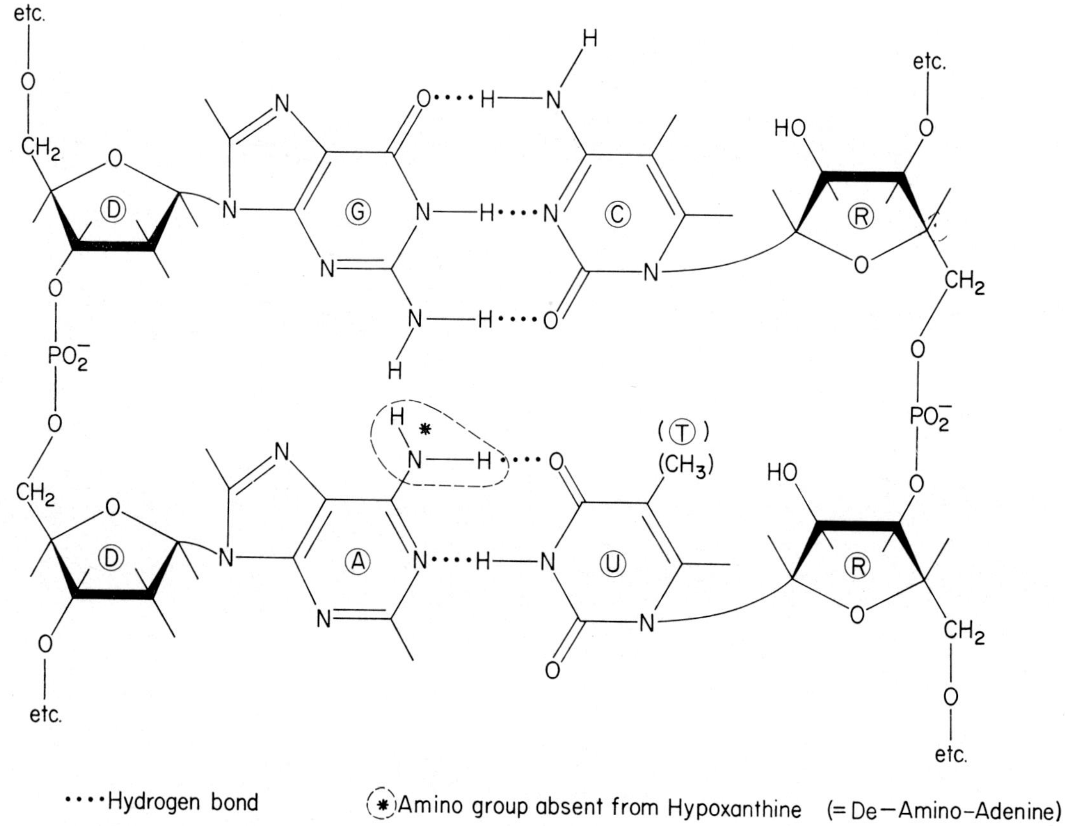

····Hydrogen bond   (✱)Amino group absent from Hypoxanthine   (= De−Amino−Adenine)

FIG. 19A. Base pairing between nucleic acids (DNA left, RNA right). Curved bonds = bases twisted into plane of paper. A = adenine, C = cytosine, D = deoxyribose, G = guanine, R = ribose, U = uracil (with additional —CH₃ where shown, becomes T = thymine).

Ribonucleic Acid Supply

The synthesis of RNA is very crudely illustrated in fig. 20. The main bulk of the nucleus makes mRNA and tRNA, whereas rRNA is made by the nucleoli (Chapter 6),

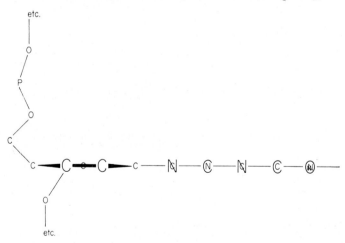

FIG. 19B. Correct orientation of Fig. 19A's deoxyguanylate residue, seen from the side of the Double Helix.

presumably because there need only be a limited number of species of rRNA, whereas the nucleus must be able to encode a different species of mRNA for every single different polypeptide (up to 5×10^6) which the cell can make. (Its total DNA—6 pg. or nearly 4×10^{12} Daltons, nearly 2 metres long—carries up to 2×10^9 anti-codons). A typical cell, however, usually contains much more rRNA and tRNA than mRNA, because the latter is often metabolized more quickly in response to the cell's varying needs for different proteins ($t_{\frac{1}{2}}$ for rRNA = 4 − 12d., for tRNA = 3 − 12d., for mRNA = 1 h. − 3d.).

The substrates of RNA synthesis, being ribonucleoside triphosphates, have all the necessary energy, and one enzyme, the Mg^{2+}-requiring **DNA-dependent RNA-polymerase** is sufficient. The Activities of these entities must affect the rate of the reaction, but its main control mechanisms remain uncertain. They cannot be simple! When an RNA is being made, it is essential that only one of the 2 DNA strands, that carrying the **anti-code** (T vs. A, A vs. U, G vs. C, C vs. G), be copied; and RNAs must be made— *i.e.* their DNA-anticodes or **cistrons** or **genes** be made available for **transcription**—when and only when required.

Histones inhibit the process, and their phosphorylation and dephosphorylation are believed to affect this inhibition, which is therefore controllable by hormones through adenyl cyclase and cAMP diesterase (*cf.* phosphorylase, fig. 11) which may also function through non-histone proteins.

Some hormones—including pituitary peptides, steroids and vitamin D—are thought to interact directly with chromatin after attachment to specific intracellular carriers, while proteins—including perhaps growth factors and insulin—may act via the plasma membrane, their direct influence being on nutrient entry or the cAMP system as above. **Thyronines** may belong to a third class of

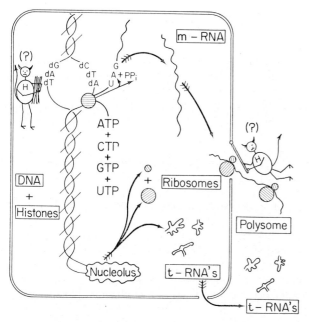

FIG. 20. How cell nuclei supply ribonucleic acids. H = hormones. The short (1 cm.) thin straight lines = histones. A = adenylate, G = guanylate, U = uridylate, dA = deoxyadenylate, dC = deoxycytidylate, dG = deoxyguanylate, dT = deoxythymidylate.

hormones increasing protein synthesis by, probably, stimulating the production of rRNA by nuclei.

Mitochondrial DNA (Table 3) encodes their few special RNAs (p. 99), but the control mechanisms are unknown.

Deoxyribonucleic Acid Replication

Cell division can only—but need not—follow the replication of nuclear (and mitochondrial) DNA. The chemistry of DNA replication is like that of RNA synthesis, except that the substrates are now the deoxyribonucleoside triphosphates (dATP, dCTP, dGTP, dTTP; figs. 3 and 19), the enzyme is DNA-dependent *DNA*-poly-

merase, and both chains are copied; but the control of the process is no better understood.

The removal or inactivation of the blocking histones may in this case involve the polyamines spermine and spermidine, which are found in relatively high concentrations, together with the enzymes and coenzymes making them from ornithine and methionine (p. 97), in rapidly growing and dividing cells. The process may need initiation by specialized "hormones," probably often proteins (see p. 104) such as **nerve growth factor** (NGF) and **erythropoietin.** In the other direction, cell division is somehow stopped both permanently by specialization, as in skeletal muscle and the CNS, and temporarily by contact with other cells and materials, as in epithelia or cartilage, or perhaps by the absence of a growth factor; but all these effects seem to be mediated by the plasma membrane.

Genes and DNA

It is now evident that a cell's whole potential composition and behaviour depend entirely on its proteins, and through them on its RNAs, and therefore on its nuclear DNA, which must accordingly be the repository of its genes; ordinary outside influences can either restrict or elicit their expression, but cannot easily modify them, as is shown by the stability of species over millions of years.

Ionizing radiations and certain chemicals can, however, induce mutations, which need not involve great chemical changes. For example, sickle-cell anaemia results from the patients' erythrocytes' HbA molecules being replaced by HbS, in which the two β-globins have the Residue 6's glutamate (code GAA, anticode CTT) replaced by valine (code GUA, anticode CAT), a very definite mutation having therefore resulted from the alteration of one base out of nearly 500 in one gene: the α-globins are perfectly normal.

Somatic cell nuclei need not each contain the entire genome; but every fertilized ovum's DNA must carry the entire prescription for the chemistry and structure of a human being, the most elaborate and therefore potentially unreliable "machine" known to us. Paradoxically, it seems to be the very complexity of this organism, its extraordinary by-product, that has so far enabled our DNA to exist in larger quantities, in more environments, and in greater security than almost any other.

8. INFLAMMATION, REGENERATION AND REPAIR

P. D. J. HOLLAND

Causes of inflammation
    Living agents
    Non-living agents

The acute inflammatory reaction
    The classical signs
    Vascular changes
    Permeability-increasing factors
    Emigration of blood cells
    Phagocytosis
    Types of exudate
    Outcome of acute inflammation

The chronic inflammatory reaction
    Irritants and the reaction thereto
    Cellular response
    Granulation tissue response
    Special characteristics

Remote effects of inflammation
    Pyrexia
    Changes in white cell count
    Rashes
    Raised erythrocyte sedimentation rate
    Changes in pulse rate
    Damage due to toxins and enzymes
    Degenerative changes
    Hypersensitivity
    Reactive hyperplasia

Circumstances which modify the inflammatory response
    Age
    Damage to the defence system
        Damage to bone marrow
        Damage to reticulo-endothelial system
    Antibiotic therapy
    Vitamin deficiency

Regeneration and repair
    Regeneration
        Labile, stable and permanent cells
    Repair
        Healing by first intention
        Factors influencing healing
        Healing by second intention
        Healing of specialized tissues.
            Bone
            Repair of nervous tissue
            Central nervous system
            Repair of peripheral nerves
            Repair of muscle
            Healing in tendons
            Epithelial repair
            Healing in liver
            Healing in kidney

INTRODUCTION

Inflammation is the term used to describe the normal expected response of healthy tissues to injury. It is therefore an essential precursor to repair. It should be regarded as a highly effective non-specific defence mechanism without which we would be unable to survive. It is necessary to stress that the injured tissues should be viable, because the medico-legal distinction between ante-mortem and post-mortem injury is the presence of an inflammatory reaction in the former.

From the beginning of time, man had been familiar with the outward manifestations of inflammation, but it took many centuries to discover that the inflammatory response could be distinguished from the injurious cause and accepted as a good thing without which the prognosis following injury would be poor. There are, however, a few exceptions to the general principle. There are some inflammatory reactions both acute and chronic that are actually harmful to patients, examples being auto-allergic and auto-immune reactions. Therapy in these cases is directed to reducing or abolishing the harmful inflammatory reaction. An older generation of doctors recognized the value of the inflammatory response and used the term "laudable pus" for the familiar expected outcome of pyogenic infections and directed their attention to promoting the acute inflammatory reaction by means of hot fomentations, poultices, dry heat, cupping and the like.

From the clinical as well as the histological viewpoint, it is possible to recognize two phases of the inflammatory reaction, *viz.* an acute phase and a chronic phase. This division, though useful from the point of view of teaching, nevertheless is a rather artificial one, and the inflammatory response cannot be so neatly subdivided but should be regarded as a spectrum of reaction having at one end the acute reaction and at the other end the chronic reaction, with an intermediate or "grey" area in between.

The type of inflammatory response evoked is determined by two factors: the nature and intensity of the irritant, and the ability of the tissues to respond, the ability being modified by many factors, *e.g.* age, immunological state, nutrition, drug therapy and the type of tissue. Inflammation should not be regarded as a purely local manifestation but may also include widespread body reactions.

CAUSES OF INFLAMMATION

The causes of inflammatory reactions may be divided into living agents and non-living agents.

Living Agents

The living agents include bacteria, viruses, mycoplasmas rickettsia, parasites, protozoa and fungi.

Non-living agents

The non-living agents include heat, trauma, ionizing radiation, infra-red, ultra-violet light, acids, alkalies, corrosives and miscellaneous foreign bodies and chemicals. It must not be forgotten that endogenous chemicals are also important causes of inflammatory reactions. The liberation of histamine during hypersensitivity reactions may cause urticarial wheals, angioneurotic oedema, erythematous rashes and vasculitis. Similarly, the liberation of fatty acids from areas of fat necrosis will evoke a characteristic chronic inflammatory reaction.

Tissue death due to ischaemia, as in infarction, also excites an inflammatory response in the surrounding living tissues. Finally, the antigen-antibody union resulting in the liberation of chemical mediators of inflammation may occur in the auto-immune diseases. The inflammatory reaction may occur *in situ*, as in Hashimoto's disease of the thyroid gland, or may result in multiple widespread lesions due to antigen-antibody complex deposition, as in systemic lupus erythematosus (SLE) or in periarteritis nodosa.

THE ACUTE INFLAMMATORY REACTION

The Roman Celsus (30 B.C.–A.D. 38) was the first to describe the classical signs of acute inflammation which have been since known as the cardinal signs of Celsus. These are *rubor* (redness), *calor* (heat), *dolor* (pain) and *tumor* (swelling). To these four signs was added a fifth, *functio laesa* (loss of function) by Galen, a Greek physician (A.D. 130–200). It would perhaps be more correct to interpret *functio laesa* as a disturbance rather than a loss of function as many inflamed tissues are hyperactive, examples being acute gastritis or acute rhinitis. The significance of these four cardinal signs of acute inflammation will be discussed in the following paragraphs.

Rubor

The redness of an inflamed part is due to a marked increase in blood supply consequent on vascular dilation. Lewis, in 1924, demonstrated that when skin is stroked firmly with the edge of a wooden spatula there occurs a dark red line corresponding to the stroke line. Shortly afterwards the red line is surrounded by a halo of lighter redness and following this the red line swells, grows pale, and forms a wheal. This sequence of events has been designated the "triple response" of Lewis. He further showed that a substance, the "H" substance, was liberated from the damaged tissues in the stroke line and that this "H" substance caused vasodilation by its action on the blood vessels in the stroke area. The duration of the inflammation could be prolonged considerably by occluding the circulation in the part, thus preventing venous drainage. The "H" substance of Lewis resembles histamine very closely, but is not identical with it. Thus anti-histamine drug therapy will not interfere with the triple response. Histamine present in many cells is undoubtedly liberated during tissue injury and is itself capable of producing a marked inflammatory response when injected into tissues. The sequence of events would appear to be:

(a) vasodilation, due to liberation of substances resembling histamine;

(b) a secondary vasodilation of arterioles in the surrounding skin resulting in the scarlet flare (fig. 1) due to the initiation of a local axon reflex by histamine-like substances; and

(c) the formation of a wheal due to fluid exudation because of increased vascular permeability in the stroke area, the pallor being due to partial obliteration of arterioles by the pressure of the exudate.

The redness of an acute inflammatory lesion can, therefore, be regarded as chemically initiated. The contribution made by the nervous system to the inflammatory response should not be overlooked, as an intact nerve supply and

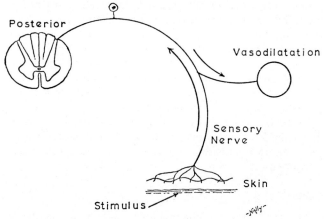

FIG. 1. The axon reflex of the triple response of Lewis.

function is probably necessary for optimum inflammatory response.

Calor

The heat produced in an inflammatory lesion is due to increased blood supply and also possibly to increased metabolic activity in the area. The appreciation of heat is only possible in those superficial parts of the body supplied with heat receptors, *e.g.* skin, subcutaneous tissues. Acute inflammation in deeper organs and structures of the body, although associated with increased heat in the area, is not associated with the perception of the increased heat.

Dolor

Pain is a manifestation of both superficial and deep inflammatory lesions through stimulation of nerve endings in the part involved, the impulses being transmitted through somatic nerves from the skin and superficial tissue, and through the autonomic nervous system from the deeper structures. All pain impulses enter the central nervous system by the lateral divisions of the posterior spinal nerve roots or the cervical nerves. The type of pain experienced depends on the extent of the stimulus rather than the type of causative agent. Pain is essentially a protective mechanism in that it draws attention to the damaging agent; trophic ulceration may occur when nerve conduction is interfered with by disease as in tabes dorsalis or syringomyelia.

Pain may be of two kinds: direct pain due to stimulation of nerve endings, and a condition of hyperalgesia or lowering of the pain threshold so that only slight stimulation is necessary to produce pain. Hyperalgesia appears to precede the directly produced pain in acute inflammatory lesions. There is a certain amount of doubt as to how pain is produced in inflammatory lesions There is little doubt that direct violence, or the pressure built up in a closed inflammatory lesion, will cause direct mechanical stimulation of the pain nerve-endings. Good examples of relatively "closed" lesions causing intense pain by pressure are acute osteomyelitis or acute dental abscess. Pain nerve endings have also been shown to be stimulated by various chemical substances released from injured tissues and present in inflammatory exudates. Examples are histamine, derived from a wide variety of cells including mast cells; 5-hydroxytryptamine derived from vascular endothelium and platelets; necrosin, a product of damaged tissues described by Menkin; a globulin or polypeptide plasma factor activated by contact with glass; and "P" factor described by Lewis and liberated from ischaemic muscles. Referred pain is due to spread of the pain stimuli along the nerves to the relevant spinal segments and relay of the pain sensation to other areas served by the same segmental distribution, examples being pain down the left arm associated with coronary ischaemia or pain in the shoulder associated with diaphragmatic inflammation.

Tumor

The swelling of an inflamed area is due to the increased vascularity and to the accumulation of fluid and cells in the damaged part. Should thrombosis of the surrounding blood vessels also occur then the swelling is greatly augmented.

Functio Laesa

As already indicated this term usually means a disturbance in function rather than a diminution in function. For example, in acute rheumatic myocarditis dilation of the heart, with heart failure, may occur. Jaundice usually accompanies acute hepatitis. Brain swelling associated with acute encephalitis may result in coma. A good example of diminution in function is the anuria which may rarely accompany acute glomerulo-nephritis.

On the other hand hypermobility of the intestine or of the stomach occurring in acute enteritis and acute gastritis manifests itself as diarrhoea and vomiting respectively.

The sequence of events which follows trauma and results in acute inflammation has been studied carefully *in vivo*, *e.g.* in the "window" preparation of a rabbit's ear or in the externalized rabbit's or guinea-pig's mesentery. Cohnheim (1882) was one of the earliest workers to study the phenomenon microscopically in the pig mesentery and in the frog's tongue. Indeed, the reader is recommended to read his vivid description of the events he observed and recorded in his "Lectures on General Pathology" (1882). The microscopic changes that occur following trauma can be seen readily by any of the above-mentioned techniques and recorded by means of cine-photography.

Vascular Changes

Calibre of Vessels

Following injury there occurs an immediate vasodilation, which not only markedly increases the size of the local arterioles and venules but also causes the opening up of dormant capillaries. The net result is a great increase of blood to the injured area.

The Formation of the Fluid Part of the Inflammatory Exudate

Escape of fluid from the dilated blood vessels into the tissue spaces takes place. This fluid, rich in protein, is known as an exudate and differs considerably from the fluid which accumulates in the tissue spaces in passive transudation. The exudate is a dynamically produced fluid while the transudate is merely a seepage of fluid from overdistended vessels. This is well seen in the analysis of excess fluid in serous cavities. In general inflammatory exudate has a high protein content, over 4 gm. per cent and a specific gravity of 1018 or higher, while the passive transudate has a protein content of 3 gm. per cent or less and a specific gravity of 1015 or lower. The cytology of the fluid is also helpful in differentiating the two fluids, there being very few cells present in a transudate.

Permeability Increasing Factors

A variety of chemical substances has now been identified in inflammatory exudates, in damaged tissues, and in the blood, which can promote increased permeability of blood vessels and lymphatics. Menkin (1936) called attention to a polypeptide which he named leukotaxine which had the property of causing increased vascular permeability. Many other workers have since confirmed the presence of permeability-increasing polypeptides in inflammatory exudates. As defined by Collier (1962) polypeptides are miniature proteins usually containing less than 100 aminoacids. The permeability-increasing polypeptides have been named kinins. Similar kinins are present in the venom of certain insects. Kinins, when applied at appropriate sites cause pain, whealing, dilation of blood vessels and contraction of smooth muscle.

Spector (1957) considered that polypeptides of a chain length of 8–14 aminoacids were responsible for the permeability-increasing effect. The permeability-increasing polypeptides are liberated from the injured cells in the inflammatory site and a polypeptide closely resembling leukotaxine has also been found in saline extracts of skin, muscle and testicle.

Apart from the permeability-increasing substances found in inflammatory exudates there are other substances present in plasma which, when activated by enzymes, also produce permeability-increasing kinins. In 1937 Werle, Gotze and Keppler in Dusseldorf demonstrated that human serum, treated with an extract of salivary glands, contained a substance capable of causing contraction of guinea pig colon. In 1948 Werle named the active substance kallidin. Later workers showed that the activating substance was an enzyme which was called kallikrein and which may be found in pancreas and salivary glands as well as in blood and in urine. Kallikrein may be activated from the inactive form, kallikreinogen, by contact with glass or by the action of proteolytic enzymes or Hageman factor XII. Another potent permeability-increasing substance, bradykinin, was first described in 1949 by Rocha e Silva, Beraldo and Rosenfeld in Sao Paulo and was isolated as a pure polypeptide containing 8 aminoacids by Elliott and his co-workers in 1960. Bradykinin may be liberated from plasma globulin by the action of trypsin. The relationship between kallidin and bradykinin was clarified when it was shown that there are two forms of kallidin, kallidin I and kallidin II, and that kallidin I is identical with bradykinin.

It is now clear that there is present in blood a substance, kallikreinogen, which can be activated into kallikrein by proteolytic enzymes or by Hageman clotting factor (XII) and which causes the formation of a permeability-increasing kinin, called kallidin or bradykinin, from the $alpha_2$ fraction of plasma globulin.

Apart from the permeability-increasing polypeptides there is some evidence to show that a permeability-increasing globulin may also play a part in the production of an inflammatory exudate. It has been shown that the serum of guinea pigs and other animals contains a permeability-increasing globulin which can be activated by dilution of the serum with saline. Spector (1957) also demonstrated the presence of both permeability-increasing and permeability-inhibiting globulins in rat plasma. The permeability-increasing globulin is present in an inactive form in plasma and can be activated by clotting in the presence of red cells, by the addition of platelet extracts and by incubation with isolated mitochondria.

Apart from the kinins and the permeability-increasing globulins, certain chemical substances are released in the injured area which also cause increased capillary permeability. These include histamine, derived from injured tissues and mast cells, and serotonin (5 hydroxytryptamine), derived from injured vascular endothelium, platelets, mast and argentaffin cells.

The prostaglandins, a group of chemically related long-chain fatty acids derived from prostanoic acid, have also been found to have a considerable vasodilatory activity in low concentration, apart from their many other functions. Prostaglandins E_1, E_2, F_{1a}, F_2 have recently been recovered from human inflammatory exudates and E_1 has been shown to behave as a histamine liberator.

Another widely distributed intracellular substance, cyclic adenosine 3′, 5′, monophosphate (cyclic AMP), has been shown to be a key intermediate in intracellular responses to a wide variety of external stimuli, including prostaglandins and many hormones, and is critically involved in the inflammatory response. High concentration of intracellular cyclic AMP appears to be associated with inhibition of many aspects of the inflammatory reaction, e.g. cellular proliferation, liberation of chemical mediators, chemotaxis, vascular and smooth muscle responses. Since cyclic AMP appears to act intracellularly and has little or no extracellular effect its role in inflammation may

be to regulate production of intracellular, short-range messengers, such as histamine and serotonin.

It will therefore be appreciated that the formation of an acute inflammatory exudate is dependent on a series of complex inter-related enzyme and chemical reactions involving kinins (kallidin, bradykinin, leukotaxine), globulin permeability factors, histamine, serotinin, Hageman factor, prostaglandins and cyclic AMP (fig. 2).

The type of fluid formed depends partly on the tissue involved and partly on the causative agent. Inflammation of serous membranes may produce a marked outpouring of fluid as in a case of "wet" pleurisy or pericarditis. In gastritis or in colitis an exudate rich in mucus will occur.

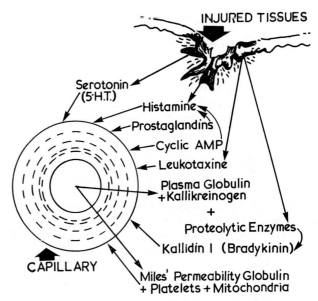

FIG. 2. Diagram to illustrate the chemical mediators of increased vascular permeability.

In other inflammatory exudates the amount of fluid formed is minimal and the production of fibrin is considerable as in the "dry" pleurisy associated with pneumonia or pulmonary infarction.

The fluid part of the inflammatory exudate has the following effects:

(a) it dilutes the irritant and renders it less harmful;

(b) it brings specific and non-specific immune substances to deal with the causative agent; and

(c) it brings fibrinogen to the area which may be converted into fibrin and help to wall off the inflamed area.

Emigration of Blood Cells

The increase in permeability of the vessel walls is accompanied by swelling and increased stickiness of the lining endothelial cells and a consequent disturbance of the axial stream of red cells and leucocytes. Normally the marginal stream in a vessel consists of plasma only. The resultant swelling of the vascular endothelium causes polymorphonuclear leucocytes to fall out of the axial blood stream and to line the walls of the vessels. This is known as "pavementing" or "margination" and is one of the earliest histological signs of acute inflammation. It is probable that the aggregations of red cells, formed because of the slowing of the blood stream, are partly responsible for forcing leucocytes into the marginal blood stream and hence facilitating margination. The leucocytes, granulocytes and monocytes alike, penetrate the vascular wall by forcing pseudopodia between the swollen and irregular endothelial cells and basement membranes and working their way through the wall by amoeboid movement, thus reaching the perivascular space. This movement is known as "emigration" or "diapedesis". The red cells also emigrate and form part of the cellular exudate, *i.e.* "haemorrhagic" exudates are sometimes seen in virulent bacterial or viral infections. Monocytes are conspicuous in many inflammatory exudates, particularly in virus infections. They are known to be phagocytic and become active macrophages when they emigrate from the blood stream into the tissue spaces. Eosinophils are the predominating cells in the inflammatory exudates associated with hypersensitivity reactions or with parasitic infestation. The presence of eosinophils in hypersensitive exudates may be related to their granules having an anti-histamine and anti-serotonin effect.

The emigration of leucocytes into the perivascular space is facilitated by the action of chemical substances liberated from the injured tissue, Menkin's leukotaxine being one of them. Similar chemically attracting substances, possibly lipo-polysaccharide in nature, may be liberated from dead bacteria. This attraction of leucocytes into the inflamed area through the action of chemical substances is known as chemotaxis.

Phagocytosis

By phagocytosis is meant the ingestion by polymorphonuclear leucocytes, monocytes, or tissue phagocytes of micro-organisms or particulate matter resulting from tissue breakdown. Small micro-organisms or particles which impinge on the surface of the cell appear to enter directly into the interior, but when larger micro-organisms or particles have to be dealt with a mass of protoplasm protrudes from the phagocyte in an amoeboid manner; this surrounds the material to be phagocytosed and engulfs it, so that it becomes incorporated into the cell body. A vacuole surrounds the ingested material and, if soluble, digestion of the material takes place. The rate and efficiency of digestion depends upon the material to be disposed of. Many bacteria may remain alive and even proliferate inside phagocytes. Indeed, bacteria may be spread throughout the blood stream by circulating leucocytes. On the other hand, virulent bacteria may kill the leucocyte that has phagocytosed them. Certain strains of streptococci possess a leucotoxic action when ingested. Quantitative or qualitative defects of granulocytes leading to a failure of phagocytosis may result in serious illness or death. Examples are drug-induced agranulocytosis and the rare genetic sex-linked defect of male children resulting in "chronic granulomatous disease" of childhood. In these children polymorphonuclear leucocytes can ingest bacteria but cannot kill them; as a result there is a chronic granul-

omatous reaction to bacterial invasion, instead of the expected acute inflammation.

Types of Inflammatory Exudates

From the foregoing it is apparent that an inflammatory exudate consists eventually of a protein-rich fluid of high specific gravity containing varying numbers and types of inflammatory cells and tissue phagocytes as well as fibrin, which varies in amount with the type of irritant. It will be appreciated that the type of exudate formed depends largely upon the tissue involved and the nature of the irritant. The following varieties of exudate are recognized:

(a) Fibrinous

In this variety the fibrinous element predominates over the fluid and cellular elements, *e.g.* the fibrinous pericarditis associated with rheumatic fever and which causes the characteristic "friction rub". Traumatic pericarditis is also largely fibrinous in type.

(b) Serous

In this type of exudate there is a massive out-pouring of fluid from serous membranes, the fluid largely obscuring the fibrinous and cellular elements. Examples of this type are exudates that occur in tuberculous pleurisy, pericarditis or peritonitis.

(c) Purulent

The essentials for the production of pus are that there should be a considerable accumulation of polymorphonuclear leucocytes in the injured area, and that there should be a good deal of tissue death, the dead materials being liquefied by proteolytic enzymes liberated from the dead leucocytes. The thickness and viscosity of pus depends largely on the amount of fibrin, nucleoprotein and nucleic acids present, the latter two substances being derived from broken down leucocyte nuclei. Purulent exudates, although characteristically produced by pyogenic bacteria, may also be caused by injurious chemical substances introduced into the tissues, *e.g.* turpentine.

The Outcome of Acute Inflammatory Reactions

The most favourable outcome for an acute inflammation is **resolution.** This is seen most dramatically when urticarial wheals are treated by anti-histamine or cortisone therapy. The exudate is resorbed quickly and tissue damage is negligible. Secondly, **localization** of the inflammation with pus production may lead to abscess formation, characteristically seen in staphylococcal skin lesions or apical dental abscesses. Thirdly, if neither **resolution** nor **localization** occurs, then **dissemination** of the process throughout the body may occur. Fourthly, if the acute inflammatory process does not succeed in destroying the irritant, then the character of the body's responses may alter and the lesion become chronic.

The amount of tissue destruction in acute inflammation depends upon the type of inflammatory agent and the duration of its activity. For instance, a common example of acute inflammation is simple sunburn which may resolve completely or lead to desquamation or "peeling" of the superficial keratinized layer of epidermis. In severe infections bacterial toxins may cause death of tissues by direct action or may cause ischaemic necrosis of tissue by thrombosing the vessels in the part. The rapid spread of gas-gangrene infection is due to a group of bacterial exo-toxins each having a specific effect on the tissues, *e.g.* lecithinase which destroys red cell envelopes, alphatoxin which is lethal for tissues and red cell envelopes, hyal-uronidase which destroys hyaluronic acid, a component of intercellular cement substances, collagenase, an enzyme which breaks down collagen, and saccharolytic enzymes which ferment the glycogen of dead muscle fibres.

THE CHRONIC INFLAMMATORY REACTION

Chronic inflammation is a distinctive response resulting from the interplay between two modifying factors, the nature of the irritant and the ability of the body to react to irritation.

There are many irritants which are harmful to the tissues but are not virulent enough to provoke the type of acute inflammatory response just described. Firstly there are groups of organisms which characteristically provoke a chronic inflammatory reaction rather than an acute one. These include *Mycobacterium tuberculosis*, *Treponema pallidum*, *Mycobacterium leprae* and a number of fungi, of which *Actinomyces israeli* is an example. These provoke a granulation tissue and mononuclear cell response and are called the chronic infective granulomata. The rather misleading term "granuloma" was introduced to describe the tumour-like mass of granulation tissue which occurs in certain chronic inflammatory lesions. Since that term was coined many more infections causing granuloma formation have been described, *e.g.* the venereal disease lymphogranuloma inguinale, caused by the lymphogranu-loma virus, and the world-wide virus diseases, trachoma and inclusion conjunctivitis, which involve the con-junctiva and cornea and lead to blindness. Coccidioi-domycosis and blastomycosis also produce granulomatous lesions.

Many industrial dusts inhaled into the lungs are known to give rise to chronic inflammatory lesions with granu-lation tissue production. Of these the best known are those lesions caused by silica, coal dust, asbestos, haematite and beryllium. Dusts of vegetable matter similarly have produced pulmonary granulomata, *e.g.* bagassosis from sugar refining residues and farmer's lung from spores from mouldy hay. Apart from these vegetable agents many foreign substances may provoke a foreign body chronic inflammatory reaction. Examples of these are unabsorbable suture material, talcum powder, and metallic and vegetable objects inhaled into the lungs. Endogenous foreign bodies such as the fatty acids liberated in fat necrosis, cystein crystals in cystinosis, and calcium deposits in hypercalcaemia, may also promote the formation of granulation tissue and ultimately fibrosis.

Occasionally pyogenic organisms which produce an acute inflammatory reaction may fail to be destroyed by the process, and the lesion becomes walled off. In these cases the body reacts by changing the acute process into a granulomatous process, the better to deal with the in-fection. Staphylococcal infections in particular may undergo this change, *e.g.* acute osteomyelitis may be con-verted into the chronic form. An acute dental abscess may be converted into a granulomatous pyogenic abscess.

Finally there are the chronic inflammatory reactions that occur in auto-immune diseases such as rheumatoid arthritis, Hashimoto's thyroiditis, and primary biliary cirrhosis, or in relation to certain type 3 hypersensitivity reactions of which farmer's lung (extrinsic allergic alveo-litis) is a good example.

Occasionally devitalized tissues such as the skin of oedematous or ischaemic extremities may fail to react to trauma with an acute inflammatory response and may instead produce a chronic granulomatous lesion. Debili-tated or elderly patients may fail to react to acute inflam-matory agents in the normal way and respond instead by a chronic inflammatory reaction. Rarely, in cases of im-paired granulocyte phagocytosis, an affected child may respond to pyogenic bacteria by producing the chronic granulomatous disease of childhood.

Just as exudation is the characteristic of acute inflam-mation so proliferation is the basic response in chronic inflammation. It is probable that the initial response to many of the previously mentioned chronic irritants is an acute one, and that the body changes its response fairly quickly when the acute inflammatory response does not deal adequately with the irritant. For example, the initial response in tuberculosis is a polymorphonuclear leucocyte exudate but this is quickly replaced by the typical epithelioid reaction. In actinomycosis also there is a leucocyte response preceding the granuloma formation. For some odd reason the leucocyte response remains around the fungus even when the granuloma is formed. In pyogenic lesions which gradually become chronic the leucocyte response may persist in a modified manner as in chronic osteomyelitis.

The chronic inflammatory response consists of two elements, the cellular response, the cell type varying with the irritant, and the granulation tissue response.

Cellular Response

The cells are derived both from the blood vessels of the part and from the tissues. The cells from the blood are for the main part lymphocytes and monocytes and, in hypersensitive states, eosinophils. Those from the tissues are mainly the cells of the reticulo-endothelial system which is stimulated to produce a variety of cells depending on the type of irritant, the cells being mainly epithelioid cells, plasma cells and lymphocytes. Non-separation of the mitosing epithelioid cells or possibly fusion of epithel-ioid cells leads occasionally to the formation of multi-nucleated cells, which have enhanced phagocytic activity. Epithelioid cells, monocytes, histiocytes and giant cells all exert their effects by phagocytosing the irritant. Plasma cells and lymphocytes are concerned with antibody production or transport.

Granulation Tissue Response

Granulation tissue is formed by the proliferation of new capillaries from the damaged blood vessels of the injured site. These are simple endothelial buds initially which grow into the injured area, become patent tubes and, finally, branching and ramifying capillaries. Diapedesis and exudation from such capillaries is a simple matter. *Pari passu* with this capillary proliferation there is a proliferation of young fibroblasts from the injured connective tissue of the part and from the injured blood vessels. Fine connective tissue fibres are soon laid down and form a firm scaffolding which supports the capillaries. As the lesion ages the fibrous tissue become collagenized and gradually forms a wall around the lesion. This granulation tissue response is the basis of the chronic inflammatory response and serves three purposes: it surrounds, tunnels into, and walls off the irritant; its rich blood supply allows phagocytic cells, enzymes, and specific and non-specific immune substances to be brought into contact with the irritant; the fibrous tissue elements allow of repair as the irritant is disposed of.

It must not be thought that the fluid part of the chronic inflammatory response is unimportant. While the fluid elements are more apparent in an acute inflammatory response, there are many chronic inflammatory lesions which produce a not inconsiderable fluid exudate. Examples of this are the "cold abscess" of Pott's spinal caries or the pus produced in a chronic osteomyelitis.

Special Characteristics

Many chronic inflammatory agents can stamp their image on the subsequent granuloma response so that they are histologically recognizable. In tuberculosis,

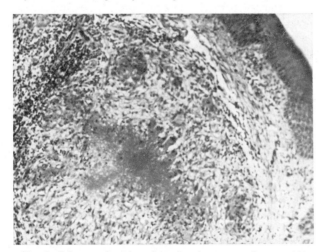

FIG. 3. Primary tuberculous focus in subcutaneous tissue. ×130.

lipid-rich necrotic tissue called caseation, and the surrounding epithelioid, lymphocytic and multinucleated Langhans type giant-cell cellular reaction are characteristic (figs. 3, 4). Plasma cell exudate, a caseous-like gumma, and the intimal proliferation of blood vessels in the part suggest a syphilitic granuloma. In tuberculoid

leprosy the presence of numerous acid-fast bacilli in the epithelioid cells helps to distinguish this granuloma from that of tuberculosis which it closely mimics. The presence of polymorphonuclear leucocytes and fat-laden phagocytes in a granuloma should make the observer suspect actinomycosis; typical "sulphur" granules in the pus consist of

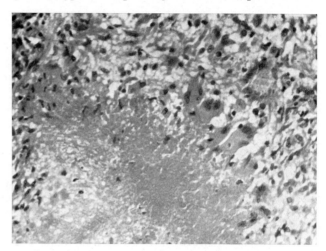

FIG. 4. Centre of the tuberculous focus showing caseation and giant cell formation. ×250.

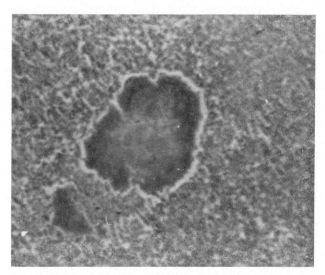

FIG. 5. Actinomycotic granuloma of the lung showing a colony of actinomyces. ×150.

colonies of fungus (fig. 5). In the foreign-body granuloma seen in the dust diseases of the lungs, around foreign bodies, around areas of fat necrosis, dead parasites and the like there are numerous multinucleated foreign-body giant cells which either contain or closely embrace the foreign particles (fig. 6). Chronic pyogenic granulomas have a less specific appearance but should be suspected when both plasma cells and polymorphonuclear leucocytes are present in the granulation tissue (fig. 7). The granuloma of rheumatism may be recognized by its distinctive Aschoff cells and Anitschkoff myocytes (fig. 8). In the collagen diseases *e.g.* periarteritis nodosa, lupus erythematosus disseminata and scleroderma, there occurs a characteristic fibrinoid necrosis of collagen fibres around which the inflammatory reaction takes place. In sarcoidosis the granuloma characteristic of the disease consists of whorled aggregates of epithelioid cells, lymphocytes and Langhans giant cells (figs. 9, 10). The appearances closely mimic those of tuberculosis but caseation is rarely seen in sarcoidosis.

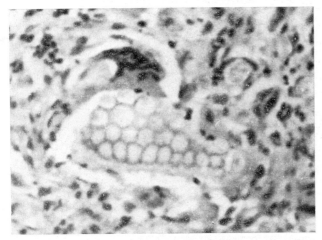

FIG. 6. Foreign body reaction surrounding vegetable matter embedded in an eyelid. ×240.

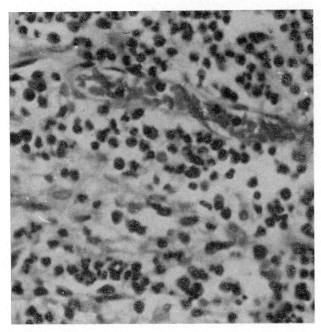

FIG. 7. Pyogenic granuloma showing multiple capillaries and cellular infiltrate. ×450.

THE REMOTE EFFECTS OF INFLAMMATION

Pyrexia

Many acute and chronic inflammations, particularly those of bacterial, viral or autoimmune origins, are accompanied by a rise in temperature and possibly by sweating, the latter being the body's method of lowering the temperature by increasing the evaporation rate from the skin surface. The causative agents are known as pyrogens and include bacterial toxins as well as products of tissue breakdown, e.g. Menkin's "pyrexin".

The temperature regulating mechanism is located in the hypothalamus, the anterior region controlling heat loss and the posterior region being concerned with heat conservation. Pyrogens are not produced by every bacterium, the Gram negative bacilli being the most pyrogenic with E. coli taking pride of place. The pyrogenic substance is a lipopolysaccharide and it is relatively heat resistant. Tissue pyrogens are destroyed by heat. The pyrogens temporarily damage the heat-regulating centre and cause a breakdown in the regulation of body temperature. In

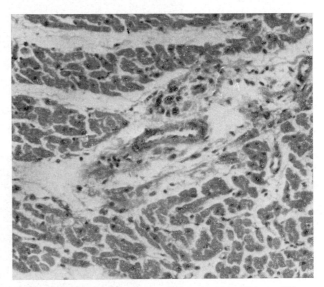

FIG. 8. Aschoff body in acute rheumatic myocarditis. ×150.

severe infections pyrexia may be accompanied by a reflex vasoconstriction of the skin vessels resulting in pallor with a feeling of coldness of the skin surfaces. This is known as the paradoxical cold sensation and is due to the fact that as skin temperature increases to 40°C the cold receptors become "triggered off", resulting in a sensation of coldness. This stage, if violent, is called a "rigor", is characteristic of the septicaemic phase of some infections, and is occasionally seen after transfusion with blood contaminated by bacterial pyrogen. Shivering is another heat centre reflex mechanism for increasing body temperature.

Changes in White Cell Count

Many acute and some chronic inflammations cause changes in leucocyte count in the blood. The pyogenic cocci and bacilli, such as staphylococci, streptococci, pneumococci, Escherichia coli, meningococci, stimulate a polymorphonuclear leucocytosis. White cell counts of 15,000–30,000 mm³ are not uncommon in pyogenic infections. Occasionally in children counts of 60,000 mm³ or more may occur and simulate leukaemia. A leucocytosis promoting factor (LPF) liberated from injured tissues has been described by Menkin. This factor, a thermolabile globulin, causes an increased output of granulocytes and megakaryocytes from the bone marrow and a rise in the

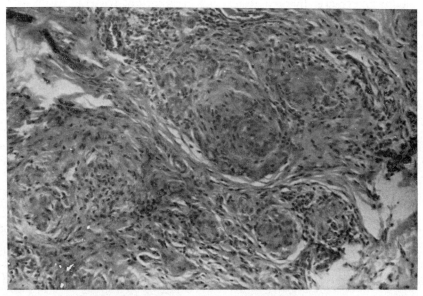

Fig. 9. Sarcoid granuloma in subcutaneous tissue. ×100.

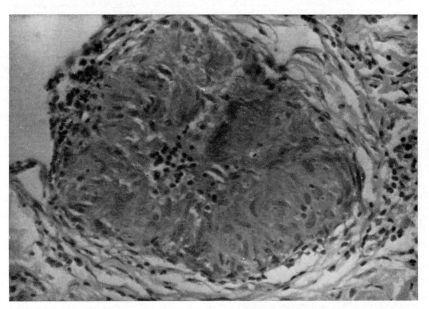

Fig. 10. Sarcoid granuloma in subcutaneous tissue. ×250.

number of circulating leucocytes. Certain infections on the other hand cause a leucopoenia, *e.g.* typhoid fever and infective hepatitis. Menkin has isolated a leucopoenia producing thermolabile pseudo-globulin from injured cells which may cause a reduction in the circulating granulocytes or mononuclear cells. He named this substance "leucopenin".

In young children, particularly, the pyogenic cocci may evoke a lymphocytic or monocytic response rather than the expected polymorphonuclear response. The characteristic lymphocytosis found in whooping cough caused by *Haemophilus pertussis* is a valuable diagnostic finding in that disease.

Virus infections characteristically invoke a lymphocytosis or a monocytosis, *e.g.* glandular fever. Many allergic, fungal or parasitic inflammations evoke an eosinophilia. Eosinophilia may thus be found in hay fever, skin diseases, asthma and hydatid disease.

Rashes

Many acute inflammations, particularly in virus infections of childhood, give rise to rashes, which are characteristic of the particular infection—for example those of measles, scarlet fever and typhoid fever.

Raised Erythrocyte Sedimentation Rate

In most inflammatory states the erythrocyte sedimentation rate is increased and this fact makes the ESR estimation a valuable aid in diagnosis. The increased rate of sedimentation of red cells is due mainly to increases in plasma fibrinogen, alpha$_2$ globulin and gamma globulin. These globulins coat the red cells and by increasing their stickiness causes the formation of rouleaux. The rouleaux, being heavier than individual red cells, sediment more quickly. The highest sedimentation rates encountered occur in those diseases which give rise to the presence of abnormal globulins, particularly macroglobulins, in the circulating blood, *e.g.* macroglobulinaemia, multiple myeloma, or rheumatoid disease.

Changes in Pulse Rate

In general the increase in temperature accompanying acute inflammation is paralleled by an increase in pulse rate, in which case a rise in pulse rate of about 10 beats per min. commonly accompanies a rise of 1°F. The increase is due to an increase in metabolic rate. Occasionally, as in diphtheria, toxic myocarditis is caused by the exotoxin. Conversely bradycardia, or slowing of the heart rate, may occur in typhoid fever. The pulse rate, therefore, is not always a reliable guide to the degree of pyrexia present.

Specific Bacterial Exotoxic or Enzyme Damage

Many tissues are damaged by specifically acting toxic substances or enzymes liberated from the bodies of the infecting bacteria. For example, haemolysins produced by beta haemolytic streptococci or lecithinase produced by *Clostridium welchii* may cause anaemia by haemolysing red cells. Many bacteria produce neurotoxins which damage the central or peripheral nervous system, examples being the exotoxin of the *Clostridium botulinum* or of *Corynebacterium diphtheriae*. The exotoxin of *Neisseria meningococcus* may cause adrenal haemorrhage and shock.

Degenerative Changes

In many acute inflammatory states, particularly generalized ones, wide varieties of cells suffer damage by toxic interference with their metabolic activities, resulting in such changes as cloudy swelling and fatty degeneration. In certain long-continued chronic inflammatory diseases such as rheumatoid arthritis, amyloid degeneration may supervene.

Development of Hypersensitivity

In many chronic inflammatory states, particularly those due to bacterial or, more rarely, viral infections, a generalized tissue hypersensitivity may develop, *e.g.* the positive tuberculin skin test in tuberculosis or the positive Frei test in lymphogranuloma inguinale. Organ sensitization may also occur during certain infections, an example being the acute glomerulonephritis that sometimes accompanies streptococcal tonsillitis.

Reactive Hyperplasia

Generalized lymph node enlargement with enlargement of the liver and spleen may accompany certain acute or chronic inflammatory states, *e.g.* miliary tuberculosis, secondary syphilis, rheumatoid arthritis, typhoid fever or infectious mononucleosis. The generalized lymphadenopathy and the organomegaly seen in many inflammatory states is due to proliferation of cells of the reticuloendothelial system in response to stimulation by the infecting agent or its toxic products. The simultaneous phagocytosis of the agent and the production of immune antibodies is the reason for such hyperplasia in most instances.

The presence of chronic inflammation with resultant increased vascularity often results in hyperplasia of epithelium in the affected area. Such hyperplasia is seen in mucous polyps in chronic rhinitis, in ulcerative colitis, and in the epithelial proliferation which occurs in an apical granuloma associated with a non-vital tooth.

CIRCUMSTANCES WHICH MODIFY THE INFLAMMATORY RESPONSE

The following circumstances alter the inflammatory response and interfere with resolution or with ultimate healing.

Age

In general terms it can be stated that the very young and the very old are less able to combat infection because of a lack of an effective inflammatory response. In infants who have died from acute infection, particularly virus infections, the histological evidence of an acute inflammatory response may be negligible. Many "cot deaths" amongst infants are of this kind. At the other end of the scale many elderly patients respond with a chronic inflammatory response to agents which in younger patients would have provoked an acute response. Such inflammations, *e.g.* pneumonia, may not resolve and the net result is organization and fibrosis.

Damage to the Bone Marrow and Reticulo-endothelial System

As the cells of the inflammatory exudate are derived from the blood stream and from the reticulo-endothelial system it is obvious that damage to or suppression of either the bone marrow or reticulo-endothelial system will seriously interfere with the inflammatory response.

Damage to Bone Marrow

Agranulocytosis may occur in susceptible persons during treatment with a wide variety of drugs, *e.g.* thiouracil, tridione, sulphonamides, amidopyrine, phenylbutazone. Occasionally, severe neutropoenia may be caused by overwhelming bacterial infection, *e.g.* pneumococcal pneumonia and tuberculosis.

A more serious condition, aplastic anaemia, may rarely occur in susceptible individuals during such forms of therapy as ionizing radiation, chloramphenicol, tridione, mesantoin, 6-mercaptopurine, folic acid antagonists, and nitrogen mustard.

In both agranulocytosis and aplastic anaemia the absence of an adequate leucocytic response in the bloodstream and in the damaged area may lead to widespread dissemination in the case of bacterial infection.

Damage to or Suppression of the Reticulo-endothelial System

The reticulo-endothelial system is the source of most of the cells of the chronic inflammatory reaction—lymphocytes, plasma cells, epithelioid cells, macrophages. Neoplasia of the system will therefore interfere with the chronic inflammatory response in conditions such as Hodgkin's disease, leukaemia, or reticulum cell sarcoma.

The reticulo-endothelial system is also the site of antibody production and damage to or a defect in the system, by preventing an effective antibody response, may prolong a bacterial inflammation. Suppression of both the cellular and immune mechanisms occurs during adrenocorticosteroid therapy. Such immunosuppression is deliberately undertaken in the treatment of auto-immune diseases or collagen disorders by steroid therapy. Another effect of adrenocorticosteroid therapy is the inhibition of granulation tissue formation, and steroids are therefore very useful in the treatment of certain collagen diseases, *e.g.* rheumatoid arthritis, periarteritis nodosa and scleroderma. Unfortunately, the inhibition of granulation tissue formation also adversely affects wound healing.

Suppression of the reticulo-endothelial system may occur as a by-product of deep X-ray therapy and, indeed, immunological paralysis may be deliberately induced prior to organ transplantation in an effort to prevent organ rejection. If suppression of the inflammatory response or antibody production is undertaken therapeutically, a careful watch has to be kept to detect occult infection.

Antibiotic Therapy

Acute or chronic inflammatory responses will be modified by antibiotic therapy or chemotherapy depending upon whether the organisms are sensitive to the drugs or not. Antisera may also have a decisive effect in limiting certain inflammatory lesions, for example immune globulin in measles and in German measles.

Vitamin Deficiency

Vitamin A is necessary for the health of epithelial surfaces and vitamin A deficient patients may fail to produce a good inflammatory response following injury. Vitamin C is essential for good granulation tissue production so that in scurvy inflammatory lesions may be slow to heal.

REGENERATION AND REPAIR

Regeneration and repair are essential concomitants of the inflammatory process. Every inflammatory reaction, all things being equal, carries within itself the impetus to repair and regeneration. The two mechanisms cannot be viewed in isolation.

Regeneration

By regeneration is meant the replacement of damaged or dead tissues by new tissues having the same function. The ability to regenerate varies from animal to animal and from tissue to tissue. Certain of the lower animals are capable of complete regeneration or reconstitution of highly specialized and functioning parts. For example, the earthworm can regenerate itself perfectly if cut in two, the newt can replace a lost limb, and the crab a claw. Higher animals have lost this facility and so regeneration is limited to replacement of specialized cells and their supporting stroma and vasculature.

This ability in man to regenerate cells is itself limited, some cells regenerating easily, some with difficulty and a few not at all. Thus it is possible to classify cells into labile, stable and permanent cells.

Labile Cells

These are cells with a limited life span and quick turnover and include squamous epithelium, transitional epithelium, columnar epithelium of the gastro-intestinal tract and respiratory tract, endometrium and the red and white cells of bone marrow.

Stable Cells

These are cells with a much lower rate of turnover than labile cells and include epithelium of the liver, of the renal tubules and of the pancreas.

Permanent Cells

These are cells not capable of regeneration; the neurone is the classic example.

The mechanism whereby specialized cells proliferate in response to injury and hence initiate regeneration has not been fully elucidated. Two factors, however, do appear to be important, one positive and the other negative. The positive factor is the increase in free RNA concentration in local cells that occurs quickly in the damaged site resulting from the breakdown of RNA protein complexes liberated from dead cells. The degraded free RNA is followed by a marked synthesis of the new RNA which probably provides the protein bricks to assist in building up of DNA and so facilitating mitosis.

The negative factor is the reduction, due to cell loss, of the mitosis-inhibiting cell specific factors (Illingworth, 1966) called chalones, which in turn leads to a rapid cell division of the surviving cells.

Repair

By repair is meant the replacement of injured tissues by proliferation of the surviving tissues in the area, specialized and unspecialized. The degree of specialized tissue replacement depends upon the extent of the injury and so it is convenient to describe the sequence of events depending upon whether the gap to be filled is small or large, *i.e.* healing by first or by second intention.

Healing by First Intention, *i.e.* Clean Incised Wounds

In such wounds the gap to be closed is small and the amount of the surface epithelial regeneration is minimal in extent. The sequence of events is as follows. Immediately following injury there is a local acute inflammatory response. Blood from the injured blood vessels fills the gap and clots on the surface to form a scab or crust (fig. 11). This protects and seals the surface and thereby limits

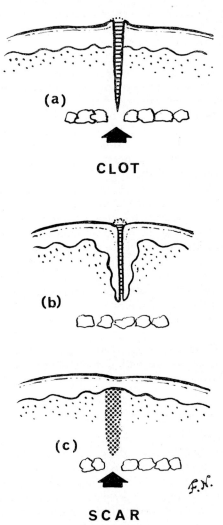

FIG. 11. Repair of an incised wound.

infection. The injured connective tissues proliferate, fibroblasts advancing from either side into the blood clot. The fibroblasts elongate into fibres which ramify with one another and by contraction tend to draw the wound edges close together. Simultaneously the cut blood vessels produce endothelial buds which ultimately form capillaries; these penetrate the blood clot and by coalescence with other capillaries produce new vessels which are supported by the connective tissue fibres. Blood and tissue macrophages move into the area and remove dead tissue or bacteria while proteolytic enzymes from the newly formed capillaries assist in dissolving other unwanted material. Thus a natural debridement takes place in the injured site.

As the fibroblast processes become collagenized they contract, drawing the wound edges together. The newly formed reparative capillaries having completed their work atrophy and disappear and the collagenized connective tissue shrinks and becomes almost indistinguishable

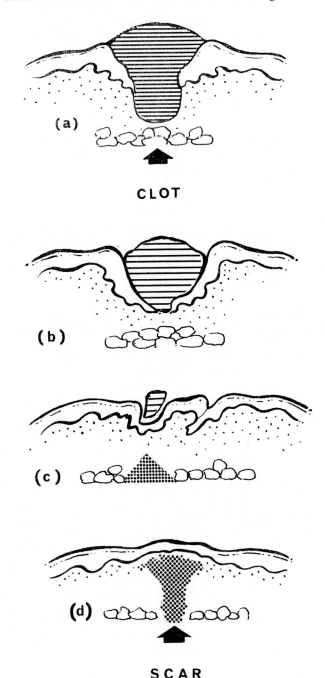

FIG. 12. Repair of a gaping wound.

from the original connective tissue of the part. Meanwhile the surface epithelium creeps in under the crust from both sides and fuses to form a new complete covering. The crust is ultimately shed, leaving a completely epithelialized surface. In the immediately adjacent tissues the acute inflammatory reaction stimulated by the injury resolves and the healing process is complete (fig. 12). This process of the healing of a clean incised wound usually takes about 5–7 days and the histopathologist has often difficulty in detecting evidence of recent healing in incised wounds 8–10 days after injury.

The circumstances described are optimal and the reader will realize that the speed and completeness of healing of an incised wound depends upon the nature and extent of the injury. These are modifying factors which influence healing and will be discussed below.

Factors which Influence the Healing Mechanism

Movement. Movement is inimical to good healing because it interferes with the proliferation of both the vascular and fibroblastic components which are the essential mechanisms of the process. Continued movement may indeed convert an incised wound into an open one, and may delay, almost indefinitely, the healing of an open wound. An appreciation of this fact is the basis for the use of bandages, adhesive plasters, plaster casts and splints. As already indicated, well placed sutures may contribute greatly to the outcome of the healing process by inducing immobilization apart from bringing closer together the edges of the wound.

Blood Supply. A good blood supply is the prequisite for good healing. Diseased blood vessels cannot be expected to produce good functioning capillaries and similarly an anaemic patient will not heal as well as a patient with normal blood. Indeed bedsores are notoriously slow to heal because, apart from the pressure atrophy which induced the skin necrosis, they almost invariably affect elderly subjects with either a degree of anaemia or else vascular disease. Varicose ulcers are similarly slow to heal because of the poor venous return from the part rendering the area hypoxic.

Vitamin C. This vitamin is concerned with the integrity of vascular endothelium, with the formation of collagen and the collagen-containing hard tissues such as bone and dentine and with the maturation of the normoblasts in the marrow; thus healing in subjects with vitamin C deficiency is notoriously slow and incomplete. Indeed trauma followed by infection of the gingivae of patients with scurvy produced the classical gingivitis seen early on in that disease. It should be noted that subclinical scurvy is not uncommon in the elderly patient who comes for dental treatment and that hypovitaminosis C is not confined to those in the lower income groups.

Wound Infection. Bacterial infection of wounds delays healing and may convert a clean incised wound, such as a surgical incision, into an open granulating wound. Postoperative wound sepsis due to the "hospital" *Staphylococcus pyogenes* or to the coliform group of bacteria may delay postoperative recovery and be an appreciable factor in prolonging hospitalization, and may occasionally lead to serious complications. While the vast majority of operative wounds are clean incised wounds which should heal by first intention, in the small percentage of inevitably contaminated wounds healing may be facilitated by judicious local or systemic antibiotic treatment. Anaerobic bacteria of the clostridia family constitute a considerable danger in soil-contaminated traumatic wounds.

Presence of Foreign Bodies. The presence in a wound of extraneous materials, or indeed of bone fragments and the like, interferes with the reparative mechanism by encouraging the persistence of the granulation tissue phase of healing. Well performed surgical debridement is essential to good healing and repair.

Drug and Radiation Therapy. Adrenal corticosteroids have an inhibiting effect on granulation tissue production and fibrous tissue organization, so that wounds heal slowly or even fail to heal in those on cortisol therapy. Spontaneous reopening of operation wounds and rupture of sutured tissues with possible necrosis are not, unfortunately, infrequent postoperative complications in those on long term cortisol therapy. Cytotoxic drugs may also inhibit healing because of their effects in depressing circulating and tissue phagocytes, thus allowing of wound infection. Radiation also has an inhibiting effect on healing, a factor which has to be borne in mind when advocating radiotherapy prior to surgery in the treatment of neoplastic disease.

General Nutrition. Adequate supplies of protein and vitamins, particularly Vitamin A, as well as a well-balanced hormonal background are essential to good healing.

Chronic Ill-health. Surgical and other wounds may be slow to heal in patients with chronic illness, *e.g.* diabetes mellitus, chronic renal failure, chronic sepsis.

Healing by Second Intention

In this type of wound there occurs tissue loss of varying degree which demands a greater reparative effort than is required for a clean incised wound. The tissue response to the injury does not differ in kind but rather in extent, and although healing will take place the end result will not be as functionally or cosmetically satisfactory as in the repair of an incised wound, and will take a great deal longer to be completed. The healing of an open wound involving skin and subcutaneous tissues will be described as this is the type of wound most commonly met with, but the principles apply to all wounds in any part of the body where there has been tissue loss of any extent. The mechanism of repair also applies equally to the disposal of dead tissue in any part of the body, *e.g.* areas of infarction, thrombi and haematomata. Regenerative capacity varies from tissue to tissue and the healing of wounds in certain tissues will be described in greater detail following the description of the general healing process.

Immediately following injury an inflammatory reaction occurs and blood clot forms in the site thus tending to seal off the area (fig. 5A). Into this clot advance the proliferating fibroblasts which traverse the clot to meet up with those from the opposite side. Ramification of the now united connective tissue fibres tends to the formation of a firm scaffolding arranged largely horizontally in the blood clot. Simultaneously capillary buds proliferate from torn blood vessels and advance along the connective tissue supports. The solid buds open up to become functioning endothelium-lined tubes which form loops by coalescing with similar vascular tubes entering the blood clot from the opposite side. The loops are so arranged that their apices project towards the surface. The clot is next dissolved and removed by a combination of proteolysis and cellular phagocytes to the healthy margin of the wound, where it is finally disposed of through the lymphatic system. Contraction of connective tissue fibres and shrinkage of the clot now bring the opposing edges close together and the looping of the capillaries supported by the connective tissue becomes more apparent; the appearance of these pink loops on the surface of the reparative tissue was the inspiration for the term "granulation tissue", which is the basic mechanism for the healing of all "open" wounds.

In the initial stage of healing surface epithelium begins to creep into the area of granulation tissue, thus forming the familiar blue margin of the healing wound. It is believed that this process is largely amoeboid in mechanism at first and that true regeneration follows later. The specialized skin appendages, i.e. sweat glands, hair follicles do not regenerate. Continued contraction of the wound occurs as collagenization proceeds. Pari passu with this the granulations begin to atrophy and re-epithelialization of the surface continues. The inflammatory reaction in the surrounding healthy tissue dies out and the blood phagocytes are replaced by tissue macrophages. Eventually the wound gap is filled with fibrifying granulation tissue and finally is converted into a mass of avascular collagenized scar tissue which projects above the surface when healing is complete. Occasionally in some patients the reparative tissue remains vascular and grows above the surface to form a soft pink tissue called "proud-flesh" which may have to be removed by cautery. A similar mass of soft granulation tissue may occur in the gingiva as a result of minimal trauma in pregnant women and is known as "pregnancy granuloma". It is axiomatic that the bigger the wound and the longer it takes to heal, the more scar tissue will be formed. This knowledge is made use of by deliberately retarding healing following gingivectomy in the hope that increased contracture of the granulation tissue may anchor the teeth more firmly to the alveolus.

By making use of the knowledge gained by studying wound healing it is possible to improve appreciably the end result of almost any kind of wound. The removal of dead tissue (debridement), of foreign particles and of pathogenic bacteria is particularly helpful in speeding up healing. Judicious suturing of the cleaned open wound may, by bringing the edges together, convert an open wound into a clean incised one, and so speed up repair and minimize scar tissue formation. In any event scars following open wound healing may be later excised, allowing of repair by first intention with a good cosmetic result. Large open granulating wounds, e.g. following burning, may be covered by split skin grafts which exercise a remarkable and little understood influence on the underlying granulation tissue so that surprisingly good end-results may be obtained. The basis for good cosmetic surgery is a thorough understanding of the principles of healing by primary and secondary intention. In some individuals densely collagenized and exuberant scar tissue forms and projects above the epithelial surface. This is known as keloid.

Healing of Specialized Tissues

Bone. The healing of bone is discussed in Chapter 47.

Repair of Nervous Tissue. As already indicated neurones are permanent cells incapable of mitotic division so that when death of such cells occurs they are not replaced. Death of a neurone is followed by degeneration and ultimate disappearance of the associated axon. Conversely if the axon is severely damaged, particularly in motor nerves, a retrograde degeneration takes place leading to histological changes in the neurone which may be reversible or which may proceed to necrosis. The neuroglial supporting and protecting cells of the brain, e.g. astrocytes, oligodendrocytes and microglial cells are capable of mitotic division and take part in repair. Because of the structural differences between the central and peripheral nervous systems the repair mechanisms of each will be described separately.

Central Nervous System. Necrosis from whatever cause in the brain and spinal cord is quickly followed by a breakdown of the myelin sheaths of the axons in the part, so that the tissue becomes soft, swollen and changes colour. The oily droplets and other tissue debris are phagocytosed by the microglial cells which proliferate, become enlarged and granular and are referred to as "compound granular corpuscles". The neurone undergoes chromatolysis, the nucleus breaks down and eventually disappears and the pale, swollen cell eventually disintegrates. The softened, necrotic nervous tissue, if extensive enough, may eventually be converted into a cavity filled with a yellow oily liquid and lined by a mass of compound granular corpuscles and proliferated astrocytes, the latter producing a profusion of fibrils which come together so that the wall of the cavity becomes relatively firm in consistency. This latter repair process is known as gliosis and represents a form of fibrous tissue repair of nervous tissue. A good example of the foregoing type of repair follows cerebral infarction in the internal capsular region of the brain. If the necrotic lesion is small, gliosis without cavitation will occur so that the end-result will be a brain scar.

Repair of Peripheral Nerves. Following damage to a peripheral nerve there occurs a change in the axon known as Wallerian degeneration. The nerve axon distal to the injury suffers breakdown of its fatty sheath into lipid droplets which are quickly phagocytosed by cells derived from the nerve covering. Simultaneously the cells of the sheath of Schwann proliferate to form cords of cells. The neurofibrils in the distal fragment undergo degenerative changes with disintegration of those fibrils which are closest to the site of injury. The axon proximal to the site of injury undergoes Wallerian degeneration up to the level of the nearest node of Ranvier. If the injury is severe enough and close to the neurone then chromatolysis or even death of the neurone may occur. Should the neurone not suffer irreversible damage, proliferation of the neurofibrils of the axon takes place, the neurofibrils penetrating into the proliferating Schwann cells and, guided and protected by them, proceed to grow into the distal proliferating Schwann cells and so establish continuity between the proximal and distal axons. Eventually, under optimal conditions, a firm union is effected, a new perineurium is established, and later a new myelin sheath. Functional continuity takes a good deal longer to be restored. It is reckoned that neurofibrils grow at the rate of about 3 mm. per day so that restoration depends on the distance to be travelled between the torn ends of the axon. While a small gap can be successfully bridged in a month or two, a period of a year may elapse before sensory or motor function is restored.

From the above facts it is obvious that surgical treatment of torn nerves should be devoted mainly to locating the torn nerve ends and reducing the gap between them by means of suturing and immobilization. Delay in surgical treatment will lead to shrinkage of the nerve endings, and the formation of granulation tissue and later fibrous or even osteoid tissue between them, will make subsequent operation more difficult and the end-result less satisfactory. Should the proximal neurone undergo necrosis, repair of the axon is impossible. Occasionally in amputation stumps there occur small extremely painful nodules which are composed of a mass of proliferated neurofibrils and Schwann cells and are known as "amputation neuroma".

Repair of Muscle. In general it is accepted that the regenerative capacity of both striated and smooth muscle is poor, and that damage to muscle is healed by fibrous tissue replacement leading to scar formation. There are, however, exceptions to this general rule. In Zenker's degeneration of muscle, particularly the rectus abdominis, in which because of bacterial toxaemia individual muscle fibres die, the dead fibres are removed by phagocytes and replaced by the ingrowth of multinucleated sarcoplasmal sprouts from the viable end of the muscle fibre; these ultimately restore continuity to the fibre. Similarly in transected areas of voluntary muscle which have been closely apposed, similar sarcoplasmal unions may occur between the cut ends leading to restoration of continuity. Surgical anastomosis of large or small bowel heals by fibrous tissue union, but there is probably also a limited muscle regeneration between the two ends allowing of functional continuity to be established.

In areas of myocardial infarction repair is by fibrous tissue replacement and there is little or no muscle regeneration, although multinucleated myocytes may be seen in the healing area. Occasionally in chronic inflammatory diseases of the lung, muscle tissue is prominent in areas of interstitial fibrosis. In these circumstances the muscle is believed to be derived from damaged blood vessels or bronchioles.

Healing in Tendons. When a tendon is damaged, bleeding occurs at the site of injury followed by a non-specific acute inflammatory reaction. From the connective tissue and blood vessels of the tendon, fibroblasts and new capillaries invade the blood clot between the torn ends. Organization follows the removal of debris by phagocytes and new connective tissue fibres produced by the invading fibroblasts link the proximal and distal tendon together. The connective tissue fibres gradually thicken and create a new fibrous tissue union. It is believed that muscle pull is important in promoting proper alignment of the reparative tissue fibres.

The process of collagenization of the repair is a slow one so that functional recovery from a torn tendon may be delayed for a long time. Suturing of the tendon and immobilization of the joint are important in determining the rate of recovery.

Epithelial Repair. As already indicated epithelial regeneration in the gastro-intestinal and respiratory tracts is both quick and effective under optimal conditions. Endometrial regeneration is a good example of cyclical repair. Regeneration in other secretory organs such as the thyroid, the pancreas, the pituitary and adrenal is rather limited.

In other tissues although regenerative capacity is good the outcome depends upon a number of factors, chief among them being the preservation of the reticular and vascular framework of the affected organ, the adequacy of the blood supply and the continuation or cessation of the action of the injurious agent. The two organs most studied in this respect are the liver and the kidneys.

Healing in Liver. It has been known for a long time that surgical removal of three-quarters of the liver in healthy animals is followed by restoration of the liver mass in a matter of a few weeks. The study of liver disease in the human by means of needle biopsy has shown that liver cell necrosis of zonal distribution, such as occurs in viral hepatitis, may be followed by complete anatomical regeneration of liver cells through proliferation of the surviving cells. This is dependent on the preservation of the reticular and vascular supporting framework of the liver lobule. Death of the framework results in connective tissue repair and liver scarring. Examples of this type of repair are "cirrhosis" and post-necrotic scarring of the liver. Persistence of the necrotizing process or the superimposition of an auto-immune mechanism, as in chronic active hepatitis, will also seriously interfere with regeneration of liver cells and result in fibrous tissue repair. Nevertheless, despite the onset of fibrosis, liver cells regenerate in a most remarkable manner and may maintain liver function despite shrinkage from the normal 1,500 gm. in an adult to 1,100 gm.

Healing in Kidney. Glomerular tufts are incapable of regeneration so that in any necrotizing glomerulonephritis healing is accomplished by fibrous tissue replacement followed by hyalinization of the tufts. Renal tubular epithelium on the other hand is capable of remarkably speedy regeneration provided that the reticular and vascular framework of the tubules is preserved.

Acute tubular necrosis arising from profound hypotension from whatever cause may be followed by complete tubular epithelial regeneration with restoration of renal function in a high percentage of cases, provided that the cause of hypotension and the disturbed fluid and nitrogen imbalance are adequately dealt with. In such cases the artificial kidney is life saving.

ADDITIONAL READING

Florey, H. W. (1970), *General Pathology*, 4th edition. London: Lloyd-Luke.

Illingworth, C. (Ed) (1966), "Wound Healing," *The Lister Centenary Scientific Meeting, 1965*. London: J. & A. Churchill.

Atkins, E. (1960), "Pathogenesis of Fever," *Phys. Rev.*, **3**, 580.

Best, C. H. and Taylor, N. B. (1961), *The Physiological Basis of Medical Practice*, 7th edition. Baltimore: Williams & Wilkins.

Cohnheim, J. (1882), *Lectures on General Pathology*, 2nd edition, pp. 247–80, London (New Sydenham Society Translation, 1889).

Collier, H. O. J. (1962), "Kinins," *Sci. Amer.*, **207**, 2, 111.

Menkin, V. (1956), *Biochemical Mechanisms in Inflammation*, 2nd edition. Springfield: Thomas.

Spector, W. G. (1957), "Activation of a Globulin System Controlling Capillary Permeability in Inflammation," *J. Path. Bact.*, **74**, 67.

SECTION III

IMMUNOLOGY

9. THE MECHANISMS OF THE IMMUNE RESPONSE

J. L. TURK AND M. F. COLE

THE NATURE OF THE IMMUNE RESPONSE

Adaptive immunity has been developed as a phylogenetic response by vertebrates to effect the elimination from the body of foreign invasive materials. It is a process of recognition and rejection of that which is foreign or "not self". The origins of adaptive cellular and humoral responses are first found in the higher cyclostomes, primitive chordate fishes, which are among the most primitive creatures to develop undifferentiated invasive tumours, and it has been suggested that the immune response evolved as a surveillance mechanism against such tumours.

The term "immunogen" is used to describe anything that induces an immune response *de novo*. Antigens are substances capable of reacting with preformed antibody or initiating antibody production in previously immunized animals. Antigens are generally protein or polysaccharide. Lipids alone are not antigenic, although they can contribute to the antigenicity of proteins or polysaccharides by forming lipo-proteins or lipo-polysaccharide molecules. Peptides of molecular weight greater than 10,000 are generally antigenic, although peptides of molecular weight as low as 1,000 have also been found to be antigens. An example of a low molecular weight antigen of clinical importance is insulin (molecular weight 6,000). Polysaccharides have to be of larger molecular weight to be antigenic; thus, while dextrans of molecular weight 100,000 are not antigenic, dextrans of molecular weight 600,000 are capable of inducing an immune response. (The dextrans used as plasma volume expanders are of molecular weight between 40,000 and 150,000 and are not believed to be antigenic.)

Molecular size, however, is not the only determining characteristic of an antigen. Complexity of the tertiary structure appears to be necessary, and a high concentration of tyrosine residues enhances antigenicity, perhaps by conferring rigidity to the molecule at the antigenic site. The physical state is another important property of an antigen; for example, albumin is a better antigen in an aggregated than a non-aggregated form.

The process of reaction with antigen to cause its eventual elimination is undertaken either by soluble circulating antibodies with recognition sites specific for each antigen, or antibody-like structures attached to the surface membrane of specifically sensitized lymphocytes. It is generally believed that antigen selects immuno-competent lymphocytes already carrying specific antibody receptors for that antigen, and that antibodies are not synthesized as a mirror image, so to speak, of the antigen being used as a template. The immune response provides a sufficient concentration of antibody receptors to effect a biological reaction. The reaction of antigen and antibody is not a function of the whole antigen but a localized area of the molecule known as the antigen determining site. The antigenic determinant may be of a relatively low molecular weight compared with the whole immunogenic molecule and can sometimes be as small as 8–12 amino acids. This fragment of an antigen capable of reacting with antibody receptors, but incapable of stimulating an immune response alone, is known as a hapten.

Body protein and polysaccharide tissue antigens are recognized as "self" because the immunological mechanism has experienced them in late fetal or early neonatal life while immature, or has been rendered "tolerant" by exposure to a particularly high concentration of them in adult life. If a hapten is bound to tissue antigens artificially the self molecules act as carriers and the whole hapten-carrier molecule becomes an "immunogen". Other than early primary antibody production, which is hapten specific, secondary humoral antibody and cell mediated responses are both hapten and carrier specific. An example of this phenomenon is chemical contact sensitivity where painting a simple chemical on the skin renders the skin (bound to the chemical) antigenic, and a reaction is mounted against the antigen, although part of it is "self", to cause its "rejection".

Such contact sensitizers are the aniline dyes, epoxy resins and hardeners used in the electronics industry, and the accelerators and antioxidants used in the rubber industry. Examples of similar substances are the halogen substituted nitrobenzenes, one of which, 2.4-dinitrochlorobenzene (M.W.203), is regularly used in clinical medicine to test the ability to develop an immune response. Other sensitizers are primulin (M.W.210) derived from the plant *Primula obconica*, potassium dichromate which causes cement dermatitis, and nickel.

There are a number of other ways in which self proteins may come to be regarded as foreign. As well as chemical changes, physical changes of the tertiary configuration of the molecule may occur. Such changes may result from exposure to ultraviolet or X-irradiation. Self molecules may also carry hidden antigenic determinants which were not available before the maturation of the immune mechanisms but may be exposed by the action of enzymes derived from infecting organisms. The term autoantigen is used to describe a self macromolecule that is not recognized as such. Failure to recognize self may occur not only as a result of changes in the chemical and physical nature of the molecule, but can also result from defects in the recognition phase of the immune response itself. This may occur in old age or during severe chronic infections such as tuberculosis, leprosy and syphilis. Such changes in antigen recognition or immune response result in the process known as autoimmunity.

The process both of recognition of a substance as foreign and its rejection is a function of the class of cells known as lymphocytes. There are two ways in which lymphocytes can effect the rejection of a foreign antigen. The first is by developing specific surface receptor sites, in which case they are referred to as "specifically sensitized lymphocytes" and the process is known as cell-mediated immunity.

The other is by the secretion of soluble serum proteins—immunoglobulins. This is called the humoral antibody response. Before secreting humoral antibodies lymphocytes differentiate into plasma cells. The reaction between specifically sensitized lymphocytes or antibody with antigen may result in the elimination or neutralization of the antigen. This is known as immunity. However, the reaction may incidentally release a sequence of enzymes which result in the local secretion of agents that can cause tissue damage. Local tissue damage occurring in the vicinity of reaction with antigen is known as an allergic or

hypersensitivity reaction. Immunity and hypersensitivity result frequently from identical immunological reactions.

DIFFERENTIATION OF LYMPHOCYTE FUNCTION

The stem cell from which all lymphocytes are derived is found in the bone marrow (fig. 1). In late fetal and early neonatal life bone marrow stem cells migrate into the thymus where they are influenced to become immunocompetent lymphocytes. These cells, called T-lymphocytes

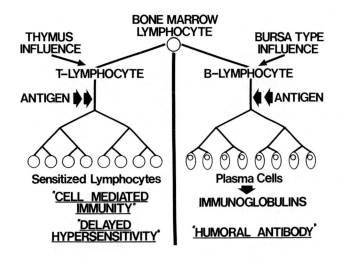

Fig. 1. Pathways of cellular differentiation.

(meaning thymus-derived), are capable of reacting with antigen to become specifically sensitized lymphocytes which mediate the cellular immune response (CMI).

The mechanism by which the thymus influences stem cells to become T-lymphocytes is not fully understood but it is possible that a thymus hormone assists cell maturation. Cells which proliferate in the thymus itself have some of the characteristics of T-lymphocytes and these can increase as thymocytes move from the cortex to the medulla. However, T-cells only achieve their full potential in cell-mediated immune reactions once they have left the thymus.

In the mouse, thymus cells carry a specific surface antigen, the θ-antigen which is also carried by all their peripheral T-lymphocytes. Human T-cells can be identified by their ability to form rosettes with sheep red cells *in vitro* due to the presence of specific receptors on their surface. There is no doubt that thymus cells can move from the thymus to the thymus-dependent areas of lymphoid tissue. However, in certain species the presence of the thymus in the adult is not necessary for the maintenance of a population of effective T-cells. There is moreover, a considerable body of evidence which suggests that the "thymus hormone" maintains an effective population of T-cells in the body in the absence of the thymus. Recently, two subclasses of T-cells have been described in mice. One population, T1, is normally present in the thymus and spleen and may decrease in numbers in secondary lymphoid tissue (spleen and lymph nodes) 2–6 weeks after adult thymectomy. The second type, T2, is not present in the thymus, nor does it decrease in numbers in secondary lymphoid tissue after adult thymectomy, but is depleted by neonatal thymectomy. It has been suggested that T1 is the progenitor of the effector cells of cellular immunity whereas T2 acts as an amplifier of the humoral immune response.

T-cells form the mobile pool of long-lived lymphocytes and migrate continuously through the thymus-dependent area of peripheral lymphoid tissue (figs. 2 and 3) (the paracortical areas of lymph nodes and the periarteriolar areas of the spleen) and appear in thoracic duct lymph. The re-circulating pool of T-lymphocytes is depleted by neonatal thymectomy in mice, congenital thymic aplasia

However, a population of long-lived B-cells is also known to exist. B-cells are depleted in bursectomized chickens and also temporarily in animals treated with large doses of cyclophosphamide. B-cells respond to antigen which is taken up first by the macrophages in the medulla of lymph nodes or in the red pulp of the spleen, and later by dendritic macrophages in the lymph follicles. In the presence of antigen, B-cells in the lymph follicles proliferate to form germinal centres whereas those at the cortico-medullary junction and in the medullary cords can proliferate and differentiate to become plasmablasts and eventually plasma cells. Plasma cells contain a network of rough endoplasmic reticulum on the surface of which polypeptide chains are assembled and secreted as immunoglobulin (antibody) molecules. B-cells can be distinguished from T-cells by the amount of immunoglobulin they normally carry on their surfaces. These accumulations of

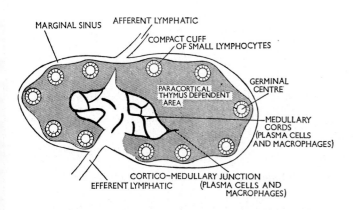

Fig. 2. Diagram of immunologically active lymph node.

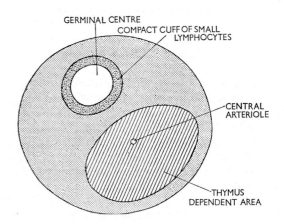

Fig. 3. Diagram of a spleen follicle.

in humans (di George syndrome and Nezelof syndrome), treatment with antilymphocyte serum (ALS), and chronic thoracic duct drainage. All these conditions are associated with a consequent failure of cell-mediated immunity—proliferation of T-cells normally occurs in the thymus-dependent areas of lymph nodes and spleen as a result of antigen stimulation during the development of cell-mediated immunity. T-cells are not found in significant numbers in the bone marrow.

In birds, bone marrow stem cells also migrate in a similar manner to the Bursa of Fabricius, a lymphoid organ lying posterior to the cloaca, where they become Bursa-derived or B-lymphocytes. (No Bursa analogue can be found in mammals but it is generally held that gut-associated lymphoid tissue serves a similar function). In response to stimulation by antigen, B-cells proliferate and differentiate into plasma cells which synthesize humoral antibody.

B-lymphocytes are found in the lymph follicles, germinal centres and at the cortico-medullary junction of lymph nodes, and in the red pulp and non-thymus-dependent areas of the white pulp of the spleen. They are mainly sessile cells with a more rapid rate of turnover than T-cells.

immunoglobulin can be seen as speckles on the B-lymphocyte cell membrane at 4°C and aggregate to form a caplike accumulation at body temperature. B-cells can also be distinguished by their receptors for complement and can therefore form rosettes when incubated with sheep red cells that have reacted with antibody and complement.

For the majority of antigens maximum humoral antibody response by B-cells cannot occur unless there is a co-existing T-cell response. However, antigens with a repeating substructure such as pneumococcal polysaccharide, endotoxin and antigens at high concentration are able to induce an independent B-cell response. The antibody produced is of the IgM class which appears to be less thymus-dependent than the other classes of antibody (immunoglobulin). There is evidence that B- and T-cell co-operation is necessary for the switch from IgM to IgG synthesis, that occurs in a secondary immune response. B-cells stimulated directly, without T-cell modulation, are easily made tolerant. It is known that B-cells are hapten specific and T-cells carrier specific, and possibly T-cell regulation occurs by means of the T-cell presenting or focussing antigen for the B-cell so that antigen forms a bridge between B-cells binding haptenic determinants, and T-cells binding carrier determinants.

However it is most widely considered that the T-cell response augments the B-cell response by the production of antigen-specific soluble mediators of relatively high molecular weight acting through macrophages. The augmentation or suppression of a B-cell response in the production of humoral antibody by a simultaneous T-cell response would appear to be an example of a natural homeostatic control mechanism. A similar control mechanism also exists in which a simultaneous B-cell response can modulate a T-cell response, resulting in a restrained cell-mediated immune response.

HUMORAL ANTIBODIES

Antibodies belong to the class of serum proteins known as immunoglobulins (Ig). On electrophoresis of serum, immunoglobulins separate into γ globulin and the slow β globulins.

All antibody molecules are thought to have a similar basic four chain structure as shown in fig. 4. This consists of two light chains of 25,000 M.W. and two heavy chains of 50,000 M.W. joined by three disulphide bonds. The molecule can be split by the enzyme papain into three fragments, two containing the antigen-combining site (denoted Fab fragment) and one which cannot combine with antigen and when purified can be crystallized (denoted Fc fragment). The antigen-binding sites are formed by the adjacent portions of the N-terminal regions of the light and heavy chains. These have a variable sequence of amino-acids which allows for the specificity of the antigen-binding capacity of the site. The variable region of the light chain consists of 107 amino-acids, and that of the heavy chain 118 amino-acids. The light chains of all immunoglobulins have either κ-antigens or λ-antigens. The rest of the molecule is relatively constant in its sequence of amino-

acids. All immunoglobulins are produced by cells of the plasma cell series. An individual plasma cell synthesizes only a single class of immunoglobulin with either κ or λ light chains.

Immunoglobulins have been divided into five classes IgG; IgA; IgM; IgD and IgE on the basis of specific antigenic differences present at the C-terminal region of the heavy chain. The concentrations of the different immunoglobulin classes in different body fluids are shown in Table 1.

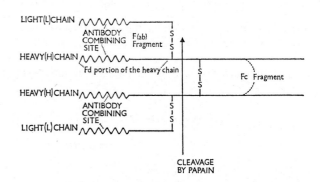

Fig. 4. Diagram of the polypeptide chains of the immunoglobulin molecule. The two antibody combining sites are formed by the end portions of the light chain and the Fd fragment of the heavy chain.

Immunoglobulin G (IgG γ Heavy Chains)

Approximately two-thirds of all immunoglobulins belong to the class known as IgG. IgG has the basic structure described above, a molecular weight of approximately 150,000 and a sedimentation coefficient of 7S when separated in the ultracentrifuge. Four antigenically

TABLE 1*

IMMUNOGLOBULIN CONCENTRATIONS (mg./100 ml.) IN SERUM AND SECRETIONS

	Immunoglobulin					Ratio	
	IgG	IgA	IgM	IgD	IgE	IgG:IgA	IgG:IgM
Serum	1,230	328	132	20	0·04	3·8	9·3
(Normal range)	800–1,680	140–420	50–190	0·3–40	0·01–0·07		
Colostrum	10	1,234	61			0·008	0·16
Stimulated parotid saliva	0·036	3·95	0·043			0·009	0·84
"Unstimulated" whole saliva N	1·44	19·40	0·21			0·07	6·86
P	6·97	37·14	0·76			0·19	9·17
Duodenal secretion	10·4	31·3	20·7			0·33	0·50
Jejunal secretion	34·0	27·6	N.D.			1·23	N.D.
Colonic secretion	86·0	82·7	N.D.			1·04	N.D.

N = Normal subjects

P = Patients with periodontitis

N.D. = Not determined

* Adapted from Brandtzaeg, P., in *Host Resistance to Commensal Bacteria*. Ed. T. MacPhee, Churchill Livingstone, Edin. and Lond., 1972.

distinct sub-classes of IgG have been identified—IgG1, IgG2, IgG3 and IgG4 which differ by small changes in the amino-acid sequences of the constant region of the heavy chain. IgG is able to fix complement, binding the Clq component through the Fc portion of the molecule. Complement activation requires two molecules of IgG in close apposition.

IgG is the only immunoglobulin which is selectively transferred across the placenta.

Agglutinating and opsonizing antibodies may be of the IgG class, but IgG antibodies are most effective at neutralization and are involved in neutralizing diphtheria toxin, lysozyme, poliomyelitis virus and in agglutinating the flagella of *Salmonella* species.

IgG can also bind to the surface of macrophages forming what is known as cytophilic antibody. Cytophilic antibody may enhance the ability of macrophages to ingest and kill virulent organisms.

Immunoglobulin A (IgA α Heavy Chains)

IgA has a higher carbohydrate content but is otherwise similar in structure to IgG except that heavy α chains replace the γ chains. Monomeric IgA molecules tend to polymerize easily into complexes with sedimentation coefficients of 9, 11, or 13S. Immunoglobulin A is the dominant immunoglobulin in external body secretions such as saliva, colostrum, tears, nasal mucus and intestinal fluid, and also in urine. Thus the concentration of IgA in parotid saliva is 100 times greater than that of IgG, and the ratio of IgA to IgG in parotid saliva is 400 times greater than the ratio in normal serum. The concentration of IgA in parotid saliva is inversely related to the flow rate. Much IgA is produced locally by plasma cells in the mucous membranes. In the parotid gland plasma cells are present in small clusters adjacent to the ducts or scattered between the acini and almost all of them secrete dimeric IgA. Apart from the local synthesis much immunoglobulin is stored in the connective tissue of the glandular stroma.

During the selective secretion of IgA molecules an epithelial glycoprotein (M.W. 50,000) known as "secretory component" (SC), "secretory piece" (SP) or "transport piece" (TP) is conjugated to each dimer. Secretory component shows great affinity for IgA dimers and some IgM polymers. The combination of IgA and SC is effected by disulphide bonds and to a lesser extent by noncovalent interactions resulting in a tightly packed quaternary structure. This compact structure may explain the unique resistance of secretory IgA (SIgA) to digestion by a variety of proteolytic enzymes. Free SC may play a part in the selective homing of IgA and IgM synthesizing plasma cells, for in the intestinal mucosa these cells are found close to secretory cells containing a high concentration of secretory component.

Recently secretory IgA and IgM have been found to contain a further polypeptide chain, the J chain (M.W. 25,000), the function of which is as yet unknown.

Antibodies of the IgA class have been found to be "natural" antibodies and to have antibacterial and antiviral activity. Local infection and vaccination are more effective in stimulating an IgA response than parenteral vaccination. The strength and duration of the response is dependent on the local persistence of antigen.

It is now considered that SIgA is capable of activating complement in the presence of lysozyme, and it is probably not without significance that SIgA and lysozyme are found together in many external secretions.

Immunoglobulin M (IgM μ Heavy Chains)

This class of antibodies is often called the "macroglobulins" because of their high molecular weight (M.W. 900,000) and valency. They are considered to be the most primitive immunoglobulins and are well adapted for highly efficient agglutination and cytolysis. IgM is particularly efficient in complement activation and only one molecule is necessary for cell lysis. Antibodies produced in the primary response to an immunogen are of the IgM class. Immunoglobulin M antibodies have antibacterial, antiviral and antitoxin activity.

Some of the ABO red cell iso-antibodies and the saline agglutinating anti-Rhesus red cell antibodies are in the IgM class (although incomplete Rh antibodies are IgG). Cold agglutinins against red cells and antibodies against the somatic antigen of *Salmonella* are IgM. The rheumatoid factor is an IgM antibody directed against IgG.

Immunoglobulin D (IgD δ Heavy Chains)

IgD has a sedimentation coefficient of 7S and a molecular weight of 185,000. It is present in only trace amount in serum (0–0·4 mg./ml.), does not fix complement, and has only been found to have antibody activity on rare occasions. IgD antibody activity has been detected to insulin, bovine albumin and penicillin, and anti-nuclear and anti-thyroid IgD antibodies have been demonstrated.

Immunoglobulin E (IgE ε Heavy Chains)

The IgE class of immunoglobulins, present in low concentrations (100–400 ng./ml.), form the greater amount of skin sensitizing or reaginic antibodies involved in anaphylactic reactions. They have a molecular weight of 200,000 and a sedimentation coefficient of 8S. The heavy chains do not fix complement but bind avidly to mast cells and basophil leucocytes.

Complement

The complement system is a series of heat labile protein factors present in fresh serum that are necessary for the lysis of erythrocytes or bacteria by specific antibody. There are nine components of complement which act in sequence although the first has three sub-units—Clq, Clr and Cls. There are also a number of inhibitors in the serum capable of controlling each stage of the complement activation cascade. The cascade is in effect a chain-reaction between the components which is amplified at every stage so that the initial activation of a single C1 molecule can result in cell lysis (fig. 5).

The first component (C1) and the second (C2) can be shown to have esterase activity, and the cascade is probably a series of biologically active enzymes and co-enzymes. The third component (C3) which, under normal circumstances, is activated by antigen-antibody complexes through

particular class of immunoglobulin. Polyclonal gammopathies occur in chronic infections such as malaria, leprosy, kala-azar and sub-acute bacterial endocarditis; and in chronic autoimmune disorders, such as rheumatoid arthritis and systemic lupus erythematosus (SLE). The condition known as benign essential hypergammaglobulinaemia has a high incidence in siblings of subjects with SLE and "purpura hyperglobulinaemia" is itself considered to be a precursor of SLE.

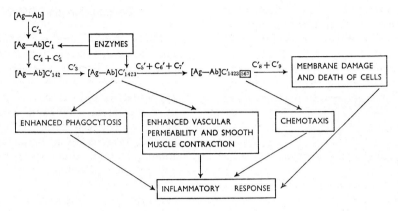

Fig. 5. Role of complement components in initiating an inflammatory reaction.
(After Lepow (1968), *Vth International Immunopathology Symposium*.)

C1, C4 and C2, is capable of enhancing phagocytosis and increasing vascular permeability and smooth muscle contraction. It can, however, be activated by an alternative pathway by bacterial endotoxin through another serum protein called properdin.

C3 is fixed at the site of allergic reactions involving complement, and the serum level is reduced in glomerulonephritis induced by immune complex deposition. C5, C6 and C7 are together chemotactic for polymorphonuclear leucocytes. The full cascade, including C8 and C9, is necessary for bacterial killing and red cell lysis.

The fixation of complement components by immune complexes is the basis of the complement fixation test used in clinical laboratories to detect antibodies to virus antigens or auto-antibodies against the lipid extract of heart muscle present in subjects with active syphilis (Wassermann reaction). An indicator system is used consisting of sheep red cells coated with horse or rabbit antibody against the red cells. If an antigen-antibody reaction has occurred the complement is fixed and is no longer available. As a result the sheep cells in the indicator system are not lysed. If either antigen or antibody are absent the complement is not fixed and is available for lysing the sheep red cells. This reaction is depicted diagrammatically in fig. 6.

Abnormalities of Immunoglobulin Synthesis

Increased concentrations of immunoglobulins in the serum may be polyclonal or monoclonal. The term polyclonal indicates a general increase in the level of immunoglobulin of a particular class and implies a general stimulation of all colonies (clones) of plasma cells making that

A monoclonal increase in immunoglobulin is indicated by a localized increase in the immunoglobulin electrophoretic pattern forming what is known as an "M" protein. This is thought to result from the mutation of a single immunoglobulin-forming cell precursor (clone). Most "M" proteins resulting from "monoclonal gammopathy" occur in elderly people and do not necessarily indicate the presence of disease. However, a monoclonal gammopathy is one of the features of multiple myelomatosis which is a proliferatory neoplasm of the plasma cell series actively producing immunoglobulins.

The immunoglobulin produced in multiple myeloma is always of one class, either IgG, IgA, IgD, or IgE; IgG is the most common form; IgD and IgE myelomas are exceedingly rare. In most cases, myeloma proteins have not been found to have antibody specificity. However, some have been found to be specific for streptococci, staphylococci and even the dinitrophenyl group. In multiple myeloma free κ or λ light chains can be found in the urine. They precipitate when the urine is heated and redissolve on boiling and are known as Bence-Jones protein. Bence-Jones proteins are a by-product of abnormal immunoglobulin synthesis.

Overgrowth of cells synthesising IgM is less malignant than that of cells making other immunoglobulins and is called Waldenstrom's macroglobulinaemia.

PRIMARY AND SECONDARY IMMUNE RESPONSES

After first contact with an antigen, a primary antibody response is induced. This is a limited response of low

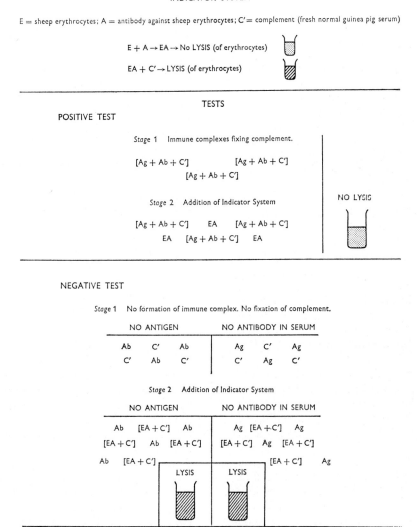

INDICATOR SYSTEM

E = sheep erythrocytes; A = antibody against sheep erythrocytes; C' = complement (fresh normal guinea pig serum)

E + A → EA → No LYSIS (of erythrocytes)

EA + C' → LYSIS (of erythrocytes)

TESTS

POSITIVE TEST

Stage 1 Immune complexes fixing complement.

[Ag + Ab + C']   [Ag + Ab + C']
      [Ag + Ab + C']

Stage 2 Addition of Indicator System   NO LYSIS

[Ag + Ab + C']   EA   [Ag + Ab + C']
      EA   [Ag + Ab + C']   EA

NEGATIVE TEST

Stage 1 No formation of immune complex. No fixation of complement.

NO ANTIGEN   NO ANTIBODY IN SERUM

Ab   C'   Ab   Ag   C'   Ag
C'   Ab   C'   C'   Ag   C'

Stage 2 Addition of Indicator System

NO ANTIGEN   NO ANTIBODY IN SERUM

Ab   [EA + C']   Ab   Ag   [EA + C']   Ag
[EA + C']   Ab   [EA + C']   [EA + C']   Ag   [EA + C']
Ab   [EA + C']   [EA + C']   Ag

LYSIS   LYSIS

FIG. 6. Complement fixation test.

intensity and short duration; it is characterized particularly by the production of low affinity IgM antibody. During the primary response, germinal centres develop in the follicles of lymph nodes and, at the same time, plasma cells begin to proliferate at the cortico-medullary junction. During the primary response, antigen is trapped by macrophages in the medulla of lymph nodes and in the red pulp of the spleen where it is processed and sometimes becomes, as a result, more antigenic. On a second or subsequent contact with antigen a secondary response develops; antigen is now localized in the germinal centres, by dendritic macrophages, as well as in the medulla of lymph nodes, and there is a much more extensive proliferation of plasma cells. This secondary or "anamnestic" response is much more extensive and of greater intensity than the primary response and as a result antibody may be produced for many months or years. This response produces molecules of the IgG class. IgM antibodies are produced on secondary contact with antigen but at the same low intensity and for the same limited period as in a primary response. The extensive secondary response occurs as a

result of "immunological memory", which is a function of T-cells. The anamnestic response of B-cells in the production of IgG can be abolished by blocking T-cell function and thereby preventing these cells from specifically augmenting the B-cell response.

Antibody–Mediated Hypersensitivity Reactions

There are two types of antibody-mediated hypersensitivity reaction. Both are referred to as "immediate-type hypersensitivity" as distinct from "delayed-type hypersensitivity" which is produced by a cell-mediated immune reaction. Immediate hypersensitivity reactions may be defined as those which reach their maximum intensity within the first 12 hr. after contact with antigen. Delayed hypersensitivities are those which reach maximum intensity at 24–48 hr. after contact. There are two types of immediate hypersensitivity reaction—those mediated by IgE antibody and referred to as "anaphylactic reactions", and those mediated by the reaction between IgG or IgM antibody and complement which result in a local vasculitis.

These conditions are sometimes referred to as "immune-complex" reactions.

Anaphylactic Reactions

The interaction between IgE antibody and antigen can result in an acute allergic reaction. This may take place within 5–10 min. of antigen contact. IgE antibodies, often referred to as reagins, bind particularly well to tissue and cell surfaces and, as mentioned previously, especially mast cells and basophils.

The reaction between antigen and IgE antibodies results in the release of certain substances. For example, the reaction between IgE and antigen causes the degranulation of basophils and mast cells which contain histidine associated with heparin. Histamine, formed from histidine by the action of the enzyme histamine decarboxylase, is thus released at the site of IgE attached to mast cells. Histamine injected in the skin causes a typical weal and flare reaction which is the result of increased capillary permeability and local vasodilation. Histamine also causes contraction of plain muscle which may result in bronchospasm. Another agent released in anaphylactic reactions is serotonin (5-hydroxytryptamine). This is a capillary vasoconstrictor found mainly in platelets. Slow reacting substance (SRS-A) is released during anaphylaxis mainly in the lung. It is recognized by its ability to provoke involuntary muscle to contract and could be one of the main causes of bronchial constriction in anaphylactic reactions. The plasma kinins, bradykinin and kallidin, are simple peptides consisting of 9 and 10 amino-acids respectively, and are formed from plasma globulins by the enzymes kallikrein, plasmin or trypsin. They cause increased capillary permeability, vasodilation and a fall in blood pressure. Once they are formed, kinins are rapidly broken down by kininases, enzymes also present in the blood, so that their accumulation at any site can be controlled. Another agent released in anaphylaxis has been shown to be prostaglandin E. Prostaglandins are fatty acids of molecular weight between 300 and 400. They act on smooth muscle and blood vessels in a similar way to kinins.

Anaphylactic reactions may be local or systemic depending on the site of contact of reagin and allergen (antigen). Reaction in the eye results in conjunctivitis and in the nose in rhinorrhoea and sinusitis. Local reaction between IgE antibody and pollen at these sites results in "hay fever". Reaction in the larynx causes laryngeal oedema and in the bronchial mucosa results in asthma. If IgE and allergen binding takes place in the gastro-intestinal tract there may be vomiting and diarrhoea. Reaction between IgE and antigen in the skin results in angioneurotic oedema, urticaria, or a maculopapular eruption. Systemically, vasodilation in the mesenteric vessels can result in a severe fall in blood pressure, shock, and anuria.

Reaginic antibodies have been detected in the IgG class of immunoglobulins as well as in the IgE class. These antibodies are not common; they are classified as reagins because they can also induce histamine mediated increased vascular permeability in the same way as IgE.

The Arthus Reaction—Immune Complex Disease

The intradermal injection of antigen into an individual with a high circulating level of IgG or IgM complement-fixing antibody results in a particularly strong skin reaction reaching its maximum intensity between 4 and 8 hr. after injection. Such an allergic reaction is called an Arthus reaction and is the result of the deposition of antigen, antibody and complement in the walls of the larger, less superficial cutaneous blood vessels. This results in fibrinoid necrosis of the vessel wall and an intense perivascular polymorphonuclear infiltrate. The ensuing increased vascular permeability and damage to the vessel walls gives rise to oedema and local haemorrhage. The antigen-antibody ratio in the complex is important because it has been shown that complexes formed in antigen excess are the most effective in producing increased vascular permeability. The complexes must also have a molecular weight of at least 900,000 before they are capable of inducing vascular damage. Maximum complex deposition also appears to depend on a prior increase in vascular permeability and can be diminished when substances known to increase vascular permeability are inhibited.

SERUM SICKNESS

Acute serum sickness can develop in response to a wide range of antigens and drugs including penicillin, streptomycin, sulphonamides and thiouracil. Acute serum sickness can be divided into two types. The first type, called primary serum sickness, occurs in individuals who have not had previous contact with the antigen and therefore have no pre-existing circulating antibodies directed against it. Symptoms occur after a latent period of about 7 days when circulating antibody directed against the foreign serum or drug antigens appears in the circulation. The severity of the illness depends on the quantity of antigen present in the circulation and the absolute and relative amounts of anaphylactic IgE and conventional IgG antibody produced in the response. Secondary serum sickness occurs in those who have had previous experience of the antigen or have existing circulating antibodies directed against it. As a result, symptoms, usually severe, develop quickly because circulating antibody is already present or is rapidly produced by an accelerated secondary anamnestic antibody response. Previous injection is not essential; for example, these more severe reactions may occur in an individual allergic to horse serum as a result of contact with horse dander, which is known to be contaminated with horse serum proteins.

The reactions which occur in serum sickness are a result of the production of both anaphylactic (IgE) antibodies and conventional circulating antibodies (IgG or IgM). The lesions which develop depend on the relative amounts of each class of antibody produced. If most of the antibodies produced are anaphylactic antibodies (IgE), the symptoms which develop will be mainly anaphylactic as a result of reactions taking place on the cell surface. If the antibodies produced are mainly IgG or IgM the lesions result from "immune complex deposition". Often the clinical features result from a mixture of anaphylactic type reactions and those due to the presence of circulating immune complexes.

CELL-MEDIATED IMMUNOLOGICAL REACTIONS (CMI)

Immunological reactions mediated by T-cells occur in a number of important biological processes (Table 2).

TABLE 2

EXAMPLES OF CELL-MEDIATED IMMUNE REACTIONS

A. Delayed hypersensitivity to microbial protein antigens
   —tuberculin
   —diphtheria toxoid—"pseudo" Schick reaction
   —vaccinia virus—"reaction of immunity"
   —fungal antigens—histoplasmin, coccidiomycin
   —protozoal antigens—Montenegro test for leishmaniasis

B. Delayed hypersensitivity to heterologous serum proteins (following small doses of foreign antisera)

C. Insect bites

D. Contact sensitivity to simple chemicals

E. The homograft reaction

F. Cellular immunity to certain bacteria (e.g. mycobacteria, brucella) fungi, protozoa and viruses

G. Collaboration between cell-mediated immunity and humoral antibody in the development of organ-specific autoimmune lesions

These include defence mechanisms against certain micro-organisms inaccessible to humoral antibody and reaction against tumours, but also allergic reactions causing severe tissue damage. In most cases the defence mechanisms and the allergic reactions are intimately associated. The allergic reactions are frequently used as both in vivo and in vitro tests for the diagnosis of infection by organisms that give rise to T-cell mediated immunological reactions (CMI). The intradermal injection of specific antigen (tuberculin) into an individual suffering from tuberculosis induces a typical allergic reaction known as "delayed hypersensitivity". Delayed hypersensitivity reactions reach their peak intensity 24–48 hr. after intradermal injection of antigen in contrast to the earlier development of hypersensitivity reactions mediated by humoral antibodies (Table 3). Macroscopically these reactions are characterized by erythema and induration. Microscopically the infiltrate is typically mononuclear consisting of an admixture of lymphocytes and macrophages with a mainly perivascular distribution. The induration observed macroscopically has been shown to be associated microscopically with the swelling of collagen. A state of delayed hypersensitivity to an antigen such as tuberculin cannot be transferred passively from individual to individual by serum as can Arthus sensitivity because the reaction is not mediated by humoral antibody. Sensitivity can however be transferred with populations of mononuclear cells containing "specifically sensitized" T-lymphocytes. These include peripheral blood leucocytes, mononuclear exudates obtained from peritoneal cavity, and suspensions of cells from lymph node or spleen. Transfer of sensitivity cannot however be obtained with suspensions of cells derived from the thymus or bone marrow.

Mechanisms of T-cell-Mediated Immunological Response

The most widely studied models of CMI reactions have been the tuberculin reaction, chemical contact sensitivity, and skin allograft rejection. A T-cell response leading particularly to delayed hypersensitivity is best induced either by an antigen fixed in the periphery (e.g. skin allograft, skin rendered antigenic by the use of a contact sensitizer, or by a living intracellular parasite, e.g. M. tuberculosis). It has been suggested that the process of T-lymphocyte activation differs from B-lymphocyte activation in that T-lymphocytes recognize antigen in the periphery ("peripheral sensitization") prior to passage to the paracortical areas of lymph nodes or the periarteriolar area of the white pulp of the spleen where they proliferate and differentiate into effector cells. This is in contrast to the humoral antibody response where antigen is taken up by macrophages in the lymphoid tissue and activates local B-lymphocytes already in the lymph nodes or spleen to proliferate and differentiate into plasma cells and produce antibody.

There is a latent period of at least 4 days between first contact with antigen and the presence of effector T-cells in the peripheral blood capable of reacting with antigen. During this time most of the cellular activity can be found in the lymphoid tissue immediately draining the site of antigen application. Local lymph nodes increase in size due to restricted egress of lymphocytes from the paracortical areas. Plugs of lymphocytes can be seen in the sinuses draining these areas into the medulla. At the same time the paracortical area is the site of massive lymphocytic proliferation. After the fourth day the lymph nodes begin to decrease in size as sensitized lymphocytes begin to pass out into the periphery. These cells are now capable of reacting with antigen (fig. 7).

TABLE 3

DIFFERENCES BETWEEN THE TUBERCULIN REACTION (CELL-MEDIATED) AND THE ARTHUS REACTION

	Tuberculin	Arthus
Time of maximum response	24–28 hours	4–8 hours
Macroscopic appearance	Erythema, induration	Oedema, haemorrhage
Microscopic appearance	Mononuclear cell infiltrate	Polymorphonuclear leucocyte infiltrate
Passive sensitization	Suspension of lymphoid tissues (containing sensitized lymphocytes)	Serum (containing antibodies— immunoglobulins)
Systemic manifestations	Fever	Deposition of "immune complexes" in organs

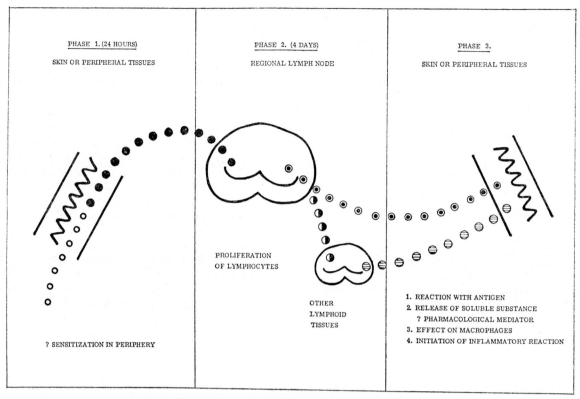

FIG. 7. The mechanism of cell-mediated immunity.

Mode of Reaction Between Specifically Sensitized Lymphocytes and Antigen

Once specific effector T-lymphocytes have been released into the circulation they may localize at the site of antigen deposition. There is no doubt that these cells can be shown to be directly cytotoxic for target cells *in vitro*. However, the extent to which protection is thus afforded against invading organisms and cancer cells, or in the production of allergic tissue damage, is not known. The intimate association between lymphocytes and macrophages in all cellular infiltrates caused by CMI indicates a significant role for macrophages in these reactions. Incubation of sensitized lymphocytes with specific antigen results in the release of agents which have been shown to modify the behaviour of macrophages. These substances have been given a number of names such as products of activated lymphocytes (PAL), lymphocyte activation products (LAP), lymphokines, and mediators of cellular immunity. These substances are proteins, mainly of molecular weight 40,000, and migrate electrophoretically in the pre-albumin range. They may be released from lymphocytes by non-specific plant mitogens such as phytohaemagglutinin (PHA) and concanavalin A (Con A) and by antigen-antibody complexes, as well as from sensitized T-lymphocytes reacting with specific antigen. *In vitro* they can be shown to inhibit the normal migration of macrophages from capillary tubes (Migration Inhibitory Factor—MIF). When injected intraperitoneally they cause macrophages to adhere to the peritoneal wall and when injected intradermally they cause erythematous indurated skin reactions resembling delayed hypersensitivi-ty (skin reactive factor—SRF). Other activities of these substances are the induction of blast cell transformation in lymphocytes (blastogenic factor—BF) and cytotoxicity for certain lines of tumour cell in tissue culture (lymphotoxin —LT).

Macrophages treated with lymphocyte activation products initially show morphological evidence of reduced metabolic activity. Later, however, there is evidence of increased metabolism and morphological resemblance to epithelioid cells with increased lysosomal hydrolase activity. The increased stickiness of macrophages which reduces their ability to migrate from capillary tubes (in the MIF test) has been found to be associated with a decrease in the electrostatic charge on the surface membrane.

Granuloma Formation

A granuloma may be defined as a focal collection of histiocytes and macrophages in the tissues. Granulomas may develop as a result of an immunological process. However, granuloma formation commonly occurs in the absence of an immunological reaction following the deposition of certain toxic materials in the tissues. Non-immunological granulomas can develop following the injection of mineral oils, colloidal aluminium hydroxide, or silica. Granuloma formation by various silica compounds parallels their direct cytotoxic effects on macrophages. Silica is taken up by lysosomes and the first effect that can be demonstrated is a diffuse release of lysosomal enzymes into the cytoplasm as a result of an increased permeability of the lysosomal membrane.

Silica can also act as an adjuvant to immunoglobulin synthesis. However, this probably does not have much relevance to its granuloma forming capacity. Macrophages in a granuloma may be long or short lived. They are derived mainly from cells in the bone marrow and, in granulomas, initially have a relatively rapid turnover due to chronic immunological stimulation.

Macrophages can under certain circumstances aggregate and form giant cells. Immunologically-stimulated granulomas can develop from cell-mediated immune reactions, antibody-induced reactions or from both. Recently it has been found that granuloma formation can be induced in tissues following the subcutaneous injection of immune complexes formed when antigen and antibody are precipitated at "equivalence". The presence of lymphocytes around a tissue granuloma indicates that this is the site of a chronic cell-mediated immune reaction. Plasma cells in the infiltrate may develop from lymphocytes arriving as part of the cell-mediated reaction in response to a local antigenic stimulus.

Granulomas due to the deposition of inorganic substances may be immunologically derived in subjects previously sensitized to the substance, an example being zirconium hypersensitivity. However, although beryllium is a powerful contact-sensitizing agent, there is no evidence that the granulomas formed by this substance in the lungs are due to a sensitization process.

Delayed Hypersensitivity Reactions in the Skin

Insect Bites

Under natural conditions typical delayed hypersensitivity reactions can develop in the skin following insect bites. The red indurated reaction in the skin which occurs 24 hr. after a mosquito bite is a manifestation of delayed hypersensitivity towards antigen present in the saliva of the mosquito. Flea bites also cause delayed hypersensitivity. Reactions to stings from bees, wasps and hornets are generally anaphylactic. Severe and fatal systemic anaphylaxis can develop as a result of stings from these insects in sensitized individuals.

Chemical Contact Sensitivity

Chemical contact sensitivity is one of the major causes of industrial morbidity. Most of these chemicals, often of molecular weight no more than 200–300, become antigenic by binding covalently to skin protein. As a result the area of the skin with which they have been in contact is no longer recognized as self but is affected as though it were a skin allograft. There is proliferation of T-lymphocytes in the draining lymph node and after 5–6 days specifically sensitized lymphocytes are released to the periphery; they are capable of reacting with specific antigen and producing substances such as skin reactive factor and macrophage activating factors. As a result a hypersensitivity reaction develops every time the sensitized individual comes in contact with the chemical, albeit at a level that normally causes no reaction. The tendency to become sensitized in this way is under genetic control and is not therefore developed to the same degree in all individuals.

Having once reacted to contact with a particular chemical, a subject is more likely to react to exposure on future occasions with a "flare up" at the original contact site. This site may then always "flare up" following systemic absorption of the specific hapten. This is one of the possible mechanisms of what is known as a "fixed drug eruption". Another type of reaction that can occur following systemic absorption of a chemical sensitizer is a generalized rash. Such an eruption can be due either to the development of circulating immune complexes containing humoral antibody as in serum sickness, or to reaction with specifically sensitized T-lymphocytes.

IMMUNOLOGICAL UNRESPONSIVENESS

Immunological unresponsiveness may be antigen specific or antigen non-specific. In the former unresponsiveness is directed towards one particular antigen, in the latter unresponsiveness is general. Specific immunological unresponsiveness includes such conditions as immunological tolerance and immunological enhancement. Specific immunological unresponsiveness is induced by injection of specific antigen and is brought about by changes in a specific population of potentially responding lymphocytes. Non-specific unresponsiveness may be due to an inherited defect in the immune response, may be secondary to other disease, or may be the result of treatment with immunosuppressive agents. In both antigen specific and antigen non-specific unresponsiveness the state of unresponsiveness may affect both T and B cells, or either type of lymphocyte individually.

Antigen-Specific Unresponsiveness

Immunological Tolerance

Immunological tolerance may be defined as an active inhibition of immune responsiveness by specific antigen. Tolerance can be produced by presenting an animal with an antigen in a form that will not induce an immune response (e.g. one that will not be taken up by macrophages) or in a high concentration. The development of a state of unresponsiveness of this type shows similarities to the development of an immune response. For example, it has been shown that the state of unresponsiveness may have a 4–5 day latent period, similar to that of a normal immune response. Moreover maintenance of a state of tolerance requires repeated exposures to antigen in the same way as the maintenance of an immune response. The development and maintenance of tolerance in T-cells and B-cells have different kinetics. T-cell tolerance is effected rapidly within 2 days of exposure to one dose of antigen and remains complete for as long as 6 months, while B-cell tolerance takes up to 7 days to develop. The mechanism by which clones of potentially responsive T or B-lymphocytes are made unresponsive by antigen is not known. As recovery is possible, unless antigen exposure is repeated, "clone elimination" cannot be postulated, although there may be a temporary reduction in the number of potentially responsive lymphocytes.

In most situations tolerance is induced by exposure to a high (supra-immunogenic) dose of antigen. However in certain situations it has been possible to induce tolerance by exposure to a low (sub-immunogenic) dose. Whereas it is relatively easy to conceive of ways in which high dose (zone) tolerance might occur, such as temporary reduction in potentially responsive lymphocytes, there have been few convincing explanations for the occurrence of low zone tolerance. One explanation suggested is that the low dose of antigen might localize preferentially in areas of high B-cell concentration, such as the lymph follicles and germinal centres, where there is naturally occurring high concentration of antigen reactive cells. Another explanation is that specific suppressor T-cells are formed, that inhibit the development of the immune response.

Antibody-mediated Unresponsiveness (Immunological Enhancement)

The term "immunological enhancement" is used to describe antibody induced T-cell unresponsiveness, and is applied to the enhancement of tumour growth. Immunological enhancement was first described by tumour immunologists and enhanced tumour growth occurs if there is specific inhibition of T-cell function. Enhancement can be induced by immunizing an animal with soluble tumour antigen which preferentially stimulates B-cell function. The production of humoral antibody is then capable of blocking a T-cell response when whole live tumour cells are injected subsequently. Humoral antibody injected passively can also be shown to suppress T-cell function and thus produce enhancement. T-cell function is affected by antibody either on the afferent or the efferent arc of the immune response. On the afferent arc blockage of the antigenic determinants on the tumour cells prevents recognition by T-cells and their subsequent proliferation and differentiation fails to occur. On the efferent arc antibody coating the antigenic determinants of tumour cells protects them from T-cell lysis. Humoral antibody can also complex with soluble tumour antigen and the complexes formed in antigen excess are also capable of combining with and blocking T-cell receptor groups.

The Role of Specific Immunological Unresponsiveness in Clinical Disease States

In certain chronic infectious diseases such as lepromatous leprosy, diffuse cutaneous leishmaniasis (kala-azar), South American blastomycosis, and muco-cutaneous candidiasis there may be a specific failure of cell-mediated immunity whereas humoral antibody production is in many cases increased. As a result there is a failure of immune mechanisms to keep the infecting organism under control, even though there is antibody in the circulation capable of reacting with antigens derived from the infecting organisms. The failure of T-cell function in the presence of normal B-cell function could arise either because of a state of immunological tolerance affecting T-cells alone, known as split tolerance or "immune deviation", or because of a state of immunological enhancement where T-cell function is suppressed by humoral antibody. In immune deviation certain types of antibody, e.g. IgG$_2$, may also be suppressed together with the cell-mediated immune response.

Non-specific Unresponsiveness

Non-specific immunological unresponsiveness may develop as a result of an inborn congenital deficiency of lymphocyte function or may be acquired as a result of disease or treatment with drugs that directly suppress lymphocyte function. Deficiencies whether congenital or acquired may affect both T and B cells or may affect T cells or B cells alone. Deficiency of both T and B cells may result from stem cell deficiency in which case there is failure both of cell-mediated immunity and humoral antibody. In pure B-cell deficiency cell-mediated immunity is unaffected and defence mechanisms dependent on T-cell function are normal, as is the ability to develop delayed hypersensitivity reactions. In pure T-cell deficiency humoral antibody is produced normally but there may be deficiencies in T-cell dependent defence mechanisms and delayed hypersensitivity reactions.

Congenital Defects of Lymphocyte Function

Combined T and B cell deficiency results from aplasia of stem cells in the bone marrow. There is an almost complete absence of lymphocytes in all lymphoid tissues. Not only is cell-mediated immunity lost, but there is also a failure of immunoglobulin synthesis with absence of plasma cells and their precursors. This condition occurs either as an autosomal recessive or sex-linked to the X-chromosome in which case it is only found in male children.

Pure T-cell deficiency with normal immunoglobulin synthesis may be due to a defect of the third branchial arch during embryonic development and is not genetically controlled. As well as thymic aplasia there is also an absence of the parathyroid glands (Di George syndrome). Another form is familial in which the thymus is very small and is replaced by histiocytes (Nezelof syndrome).

Acquired Defects of Lymphocyte Function

Defects in T-lymphocyte function as assessed by inability to demonstrate delayed hypersensitivy reactions in the skin, prolonged rejection of skin allografts, and decreased responsiveness of lymphocytes to PHA in vitro can be found associated with a number of diseases. These include tumours and granulomatous conditions of the reticulo-endothelial system such as lymphosarcoma, Hodgkin's disease, sarcoidosis, and gastric carcinoma but not bronchial carcinoma.

Defects in T-lymphocyte function have also been described in states of protein-calorie malnutrition. Defects in B-lymphocyte function (hypogammaglobulinaemia) can occur secondarily to a number of conditions. These include catabolic states where there is an increased turnover of protein such as the nephrotic syndrome, protein losing enteropathy and severe malnutrition, bone marrow disorders including marrow hypoplasia, extensive bony metastases, and as a result of toxic factors produced in renal failure, thyrotoxicosis and diabetes mellitus. B-lymphocyte function may also be defective in primary neoplasms of the reticulo-endothelial system. Hypogammaglobulinaemia may also occur physiologically in premature babies and in states of delayed maturity.

10. IMMUNOLOGICAL ASPECTS OF INFECTION

J. L. TURK AND M. B. EDWARDS

Innate and acquired immunity
  Natural resistance
    Genetic and environmental factors
  Development of acquired immunity
    Passive—maternal antibody
    Active— fetal infection
        antibody maturation
        origins of natural antibody

The immune elimination of micro-organisms
  Bacteria
    Complement-mediated reactions
      Bacteriolysis
      Alternate pathway
      Opsonization, adherence
      Inflammatory mediators
    Phagocytosis, phagocytolysis
      Resistance to ingestion and digestion
      Facultative parasitism
      The macrophage and cell-mediated immunity
    Specificity of cell-mediated immunity
  Viruses
    Antibody and complement
      Neutralization
      Virolysis
    Macrophage and antibody
      Experimental immunosuppression
    Cell-mediated immunity
    Antibody-dependent, cell-mediated cytotoxicity
  Fungi and Protozoa
    Influence of structure and life-cycle

Immune elimination at seromucosal surfaces
  Secretory antibody, local immunity
  Dental caries
    Immunization
    Possible mechanisms

Immunodeficiency and infection
  Primary deficiency states
  Secondary deficiency states
    Lymphomas, leukaemias
    Immunosuppressive therapy
  Deficiency arising from infection
    Non-specific
    Antigen-specific unresponsiveness
      Disease spectra
      Leprosy, leishmaniasis
    Chronic mucocutaneous candidiasis
      MIF abnormality
      Serum iron kinetics
    Syphilis
  Mechanisms of tolerance and immune deviation
  Chronic periodontal disease

Allergy and hypersensitivity
  Immune-complex disease
    Pathology of lesions
      Problems of diagnosis in AUG
    Examples: bacterial, viral, mycotic
    Comparison with Shwartzman phenomena
      Role of endotoxins
  Delayed hypersensitivity

The body is continually exposed to a wide range of micro-organisms only a minority of which are true pathogens. These vary considerably in their invasiveness and rate of proliferation. Some can proliferate in an extracellular milieu, whereas others need an intracellular environment for replication. As well as having random contact with exogenous micro-organisms the skin, oral cavity, upper respiratory tract and parts of the alimentary canal support a permanent flora of numerous species of organism. These organisms may be specially adapted to various micro-environments and able to survive in the presence of both non-specific factors such as lysozyme (muramidase) and the specific secretory antibodies which form part of the first line of defence at seromucosal surfaces. It is probable that these factors and interactions between different microbial populations exert a regulatory influence over the total flora. The relationship between host and commensal flora is complex and may include both beneficial symbiosis and opportunistic pathogenicity arising in conditions of altered host resistance. The topic of microbial pathogenicity is considered in detail in Chapter 16 and the present purpose is to discuss the immunological aspects of resistance to infection and the nature of the reactions between infective agents and the immune system.

INNATE AND ACQUIRED IMMUNITY

It is clear that much of host resistance is innate or inborn and that such immunity is genetically controlled. There is of course a broad distinction to be made between innate immunity and immunity acquired by contact with the antigens of micro-organisms and their metabolites. Both innate and acquired immunity will in most cases be boosted by further contact with antigen. Innate immunity to infection may vary from species to species and in the animal world between strains of the same species. In man there are occasional genetic traits associated with variation in resistance. An important example is the increased resistance to malaria associated with the sickle-cell trait. It has also been suggested that people with blood group O or B are more resistant to smallpox than those with group A. Possibly of more far-reaching importance is the intra-species variation in both innate and acquired immunity which depends upon environmental factors such as climate and diet. Immunity may also be conditioned by influences in the internal environment, particularly the presence of intercurrent infection and the balance of hormones. Immunological processes depend on protein synthesis which is susceptible to changes in both the dietary and endocrine status of the individual. There is also evidence that endocrinological and immunological maturation occur in parallel and that the latter too is under the overall influence of the pituitary gland.

The maturation of antibody-mediated immunity can be monitored to some extent by the sequential measurement of immunoglobulin levels in the serum and external secretions after birth. The development of cell-mediated immunity cannot be assayed so readily but it is clearly functional in the neonate. Serum levels of IgG rise rapidly during the final trimester of fetal life to approach or exceed normal adult levels at birth. This acquisition of a wide range of antibodies is passive; IgG is actively transported across the placenta from the maternal circulation. Fetal lymphoid tissue, which is normally sequestered from microbial antigens, may be stimulated to produce antibody after week 18—20 of IU life by fetal infection such as may occur in rubella, syphilis and toxoplasmosis. Antibody so produced is usually in the IgM and IgA classes. Uninfected neonates also have a low but detectable level of IgM in cord serum which may indicate a response to maternally derived antigen. After birth the human infant passively acquires secretory IgA (SIgA) from colostrum and breast milk. Maternal IgG is catabolized more rapidly than the infant can synthesize its own and serum levels of this immunoglobulin fall rapidly between birth and three months of age. At the same time there is a rapid rise in IgM levels which may reach adult values before the age of one year. There is some evidence to suggest that SIgA levels also mature rapidly. IgG again increases after three months and may approach adult levels at three years. Serum IgA, IgD and IgE may not gain full maturity until adolescence.

The origin of the stimulus to a wide range of agglutinating and bactericidal, "natural" antibodies in the serum of young individuals is a source of controversy. Numerous antibodies sometimes known as "copro-antibodies" can also be found in the intestinal lumen and natural secretory antibodies are found in saliva. It is true that many natural antibodies are directed against saprophytic bacteria. Others, however, may be directed against such pathogens as *Shigella* and *Salmonella*, organisms which are associated with enteric infection, and even against the cholera vibrio. The range of natural antibodies may far exceed the known extent of previous infection in the individual concerned. This finding prompted the suggestion that they develop as a genetic function, especially as the pattern of natural antibody occurrence appears to be specific to a particular species. However, germ-free laboratory animals fail to develop these antibodies. They have a low level of circulating immunoglobulin and poorly developed lymphoid tissue. This evidence suggests that in the normal individual natural antibodies develop as a result of antigenic stimulation in early infancy. The source of antigens may be intestinal bacteria or foodstuffs. Natural antibody to pathogens with which the individual is unlikely to have had contact may derive from cross-reaction with closely related antigens on the surface of non-pathogenic commensals. There is, however, little doubt that the presence of natural antibodies is to some extent under genetic control which may influence the extent of the response of host lymphoid tissue to the indigenous flora of micro-organisms. The part played by natural antibacterial antibodies in protection from infection will vary from organism to organism. It is probable that in certain cases they contribute significantly to such protection. However, there are recorded examples of animals which are highly susceptible to infection with a particular organism despite the presence of a relatively high concentration of natural antibodies in the serum against the organism in question. In this context a distinction may perhaps be made between natural antibody and antibody stimulated by subclinical infections which pass undetected. In most circumstances such antibody would be expected to confer some degree of acquired immunity against reinfection.

THE IMMUNE ELIMINATION OF MICRO-ORGANISMS

The elimination of infection may clearly be enhanced in an immunized host. Micro-organisms may, however, be killed and then expelled from the host by mechanisms without immunological specificity. In fact immunological reactions may largely serve only to generate and augment non-specific effector mechanisms of elimination. These include at the cellular level phagocytes—polymorphonuclear leucocytes and macrophages—and at the humoral level agents either activated or released from cells during immunological reactions. Among these are the **complement** (**C′**) cascade, lysosomal enzymes, and the pharmacological mediators of cellular immunity (the **lymphokines**). Some micro-organisms require cell-mediated immunity for their elimination. However, antigens other than those that stimulate cell-mediated immunity may also induce the production of antibody during the course of an infection. These antibodies may have little influence on the elimination of the organism but may be the cause of damaging hypersensitivity reactions. In the case of bacteria which produce disease by the effect of their exotoxins, *e.g.* diphtheria and tetanus, effective immunity may depend upon the presence of antitoxin and the elimination of local infection may be a secondary feature. This discussion will, however, be concentrated upon the elimination of micro-organisms rather than antitoxic activity. Though logic might dictate that mechanisms of immune elimination at the body surfaces should be discussed first, these rather than the non-specific factors operative at the first lines of defence are still poorly understood. Therefore the elimination of infection which has penetrated the epithelial surfaces will first be considered and the mechanisms involved will then be discussed in relation to the expression of immunity at those surfaces.

Two important points should be emphasized at the outset. Firstly, although a clear division may appear to exist between the two limbs of the immune system it is now known that antibody production to many antigens is enhanced by the synergistic activity of T-cells, sometimes called "helper cells" (see Chapter 9). Secondly, it is necessary to make a clear distinction between the results of *in vitro* experiments, experiments upon laboratory animals and data derived from the investigation of human disease. In a rapidly expanding subject such as immunology, extrapolation between these three modes of research requires caution and at best the connection between different phenomena may be suggested rather than proved.

Bacteria

Few bacteria are killed or undergo lysis *in vitro* by serum rich in antibody but in which heat-labile substances have been inactivated. Of these substances C′ may be regarded as the most important and there is now evidence of the precise way in which interaction between C′, and antibody in combination with bacterial antigen, can lead to **bacteriolysis.** The biochemical activation of the C′ cascade has been described in Chapter 9. Bacteriolysis is a terminal event of this sequential activation, involving components C8 and C9 generated at the bacterial cell surface. The essential step preceding this event is the deposition of modified C3 on the surface of the bacterium. This step, which may be promoted through the activation of C142 by a complex of surface antigen and antibody, is fundamental to the further elaboration of various reactions attributable to C′ fixation. However, C′ fixation can occasionally be by-passed so that, for example, C8 present on the lymphocyte cell membrane may be directly activated in the cytotoxic reactions of the cell-mediated response. Of the components C8 and C9 it appears that C8 is the cytolytic agent but C9 may enhance its function. C8 has phospholipase activity and the formation of negatively stained pits in bacterial cell walls as observed by electron-microscopy is interpreted as indicating the site of this enzymic activity. In the case of C′ bound by IgM at the cell surface each pit is thought to correspond to the site of combination with a single immunoglobulin molecule. There remains speculation as to the final mechanism of lysis after cell-wall damage. The exposed cell membrane contains the mucopeptide substrate of lysozyme and sites susceptible to this enzyme also occur in the altered cell wall. The penetration of the cell wall by the synergistic activity of C′ components and lysozyme could lead both to collapse of support for the cell and membrane leakage, both of which events will produce an osmotically fragile organism. C′-dependent bacteriolysis as demonstrated in the laboratory is limited to Gram-negative organisms such as *E. coli*, the cholera vibrio and *Shigella dysenteriae*. The relative resistance of Gram-positive organisms has been attributed to the absence of cell-wall lipids which incorporate the substrate for C8 phospholipase.

Until quite recently the activation of the C′ cascade was thought to be initiated only by the combination of antigen and C′-fixing antibody. It is now known that activation can occur through an **"alternate" pathway**, sometimes called the properdin pathway, which is not triggered by an immune complex although the reaction is apparently enhanced in the presence of specific antibody. The cascade is activated directly at the level of C3 through a pro-activator substance so that the basic reactions associated with C3 fixation can develop as they do in the conventional pathway. Properdin itself is derived from normal plasma by absorption and elution from zymosan, a component of yeast cell walls. In appropriate experimental systems it can promote the lysis of a number of micro-organisms although doubts have been raised as to its function *in vivo*. Currently there is a body of opinion to suggest that properdin-like factors are involved in the activation of the alternate pathway in natural infection. Of particular relevance to infectious disease is the finding that bacterial surfaces may activate the alternate pathway and that a number of substances derived from the cell walls of Gram-negative organisms, and conventionally known as endotoxins, may do likewise. Among the bacterial endotoxins able to elicit this reaction are those derived from several of the constituent organisms of dental plaque including *Veillonella alcalescens*, *F. fusiformis* and *Actinomyces viscosus*. Though susceptible organisms present in the extravascular fluid and in the blood stream may undergo lysis by C′ activity following the conventional or the alternate pathway, it is clear that the elimination of most bacteria is finally dependent upon effective phagocytosis. It is by this process that the body ultimately disposes of the majority of infections.

That there are serum factors which enhance phagocytosis was postulated at the turn of this century, and has since been authenticated by numerous experiments. These factors are commonly termed **"opsonins"** to indicate that in some way they prepare material for phagocytosis. Opsonic activity resides in both heat-labile and heat-stable components in plasma; the principal opsonin in the former category is C′, and in the latter, antibody. The current interpretation of the mechanism underlying opsonization is of a process which improves contact and adhesion between the surface of the phagocyte and the micro-organism. This adherence has been shown to depend upon the presence of receptor sites on the phagocyte cell membrane which can give specific attachment either to a modified molecule of C3 or to the Fc component of certain subclasses of IgG molecule. As in the case of C′-mediated cytolysis it appears that the deposition of the active component of C3 on the bacterial cell surface is the most important step in opsonic adherence reactions, for once this occurs many C3 fragments can be bound to the complex over the bacterial surface. These in turn provide multiple sites for binding to the special receptors on the phagocyte. Whilst the Fc region of IgG in an immune complex, or unbound IgG coating a bacterium, may directly engage the specific receptor sites, adherence promoted by IgM alone is thought to be non-specific and weak. IgM may, however, promote opsonic adherence through C′ fixation. The binding of free IgG to the phagocyte can occur, though it appears that binding occurs more readily after complexing with antigen. Therefore, although phagocytes may carry uncomplexed IgG on their surfaces in the form of "cytophilic" antibody, it is uncertain how important this may be in promoting adherence after random contact with bacteria.

Investigators have found reason to dispute the relative

importance of heat-labile factors such as C′ and more stable factors such as antibody in opsonization during the course of disease. *In vitro* phagocytosis of many organisms can be effected in the absence of serum, but it seems likely that immune factors enhance their elimination during natural infection. Conversely some species, notably those that form a capsule such as pneumococci, are ingested only in the presence of specific antibody. This requirement influences the course of pneumococcal infection, conferring upon the capsular polysaccharide the properties of an aggressin which, when present in excess, can complex much of the circulating antibody leaving the bacterial population intact. In this now classic example of the conflicting activity of an opsonin and aggressin the role of antibody is distinct. There is, however, a group of organisms, *e.g.* staphylococci, in which specific and non-specific opsonization is observed. Opsonization as measured in the serum of a patient with staphylococcal endocarditis can be shown to depend upon specific antibody with C′ having an augmenting effect, but in normal serum opsonization is destroyed by heating which suggests a dominant role for C′. However, recent investigations have indicated that absorption of the small quantities of natural antistaphylococcal antibody equally inhibits opsonization, emphasizing that C′ fixation by this antibody may occur in normal serum.

Except in the case of virulent, encapsulated bacteria the clearance of micro-organisms from the bloodstream by the reticulo-endothelial system is usually rapid and effective in the normal host. Few infections are accompanied by more than a transient bacteraemia so that in real terms the immune elimination of infection requires the effective delivery of serum factors and phagocytes to extravascular sites. This facility is traditionally ascribed to the **inflammatory response,** which is discussed in detail in Chapter 9. It is relevant to emphasize here that the activation of C′ generates factors chemotactic for polymorphonuclear leucocytes and anaphylatoxin which, by promoting histamine release, indirectly affects vascular permeability. In this way it seems likely that immune reactions can influence the evolution of the inflammatory response early in the course of a local infection. The same mediators of the acute inflammatory response are, of course, released in the alternate pathway of C′ fixation, which is not directly dependent upon immunological activity.

While it is clear that the elimination of infection depends upon phagocytosis, the ingestion of bacteria is not always followed by intracellular killing and digestion. Several bacterial characteristics are involved in resistance to phagocytolysis but two are of special significance. The first is exemplified by groups such as α-haemolytic streptococci which are ingested in an unimmunized host only to multiply within the phagocyte and then be released from it. Resistance to phagocytosis in this instance depends upon a constituent of the cell surface, the M protein, but in the presence of antiserum to this protein phagocytosis is enhanced and phagocytolysis can occur. The second characteristic is that of **facultative intracellular parasitism,** in the most extreme forms of which, exemplified by *Mycobacterium tuberculosis* and *Mycobacterium leprae,*

the principal parasitized cell is the macrophage. The distinction between temporary antiphagocytolytic activity and intracellular parasitism is not absolute, for several micro-organisms such as *Brucella,* some strains of *Salmonella,* and *Treponema pallidum,* may survive for part of the course of an infection in a variety of cells, including macrophages.

In all these infections an important feature is a shift away from humoral to cell-mediated factors as a mechanism of immune elimination so that in the case of tuberculosis antibody appears to play no part in immunity. The mechanisms by which enhanced elimination of these organisms during the course of infection, and immunity against reinfection, are conferred have remained obscure until recently, although clearly the sensitized T-lymphocyte and the macrophage were likely to be implicated. Observations upon the course of experimental infection in mice with *Listeria monocytogenes,* a bacterium able to live freely in murine phagocytes, have shown that in animals which survive the initial infection there is a change in phagocytic capacity with respect to the bacteria after about five days. Macrophages then become able to break down *Listeria* and it has been shown that this state of enhanced phagocytic capacity extends to other parasitic micro-organisms such as *Brucella* and *Mycobacteria* if they are introduced into the animal. There is substantial evidence that these changes in the activity of macrophages are brought about by lymphokines produced by activated T-lymphocytes. The activity of these products in disease is thought to be similar to that of the factor (MIF) released from lymphocytes in culture which inhibits the migration of cultivated macrophages from capillary tubes.

The observation that the enhanced elimination of both *Listeria* and other intracellular parasites develops as part of immunity in experimental listerosis has given rise to the concept that cell-mediated immunity against these and other organisms is specifically engendered and recalled but is non-specific in its action. There is, however, an extensive series of experiments in tuberculosis which have been interpreted as suggesting that such immunity is largely specific in action. In essence these experiments have shown that there are several substances in the mycobacterial cell capable of conferring increased resistance to tuberculosis and that different grades of resistance to these arise. One such substance is heat-labile and found in the ribosomal fraction of disrupted mycobacteria. It has been shown to be highly immunogenic. Immunity to infection by virulent mycobacteria only is conferred through this specific immunological process. This immunity is probably expressed through activated macrophages responding to sensitized lymphocytes. Of great interest is the finding that animals immunized by this substance do not show delayed hypersensitivity to tuberculin. Other immunizing components appear to reside in the cell wall; these induce a low-grade resistance which may be associated with tuberculin hypersensitivity. This state of resistance extends to heterologous organisms and may be regarded as non-specific. The non-specific activity is thought to be a function of the cell-wall components in directly attracting and activating macrophages to produce a marked granulomatous response. These activated macrophages can ingest and break down bacteria regardless of species. The apparent dissociation revealed between delayed hypersensitivity and cell-mediated immunity in tuberculosis is discussed in a later section.

Viruses

The role of the immune response in recovery from a primary viral infection remains problematical. In many instances the production of antibody lags behind the natural course of the infection. Indeed some children with hypogammaglobulinaemia can recover from certain virus infections, such as measles and herpes, without producing antiviral antibody. There is, however, little doubt of the protective function of antibody against second and subsequent infections, particularly those which produce a disseminated, systemic disease with viraemia. There is also clear evidence that viral infections which develop through seromucosal surfaces, such as poliomyelitis and influenza, stimulate the local production of SIgA and that this antibody may confer immunity more effectively than a high titre of serum immunoglobulin.

The activity of antibody in the immune elimination of virus is essentially that of **neutralization** and any opsonizing effect of the immune reaction upon phagocytosis appears less important than in bacterial infection. A number of mechanisms of viral neutralization have been postulated but the underlying factor is thought to be that antibody coating the virion interferes with the attachment, penetration, or uncoating of the particle at the surface of the target cell. However, antibody-virus combinations may remain infectious and can be found in the circulation in experimental chronic viral infections in animals, for example, murine lymphocytic choriomeningitis (LCM), where they may promote disease by dissemination or become involved in the formation of immune complexes which indirectly damage the host. Any activity of C' components in virus neutralization has commonly been attributed to their supplementation of the protein aggregates coating the virus. There is recent evidence from studies of herpes simplex virus that neutralization is indeed enhanced by the selective addition of the early components of the C' cascade as well as by the addition of anti-immunoglobulin directed against antiviral antibody, both of which procedures increase the bulk of the protein complex at the virion surface. However, a role for C'-mediated "virolysis" cannot be discounted in the case of enveloped viruses rich in lipoprotein and there is some evidence for virolysis of rubella and influenza viruses.

Neutralizing antibody can only attack virus directly when it is outside the target cell. Antibody cannot thus interfere with intracellular virus replication. Moreover, viruses such as the herpes simplex virus can spread from cell to cell without passing through the extracellular fluid. Therefore other mechanisms must exist for the elimination of virus infection and it is logical that these should be sought both amongst non-specific defence reactions and those immune reactions which affect host cells in which virus replicates. Of the former non-specific factors the inherent resistance of target cells is obviously important. However, once infection is established, but before a significant immunological reaction can be mounted, a part may be played by interferon. Discussion of this virus-induced inhibitory factor is largely outside the scope of this chapter but it is reasonable to state that its exact role during the course of natural disease is unknown and that many viruses are eliminated without the production of detectable amounts of interferon. However, the fact that *in vitro* interferon-like substances may be produced by macrophages and during lymphocyte transformation suggests that a link may exist between interferon activity and cell-mediated immune processes.

There is, of course, ample evidence that virus infections are associated with the development of the classic responses of cell-mediated immunity and that viral antigens may induce cutaneous delayed-hypersensitivity reactions and lymphocyte transformation. Cell-mediated immunity appears to be essential in the immune elimination of viruses such as herpes virus, poxvirus and myxovirus that infiltrate and alter the target-cell membrane. Experimental evidence for the relative importance of antibody, cell-mediated immunity and non-specific macrophage activity in the elimination of virus has been obtained by their **selective suppression** and **reconstitution.** Cyclophosphamide preferentially suppresses B-cell activity and therefore can be used to suppress antibody formation, though there is evidence that cell-mediated immunity and macrophage activity are also inhibited to some degree. The Coxsackie B-3 virus may be used in mice as a model of enterovirus infection. Infection in normal adult mice is not fatal and only a transient viraemia is produced which disappears with the appearance of specific antibody. Cyclophosphamide treatment drastically modifies the course of infection and viraemia is persistent; fatal lesions are produced in the heart and pancreas. If the immunosuppressed animals are passively immunized with specific antibody, protection against fatal infection may again be conferred. In normal suckling mice, Coxsackie virus infections are lethal. However, these immature animals can recover from infection if they are given both specific antibody and syngeneic peritoneal macrophages from adult animals. The inactivation of Coxsackie B-3 virus has been demonstrated in adult murine macrophages *in vitro*. These findings suggest that macrophage-antibody interactions may be important in the elimination of at least some virus infections associated with viraemia. Further evidence for the role of macrophages in experimental infection comes from the effects of intravenous injection of colloidal suspensions of, for example, silica, which is selectively ingested by macrophages. The intracellular silica then impairs macrophage function and adult mice so treated become more susceptible to infection with Coxsackie virus. A similar effect can be elicited in yellow-fever virus infection in mice. Adult mice are normally resistant to infection but pre-treatment with silica promotes a lethal encephalitis. This can be prevented, however, by the subsequent passive administration of antibody up to 48 hr. after infection.

T-lymphocyte function is suppressed by neonatal thymectomy or treatment with antilymphocyte serum.

These experimental procedures greatly enhance herpes virus and poxvirus infections but have little effect on arbovirus and enterovirus infections. Normal adult mice are resistant to herpes simplex infections by the intra-peritoneal route but cyclophosphamide treatment can lead to a fatal infection. However, protection against this effect cannot be conferred by the passive reconstitution of antibody but can only be effected by the transfer of T-cells from immune animals. At this point it should be mentioned that T-cell suppression involves the "helper cell" effect on B-cell activity. For this reason procedures such as neonatal thymectomy may be followed by the production of far less antiviral antibody than is normally found during the course of an experimental infection. Antibody levels may rise after reconstitution with T-cells. The mechanisms by which cell-mediated immunity might reduce viral infection have remained hypothetical and only partly substantiated by experiment. The T-cell induced "activation" of macrophages infected by virus could produce enhanced intracellular killing and a degree of macrophage activation has been measured during the course of LCM in mice. *In vitro* studies have also demonstrated the direct cytotoxic activity of sensitized T-cells against virus-infected cells in which virus antigen appears on the cell membrane. However, such cytoxicity may be of little benefit unless the cell is destroyed before replication is complete as cytolysis is an essential part of the dissemination of virus progeny. Similar considerations arise in relation to the cytolytic activity of antibody and C' against cells bearing virus antigen though such activity has been clearly demonstrated *in vitro*.

A further mechanism of cytolytic activity which may be directed at cells with virus antigen at their surface has only recently been examined and there is no conclusive evidence of its function during the course of natural infection. This mechanism, known as **antibody-dependent, cell-mediated cytotoxicity** has also been considered as promoting immune elimination in protozoal infections. The essential steps in this process as observed *in vitro* are, firstly, the coating of the target cell with specific antibody in amounts which may be too low to promote C'-dependent cytolysis. This is then followed by the attachment of an effector cell, sometimes known as a K (killer)-cell, which is not itself specifically sensitized to antigen at the target-cell surface but which produces a cytotoxic effect. The effector cell is known not to be identical with either T- or B-lymphocytes or mono-cytes but it does carry surface receptors for modified Fc, which are presumably involved in binding the cell to the antibody-coated target.

Fungi and Protozoa

Pathogenic fungi may produce disease as wide and varied as do bacteria and many of the mechanisms of immune elimination which have been discussed in relation to bacteria apply in the case of mycoses. In the normal host the elimination of highly infectious fungi such as *Histoplasma capsulatum* appears to be efficient. The majority of subjects in endemic regions show evidence of past infection, as indicated by a positive skin test, but only few develop disease. Conversely, overt infection by *Candida albicans*, which is a frequent member of the commensal flora, may only occur after alteration of susceptible tissues by local or systemic factors.

Many mycotic infections are largely confined to cutaneous sites. Here the most superficial infections, *e.g.* tinea, may be associated with negligible antigenic stimulation and it is not likely that immune factors play any great part in their elimination. In superficial candidiasis, fungal invasion is usually confined to the upper layers of the epithelium. Here the hyphae may be inaccessible to antibody though the development of infection at mucosal surfaces could in theory be influenced by secretory antibody which is known to have anticandidal activity. Serum antibodies to *Candida* also develop during the course of mucocutaneous infection so that it appears that antigen is available for the stimulation of regional lymphoid tissue. However, in experimental circumstances the passive immunization of animals with antibody may not protect against challenge with *C. albicans*, *Cryptococcus neoformans* and *H. capsulatum*. Such findings in part may reflect the intrinsic susceptibility of certain laboratory animals and may be influenced by the route of challenge and the dose. In man, it is likely that antifungal antibody may to some extent limit the dissemination of infection through the vascular system. The major function of antibody in this respect may be opsonization. Observations *in vitro* upon the uptake of *C. neoformans* by human phagocytes have shown that serum and a heat-labile substance, probably C', are required.

The large size and the formation of mycelia by certain fungi may inhibit effective phagocytosis and phagocytolysis. The appearance of atypical and prolonged infection with *Candida* in the rare congenital absence of myeloperoxidase, an important bactericidal enzyme present in neutrophils, suggests that the activity of this enzyme is important in the phagocytolysis of fungi as well as bacteria. During the breakdown of the fungal cell wall within the phagocyte new antigenic determinants may be revealed and antigenic material may be released from disrupted phagocytes. This antigenic variety may lead to the formation of antibodies with differing serological properties during the course of an infection. Many fungal diseases are, however, characterized by the retention of the micro-organism in histiocytes and phagocytic giant cells. In some instances, *e.g. H. capsulatum*, this may represent a state of prolonged, facultative parasitism of the reticulo-endothelial system. In addition, both deep-seated and superficial mycoses may be associated with the formation of chronic, granulomatous lesions. These characteristics, as in the case of mycobacterial infections, are likely to be associated with cell-mediated mechanisms of immune elimination operating through the interaction of lymphocytes and macrophages, and with the development of delayed hypersensitivity. The relationship between certain mycoses and immunodeficiency affecting T-cell reactivity is discussed below.

The localization and persistence of parasitic protozoa such as *Toxoplasma* and *Leishmania* within phagocytic cells, during at least part of the course of natural infection, suggest that the organisms may become sequestered from antibody and that the host may depend upon cell-mediated factors for successful defence. Leishmaniasis may provide an important example of disease associated with cell-mediated immunodeficiency (see below). However, the complexity of structure and life-cycle in protozoa may give rise to a variety of immune responses. There is some evidence to suggest that immune elimination in trypanosomiasis depends on the activity of antibody and C′ in promoting cytolysis and immune adherence to macrophages. There are high levels of IgM in the blood and cerebrospinal fluid. Humoral and cell-mediated factors may be involved in immunity to malaria, though the life-cycle of the parasite renders it inaccessible to immune processes for all but short periods. In experimental plasmodial infections in rodents, immunity can be transferred both by the IgG fraction of serum and by preparations of lymphoid cells. There is evidence that more severe infections occur in thymectomized animals.

IMMUNE ELIMINATION AT SEROMUCOSAL SURFACES

Antigenic stimulation at certain seromucosal surfaces including the oral cavity, parts of the intestine and the respiratory tree can give rise to an immunological reaction in local lymphoid tissues. Distinct populations of B-cells are found in sites such as the lamina propria of the gut, and in the interstitial tissue of salivary glands. Much of the immunoglobulin formed by these cells is of the IgA class and appears in the secretion as a specialized dimeric molecule, SIgA. The strength and duration of local antibody formation is dependent upon the local persistence of antigen. In addition, there is now evidence that cell-mediated responses can be elicited at mucosal surfaces. The immunological activity of local lymphoid aggregations is apparently dissociated from that of more distant tissues particularly in respect to the B-cell response. Parenteral inoculation of antigen may often fail to produce secretory antibody though in some instances sites of local antibody production may be stimulated by circulating antigen. Conversely, experimental infections of the intestinal tract and peroral immunization may produce only secretory antibody. When serum antibody is also produced by these procedures its appearance may lag behind that of SIgA. More important is the finding that adequate immunity to certain infections, e.g. poliomyelitis, experimental cholera and Shigella infections, correlates better with secretory than serum antibody production, and that immunization to these and related infections can be effected by the oral route.

These observations have lead to the definition of "**local immunity**", both as an important part of the first line of defence against invasive pathogens, and as a major feature in the elimination of infection at seromucosal surfaces. **Dental caries** is a unique example of a largely external infection and evidence is accumulating which suggests that immunological factors may affect cariogenic bacteria. It is clear that avascular tooth enamel is not an immunologically reactive tissue and that the source of antibody to plaque organisms may be either saliva or crevicular exudate. There is some evidence to suggest that adults with a high caries rate have significantly lower concentrations of salivary SIgA than those with little caries but this observation requires confirmation. However, the results of immunizing experimental animals with various preparations of cariogenic bacteria leave little doubt that caries can be influenced by immunological reactions, for studies have shown protection against caries in vaccinated animals. Subcutaneous, intravenous and submucosal routes of administration have been employed; each of these routes can give rise to serum antibody formation against the immunogen. There is evidence to suggest that secretory antibody is also stimulated, particularly by submucosal vaccination. It is likely that secretory antibody in saliva, rather than serum antibody, has a cariostatic effect, but this is not yet proven. In dental caries, as in other infections in which secretory antibody more clearly confers immunity, the problem is to elucidate the mechanisms of immune elimination or inhibition.

Secretory antibody is functional outside the tissues, separated from many of the effector mechanisms of serum and subject to continual dilution. It is conceivable that antibody is to some extent retained at the surface of epithelial cells. Recent findings suggest that SIgA is one of the first proteins to be absorbed on to newly exposed enamel surfaces where it may in some way influence bacterial colonization and metabolism. SIgA complexes readily with protein; several species of oral bacteria have been shown to be coated with SIgA in vivo but difficulty has arisen in distinguishing non-specific coating from the specific complexing of antibody with cell-surface antigen. Even if such immune complexes can form in vivo it is not clear how immune elimination can proceed. Very little C′ can be detected in external secretions such as saliva, but C′ components can appear in inflammatory exudates from mucosal surfaces, for example in the gingival crevicular fluid. However, SIgA is not in the classic sense a C′-fixing antibody. An unconfirmed study has shown that in vitro colostral SIgA can fix C′ in the presence of lysozyme and that lysozyme appears to be a key factor in the system. Aggregated SIgA has also been shown to activate the alternate pathway and it is possible that micro-organisms coated with secretory antibody may do likewise. It is not clear whether secretory antibody alone or in combination with C′ has opsonic activity. Some experiments have suggested that in vitro the phagocytosis of cariogenic streptococci may be enhanced by specific SIgA of salivary origin but observations upon the opsonic activity of SIgA from other sites have not shown a marked opsonic effect. There is also some doubt as to whether phagocytic cells remain fully viable outside the tissues and whether they are concentrated by chemotactic factors to the same extent as obtains in tissue spaces.

It is possible that the coating of bacteria by SIgA alone is one of the most important activities of this antibody. Such coating may inhibit bacterial growth and the aggregation of coated organisms may promote their removal by the flow of mucus and by peristalsis. Evidence is now emerging to show that the degree of virulence of certain organisms such as gonococci and pathogenic E. coli may depend upon a superior ability to adhere to epithelial surfaces. Adherence may be inhibited by specific secretory antibody. However, it could be argued that the colonization of tooth surfaces by cariogenic streptococci is promoted by the aggregation of plaque-forming micro-organisms. Recently it has been shown that SIgA can be produced against glucosyl transferase, an enzyme involved in the formation of extracellular polysaccharides by cariogenic organisms. If this enzyme were inhibited by antibody activity *in vivo* the adhesion of bacteria to enamel could be reduced and this could conceivably influence the formation of plaque and the pathogenesis of caries.

IMMUNODEFICIENCY AND INFECTION

Immunodeficiency may arise through a primary defect in development of the lymphoid tissues. In the previous chapter a broad distinction was made between **primary deficiencies** which affect only one limb of the immune system, either B- or T-cells, and those which arise from a stem-cell defect leading to a combined immunodeficiency state. The infections which arise in association with immunodeficiency are regarded as providing additional evidence of the relative importance of either humoral or cell-mediated immunological reactions for their elimination in the normal host. Primary T-cell deficiency states are rare and may be determined by genetic and familial factors. Until recently they were regarded as untreatable and affected infants died as a result of increased susceptibility to systemic fungal infections and to certain virus infections such as vaccinia. These infections also predominate in the equally rare stem-cell deficiency states. Primary B-cell defects, which lead to hypogammaglobulinaemia, are more common and not necessarily incompatible with life. Affected patients may develop recurrent pyogenic infections and infections with certain Gram-negative organisms.

These differences in susceptibility to infection also occur in diseases of the lymphoid system which give rise to **secondary immunodeficiency.** An important example of secondary T-cell deficiency is Hodgkin's disease, a condition that appears specifically to affect thymus-dependent tissues. Patients with untreated Hodgkin's disease are prone to infection by organisms which flourish in an intracellular environment such as tubercle bacilli, *Brucella*, *Cryptococcus* and vaccinia. They may show defective development of cutaneous delayed hypersensitivity to new antigens and to those to which they are known to have been previously exposed. At a cellular level their lymphocytes may show a depressed level of transformation when exposed to both non-specific mitogens such as phytohaemagglutinin (PHA) and specific antigens. Secondary immunodeficiency involving B-cells occurs in myeloma, in which the circulation is loaded with atypical globulins and in which neoplastic plasma cells displace normal B-cells. Secondary hypogammaglobulinaemia is also found in chronic lymphatic leukaemia (but this neoplastic proliferation may also involve T-cells). Both diseases may be complicated by pyogenic and pneumococcal infections. Acute myeloid leukaemia may also predispose to pyogenic infection through a gross reduction in the number of mature polymorphonuclear leucocytes. However, the prolonged treatment of leukaemia with corticosteroids may suppress normal cell-mediated immunity, and infections whose elimination requires intact T-cell function may assume atypical features. Thus measles may be followed by giant-cell pneumonia in which the giant cells often found in hyperplastic lymphoid tissue during measles occur in the lungs during the course of the disease. This atypical extension of measles may also arise in primary stem-cell deficiency states. The use of steroids, cytotoxic drugs and irradiation as therapeutic or palliative measures may frequently lead to an induced immunodeficiency affecting both T- and B-cells. This compounds the reduced resistance to infection already attendant upon severe disease. Opportunistic infection may cause not only persistent local disease such as oral candidiasis but disseminated and fatal infections by *Aspergillus, Pneumocystis carinii* and cytomegalovirus.

Abnormalities of lymphoid tissue are not, however, the only factors which determine immunodeficiency and predispose to infection. It is now well-recognized that alterations, particularly in cell-mediated immunity, can be brought about by infection itself. These changes may be **non-specific,** or apparently specific, taking the form of **antigen-dependent unresponsiveness.** Non-specific changes form a heterogeneous group and it is not entirely clear whether abnormalities recorded by the available laboratory and clinical tests are always relevant to the course of the disease. For example, a substantial number of patients with lepromatous leprosy cannot be sensitized with the contact agent dinitrochlorobenzene (DNCB) but sensitization can be effected in the majority of cases by injection of a more potent agent, keyhole limpet haemocyanin. Reports that lymphocytes from these patients are unresponsive to non-specific mitogen such as PHA have been variable whereas there is little doubt that specific unresponsiveness to *M. leprae* antigen does develop (see below). However, there is no apparent increase in the incidence of other infections or of tumours, suggesting that mechanisms of immunological surveillance are unimpaired in this disease.

In primary and secondary syphilis diminished lymphocyte transformation to PHA can be demonstrated. A factor may also be present in the patient's serum which can reduce the response to PHA of lymphocytes from an uninfected individual, suggesting that in some instances humoral factors may promote non-specific unresponsiveness. In addition, the profound effect of certain infections upon the structure of lymphoid tissues must influence the expression of cell-mediated immunity. For example, a marked depletion of lymphocytes is found in the spleen and lymph nodes of neonates suffering from congenital syphilis and a similar depletion can be induced in rabbits infected with *T. pallidum* at birth. The direct cytolytic effect of virus upon lymphoid cells has been shown to lead to non-specific immunodeficiency in animal diseases such as Newcastle disease of fowls, and has been implicated in the similar deficiency which accompanies some human viral infections such as measles. In measles there may be a loss of delayed tuberculin hypersensitivity and a failure of lymphoblastic transformation to PHA. The defects in this instance can be correlated with clinical manifestations such as the aggravation of concurrent tuberculosis or malaria.

A final but especially important aspect of non-specific unresponsiveness is the interrelationship between malnutrition, infection and immunodeficiency. Malnutrition arising as a primary state due to dietary insufficiency may lead to a reduction in cell-mediated responses, and specific states of malnutrition may be initiated by infection, particularly of the upper respiratory tract or gut. Thus measles tends to precipitate kwashiorkor and a cyclic interdependence between the two conditions may exist, for children suffering from kwashiorkor often develop a lethal measles infection. This special form of malnutrition is also linked with impairment in cell-mediated immunity. Atrophic changes in the lymphoid tissues may also be found in this condition. The dual role of malnutrition and intercurrent infection in promoting exacerbation of chronic disease such as leishmaniasis (see below) may also be of great importance.

Antigen-specific Unresponsiveness

In certain diseases, many of which are caused by intracellular parasites, a specific defect in cell-mediated responses to antigens of the causative organism may be

Leprosy and Leishmaniasis

Leprosy is a disease of little direct importance in dentistry apart from frequent involvement of the facial nerve and facial bones in the chronic granulomatous process. There is, however, no more appropriate example of the horizontal spectrum. The polar forms of leprosy are the tuberculoid (high resistance) and the lepromatous (low resistance) form. Between these is an arbitrarily defined "borderline" category into which the majority of cases fall and from which two-way movement across the disease spectrum is exemplified by frequent variations in symptomatology. Tuberculoid leprosy is associated with marked cell-mediated immunity: the lepromin skin test is positive, lymphocyte transformation to *M. leprae* antigen is demonstrable (fig. 1). The granulomatous lesions contain macrophages that show epithelioid changes and have few intracellular mycobacteria. The macrophages are accompanied by a dense, lymphocytic infiltration. Antimycobacterial antibody is detectable in only a minority of patients. Crossing the spectrum toward the lepromatous pole there is an inverse relationship between the lymphocyte content of the lesion and the number of bacteria (fig. 1), so that polar lepromatous lesions are dominated by lepra cells, undifferentiated macrophages containing undigested bacilli, and negligible infiltration of lymphocytes. The transformation of cultured lymphocytes at this pole of the

Characteristics	Indeterminate ↙ ↓ ↘ Tuberculoid ⇌ Borderline ⇌ Lepromatous		
Mycobacterium leprae in tissues	− or ±	+ or ++	++++
Lymphocytic infiltration	+++	+	−
Lepromin test	+++	−	−
Antimycobacterial antibodies (% patients with precipitins in serum)	11–28	82	95
Plasma cells in lymphoid tissue	±	+	+++
Immune complex disease (erythema nodosum leprosum)	−	±	+++
Delayed hypersensitivity (%) to			
Dinitrochlorobenzene	90	75	50
Haemocyanin	100	100	100

FIG. 1. The immunological features of the spectrum of leprosy.

demonstrated, whereas humoral antibody production may be relatively intact and have little influence on the course of the infection. In the most clear-cut examples of this antigen-specific unresponsiveness a correlation may be demonstrated between variations in the severity of the defect and the spectrum of clinical manifestations of the disease. These spectra can be conveniently described as "horizontal" or "vertical", each with a pole of high and low resistance. In the **horizontal spectrum,** which is especially exemplified by leprosy, leishmaniasis and South American blastomycosis, there is potential for two-way movement between the poles. In the **vertical spectrum,** such as is found in syphilis and Chagas disease, movement is unidirectional from low through high resistance and finally to low resistance again in the tertiary disease.

disease shows variation with respect to PHA but there is a distinctly depressed transformation to *M. leprae* antigen. In many cases the response to unrelated antigens such as *M. tuberculosis* is intact.

Histological and immunological observations have suggested that the state of high resistance to the leprosy bacillus which occurs at the tuberculoid end of the spectrum is a function of sensitized T-cells effected through activated macrophages. Conversely, the low resistance lepromatous disease appears to demonstrate a specific T-cell defect that depends upon the high load of antigen within phagocytic cells. The importance of the T-cell in leprosy has been confirmed by animal studies. A disease with the salient features of lepromatous leprosy can be produced in mice if bacilli are administered after the ablation of T- and B-cells by thymectomy and whole-body irradiation, followed by the selective reconstitution of only B-cells by bone-marrow grafting. Some of the ability to reject the infection can be shown to be regained after the injection of viable lympho-cytes which will restore T-cell function.

The precise reasons for T-cell suppression in lepromatous leprosy remain unknown, although the possibility of an underlying genetic or familial predisposition cannot be entirely excluded. There are at least two possible ways in which the antigen-specific unresponsiveness may occur. In the first a high concentration of antigen may directly suppress potentially responsive clones of T-lymphocytes producing **immunological tolerance** of the **high-dose** type. This is sometimes referred to as high zone, antigen-dependent clone elimination. The second possibility is that a clone of specific **suppressor cells** (which might be either B- or T-cells) proliferates and competes with effector T-cells thus blocking the cell-mediated response. The compati-bility of these theories, particularly the former, with the fact that in polar lepromatous leprosy the T-cell defect is permanent, and unaffected by reductions in bacillary load after chemotherapy, is uncertain. In cases less severe than the polar form such treatment can, however, promote a restoration of cell-mediated immunity and movement toward the tuberculoid pole.

Since lepromatous leprosy occurs in the presence of high titres of antibody it has also been suggested this may block T-cell function by the process which in tumour immunology is known as "immunological enhancement" (see Chapter 13). However, the impairment of T-cell function *in vitro* is demonstrable both in the presence of autologous serum or in serum free of antibody. Also the serum from lepro-matous patients does not block the reactivity of T-cells from subjects normally responsive to *M. leprae* antigens. While these findings fail to confirm the role of antibody in T-cell suppression in leprosy there is some experimental evidence from infections with *Leishmania* implicating B-cells and serum factors in the active elimination of this infection, which otherwise has a similar immunological spectrum to that of leprosy. Guinea pigs infected with *L. enrietti* develop a local lesion resembling the "oriental sore" which in human disease appears to occupy a border-line position in the horizontal spectrum. If either antilymph-ocyte serum, or cyclophosphamide is then administered to the animal, delayed healing and a more diffuse disease ensue. In addition, it has been shown that serum from animals recovering from an infection contains a factor which inhibits the growth of *Leishmania* in culture. It is therefore possible that immunity in some stages of human leishmaniasis will be found to depend upon synergistic activity between T- and B-cells.

Chronic Mucocutaneous Candidiasis

A number of defects in cell-mediated immunity have been demonstrated in patients suffering from various forms of candidiasis, particularly chronic mucocutaneous candid-iasis (CMCC). Contemporary classifications of CMCC suggest that there are at least four types of the disease with characteristics sufficiently different for them to be regarded as separate entities. All of them commonly exhibit oral candidiasis. In three of the groups, lesions occur early in life and tend to be florid and intractable. Two of these groups appear to be linked with an autosomal recessive trait; in one, mucocutaneous lesions are a major feature, while the other is characterized by the multifocal endo-crinopathy sometimes called the endocrine-candidiasis syndrome. There is, however, no distinct evidence of a genetic defect in the immune response. The third group of early-onset CMCC has not yet been shown to have a genetically determined background. It may be associated with extensive pseudo-granulomatous skin lesions together with an increased susceptibility to other fungal and bacterial infections. The fourth group occurs much later in life and again there is no genetic trait; oral lesions predominate and this grouping may embrace a variety of lesions including some otherwise known as candidal leukoplakia. In each of these four groups many patients have been shown to have defects in the expression of cell-mediated immunity. While in many instances a high serum titre of anticandidal antibody may be present, some cases may show a deficiency of humoral antibody or selective deficiency of SIgA.

An important feature of the immunodeficiencies is that they are found to be scattered randomly across the clinico-genetic groups so that any one form of the disease is not exclusively marked by a characteristic deficiency. It has, however, been suggested that there is a discernible correla-tion between the degree of immunodeficiency and the severity of infection so that a disease spectrum may be present in CMCC. In some subjects the deficiency corresponds to that found in other examples of antigen-dependent unresponsiveness. Thus lymphocyte trans-formation to candida antigen may be impaired while transformation to PHA is variable. The former activity may be influenced by a serum factor. These findings may be explained in terms of high-zone tolerance and, in the least severe forms of the disease, reduction of antigen load by chemotherapy may lead to clinical improvement and a restoration of cell-mediated responses. Recently, treat-ment has also been effected by the injection of "transfer factor", a substance which is extracted from the sensitized lymphocytes of a donor and can transfer cell-mediated sensitization to a host previously unresponsive to the particular antigen. The relative success of this treatment may be taken as additional evidence for the role of cell-mediated immunity in controlling candidal infection.

There is, however, substantial evidence that a separate and unusual defect occurs in another group. In these patients lymphocytes transform normally to non-specific mitogen and candida antigen but transformation is not associated with the formation *in vitro* of the mediator (MIF) which inhibits the migration of macrophages in tissue culture. It is tempting to relate this deficiency to the cutaneous anergy which may be found in these patients as it is possible to regard MIF as a mediator of cutaneous delayed hypersensitivity. However, cutaneous anergy or the specific absence of delayed hypersensitivity to candidin occurs frequently in CMCC, both in cases which have a normal MIF response and in some cases with impaired lymphocyte transformation. These findings emphasize that the *in vitro* responses of lymphocytes do not always correlate well with the state of delayed hypersensitivity and they also suggest that any functional significance should with caution be ascribed to MIF deficiency in CMCC. It is, however, of interest that the localized chronic candidiasis of the palate known as "denture stomatitis" has been associated in some patients with similar abnormalities of cell-mediated immunity. These may be expressed as a low incidence of delayed hypersensitivity to candidal extracts and decreased inhibition of leucocyte migration *in vitro*. The restoration of these responses after topical antimycotic therapy has been demonstrated. Since this form of candidiasis is seldom associated with a demonstrable invasion of the epithelium by the organism, the immunological findings appear to indicate that the cell-mediated immune response can be affected by superficial infection. It is therefore possible that the potency and persistence of antigen, rather than the extent of the infection, are influential in the alterations in cell-mediated immunity which occur in CMCC.

Any interpretation of the nature of the immunodeficiency in this mycotic disease must, however, take into account the frequent occurrence of **latent iron deficiency** without anaemia in these patients. Whether this deficiency is fundamental and perhaps determined by genetic factors remains to be shown, but the deficiency may certainly occur in those forms of CMCC which do not appear to be linked to a genetic trait. It is possible that iron deficiency, acting through a depletion of iron-rich enzymes, initiates epithelial dystrophy which in turn predisposes to candidal infection. However, a reduction in the iron available for enzyme activity and for normal DNA synthesis may also have a direct effect on the function of lymphoid cells. While this could account for the persistence of infection in CMCC, and might in some way influence the apparent immunodeficiency, it cannot readily explain the fact that the deficiency often appears to be antigen-dependent. Of some value in unifying these apparently unconnected data is the observation that chronic inflammation may influence iron metabolism and particularly serum iron kinetics. It appears that the activity of macrophages during the inflammatory response results in a redistribution of iron to the reticuloendothelial system and that this may be an essential part of a normal response. Whether in the special circumstances of candidal infection this shift in iron metabolism predisposes to persistent infection and even to an immune defect is as yet hypothetical. What is clear is that infection may regress during iron-replacement therapy but even this is a paradox for iron is an important growth factor for *Candida* in culture. Nutrient depletion may, however, promote the change from yeast to mycelial forms in these fungi, and in CMCC pathogenicity is associated with the invasive hyphal form. *In vitro* this form may arise in adverse cultural conditions. Though the example of CMCC raises as yet unanswered questions about host-pathogen interaction it clearly illustrates the probability of direct and indirect relationships between altered metabolism and altered immunity.

Syphilis

A final example of disease in which a specific defect in cell-mediated immunity may be found is that of syphilis. It has been mentioned above that the clinical manifestations of syphilis move over a spectrum which may be notionally called "vertical". Unlike the horizontal spectrum, progress away from the initial lesion is relentless and unidirectional. Concurrently with the clinical spectrum an immunological spectrum may be visualized with a low-resistance pole represented by the primary and early secondary disease (fig. 2). At this stage cell-mediated immunity is defective: there is an absence of delayed hypersensitivity to treponemal antigen and lymphocyte transformation to PHA is impaired. In addition, a factor in the patient's serum has been shown to reduce the response to PHA of lymphocytes from an uninfected subject. This impairment of cell-mediated immunity, which is not distinctly antigen-specific but is possibly related to a high antigen load, is associated with uncontrolled proliferation of the spirochaete in the face of significant levels of treponemal antibody. A progressive restoration of cell-mediated immunity may be apparent during the latter stages of secondary syphilis. Infectivity decreases, lesions may become tuberculoid and delayed hypersensitivity to treponemal antigen may be demonstrable. A variable latent period then ensues during which the organism may be difficult to find but antibody is still produced. There appears to be a state of equilibrium between host and pathogen but if this balance is upset, perhaps by events such as intercurrent infection, the disease may enter its tertiary phase. Unlike the horizontal spectrum, cell-mediated immunity at this pole of the vertical spectrum is not necessarily maximal. Therefore, while gummatous disease is associated with marked delayed hypersensitivity and modest levels of antibody, some forms of neurosyphilis are associated with depressed delayed hypersensitivity and a high antibody titre; organisms may again be detectable within the lesions (fig. 2).

These examples of infection associated with immunodeficiency illustrate the way in which immunological investigations may help to explain variations in host response seen in chronic disease. The data do not lead to a unifying concept of the cause of immunodeficiency and it is likely that many unknown factors are also involved. In each example there is, however, some evidence of **immune deviation.** Tolerance occurs with respect to cell-mediated activity but antibody production is not reduced. The mechanisms which may induce tolerance have been discussed; these may be antigen-dependent and influenced by antigen load, though it should be emphasized that several different antigens may arise during the course of a disease. It has been suggested that high-zone tolerance is effected by antigen acting directly upon lymphoid cells without the prior processing of antigen by macrophages, which is thought to be the more usual process. At the same time it is clear that macrophage activity is important in immune elimination in these diseases, although parasitization of macrophages is not an essential feature of candidiasis or syphilis. Some workers believe that cell-mediated cytotoxicity rather than macrophage activation is an important effector mechanism in leishmaniasis. In addition, although it is known that serum factors can influence the transformation characteristics of cultured lymphocytes in an apparently specific fashion, these factors largely remain to be characterized. From time to time it has been suggested that the factors are enzymes, a product of the micro-organism, immune complexes, or antibody.

Chronic Periodontal Disease

The uncertainty which surrounds the interpretation of immunological phenomena in chronic infection by a single

ation of lymphocytes might also indicate that cell-mediated hypersensitivity phenomena are involved in its pathogenesis. There may be similarities between the production of destructive lesions towards the poles of high resistance in horizontal disease spectra, which is discussed in the next section, and the chronic tissue response to plaque antigens. Many more studies, however, are required to confirm the role of immune reactions in chronic periodontal disease.

ALLERGY AND HYPERSENSITIVITY

The pathways by which immunological reactions may promote an inflammatory response have been outlined in

Stage of Disease	B-cell Function		T-cell Function		
	Plasma Cells	Antibody	Presence of T. pallidum	PHA Transformation	Luetin Skin Test
1°	++	+	++	−	−
2° early	++	+++	+++	−	−
2° late	+	+	+	+	++
Latent	?	+	−	+	+ or −
3° Gumma	++	+	+	+	+++
3° GPI	++ (In CSF)	+++	+++	?	±

FIG. 2. The immunological features of the clinical spectrum of syphilis.

micro-organism extends to findings so far presented in relation to chronic periodontal disease. In this condition the aetiology appears to be multifactorial and the mixed infection of plaque is only superficially related to the gingival tissue. Several studies have shown that lymphocyte transformation can be induced by fractions extracted from dental plaque. Separate preparations of Gram-negative bacteria commonly found in plaque also cause transformation, and there is evidence to suggest that the degree of transformation activity increases in relation to the clinical severity of disease as measured by available indices. One study has apparently shown a decrease in transformation in severe periodontal disease. Lymphocyte transformation in these experiments has also been shown to produce MIF activity and cytotoxic activity against chicken erythrocytes. Serum factors appear to influence transformation; serum from subjects with early periodontal disease strengthened the response of lymphocytes from subjects with advanced disease, and serum from this latter group was inhibitory in respect of lymphocytes from cases of early disease. The decrease in transformation described in severe disease may therefore depend upon serum factors or it may conceivably represent a developing form of tolerance. The apparent relationship between increasing severity of periodontal disease and the increased stimul-

the previous sections. It is evident that tissue damage may result from inflammation and the extent of this damage may exceed that which might be elicited by microbial products alone. Many of the manifestations of hypersensitivity or allergy are attributable to the inflammatory response induced by immunological reactions. The concept of allergy is derived from the observation of apparently excessive reactions to antigenic challenge in a previously immunized host. Certainly the morbidity and occasional mortality associated with allergic disease evokes a picture of excessive and paradoxical response. This paradox is seen in hypersensitivity occurring as a result of infection, the lesions of which may be far more damaging and extensive than those of the infection. A classic example of this is the association between streptococcal pharyngitis and rheumatic fever. In many infectious diseases, however, the manifestations of hypersensitivity bear a complex relationship to the course of the infection and the circumstances in which they occur cannot be so readily interpreted as bizarre immunological hyperactivity. Hypersensitivity without overt symptoms may occur in many diseases and may occasionally benefit the host. Because of the connections between immune reactions and inflammation there may be no clear dividing line between normal response and hyperactivity. Instead there may be a spectrum of changes with a shifting point of equilibrium between immune elimination and tissue damage.

Of the immediate-type hypersensitivities, which arise from the combination of antigen and humoral antibody, the **complex-mediated** type appears to be of greater importance in infectious disease. The combination of soluble antigen, antibody, and fixed C′, which gives rise to an immune complex, generates the release of mediators of acute inflammation at the level of C3 and C5. These are responsible for an increase in vascular permeability and the attraction of polymorphonuclear leucocytes, often in large numbers. Vascular changes are intimately involved in the pathogenesis of lesions caused by immune complexes since complexes tend to localize in vessel walls, particularly in plexi of small vessels such as are found in the dermis, the renal glomerulus, the synovial fringes of joints, and in the iris and sclera. Several factors appear to determine whether a complex will localize readily. The mean size of soluble complexes has been shown to decrease as the antigen: antibody ratio increases so that the soluble complexes formed in antigen excess, which are known to be retained in the circulation, are probably smaller than complexes formed at equivalence which are rapidly eliminated. There is, however, a minimum size of complex capable of initiating damage. In contrast to the soluble complexes which cause disseminated lesions such as are found in serum sickness, complexes formed in gross antibody excess may precipitate rapidly at the source of antigen. Lesions formed in this way in disease states may, if subcutaneous, resemble the experimental Arthus reaction. The extent of vascular damage in immune-complex disease may depend upon the activation of several systems apart from the mediators of activated C′. The Hageman factor is thought to be activated by complexes so that the kinin system of inflammatory mediators may become involved in the response. Similarly, platelet aggregation may yield vasoactive amines and induce local thrombosis. Another important factor in tissue damage, particularly in lesions which proceed to necrosis, is the activity of hydrolytic enzymes derived from polymorphonuclear leucocytes. Some measure of the clinical features associated with the extent of the lesion may be obtained from skin diseases where the deposition of circulating immune-complexes would be expected to cause (in increasing order of severity) erythema, oedema, purpura and necrosis.

In man, evidence for immune-complex formation in the causation of disease should ideally include the demonstration of the components of the complex in the lesion and, in the case of circulating complexes, the demonstration of such complexes in serum preferably together with a fall in serum C′ level. Although the demonstration of deposits of immunoglobulin and C′ in vessel walls by immunofluorescence is often taken as evidence of immune-complex disease, it should be noted that a similar appearance can occur in vascular injury of unrelated aetiology, particularly if the leakage of serum proteins is extensive. Conversely, in experimental situations immune complexes may disappear rapidly from a lesion so that their absence in suspect lesions does not necessarily mean that they are uninvolved. An example of these diagnostic problems is

found in oral disease. Some features of **acute ulcerative gingivitis** (AUG) are reminiscent of an Arthus reaction although the large number of organisms present suggests that local antigen excess is likely to occur. Also the overall histological appearance is not convincingly similar to an experimental, Arthus-type lesion. Yet by immunofluorescence both IgG and C′ components have been found in vessels in biopsies taken from AUG. However, the fluorescent material is not in the "lumpy" distribution said to be typical of complex formation and it can be readily dispersed by elution with saline. It has been suggested that these findings add to the evidence against the formation of complex-mediated lesions in AUG. In other conditions, the limitations of experimental procedures may dictate that evidence for immune-complex disease is incomplete, and suggestive rather than conclusive.

There are, however, several human diseases which exemplify immune-complex phenomena, and some of them are of infectious origin. There is much evidence to suggest that disseminated lesions in the joints, skin and heart in rheumatic fever result from immune-complex formation. The sequential association of this disease with a localized throat infection by Group A streptococci suggests that complexes form around streptococcal exotoxin in a previously sensitized individual. In subacute bacterial endocarditis (SABE) showers of mucosal, conjunctival and cutaneous petechiae or splinter haemorrhages may occur, and Osler's nodes are commonly found. Although these lesions may be embolic, there is evidence to suggest that circulating immune complexes are responsible for some of the manifestations. For example, an Osler's node appears histologically as an acute, leucocytoclastic necrotizing vasculitis of the glomus arterio-venous anastomosis; bacteria are not detectable nor is there evidence of thrombus or embolism. The glomerulonephritis which may occur in SABE has histological features consistent with circulating immune-complex disease and is associated with a low serum C′ level. The separate condition known as post-streptococcal glomerulonephritis may arise in a fashion similar to rheumatic fever and appears to be of immune-complex origin. There is recent evidence to suggest that the arthritis and cutaneous vasculitis which can occur five or more days after the onset of severe meningococcal meningitis may also be an example of immune-complex disease, though in this case it is not clear whether the skin lesions arise from the deposition of circulating complexes or from a direct Arthus reaction. Proven examples of Arthus-like phenomena in human infectious disease are few, but a striking instance is seen in erythema nodosum leprosum (ENL). This condition arises in cases of lepromatous leprosy slightly removed in the spectrum from the intractable polar form (fig. 1). It usually occurs during chemotherapy rather than spontaneously and the clinical presentation is a red, painful, nodular rash which may coalesce to form plaques or ulcerations. Histologically the lesions show vessel damage and an intense polymorphonuclear infiltrate; mycobacteria, usually degenerating, can be found at most sites. These would provide a source of antigen to react across the vessel walls with the high levels of mycobacterial antibody present in this part of the leprosy spectrum and thereby produce an Arthus reaction. Since ENL is sometimes associated with arthritis, iridocyclitis and nephritis, it is possible that the large amounts of soluble antigen released into the circulation during chemotherapy also combine there with antibody to form soluble complexes and disseminated lesions.

A number of viral and mycotic diseases also give rise to symptoms suggestive of immune-complex pathology. The prodromal phase of virus hepatitis, particularly of the type associated with the Australia antigen, may be associated with an illness resembling serum sickness. Immune complexes have been demonstrated in the serum in viral hepatitis and low C' levels have also been found. In some patients a mild hepatitis may occur together with polyarteritis nodosa. Complexes of Australia antigen and immune globulin have been found in serum in these cases, as well as deposits of the antigen, IgM and C' in the vessel walls. Rarely a syndrome of polyarteritis, urticaria and angioedema may be associated with rubella, variola, or mumps. However, in exanthemata where virus can be recovered from the typical skin lesions, as in variola and varicella, it should be noted that the pock probably arises as a direct toxic effect of the virus. The typical rash of measles can be found in agammaglobulinaemic patients suggesting that circulating antibody is not involved. Glomerulonephritis, with some evidence of immune-complex deposition, may complicate infectious mononucleosis but the cause of the typical palatal petechiae is not clear. In some 5 per cent of mycotic infections by *Coccidioides immitis*, erythema nodosum and erythema multiforme may arise as a manifestation of hypersensitivity thought to be of immune-complex origin. The aetiology of **erythema multiforme** remains, however, problematic. The presence of immune-complex formation is an attractive hypothesis to explain the occurrence of this disease after a number of infections, including herpes simplex, mycoplasma and non-specific infection of the upper respiratory tract. However, immunofluorescent microscopy has not unequivocally demonstrated complex deposition and low serum C' levels have not been found.

Before leaving the topic of hypersensitivity involving the fixation of C' some mention should be made of the inflammatory lesions attributable to bacterial endotoxin. These include the experimentally-induced phenomena grouped under the general heading of the **Shwartzman** reaction. It should be emphasized at once that there is no direct evidence to suggest that these events are immunological hypersensitivity reactions. They may, however, occupy a field of action analogous to hypersensitivity where the damaging effect of the inflammatory response may outweigh its benefit in eliminating infection. If an endotoxin preparation is injected subcutaneously an inflammatory lesion can be produced: it is probable that the alternate pathway of C' activation is involved. If 24 hr. later the animal is challenged intravenously by endotoxin, necrosis occurs at the site of the skin injection. This reaction is known as the local Shwartzman phenomenon; a general effect, sometimes known as the Sanarelli-Shwartzman phenomenon, can be produced if both administrations are intravenous. In this instance a state of endotoxin

shock is induced with the widespread, intravascular deposition of fibrin and cortical necrosis of the kidneys. The interaction of platelets with endotoxin and the activation of the alternate pathway may be involved in these pathological effects. This apparent hypersensitivity is, however, non-specific and without any clear-cut immunological basis, for the second endotoxin used in challenge need not to be the same as the first. There is little direct evidence that these phenomena play a part in infectious disease although they cannot be lightly discounted. It will be remembered that many of the bacteria in dental plaque contain endotoxin; there can be little doubt that there is an aetiological association between plaque and chronic gingivitis. However, bacterial penetration of the tissues is not common in gingivitis and it has been suggested that some of the inflammatory events in the gingivae result from the action of endotoxin liberated from plaque. Both the conventional and alternate pathway of C' activation may be engaged by endotoxin in chronic gingivitis, though evidence for this is as yet largely circumstantial. However, in AUG, which frequently occurs as an infection superimposed upon chronic gingivitis, there is a local tissue invasion by organisms which can yield endotoxin, possibly in large quantities. The evidence against an Arthus-like hypersensitivity in AUG has already been discussed. Aside from any direct toxic effect it has also been proposed that endotoxin in AUG may give rise to a local Shwartzman phenomenon but in the absence of a satisfactory experimental model this is unproven.

In **delayed hypersensitivity** the paradox of damaging immunological reactions is aptly illustrated for defence mechanisms and allergy appear to be intimately associated. Unlike hypersensitivity mediated by antibody the lesions are usually not disseminated but are closely associated with the source of infection. However, it is this close link which leads to the conclusion that in cell-mediated immunity, allergy and immune elimination may be part of the same spectrum of changes. Delayed hypersensitivity to tuberculin is a classic manifestation of allergy dependent upon cellular rather than humoral factors. In the course of human tuberculosis the state of increased resistance or partial immunity appears to be correlated with the development of a positive tuberculin skin test. It may, however, be shown that cellular immunity to mycobacteria can exist in the absence of allergy to tuberculin, following desensitization, and that a high degree of tuberculin allergy can be produced without the development of immunity. This apparent dissociation between delayed hypersensitivity and acquired immunity has been described in a previous section and it has been suggested that the basis for it lies in the activity of several different mycobacterial antigens. Undoubtedly the discovery of this dissociation resolves in part the paradox of how a destructive process appears to promote a protective effect, for it seems the two may run parallel but separate courses dictated by different antigens. Cutaneous delayed hypersensitivity reactions may be a feature of natural human tuberculosis in lupus vulgaris. It is also probable that the tissue reactions to superficial fungal infections are similarly produced.

There is a considerable body of evidence to suggest that

lymphokine production by the sensitized T-cell is responsible for the tissue damage associated with delayed hypersensitivity. Therefore, in those diseases with a spectrum of cell-mediated responses, hypersensitivity phenomena may arise in that part of the spectrum associated with the effective expression of cell-mediated immunity. The lesion of tuberculoid leprosy is an example. In it macrophages become activated by lymphokines and acquire epithelioid characteristics that can be associated with the elimination of a large proportion of infecting mycobacteria. However, the accumulation of macrophages and lymphocytes continues in response to residual antigenic stimulus, and the lesion is associated with tissue damage which must be regarded as hypersensitivity since few viable organisms remain. A similar process is seen in a mature focus of tuberculosis. If macrophages are indeed the effector cells in these hypersensitivity reactions it could be that one of the major mechanisms of tissue damage is the release of hydrolytic enzymes. In this respect cell-mediated hypersensitivity and complex-mediated hypersensitivity have a common feature for in the latter the overspill of lysosomal enzymes from polymorphonuclear leucocytes could also be a major cause of tissue damage.

FURTHER READING

Allison, A. C. (1972), "Immunity and Immunopathology in Virus Infections," *Ann. Inst. Pasteur*, **123**, 585.

"Cell-mediated Immunity and Resistance to Infection" (1973), *World Health Organization Technical Report Series*, No. 519. Geneva: W.H.O.

Cream, J. J. and Turk, J. L. (1971), "A Review of the Evidence for Immune-complex Deposition as a Cause of Skin Disease in Man," *Clinical Allergy*, **1**, 235.

Lehner, T. (1972), "Cell-mediated Immune Responses in Oral Disease: A Review," *J. oral Path.*, **1**, 39.

Notkins, A. L. (1973), "Immunological Defense and Immunological Injury in Herpes Simplex Virus Infection," in *Comparative Immunology of the Oral Cavity*, p. 192 (S. E. Mergenhagen and H. W. Scherp, Eds.). U.S. Department of Health Monograph.

Shearman, D. J. C., Parkin, D. M. and McClelland, D. B. L. (1972), "The Demonstration and Function of Antibodies in the Gastrointestinal Tract," *Gut*, **13**, 483.

Stossel, T. P. (1974), "Phagocytosis," *New Engl. J. Med.*, **290**, 717.

Turk, J. L. and Bryceson, A. D. M. (1971), "Immunological Phenomena in Leprosy and Related Diseases," *Advanc. Immunol.*, **13**, 209.

Valdimarsson, H., Higgs, J. M., Wells, R. S., Yamamura, M., Hobbs, J. R. and Holt, P. J. L. (1973), "Immune Abnormalities Associated with Chronic Mucocutaneous Candidiasis," *Cellular Immunol.*, **6**, 348.

Youmans, G. P. and Youmans, A. S. (1969), "Recent Studies on Acquired Immunity in Tuberculosis," *Current Topics in Microbiology and Immunology*, **48**, 129. Berlin: Springer-Verlag.

11. TISSUE TRANSPLANTATION

ARNOLD R. SANDERSON

INTRODUCTION

It is the intention in this chapter to outline the present state of knowledge in transplantation. The underlying principles have recently been shown to apply also to tooth germ transplantation although the fundamental work was done with other tissues. For this reason, considerations of dental material are delayed to the end of the review, by which point it is hoped that the reader will be familiar with the basic tenets.

Transplantation of kidneys in man has now reached a sufficiently successful level for it to be of major therapeutic consideration in renal disease. There is much less experience of homovital human grafts of bone marrow, heart, skin, liver, lung and endocrine tissues. The logistics of supply, ethical considerations, organ storage or support mechanisms, and alternative forms of therapy for the disease in question, are major factors in the continuing debate. It is the intention to review particularly the immunological and genetic basis of tissue transplantation.

Given adequate surgical technique, the principal problem to be overcome in tissue grafting is the immune response, which occurs as a result of genetic differences between donor and recipient. The most compelling evidence for this is that genetically identical animals (*e.g.* inbred lines of rodents; identical twins) do not reject one another's grafts. The same basic principles have been found to apply to transplantation within species as diverse as earthworms, fishes and man. Since the accepted terminology of transplantation immunogenetics is often confusing due to its evolution, and is somewhat different from that commonly employed in classical immunology, a glossary is given at the end of this chapter. Such a vast body of literature on the subject has accumulated during the past fifteen years that no attempt is made to interpolate specific references in the text. Instead, a suggested further reading list is appended following the glossary.

IMMUNOLOGICAL BASIS OF HOMOGRAFT REJECTION

Much of what is now understood about transplantation immunogenetics rests on the firm foundation provided by inbred lines of mice. No two randomly bred laboratory animals are genetically identical. However, because almost half a century ago biologists required genetically uniform and reproducible animals for the study of transferable malignancies, inbred lines were produced. They began, curiously enough, with Japanese "waltzing mice" which had been kept for many years in circuses. Selective breeding was practised to maintain the inherited characteristic of a defective gait.

Skin grafts exchanged between sexually identical members of any inbred strain of mice are invariably successful: skin grafts from one strain to another invariably fail. Skin is used because the technique is relatively simple, the progress of the graft is clearly visible, and the tissue is exquisitely sensitive to the rejection process. For a few days a first graft clearly remains viable, but then rapidly becomes necrotic. A second graft from the same, or a genetically related, donor is rejected much more quickly, while subsequent grafts may fail to show any initial healing-in, but be sloughed-off very rapidly (some hours) with a pallor ("white graft") which indicates a lack of vascularization.

Several features of the phenomenon of homograft rejection are indicative of an immune response. Firstly, the initial healthy state of a first graft indicates an acquired state of the host as responsible for subsequent tissue destruction. Secondly, there is the demonstration of memory in that the recipient remembers its prior insult and appears to be equipped to deal more promptly with a second confrontation. This memory is of course demonstrated by the whole host, and is not confined to the area of the initial sensitization. Thirdly, the phenomenon is specific: that is to say, the second graft only shows accelerated rejection when the donor(s) of the two grafts are related. An unrelated graft behaves like the first graft. Rejection is also accompanied in most cases by the appearance of antibodies in the serum of the recipient. As will be explained later, these mirror the difference between donor and host. At this stage, however, it is important to emphasize that neither the appearance nor specificity of these immunoglobulins should be assumed to imply any role which they may play in graft rejection. Finally, the rejection can be shown, with some

care, to be dose-dependent in that larger homografts survive somewhat less well than smaller ones.

These findings constitute an impressive body of evidence that homograft rejection within a species is brought about by an immunological mechanism, and is characterized by the twin features of memory and specificity. Furthermore, the sensitized state can be transferred to an animal that has received no grafts. This transfer of adoptive immunity is achieved by sensitizing an animal, and then transferring lymphocytes to a second, genetically identical, but non-immune host. This second animal now manifests the sensitized state and will reject grafts in an accelerated fashion. Humoral antibodies totally fail to confer immunity on a second host, which thereby formally places graft rejection in the category of cellular, as opposed to humoral, immune processes.

TRANSPLANTATION ANTIGENIC STRENGTH AND GENETICS

Although we know that it is genetic differences between host and graft which provoke rejection, it is evident from research with inbred lines of mice that the vigour of the response depends on the kind of genetic disparity. Thus, the difference between two strains of mice, A and B, may be such that grafts survive as long as 20 days, and when performed under the cover of immunosuppressive drug therapy, they may survive longer or permanently. In contrast, two other strains, A and C, reject skin within 9–10 days and the prolongation noted under immunosuppression is not remarkable. We say then that the A–B antigenic or histocompatibility difference is weak, compared with the A–C difference. Mouse geneticists, seeking to explain the failure to transplant tumours between in-bred lines of mice, and their F1 or F2 generation hybrids, discovered that a large number of genes determine histocompatibility (H) antigens. There are at least 14 H genes in mice and there is good evidence that similar systems operate in all species so far tested. However, the interesting (and refreshingly simple) fact has emerged that in every species, one out of the many H genes determines H antigens of unquestionably greater importance than the remainder. This is the strong H locus (H–2 in mice; HL–A* in man); the remainder are weak. Thus, in the example used earlier, the more vigorous rejection may be attributed to strong H locus differences between strains A and C, and the less vigorous rejection to weak H locus differences between strains A and B† (see Table 1).

It is of the utmost importance to appreciate that antigenic strength, as applied here to transplantation antigens, is

---

* Nomenclature in mouse histocompatibility systems is H–1, H–2, H–3 and so on. The H–2 genetic locus is the strong locus. Nomenclature in man is less clearly defined. For example, some systems such as ABO, Rhesus, had already been well-established with their trivial names before the strong locus system was discovered and characterized. The strong locus has been called HL–A (Human Leukocyte antigen system—*A*) in recognition of the cell type upon which its discovery was dependent. *A* anticipates, in an optimistic but commendable fashion, the revelation of other systems, *B*, etc., on leukocytes.

† A qualifying rider is that multiple weak locus differences can exert a cumulative effect. Immunosuppressive therapy nevertheless appears to distinguish between weak (suppressible) and strong (much less suppressible) H locus differences.

TABLE 1

STRENGTHS OF ANTIGEN IN PRIMARY RESPONSE
TO MOUSE SKIN GRAFTS

Loci Same	Loci Different	Rejection Time
H–1, H–2, H–3 to H–13	—	Indefinite survival
H–2, H–3 to H–13	H–1	+ (20–124 days)
H–2	H–1, H–3 to H–13	++++ (9–11 days)
H–1, H–3 to H–13	H–2	++++ (9–11 days)

Conclusions
 1. H–2 is the most important single difference.
 2. Multiple "non-H–2" differences are important.
 3. Any single "non-H–2" difference is less important.

defined strictly in terms of the first contact between host and graft. All subsequent contacts are influenced by prior sensitization. The recipient is now "armed", so to speak, and promptly marshalls its defences to deal a more resounding

area, each of which is called a genotype. This is reflected in the diversity of antigens determined by the locus throughout the species concerned. Within each strong locus area on the chromosome, the genetic information codes for two strong antigens. A heterozygous individual will thus possess four such antigens. The unravelling of this complexity has depended entirely on careful serology. As mentioned earlier, graft rejection is accompanied by the appearance of anti-graft antibodies in the recipient's serum. These antibodies reflect strong locus differences (fig. 1). Thus, if A rejects B, and produces A anti-B antibodies, which are found to react with cells of a third individual C, then the simple conclusion is that B and C share an antigenic factor lacked by A.

The reality is unfortunately more complicated, but antibody absorption studies, massive computer analysis, and co-operation between worldwide groups of serologists in the last decade has enabled big strides to be made. Since the genes determine the antigens, which in turn provoke antibodies upon transplantation, the latter serve as identifying markers for genetic similarity or identity. It is important to distinguish between this apparent and real identity. An

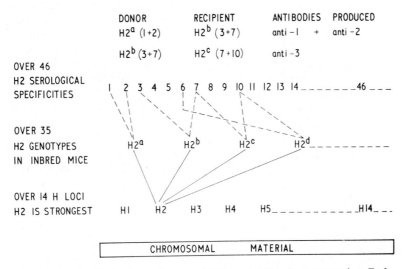

FIG. 1. A simplified view of mouse histocompatibility immunogenetics. Each genotype determines 2 antigens. This is because strains are inbred to homozygosity. A hybrid will possess 4 antigens and thereby resemble an outbred animal. These antigens are selected from a total, so far discovered, of 46.

blow. Thus, what were recognized *ab initio* as weak rejections due to weak differences, will be dealt with as if they were strong upon re-presentation. This argument is considered in some detail here because it is important in understanding the role of blood group ABO antigens in human transplantation. ABO differences would be of much less importance in transplantation than the strong locus HL–A antigens were it not for the fact that all adult humans have already been sensitized, due to environmental or dietary exposure to similar (cross-reacting) microbial antigens. To transplant across an AB or O barrier therefore presents antigens, albeit weak, to a presensitized host.

There are other notable features of strong locus systems. Firstly, they are extremely polymorphic: that is, there are many alternative forms (alleles) of the one chromosomal

antibody may fail to make a distinction between two closely similar antigens, thereby obscuring a real difference under a cloud of cross reaction. Only in families is real identity unequivocal, because of genetic inheritance. Bearing this in mind, it is nevertheless possible, by using antibodies, to tissue type many of the world's major populations for HL–A antigens and thereby establish the antigenic and infer the genetic similarity between individuals.

By selecting donor-recipient pairs with a close serological relationship, it is possible to keep immunity to other histoincompatibilities at bay with immunosuppressive therapy. The greatest surgical experience has been with renal grafting. The situation within families is clear. Figure 2 illustrates a typical HL–A inheritance pattern in a family. Children 1 and 5 inherit the same chromosomes by which the HL–A antigens are determined; children 1 and 2 have one HL–A chromosome in common, as do 1 and 3, 2 and 4, 3 and 4; children 1 and 4, 2 and 3 share no HL–A antigens. The pair of HL–A antigens determined by a single chromosome are called a **haplotype**, and individuals in a family who share a **haplotype** are said to be **haplo-identical**, such as children 1 and 3. By the same token, those who inherit the same chromosomes (1 and 5) are said to be HL–A

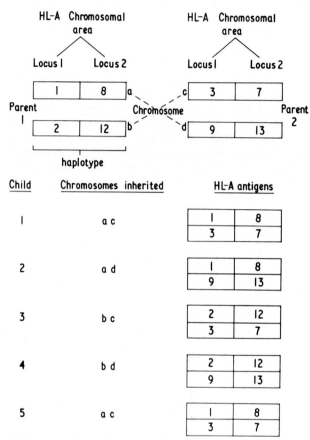

Children 1 and 5 are HL–A identical siblings

FIG. 2. HL–A antigen inheritance in a family.

identical and those who share no HL–A antigens are **non-identical**. Renal grafting and skin grafting have shown unequivocally that HL–A identical siblings enjoy superior graft survival over the other combinations possible within the family (*e.g.* parents must be haplo-identical with all children), while grafts between HL–A non-identical pairs fare worst of all. Without doubt, this constitutes the most important piece of evidence that it is HL–A matching, and thereby selection for HL–A antigen identity or not, which is the crucial factor in graft survival in man. In inbred lines of mice, where several genetic markers have been mapped, and where strains exist with defined H–2 and non-H–2 differences, all available evidence would have predicted this result.

When dealing with survival data of transplant recipients and unrelated donors, the picture is less clear. It is possible

to place donors into five groups, *viz.* those who are serologically identical with, or have one, two, three, or four serological mismatches with their recipient. There is no argument about the difference in survival rates between recipient-donor pairs who type as HL–A identical, and those who have three or four mismatches. The former group clearly shows superior graft survival compared with the latter. The intermediate groups, however, show no clear pattern and the data must be viewed as ambiguous at present. There are several parameters which probably affect the results, but whose weighting is difficult to assess. These include: (a) quality of clinical management and particularly of the immunosuppressive therapy involved; (b) the prior sensitization of the patient via blood transfusion, either to graft HL–A antigens, antigens which cross-react with HL–A antigens, or to non-HL–A antigens (such as the ABO antigens mentioned earlier); (c) non-identity concealed as apparent identity because of serological cross reaction. All of these possibilities serve to explain why some patients predicted to do well, in practice do not. Rather more difficult to account for are those patients who are clearly neither related nor serologically HL–A identical yet continue to have good and prolonged renal function (over a decade in some cases). Recently, however, a possible explanation has been forthcoming which is important not only in transplantation immunology, but which also forms a corner-stone in basic immunological theories.

Work initially carried out with inbred lines of guinea-pigs, and subsequently expanded with mice, has established that different strains have entirely different abilities to respond to the same antigen. This ability is genetically determined and these loci have been called Ir loci (Immune response genes). Where mapping studies have been possible, the interesting fact emerges that in several cases these Ir loci are situated within the H–2 locus of mice, and the analogous locus in guinea-pigs. Furthermore, it is also known that this ability to respond can also apply to a transplantation antigen. Therefore, in addition to being of different strong locus genotypes, in mice, guinea-pigs, and by analogy in man, in order to mount a rejection, it is necessary also for there to be differences at the Ir locus controlling the response to strong histocompatibility antigens.

Work in man is more difficult because of the impossibility of conducting critical experiments. However, it is believed that the blastogenic reaction invariably observed when lymphocytes from unrelated individuals are cultured together (MLC reaction: **Mixed Lymphocyte Culture**) is concerned with the initiation or "recognition" phases of an immune response and may therefore reflect an Ir difference. Lymphocytes from HL–A identical siblings do not stimulate one another in the overwhelming majority of cases. Provided the hypothesis is correct that the MLC reaction really does represent an *in vitro* immune recognition, then the failure to stimulate found with HL–A identical siblings constitutes very strong evidence that the HL–A locus and the Ir genes to HL–A antigens themselves are strongly associated. Genetic "back-cross" experiments in mice have clearly demonstrated that H–2 and the MLC loci are linked.

Recently, a number of human "crossover"* families have been discovered in which HL–A identical siblings stimulate one another in the MLC reaction. In the same families siblings are found who type as unequivocally HL–A different, yet they fail to stimulate in the MLC reaction. The inference is, of course, that in the former case the HL–A identical children inherited different Ir genes, while in the latter situation the HL–A non-identical children inherited the same Ir genes controlling the immune response to HL–A. Now, if we assume that this Ir locus is highly polymorphic within the species, then most randomly selected donor-recipient pairs will be different at Ir anyway, and therefore the requirement for very careful HL–A matching is emphasized. The assumption is probably justified because of the almost invariable MLC reaction which occurs between unrelated humans. Nevertheless, a proper understanding of immune response genes is a fundamental part of modern immunology in general. Appreciation of transplantation immunogenetics also requires familiarity with Ir genes to strong histocompatibility antigens, and the MLC reaction.

It will be evident from the foregoing section that identity at the Ir locus to HL–A antigens is unlikely to account for every long survival noted in mis-matched cadaveric transplants. However, a possible further explanation lies in the phenomenon of **immunological enhancement**, which will be discussed at length later in this chapter.

CURRENT METHODS FOR TESTING HISTOCOMPATIBILITY

There are two phenomena which may be exploited to establish identity or difference between two individuals at their strong histocompatibility locus. The phenomena are: (1) the MLC reaction; and (2) serological typing: both have their champions and respective drawbacks and advantages. During the MLC blastogenic reaction there is mutual stimulation of both kinds of lymphocytes (from two people) which results in the turnover of DNA within the cells, and concomitant uptake of nuclear precursors (*e.g.* nuclides such as ^{3}H-thymidine). Thus, a culture of mixed lymphocytes takes up much more nuclide than the sum of the uptakes of either type of lymphocyte cultured separately. If the turnover of one lymphocyte type is prevented or arrested by its previous incubation with a DNA inactivator (*e.g.*, mitomycin C), its contribution to subsequent mixed culture uptake of ^{3}H-thymidine is negligible. Under these circumstances, referred to as "one-way" MLC, the stimulation of either type of lymphocyte by the other can be measured. As has been mentioned, however, the almost invariable

finding in MLC reactions is stimulation between unrelated individuals. There appears to be no simple way, either, of relating the degree of stimulation, *e.g.* nuclide uptake per cell or per culture, to the degree of histocompatibility difference. With the few exceptions mentioned, of "cross-over" families, lack of stimulation between lymphocytes of siblings is, nevertheless, almost irrefutable evidence of strong locus (HL–A) identity. The principal practical drawback to MLC reactions is that they usually take 4–6 days to complete. In any event, simple serological assays with only a few sera are enough to establish HL–A inheritance patterns in families. In renal transplantation within families there is no immediate urgency for surgery. The serological analyses are supplemented by MLC reactions to confirm that an HL–A identical sibship pertains between donor and recipient (the MLC reaction should be negative). In cases where cadaveric organs are used, speed is necessary to establish which of several possible recipients* has closest HL–A similarity to the donor. Serological assays offer the required simplicity and rapidity and are invariably used. Their interpretation is not always easy and the reasons for this have already been discussed.

A. Leukoagglutination Techniques

The principle here is that leukoagglutinins will agglutinate leukocytes (granulocytes and lymphocytes) when they possess the corresponding antigen. All methods presently used in tissue typing recognize that antisera are in short supply. Apart from deliberately immunized volunteers (a euphemism for one's laboratory colleagues and assistants), the principal source of typing sera is multiparous women. Pregnancy is of course the only natural circumstance in which a human is in contact with foreign tissue of the same species under conditions which could provoke an immunity. The use of small volumes of reagents (0·001 ml.) requires the analyst to overcome evaporative losses, which would result in destructive conditions during the test when solutions became hypertonic. Reactions are therefore conducted under oil. Buffy coat leukocytes are prepared, mixed with antiserum, and microscopically examined for agglutination after a suitable incubation period. The leukocyte agglutination technique has now been largely superseded because of high numbers of false positive or negative reactions. It also suffers from the additional drawback that it it not quantifiable.

B. Lymphocytotoxicity Tests

The principle is that when lymphocytes are incubated with cytotoxic antibodies in the presence of complement, lysis ensues when the target cells possess the corresponding antigen. Peripheral lymphocytes are simply prepared in highly purified suspension from defibrinated or heparinized

---

* When two loci are known to be carried on the same chromosome they are said to be linked. The closer the loci are together, the closer the linkage. Two alleles whose loci are closely linked may travel together through many generations without being separated. However, alleles at loci linked but sited at some distance from each other will often be separated by crossing-over, which happens at the first meiotic division of gametogenesis. The effect is as if the homologous chromatids broke symmetrically and rejoined crosswise. The chance of crossing-over happening between two linked loci is greater the further apart they are, so the frequency of cross-over offspring can be used as a measure of the distance separating the loci. The cross-over frequency of the two HL–A loci in man is about 1 per cent.

* Logistics demand that pools of recipients be typed, and then, when a cadaveric graft becomes available, it is used in the patient with whom it most closely matches. Obviously, the larger the recipient pool, the more likely that a compatible situation will be revealed. Several co-operative organ-sharing schemes exist in Great Britain, France, Holland, Scandinavia, and other countries, where typing information is held in a central computer mass memory.

blood, by density centrifugation. Rabbit complement is the most efficient for lysing human lymphocytes. The proportion of damage in a cell population is easily measured by vital staining and microscopic examination. This is the most common technique used for tissue-typing today. It is possible to complete a typing assay within 2 hr. of receiving the blood sample, and there is high reproducibility between different observers. Lymphocytes can be stored indefinitely in liquid nitrogen at −196°C, and shipped between laboratories, which has facilitated collaboration and validation of results.

C. Complement Fixation Tests

The principal involved is analogous to that generally involved in complement fixation. A test system is used in which rabbit antibody causes lysis of sheep erythrocytes in the presence of a limited amount of complement. Any agent which, when added to the test system, "fixes", *i.e.* utilizes, some complement, will leave less to cause lysis in the test system. Therefore, if HL–A antibodies combine with their respective antigen on, say, platelets, or lymphocytes, the combination fixes complement, and upon adding the test system of rabbit antibody and sheep cells, reduced haemolysis is observed. This system is quantifiable, and does not necessarily require lymphocytes from the human individual under examination. Platelets, which are easier to prepare and store, are equally good. Not all HL–A antibodies fix complement with equal efficiency, and most typing groups rely somewhat more heavily on lymphocytotoxicity as their prime assay for HL–A antigens. Nevertheless, fixation by platelets forms a valuable adjunct to the other test methods. Leukoagglutination and complement fixation currently enjoy less favour than lymphocytotoxicity for tissue typing.

When the gene frequencies of the various HL–A antigens detected are added together, the sum comes very close to 1 for many ethnic groups. (The theoretical sum for a truly allelic system must of course be 1, provided there is no "null" allele). The separation of the HL–A chromosomal region into 2 distinct areas, and the established inheritance patterns of haplotypes, taken together with the overwhelming occurrence of a maximum of 4 HL–A antigens in heterozygous individuals, give one confidence in the correctness of present views of the HL–A system. Purported "third" HL–A loci, the interpretations of cross-reactive groups of antigens, and problems in going from one ethnic group to another where not exactly the same antigens seem to be recognized, excite the curiosity of all scientists in this field. Their clarification is unlikely to shatter the principles on which current understanding is based.

MICROSCOPIC AND CELLULAR EVENTS IN HOMOGRAFT REJECTION

The mechanisms of immune recognition and effector systems have been covered in Chapters 9 and 10. There is now an impressive body of evidence which suggests strongly that homograft sensitivity is closely related to delayed hypersensitivity phenomena. Similar cellular reactions are seen in the thymus-dependent areas of regional lymph nodes, and both types of response are ablated by neonatal thymectomy. There is a similar activation of lymphocytes to pyroninophilic lymphoblasts which divide to produce a population of effector cells capable of transferring the sensitive state to other normal (unsensitized) animals of identical genetic makeup. That homograft rejection resembles delayed hypersensitivity is convincingly demonstrated by the fact that when a sensitized (skin-grafted) guinea-pig receives an intradermal injection of living donor cells, it responds with a delayed inflammatory rejection. Furthermore, lymphoid cells from the specifically sensitized recipient produce an identical reaction following intradermal injection into the donor.

Histology and Physiology

An autograft of whole-thickness mouse skin heals into position within 12 days. At this time the new epidermis forms a continuous covering over the underlying dermis and new hair follicles are well advanced in development. Vessels are normal and so is the cell population when compared to normal skin. During primary graft rejection, there is an initial period, about 2 days, which is identical to the autograft case, where polymorphonuclear neutrophils infiltrate the graft bed. However, between the 3rd and 9th day, there occurs an increasing infiltration of monocytes and lymphocytes. This begins around the vessels in the graft base dermis, and then extends through the dermis and into the epidermis. Mature plasma cells are not frequently seen, although some usually appear after about 7 days. Histologically recognizable necrosis begins about day 7–8, and is macroscopically visible within a further 2 days. Even before this, intracellular oedema of epidermal cells is observed.

During rejection of skin by a previously sensitized animal, the graft does not become truly vascularized. The cellular infiltration of the graft itself may therefore not occur. However, a massive accumulation of cells is seen along the line of the graft dermis but in the host tissues. Histiocytes and immature plasma cells feature prominently.

The example of skin has been cited because it is the usual tissue used in experimental transplantation. There is much evidence to suggest that the same, or closely similar principles and processes are used by a host to destroy other foreign grafts. Two factors should be borne in mind, however, which may modify this situation. Both are to some extent concerned with the two arcs of the immune response. The afferent arc is the means by which a graft succeeds in sensitizing its recipients, *i.e.* the liaison which is arranged between immunologically competent cells and graft histocompatibility antigens. Skin rapidly acquires a vasculature, and it is known that when flaps of host skin are constructed which are devoid of lymphatic connections, homograft skin placed within such flaps is not rejected. Kidney transplants of course have their vasculature immediately. Therefore, the speed with which the afferent arc is established, if at all, can play an important role in the kinetics of rejection. This will be referred to again later when considering "privileged" sites, which are important in certain kinds of grafts, *e.g.* cornea. The efferent arc is the means by which host mechanisms actually destroy the graft. Again mechanical access is clearly necessary, and it is known that homografts are destroyed by a cellular rather than humoral mechanism. "Killer" cells, as they have come to be known, can be obtained from spleen, lymph nodes, peripheral blood or thoracic duct drainage. When an animal is sensitized by a graft, and the potential of its killer cells is examined, they appear to be fully armed, so to speak, within 4–5 days. At this time killer lymphocytes will cluster around cells of the graft donor if grown *in vitro*, and effect destruction within 20 hr. of contact.

The role of functionally different kinds of lymphocytes (B cells of bone-marrow origin, and T cells of thymic origin, lineage, or processing), of macrophages, and of immune alloantiserum or its complexes with antigen is crucial to a sophisticated understanding of the whole mechanism of graft sensitization and ultimate demise. However, this is not the place to discuss them in detail, and in any event this is an area of intensive present study and consequently a graveyard of hypotheses.

The classical small lymphocyte, nevertheless, has been shown to possess all the properties necessary for the primary effector cell in homograft rejection. Subversion of this function is the major aim of the clinical transplanter and will be considered later.

THE CHEMICAL NATURE OF TRANSPLANTATION ANTIGENS

To determine the nature of transplantation antigens, it is obviously necessary to have a means of measuring them and thereafter to exploit the assay in order to purify the responsible substances. The whole cell may be considered as the raw material, and upon its rupture various fragments may be examined to discover which possesses the relevant activity.

Biological assays aim at inducing a specific state of immunity in a test animal. That animal is then grafted and the fate of the graft indicates, by its speed of rejection, the immune status of the host. That fraction which contains the transplantation antigens is the one capable of inducing specific sensitivity. Such assays are exquisitely sensitive and clinically relevant, but lack the requirement of speed and quantitation.

Serological assays are based on the principle that the transplantation antigen will combine with its antibody. This combination leaves less antibody to bind to a test cell which is subsequently added. If lymphocyte lysis is the end result of such an assay, then reduced lysis is seen when specific antigen has been added. The system is illustrated in fig. 3.

It is important to realize that while biological assays directly measure the transplantation antigen, serological assays quantify the epitope (immunochemical determinant) region of the antigen molecule. However, the latter are

speedy and precise: they are also sensitive and specific and have been employed most frequently in following the purification of antigen. There is little argument today that the transplantation antigens are glycoproteins which, when released from cell surfaces by proteolysis, have molecular weight about 45,000. Their native form on the cell may be somewhat larger. The study of the detailed structure is currently under intensive investigation in several laboratories. The question of whether antibody binding specificity resides exclusively in the amino-acid sequence remains unproven, although its exclusive residence in the carbohydrate moiety seems to be ruled out. Some compromise

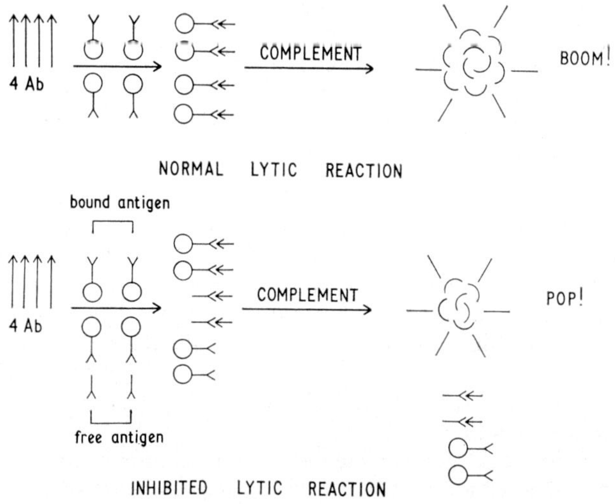

FIG. 3. Principle of the inhibition assay. Reduced lysis is obtained when free (usually soluble) antigen is added to antibody plus the test cell bearing the same antigen. A specificity control to establish that free antigen does not inhibit the action of an indifferent antibody is essential.

involving those amino acids in the neighbourhood of the large carbohydrate moiety may prove to be the crucial portion of the molecule.

Metabolic studies have shown that a living cell has a remarkable synthetic apparatus for manufacturing its transplantation antigens. Lymphocytes, which have the heaviest density of these particular markers, can re-express them completely within 6 hr. following their total removal by proteolysis.

METHODS OF SECURING PROLONGED SURVIVAL OF GRAFTS

The first agents to be discussed are those which were initially developed for their anti-mitotic activities in inhibiting neoplastic growth. Many of their unwanted side-effects depend on their ability to inhibit cell regeneration in the bone marrow and gut epithelium as well as in wound healing. Since the provocation of an immune response involves cellular proliferation, these agents are of value, but it is also necessary to consider their effect on immunogenicity, immunological memory, and cellular versus humoral immunity.

X-ray Irradiation

Immunological changes are summarized as follows:

(a) Primary response is severely depressed or abolished for a prolonged period (up to 50 days in rodents) after irradiation. Antibody production is more drastically affected than delayed hypersensitivity, and the most marked effect is seen when antigen is given shortly (24–28 hr.) after irradiation;

(b) X-rays have little effect if given when the immune response has been mounted (3–4 days after immunization);

(c) augmented levels of antibody are produced if sensitization precedes irradiation by up to 3 days;

(d) the secondary response to an antigen is much less radiation-sensitive than the primary; and

(e) if irradiation is closely followed (1 day) by large amounts of protein antigen, a long-lasting and specific unresponsiveness is obtained.

The above results are obtained when an animal is given sublethal doses (300–600 r.) of whole body X-rays. The cellular changes which are seen include massive distintegration of lymphocytes followed by the clearance of debris by phagocytosis. Lymphoid tissue then regenerates to completion within some weeks. Other lymphoid elements such as macrophages or Hassall's corpuscles appear to be radiation-resistant at these X-ray levels, as are mature and immature plasma cells.

Supralethal doses of irradiation can of course be followed by transplantation of stem cells in haemopoietic tissue, and where this is genetically identical, can result in complete restoration of immune responsiveness. When the transplant is not genetically identical with its host, a chimera results, because the recipient is unable to reject the graft. Immunologically competent cells in the graft are, however, able to react against the host, and radiation chimeras are usually permanently impaired in immune competence if they survive at all for a long time. It is this recovery of competence when the radiation dose is sublethal, resulting in graft destruction, and the inadequacy of radiation chimeras when the dose is supralethal that makes X-rays a poor candidate for human immunosuppressive therapy.

Antimetabolites

The action of several of the drugs used in immunosuppression is to inhibit synthesis or expression of nucleic acids. Nuclear turnover is an obvious requirement for cellular proliferation and there are various points in the biosynthetic chain where an antimetabolite can interfere. The unpleasant side-effects of these agents are all too well known to clinicians. Like X-rays, it is the non-specific nature of their effect on cell metabolism which is the drawback. Despite this criticism, they are currently of great value in assisting the acceptance of grafted tissue in foreign hosts, and sophisticated regimens of therapy are one of the most powerful weapons in the armoury of the transplanter. Likewise, the use of corticosteroids to suppress the inflammatory response is widely and usefully exploited in promoting graft acceptance: any discussion of their mechanisms of action is beyond the scope of this chapter, except to note in passing that lymphocyte levels are known to be reduced under corticosteroid action.

Antilymphocyte Serum (ALS)

ALS has been extensively investigated and exploited. It is produced by immunizing an animal of a different species with lymphocytes from the species under investigation. A short course of immunization seems to be preferable, as longer schedules do not necessarily produce a more effective reagent. Although antibodies may be produced against cells other than lymphocytes in the injected material (*e.g.* erythrocytes), these are easily removed by absorption of the resultant serum. Lymphocyte (or thymocyte) membranes serve equally well to produce a potent ALS and it is believed therefore that the action is principally against lymphocyte surface antigens. ALS, in moderate doses, prolongs graft survival, even xenografts, significantly. It abolishes tuberculin reactions or skin reactions in previously sensitized animals, and seems in general to be directed against cell-mediated or delayed-type hypersensitivity reactions. Although more dramatic against a primary homograft response, it also exerts a significant effect in a previously sensitized animal. Such a recipient, when treated with ALS and then regrafted, behaves as if the second transplant were to a previously unsensitized host. Histological examination of treated animals reveals that the lymphoid tissue most affected is in the "thymus-dependent" areas of nodes. There is transient but marked depletion in the population of peripheral circulating lymphocytes. Cortical areas of lymph nodes, the Malpighian bodies of the spleen and germinal centres are not particularly impaired. Of the two different kinds of lymphocyte (T and B) which currently occupy the centre of the immunological stage, it is T cells which appear to be affected by ALS. Antigens appear presently to be rather broadly separable into two classes: T cell-dependent and T cell-independent. Transplantation antigens fall in the former category. Co-operation between a T cell and a B cell is necessary for a T cell-dependent antigen to initiate antibody production. Other antigens may be able to interact directly with B cells. In addition, a T cell, having reacted with an antigen, may also divide to produce direct killer cells, or go on to produce memory cells. In any event, if ALS acts principally on T cells, antibody production to T cell-independent antigens may not be affected. This is in fact what is found, *i.e.* antibody production is much less affected by moderate doses of ALS than are the delayed-type hypersensitivity responses mentioned previously. In fact, even when a homograft is accepted under an ALS cover, antibodies against the graft are sometimes detectable. The precise meaning of this finding is not clear unless it has something to do with recovery of a particular portion of the immune apparatus against H antigens.

ALS, then, has the capability of dissecting cellular from humoral immunity and this feature has been exploited in the use of this agent in human renal transplantation. Its significant, and somewhat sinister, association with an increased incidence of certain kinds of tumour in survivors under the treatment requires critical examination, however. This may result from its non-specific ablation or reduction of all cellular immune effects, including those which combat neoplasms.

Enhancement

It is by no means impossible that antibody could play a role in accelerating the rejection of a solid tissue homograft. Indeed, xenografts (*e.g.* rat skin on a mouse) accepted under ALS therapy, are dramatically rejected within hours when mouse anti-rat serum is administered within some days of graft establishment. Furthermore, recipients of human renal grafts who are ascertained to be presensitized against graft antigens by detection of donor-specific antibodies (a cross match) often reject the graft within an hour or two of its transplantation; too fast, in fact, for the phenomenon to be readily attributable to a marshalling of cellular forces.

Nevertheless, one of the most significant properties of H antibodies is their capacity to facilitate homograft persistence when they are passively administered shortly before or after grafting. This is the phenomenon known as **immunological enhancement**. It was discovered in relation to the transplantation of tumours. Many tumours are known which grow specifically only in the respective mouse strain in which they arose. They possess the full or at least the majority of H antigens of their "home" strain, and consequently are rejected promptly by genetically different inbred mice. Let us say a tumour specific for A strain mice is transplanted into strain C. It will be rejected. If, however, transfer is accompanied by the injection of antiserum prepared in other C animals against A tissue, then the tumour persists, grows, and eventually kills its host. This is at first sight a most puzzling observation, because it suggests that antibody prepared against a graft and used passively in an animal not previously sensitized, far from promoting graft destruction, actually confers protection against the host's cellular defences. The same phenomenon can be shown to apply for normal tissue, such as skin (under special circumstances where the H difference is minimal) and is particularly well documented for renal grafts in rodents.

What is so attractive about graft prolongation using enhancing antisera is the specificity of the phenomenon. Only tissue which interacts with antiserum enjoys promotion. The animal's other immune functions are in no way impaired so that, for example, the antibiotic therapy necessary to combat pathogenic microorganisms encouraged under other immunosuppressive treatments, is completely unnecessary. The mechanism by which enhancement operates has not yet been fully elucidated. It is clear, however, that a simple "masking" of graft antigens so as to conceal them from recognition by host cells which initiate cellular immunity is not the answer. Enhanced grafts have been shown to absorb further administered specific antibodies long after the promoting dose has fallen below a detectable level. Grafts established with enhancing antisera ultimately provoke antibodies having the same specificity in their host—a sort of autoenhancement. This is reminiscent of the situation existing with ALS, and confers the further advantage

that once established with an initial injection of enhancing antibody, a graft can induce conditions which engender its indefinite survival. Current hypotheses favour a mechanism by which specific antigen-antibody complexes, possibly shed from the graft, abrogate only T-cell killer induction in the host. Enhancement provides a most promising avenue of exploration towards the goal of specific graft acceptance. It may also provide the explanation for the long survival of some renal grafts which are known to be serological mismatches (chance Ir gene identity between host and graft has already been discussed as an alternative). Immunosuppressive therapy may permit the initial graft acceptance; then, a partial recovery of the host's immune process could elicit antibodies which promote prolonged acceptance by autoenhancement.

Tolerance

Neonatally induced specific unresponsiveness has been known for many years. As long ago as 1953 it was shown that mice exposed *in utero* to allogenic cells would fail to recognize those same cells throughout their subsequent life. That is to say, foreign cells would be recognized as "self" because of the host's embryonic exposure to them. The principal other method by which specific tolerance can be induced by antigen alone in the absence of chemical or serological agents is by administration of very large or very small doses of soluble antigen. These are the areas of so-called "high zone" or "low zone" tolerance and have been convincingly demonstrated only for protein antigens and not for transplantation antigens. There is considerable dissent about the exact meaning of the words "true tolerance" and as to whether the expression should be reserved for induced indefinite inability to respond to an antigen. Graft prolongation may be a different matter. It is not easy to summarize opinions at this stage, nor to go further than state that specific antigen-antibody complexes have been alleged (and denied) to be responsible for all states of specific unresponsiveness to transplantation antigens.

IMMUNOLOGICALLY PRIVILEGED SITES

In Animals

Tissues, including xenografts, soon establish a blood supply and survive over long periods when transplanted into the cheek pouch of the Syrian hamster. If the recipient has previously been or is subsequently deliberately sensitized (*e.g.* by a skin graft), then the cheek pouch graft is rapidly destroyed. The explanation seems to be that, while the efferent arc of this animal is perfectly normal, an afferent arc is not established from that particular site, which is termed "privileged".

In Humans

Other sites in different animals, *e.g.* the brain and anterior chamber of the eye, enjoy a similar status. A major part of the explanation of this is the failure to establish lymphatic drainage from the site. In the case of full thickness corneal grafts the transplanted tissue is nourished by diffusion through epithelium and endothelium. There is usually also a failure to establish an effective efferent arc, so that such grafts remain isolated from immunologically competent, and sensitized, cells. The small size of the corneal graft itself is important, in that antigenic stimulus is minimal. When corneas are, or become, well vascularized following transplantation, the situation is different and rejection (clouding) is common. Preliminary evidence has been obtained which suggests, perhaps predictably, that under these circumstances where vasculature is established, matching for HL–A antigens is a prime consideration, with close matches faring better than multiple mis-matches.

There is also some reason to believe that cartilage, like cornea, being an avascular tissue, enjoys privilege because it is segregated from contact with its host's immune apparatus. Grafts may be made with living tissue, yet they persist readily between unrelated individuals. The milieu of sulphated mucopolysaccharide (which is itself non-immunogenic) in which the chondroblasts are embedded may also be an important factor in survival.

In Pregnancy

The fetus as a homograft deserves special consideration. It is the one natural circumstance under which mammals are confronted with foreign tissue. The fetus and fetal membranes contain transplantation antigens because they can be used to induce an accelerated rejection of a subsequent transplant of paternal skin. In addition, serum from multiparous females is a major source of typing antibodies. However, only about a fifth of such women have detectable levels of these serum antibodies. Pregnancy may induce in the female a reduction in her immunological responsiveness towards the specific paternally derived alloantigens of her offspring. Enhancement may also play a part. Whether only those women who show antibodies have been sensitized, and the remainder not, or whether all are sensitized but only some to a detectable level, is not clear. The question exists as to whether the "killer" cell response is switched off or never even stimulated and if so by what means this is achieved. It is clear that the immune response can be initiated (the afferent arc) but that the efferent arc is ineffectual. This being so, the maternal uterus may be considered to be a privileged site. Distinction must be made between this form of privilege and the one previously discussed, when a failure to establish the afferent arc is responsible. So far there is no evidence to suggest that deliberate presensitization of the mother to paternal H antigens has any influence on the successful outcome of subsequent pregnancies.

Homostatic Grafts

Bone and blood-vessel transplants, as presently constituted, must serve a purely mechanical function, if only because they are frequently boiled, lyophilized or formaldehyde treated before use, which precludes any living cells being transferred. As such they should be considered as homostatic grafts, providing a framework into which host cells can grow. The principles of transplantation heretofore considered apply to homovital grafts wherein cells must remain alive if the tissue is to function. Although full thickness corneal grafts are homovital, lamellar grafts of cornea may be considered homostatic. In the full thickness case, leakage of aqueous humour must be prevented which requires a functioning endothelium.

TOOTH TRANSPLANTATION

It would be singularly inappropriate if a chapter in this particular book were to ignore tooth transplantation. This aspect is best separated into two distinct areas, whole developed teeth, and tooth germs.

Transplantation of a developed tooth involves severance of all vascular and nervous connections. It is well known both in experimental animals and in man, that teeth which have been removed and immediately reinserted in the same, or even in different sockets, can become firmly re-attached by regeneration of the periodontal membrane. Although part of the tooth (enamel and possibly dentine) may be regarded as homostatic, the pulp clearly cannot. Allotransplantation of developed teeth would therefore presumably fail because of rejection mechanisms which would operate against pulp structures. As will be explained later, teeth unequivocally contain cells which bear H antigens and there is no reason to believe that the socket is a privileged site. As with corneal grafting, however, perhaps an era lies ahead when success in developed tooth transplantation will be shown to depend on the degree of matching at the strong H locus. An additional, but major factor, is to determine why autotransplants of developed teeth so often fail. The principal difficulty seems to be that of root resorption. When the transplant is heterotopic, parameters such as tooth and socket size also warrant consideration. Careful attention to extraction and socket preparation, particularly with regard to the condition of the periodontal membrane, is generally thought to be essential. Considerations such as storage of typed teeth in a bank are obviously impractical at present, especially at a time when proper dental hygiene and prostheses offer so much simpler a solution.

Autotransplantation of tooth germs is another matter, because prior to eruption the nutrition is provided by an abundant network of capillaries. Considerable success has been reported with autotransplantation of the third molar tooth germ in cases of loss, or threatened loss, of the first permanent molar in teenage patients. Satisfactory eruption and occlusion is claimed.

In mice, it has been shown that heterotopic transplantation of tooth germs across the strong H-2 barrier, or a cumulation of several weaker H loci, resulted in a relatively strong rejection. The grafts were heavily infiltrated with mononuclear cells and their further development was either completely arrested, or seriously distorted. Transplantation across a single weak H barrier behaved identically with a syngeneic graft, in that there was no evidence of immune allograft rejection. It must always be borne in mind, of course, that rodent incisor teeth have pulps with open apices, which allow continuous eruption, as opposed to the human situation. Deliberate sensitization with allogeneic heterotopic tooth germ grafts was moderately successful, subsequent skin grafts showing accelerated rejection, which is good evidence for tooth germs bearing their expected complement of H antigens.

There would seem to be a good case for the establishment of a proper model system in which autotransplantation of developed teeth can be accomplished without a high incidence of resorption. Allogeneic transplantation between siblings differing or not at the strong histocompatibility locus would then reveal any immunological impact on the transfer. Teeth may predictably turn out to be subject to the same transplantation principles as other tissues. Once this is adequately determined, practical implications would obviously deserve serious consideration.

GLOSSARY

Allele: Alternative characteristic, due to alternative genes acting at the same locus on the chromosome.

Alloantibody: An antibody which reacts with an alloantigen. Synonymous with **isoantibody**.

Alloantigen: A constituent of one animal which can elicit specific sensitization in another, but genetically different, member of the same species. Synonymous with **isoantigen**.

Allogeneic: Of different genetic constitution. Now usually taken to be within the species; when outside the species the term **xenogeneic** is used.

Allograft: Synonymous with **homograft**.

Autograft: Graft derived from one animal to another site or the same site on the same animal.

Epitope: Specific antigenic determinant site or area on a molecule; the remainder of the molecule is called the **paratope**.

F–1 hybrid: The first generation offspring of a mating between members of two inbred strains. **F–2** generations result from mating F–1 hybrids. **Back-crosses** are derived from mating F–1 hybrids back with parents.

Haplotype: In HL–A immunogenetics, one chromosomal area determines two serologically detectable antigens which are known collectively as a haplotype.

Heterotopic: Grafting tissue into a site anatomically different from that of its origin.

Heterozygous: In which both chromosomes carry different alleles at a locus.

Histocompatibility antigens: Material which is genetically determined and occurs on the surface (and possibly other structures) of cells and which is able to immunize another animal of the same species so that subsequent grafts of tissue from the donor are destroyed by a specific immunological mechanism.

Homozygous: In which both chromosomes carry the same allele at a locus.

Homograft: Graft derived from one animal to an animal of the same species, but differing in genetic constitution.

Ir genes: Genes which determine an animal's ability to respond to a particular antigen.

Iso-: Classically (Gk.: *isos*, equal) this prefix should mean derived from animal of the same genetic constitution, hence **isogenic, isograft**. However, its particular use in transplantation terminology is, for example, **isoantigen; isoantibody** (*q.v.*) means something different. To avoid confusion, it is commoner now to avoid **iso-** altogether, and use **allo-** (Gk.: *allos*, other), **syn-** (Gk.: *syn*, alike), and **xeno-** (Gk.: *xenos*, foreign). Similarly, there is confusion with the prefix **homo-** (Gk.: *homos*, same), although it has proved difficult to dislodge **homograft** from common usage in the field.

Orthotopic: Grafts transferred to positions formerly occupied by tissue of the same kind.

Syngeneic: Of the same genetic constitution. Synonymous with **isogenic**.

Xenograft: Graft derived from one animal to another animal of a different species (synonymous with **heterograft**).

FURTHER READING

Albert, F. and Medawar, P. B. (Eds.) (1959), *Biological Problems of Grafting*. Oxford: Blackwell.

Antilymphocytic Serum (1967), Ciba Foundation Study Group No. 29, London: Churchill.

Calne, R. Y. (1967), *Renal Transplantation*, 2nd edition. London: Arnold.

Histocompatibility Testing, 1964, 1965, 1967, 1970, 1972. Copenhagen: Munksgaard.

Humphrey, J. H. and White, R. G. (1970). *Immunology for Students of Medicine*. Oxford: Blackwell.

Woodruff, M. F. A. (1960), *The Transplantation of Tissues and Organs*. Illinois: Springfield.

For a Review of Tooth Transplantation in Man, *see* Natiella, J. R., Armitage, J. E. and Greene, G. W. (1970), *Oral Surg.* **29**, 397.

Original papers in the *Journal of Experimental Medicine, Transplantation, Journal of Immunology, Immunology* and *Tissue Antigens*; review articles in *Advances in Immunology, Transplantation Reviews* and *Progress in Allergy*.

12. THE CONCEPT OF AUTO-IMMUNITY

J. L. TURK

Possible causes
- Failure to eliminate abnormal clones
- Chronic stimulation by non-specific antigens
- Antigenic modification of host cells by micro-organisms
- Cross reaction between antigens of micro-organisms and tissues
- Physical or chemical modification of antigens
- Naturally occurring auto-antibodies

Early immunologists at the turn of the century, following the teaching of Paul Ehrlich, could not conceive that the body could react against components of its own tissues with an immune response. At that time, it was considered that all immunological reactions were potentially damaging and that the production of an auto-immune state would naturally result in the destruction of the target tissue. This concept was described by Ehrlich as "horror autotoxicus". It is now known that under certain circumstances, the body can overcome this horror autotoxicus and develop auto-antibodies or an auto-immune cellular reaction against its own tissues.

Recent interest in auto-immune processes in clinical medicine started between 15 and 20 years ago, with the demonstration of antibodies directed against red cells in idiopathic haemolytic anaemia and against nucleoproteins in systemic lupus erythematosus. This was followed by the demonstration of antibodies against thyroid tissue in Hashimoto's thyroiditis. These observations were enlarged conceptually by Burnet's notion of antibodies directed against "self" in pathological immune responses, as opposed to those directed against "non-self" in normal immune responses. At the same time, a number of auto-immune conditions were being produced in experimental animals which appeared to parallel a number of clinical conditions the aetiology of which had previously been unknown. Auto-immune thyroiditis in rabbits and rats paralleled Hashimoto's thyroiditis. Auto-immune allergic encephalomyelitis had many features in common with multiple sclerosis and other demyelinating diseases. An auto-immune adrenalitis could be produced, mimicking idiopathic Addison's disease, and auto-immune allergic orchitis mimicked aspermatogenesis of unknown aetiology in the human. In addition, the discovery of a strain of mice, the NZB strain, which developed many of the features of systemic lupus erythematosus—haemolytic anaemia, immune complex nephritis and antibodies against nucleoproteins in the circulation—confirmed the concept than an immune reaction against "self" antigens might underlie the pathogenesis of a number of disease states in man.

POSSIBLE CAUSES OF THE DEVELOPMENT OF AN IMMUNE REACTION AGAINST "SELF" ANTIGENS

Two main means have been considered by which the body can be induced to develop antibodies against its own antigens. The first, and one which has been favoured most until recently, has postulated a defect in the antibody producing mechanism: "the failure to eliminate abnormal clones (colonies) of antibody producing cells". Little data have, however, been produced in support of this highly attractive hypothesis. The second hypothesis, for which certain parallels exist in experimental situations, suggests that the body's immunological mechanisms are intact, but are receiving an abnormal antigenic stimulus. These two hypotheses will be discussed separately.

Failure to Eliminate Abnormal Clones

Burnet has postulated that the body is capable of producing a large number of clones of lymphocytes, each of which has the potential of proliferation when in contact with the appropriate antigens. These clones are directed against all possible antigens, both "self" and "non-self". However, the clones directed against "self" antigens are eliminated in late fetal and early neonatal life, before the body has developed its full capacity to produce an immune response. This process of immunological tolerance to "self" antigens would only develop during the period of immunological immaturity and in response to a massive dose of antigen, such as that present in the whole body. If this inborn defensive mechanism against "forbidden" clones directed against "self antigens" were to break down, lymphocytes would proliferate with the ability either to produce cell-mediated immune reactions, or to develop into plasma cells secreting antibodies against the body's own tissues. The result would be a multi-organ auto-immune disease such as systemic lupus erythematosus. It was considered by the protagonists of this hypothesis that the thymus played a key physiological role in deleting "aberrant" or "forbidden" clones of lymphocytes which might develop later in life, possibly by somatic mutation, and react against constituents of the body's own tissues. In support of this concept, abnormalities of the thymus were found in a wide range of "auto-immune diseases". In systemic lupus erythematosus (SLE) and rheumatoid arthritis there is a loss of differentiation between the cortex and the medulla, the presence of germinal centres and an increased number of plasma cells as well as changes in Hassall's corpuscles. Germinal centres, not normally found in the thymus, are seen in patients with thyrotoxicosis and other diseases of the thyroid associated with auto-immune phenomena, as well as in myasthenia gravis. They are also seen in the NZB strain of mice which develop the multi-organ auto-immune disease resembling systemic lupus erythematosus.

It has been suggested that the germinal centres in the thymus in SLE, rheumatoid arthritis, myasthenia gravis and in the auto-immune disease of NZB mice are the actual site of the proliferation of the abnormal or "forbidden" clones. However, the disease in mice still develops even if the thymus is removed at birth and in man thymectomy does not affect the course of SLE and rheumatoid arthritis. Both SLE and thyroiditis with associated auto-immune antibodies have been reported as developing even after the thymus has been removed for myasthenia gravis. The relation between the thymus and auto-immune processes is complex. No real evidence has so far been brought to show either that the function of the thymus is to destroy "forbidden" clones, or that in diseases with associated auto-immune processes "forbidden" clones are allowed to proliferate in the thymus.

Chronic Stimulation by Non-specific Antigens in Infectious Diseases

Evidence has been accumulating over a number of years that auto-antibodies can develop against components of the body's own tissues in a wide range of chronic infectious states. For over 60 years it has been known that antibodies against a non-species-specific antigen present in heart muscle occurs in the serum of patients with syphilis and in a wide range of other infectious diseases including malaria. This antibody is the basis of the Wasserman and similar reactions, and its presence in diseases other than syphilis is referred to as a "biological false positive reaction". Rheumatoid factor, an antibody directed against antigens on the immunoglobulin molecule, is also present in the sera of 10 per cent of patients with syphilis. Cryoglobulins, which indicate the presence of immune complexes formed between immunoglobulins and anti-immunoglobulin molecules in the circulation, also occur in 15 per cent of patients with this disease.

Auto-antibodies to a wide range of antigens have been described in leprosy. These include anti-immunoglobulin factors such as the rheumatoid factor and the presence of cryoglobulinaemia, anti-nuclear factors, anti-thyroglobulin antibodies and antibodies which react with the antigens used in the Wasserman and similar tests associated with the diagnosis of syphilis. These occur in 30–50 per cent of patients with lepromatous leprosy and in 3–10 per cent of patients with tuberculoid leprosy. Three patients with lepromatous leprosy have also been described with the LE cell phenomenon typical of systemic lupus erythematosus. A high incidence of rheumatoid factor has been described in the serum of patients with kala-azar and also in subacute bacterial endocarditis, and 27 per cent of patients infected with *Schistosoma haematobium* have auto-antibodies against liver or lung, or both, in the serum. The presence of auto-antibodies against lung and other tissues has been described in the serum of patients with chronic pulmonary tuberculosis. Similar auto-antibodies can be found to develop in rabbits within 12 weeks of infection with *Mycobacterium tuberculosis* or *Pasteurella pseudotuberculosis*. An increase in titres of similar auto-antibodies occurs in rabbits as a result of infection with the protozoon *Eimeria stiedae*, the agent which causes coccidiosis. The association of virus infection with development of auto-immune processes comes mainly from studies in experimental animals. Virus-like particles have been demonstrated by electron microscopy in the tissues of mice of the NZB strain which develop many of the auto-immune phenomena found in systemic lupus erythematosus in man.

Antigenic Modification of Host Cells by Micro-organisms

The possibility has been considered that micro-organisms, especially viruses, can modify the antigenic nature of host cells, so that they fail to be recognized as "self" and an immune reaction is mounted against the tissue, as though it contained foreign antigen. Influenza virus and mumps virus possess an enzyme, neuraminidase, which is capable of modifying cells antigenically. Similar enzymes are carried by bacteria such as *Clostridium welchii* and *Vibrio cholerae*. Neuraminidase and similar enzymes are capable of exposing antigens on cell surfaces which would not normally be exposed to the body's immune recognition system. Contact of cells with viruses can cause them to be modified antigenically in a manner independent of enzyme action. Virus antigens can be incorporated in, or associated with, the cell wall, so that the tissue becomes antigenically modified. This however, is not true auto-antigenicity, for the immune reaction is directed against virus antigens, and not the body's own antigens modified by the infecting organism. Another process by which virus could cause auto-immune reactions is by the well-known phenomenon of incorporating host tissue antigens during intracellular replication. It has been suggested that meningoencephalitis and orchitis, following infection with mumps or measles viruses, could be the result of auto-immune processes against antigens in the brain or testis which are normally separated from the host's immune apparatus by physiological barriers, and therefore regarded as foreign. During viral assembly, these foreign host antigens could be incorporated into the virus particle. The virus is then released into the circulation and travels to the central lymphoid tissue, where it is in a position to stimulate an immune response, not only to its own viral antigens but to the host tissue antigens which it has incorporated.

A further possibility is that normal tissues are damaged by the infective agent as a result of which there is liberation of normal unaltered tissue components into the circulation. If these components have not previously been in contact with the body's central immune apparatus (hidden antigenic determinants) they would now be in a position to stimulate an "auto-immune response". Examples of this phenomenon, not however due to micro-organisms, are the auto-antibodies against liver found in carbon tetrachloride poisoning and against heart muscle after myocardial infection or cardiotomy.

Cross Reaction Between Antigens Carried by Micro-organisms and Normal Tissue Components

Antigens on micro-organisms may cross react with antigens in the body. Examples of this are the antigenic relationship between the cell walls of Group A, β-haemolytic streptococci and human heart muscle, and between type 12, Group A, β-haemolytic streptococci and human glomeruli. Another example is the antigenic relationship between *E. coli* 014, and certain other *E. coli*, with antigens in the colonic mucosa. There is little evidence that these antibacterial antibodies can cause direct tissue damage. However, they could well account for the presence of anti-tissue antibodies which are not directly cytotoxic *in vivo*.

Antigenic Modification by Physical or Chemical Means

DNA, after irradiation with ultra-violet light, has been shown to be immunogenic in rabbits and elicits antibodies reacting specifically with UV-irradiated DNA. Such antibodies can be shown to react with the nuclei of epidermal cells damaged by UV-irradiation. Moreover, mice irradiated with UV light develop anti-nuclear antibodies which react with normal nuclear material. These studies bear particular relevance to systemic lupus erythematosus in man, which may be either initiated or aggravated by exposure to sunlight. An allergic reaction to DNA altered by UV light could also underlie certain types of photosensitivity in the skin.

It has also been suggested that some forms of hypersensitivity reactions to cold could be due to an immunological reaction directed against skin proteins in which the tertiary structure has been modified by physical means, so that it becomes antigenic *in situ*.

The alteration of skin proteins by the attachment of foreign chemical groups of small molecular weight is the basis of the well-known phenomenon of contact sensitivity to such chemicals. However, it is well known that immunological response of the cell-mediated type to such hapten-protein complexes is usually not directed only to the small molecular weight chemical but also to the carrier protein itself. It has also been shown that a similar carrier specificity may occur with circulating antibodies and that antibodies can exist where specificity is directed to the linkage group between the hapten and the carrier protein. This suggests a further possible route by which auto-immunization might occur. If a person is immunized by his own protein linked to a foreign chemical grouping, the immune reaction could be directed to his own tissue acting as the carrier, as well as to the hapten chemical group which initially changes the three-dimensional configuration of the molecule, so that it is no longer recognized as "self".

Naturally Occurring Auto-antibodies

Auto-antibodies are now known to occur in the circulation of normal animals and people against a wide range of antigens, without causing any harmful side-effects. These range from antibodies against components of tissues such as the lens of the eye to antibodies against determinants on the immunoglobulin molecule. Antibodies have been described in normal rabbit serum which react with extract of homologous skin. Moreover, anti-nuclear antibodies are present in the sera of normal people and the incidence of these antibodies in the population increases as a function of age. Over the age of 60, more than 50 per cent of normal subjects have one or more of the following auto-antibodies in their serum: anti-nuclear antibody, rheumatoid factor, smooth muscle antibody, antimitochondrial or anti-microsomal antibody, or antibody to adrenal, thyroid, or gastric cells. Many of these naturally-occurring anti-tissue auto-antibodies are macrogobulins (IgM), rather than IgG, and are not tissue or species specific. It is thought that these antibodies arise as a result of antigenic stimulation, possibly as a result of immunization with cross-reacting antigens derived from micro-organisms or even from ingested foodstuffs. Although anti-tissue autoantibodies of this type can be found in normal people, there is a marked increase in their incidence in certain disease states, particularly liver and kidney diseases, and especially in systemic lupus erythematosus and paraproteinaemias or during infection with trypanosomes. The increased incidence of natural auto-antibodies as a function of age appears to be inversely related to the presence of natural antibodies to certain extrinsic antigens of bacterial origin, which decreases with age.

13. IMMUNOLOGICAL ASPECTS OF CANCER

T. LEHNER and E. SHILLITOE

INTRODUCTION

The principal aims in studying immune responses to malignant disease are to understand the defects in host immunity which permit tumour establishment and progress, and to devise methods of eradicating tumours by immunotherapy. The earliest studies became possible with the development of inbred strains of mice, which were genetically so similar that they would accept skin or organ grafts from one another indefinitely. Thus, if a tissue graft was rejected, this was evidence that the tissue had acquired new antigens. A crucial experiment showed that a sarcoma induced by methylcholanthrene in one mouse was rejected when transplanted into a syngeneic recipient. Normal skin from the donor was then transferred to the same recipient and was accepted indefinitely, showing that the rejection of the tumour had been due to a new, tumour-associated antigen. The concept, therefore, arose of tumour-specific transplantation antigens and this has been the basis of most of the work in tumour immunology.

There are two important groups of oncogenic agents; chemicals, such as methylcholanthrene, and the RNA and DNA viruses. Chemically-induced tumours carry individually distinct antigens, and immunity against one tumour does not protect an animal from any other tumour induced by the same chemical at another site. However, all tumours induced by a particular virus carry a common antigen. Animals immunized with a virus-induced tumour are protected against transplants of tumours induced by that virus at any site or in donors of other species.

The nature of these newly acquired antigens is largely unknown, as they have not yet been isolated. Some are embryonic antigens which were expressed during an early stage of ontogeny but were then replaced by adult antigens, before the immune system had matured. If embryonic antigens are re-expressed in a tumour, they will be recognized as being foreign and an immune response will be mounted against them. Virus-induced tumour antigens vary according to whether RNA or DNA viruses are involved. Tumours induced by RNA viruses have a common surface antigen which appears to be identical with the viral envelope. However, tumours induced by DNA viruses have a cell surface antigen which can be quite distinct from that of the virus, but which probably is coded for by the virus rather than by the cell; the same antigen is found in tumours elicited in different species by the same virus. Some tumours induced by DNA viruses, such as Burkitt's lymphoma in which the Epstein–Barr virus is implicated, do not manifest virus antigen unless the cells are cultured. In Herpes simplex virus transformed cells, viral antigen can also be found. The antigenic strength of animal tumours is known to vary; those arising most rapidly after induction, or those which appear spontaneously, have weak or undetectable antigens.

Tumour transplantation experiments in humans are clearly not ethical and evidence for tumour antigens and their immune responses are based largely on *in vitro* studies. These studies have also detected tumour antigens which cross react between different individuals in the same way as virus-induced tumour antigens do in animals. As man is also capable of mounting an immune response to tumours, the aims of tumour immunology are to manipulate the patient's immunity in such a way as to reject the tumour.

IMMUNOLOGICAL SURVEILLANCE

The concept of cell-mediated immunity in the development of neoplasia was expressed in the immuno-surveillance hypothesis by Burnett (1970). The mechanisms of cell-mediated immunity in higher animals may have developed with the primary function of defence against antigenic tumours. It has been postulated that malignant cells may arise at regular intervals in all normal individuals, but are rejected by an immune response. It follows from this that a tumour could develop only if the immune response were in some way defective, and this should be demonstrable at the initial stages of tumour development. Furthermore, immunodeficiency whether due to congenital defects or drug-induced, should be accompanied by an increased incidence of malignant tumours. Immunodeficiency states have been investigated in man in some detail, and the evidence will now be examined.

Malignant Disease in Immunodeficiency Diseases

Congenital immunodeficiency diseases are rare, but are extensively studied because they help in the understanding of normal immune functions. An analysis of reported cases showed that the incidence of malignant disease in patients with congenital immunodeficiencies was about 10,000 times higher than in the normal population, matched for age. Patients suffering from Bruton's agammaglobulinaemia lack plasma cells and cannot form antibody; of about 50 reported patients, 5 (10 per cent) have developed leukaemia. In the Wiskott–Aldrich syndrome and in ataxia telangiectasia, which are characterized by disorders of humoral and cell-mediated immunity, about 10 per cent of the reported cases have developed tumours. These have generally been reticulum cell sarcomas, lymphomas or leukaemias, although occasionally carcinomas have occurred. In immuno-deficiency diseases of late onset, again a prevalence of about 10 per cent of malignant tumours has been found and these have usually been tumours of the lymphoreticular system.

Malignant Disease in Drug-induced Immunosuppression

Patients receiving immunosuppressive therapy for an organ transplant also have a high incidence of malignancy, up to 100 times the expected rate. The majority of these tumours have been lymphomas, although carcinomas have also been found more frequently than in the general population. However, immunosuppression in patients with other diseases resulted in a malignancy rate only marginally higher than that found in the normal population, and significantly lower than the rate in suppressed graft recipients. The prevalence of lymphoid tumours compared to carcinoma in immunodeficiency states shows an inverse relationship to that found in the general population. Although the link between immunodeficiency and tumour development may be interpreted in favour of the immuno-surveillance hypothesis, an alternative explanation must be considered.

There is evidence that prolonged activation of lymphocytes in animals can result in the development of lymphoid malignancies. The mechanism is unknown but activation of latent RNA oncogenic viruses in lymphocytes has been suggested. In man prolonged lymphocyte activation occurs in individuals with congenital immunodeficiencies, whose inability to remove antigens effectively causes lymphoid hyperplasia. In organ recipients the immunosuppressive drugs prevent rejection of the graft, which then provides a persistent antigenic stimulus. If the lymphocyte activation in these instances leads directly to the observed malignancy, then the association between cancer and immunodeficiency does not necessarily favour the immuno-surveillance hypothesis.

Immunodeficiency in Cancer

Many investigations have been carried out to find if patients with carcinoma have an immunological defect. It has been reported that patients suffering from advanced cancer were unable to reject skin grafts from unrelated donors. Furthermore, grafts of malignant tissue, although rejected by normal individuals, were accepted by patients suffering from a malignant disease; the latter must therefore have an immunological deficiency. The nature of this deficiency has been studied intensively, and it is now known that both humoral and cell-mediated immune defects may exist. Immunoglobulin levels in cancer patients are either within normal limits or increased. The ability of patients to produce antibodies to an antigen, such as tetanus toxoid, is however impaired and this increases in severity as the disease progresses.

Skin Delayed Hypersensitivity

Cell mediated immunity has been assessed by delayed hypersensitivity skin responses to unrelated antigens. This is impaired in cancer patients and the degree of impairment correlates with the clinical stage of the tumour. A series of 100 patients with various carcinomas and some sarcomas, but otherwise in good health, were treated with the contact sensitizing agent di-nitro-chloro-benzene (DNCB). Only 60 per cent of these patients were sensitized, compared to 95 per cent of a control group. Furthermore, 92 per cent of the sensitized patients were apparently free of cancer six months after surgical treatment, whereas 93 per cent of the non-responders were either inoperable or had developed metastases within six months. A group of 12 patients who had been free of carcinoma for at least five years after treatment were all sensitized to DNCB, as were four patients with apparent spontaneous regression of the tumours. A similar pattern of delayed hypersensitivity was found when skin tests were performed with common microbial antigens (e.g. PPD, mumps, histoplasmin). A response to at least one of the antigens was seen in 90 per cent of normal individuals, but in only 39 per cent of patients with carcinoma. Of those patients responding to one or more antigens, 55 per cent were free of disease after six months, in contrast to those negative to all antigens, of whom 79 per cent had a recurrence or developed metastases during that time. Long-term follow up was also correlated with the delayed hypersensitivity response to microbial antigens.

The ability of patients to respond to DNCB and, to a lesser extent, to common microbial antigens, correlated with the prognosis, and can be used to predict the clinical course of the disease. If tumours had developed as a consequence of impaired delayed hypersensitivity, this would be expected to remain impaired even in cured patients. The presence of normal responses in long-term survivors suggests that impairment is a result rather than a cause of development of carcinoma. However, skin testing is an insensitive test detecting gross changes, and yielding reliable results only when standardized antigens and procedures are used in large groups of patients. Hence, various *in vitro* markers of cell-mediated immunity have been used.

Lymphocyte Transformation by Phytohaemagglutinin

One of the most frequently used *in vitro* tests for general evaluation of cell-mediated immunocompetence is the ability of lymphocytes to respond to phytohaemagglutinin (PHA). Stimulation of normal lymphocytes by PHA results in their transformation into large blast cells and this can be assessed by counting the percentage of blast cells present after a given time or, by means of radioactive labels, measuring the rate of DNA or RNA synthesis. In patients with malignant disease, the response to PHA has frequently been observed to be lower than in normal subjects. The cause of this is unknown, but inhibitory serum factors from some patients with cancer can depress the PHA response of lymphocytes from normal individuals. The nature of the inhibitory factor has not been elucidated; there is some evidence that it may reside in the IgG fraction, and that an antigen-antibody complex may be involved. There is no doubt however, that quite apart from serum inhibitory factors, lymphocytes can be intrinsically impaired, for if they are cultured in normal human or animal serum their response to PHA may remain inhibited. Experimentally, the development of sarcoma in mice is accompanied by a fall in the response of lymphocytes to PHA, and removal of the tumour is accompanied by a return of the PHA response to normal values. A similar sequential response has been observed recently in some patients. Why a tumour should be immunosuppressive is not known, but it is noteworthy that in animal experiments, those chemicals or viruses that act as carcinogens are also immunosuppressants, whilst closely related but non-carcinogenic agents are not immunosuppressive. These observations raise the possibility that in man neoplasia and immunosuppression may be caused by the same agent and that this may be a necessary property of some carcinogenic agents.

TUMOUR IMMUNITY

In Vivo Immune Responses

Delayed hypersensitivity skin responses to extracts of malignant tumours are frequently found in cancer patients. The antigen responsible for this appears to be located on the plasma membrane of malignant cells, and is not found in normal tissue of the same type. The skin response reaches a maximum 48 hr. after injection of the extract, indicating that the patient is pre-sensitized by his own tumour. The intensity of the response varies with the course of the disease, and fades as the disease progresses.

Histological examination of tumour sections frequently shows a marked infiltration with mononuclear cells which are mainly lymphocytes and a variable proportion of monocytes and plasma cells. The intensity of infiltration varies, and several studies have shown a correlation between the number of mononuclear cells and the length of survival of patients with carcinoma of the breast, stomach, testis and larynx. The degree of lymphoid hyperplasia in the regional lymph nodes has also been correlated with the survival in patients with various carcinomas. The existence of delayed hypersensitivity skin reactions to tumour extracts, and the importance of the mononuclear cell response in the growing tumour provides evidence of an immune response to the tumour, which is similar to that mounted against an allograft. For quantitation of this response, and detailed information as to its mechanism, it is necessary to turn to laboratory tests of cell-mediated immunity.

Lymphocyte Cytotoxicity

The most important evidence for an immune response against tumours in man has come from specific cytotoxicity tests. These tests require successful separation of viable malignant cells from other cells in the tumour, and selective cultivation of the malignant cells. The cells are then plated out into petri dishes or the wells of small plastic plates, and exposed to lymphocytes from the tumour-bearing patient. The test was developed in animals, and under optimum conditions lymphocytes from animals rendered immune to a tumour by transplantation, killed cells from that tumour. Normal cells, or cells from a different type of tumour were not killed, indicating that the cytotoxic effect was immunologically specific, and that it was associated with tumour immunity. The cytotoxicity test was then applied to a variety of human neoplasms and the results of animal studies were largely confirmed in man.

Cytotoxic lymphocytes have now been found in the peripheral blood of most patients with malignant tumours; carcinoma of bladder, breast, bronchus, cervix, colon, mouth, malignant melanomas, neuroblastomas and sarcomas. The lymphocytes do not kill normal cells from the same patient, or cells from benign tumours, but they kill cells from a histologically similar tumour from any other unrelated patient. It may be inferred, therefore, that all malignant melanomas carry a common antigen, all cervical carcinomas carry a common antigen, and all sarcomas carry a common antigen. This is analogous to virus-induced tumours of animals, which all carry the same tumour-associated antigen. The identity of lymphoid cells and the mechanisms responsible for the cytotoxic effect are as yet not clear; for further discussion, see Chapter 9.

Lymphocyte Transformation and Macrophage Migration Inhibition

In vitro markers of cell-mediated immunity, other than cytotoxicty, have not been studied comprehensively. Blast cell transformation of lymphocytes in response to *in vitro* stimulation by autochthonous carcinoma can be detected, but in fewer patients than those with cytotoxic lymphocytes. A response to a tumour from another patient does not occur. It seems likely that the strength of this response decreases as the disease advances. Macrophage migration inhibition activity is also found in patients whose lymphocytes are cultured in the presence of their autochthonous tumour, but as this test has as yet been applied to few patients, the incidence and significance of the response are not clear. The leukocyte migration inhibition test has detected immune responses in patients with carcinoma of the breast or malignant melanoma to their own, as well as to allogeneic tumour tissue.

Stimulation of lymphocytes from cancer patients with an appropriate antigen also results in the release of a factor which reduces the rate of mobility of macrophages in an electrical field. The nature of the antigen is obscure, though it is a basic protein which is found not only in malignant tissue, but also in normal human brain. The lymphocyte response is seen in patients with a variety of malignant diseases so that it can be used as a screening test for cancer. Since a number of other diseases can also give positive results, the clinical value of this test, as well as its relevance to specific tumour immunity, remain to be evaluated.

Antibodies

In addition to cell-mediated immunity, antibodies have been found in the serum of cancer patients, but have been studied comprehensively only in malignant melanoma. Most patients have antibodies which react with some component of the melanoma-cell cytoplasm and also with melanoma from other patients. They may also have complement-fixing and cytotoxic antibodies which will kill melanoma cells from that patient. These antibodies are present only when the tumour is localized, and are not found when metastases have developed. Furthermore, complement-fixing antibodies to sarcoma cells are present in a high proportion of patients with sarcoma but tend to decline as the disease advances. It is therefore possible that antibodies prevent blood-borne spread of tumours. This is supported by evidence from animal experiments showing that sarcoma-bearing rats have a specific serum factor, which might be antibody, preventing the development of lung metastases. Passive transfer of immunity to metastatic tumours can be achieved by serum, but to produce immunity to a localized subcutaneous or intramuscular tumour, lymphocytes are required. It is generally thought that in man, cell-mediated immunity probably plays the most important part in the control of carcinogenesis.

Blocking Factors

It is evident that malignant tumours continue to grow despite the presence in the blood of cytotoxic lymphocytes, and this paradox was unresolved until serum-blocking factors were found (Hellström and Hellström, 1970). Serum from an animal or a patient with a growing tumour may prevent cytotoxic lymphocytes from killing tumour cells *in vitro*, whereas serum from a normal or cured individual will not affect the lymphocytes. This blocking activity is highly specific, as it blocks lymphocyte cytoxicity to similar tumours from other patients but not against other types of tumour. Most, but not all patients, lose the serum-blocking factor after removal of the tumour. Such patients tend to have a lower rate of recurrences or metastases, thus supporting the concept that the blocking factor prevents rejection of tumour cells. The nature of blocking factors in cancer patients is uncertain, but the evidence suggests that

they are either soluble, tumour-associated antigens (Baldwin, Price and Robins, 1973), or complexes of such antigens with antibody. The mechanism by which blocking factors prevent killing of tumour cells by lymphocytes is unknown; it has been proposed that the factors become attached to tumour cells, and other work suggests that they affect lymphocytes directly. However, an intrinsic weakening of the cytotoxic response may occur, in addition to the serum-mediated loss of cytotoxicity in tumour-bearing patients. A larger number of lymphocytes may be required to kill tumour cells if the lymphocytes are taken from patients with an advanced tumour.

IMMUNOTHERAPY

The wealth and diversity of immunological information has opened up a number of new methods of controlling cancer. These can be divided into passive, active and non-specific immunotherapeutic methods (Currie, 1972).

Passive transfer of serum from patients who have undergone tumour regression was not successful until the existence of serum blocking factors was appreciated. De-blocking factor has been found in the serum of tumour-immune animals and this can counteract blocking factor in tumour bearers and cause rejection of the tumour. This approach has been successfully utilized in controlling renal carcinoma in a few patients. Passive transfer of immune lymphocytes has recently been attempted in malignant melanoma, carcinoma of bladder and leukaemia. Although some tumours have regressed, difficulties arise from histocompatibility antigens, and this method needs to be explored further. Cell-free transfer factor from a leukocyte lysate, can transfer specific cell-mediated immunity without stimulating an immune response against itself, and could prove beneficial in correcting cell-mediated immune defects in patients with cancer.

Active immunization of tumour-bearing patients, with live or irradiated tumour cells or extracts of their own tumours, with or without adjuvants, results in the development of circulating tumour antibodies, cytotoxic lymphocytes, delayed hypersensitivity skin reactions and infiltration of the tumour with lymphocytes. Clinical responses have usually been found only in patients with early tumours or small residual tumours following other treatment.

Non-specific stimulation of immunity can be achieved by injection of live BCG (Bacille Calmette–Guerin), and in rodents this can result in complete elimination of tumour cells. In man BCG therapy has been tried, particularly in acute leukaemia. Remission has first been induced by chemotherapy, and prolonged by BCG administration designed to encourage immune elimination of the remaining malignant cells. The exact role of BCG is not clear, as in addition some patients have been immunized with allogeneic leukaemic cells and it seems that in this disease a combination of agents is required in order to produce a useful clinical result. In malignant melanoma BCG therapy can also improve the survival rate.

Basal-cell carcinomas and keratoacanthomas have been successfully treated by sensitization of the patient to DNCB, followed by application of DNCB to the tumour. This form of treatment may be particularly suitable for tumours of low-grade malignancy, multiple tumours and pre-malignant lesions, and may be developed further for tumours of skin and mucous membranes.

Although immunotherapy has reached only an early stage of development, preliminary results suggest that significant advances in cancer treatment can be envisaged in the next decade. Much work will have to be carried out, for only reliable and discriminating immunological criteria will make it possible to select the appropriate immunotherapy for a particular tumour, and responses will need to be monitored before and after threatment.

ORAL LEUKOPLAKIA AND CARCINOMA

It has long been appreciated that some forms of leukoplakia may undergo carcinomatous change. The incidence of carcinomatous transformation varies with age, sex and length of the follow-up period, though recently published large series indicate an overall incidence of about 5 per cent. However, the incidence increases to about 30 per cent in those lesions which show histological evidence of epithelial atypia. Leukoplakia may therefore serve as a useful model for studying carcinomatous transformation.

The term leukoplakia is defined here as a white plaque that from the clinical and histological features cannot be assigned to any other disease. The aetiology of most oral leukoplakias is unknown, but among the variety of agents suggested, smoking, friction, use of betel nut, syphilis, chronic candidiasis and possibly latent Herpes simplex type 1 infection have been supported by clinical, epidemiological, pathological and immunological evidence. An important point to have evolved is that leukoplakia can be caused by microbial, fungal, and probably viral agents so that immune responses might play a decisive part in the development of leukoplakia and its transformation to carcinoma. Furthermore, smoking is also associated with immunological changes, suggesting that both chemical and microbial agents related to leukoplakia might induce their effects, to some extent, by way of the immunological responses.

Mononuclear Cell Infiltration in Leukoplakia and Carcinoma

A chronic inflammatory cell infiltrate, consisting of a variable proportion of lymphocytes, monocytes and plasma cells, can usually be observed in the lamina propria of leukoplakia and carcinoma. Differential counts of the mononuclear cell infiltration in biopsies of leukoplakia, candidiasis and lichen planus revealed significant differences between these diseases. Hyperkeratotic (or para-keratotic) lesions without acanthosis showed a significantly smaller number of non-pyroninophilic mononuclear cells (mostly lymphocytes) than any of the other lesions, and less than 10 pyroninophilic cells per mm² (mostly plasma cells) were found (fig. 1). There was a significant increase in the number of lymphocytes and plasma cells with the development of acanthosis (with or without hyperkeratosis) and a progressive increase in the number of both types of cells

continued through epithelial atypia and carcinoma *in situ* until a maximum was reached in carcinoma. The histological grading, lymphocyte and plasma-cell counts were correlated with the risk of carcinomatous transformation in leukoplakia. It is significant that an increased number of Russell bodies has been observed in lesions that subsequently changed to carcinomas.

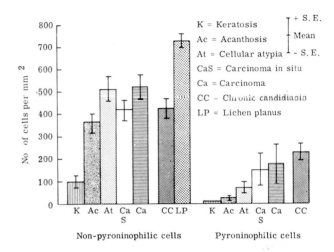

Fig. 1. Non-pyroninophilic (lymphocytes) and pyroninophilic (plasma cell) counts in 7 pathological types of white lesions of the oral mucosa.

Cell-mediated Immune Response to Tissue Homogenates

The correlation between lymphocyte and plasma-cell infiltration, and the different stages of leukoplakia and carcinoma, suggests that immunological factors may be involved in the development and progress of this disease. Saline homogenates of excised leukoplakia were used to study the response of lymphocytes from these patients. This revealed a significant negative correlation between transformation of lymphocytes stimulated with autologous homogenates of leukoplakia and the lymphocyte infiltration in biopsies. Hyperkeratotic tissue without acanthosis appeared to be associated with the highest rate of lymphocyte transformation and the lowest intensity of mononuclear cell infiltration, and there was a decrease in the former and an increase in the latter as the histological grading changed to acanthosis, epithelial atypia and carcinoma (see fig. 5). The results suggest that a new or altered antigen is detected in leukoplakia and that carcinomatous transformation is accompanied, either by loss of or change in antigenicity, or by a specific depression in cell-mediated immunity to this antigen. Alternatively the antigen may be concealed by blocking factors.

A factor is also released by sensitized lymphocytes from patients with carcinoma or leukoplakia in the presence of tumour antigen and this inhibits migration of guinea-pig macrophages in an electrical field. A serum factor depressing the lymphocytes has been detected and the titre in sera from patients with leukoplakia is intermediate between those from carcinoma and normal controls. Leucocyte migration can also be inhibited by homogenates of leuko-plakia but not of normal mucosa in patients with leuko-plakia. These findings are consistent with the concept that cell-mediated immune responses may play a part in the development and progress of leukoplakia.

Immune Responses to Microbial Agents in Leukoplakia and Carcinoma

Syphilis

Leukoplakia is found in tertiary syphilis and may develop 4–20 years after the primary and secondary stages of the disease. Carcinomatous transformation is said to occur more often in syphilitic than other types of leukoplakia.

Cell-mediated immunity to treponemal antigens in prim-ary and particularly early secondary syphilis is impaired, but in some patients in late secondary and especially latent syphilis the cell-mediated responses are intact. Leukoplakia becomes clinically detectable in tertiary syphilis and it is likely that the cell-mediated immune responses at those stages are therefore intact (see also Chapter 10).

Chronic Hyperplastic Candidiasis (see also Chapter 41)

The association of a specific type of leukoplakia with Candida has been appreciated only recently. Although there has been little doubt about Candida causing chronic muco-cutaneous lesions with oral manifestations of leuko-plakia, the extension of this relationship to cases with exclusively oral candidal leukoplakia does not necessarily indicate an aetiological relationship. The oral carrier rate of Candida is about 30 per cent and the presence of hyphae of Candida in leukoplakia might result from secondary infection by Candida of a suitably altered tissue. The clinical and pathological diagnosis of chronic hyperplastic candidiasis has now undergone the test of time and can be summarized as follows:

(a) the lesions appear as diffuse, irregular, white patches which cannot be scraped off, with intervening circular areas of normal or inflamed mucosa affecting most commonly the post-commisural part of the cheeks and adjacent lips, and dorsum of the tongue;

(b) cultures from the lesions usually yield *Candida albicans* and cytological examination of direct scrapings show hyphae of Candida;

(c) biopsy examination shows epithelial hyperplasia, sometimes with intervening areas of atrophy and an infil-tration of the superficial layers of epithelium by hyphae of Candida. Inflammatory changes, mainly oedema and polymorphonuclear cells are found commonly between the parakeratinized cell layer and stratum spinosum adjacent to the Candida hyphae. The lamina propria is densely infiltrated by lymphocytes and histiocytes, with a larger number of plasma cells which can be the predominant cell;

(d) antibodies to *C. albicans* have been particularly studied by the fluorescent antibody test; increased salivary IgA and serum IgG antibodies are found in most

patients, but serum IgA antibodies are decreased in some and IgM antibodies in most patients;

(e) cell-mediated immune investigations show a negat-ive cytotoxic response in all and macrophage migration inhibition in most patients. A positive skin delayed hypersensitivity reaction is found in about half the patients and a significant, though low stimulation of lymphocyte transformation in most patients; and

(f) antifungal agents may eradicate chronic candidiasis, though the lesion recurs after the drug is discontinued. This can be achieved only occasionally by topical nystatin, more often by using clotrimazole, but intravenous Am-photericin B has proved most effective. Clearance of leukoplakia by drugs effective against Candida and other fungi is found only in chronic candidiasis and can be used as a diagnostic test.

Although the evidence for Candida causing a specific type of leukoplakia can no longer be in doubt, there is little firm evidence as yet to suggest that Candida can induce carcinomatous transformation. This view arose from the increased frequency of association of Candida hyphae with epithelial atypia as compared with other types of leuko-plakia. As Candida thrives particularly well in altered tissues, its presence might indicate a secondary infection. An alternative interpretation of the presence of Candida in leukoplakia is that an impaired immune response to Candida in patients with epithelial atypia and carcinoma enables the fungus to proliferate.

Latent Herpes Simplex Virus Type 1 Infection

There is increasing evidence that the genital strain of Herpes simplex virus type 2 is associated with cervical can-cer. The oro-facial strain, Herpes simplex virus type 1 (HSVI) has been implicated in cancer of the head and neck and the evidence will be briefly presented. A relationship between recurrent herpetic infection and carcinoma of the lip was suggested in the past, though HSVI had no demon-strable oncogenic properties. However, it was recently found in mice that HSVI can enhance papilloma formation when administered with methylcholanthrene and that it can enhance carcinomatous transformation of papilloma.

Evidence has recently been presented to suggest that the oncogenic properties of HSVI could be related to a non-virion antigen and can be differentiated immunologically from virion antigen which is associated with infective and cytopathic functions of the virus (Tarro and Sabin, 1973; Hollinshead and Tarro, 1973). Significant complement fixing antibody titres to the non-virion antigen were found in patients with cancer of the head and neck, as compared with normal and diseased controls. Furthermore, soluble membrane antigens from carcinoma of the lip reacted specifically with an antiserum to non-virion antigen of HSVI, suggesting that a cross-reacting antigen, or the non-virion antigen is present in the tumour. That inactivated HSVI can impart genetic information to cells has been shown by transferring thymidine kinase to cells lacking this enzyme. It can be readily seen that transfer of genetic information by HSVI might occasionally lead to neoplastic conversion. Indeed, ultraviolet light inactivated HSVI can cause transformation of hamster embryo fibroblasts and when these cells are injected into newborn Syrian hamsters they induce metastasizing fibrosarcomas. The epidemiological relationship between sunlight and carcinoma of the lips and face in some patients, as well as sunlight and activation of HSVI lesions of the lips and face in others might therefore be relevant.

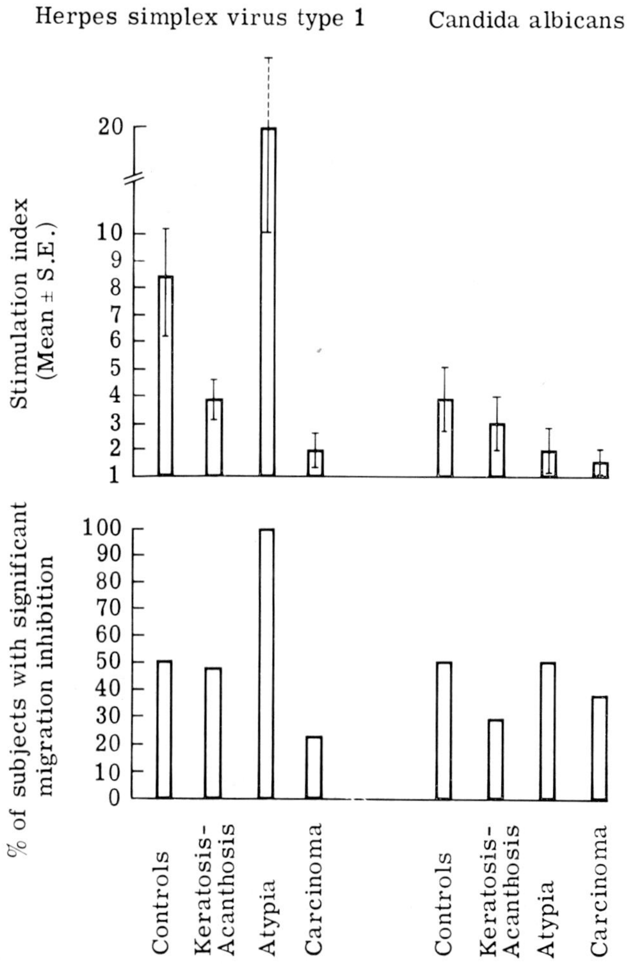

FIG. 2. Mean stimulation indices and percentage of subjects with significant migration inhibition indices elicited by *Herpes simplex virus type 1* and *Candida albicans*.

The possibility that HSVI might be involved in some cases of leukoplakia and carcinoma has been raised recently on the basis of immunological investigations (Lehner, Wilton, Shillitoe and Ivanyi, 1973). Cell-mediated and humoral immune responses to HSVI and *Candida albicans* were studied in patients with leukoplakia, showing a histological spectrum of changes from epithelial keratosis to acanthosis and atypia and in patients with carcinoma. The results showed that patients with epithelial atypia had the highest indices of lymphocyte transformation and migration inhibition to HSVI and this relationship was not evident with *C. albicans* (fig. 2). In patients with keratosis and acanthosis there was a significant lack of correlation between lymphocyte transformation and migration inhibition

to both HSVI and *C. albicans*. In carcinoma, these indices were depressed and a significant negative correlation was found between lymphocyte transformation and migration inhibition to HSVI, unlike the positive correlation in control subjects. Complement fixing antibodies to HSVI and HSV2, and fluorescent antibodies to *C. albicans* failed to show a significant change in titre in any one group of subjects tested.

It is assumed that an intact cell-mediated immune response is required for protection against HSVI, so that a dissociation between lymphocyte transformation and macrophage migration inhibition to HSVI, as is found in the keratosis-acanthosis group, may permit viral replication. It is, however, surprising that recurrent herpetic infection does not appear to be more common in these patients; only 3/13 (23 per cent) gave a history of recurrent herpetic infection of the lips.

An increase in both lymphocyte transformation and macrophage migration inhibition to HSVI in patients with epithelial atypia suggests that the virus should be effectively controlled, yet it is at this stage of leukoplakia that carcinomatous transformation occurs most commonly. However, this mechanism may control HSVI only at an extracellular and not an intracellular site. Although the number of patients with epithelial atypia was small, quantitative changes observed in the three groups of patients were borne out by sequential studies. Some fluctuations of the response of lymphocytes to HSVI were found over a period of three years in the keratosis-acanthosis group. However, only patients with atypia showed a fall from a high stimulation index (>7) to a negative value (<2) and this was observed in patients who developed carcinoma or severe epithelial atypia bordering on carcinoma *in situ* (fig. 3). The pattern of lymphocyte transformation by *C. albicans* was much more steady and, except for one patient in each of the three groups, unremarkable. It has been postulated that HSVI might cause neoplastic transformation of epithelial cells, for the cell-mediated immune responses could inactivate HSVI in such a way as to prevent replication but induce oncogenic properties of the virus, as has been shown with ultraviolet light. Alternatively, an enhanced and prolonged cell-mediated response to HSVI might activate repressed RNA oncogenic viruses, resulting in epithelial atypia.

The subsequent development of invasive carcinoma has been associated with a decrease in sensitized lymphocytes in peripheral blood and as these might have been sequestrated by the carcinoma, an insufficient number remains available in peripheral blood to yield significant lymphocyte transformation. This view is consistent with the high lymphocyte count at the site of a carcinoma and a low count in keratosis without acanthosis. Apart from an association between malignant change and impaired cell-mediated immunity to HSVI, the depression of lymphocyte transformation to HSVI can serve and is used as a marker in prognosis and management of leukoplakia and carcinoma.

The HSVI used in the cell-mediated studies was grown in kidney cell cultures and the antigen was prepared by ultrasonication. It is possible, therefore, that both virion and non-virion antigens are present, and that the differences in response at various stages of leukoplakia and in carcinoma could be due to the virion antigen participating in one response and non-virion antigen in another. This possibility is now being explored and could prove of some importance in interpreting immune responses to HSVI in man.

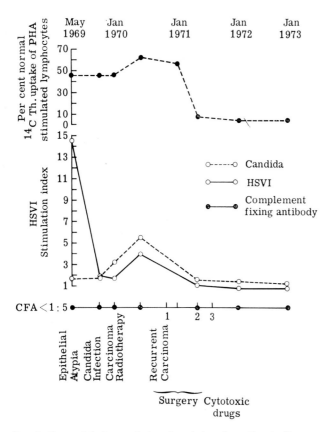

Fig. 3. Sequential changes in lymphocyte transformation to *Herpes simplex virus type 1, Candida albicans* and phytohaemagglutinin in a patient where epithelial atypia changed to carcinoma.

If the population with leukoplakia and carcinoma is no different from the population at large in acquiring HSVI infection, then the latent period between first infection with the virus and subsequent development of leukoplakia could be of the order of 30–50 years. Latency with HSVI, as with other DNA viruses, implies that the virus is maintained in cells in an undetectable, dormant state, from which it may be reactivated. A long latent period of 5–25 years, from the time of exposure to a carcinogenic agent to the appearance of the neoplasm, is one of the characteristic features of occupational cancer. Nevertheless, some co-factor might be required, for only a very small proportion of subjects with HSVI infection develop leukoplakia and carcinoma. Clinically associated factors, such as smoking and a variety of local irritants, have been postulated in the past, though the evidence is unsatisfactory. It is possible that immunological adjuvants and suppressors present in the mouth, particularly dental bacterial plaque, may modulate immune responses to viruses. There is some indication that the bacterial flora of dental plaque might enhance immune responses (Lehner, Wilton, Challacombe and Ivanyi, 1974).

Furthermore, the effect of smoking on the response of lymphocytes to HSVI is age-dependent.

Cell-mediated Immune Responses in Oral Carcinoma

A progressive impairment of the capacity of lymphocytes to respond to antigens and mitogens has been evident only on sequential studies in patients with early carcinoma and leukoplakia. This is best illustrated by phytohaemagglutinin, for a response of lymphocytes under 50 per cent of normal on one or more occasions during a three-year period was found in two out of four patients with keratosis and/or acanthosis, three out of four patients with epithelial

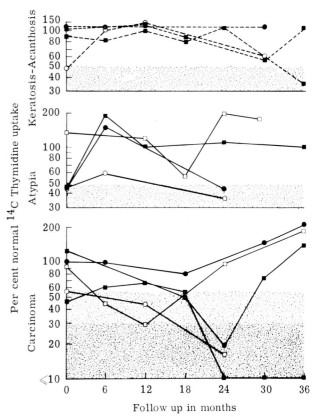

Fig. 4. Sequential changes in lymphocyte transformation to phytohaemagglutinin in patients with leukoplakia and carcinoma.

atypia and four out of five patients with carcinoma (fig. 4). Furthermore, values under 30 per cent of normal were recorded only in carcinoma, and were found in four out of five patients, two of whom died later.

Single estimation of lymphocyte transformation may not give a true indication of the response of lymphocytes in cancer, as there are many variables that cannot be controlled. Sequential data are much more informative, for comparisons can be made, if the technique is standardized. A progressive decrease in the phytohaemagglutinin-responding, and therefore predominantly T lymphocyte population in pre-cancerous patients suggests that some impairment of T lymphocytes may occur during carcinomatous transformation. Subsequent depression of T lymphocytes in patients with carcinoma can be due to treatment by radiotherapy or cytotoxic drugs.

Cytotoxicity tests have also been applied to oral carcinoma. The target cells used are continuous cell lines of squamous carcinoma, such as Hep-2 cells, Although these studies are at a preliminary stage they indicate that cytotoxic

modulating activity of antibodies. A cell-mediated immunodeficiency may play a part in chronic candidiasis, syphilis, HSVI infection and the effects of smoking at the initiating stage and during carcinomatous transformation.

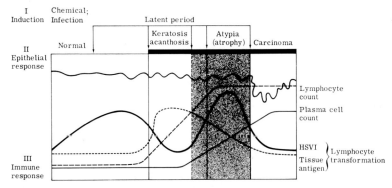

FIG. 5. Diagrammatic representation of the induction and development of leukoplakia and carcinoma. During the pre-cancerous phase (shaded), major pathological and immunological changes take place. (HSVI = *Herpes simplex virus type 1*)

lymphocytes are detectable in patients with carcinoma and with leukoplakia showing evidence of epithelial atypia.

Prognosis

In assessing the probability of leukoplakia transforming into carcinoma, there is no single definitive factor but a number of features should be considered in each case.

Serial assessments, using clinical, histological and immunological criteria are the best means available in the prognosis of leukoplakia.

Sequential changes in cell-mediated immunity to HSVI, phytohaemagglutinin and the leukoplakia tissue antigens can offer advance warning of imminent change or of actual malignant transformation having taken place.

Unified Concept of the Pathogenesis of Leukoplakia and Carcinomatous Transformation

A working hypothesis has evolved from the immunopathological investigations of leukoplakia (fig. 5). The initial development of leukoplakia and subsequent transformation to carcinoma is induced by microbial and/or chemical agents. The induction phase usually has a long latent period, a matter of years, during which time prolonged exposure to the chemical agent (*e.g.* smoking), chronic infection (*T. pallidum, C. albicans*), or latent viral infection (*Herpes simplex* Type 1), may initiate a local epithelial reaction as well as local and systemic immune reactions. The epithelial changes of keratosis, acanthosis, atypia and carcinoma may develop sequentially in some but may appear at any one stage and remain unchanged in others. This may be associated with a newly acquired or altered epithelial antigen. The initiation and development of any stage of leukoplakia and carcinoma could be dependent on cell-mediated immune responses, with

Epithelial atypia, however, appears to be associated with enhanced cell-mediated immune responses to HSVI. These changes are associated with an increase in lymphocyte, plasma cell and probably in monocyte infiltration at the pathological site. Initiation of neoplastic changes may occur in leukoplakia with epithelial atypia and to a lesser extent with acanthosis irrespective of the presence of hyperkeratosis. A number of markers are now available in defining the premalignant stage and these can be utilized in assessing prognosis of the lesion.

REFERENCES

Baldwin, R. W., Price, M. R. and Robins, R. A. (1973), "Significance of Serum Factors Modifying Cellular Immune Responses to Growing Tumours," *Brit. J. Cancer*, **28**, suppl. 1, 37.

Burnet, F. M. (1970), "The Concept of Immunological Surveillance," *Pro. exper. Tum. Res.*, **13**, 1.

Currie, G. A. (1972), "Eighty Years of Immunotherapy: a Review of Immunological Methods Used for the Treatment of Human Cancer," *Brit. J. Cancer*, **26**, 141.

Hellström, K. E. and Hellström, I. (1970), "Immunological Enhancement as Studied by Cell Culture Techniques," *Ann. Rev. Microbiol.*, **24**, 373.

Hollinshead, A. C. and Tarro, G. (1973), "Soluble Membrane Antigens of Lip and Cervical Carcinomas: Reactivity with Antibody for Herpesvirus Nonvirion Antigens," *Science*, **179**, 698.

Lehner, T., Wilton, J. M. A., Shillitoe, E. J. and Ivanyi, L. (1973), "Cell-mediated Immunity and Antibodies to Herpesvirus Hominis Type 1 in Oral Leukoplakia and Carcinoma," *Brit. J. Cancer*, **27**, 351.

Lehner, T., Wilton, J. M. A., Challacombe, S. J. and Ivanyi, L. (1974), "Sequential Cell-mediated Immune Responses in Experimental Gingivitis in Man," *J. Clin. exp. Immunol.* **16**, 481.

Tarro, G. and Sabin, A. B. (1973), "Non-virion Antigens Produced by Herpes Simplex Viruses 1 and 2," *Proc. nat. Acad. Sci (Wash.)*, **70**, 1032.

14. THE CLINICAL APPLICATIONS OF IMMUNOLOGICAL TECHNIQUES

P. D. J. HOLLAND and ORLA BROWNE

Investigation of humoral antibody
    Precipitation of antigen/antibody complexes
        Single radial diffusion
        Double (Ouchterlony) diffusion
    Agglutination techniques
    Immunoelectrophoresis
    Complement fixation
    Immunofluorescence
        Direct
        Indirect
        Examples of autoantibodies associated with disease
    Antiglobulin test

Cellular immune mechanisms
    Skin tests
    Blast transformation
    Rosette formation
    Leucocyte migration inhibition
    Macrophage migration inhibition
    Mixed lymphocyte reaction

In this chapter it is proposed to classify immunological tests, to outline briefly the underlying mechanism of each test and to indicate its clinical application. By "immunological" is meant any test which is based directly or indirectly on the reaction of antigen with antibody or cells of the immune system. In general the body deals with non-self antigens both specifically and non-specifically. The vast majority of immunological tests are based on the detection of specific defence mechanisms. These will be dealt with in some detail from the practical point of view and their applications to clinical medicine and dentistry stressed. It must not be forgotten, however, that non-specific defence mechanisms both humoral and cellular are of great importance as first-line protection against disease.

Specific immune mechanisms are based on either (a) humoral antibody activity or (b) cellular activity (see Chapter 9). Both of these immune activities are lymphocyte derived. Humoral antibodies are produced by B lymphocytes which on activation by contact with antigen become converted into plasma cells; these function as little factories for the production of the various immunoglobulin antibodies which can combine with and destroy the offending antigen. Cellular immune defence mechanisms, on the other hand, are conducted by thymus indoctrinated (T) lymphocytes which, on antigenic stimulation, become specifically activated and capable of blast transformation and mitotic division, thereby producing clones of specifically conditioned T lymphocytes; these, either by direct action or through the secondary specific activation of tissue and blood phagocytes, can destroy the antigen. In this context it must be emphasized that both the T cell and B cell systems will react with antigens whether exogenous, *e.g.*

microbiological agents or allergens, or endogenous, *e.g.* antigenic alteration of self-proteins, as in autoimmune disease or in neoplasia.

It is proposed to discuss separately immunological procedures based on these two interdependent defence systems.

INVESTIGATION OF HUMORAL ANTIBODY

The logical starting point is an assessment of the patient's ability to produce protecting antibodies, *i.e.* immunoglobulins. These are present largely in the gammaglobulin fraction of serum and may be roughly calculated by serum electrophoresis. In this technique, serum protein molecules travel in an electric field on buffered wet cellulose acetate paper or other suitable media and take up positions on the paper relative to their molecular mobilities (fig. 1a). Staining of the protein bands thus produced allows of both a qualitative and a quantitative assessment of the various protein fractions. Hypogammaglobulinaemia (fig. 1b) may be detected in this way in the majority of cases. It must be stressed that a "normal" gammaglobulin estimation may mask a qualitative defect in immunoglobulins, *e.g.* isolated IgA deficiency, so that where doubt exists it is mandatory to undertake qualitative immunoglobulin analyses. A normal or only slightly raised gammaglobulin value may also be present in the gammopathies, *e.g.* myeloma and macroglobulinaemia, but the experienced immunologist will be able to detect these sharply defined "M" bands of abnormal protein on the electrophoresis strip (fig. 1c). A hypergammaglobulinaemia of polyclonal type will be present in chronic pyogenic infections, in autoimmune and connective tissue disorders, and in chronic liver disease.

If a hypogammaglobulinaemic state is uncovered, particularly in a child, it is important to determine whether this is a primary or secondary phenomenon. Primary hypogammaglobulinaemia is an inherited condition in which there is a defect in the production of the immunoglobulin-producing plasma cells. The patient, usually a male child, suffers repeated serious pyogenic infections, with failure to thrive and possibly an associated enteropathy or bronchiectasis. Late-onset hypogammaglobulinaemia of inherited type may occasionally occur and become manifest in adult life.

The investigation of such a case is concerned with determining the presence or absence of an adequate number of plasma cells. This may be assessed in one of two ways. The patient may be "challenged" with an injection of TAB vaccine and the response determined two weeks later by means of the Widal test for the presence of agglutinating antityphoid antibodies in the serum. In true congenital hypogammaglobulinaemia there will be no response. The

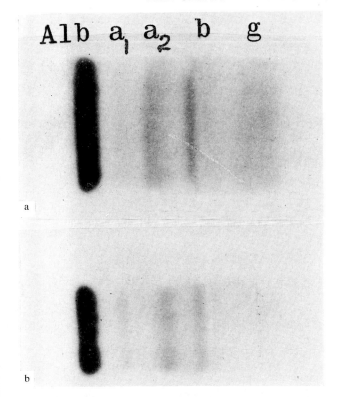

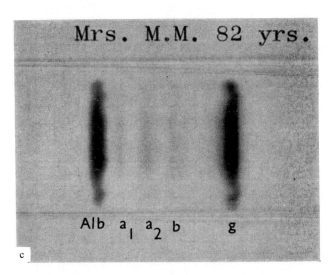

FIG. 1. (a) Electrophoretogram of normal serum. (b) Electrophoretogram of hypogammaglobulinaemia. (c) Electrophoretogram from a case of myeloma showing abnormal protein.

It should be stressed that the most common congenital immune deficiency disorder is hypogammaglobulinaemia. Secondary hypogammaglobulinaemia is due to depression or replacement of the normal lymphocyte system, *e.g.* drug immuno-suppression or acute leukaemia.

The tests so far described have been concerned with the ability or otherwise of the patient to produce immunoglobulins. There are also several valuable techniques for determining the type and activity of the immunoglobulins present, and these will now be briefly described.

Techniques Used in Antibody and/or Antigen Identification

Precipitation of Antigen/Antibody Complexes

This technique was originally performed by carefully layering the anti-serum on top of a solution of antigen and allowing a whitish precipitate to develop at the interface. It still forms the basis for Lancefield's grouping of *Streptococcus pyogenes*, and is useful for detection of several antigens of the oral flora (*e.g. A. israeli, Strep. mutans*). Gel diffusion techniques have largely replaced the layering method and are extremely valuable additions to immunological bench tests as they may be used either qualitatively or quantitatively. Gel diffusion may be employed in two ways, *viz.* single radial immunodiffusion, and double diffusion (Ouchterlony).

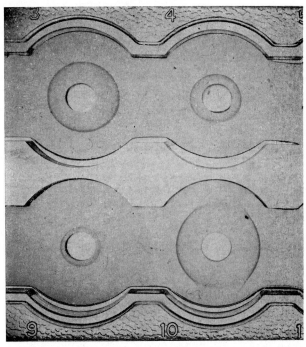

FIG. 2. Single Radial Diffusion; note differing diameters of precipitin rings.

(a) **Single Radial Diffusion (SRID).** Principle: In this technique the antigen is incorporated into the agar-gel and the test serum added to a circular well cut in the medium. Diffusion outwards of the serum is allowed to continue until a white precipitin line of antigen/antibody complex forms a ring around the well, the concentration of antibody determining the diameter of the precipitin ring (fig. 2).

second method of investigation is to examine histologically lymphoid tissue either with or without prior local injection of TAB vaccine into tissues distal to the lymph node group. Opportunity may also be taken at appendectomy to ascertain the presence or absence of plasma cells in the lymphoid tissue of the submucosa. Plasma cell precursor B lymphocytes from the peripheral blood may also be identified by demonstrating a thin rim of immunoglobulin on the cell surface by means of immunofluorescent staining.

Control-quantitated antisera are included in the test plate and comparison of the diameters of known and unknown antisera allows accurate quantitation of the unknown serum.

This technique is extensively employed in quantitating immunoglobulins IgG, IgA, IgM, IgD or IgE, in both serum and cerebrospinal fluid. Transferrin, the third component of complement (B_{1c} globulin) and C reactive protein may also be quantitated in similar manner.

(b) Double diffusion (Ouchterlony) Technique. Principle: Antigen and antibody solutions are placed in contiguous wells cut in agar-gel plates or slides and diffusion outwards is allowed to take place. Where antigen and antibody meet in optimal proportions, white precipitin lines are formed

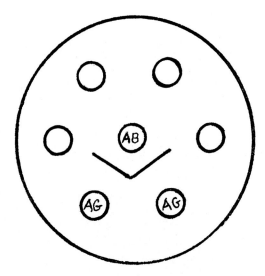

FIG. 3. Ouchterlony double-diffusion technique.
AB = Specific antibody
AG = Specific antigen

(fig. 3). This test allows of identification of either antigen or antibody, depending upon which is the known solution. Positive and negative controls must be included in the test plate. The technique is mainly used for the identification of precipitating antibodies in serum. It is particularly useful in diagnosing hypersensitive (type III) organic dust diseases, e.g. farmer's lung or aspergilloma (mycetoma) of the lung.

Agglutination Techniques

Principle: Agglutination is the result of the interaction of antibody molecules with antigen in the form of particulate matter. The antibody combines with surface antigens, linking them together to form visible aggregates. The test may be performed in tubes or as slide agglutination. Agglutination forms the basis for blood group identification and is also used in the identification of bacteria and for the detection of antibacterial antibodies in serum as in typhoid and brucellosis (Widal test). The titre of antibody present is the reciprocal of the highest serum dilution showing unequivocal agglutination. A rising titre of antibody is more significant in detecting infection than a single

positive test. It is possible to improve upon the Widal test by testing the well-washed agglutinate of bacteria with antihuman gammaglobulin to detect weak or incomplete antibody union. This is the basis of the Kerr-Coombs test for antibody detection in brucellosis.

Antigens in molecular form may be tested for by coating them on to carrier particles such as inert polystyrene latex particles (latex agglutination test), or on to sheep red-blood cells previously treated with tannic acid (tanned red cell haemagglutination test). The union of such sensitized particles with antibodies in serum will result in rapid agglutination of the particles.

Examples of uses of latex slide tests are in glandular fever, rheumatoid disease and for detecting antithyroid antibodies. The tanned sheep red-cell technique is used commonly in identifying antibodies to thyroglobulin in thyroid disease.

Flocculation is a form of agglutination that occurs when a very fine suspension of antigen clumps together on coming into contact with specific antibody. Good examples of this form of antigen/antibody reaction are the Kahn and VDRL flocculation tests for syphilis or other closely related treponemal diseases.

Immunoelectrophoresis

This is a technique which makes use of two immunological procedures. Firstly, the patient's serum is separated electrophoretically on an agar-gel slide, and then human serum antibody created in a laboratory animal is allowed

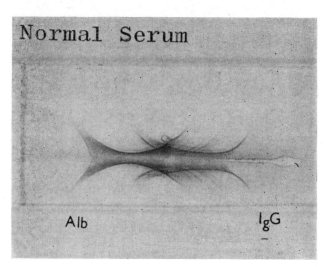

FIG. 4. Immunoelectrophoresis.

to diffuse from a long gutter cut in the agar-gel parallel with the separated proteins. Precipitin lines of antigen/antibody complex are formed for each individual fraction of the human-serum and can be compared with a normal serum control set up on the other half of the slide (fig. 4). In this way, abnormal globulins may be detected as in myeloma or macroglobulinaemia, or the absence or accentuation of individual immunoglobulins may be revealed.

Complement Fixation

Principle: Certain antibodies when combined with antigen have the ability to utilize or "fix" complement and so inactivate it. As this reaction is not visible to the naked eye an indicator system must be added consisting of a second complement fixing antigen/antibody combination, *e.g.* sheep red cells with sheep red cell antibody prepared in another animal. If the antigen is bound by the antibody in the first or test system, then the complement provided will be fixed and none will be available for the indicator reaction, so that haemolysis of the sheep red cells will not take place. Conversely, if specific antibodies are not present in the patient's serum, complement will be available for the indicator system and haemolysis will occur.

Complement fixation tests are widely used in the diagnosis of syphilis (and other treponematoses), in a wide variety of virus infections, in hydatid disease and in trichinosis.

Immuno-fluorescent Techniques

Principle: The basis of this type of immunological technique is the ability to make visible antigen–antibody union in tissues by the incorporation of a fluorescent dye in the reaction. The test can be used in two ways, *i.e.* the direct and the indirect test (figs. 5a, 5b).

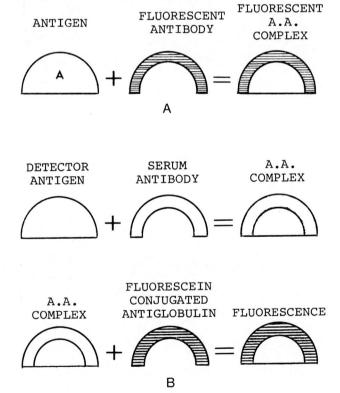

FIG. 5. Immuno-fluorescent Techniques. (a) Direct test—antigen identification. (b) Indirect test—antibody identification.

The Direct Test. This is used for the identification and localization of immune antigen–antibody complexes or of autoantibody in tissues.

As all antibody activity is confined to the globulin fraction of serum, an antibody directed against human globulin is prepared by animal inoculation. The anti-human-globulin so produced is labelled with a fluorescent dye and is used to detect the presence of antibody in human tissues.

Biopsy material is suitable for this examination provided that it is fresh and has not been placed in a fixative solution. It is best transported to the laboratory in a clean dry container or, if very small, should be floated in a few drops of physiological saline to prevent dehydration. Frozen sections are cut from this material and are incubated with the labelled antihuman-globulin for 30 min. The sections are then thoroughly washed to remove all unreacted antiserum. They are then viewed under an ultraviolet light microscope, and the sites of immune complex or autoantibody attachment are seen to glow with a brilliant fluorescence.

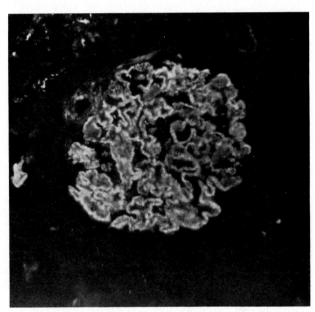

FIG. 6. Antigen-Antibody Complex deposition on glomerular basement membrane. × 260.

Examples of this test are the identification of immune complexes in the glomeruli of patients with glomerulonephritis using needle biopsy of renal tissue (fig. 6), or the examination of gingival biopsy material for the presence of basement membrane antibody in cases of pemphigoid.

The Indirect Test. This test is designed to show the presence of specific autoantibody in serum; for example, to test for the presence of thyroid antibodies the serum is incubated with frozen sections of thyroid tissue for 30 min. at 37°C followed by repeated washings. Should thyroid antibody be present in the serum, it will remain firmly bound to the thyroid tissue. As this bound antibody is a globulin it can be made visible by a second incubation, this time using labelled anti-human globulin as described in the direct test (figs. 7a and 7b).

A wide variety of autoantibodies can be detected simply by varying the tissue antigen employed, *e.g.* gastric, renal, liver, salivary gland, adrenal.

It should be noted that the presence of an autoantibody in the blood stream does not necessarily establish the diagnosis of a disease. Autoantibodies in low titre may be present in perfectly healthy adults, *e.g.* about 8 per cent of healthy adults over the age of 40 years will have anti-thyroid or anti-gastric antibodies in their serum. Statistically there is an increased incidence of these autoantibodies in close relatives of patients with either Hashimoto's disease of the thyroid or with Addisonian pernicious anaemia.

Examples of Autoantibodies Associated with Disease

Disease	Relevant Antibody
Pemphigus vulgaris	Epidermal intercellular
Pemphigoid	Skin basement membrane
Systemic lupus erythematosus	
Discoid L.E.	
Scleroderma	Antinuclear factor (ANF)
Dermatomyositis	(see fig. 7c)
Rheumatoid arthritis	
Sjögren's disease	
Sjögren's syndrome	Salivary gland and ANF
Addisonian pernicious anaemia	Gastric parietal cell
Atrophic gastritis (autoimmune)	
Hashimoto's thyroiditis	(Thyroid microsomal and Thyroglobulin
Idiopathic Addison's disease	Adrenal
Idiopathic hypoparathyroidism	Parathyroid
Premature menopause (some cases)	Steroid-producing cells ovary and adrenal
Myasthenia gravis	Voluntary muscle
Active chronic hepatitis	Smooth muscle and ANF
Primary biliary cirrhosis	Mitochondria
Coeliac disease	Reticulin
Goodpasture's syndrome	Glomerular and lung basement membrane

Antiglobulin Test (Coombs)

This is an extremely valuable technique for detecting weakly acting (incomplete) antibodies in or attached to cells.

Principle: Anti-human-gammaglobulin when mixed with a well-washed suspension of red cells in saline will cause immediate agglutination of the cells if incomplete antibody, usually IgG, is attached to the red cell surfaces. This is known as the direct Coombs test and is diagnostic for acquired haemolytic anaemia of autoimmune type, or haemolytic disease of the newborn due to Rhesus incompatibility. In the latter disease the antibodies may be detected in the Rh negative mother's blood before the birth of the Rh-positive baby; this is done by incubating a suspension of Group O Rh-positive red cells with the mother's serum to pick up the antibodies, and then performing the Coombs test on a saline suspension of the well-washed red cells as described above. This is known as an indirect Coombs test.

CELLULAR IMMUNE MECHANISMS

The investigation of cellular immune mechanisms in disease has lagged a long way behind investigation and understanding of the humoral antibody immune system, mainly because it is much more complicated and because it is less amenable to laboratory investigation and measurement. The handling of living cells is a slow and tedious process hampered by contamination, thermal susceptibility and the necessity to maintain cellular metabolism.

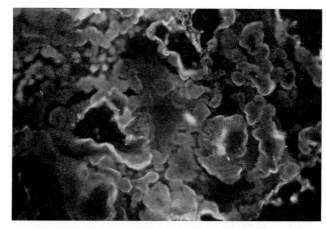

FIG. 7a. Thyroglobulin Auto-antibody. × 260.

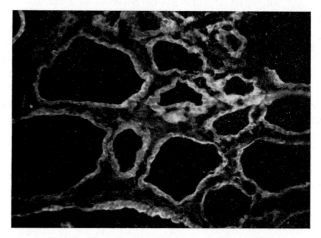

FIG. 7b. Thyroid microsomal auto-antibody. × 320.

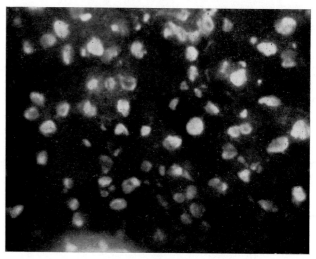

FIG. 7c. Antinuclear factors. × 560.

Cellular immune mechanisms depend upon the activity of T lymphocytes and tissue and blood phagocytes controlled by the lymphocytes. Depressed T-cell function and depressed or absent humoral antibody function results in the most serious immune-deficiency disorders, *e.g.* lymphopoenic or Swiss-type immune-deficiency syndrome. It has been more recently recognized that isolated cellular immune-deficiency may exist in the presence of an intact humoral antibody system. This isolated cellular defect (di George type) is associated with depressed or deficient thymus activity due to thymic maldevelopment or acquired disease (see also Chapter 9). One of the striking advances in immunology during the past few years has been the success in correcting this cellular immune-deficiency by the implantation of compatible thymic tissue in the tissues of such patients.

In cellular deficiency syndromes the patient suffers from chronic viral, protozoal or fungal infections, particularly due to *Candida albicans*, and children may be seen with chronic granulomatous disease or muco-cutaneous candidiasis. Hypersensitivity reactions are depressed so that skin tests such as the tuberculin test are negative, absolute lymphocyte counts show a reduction, and homografts are usually accepted.

Investigation of Cellular Immune Mechanisms

T lymphocytes have the ability to respond to antigenic and mitogenic stimulation by undergoing blast transformation, followed by mitotic division and the development of clones of specifically sensitized cells. Apart from cell division, antigen-stimulated T lymphocytes also produce a variety of products (lymphokines) that affect the function of other cells, *e.g.* macrophage chemotactic factor, macrophage migration inhibitory factor, macrophage aggregation factor, lymphotoxin and interferon. The ability to respond to mitogens and the production of a variety of lymphokines form the basis for tests of T cell activity in the body.

Tests of T Lymphocyte Activity

Skin Test Reactions. Delayed or cell-mediated hypersensitivity skin test reactions are absent or greatly diminished whenever T lymphocyte function is depressed. This is known as anergy. The test antigens mostly used are *Candida* and Streptokinase/Streptodornase as experience has shown that the majority of patients have been sensitized to these antigens. Also used is PPD in patients known to have been exposed to tuberculo-protein. Dinitrochlorobenzene (DNCB) has been shown to be antigenic and most subjects become sensitized to it seven days after injection of the sensitizing dose. The DNCB skin test is therefore extremely useful in assessing cell-mediated skin responsiveness. Anergy is a feature of patients with immune-deficiency syndromes of cellular type; it is also seen in patients with widespread malignant tumours and is a feature of sarcoidosis. Anergy may also be induced as a complication of immunosuppressive or cytotoxic therapy and, in patients so treated, may lead to systemic fungal or protozoal invasion, *e.g.* systemic candidiasis, coccidioidomycosis or *Pneumocystis carinii* infections.

Blast Transformation Test. Principle: When lymphocytes are cultured in the presence of a plant mitogen such as phytohaemagglutinin (PHA) the T cells proliferate and transform into larger blast-like cells with pale staining nuclei and basophilic cytoplasm. The blast cells may be counted directly or, following the addition of radioactive thymidine

to the culture medium, the amount of thymidine (DNA precursor) incorporated in the newly synthesized DNA is measured. Specific sensitization to a particular antigen may be demonstrated by substituting the antigen for PHA in the test and measuring the degree of blast transformation induced.

Rosette Formation Test. Principle: By a happy chance it has been found that washed sheep red cells in suspension will adhere in the cold to the membranes of T lymphocytes and form clusters or rosettes which may be counted in a haemocytometer (fig. 8). They will not adhere to B lymphocyte membranes under these conditions. The test allows of

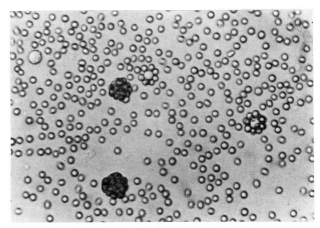

FIG. 8. T cell rosettes. × 325.

a reasonably good assessment of the percentage of T cells present in the lymphocyte population separated from the buffy cell layer of freshly taken blood. The test may also be used to monitor the effectiveness of immunosuppressive therapy in organ transplantation, *i.e.* Rosette Inhibition Test.

Leucocyte Migration Inhibition. Principle: Washed leucocytes from the buffy layer of freshly taken heparinized blood are aspirated into capillary tubes and the tubes carefully inserted into tissue culture medium in culture chambers. Normally migration of cells from the mouths of the capillary tubes is visible in 24 hr. Addition of specific antigen to the culture medium inhibits the movement of the leucocytes if the T lymphocytes are specifically sensitized to the antigen. The inhibiting substance is produced following antigen–antibody union in the medium. By means of this test, specific lymphocyte sensitization to tuberculoprotein, brucella antigen, and to a variety of tissue antigens in autoimmune disease has been demonstrated, *e.g.* ulcerative colitis, thyroiditis, primary biliary cirrhosis.

Macrophage Inhibition Test. Principle: When sensitized lymphocytes react with specific antigen some factor or factors are released which produce a slowing of macrophage movement in an electric field. The mobility rate of normal guinea-pig macrophages when mixed with the test lymphocytes is measured in a cytopherometer under phase contrast microscopy. This measurement serves as a control. The test is repeated with the addition of specific antigen and slowing ot the mobility rate confirms a specific sensitization of the test lymphocytes.

This test is particularly useful in investigating diseases with a possible autoimmune or autoallergic basis using tissue extracts as antigens.

Mixed Lymphocyte Reaction: This is a similar but possibly more sensitive assessment of immunological competence than the PHA blast transformation test. The test lymphocytes are cultured with lymphocytes from a normal histo-incompatible donor and the degree of blast transformation is measured as previously described. The donor lymphocytes are pre-treated by irradiation or mitomycin "C" to prevent a two-way reaction so that only the test lymphocytes undergo blast transformation.

FURTHER READING

Clinical Aspects of Immunology, 3rd edition (1975) (P. G. H. Gell and R. R. A. Coombs, Eds.). Oxford and Edinburgh: Blackwell Scientific Publications.

Autoimmunity—Clinical and Experimental, Anderson, J. R., Buchanan, W. W. and Goudie, R. B., American Lecture Series. Illinois U.S.A. Charles C. Thomas.

Asherson, G. L. (1972), "The Development of Lymphocyte Function Tests," *Brit. J. Hosp. Med.*, **8,** 665.

15. MECHANISMS OF BACTERIAL, VIRAL AND FUNGAL INFECTION

H. SMITH

INTRODUCTION

The proof that micro-organisms cause disease, and the subsequent recognition of the species involved, have had a dramatic effect on human affairs. The worst effects of infectious disease have been controlled in many countries by the resulting hygienic measures. However, these measures, and the drugs and vaccines which have played a significant but smaller part in controlling infection, were developed largely by empirical methods requiring little or no knowledge of the mechanisms of microbial infection. It is not surprising, therefore, that these mechanisms remain obscure. For example, effective procedures of dental hygiene are known and if applied can go far towards preventing caries and periodontal disease, but we know very little about the complex biochemical interactions of oral microbes that initiate these diseases and even less of the processes determining their persistence in chronic states.

A student might question the need to investigate mechanisms of microbial pathogenicity if the diseases can be controlled. Despite the advances of the past century, infectious disease remains a major problem in human and veterinary medicine, with the economically important nuisance and chronic aspects gaining prominence as the fatal consequences become less frequent. Drug resistance of bacteria and fungi is increasing. Effective chemotherapy of troublesome virus diseases is still lacking. Many vaccines remain unsatisfactory, either because they afford incomplete protection or because of the hazard of injecting live organisms.

The alarming increase in gonorrhoea is a current reminder of the ability of a once-regulated disease to rebound with changing social conditions. New methods of attacking infectious disease are needed and one method is to attempt to recognize and then neutralize the determinants of microbial pathogenicity.

This chapter summarizes present knowledge of microbial pathogenicity and emphasizes the gaps in this knowledge. Only broad principles will be covered and there is no special orientation to dental disease, but, where relevant, some examples are cited from this field. Bacteria form the main subjects; they have received most attention in studies of microbial pathogenicity, and although many aspects are still unexplained in biochemical terms far more is known about them than other pathogenic microbes. Furthermore, effort in the bacterial field has revealed difficulties of investigation and produced broad concepts of pathogenesis which probably apply to studies of other microbes. Towards the end of the chapter the lesser-known mechanisms of pathogenicity of viruses and fungi are discussed briefly in the context of concepts used for bacterial pathogenicity.

The nearly synonymous terms pathogenicity and virulence mean the capacity to produce disease; the former is generally used with respect to species and the latter with respect to degrees of pathogenicity of strains within a species. In the three sections that follow, a description of the methods and difficulties of research in this field form a prelude to a discussion of five main aspects of pathogenicity: (a) entry to the host by surviving on and penetrating surface membranes (or structures such as teeth); (b) multiplication *in vivo*; (c) inhibition of host defence mechanisms; (d) damage to the host; and (e) the reasons for tissue and host specificity. References for the work described and greater detail of the problems of dental disease will be found in books and reviews cited in the bibliography.

BACTERIAL PATHOGENICITY

Pathogenic bacteria are peculiarities. The great majority of bacteria are harmless and often beneficial. Obviously, pathogenic bacteria have a chemical armoury which enables them to invade a host and produce disease. The problem is to identify the weapons in this armoury, their chemical nature, mode of action and order of importance.

Methods and Difficulties of Studying the Determinants of Pathogenicity

The fact that the pathogenicity of most organisms such as oral streptococci is determined by a number of products and not a single powerful toxin as in tetanus provides one difficulty in biochemical studies. But the main factor contributing to difficulty in this field is that virulence, the disease-producing capacity of a microbial population, can be measured only *in vivo* (by determining the minimum number of organisms needed to kill half of a group of animals—LD_{50}, or to produce a lesion of a certain size), and it is markedly influenced by changes in growth conditions due to selection of types and to phenotypic change. Bacterial virulence is at its maximum in bacteria obtained directly from an infected host. Usually it is reduced by sub-culture *in vitro* because, under laboratory conditions, bacteria lose the capacity to form one or more of the full complement of virulence attributes manifested in the infected host. Also *in vitro*, apparent virulence factors might be produced which are not formed, and therefore have no relevance, *in vivo*. There is now abundant evidence for many species including streptococci, staphylococci, gonococci, anthrax bacilli and tubercle bacilli that organisms grown in infected animals are different chemically and biologically from those grown *in vitro*. Thus, although most studies are made on bacteria grown *in vitro*, such bacteria can give incomplete or misleading information as regards the possession of virulence attributes. This is the essence of the difficulties encountered in studies of pathogenicity.

How then can the various factors governing pathogenicity be identified? Obviously, these factors can be produced in laboratory cultures if the correct nutritional conditions can be found. This has already happened for the classical bacterial toxins and some antiphagocytic substances. However, for problems of pathogenicity which have defied solution by conventional procedures using cultures *in vitro*, one approach would be to study bacterial behaviour *in vivo*. There are no vitalistic leanings behind this suggestion, but merely a realistic assessment of an approach likely to reveal aspects of pathogenicity which later could be reproduced *in vitro* by appropriate changes in cultural conditions. This chapter describes several examples of virulence factors that were recognized in this way.

Information on bacterial behaviour *in vivo* can be gained by several methods. Bacteria and their products can be separated directly from the diseased host for biological examination and for chemical and serological study *in vitro*. The behaviour of organisms growing *in vivo* and their effects on the host can be examined either in the whole animal or in tissues. The largest gaps in our knowledge of pathogenicity occur here; detailed experimental pathology and precise biochemical determinations are not easily and safely accomplished during infection and only in a few cases have such detailed studies supplemented the clinical findings. Yet this information is vital, if mechanisms of pathogenicity are to be understood and relevant biological tests for potential virulence factors designed. A cardinal requirement is a suitable laboratory animal in which a natural infection of man can be simulated (*e.g.* the production of dental caries in germ-free rats by streptococci). Some light can be shed on particular phases of microbial behaviour *in vivo* by making observations in tissue or organ culture. Finally, tests *in vitro* can often be made more relevant to microbial behaviour *in vivo*.

Investigating mechanisms of pathogenicity is difficult enough when only one type of organism is involved. But clinical disease is often due to mixed infection, sometimes with organisms that are normally commensals. It is well known that one infection can have a profound effect on another, for example the promoting effect of influenza on pneumococcal and staphylococcal infections. However, the difficulties of investigation are such that we have only a superficial knowledge of the complex interactions occurring in mixed infections. Comparative experiments with single and mixed cultures must be conducted *in vitro* and *in vivo* and here there may be scope for methods already used for studying other mixed culture conditions such as those in the rumen. A few detailed investigations of mixed infections have been carried out and provide templates for future work. Invasion of the periodontal tissues, which was simulated by subcutaneous infection of guinea-pigs, occurred only in the presence of four oral organisms, namely, *Bacteroides melaninogenicus*, another bacteroides species, a motile Gram negative rod and a facultatively anaerobic diphtheroid. *B. melaninogenicus* was regarded as the primary "pathogen" and the diphtheroid produced for it an essential growth factor, vitamin K. The roles of the other two organisms have not been defined. A similar situation occurs in heel abscess of sheep where a mixture of *Corynebacterium pyogenes* and *Fusiformis necrophorus* is needed for pathogenesis. The former provides a growth factor and an anaerobic environment for the latter which produces an aggressin that prevents phagocytosis of both organisms.

Finally, a comment on the classical method of studying bacterial virulence: that is, comparing the propetires of virulent and avirulent strains. Properly used, this method of bacteriology is a powerful tool which could be applied to studies of pathogenicity of other micro-organisms. The techniques of microbial genetics have increased the scope of the method; and studies *in vitro* on enzymes, metabolic characteristics, and antigens of different bacterial strains have indicated many virulence markers, *i.e.* factors associated with virulence. Some of these factors have been shown to be virulence determinants, *i.e.* produced during infection and having biological activities directly connected with virulence, *e.g.* the power to inhibit or destroy phagocytes. Studies on virulence can benefit from a comparison of the behaviour and properties of virulent and avirulent strains, and from examinations of the influence of the products of a virulent strain on the behaviour of an avirulent strain, provided tests are carried out *in vivo* or in simulant conditions *in vitro*. These methods have been used to good effect in bacteriology in identifying cell-wall and capsular materials which inhibit humoral and cellular defence mechanisms.

Entry: Survival on and Penetration of Surfaces

Defence of surface membranes and structures against microbial attack relies on: (a) the mechanical flushing action of moving mucus or lumen contents; (b) competition with and interference by surface commensals; and (c) the presence of bactericidal or bacteriostatic materials in local secretions. These defences are overcome in infectious disease but it is important to determine how this is accomplished. Electron and light microscopy indicate at least three types of early attack on surfaces. First, bacteria attach to the surface and multiply on it but do not penetrate to any significant extent; this occurs in dental caries, in respiratory infections with *Bordetella pertussis* and in some *E. coli* enteric infections. Second, there can be attachment and subsequent phagocytosis by mucosal cells with consequent surface damage as occurs in bacillary dysentery. Finally, there can be attachment and passage into the underlying tissues either through the mucosal cells or between them as occurs in streptococcal infections such as erysipelas, in acute ulcerative gingivitis, and in enteric fever. The precise mechanisms underlying the three types of attack are not yet clear but there is much recent work on the problems.

In some cases we know a little of the nature of materials produced by bacteria which stick them to surface membranes and structures, despite the flushing action of lumen contents, thus allowing bacterial proliferation at certain sites. Two of the most prominent organisms in dental caries, *Streptococcus mutans* and *Streptococcus sanguis*, produce from sucrose *in vivo* and *in vivo* sticky glucans which are important components of dental plaque. Genetic transfer and other experiments with *E. coli* strains indicate the importance of the K88 protein antigen in attaching enteropathogenic strains to the brush border in the upper small intestine. In addition to being antiphagocytic (see below) the M protein of *Streptococcus pyogenes* may help its attachment to epithelial surfaces in the mouth and throat. Gonococci appear to adhere strongly to urethral epithelial cells and possibly this is due to thread-like projections called pili, from the gonococcal surface.

In trying to understand the complex ecology of different microbes on mucous membranes and surface structures in relation to disease, there are two essential questions to be answered. First, how do small inocula of extraneous pathogens, *e.g.* the cholera vibrio survive and grow in competition with the normal commensals? Second, in what circumstances and by what mechanisms do normal commensals adopt a pathogenic role? The second question is particularly relevant to caries and periodontal disease. Unfortunately, in most cases the answers to both questions are not known although there have been some interesting peripheral studies. Many qualitative and quantitative assessments of the different members of bacterial populations on different mucous surfaces in animals of different ages, in animals on different diets and in animals treated with antibiotics have shown that the normal flora varies with site, age and diet and that one organism can be antagonistic to another. For example, the removal of bacteria, especially lactobacilli, from the alimentary tracts of animals with penicillin usually results in an increase of *Candida* infection. The biochemical bases for these changes in flora are largely unknown. These population experiments have emphasized that the environment in many areas of mucous surfaces is anaerobic since only anaerobes survive as commensals; they have thus underlined the difficulty of aerobic pathogens initiating infection in these areas. Commensal competition with some extraneous pathogens has been investigated *in vitro* and in germ-free and normal animals and the nature

of some bacteriostatic materials is known. In a reducing environment the fatty acids produced by intestinal fusiform bacteria are inhibitory to typhoid and dysentery organisms, but how these inhibitory acids are overcome in the initial stages of dysentery and typhoid is still unknown. Concentration of potentially pathogenic commensals in one place by dietary influences may start pathogenic processes, *e.g.* the influence of a sucrose diet on dextran production by dental plaque organisms. Also, as discussed previously, the correct mixture of otherwise non-pathogenic commensals may be needed in some cases.

The manner in which pathogenic bacteria inhibit the third defence mechanism of surfaces, the bactericidal or bacteriostatic materials in local secretions (*e.g.* lysozyme) is discussed later.

Multiplication *In Vivo*

In order to produce disease, virulent bacteria must multiply in the host tissues either by increasing locally or by spreading throughout the host. Two qualities are needed for multiplication. Firstly, an inherent ability to multiply in the biochemical conditions of the host tissue and secondly, an ability to inactivate or not to stimulate host defence mechanisms which would otherwise kill or remove them. The effects of these two qualities *in vivo* are not easy to separate and often it is difficult to assess their relative importance in the increase of a single infecting population, in the interactions between mixed populations, in the differential behaviour of virulent and attenuated strains and in the different susceptibilities of tissues or hosts to infection. In this section the first quality, ability to multiply, is discussed.

Avirulence can arise from inability to grow and divide in the environment *in vivo*. Thus, nutritionally deficient mutants of pathogenic species have been shown to be avirulent unless injected with their required nutrients. However, for most bacteria the tissues and body fluids probably contain sufficient nutrients to support some growth. Few naturally occurring strains will be avirulent due solely to inability to grow in the host. Nutritional considerations will, however, affect rate of growth *in vivo*. The more rapid it is, the greater the chance of establishing the infection against the activity of the host defence mechanisms. What is known about multiplication rate *in vivo*? The numbers of viable bacteria in the tissues of an infected host can be counted at any time after inoculation, but these numbers are only the resultants of multiplication and destruction or removal. Only recently has a method been evolved for measuring true bacterial division rates *in vivo*. Pathogenic bacteria, genetically labelled with biochemical markers retained by a known proportion of the progeny at each division were used. The division rate was determined by measuring the proportion of organisms with the marker at various times after inoculation into animals. Remarkable results were obtained. In the spleens of mice *Salmonella typhimurium* divided at only 5–10 per cent of the maximum rate *in vitro*. This type of approach may be used for measuring true division rates of other microbes *in vivo*. Examples will be given later of how variation in the biochemical conditions for bacterial multiplication can explain some instances of tissue preference of pathogenic bacteria.

Inhibition of Host Defence Mechanisms

To increase within the host tissues, metabolic ability to multiply in the nutritional environment is not enough. Pathogenic bacteria must also be able to inhibit host defence mechanisms which otherwise would destroy them. The bacterial compounds which inhibit these mechanisms are called "aggressins", an old term which well describes their biological role.

Aggressins act in the decisive, primary lodgement period of infection, that is, during the first hours when the few invading bacteria are most vulnerable to the protective reaction of the host. At this early stage, aggressins must inhibit non-specific bactericidal mechanisms; not only those already existing in or on the tissues but also those agencies, especially phagocytic cells that are mobilized by inflammatory processes soon after the tissues are stimulated. If some bacteria survive the primary lodgement and grow, spread of infection is opposed by the fixed phagocytes of the reticulo-endothelial system (lymph nodes, spleen, liver); and again to make headway bacteria need aggressins, possibly different from those operating during the early lodgement phase. To break through the protection of previously immunized animals, or of animals several days after infection, bacteria must either be numerous or well-endowed with aggressins since the host defence mechanisms are of increased efficiency and are supplemented by antibodies capable of direct neutralization of microbial products. The clinical outcome of the disease depends on the interplay between the bacterial aggressins and the defensive reactions of the host; this outcome varies from complete subjugation of the host to complete destruction of the bacteria and includes the shifting balance that exists in chronic infections such as periodontal disease.

Inhibitors of Blood and Tissue Bactericidins

Body fluids (such as blood, saliva, mucus) and tissue contain a variety of bactericidal factors such as basic polypeptides, lysozyme, complement (acting with antibody or possibly non-specific substances), and perhaps a system involving the iron-binding protein transferrin. Since clearly there are several different types of bactericidins, virulent bacteria must produce different type of aggressins to inhibit them. Resistance to these bactericidins has been associated with virulence in strains of many bacterial species such as streptococci, enteric pathogens, staphylococci, anthrax bacilli, brucellosis bacilli and recently gonococci isolated directly from patients and tested without subculture. But only rarely have the aggressins been chemically identified. Those from anthrax bacilli are capsular poly-D-glutamic acid and the three-component anthrax toxin. Resistance of *Brucella abortus* to the bactericidal action of bovine serum is due to a cell-wall component containing protein, carbohydrate, formyl residues and much (35–42 per cent) lipid. The acid polysaccharide K antigens of *E. coli* act in a similar manner.

Inhibitors of the Action of Phagocytes

Once a microbe has penetrated into the tissues the phagocytic activity of the wandering and fixed cells of the reticulo-

endothelial system forms the main protective mechanism of the body: a mechanism which acts nonspecifically but which is greatly enhanced by immunization. Phagocytes vary in origin, morphology, constituents and bactericidal function. There are two main types, each having two subdivisions: polymorphonuclear (neutrophils and eosinophils) and mononuclear (blood monocytes and tissue macrophages). Polymorphonuclear phagocytes are end cells with a short life; they are derived from different stem cells from the long-lived mononuclear phagocytes. Inflammatory exudates contain cells of all types, the polymorphonuclear cells predominating initially but later dying to leave the mononuclear phagocytes in the majority. Macrophages form the fixed phagocytic system in the lymph-nodes, spleen and liver.

Phagocytosis of bacteria involves three stages, contact, ingestion and intra-cellular killing and digestion. Virulent bacteria may produce aggressins which inhibit any of these stages.

Inhibitors of Contact. Contact with bacteria is effected by random hits, by trapping on uneven surfaces in confined tissue spaces, by filtration systems in lymph nodes, spleen, and liver and by chemotaxis. Bacterial products could hardly interfere with the mechanical processes, but they can inhibit chemotaxis. Certain fractions from tubercle bacilli and a cell wall material from staphylococci inhibit leucocyte migration.

Inhibitors of Ingestion. Ingestion of bacteria involves engulfment within a phagocytic vacuole—the phagosome —the wall of which is derived by invagination of the phagocyte membrane. Specific and non-specific opsonins (serum factors) enhance this process of ingestion. Once inside phagocytes, many bacteria (*e.g.* streptococci, pneumococci and meningococci) are rapidly killed and digested. Resistance to ingestion thus avoiding intracellular bactericidins, is therefore essential for the survival of virulent strains of these species. Aggressins that inhibit ingestion fall into two main types: surface and capsular products which do not harm phagocytes, and toxic materials producing direct damage. Examples of the first are the capsular polysaccharides of pneumococci, the cell-wall M protein and capsular hyaluronic acid of streptococci, the capsular poly-D-glutamic acid of *Bacillus anthracis* and the O-somatic antigens of some Gram negative organisms. Dextrans and levans also prevent ingestion by phagocytes and these materials produced by *Strep. mutans*, *Strep. sanguis* and *Strep. salivarius* may play a contributory part in the development of dental disease. An example of a toxic aggressin is the leucocidin of staphylococci.

Investigations of the relation between structure and antiphagocytic activity have begun using the known chemical structure of the O antigens of mutants of the enterobacteriaceae. Resistance of *E. coli* to phagocytosis by mouse polymorphonuclear leucocytes appears to depend on a complete saccharide component of the cell-wall lipopolysaccharide; a mutant lacking only colitose in its side chain was significantly more susceptible to phagocytosis (and less virulent) than the wild type, and a mutant lacking galactose, glucose, N-acetyl glucosamine and colitose was even more so. Similarly, work with mutants and with media inducing phenotypic change has indicated that not only a complete sugar sequence in the core but also a complete O-specific polysaccharide side chain in the O antigens are necessary for full phagocytosis resistance and virulence of *Salmonella typhimurium* for mice; the tetrasaccharide sequences absequosyl-mannosyl-rhamnosyl-galactose have been suggested as the determinant group, acetyl and glucosyl groups being less important.

Although knowledge of the connection between structure and aggressive activity is developing, the mode of action of these aggressins is still not clear. Non-toxic aggressins may interfere with ingestion by purely mechanical means, by inhibiting the adsorption of serum opsonin as seems to occur for *B. anthracis* and staphylococci, and possibly by rendering the bacterial surface less foreign to the host. Toxic aggressins probably harm phagocytes in the same way as they affect ordinary cells; for example, interference with membrane function by the leucocidin of staphylococci.

Inhibitors of Intracellular Bactericidins; Promotion of Intracellular Growth. When bacteria are phagocytosed, granules from the cytoplasm of the phagocyte discharge into the phagosome. The granules contain the bactericidins which normally kill and digest phagocytosed organisms. Virulent strains of some bacteria resist the phagocytic bactericidins which destroy other bacteria and thus they can survive or grow intracellularly. Within the cells, the bacteria are protected from natural and injected antibacterial agents and hence they produce diseases which are often chronic and beset with the complications of hypersensitivity. Tubercle bacilli, leprosy bacilli and brucellae are the typical "intracellular" pathogens and ability to grow within phagocytic and other cells is probably the most important aspect of the pathogenicity of these bacteria. It can be seen both in infected animals and in cell maintenance culture *in vitro*. In addition, bacteria whose virulence is determined in part by resistance to phagocytic ingestion can, when ingested under certain circumstances, survive and grow intracellularly. Examples are salmonellae, shigellae and staphylococci.

Although much has been learned of the many and different bactericidal mechanisms of polymorphonuclear and monocytic phagocytes practically nothing is known of what happens to the bacteria when they are killed by these mechanisms. However, studies of how virulent intracellular pathogens resist the phagocytic bactericidins have begun. By making observations first on brucellae isolated directly from infected animals, a cell-wall antigen from virulent brucellae has been recognized which inhibits the bactericidal action of bovine phagocytes as evidenced by promotion of increased survival and growth of an attenuated strain of brucellae in phagocytes pretreated with preparations containing the virulence antigen. It appears that virulent tubercle bacilli inhibit intracellular bactericidal mechanisms by preventing phagocytic granules discharging into phagosomes, whereas leprosy bacilli allow the discharge but are unaffected by the liberated bactericidins; the aggressins responsible are unknown.

Damaging the Host

There are two methods whereby pathogenic bacteria can damage the host, directly by the production of poisons or toxins and indirectly by sensitizing the host to bacterial products so that subsequent immunological reactions of the host cause tissue damage.

Bacterial Toxins

This is the one area in microbial pathogenicity where biochemical studies in depth have been made both on the nature of the toxins and their mode of action at cellular and subcellular levels. Only the main outlines and a few highlights can be covered here. The toxic activities of bacteria can be divided into five categories.

(i) **Toxins Responsible for Non-infectious Disease Because They are Produced in Food.** The toxin of *Clostridium botulinum* and the enterotoxin of staphylococci are the main examples. The disease that occurs on ingestion of infected food material is a chemical poisoning. It is not an infectious process but clearly the microbial toxin is responsible. Botulinum toxin is a protein neurotoxin acting on the autonomic system by interfering with acetylcholine synthesis or release. Staphylococcal enterotoxin is the one microbial toxin for which a full amino acid sequence is available.

(ii) **Toxins of Over-riding Importance in Infectious Disease.** *Clostridium tetani* and *Corynebacterium diptheriae* produce *in vitro* powerful exotoxins which have been well characterized. These toxins are produced *in vivo* and are responsible for almost the whole disease syndrome. Both are proteins with no toxic moieties or abnormal aminoacids. Tetanus toxin is a neurotoxin acting on the brain and diphtheria toxin interferes with protein synthesis. Immunization with toxoid (formalin treated, detoxified toxin) protects against disease.

(iii) **Toxins Which Are Significant But Not the Only Factors Responsible for Infectious Disease.** These toxins were originally recognized in cultures *in vitro* and then shown to be produced *in vivo*. They can be responsible for some pathological effects of infection. However, they are not the sole determinants of disease for often as much toxin is produced by avirulent as by virulent strains, sometimes injection of toxin does not produce all the pathological effects of disease, and usually immunization with toxoid does not confer complete protection against infection. Some can be small molecular materials: examples are the collagenase of *Bacteroides melaninogenicus* which may destroy the structural fibres in periodontal disease and the α-toxin of staphylococci which is dermonecrotic and haemolytic. Perhaps the most important representatives of these toxins are the endotoxins, lipopolysaccharides intimately associated with the cell-walls of many different Gram-negative bacteria. When extracted from cell-walls by fairly drastic means (treatment with trichloracetic acid or warm aqueous phenol) and injected into animals they produce toxic manifestations—pyrexia, diarrhoea, prostration and death. In some infections, there is little doubt that endotoxins are liberated from the cell-wall of the invading bacteria and are responsible for pathological effects, such as pyrexia, leucopenia, shock and death in typhoid fever. On the other hand, in some diseases the pathological effects are due to easily liberated toxins and not cell-wall endotoxins which are never liberated from the cell-wall in significant quantities.

(iv) Toxins Produced *In Vitro* But of Unknown Importance in Disease. Many substances, producing toxic effects related or unrelated to disease syndromes, have been isolated from cultures. Some of these products may be laboratory artefacts having no relevance to disease *in vivo*. Even if formed *in vivo*, the question is whether they play significant roles in infection. Examples are some of the many enzymic and haemolytic products of streptococci and staphylococci.

(v) Hitherto Unknown Toxins Recognized By Studying Bacterial Behaviour *In Vivo* or in Biological Tests Relevant to the Disease. Several important bacterial toxins have been recognized in this way. The first was the anthrax toxic complex now generally accepted as the cause of death in anthrax; it was found originally in the plasma of guinea-pigs that had just died of anthrax. Later it was reproduced *in vitro*, purified and shown to consist of three synergistically acting components, two proteins and one a metal chelating agent containing protein, some carbohydrate and phosphorus.

In the past decade there have been spectacular advances in our understanding of the role of toxins in the acute diarrhoeal diseases of man and animals, the so-called "enterotoxic enteropathies". This has been due to discarding mouse toxicity tests for other biological and animal tests in which organisms and their products were put into the gut lumen and their effects in this site observed. Investigations on cholera formed the template for those on other diseases.

An enterotoxin from *Vibrio cholerae*, responsible for the gross and fatal fluid loss from the intestine which occurs in cholera, was recognized by using two tests. Firstly, a ligated segment of small intestine in a living rabbit would fill with fluid following intra-luminal injection of *V. cholerae* and its products. Secondly, *V. cholerae* and its products caused fluid accumulation and diarrhoea in sucking rabbits when introduced into the gut lumen by a gastric tube. The extra-cellular enterotoxin has been purified and its mode of action studied. It is a heat labile, trypsin resistant, antigenic protein with a molecular weight of 90,000; it is different from the cell-wall endotoxin. It acts by increasing the normal secretion of the small intestine, possibly by activating adenyl cyclase present in the intestinal epithelial membrane, thereby raising intra-cellular cyclic adenosine monophosphate (CAMP) levels which in turn would affect electrolyte transport. Simple replacement of fluid and electrolytes usually leads to rapid and complete recovery from the disease.

Using similar "gut reaction" tests, enterotoxins have now been demonstrated for the following diarrhoea-producing organisms: certain strains of *E. coli* (scours in young pigs and calves, and diarrhoea in babies; enterotoxin production is plasmid-transmitted and the enterotoxin activates adenyl cyclase), *Vibrio parahaemolyticus* (a marine vibrio which in the summer causes the majority of the food-poisoning cases in Japan), *Clostridium perfringens* (food poisoning in man) and *Shigella dysenteriae* (human dysentery).

These recent discoveries of relevant toxins in several important diseases are a warning against attributing damage in other microbial disease to causes other than direct toxicity until the possible production of toxins has been thoroughly investigated using realistic biological tests.

The Role of Immunopathology in Bacterial Disease. Although usually protective, the immunological reactions of the host can sometimes have unpleasant consequences. Classical work with *Mycobacterium tuberculosis* in guinea-pigs showed that hypersensitivity to bacterial products can be dangerous and even fatal for the host. Furthermore, skin tests show that hypersensitive states occur in many bacterial diseases. The hypersensitive reactions are usually of the delayed type, indicating that cellular mechanisms are involved, but antibody-mediated, Arthus-type reactions can also occur, *e.g.* against bacterial polysaccharides. Thus, potentially in many diseases, non-toxic bacterial products could produce harm by evoking hypersensitivity reactions. But, just as production of a toxin *in vitro* does not necessarily mean that it is relevant *in vivo*, mere demonstration of a state of hypersensitivity by a skin test is no proof of the implication of hypersensitivity reactions in the main pathological effects of the disease. More extensive investigations are needed; the main systemic and local effects of the disease must be simulated by hypersensitivity reactions evoked in a sensitized host by products of the appropriate microbe. The prolonged work on tuberculosis and rheumatic fever emphasizes the difficulties of obtaining precise biochemical knowledge in this field. There seems little doubt now that the pathological changes seen in tuberculosis are largely due to hypersensitivity to the products, particularly the waxes, of *M. tuberculosis*. Hypersensitivity also appears to play a role in the cardiac and kidney lesions following infection with streptococci, although acute effects seem to be due to direct toxicity of streptococcal products on the susceptible tissues.

Tissue and Host Specificity in Bacterial Infections

Why, in man, do *Strep. mutans*, diphtheria bacilli, pneumococci and meningococci show predilections for the teeth, throat, lung and meninges respectively? Why is gonorrhoea confined to man and Johne's disease to cattle and related species? The two most likely explanations for differences in susceptibility to infection between different tissues or hosts, are differing distributions of bactericidal mechanisms and differing distributions of nutrients for which the metabolism of the parasite is especially adapted. Despite much effort, attempts to lay the responsibility for specificities of single infections unequivocally on variation of defined bactericidal mechanisms have so far failed. There is some evidence however, that kidney tissue is prone to a number of infections due to inhibition of complement and of phagocytosis by the high pH and salt concentrations respectively in this site.

More success has been achieved in investigations of the influence of nutrition. *Corynebacterium renale* and *Proteus mirabilis* persist in and cause severe damage to the kidney of cattle and man respectively. These localizations appear to be due to the possession of ureases which enable the bacteria to use urea for growth and for the production of ammonia which damages the tissue. Brucellosis in many animals (*e.g.* man, rats, guinea-pigs and rabbits) is a relatively mild and chronic disease; the causative organisms do not grow prolifically and have no marked affinity for particular tissues. However, in pregnant cows, sheep, goats and sows there is an enormous growth of brucellae in the placentae, the fetal fluids and the chorions, leading to the characteristic climax of the disease—abortion. The presence of erythritol, a growth stimulant for brucellae, in tissues of susceptible species explains this tissue specificity in brucellosis. *Strep. mutans* and *Strep. sanguis* localize in dental plaque in part because of a nutritional influence, that of sucrose in the diet. In this instance, however, the cause is not so much a direct stimulation of growth, as in the two examples above, but the production of polyglucans which enhance the ability of the organisms to adhere to certain surfaces. Polyglucans may also contribute to the localization of these organisms on damaged heart-valves in endocarditis.

A recent example of host resistance being determined by nutritional influences involves Brazilian strains of the plague bacillus. These did not kill guinea-pigs which are killed by normal strains because, unlike the latter, they require asparagine to grow well and guinea-pig serum contains a powerful asparaginase.

VIRUSES

Viruses differ from other microbes in having a unique method of replication. But viral like bacterial pathogenicity is not determined solely by biochemical ability to replicate in the host tissues. Virulent and attenuated strains replicate in host cells *in vitro* yet they differ fundamentally in behaviour *in vivo*, presumably—as for bacteria—due to different capacities to counteract host defence mechanisms and to damage tissues. Also, the fact that viral factors responsible for virulence mechanisms are induced within host cells does not confer uniqueness on viral pathogenicity; although replicating by different processes many pathogenic microbes, including bacteria, are intracellular parasites producing their virulence factors intracellularly.

Studies on mechanisms of virus pathogenicity suffer the same difficulties as in the bacterial field, namely, that pathogenicity is determined by more than one factor and can only be studied *in vivo*, where viruses often behave differently from the way they do in the more convenient tissue culture systems. In addition, the first essential for studying the subject, quantitative comparison of the virulence of different strains, is inaccurate. Disease effects in animals (LD_{50}; lesion size) must be related to amounts of virus particles indicated by, for example, plaque formation or egg infection. These assays detect only a small proportion of the total virus particles and therefore may not measure the number of particles capable of multiplying in the experimental animals. Hence, only strains for which the presently available tests have indicated the greatest possible difference in virulence should be compared to recognize virulence markers and determinants. Only in a few virus systems, such as Newcastle disease virus, are such strains available.

Early virus attack of the respiratory tract has received some attention and the site of membrane lesions and the preferentially attacked cell types have been observed in Newcastle disease of chickens and influenza of experimental animals and man. Nevertheless, there appear to be few deeper investigations, for example, on the influence of oxygen tension, temperature, pH, commensals and mucus on virus survival on, and replication in, membranes; and also on the mechanisms of entry of various viruses into the particular epithelial cells they select for attack.

A virulent virus must be able to replicate in host cells and to spread from one to another; any change in these abilities will almost certainly result in changes in virulence. Investigations of the biochemistry of virus replication in animals are complicated by the obligate parasitism involved, which not only entails complexity of the factors required for replication but increases the difficulty of distinguishing the influence of their absence from that of host factors (defence mechanisms) which actually destroy virus or inhibit replication. The ability of a virus to replicate in a particular cell depends on inherent features of that cell. These features can be involved in one or more stages of replication; attachment and penetration of virus, uncoating, provision of energy and precursors of low molecular weight, synthesis of viral nucleic acid and proteins, assembly and release. The characteristics of the host cell which determine these stages of replication might be called "replication factors" and seem to be the counterparts in virology of such environmental factors as low molecular weight nutrients, necessary for bacterial multiplication in host tissues or fluids. Tissue culture experiments show that "replication factors" vary from cell type to cell type and are influenced by changes in the environment of the cell. In animal infection, variation in the availability of "replication factors" in particular hosts or tissues and under different conditions will affect virus pathogenicity. Attenuated viruses may have a decreased capacity to use the factors. But few investigations of the influence of such factors comparable in depth to the experiments in tissue culture, have been conducted either in animals or organ culture. Nevertheless, there are signs of this influence in the available studies. There is some parallel between the ability of homogenates of various primate tissues to attach polio-virus and their susceptibility to virus replication and damage in infection, and some attenuated strains attach to susceptible nerve tissue less strongly than virulent strains. The effect of temperature on virus virulence probably reflects a temperature sensitivity of the enzymes used in virus synthesis rather than an influence on host defence mechanisms. And virus replication *in vivo* can be affected by low molecular-weight materials; vaccinia virus infection of mice, like that in cell culture, is enhanced by injection of leucine.

There has been much work on host defence against viruses but very little on the mechanisms whereby viruses overcome this defence. Host defence includes inhibitors in serum, interferon (a virus inhibitor induced in host cells) and macrophages, but polymorphonuclear leucocytes may be less important than in bacterial infections. In the immunized host, or several days after primary infection, antibody and cellular immunity play their part. It is clear that virulent viruses inhibit, or do not induce, host defence mechanisms. Virulent strains of influenza virus resist serum inhibitors more than avirulent strains and virulent strains of some, but not all viruses, induce less interferon formation than avirulent strains. Macrophages are more readily infected by virulent than avirulent strains of some viruses. But what virion constituents or virus-induced products determine the superior resistance to host defence or virulent strains? Is some peculiarity of the envelope protein responsible for interference with serum and phagocyte inhibitors? Could host nucleases (which could destroy an invading virus) be inhibited by a particular folding of the viral nucleic acid or by an internal protein? What chemical difference determines induction of interferon by an avirulent strain in contrast to a virulent strain? Some viruses, such as Newcastle disease virus, appear to produce interferon antagonists, and these may be the viral counterparts of the bacterial aggressins.

Viruses produce cytopathic effects in cells both in tissue culture and in disease. These effects could result from a passive role of the virus; cells might burst after acting merely as hosts for virus replication or they might die from the profound re-direction of metabolic processes required by such replication. Cell damage might also occur as a consequence of cessation of host cell macromolecular synthesis, and even by direct "toxic" action of viral products. Thus, massive doses of some viruses, such as influenza and pox viruses, produce rapid toxic effects in animals and virion components such as the penton of adenovirus produce morphological damage in tissue culture. Furthermore, in tissue cultures of polio-virus, Newcastle disease virus and vaccinia virus, replication of virus is not essential for cytopathic effects which require, however, virus-induced protein synthesis. Evidence is increasing that the virus-induced proteins which accompany these cytopathic effects are cytotoxins. Virus-free products from HeLa cells infected with vaccinia virus have produced cytotoxic effects in fresh uninfected HeLa cells in the presence of magnesium sulphate solution to increase membrane permeability, thus allowing entry of the virus products. Hypersensitivity also enters into the pathology of virus infections and auto-allergic sensitization of the host to host components is more likely to occur in virus infections than in bacterial disease because many viruses incorporate host components into their structure. Deciding whether evocation of hypersensitivity reactions or direct toxicity is responsible for the main pathological effects of virus disease is not made easier by the present lack of knowledge of virus toxicity. Nevertheless, clinical observations and experimental studies in which pathological effects of virus diseases have been provoked or made worse by introducing into an infected host antibody or immune cells, indicate that hypersensitivity or autoallergic reactions may be involved in the pathology of encephalitis and rashes in man and lymphocytic choriomeningitis in mice.

Tissue and host specificities occur in virus infections and are largely unexplained. Variation of host defence mechanisms and variation of "replication factors" from tissue to tissue and host to host are the most likely reasons for the phenomena. Only in the classical work on polio-virus is

there clear-cut evidence. The susceptibility of appropriate (brain, anterior horn of spinal chord, intestine) primate tissues and the resistance of non-primate and some primate tissues to infection with polio-virus was correlated with the presence and absence of surface receptors. If the receptors were by-passed by using infectious polio-virus nucleic acid the virus grew in "resistant" tissues.

FUNGI

Examples of common diseases caused by fungi are thrush, "athlete's foot", "farmer's lung", and mycotic abortion. Some have mycelial (arthrospore) and yeast forms differing in virulence and thus they seem particularly appropriate for comparative studies which might reveal mechanisms of virulence. A quantitative comparison of the virulence of yeast and arthrospore forms should be relatively easy, since both forms are easily counted *in vitro*. Nevertheless, we know little about fungal pathogenicity; this perhaps is due more to lack of study than to the difficulty of such studies.

Antifungal mechanisms operative on mucous and other body surfaces include inhibitory activity of bacterial commensals (since antibiotic treatment can result in fungal infection) and fungistatic materials in various secretions such as those of the conjunctiva and saliva, and the fatty acids in teat secretions of domestic animals. Within the tissues, humoral antifungal factors including complement have been noted, and killing by phagocytosis also appears important in resistance to some mycoses. The factors which determine the survival of fungi on mucous membranes are not known, nor are those which determine replication in animal tissues. Many fungi are larger than phagocytes and mere size may prevent ingestion, so that rapid growth alone can be an aggressive mechanism. A capsular polysaccharide prevents the phagocytic ingestion of virulent strains of *Cryptococcus neoformans* whilst *Candida albicans* and *Histoplasma capsulatum* like brucellae and tubercle bacilli can survive and grow within phagocytes. Inhibition of intracellular killing may be due to fungal aggressins comparable to those produced by brucellae. Production of aggressins may be related to yeast forms; the non-invasive mycelial dermatophytes probably lack the powerful aggressins of the yeast-like fungi causing the deeper mycoses.

In some mycotic diseases, mechanical blockage by large mycelia probably damages the host. Fungi produce, in foodstuffs, powerful toxins such as aflatoxin and sporidesmin. The chemical constitutions of these toxins are known and their actions in various hosts have been studied. Nevertheless, at present they are comparable to botulinum toxin in being produced outside the host and only being proved responsible for a non-infectious disease. They may well be produced in mycotic infections but this has yet to be demonstrated. Peptidases, collagenase and elastase appear to be involved in dermatophyte damage but hypersensitivity to ill-defined glycopeptide cell-wall products probably explains to a large degree the lesions of most fungal skin diseases. Whether or not hypersensitivity is an important factor in oral or deeper mycoses is largely a matter of speculation.

Recently one example of tissue specificity in fungal infections, namely the growth of *Aspergillus fumigatus* in placental tissue, which causes mycotic abortion in ewes and cattle, may have been shown to have a nutritional basis. A material which stimulates spore germination is concentrated in bovine placenta but its nature is yet unknown.

This survey over the field of mechanisms of microbial pathogenicity shows that much remains to be learned, especially in regard to microbes other than bacteria.

BIBLIOGRAPHY

Ajl, S. J., Kadis, S. and Montie, T. C. (1970), *Microbial Toxins*. London and New York: Academic Press.
Burnett, G. W. and Scherp, W. W. (1968), *Oral Microbiology and Infectious Disease*, 3rd edition. Baltimore: The Williams and Wilkins Co.
Dubos, R. J. and Hirsch, J. G. (1965), *Bacterial and Mycotic Infections of Man*, 4th edition. Philadelphia: Lippincott.
Dunlop, R. H. and Moon, H. W. (1970), *Resistance to Infectious Disease*. Saskatoon: Modern Press.
Howie, J. W. and O'Hea, A. J. (1955), *Mechanisms of Microbial Pathogenicity*. Cambridge: Cambridge University Press.

Mims, C. A. (1964), "Aspects of the Pathogenesis of Virus Disease,' *Bact. Rev.*, **28**, 30.
Smith, H. (1960), "The Biochemical Response to Bacterial Injury," in *Biochemical Response to Injury*, p. 341. Oxford and Edinburgh: Blackwell.
Smith, H. (1968), "The Biochemical Challenge of Microbial Pathogenicity," *Bact. Rev.*, **32**, 164.
Smith, H. (1972), "Mechanisms of Virus Pathogenicity," *Bact. Rev.*, **36**, 291.
Smith, H. (1975), "Microbial Interference with Host Defence Mechanisms," in *Prophylaxis of Infectious and Other Diseases* in *Monographs in Allergy* Vol. 9 Basel: Karger.
Smith, H. and Pearce, J. H. (1972), *Microbial Pathogenicity in Man and Animals*. Cambridge: Cambridge University Press.
Smith, H. and Taylor, J. (1964), *Microbial Behaviour* In Vivo *and* In Vitro. Cambridge: Cambridge University Press.
Smith, W. (1963), *Mechanisms of Virus Infection*. London and New York: Academic Press.
Tamm, I. and Horsfall, F. L. (1965), *Viral and Rickettsial Infections of Man*, 4th edition. Philadelphia: Lippincott.
Wilson, G. S. and Miles, A. A. (1964), *Topley and Wilson's Principles of Bacteriology and Immunity*, 5th edition. London: Edward Arnold.

16. PRINCIPLES OF STERILIZATION AND DISINFECTION

E. M. DARMADY

Sterilization by steam
  Downward displacement steam sterilizer
  Pre-vacuum high pressure steam sterilizer
  Sterilizing cycle
  Methods for testing steam sterilizers
    Instrument sterilizer
    Dressing sterilizer

Sterilization by dry heat
  Hot air ovens
  Conveyor oven
  Sterilizing cycle
  Methods for testing dry heat sterilizers
    Use of Brown tubes

Other methods of sterilization
  Formaldehyde
  Ethylene oxide
  Boiling water
  Hot oil

Use of chemical agents
  For application to skin
  For application to oral mucous membrane
  Sterilants
  Disinfectants

Special problems
  Instruments
  Infectious hepatitis

INTRODUCTION

The terms sterilization and disinfection have been variously defined by many previous authors. However, it has now been generally accepted that sterilization should be defined as the destruction of all forms of life, including sporing forms of micro-organism such as *Clostridium tetani* as well as the pathogenic viruses, whilst disinfection on the other hand is a method of destroying pathogenic vegetative or non-sporing organisms. In the past, this latter process has been largely associated with chemical agents (disinfectants), but recent work has shown that other methods such as heat are more reliable. In practice, most articles have to be packaged prior to sterilization in such a way as to prevent the penetration of organisms before use. Disinfection, on the other hand, is usually concerned with the destruction of pathogenic organisms on instruments immediately after use to prevent the transfer of such organisms to the patient or even the operator.

In recent years another group of organisms has come to the fore—in particular the virus of hepatitis which is found in the blood of carriers and which, if transferred to a susceptible patient or operator, can produce severe jaundice or hepatitis some 60–100 days later. Some of these patients can be detected, and are known as Australia antigen positive; their blood should always be handled with special precautions (*see* p. 195). Although the virus is not perhaps as difficult to destroy as the sporing organism, precise information on this point is not available. It has been established that minute quantities of body fluids or blood from a carrier can be introduced via an abrasion or by injection, and are capable of causing hepatitis. For example, the use of improperly sterilized syringes for local anaesthesia in dentistry has been followed by hepatitis. Of the 15 cases reported in one series, 3 were fatal (Foley and Gutheim, 1956).

GENERAL CONSIDERATIONS

The most successful method of sterilization and disinfection is by heat, with or without steam. Chemical agents are often suggested as disinfectants or sterilants, but their killing power varies enormously and often unpredictably, with changes of concentration, temperature, pH, and in the presence of blood, pus or body fluids. Some gases, particularly formaldehyde, when combined with low temperature steam, provide both sterilization and disinfection conditions. Ethylene oxide is another agent which may be useful for sterilization of thermolabile materials, but requires careful control of temperature, humidity and exposure time. The gas is inactivated by serum, blood or biological fluids. Probably its principal value is for sterilization of articles manufactured from plastics, or fabrics which are relatively free from organisms at manufacture, and where the conditions can be adequately controlled while speed is not a major factor.

Another method which is suitable for manufactured thermolabile goods such as rubber gloves or catheters, syringes and various plastics, is sterilization by ionizing radiation produced either by degradation of a radioactive isotope such as cobalt 60 or by high energy electrons produced by linear accelerators. However, these methods are appropriate to factory conditions rather than hospital practice, so that suitably packed sterilized articles are provided by manufacturers. Finally, although boiling of instruments or syringes is widely practised, it cannot be considered reliable or satisfactory as a method of sterilization or disinfection.

The reason why vegetative organisms are more susceptible to destruction by heat is that about four-fifths of their substance consists of water, which is enclosed in an envelope containing a colloidal suspension of protein in a solution of salts. If such a system is heated in a moist atmosphere at a comparatively low temperature (less than 100°C), the equilibrium of capsular colloidal suspension is upset, the protein coagulated, and the organism destroyed. Thus it is found that the vegetative organism can be destroyed by moist heat at 80°C for 1 min., whilst the spores which contain less water can withstand temperatures of 120°C for the same length of time, and indeed are only killed when exposed to this temperature in moist heat for approximately 10 min. Therefore, both sterilization and disinfection depend upon a time-temperature relationship, provided of course the temperature is not too low, and is capable of upsetting the colloidal suspension to an extent that leads to death of the organism. Furthermore, it will also vary with the type of condition obtaining. For example, when organisms are exposed to moist heat, the temperature required is considerably less than when dry heat is used; it must, however, be remembered that steam can only destroy organisms if it comes into direct contact: for example, steam is unsuitable for the sterilization of an assembled syringe or articles enclosed in a sealed tube, where steam cannot penetrate to all the surfaces.

STERILIZATION BY STEAM

Steam has certain properties which must be understood if steam sterilizers are to be operated successfully. The temperature at which water boils depends on the pressure to which it is subjected; thus the higher the pressure, the higher the temperature of the steam. For this reason a vessel which will withstand high steam pressure is required to produce the conditions necessary to kill spores.

Two other conditions are required to ensure sterilization. Firstly the steam must be at its "boundary phase", that is to say the temperature of the steam must be at a point when it will condense from vapour to liquid, releasing its latent heat as soon as it comes into contact with any object which is at a slightly lower temperature. If steam under pressure is heated in a chamber to a temperature above that of its boundary phase, it is said to be in a state of "superheat". This will prevent it from condensing and thus cause a failure of sterilization. Such conditions sometimes prevail in a chamber where the surrounding jacket is at higher temperature. Secondly, the steam must be pure and contain the minimum quantity of air. For example, if the sterilizer chamber is closed and steam at 15 lb. pressure of 121°C admitted, none of the residual air having been removed, the temperature will be only 100°C. If half the air is removed then the temperature will be 112°C. This will mean either that sterilization could not be carried out or that a long exposure would be required. Furthermore, as steam and air do not mix readily, layering may occur with the result that the temperature may vary from one part of the chamber to another. The presence of air in the chamber has also another disadvantage, in that it will prevent steam penetrating into the load of dressings since it acts not only as an insulator but also becomes entrapped within the dressings. The thicker or more tightly packed these are, the more difficult will the removal of air become. It is therefore seen that the removal of air from the chamber is the first essential to successful sterilization. How this is to be done is largely a question of the type of equipment to be sterilized. For this reason, two types of sterilizer are available.

Downward Displacement Steam Sterilizer

Earlier it was stressed that steam can only kill organisms if it comes into direct contact with objects to be sterilized or disinfected. In this piece of equipment, steam under pressure is introduced at the top of the chamber and pushes the air downwards through a vent at the bottom. At the same time, during the course of the process, steam will condense to water and collect at the bottom of the chamber lowering its temperature. To remove the condensate and the air, either a continuous steam bleed or a near-to-steam trap is fitted to the discharge line at the base of the chamber. The near-to-steam trap is operated either by bellows or a spring which, when cooled, contracts and opens the valve, allowing water and the air to be discharged. As soon as this is completed, the steam restores the temperature and the valve shuts. It is important that the valve closes at the correct steam temperature, and for this reason a temperature measuring device is fitted to the discharge line which in turn controls the sterilizing cycle (see later). In sterilizers of this type a partial vacuum can be obtained by means of a steam injector or venturi tube which helps to quicken the discharge of air or steam. This type of apparatus is particularly useful for surface sterilization or disinfection of unwrapped instruments such as are commonly used in dentistry. It is not entirely suitable for the sterilization of fabrics since the penetration rate of the steam may be variable and will result in delay and uncertainty in reaching the sterilizing temperature.

A variation in the design of the small downward displacement steam sterilizer is that fitted with its own distilled water reservoir which in turn feeds a chamber connected to the sterilizing chamber which has its own immersion heater. As soon as the steam is generated the chamber is shut, the cycle started and the air and excess water discharged through special safety valves. When the steam achieves the desired sterilizing temperature (usually 134°C) the timing device commences. At the end of exposure time, a valve opens and the excess steam is then discharged to the water reservoir where it condenses for re-use, and the immersion heaters cut off.

This machine is particularly suitable for sterilization or disinfection of dental instruments and where there is no piped steam supply.

Prevacuum High Pressure Steam Sterilizer
(Dressings Sterilizer)

A reliable method of removing air from the centre of packages, particularly dressings, was first described by Knox and Penikitt (1958) who showed that an initial vacuum of 20 mm. Hg absolute allowed an instantaneous penetration of steam to all parts of the load. They also showed that provided a vacuum of 20 mm. absolute had been obtained the temperature taken in the discharge line gave an exact indication of the temperature achieved in the load and, as a result, a shortened cycle of sterilization could be obtained.

However, over the years it has been demonstrated that if a single package is placed in a standard high pressure sterilizer and a vacuum of 20 mm. drawn as before, injected steam may fail to penetrate the centre of the load ("the small package effect"). To overcome this, it has been found that a prevacuum of 20 mm. absolute with a continuous steam bleed, or a prevacuum of 20 mm. followed by a series of steam bursts to atmospheric pressure, followed by a vacuum of 20 mm. or less, will ensure instant penetration of steam to the centre of a single challenge pack. Furthermore, the temperature in the discharge line could be relied upon to reflect accurately that in the centre of the pack. Most modern prevacuum high pressure steam sterilizers or dressing sterilizers use the pulsation system to ensure the removal of air and to achieve a satisfactory sterilization cycle.

Sterilizing Cycle

In order to ensure that all micro-organisms are killed, including spores in all parts of the load, a correctly timed sterilizing run must be provided whether this is by dry heat or by steam. The sterilizing cycle is made up of three phases—first the penetration time, second the holding time, and third the safety period with discharge of the steam to the atmosphere. The penetration time is the time taken for the steam or heat to reach the required sterilizing temperature. In the case of steam where the procedure mentioned above has been carried out, the discharge line temperature can be regarded as being the sterilizing temperature. With dry heat, on the other hand, a temperature-measuring probe placed in the centre of the representative object can be used to determine the sterilizing temperature. The penetration time will vary from sterilizer to sterilizer according to its size and the kind of load. The holding time is the time taken to kill the test

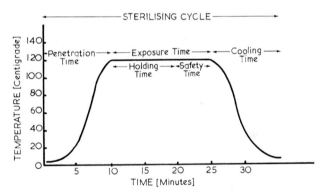

Fig. 1. Diagram showing the different phases of the sterilizing cycle in a steam sterilizer.

spores at the sterilizing temperature selected. The safety time is 50 per cent of the holding time and allows for variation in the apparatus and the method of packing. Thus, as soon as the drain or simulator temperature reaches the sterilizing temperature, the exposure time commences, which consists of the sum of holding + safety time or exposure time. For example, if steam under pressure will kill spores in 10 min. at a temperature of 121°C, (the holding time) then the safety time will be half of the holding time—e.g. 5 min. at 121°C. Thus, the total time of the sterilizing cycle at 121°C might be:

Penetration time 10 min + holding time 10 min
+ safety time 5 min = a total of 25 min (see fig. 1).

The pressures, corresponding temperature and exposure times recommended by the Medical Research Council

Working Party on high pressure steam sterilizers are as follows:

121°C	(15 lb. p.s.i.)	20 min.
126°C	(20 lb. p.s.i.)	10 min.
134°C	(30 lb. p.s.i.)	3 min.

More recently some instrument sterilizers have come on the market which work at the higher pressure of 50 lb. p.s.i. (148°C) and it is recommended that the sterilizing time should be at least 30 sec. Normally, the dental surgeon would not be expected to undertake the sterilizing of dressings or fabrics—they would be provided through the hospital Central Sterile Supply Service or commercial sources; but it is essential that the principles are understood.

Methods for Testing Steam Sterilizers

Most sterilizers now work on an automatic cycle, controlled from the drain temperature or simulator. Nevertheless, it is important to ensure that the autoclave is working satisfactorily; this should normally be under the care of a bacteriologist and engineer.

Instrument Sterilizer

In the downwards displacement sterilizer, the easiest method is to place a Brown Tube No. 1 in the jaws of a pair of forceps and note whether there is a complete change in the colour of the tube after completion of the sterilizing cycle.

Dressing Sterilizer

For the dressing sterilizer, three tests should be employed: (a) a vacuum should be drawn to 20 mm. absolute and tested either by a U tube or by a properly compensated vacuum gauge to see whether there is a leak; (b) a Brown Tube No. 2 should be placed in the centre of a pack or combined with a Bowie Dick Test; and (c) a Bowie Dick Test should be carried out. This is the most informative test since it ensures that there is instant steam penetration, that air is removed and that there are no air leaks. It is carried out as follows: diagonal crossed autoclave tapes are placed on a sheet of unglazed paper and enclosed in the centre of a stack of 29 recently laundered huckaback towels of standard size and enclosed either in a square drum or in an outer cover of the same material. The pack is now submitted to the sterilizing cycle, and at the end of the cycle the tape examined. This should show a similar degree of colour change throughout the length of the tape. However, if there is partial or uneven change the autoclave should be examined for faults. The penetration time both in the downward displacement autoclave and the dressing sterilizer can be determined by temperature readings taken from the discharge to see whether the temperature is consistent with the steam pressure. This, however, should be checked by thermocouples.

As a further test, spore strips of *Bacillus stearothermophilus* should be placed in strategic positions within the sterilizer and subsequently cultured.

STERILIZATION BY DRY HEAT

Sterilization by dry heat is dependent upon penetration of heat to all parts of the load. It is particularly suitable for sterilizing delicate instruments and for glass syringes and needles already assembled and sealed in containers. The disadvantage of dry heat, as explained earlier, is that higher temperatures and a longer exposure time are required than is necessary with steam.

Hot Air Ovens

The most commonly used method for dry heat sterilization has been the hot air oven, but tests have shown that many were unreliable as there was considerable variation in temperature from one point to another. However, the British Standards Institution has now laid down a specification which requires that when loaded, ovens must show an overall variation on testing of less than 5°C (B.S. 1/3421). In order to achieve this, the ovens are normally fitted with a fan to ensure a forced flow of air within the chamber. At the same time, it is essential that the articles to be sterilized should be loosely packed and separated so that the heat can penetrate to all parts of the load. The heat of the oven should be accurately controlled by a sensitive thermostat or by a probe in a representative article. It is, therefore, important before purchasing such an oven to make sure that it conforms with the B.S.I. specification.

Conveyor Oven

This piece of equipment is normally used in Central Sterile Supply Departments where large numbers of articles of the same type are to be sterilized. The articles, normally glass syringes in their containers, are loaded on to a moving belt which carries them under a series of infra red heaters, normally set to work at 180°C. One of the advantages of this piece of equipment is that, since the heat source is near to the infra red band, the articles take up the heat more quickly than in an oven and the holding and safety times can be reduced so that the total sterilizing cycle can be achieved in less than 20 min.

Dry Heat Sterilizing Cycle

The temperature and time of exposure needed to ensure sterility, as determined by The Medical Research Council Working Party on the Sterilization Use and Care of Syringes (1962), are as follows:

Sterilizing Temperature	Exposure Time
°C	min.
160	45
170	18
180	7½

However, the Committee felt that 160°C for 1 hr. should be recommended as it gives an additional safety margin and has been in general use for some time. For further details for both steam and dry heat, see M.R.C. Council Report No 41. It should be noted that the thermometer provided with the oven does not always give an accurate guide to the temperature of the oven, particularly as the heat penetration time will vary with the load. It is therefore important to check the time taken to reach sterilizing temperature before commencing the sterilizing exposure time.

Method of Testing Equipment for Dry Heat Sterilization

In order to test the temperature within the hot air oven or conveyor arm, thermocouples should be placed in a number of dummy test syringes sealed in the containers or attached to a large instrument in a sealed instrument set. Bacteriological tests require special techniques and are not recommended. Probably the Brown Tubes are the most practical of those tests available. The Brown Tube consists of a sealed glass capsule containing fluid which changes from red to green according to the exposure time and the temperature of the tube concerned. There are four types of Brown Tube, and their characteristics are set out in Table 2.

TABLE 2
BROWN TUBES FOR TESTING
STERILIZING TEMPERATURE

Proposed Sterilizing Temperature	No. 1 (Black Spot)	No. 2 (Yellow Spot)	No. 3 (Green Spot)	No. 4 (Blue Spot)
120°C	160	9		
125°C	10	5½		
130°C	6½	3½		
160°C			60	45
170°C			31	23
180°C			16	12
190°C			8	6½

The figures denote the time taken in minutes to produce the complete change in colour from red to green.

As the tubes are heat sensitive, it is important that they should be stored in a refrigerator until required. No. 1 and No. 2 are suitable for steam sterilization for temperatures up to 126°C and 134°C respectively; No. 3 and No. 4 for dry heat for temperatures at 160°C and for conveyor ovens at 180°C respectively. It must be clearly understood that these tubes measure heat only and provide no guarantee that steam has penetrated to the surface of the articles to be sterilized.

Method of Use of the Brown Tube

Care should be taken to insert the appropriate Brown Tube in the centre of a dummy load or when combined with the Bowie Dick Test by fixing the tube in the centre of the crossed heat-sensitive tapes. For dry heat sterilization the tubes can be inserted either in the barrel of the syringe or in the plunger of the larger syringes and sealed in the normal way.

OTHER METHODS OF STERILIZATION

The most satisfactory methods of sterilization have been outlined earlier. There are, however, some new methods, particularly those for thermolabile materials; these materials can be satisfactorily disinfected, and in some instances, when steam is combined with formaldehyde, sterilization can be achieved. Such methods could be of value in dental practice.

Formaldehyde

Many plastic or heat sensitive articles, such as cystoscopes and endoscopic instruments, need to be disinfected between use. In the past, neither boiling in water nor chemical disinfection proved to be satisfactory, and this has lead to the introduction of low temperature autoclaves working at subatmospheric pressures (Alder, Brown and Gillespie, 1966). The addition of formaldehyde to the steam under subatmospheric pressure has also provided a method of sterilization. After evacuating as much air as possible before introducing steam, temperature is normally maintained at 80°C and, using pulsating steam for periods up to 10 min. or even as short as 6 min., instruments have proved to be reliably disinfected.

Recently Line and Pickerill (1973) have demonstrated that steam and formaldehyde in a pulsating system within a subatmospheric autoclave can sterilize a test helix satisfactorily, using a variety of organisms in a cycle of approximately 100 min. at temperatures of both 75°C and 80°C. They also proved that evacuation of the system at the end of the cycle reduces the residues of formaldehyde. Unfortunately there is no indicator available to ensure that the sterilization cycle has been completed successfully. This system which uses both steam and formaldehyde has undoubtedly provided a satisfactory method of disinfection and sterilization particularly since formaldehyde is relatively cheap as compared with other gases; there are no explosion risks and it is claimed that formaldehyde residues in the sterilized articles are negligible.

Ethylene Oxide

Earlier a short survey of sterilization and disinfection by ethylene oxide was referred to; here its properties are considered in greater detail. Experience shows that when proper conditions are maintained, it is bactericidal, sporicidal and viricidal, even at room temperature, although raising the temperature does shorten the time required to achieve sterilization. It is soluble in water and is absorbed by rubber and many plastics and its residues may be toxic. It is therefore essential to remove residues of the gas after sterilization. The gas is capable of penetrating paper, fabrics and some plastics. Thus, it is possible to pack the article prior to sterilization.

The principal difficulty is one of control during the sterilizing cycle. Ethylene oxide is highly explosive when more than 3 per cent is mixed with air. This can be overcome by mixing up to 12 per cent by weight with carbon dioxide or with freon gas. Humidity must be maintained at about 30 per cent. Unfortunately no hard and fast rules can be laid down as to time and temperature and it is essential that each batch should be tested individually to ensure that the test organism, *B. subtilis* var *globigii* is destroyed. Unfortunately the culture procedure may take up to 5 days but no other test object, such as a Brown Tube, is available for the control of sterilization. Although this method has been used for disinfection of high speed drills, its use is not recommended unless competent supervision is available.

Boiling Water Bath

The use of boiling water, although widely practised, has many disadvantages. Boiling water will destroy vegetative organisms, but not spores, and therefore cannot be regarded as a sterilizing agent. Although it is probable that hepatitis virus can be destroyed by boiling water, there is no reliable information on this point. The World Health Organization recommends that at least 10 min. boiling is necessary to kill the hepatitis virus. Apart from its unreliability another disadvantage of this method is a practical one—*viz.* assembled syringes cannot be disinfected. The plunger is difficult to fit into the barrel after boiling, and in any case, hot syringes and instruments are difficult to handle and may be dropped or remain wet which may result in recontamination.

If no method more reliable than boiling in water is available, it is essential that instruments or syringes should be handled with sterile dry forceps or with clean dry hands. It is also important that the syringe or instrument should not be rinsed or cooled by "sterile water" and/or transferred to a bowl which may contain liquid, both of which may be contaminated. If none of the methods given earlier is available, the use of a domestic pressure cooker might provide a more reliable form of disinfection and possibly sterilization. It should be tested before use with a dummy run with a Brown Tube No. 1 which should change colour after 20 min. If a longer period than this is necessary the pressure cooker is probably unreliable and should be discarded. However, the principal disadvantage of this method is that the instrument and/or syringe remain wet and may become recontaminated.

Hot Oil Baths

In some dental clinics, low speed hand-pieces are immersed in a tank of hot oil, normally held at 145° or 150°, for 10 min. This time varies as does the temperature recommended. However, the temperature of hot oil cannot be guaranteed to kill sporing organisms, and in any case after this treatment, handpieces have to be drained by gravity or centrifuged before use. In either case there is a danger of recontamination as described with the boiling water method. This system is therefore not recommended.

CHEMICAL AGENTS

Most chemical agents vary in their ability to kill non-sporing organisms, and only a few destroy spores. Their method of action seems to be due to an interaction with protein and nucleic acid of the bacterial cell itself. Unfortunately this interaction is non-specific and also occurs with tissue cells, so that chemical agents may prove toxic if brought into direct contact with skin or mucous membrane. Nevertheless, bearing in mind that heat still remains the method of choice, there are situations where chemical agents have to be used as alternatives. These will be discussed later. A critical assessment of the large number of chemical agents commercially available would occupy more space than is available, and those wishing to study them in greater depth are referred to *Disinfection and Sterilization* by G. Sykes (1958).

Skin

The dental surgeon's and nurse's hands, unless proper protective care is taken, may be one of the principal causes of cross-infection. This is sometimes accentuated by constant hand washing between patients causing small abrasions and roughness of the skin which may become chronically infected with pathogenic organisms. Two substances may be useful in protecting the dental surgeons' hands—hexachlorophane and chlorhexidine—both of which are more active against Gram positive than Gram negative organisms. Both substances have been incorporated into soaps and hand lotions and provide protection by their accumulative action, provided that the soap or hand lotion is constantly used. Disinfection of the patient's skin prior to injection or incision raises two considerations—firstly, mechanical action of applying the disinfectant may remove visible dirt and destroy the bacterial flora on the skin surface; secondly, the mechanical action may, in turn, force other organisms from the depths of the skin to the surface, necessitating further treatment. In order to obtain immediate effect, the area should be treated with a 70 per cent solution of alcohol or 1 per cent alcoholic solution of chlorhexidine or with an alcoholic solution and iodine, provided the patient is not sensitive to iodine. All these substances have rapid disinfectant action that will last up to a few hours against a wide range of organisms, but will not necessarily destroy organisms trapped in a depth of skin.

Oral Mucous Membrane

Disinfection or sterilization of the mucous membrane before surgery or injection can be rapidly achieved by the application of isopropyl alcohol 60–90 per cent, or combined with iodine. Iodophors (1·0–0·75 per cent available iodine) can also be used which have the advantage that they normally contain a detergent which has an added cleaning action. However, although the disinfection may be immediate, there is a danger in the oral cavity that the area may be recontaminated with infected saliva. The dental surgeon may, therefore, consider the application of disinfectant to the mucous membrane an unnecessary step, particularly as there does not seem to be a satisfactory method, even by the use of antiseptic lozenges or mouth washes, of clearing or reducing the number of organisms from infected tonsils or mucous membranes. However, during incision or the injection process, it is possible for a portion of infected mucous membrane to be carried into the deeper tissues, which may result in an abscess if the superficial tissue has not been treated with a disinfectant prior to injection. It is, therefore, considered a wise precaution to sterilize or at least reduce infection on the mucous membrane prior to incision or injection. Bacteraemia of oral origin is dealt with in Chapter 17.

In cases where extensive trauma to the oral tissues is unavoidable, there is always a danger that such areas may become secondarily infected either by the surgeon's hand or by aerial contamination. It is considered essential for dental surgeons to wear a satisfactory mask, and sterile rubber gloves.

Sterilants

Only two chemical agents are known to be sporicidal and viricidal—glutaraldehyde and formaldehyde. Both are difficult to handle and their residues on treated instruments may be toxic. Glutaraldehyde and formaldehyde can be used as buffered 2 and 4 per cent solutions respectively. The exposure time is long, although it can be improved with heat, but as far as glutaraldehyde is concerned, it will only penetrate organic matter slowly and therefore absolute cleanliness of the instrument is essential if glutaraldehyde is to be successful. Formaldehyde solution is less effective against spores and repeated treatment of instruments with this substance may cause severe irritation to the operator or his assistant. Formaldehyde and glutaraldehyde are probably better considered as disinfectants.

Disinfectants

Chemical disinfection of instruments depends largely on the cleaning method employed. If the instruments are throughly cleaned, they can be disinfected satisfactorily either by soaking in 0·5 per cent alcoholic chlorhexidine solution for two or more minutes or in 2 per cent aqueous glutaraldehyde for 15 min. or more. The instruments should be rinsed with two or more changes or sterile water before use.

SPECIAL PROBLEMS

The decision as to whether a full aseptic procedure should be used or merely the disinfection of instruments between patients may pose some difficulties to the dental practitioner. The oral cavity may carry many types of pathogenic vegetative organisms without showing any obvious infection. Danger to the patient or operator occurs when such organisms are introduced into the tissue. Fortunately, spore bearers are not found in the oral cavity. It would seem then that most dental procedures should depend upon cleaning and disinfection between cases, and

that full surgical aseptic techniques should be reserved for those cases in which actual incision of the tissues is contemplated.

Instruments

It should be stressed that whatever method is contemplated, the destruction of such organisms must depend in part on the level of cleanliness achieved, for cellular debris or body fluids may prevent the heat or the chemical agent from reaching the organisms; in dentistry, instruments such as burs, may get clogged and only careful cleaning will free them. For the larger pieces of equipment, a mechanical washing machine using a high temperature detergent or caustic wash may be entirely satisfactory. For the smaller and more delicate instruments, a small ultrasonic bath will prevent damage to the equipment and loosen debris from the interstices of instruments, such as burs or drills. It is important that sharp instruments are supported in a holder or tray so that vibration does not cause them to touch a hard surface and get damaged.

Special instruments, such as air turbine handpieces may present difficulties in deciding which method of disinfection or sterilization should be adopted, but as their use is restricted to the tooth itself and not the mucous membrane the danger of cross-infection is minimal. Some makers recommend disinfection by ethylene oxide, but a busy practice suffers from the disadvantage that the length of exposure to the gas should be at least 4 hr., and bacteriological control is desirable.

Perhaps a more practical method is to clean the chuck thoroughly and soak in 0·5 per cent alcoholic solution of chlorhexidine for 2 min. or more, as recommended by Rubbo and Gardner (1965).

As far as low speed handpieces are concerned, sterilization by dry heat is far the easiest method, as described earlier. The temperature selected for sterilization may have to be decided after consultation with the makers. Obviously, the higher the temperature the shorter the sterilization cycle and time needed. However, the care of these instruments, including cleaning and lubricating, has in many instances been placed under the control of the Central Sterile Supply Service or Hospital Sterilizing and Disinfecting Unit, thus removing anxiety from the dental surgeon.

The Problem of Infectious Hepatitis

Earlier the risk of hepatitis to operators from saliva and small quantities of blood entering small skin abrasions has been stressed. It is, therefore, of extreme importance to both dental surgeon and nurse to take special precautions when dealing with known carriers; such patients should be referred to hospital dental units where special equipment required is at hand.

The patients likely to be risks are those who are under treatment for renal disease or disease requiring multiple transfusions. Before dental treatment is commenced, such patients should be tested by the laboratory to see whether they are Australia antigen positive. Positive cases must be treated as a potential risk to the operator.

In the event of such cases requiring treatment, both the dental nurse and surgeon should change into unit dress (preferably trouser suits with long sleeves and disposable overshoes). Over this should be worn protective clothing such as a light impermeable apron covered by a sterile gown, as well as sterile gloves, masks and safety spectacles.

As far as possible disposable syringes, needles, plastic sheets and tubing should be used throughout. Immediately after use, these should be placed in containers, which should be sealed, autoclaved and incinerated. Instruments, gowns, and other non-disposable items should be sealed and autoclaved before being washed or cleaned. Any spilt blood, saliva, or mucus should be treated with hypochlorite solution yielding 10,000 parts per million of available chlorine, before being mopped with a disposable swab.

Biopsy specimens for histological examination should be placed in a large screw-capped rigid container filled with 10 per cent neutral formol saline or other suitable fixative, and the specimen introduced. Care should be taken to see that the outside and top edge of the container are not contaminated with blood or saliva. The sealed container should then be placed in an individual plastic bag, heat sealed, and marked with a self-adhesive label.

Request forms should not be included with the container. Care should be taken to mark the request form and container with a red label to show that the specimen comes from an infected patient.

REFERENCES

Alder, V. G., Brown, A. M. and Gillespie, W. A. (1966), *J. clin. Path.*, **19**, 83.
Foley, F. E. and Gutheim, R. N. (1956), *Ann. intern. Med.*, **45**, 369.
Knox, R. and Penikitt, E. J. K. (1958), *Brit. med. J.*, **1**, 680.
Line, S. J. and Pickerill, J. K. (1973), *J. clin. Path.*, **26**, 716.
Rubbo, S. D. and Gardner, Joan F. (1965), *A Review of Sterilization and Disinfection*, p. 200. London: Lloyd Luke.
Sykes, G. (1958), *Disinfection and Sterilization*, pp. 6–7. London: Spon.

17. ANTIMICROBIAL DRUGS

J. G. WALTON AND J. W. THOMPSON

INTRODUCTION

Chemotherapeutic agents are substances which are used to kill infective organisms or neoplastic cells. This chapter will be concerned with antimicrobial drugs, which are agents used against micro-organisms, and with the principles underlying their use. The term antibiotic refers to substances produced by micro-organisms which, in high dilution, will prevent the growth of, or kill other micro-organisms. As many antibiotics are now synthesized, this restricted meaning may be somewhat academic.

Until the advent of the sulphonamides in 1935, the

search for systemic chemotherapeutic agents to treat infection had met with little success. The introduction of sulphonamides heralded an era prolific in the discovery of new substances capable of acting on infective organisms. Great successes can be claimed for antibacterial chemotherapy, for example the use of penicillin in the treatment of infections with haemolytic streptococci. On the other hand, the number of substances available for use against viral infections is relatively small.

The object of chemotherapy is to kill, or to prevent the multiplication of invading organisms with minimal damage to the host. Unfortunately, valuable though these powerful chemotherapeutic agents are, they can also produce unwanted effects in the individual, and in the community. It is clearly important that these powerful agents be used with discrimination.

Although it is impossible to make definitive rules for the prescribing of chemotherapeutic agents, there are certain guiding principles.

GENERAL PRINCIPLES OF TREATMENT

Diagnosis

There must be some clear indication that chemotherapy is necessary. It is indefensible to prescribe antimicrobials for conditions not due to infection; nor indeed, should trivial and self-limiting infections be treated with antimicrobial drugs.

Choice of Drug

Ideally this should depend upon bacteriological identification of the causative organisms, and sensitivity tests to establish the susceptibility of the particular organism to the antimicrobial of obvious choice. In dental practice such specialist services are not usually available and are mostly unnecessary. Clinical experience has shown that most acute oral infections respond to penicillin and it remains the antibiotic of first choice. Exceptions to this general statement will be discussed later. It should be kept in mind that severe infections should not be treated without bacteriological assistance and the position has been well summed up by O'Grady (1973) in the following words: "Blind treatment of severe infections without bacteriological assistance, and delay of treatment while the wheels of the bacteriological machine slowly turn, are both wrong. Adequate specimens should always be obtained before therapy of dangerous infections begins. However, treatment should then be instituted with what appears to be the most appropriate agent."

Dosage and Route of Administration

The object of treatment is to maintain a sufficiently high concentration of the drug in the infected tissues for as long as is required to overcome the infection. The actual concentration in the blood is not so directly important, except in the instance of septicaemia. In clinical practice, it has been suggested by Chisholm et al. (1973), that to achieve effective tissue levels "most anti-bacterial agents

which are excreted rapidly should be administered either frequently or in sufficiently large doses to ensure that adequate blood levels are maintained and the tissue levels equilibrate". An example of such a drug is benzylpenicillin, the half-life of which is less than an hour.

The duration of therapy depends on several factors, not least being the precise nature of the infection and the response to treatment. Patients should be impressed with the importance of adhering to the therapeutic regime advocated and not to discontinue therapy at their own discretion. Treatment should be continued until the infection is overcome and the early response monitored. In general terms, if there is no response to treatment within 48–72 hr. the antibacterial substance is unlikely to prove effective.

Systemic antimicrobial agents are usually given by the oral route or by intramuscular injection. Where there is a choice, administration by injection is to be preferred in severe infections as absorption is more certain and it produces a more immediate effect. Sometimes treatment can be started by injection and followed up by oral administration.

Use of Antimicrobial Agents in the Presence of Renal Failure

When it is essential to prescribe an antimicrobial agent in the presence of renal disease, it is mandatory to consider what effect any impairment of renal function may have on the dose regime to be employed. For those drugs which are excreted predominantly by the kidney it may be necessary to modify therapy under those circumstances. In some instances it may be essential to check that plasma levels of the drug are within safe limits, especially when there is the risk of ototoxicity. Some antimicrobial drugs should be avoided altogether in the presence of renal disease.

The table below divides the more commonly used agents into four categories (see also Smith and Rawlins, 1973):

Group I: No dosage modification.
Ampicillin, cloxacillin, erythromycin, fucidin, novobiocin, sulphadimidine.

Group II: Minor dosage adjustment (reduction).

Benzylpenicillin, carbenicillin, cephalothin, co-trimoxazole (trimethoprim and sulphamethoxazole), lincomycin, clindamycin.

Group III: Major dosage adjustment (reduction) (Serum concentrations should be monitored).
Colistin, gentamycin, kanamycin, streptomycin, vancomycin, amphotericin B (when used systemically).

Group IV: To be avoided altogether.
Cephaloridine, chloramphenicol, nitrofurantoin, tetracyclines (with possible exception of doxycycline).

Accompanying Treatment

Antibiotics are not a substitute for necessary surgery; where pus is present, drainage should be established. It is unjustifiable to rely on antibiotics alone when drainage is obviously necessary; to do so may cause the formation of a tumour-like cold abscess surrounded by fibrous tissue. In many instances drainage of an infected area will suffice in itself without recourse to antibiotics.

Combination of Drugs

Anti-microbial drugs are basically bacteriostatic or bactericidal: bacteriostatic drugs inhibit multiplication of organisms and bactericidal drugs kill organisms. Some bacteriostatic drugs exhibit bactericidal activity when used in high concentrations.

Drug combinations can sometimes reduce the development of resistant organisms, a well-known example being the use of streptomycin and isoniazid together in the treatment of tuberculosis. Used alone, resistance quickly develops to either of these drugs, but is much reduced when they are combined. However, combined drug therapy is not always beneficial and may be harmful. For example, many bactericidal drugs only kill rapidly multiplying cells and, in the presence of a bacteriostatic agent, their killing effect is antagonized (e.g. penicillin in the presence of tetracyclines). Such combinations should, therefore, be avoided.

Topical Administration

The principal arguments against the topical use of antibiotics are:

(a) the risk of sensitizing patients; and
(b) the risk of development of resistant strains.

It is generally accepted that antibiotics for topical use should be selected from those which are unlikely to be used systemically, possibly because they are not absorbed or because they are liable to produce unwanted effects. Common examples are bacitracin, neomycin, and polymyxin B, but it would be unwise to assume that such antibiotics would never be used systemically; the severity of a situation may demand the employment of an agent which would otherwise be regarded as too dangerous. Nevertheless, the topical use of antifungal agents (e.g. nystatin) has proved most valuable in dentistry and their usage will be considered later.

Previous Hypersensitivity

If a patient gives a history of hypersensitivity to any particular antimicrobial agent, then drugs of similar structure should not be administered because of the likelihood of cross allergenicity. Although some patients provide doubtful evidence of previous reactions, it would be unwise to ignore the history however seemingly improbable. Drug hypersensitivity reactions are likely to occur more commonly in patients with an allergic diathesis.

INDICATIONS FOR THE USE OF SYSTEMIC CHEMOTHERAPEUTIC AGENTS IN DENTISTRY

Treatment of Infections

Chemotherapeutic agents should not be used in the normally healthy patient for minor infections which are likely to respond to treatment by other means. Needless to say, if local measures appear to be inadequate, or in the presence of severe infection, antimicrobial therapy should be instituted. A number of indications for the use of antimicrobials in dental practice are indicated below:

(i) severe acute ulcerative gingivitis, especially there if are signs of systemic involvement. In less severe cases, but where systemic chemotherapy is deemed to be necessary, metronidazole (Flagyl) is the drug of choice;
(ii) severe infections of dental origin, e.g. cellulitis, acute osteomyelitis, severe pericoronitis, deep infections implanted by local anaesthesia; and
(iii) sinus infection complicating oro-antral fistula.

General Prophylaxis

Chemotherapeutic agents may be used prophylactically in an attempt to prevent infection following surgery. There is not a great deal of evidence to suggest that antibiotic prophylaxis will prevent post-operative infection, although there are circumstances where it is generally agreed that such chemoprophylaxis should be provided. Of course, a different situation exists when the patient has some underlying medical condition, but even then the exact position of chemoprophylaxis is uncertain. However, prophylactic antimicrobials may well be considered for:

(a) debilitated patients who are to have surgery, e.g. patients with severe anaemia, blood dyscrasias or diabetes. Some diabetic patients show a lessened resistance to infection, and this is especially true with uncontrolled diabetes mellitus;
(b) patients who have had radiation to the jaws and for whom, unfortunately, oral surgical procedures are required. Any irradiated area must be considered as one with lowered vitality and with poor resistance to infection; and
(c) patients on prolonged steroid therapy for whom oral surgery is to be undertaken. Prolonged use of steroids weakens natural defence mechanisms against infection. Antimicrobial cover is certainly not required for all such patients; much will depend on circumstances at the time (e.g. the extent of the operation).

It must be emphasized that the prophylactic use of antimicrobial agents to prevent post-operative infection is an uncertain measure, even in the conditions listed above. If it is to be used, the agent of choice should be given just prior to surgery in order to allow peak plasma concentrations of the chosen antimicrobial agent to be reached at the time of operation. The cover should be continued for 3–7 days; exactly how long must depend on the clinical judgement of the operator.

Particular Prophylaxis: Prevention of Bacterial Endocarditis

This is an especially important subject for the dental surgeon and will be considered later in this Chapter, after consideration has been given to individual antimicrobial agents.

MECHANISMS OF ACTION OF ANTIMICROBIAL DRUGS

Elucidation of the way in which antimicrobial agents interfere with micro-organisms has followed only slowly upon their clinical use and has characteristically depended upon the discovery of the structure and function of cells in general, and of pathogenic micro-organisms in particular. Only as this information has become available has it been possible to begin to understand the way in which different antimicrobial agents interfere with the normal functions of micro-organisms. This knowledge has also pointed the way to an understanding of the mechanisms responsible for the phenomena concerned with the clinical problem of drug resistance. To be clinically acceptable an antimicrobial agent must possess a high degree of selective toxicity in order that the damage produced to the infecting organism is much greater than that produced to the host. Antimicrobial agents exhibit varying degrees of selective toxicity so that, for example, penicillin shows a high degree of selectivity whilst chloramphenicol and the polymyxins can produce serious damage to the host. These differences depend to a large extent on whether or not the system upon which the particular antimicrobial agent acts is peculiar to the micro-organism or is also present in the human host and, if so, the degree of differential sensitivity of the system in the two species.

Site of Action of Antimicrobial Agents

An antibiotic may interfere with the normal function of a micro-organism at one, or more, of four sites:

(1) cell wall;
(2) cell membrane;
(3) protein synthesis and ribosome function; and
(4) nucleic acid synthesis or metabolism.

Interference with the Bacterial Cell Wall

Before discussing the different ways in which certain antimicrobial drugs interfere with the bacterial cell wall, it is important to realize that there is a striking difference between the cell walls of bacteria and those of mammalian cells. Unlike the mammalian cell wall, the bacterial cell wall is a tough thick structure which is situated external to the cytoplasmic membrane and so acts as a rigid external casing to the organism; this accounts for its remarkable resistance to osmotic damage. If there existed an antimicrobial agent which acted exclusively on the bacterial cell wall, it would have no effect on the mammalian host since there is no counterpart to the bacterial cell wall in the mammal; the nearest example to this ideal is penicillin.

A further important point is the difference between the composition of the bacterial cell walls of Gram positive and Gram negative organisms, a fact which accounts in some instances for the different sensitivities of these two main groups of micro-organisms to particular antibiotics (Lorian, 1971).

Gram positive micro-organisms have a thick cell wall which contains a rigid layer of mucopeptide which represents at least 60 per cent of the cell wall. The mucopeptide is coated with magnesium ribonucleate.

Gram negative micro-organisms have a thin layer of mucopeptide which represents not more than 10 per cent of the cell wall, the main components of the cell wall being lipopolysaccharides and lipoproteins.

The different structure of the cell walls of Gram positive and Gram negative organisms is important in regard to the penetrability of the antibiotic into the micro-organism. For example, polymyxin is inactive on Gram positive organisms because it is unable to penetrate the magnesium ribonucleate coating on the cell wall, whilst it is active on Gram negative organisms which do not contain this substance in the cell wall.

Another contrasting feature between Gram positive and Gram negative organisms is that the osmotic pressure is about 20 atmospheres in the Gram positive organisms, whereas it is only about one-quarter of that in the Gram negative organisms. This difference has considerable relevance since a drug which weakens the cell wall of an organism with a high osmotic pressure will result in considerable damage to that cell.

Formation of the cell wall: The first step is concerned with the conversion of natural L-alanine into the D form with subsequent linking of two D-alanine molecules, steps which are under the control of the enzymes alanine racemase and D-alanyl-D-alanine synthetase, respectively. The antibiotic cycloserine is a close analogue of alanine and both these steps are competitively inhibited by cycloserine.

In the second step D-alanine is linked with other amino acids, and also with acetylmuramic acid, a sugar which is characteristically found in the bacterial cell wall. This complex is coupled to a molecule of acetylglucosamine which together form a glycan unit, the basic building brick of the bacterial cell wall. The glycan units are then carried across the cytoplasmic membrane of the bacterial cell by means of a lipid carrier and are laid down in layers until the appropriate thickness of wall is achieved.

The final step involves the linking of the peptides of one layer to the peptides of the next and this is achieved through a peptide link which couples the first of the two alanines (of the D-alanyl-D-alanine) with the lysine of the adjoining peptide chain (with the liberation of free D-alanine).

Vancomycin, ristocetin and bacitracin prevent the incorporation of new glycan units either by interfering with their release from the lipid carrier (vancomycin and ristocetin) or with the subsequent regeneration of the carrier (bacitracin).

The penicillins and cephalosporins prevent the cross linking of peptide strands, which is the final and vital step. This is achieved by blocking the transpeptidase enzyme which is responsible for this final step. This effect is due to the fact that penicillin is a structural analogue of D-alanyl-D-alanine and the cephalosporins are also closely related chemically to the dipeptide. The penicillins and cephalosporins are the most important members of the group of antibiotics which act on the bacterial cell wall and (with the exception of the broad spectrum penicillins) are narrow spectrum antibiotics which interfere only with actively growing organisms. They are inactive against Gram negative organisms, probably because the more complex wall of the Gram negative organisms prevents them from reaching the site of the transpeptidase enzyme on which they normally act.

Interference with the Cytoplasmic Membrane

The cytoplasmic membrane of bacteria corresponds to the membrane of mammalian cells. It consists of three layers, an outer and inner layer of protein, between which is a layer of lipid. The whole membrane is about 8 nm. thick. The most important antimicrobial agents which act on the cytoplasmic membrane of bacteria are the polypeptides (polymyxins, including colistin) whilst the polyenes, examples being nystatin and amphotericin B, act on the cytoplasmic membrane of fungi.

The polymyxin molecule is a peptide and whilst one end of it is lipid-soluble, the other is water-soluble. When it comes into contact with the cytoplasmic membrane, the polymyxin molecule inserts itself between the lipid and protein layers so that the lipid-soluble end of the molecule is dissolved in the lipid layer and the water-soluble end is dissolved in the protein layer. This causes a disruptive separation of the lipid and protein layers of the cytoplasmic membrane with the result that selective permeability of the membrane is abolished, so enabling substances to pass freely to and fro with consequent rapid death of the organism. It is due to this mechanism that polymyxins are rapidly bactericidal irrespective of whether the cell is in a metabolically active state. Whereas the polymyxins are active against Gram negative organisms, they are virtually inactive against Gram positive organisms because they are unable to cross the magnesium ribonucleate coating of the cell wall present in the latter type of organism. Certain Gram negative organisms are resistant to polymyxins which are probably not able to penetrate to the cytoplasmic membrane.

The polyenes, nystatin and amphotericin B, are active against fungi and yeasts but inactive against bacteria. This selective toxicity is due to the presence of ergosterol in the cytoplasmic membrane of fungi and yeasts which is not present in bacterial membranes. The hydrophobic interaction between the polyenes and the ergosterol molecule of the cytoplasmic membranes of fungi and yeasts disrupts the osmotic function of the membrane (Gale, 1973). In other words, the end result is similar to that produced by the polypeptide antibiotics in the cytoplasmic membrane of bacteria.

Interference with Protein Synthesis

The majority of the broad spectrum antibiotics act by interfering with the synthesis of protein by bacteria. They achieve this by interrupting one or more of the critical steps in the process of protein synthesis which depends upon the sequential coupling of amino acids brought about through the beautifully co-ordinated activities of messenger RNA (mRNA), ribosomal RNA (rRNA), and transfer RNA (tRNA). In order to describe the various

ways in which different antibiotics interfere with protein synthesis, it is necessary to review briefly the normal mechanism of bacterial protein synthesis.

The primary information for protein synthesis is stored by DNA which is transmitted to mRNA during transcription. The actual process of protein synthesis takes place on ribosomes which consist of rRNA and protein, and which either lie free in the cytoplasm or attached to the cytoplasmic membrane. Each ribosome, which consists of a 30S and a 50S component (the "S" refers to Svedberg unit which is a measure of the relative density as determined by speed of centrifugation), threads itself on to the end of a strand of mRNA where it contains two attachment sites for amino acids. At the same time, the available amino acids become temporarily attached to tRNA, each amino acid having its own specific tRNA, thus ensuring the correct assembling of the amino acids to form the peptide chain. Thus, mRNA consists of a long chain of four nucleotides joined in such a way as to provide a codon triplet, each one of which represents a code for a specific amino acid. Similarly, each amino acid is "recognized" by its specific anticodon triplet which couples to it and transports it to the appropriate codon triplet site on mRNA when the appropriate acceptor site becomes available. Transpeptidation then takes place whereby the peptide chain already attached (by means of tRNA) is transferred to the next amino acid thus freeing the carrier tRNA. Translocation of the ribosome now takes place and it moves along mRNA and opens a new acceptor site which contains another codon for the next amino acid in the chain. The whole process is then repeated.

There are four main stages at which different antibiotics interfere with this process.

(a) Block of Amino Acid Transfer. The tetracyclines interfere with the transfer of amino acids because they bind to the 30S component of the ribosome and thereby block the binding of the tRNA amino acid complex to the ribosome and thus prevent polypeptide synthesis. The tetracyclines are broad spectrum antibiotics which are bacteriostatic.

(b) Block of Transpeptidation. By contrast with the tetracyclines, chloramphenicol acts on the 50S component of the ribosome and blocks peptidyl transferase so preventing the transfer of amino acids on to the growing polypeptide chain. Chloramphenicol is bacteriostatic and the dose-related depression of haemopoiesis which may occur is probably due to inhibition of mitochondrial protein synthesis. By contrast the aplasia of bone marrow is an idiosyncratic response.

(c) Interference with mRNA Function. The aminoglycosides include streptomycin, gentamycin, neomycin, and kanamycin and act directly on the 30S ribosome interfering with the function of mRNA and, in high concentrations, causing mis-reading of the codon with production of non-functional (nonsense) protein. Streptomycin, a bactericidal antibiotic, may possibly interfere with the ribosomes of the sensory epithelium of the inner ear and thereby cause vestibular damage.

(d) Block of Translocation. The macrolides (*e.g.* erythromycin), lincomycin, clindamycin and fusidic acid, bind to the ribosomal units and prevent translocation with subsequent blocking of polypeptide synthesis. Erythromycin is a bacteriostatic drug but in high concentrations may exert bactericidal activity. Drugs which affect translocation are, for some reason, especially liable to give rise to resistant mutants. In general, Gram positive organisms are more sensitive than Gram negative organisms because the cell wall of the former is more readily permeable to these drugs.

Interference with Nucleic Acid Metabolism

Antimicrobial drugs may interfere at one or more stages in the production of DNA or RNA or both. Interference may take place at an early stage, such as the production of co-factors required in the elaboration of nucleic acid, or at a much later stage such as the replication of DNA.

Although the sulphonamides and trimethoprim are not antibiotics, they ultimately interfere with the production of nucleic acid. Sulphonamides act as competitive antagonists to *p*-amino-benzoic acid which is essential for the bacterial synthesis of folic acid. They are bacteriostatic agents which in general terms have a broad spectrum of activity.

Trimethoprim blocks the conversion of folic acid to folinic acid by inhibiting bacterial dihydrofolate reductase. Trimethoprim thus acts at a later stage in the synthesis of bacterial folic acid and when used in combination with a sulphonamide potentiates the effect. In addition, the combination is bactericidal whereas the individual drugs are bacteriostatic. Since bacteria cannot utilize preformed folic acid and the mammalian host cannot synthesize folic acid, this explains the selective toxic effect of these two drugs. On the other hand, the mammalian host also requires dihydrofolate reductase but fortunately the mammalian enzyme is about 50,000 times less sensitive to trimethoprim than is bacterial dihydrofolate reductase, which explains the selective toxicity.

Antiviral Drugs. Viruses can be divided into two classes on the basis of nucleic acid content, namely DNA or RNA. DNA viruses of clinical importance include herpes simplex, zoster, varicella, variola, vaccinia, verruca, adenoviruses and molluscum contagiosum. A drug being used with some success is idoxuridine which is an analogue of thymidine. Idoxuridine blocks the utilization of thymidine in the synthesis of DNA.

The RNA viruses include many of clinical importance such as colds, influenza, and enteroviruses. Unfortunately, with the exception of amantadine for the treatment of certain types of influenza, diseases due to the RNA group of viruses are not as yet amenable to pharmacological treatment. Amantadine is effective in conferring some degree of protection against type A2 influenza and will also reduce the duration of fever and illness once the infection has become established. It appears to act by blocking the entry of the RNA type influenza A2 virus into the cell.

DRUG RESISTANCE

Antimicrobial drugs are not active against all micro-organisms. Each drug has its own spectrum of activity which depends to a large degree on its mechanism of action. The phenomenon whereby certain micro-organisms are resistant to a particular antimicrobial agent—drug resistance—is an important and complex one. Bacteria which are drug resistant can be divided into two main groups (Garrod, Lambert and O'Grady, 1973):

(a) **Drug tolerant bacteria** are those which are able to grow in the presence of the antibiotic to which they are tolerant. The presence of the antibiotic has little or no effect upon the growth of these bacteria. Occasionally, the bacteria may become physically dependent upon the antibiotic, for example streptomycin, just as some human individuals become physically dependent upon morphine.

(b) **Drug destroying bacteria** are those which are able to grow in the presence of the drug because they possess mechanisms which inactivate the drug. The main example of this type is the penicillinase-producing staphylococci.

Various mechanisms may be concerned with the development of drug resistance in the therapeutic use of antimicrobial agents and these can be divided into three main groups.

Therapeutic Selection

In certain instances a bacterial population consists of some strains which are naturally resistant to a particular drug whilst other strains are sensitive. In the course of therapy the sensitive strains are eliminated leaving the resistant strains to flourish. The strains may be resistant because they are drug tolerant or drug destroying. Respective examples are gonococci which are resistant to sulphonamides, and penicillinase-producing staphylococci.

Mutation

It seems beyond dispute that the exposure of certain organisms to certain antibiotics leads to a degree of drug resistance; what is not yet settled is how this comes about. In the earlier days of antibiotic therapy it was generally believed that the development of drug resistance was due to mutation and the best known evidence to support this idea is that which results from the method of replica plating (Lederberg and Lederberg, 1952) in which successive replica plating of a particular culture, followed by sensitivity testing, showed that organisms which had never been exposed to a particular antibiotic nevertheless contained some insensitive cells. However, other evidence (Dean and Hinshelwood, 1964) indicates that drug resistance by bacteria can arise by adaptive mechanisms. Whatever the ultimate picture, one fact seems clear, namely, that with some antibiotics, for example, polymxyin, drug resistance does not develop, and this may reflect the particular mechanism of action (see section on Cell Wall).

On the other hand, when it is liable to occur, for example with streptomycin, then special steps must be taken to reduce the risk to a minimum, such as by the use of a combination of chemotherapeutic agents. Some organisms may develop drug resistance within a matter of hours (to streptomycin) or days (to erythromycin) but fortunately, in the majority of organisms, resistance develops more slowly.

Transmission of Genetic Material from One Organism to Another

The genetic control of the activity of a cell may be altered if the genetic composition of that cell is changed. Thus, the genetic composition of a bacterial cell may be altered by the arrival of genetic material from external sources and this may occur mainly in one of two ways.

In **transduction,** plasmids, which are extra-chromosomal particles of genetic material, are transferred to the micro-organism by means of bacteriophage (a virus which infects bacteria). This mechanism was first demonstrated in a staphylococcus which had been originally sensitive to penicillin and was transduced to produce penicillinase and thereby became penicillin resistant. It has since been shown that simultaneous transduction of resistance to more than one chemotherapeutic agent may occur. However, the mechanism depends on the existence of a suitable host for the bacteriophage which, because of its fastidiousness, in general confines the transduction between organisms of the same species.

In **episomal** transference by conjugation (infectious resistance) it has been found that by means of conjugation, transfer of drug resistance can occur between organisms of all genera of the Enterobacteriaceae. As with transduction, the genetic material which is transferred consists of plasmids or episomes which themselves consist of extra-chromosomal genetic particles. These are transferred by conjugation, and in contrast to the more selective transfer of drug resistance can be transferred from one species to another. However, it appears that this type of transference does not occur either to or between Gram positive organisms but appears to be restricted to Gram negative species. It has since been found that bacteria which are capable of transmitting drug resistance by this mechanism can only do so when a second factor is present known as the 'resistance transfer factor' (Anderson, 1965).

The mechanism whereby an organism, previously drug sensitive, becomes drug resistant as a result of episomal transference by conjugation is due to the formation of an enzyme which inactivates the antibiotic to which the organism was previously sensitive. Thus, the following enzymes appear to be responsible for producing infectious resistance to the particular drugs concerned (Davies, 1971).

Substrate	Enzyme
chloramphenicol	chloramphenicol acetyl transferase
ampicillin	β-lactamase
streptomycin	streptomycin phosphotransferase
kanamycin, neomycin and gentamycin	kanamycin phosphotransferase

Other drugs to which resistance can be transmitted include cephalosporins, fusidic acid, sulphonamides, trimethoprim and nalidixic acid.

It is of course of fundamental importance to know whether infectious drug resistance is a permanent feature or whether it is reversible. Fortunately, it appears that provided the affected organism is removed from further exposure to the antimicrobial agent, infectious resistance disappears within a matter of weeks or months. Indeed, if this were not so it would be difficult to understand how the organisms concerned had retained any sensitivity to the drugs which are commonly used to treat the infections they cause. It is alarming to learn that over 50 per cent of cultures tested have been shown to exhibit infectious resistance. This finding obviously demands that the greatest care be taken in deciding to use an antimicrobial drug and also in the prevention of cross-infection between patients. The only redeeming feature about this serious situation is that Anderson *et al.* (1972) found that when they examined 95 strains of *Ps. aeruginosa*, and also 429 strains of enterobacteria from a variety of infections in a general hospital, there were no strains which were not sensitive to at least one antibiotic. Nevertheless, this finding leaves no grounds for complacency.

PENICILLINS

A wide variety of penicillins is now available. Of those originally isolated, benzylpenicillin was found to be the most suitable for use and its basic properties will be described.

Benzylpenicillin

Benzylpenicillin has a relatively narrow spectrum of antibacterial activity. It is effective against many species of Gram-positive cocci and bacilli, Gram-negative cocci, and also against *Treponema pallidum* and other treponemata. Most Gram-negative bacilli are resistant.

Amongst susceptible organisms naturally occurring resistant strains are found. Naturally resistant strains of *Streptococcus viridans* may occur in the mouth together with a majority of sensitive strains, and this poses a hazard for patients with valvular defects of the heart.

Resistant strains of *Staphylococcus aureus* exist, resistance being due to their action in forming beta-lactamase (penicillinase) which destroys penicillin. These strains existed before the era of antibiotics but, in the early days of penicillin, were probably few compared to those staphylococci sensitive to the antibiotic. The widespread use of penicillin has encouraged the few originally resistant strains to increase and this has led to serious problems in some hospitals where the proportion of strains resistant to benzylpenicillin could be as high as 90–95 per cent. Outside of hospitals the figure may be in the region of 15–20 per cent.

Mode of Action of Penicillins

Penicillins are bactericidal and interfere with bio-synthesis of the bacterial cell wall in susceptible organisms.

Absorption, Fate and Excretion

Benzylpenicillin is unstable in an acid medium and therefore cannot be relied upon to produce satisfactory results if given by mouth because a high proportion of the original drug is rendered inactive by the acid contents of the stomach. When given by intramuscular injection it is quickly absorbed, the maximum plasma concentration being reached within half an hour and then rapidly falling. In order to maintain a satisfactory plasma level, at least 300 mg. of benzylpenicillin should be adminstered intramuscularly every 4–6 hr. It should always be remembered that tissue levels take time to equilibrate with plasma levels.

The drug readily diffuses from the maternal to the fœtal circulation. It is partially bound to plasma protein (46–58 per cent) and although it passes into serous cavities the concentration is low, especially in the cerebrospinal fluid and joint cavities. Inflammation increases the penetration of the drug.

The half-life of benzylpenicillin is less than an hour. The major part (80 per cent) of any dose is excreted rapidly by the kidney due to extensive tubular secretion, the remaining 20 per cent being via glomerular filtration. Excretion through the kidneys can be delayed by the administration of substances which compete with penicillin for active tubular secretion. Such a drug is probenecid (Benemid) and by delaying excretion it prolongs therapeutic blood levels.

Less soluble compounds of penicillin delay absorption from the site of injection and a commonly used preparation for this purpose is procaine penicillin, prepared by the interaction of procaine hydrochloride and benzylpenicillin. The peak level of procaine penicillin is reached in 4 hr. and thereafter falls over the next 24 hr. Even less soluble compounds are available, such as benethamine penicillin and benzathine penicillin, the effects of which are prolonged up to days or weeks. Unfortunately, the less soluble compounds produce lower plasma concentrations than benzylpenicillin.

Phenoxymethylpenicillin

Phenoxymethylpenicillin is an oral penicillin which resists destruction in gastric juice and is absorbed from the upper part of the small intestine, although incompletely. About one-third of the dose is absorbed from the gastrointestinal tract. Maximum blood concentration is reached in 1 hr. and excretion is as rapid as with benzylpenicillin. Administration every 4–6 hr. is necessary to maintain therapeutic levels.

The range of antibacterial activity is similar to that of benzylpenicillin, but it is somewhat less active against streptococci and more active against resistant staphylococci.

Other acid resistant penicillins have been introduced and include phenethicillin (Broxil) and propicillin (Brocillin, Ultrapen). Although more effectively absorbed than phenoxymethylpenicillin, these latter acid resistant penicillins do not seem to offer any real advantages. Phenoxymethylpenicillin is less protein bound than these later penicillins and consequently there is more antibiotic freely available to diffuse to the site of infection. Phenoxymethylpenicillin remains the acid resistant penicillin of choice.

Unwanted Effects of the Penicillins

Penicillin therapy is remarkably free from unwanted effects except for the production of hypersensitivity reactions. Sensitization is often produced by previous treatment but sometimes no such contact can be established. On the other hand previous exposure to penicillin may not be obvious, such as the drinking of milk from cows treated with the drug. Penicillin is thought to be the most common cause of drug allergy, but this must be considered against the background of its extensive usage. The allergic reactions range from a mild urticaria to occasionally a serious anaphylactic shock leading to death. The estimated incidence of allergic reactions to penicillin in various areas of the world ranges from 0·7 to 10 per cent.

All preparations of penicillin can bring about hypersensitivity reactions. Although oral preparations are thought to produce reactions much less frequently than parenterally administered penicillin, it must be emphasized that serious reactions have occurred following oral administration. Procaine penicillin is probably the most common offender. All patients who are to receive penicillin, by whatever route, should be questioned as to any previous untoward experience with this drug and offered an alternative antibiotic when necessary.

Therapeutics

Extremely serious infections of dental origin should be treated by means of benzylpenicillin intramuscularly, 300–600 mg. every 4–6 hr., and continued until the infection is overcome. Such a regime would require in-patient care and usually a dose of 300 mg. 6-hourly will be found to be adequate.

Most susceptible infections of dental origin can be controlled by the initial intramuscular injection of 2–3 ml. of fortified procaine penicillin; this should be followed by daily injections of a similar amount for 4–5 days. (Fortified Procaine Penicillin Injection contains in each ml. procaine penicillin 300 mg. and benzylpenicillin 60 mg.) Benzylpenicillin provides a maximal concentration of the antibiotic in the blood within 30 min. and the procaine penicillin sustains a therapeutic level over a period of 24 hr.).

For the less severe infections an oral penicillin, i.e. phenoxymethylpenicillin, 250 mg. 4–6 hourly will often suffice. The drug should be taken not later than 30 min. before a meal.

Because of the incomplete absorption of the oral penicillins, parenterally administered penicillin is more certain in its effects and should be used for severe infections. As a rule, if the patient treated with penicillin is showing no response within 48–72 hr., continued use of the drug is unlikely to be effective.

Penicillinase Resistant Penicillins
(*e.g.* Methicillin, Cloxacillin and Flucloxacillin)

These penicillins are reserved for the treatment of staphylococcal infections and treatment of severe staphylococcal infections should be started with one of these drugs unless the antibiotic sensitivity of the strain is known. Methicillin must be administered by injection as it is not acid resistant, whereas cloxacillin and flucloxacillin can be given orally or by injection. The degree of protein binding is much higher with the acid resistant compounds than with methicillin and this would point to the advantage of using methicillin. On the other hand methicillin is much less active against staphylococci and so the value of these three antibiotics against resistant staphylococci is probably little different.

Broad Spectrum Penicillins
(*e.g.* Ampicillin and Amoxycillin)

Ampicillin is effective against Gram-positive organisms, although slightly less so than benzylpenicillin. However, it has much greater activity against Gram-negative bacteria. It is destroyed by penicillinases and should not, therefore, be used to treat resistant staphylococcal infections.

Ampicillin is acid resistant and can be administered orally, but for maximal effect it should be given parenterally. Its main use seems to be in the treatment of urinary infections and bronchitis, and there seems little place for it in dental practice.

Skin rashes appear to be more common with ampicillin than with other penicillins, with an incidence of about 7 per cent. Most of these rashes are of the maculopapular type and seem unrelated to those of true penicillin allergy.

The rashes may develop during the course of treatment with ampicillin or sometimes days after treatment has stopped. Ampicillin rashes tend to occur more frequently in patients suffering from viral infections and this drug should not be administered to patients with mononucleosis.

Cross hypersensitivity probably exists between all penicillins in the susceptible patient. However, the maculopapular rash of ampicillin does not necessarily contraindicate later treatment with other penicillins.

The antibacterial spectrum of amoxycillin is similar to that of ampicillin. It is well absorbed when taken orally and is unaffected by food. Serum concentrations of amoxycillin are twice as high as those produced by the same dose of ampicillin. It is probable that amoxycillin will prove to be a more useful drug than ampicillin.

Carbenicillin

Carbenicillin is not likely to be required by the dental surgeon but it is of importance because of its usefulness in the management of Pseudomonas infections.

TETRACYCLINES
(*e.g.* Tetracycline, Chlortetracycline, Oxytetracycline, Demethylchlortetracycline, Methacycline, Lymecycline, Clomocycline, Doxycycline).

The tetracyclines comprise a group of closely related antibiotics which provide a "broad spectrum" of activity against organisms. Susceptible species include Gram-positive organisms which are also sensitive to penicillin, and many Gram-negative organisms which are insensitive to penicillin. Tetracyclines are also active against rickettsia (*e.g.* typhus) and diseases due to the larger viruses (*e.g.* lymphogranuloma venereum), as well as against *Treponema pallidum* and other treponemata.

Bacterial Resistance

The development of resistance to tetracyclines is slow but now includes strains of staphylococci and coliform bacilli. Estimates vary, but as many as 32 per cent of strains of haemolytic streptococci may be resistant. However, Robertson (1973) reported a fall in the incidence of tetracycline resistant beta-haemolytic streptococci in south-west Essex over a period of 10 years up to 1972. It is hoped that this decline of the tetracycline resistant streptococcus is due to greater selectivity in the prescribing of tetracycline. Resistant strains of the pneumococcus are also developing and may limit the future usefulness of the tetracyclines in this field. An organism resistant to one of the tetracyclines is most likely to be resistant to all members of the group.

Mode of Action

The tetracyclines are bacteriostatic; that is they inhibit the multiplication of organisms so that natural defence mechanisms are not overwhelmed. The tetracyclines act by interfering with protein synthesis.

Absorption, Fate and Excretion

The tetracyclines are generally administered orally, but occasionally by intravenous or intramuscular injection.

Absorption from the gastro-intestinal tract is fairly rapid, but significant amounts are retained in the bowel. Absorption is reduced if the drug is taken with milk or substances containing calcium, magnesium, iron, or aluminium which chelate with tetracyclines.

The maximal concentration in the plasma is reached in 2–4 hr. after oral administration, and gradually falls to about half this amount in 9–12 hr., and to a very low concentration at 24 hr. The original tetracyclines, *i.e.* tetracycline, chlortetracycline and oxytetracycline, produce adequate and maintained plasma levels by the administration of 250 mg. at 6-hourly intervals. The dosages for the newer tetracyclines are somewhat different; for example, clomocycline is given 170 mg. 6-hourly and doxycycline is given 200 mg. on the first day, and then 100 mg. daily.

Tetracyclines are widely distributed in the tissues and they also enter the cerebrospinal fluid. As they chelate with calcium ions they are localized in bone and teeth. Excretion of the tetracyclines is in the bile and urine, with a variable amount in the faeces.

Unwanted Effects of the Tetracyclines

Hypersensitivity reactions are rarely encountered but, if they are, cross hypersensitivity between the various members of the group will be present.

Large doses of tetracyclines given parenterally can damage the liver.

Immediately after absorption tetracyclines are built into calcifying tissues and this becomes a permanent feature in the teeth. There is a clear linear relationship between the number of courses of treatment with tetracyclines and the discolouration of developing teeth. If at all possible, the use of tetracyclines should be avoided during the formative period of the crowns of the teeth. If a tetracycline has to be used, then oxytetracycline is to be preferred, as it produces the least objectionable staining.

In infants increased intracranial pressure with bulging fontanelles has been observed. This is not a common occurrence and all signs clear up on cessation of treatment.

Gastrointestinal disturbances may complicate therapy with the tetracyclines, some patients complaining of abdominal discomfort, a feeling of nausea, or vomiting. These effects probably result from the direct irritant action of the drug on the gastric mucosa. Diarrhoea may also be a direct result of this irritant action, but it could be due to superinfection with organisms resistant to tetracyclines. All antibiotics have the power to alter the normal microbial population of the upper respiratory, intestinal, and genitourinary tracts in patients receiving them, and probably do so to some extent in each individual. Unfortunately, as a result of this change, some patients develop disease due to overgrowth of resistant organisms which are normally balanced by naturally occurring sensitive strains. Such superinfection, as it is called, is more likely to occur with broad spectrum antibiotics and tetracyclines have the widest antimicrobial spectrum of any antibiotics.

Tetracyclines produce a marked depression of the normal bacterial flora of the mouth, throat and colon, and tetracycline resistant organisms, if present, can proliferate in the altered microbial environment. Under certain circumstances this may lead to infection, the organisms involved being:

(a) various *proteus* and *pseudomonas* species which may proliferate in the bowel and cause diarrhoea;

(b) *Staphylococcus aureus*—superinfection with this organism being serious; the resistant staphylococcus predominates in hospitals and any clinical condition caused is mainly found in post-operative surgical cases; and

(c) *Candida albicans*—overgrowth of which is of immediate concern to the dentist. Most individuals harbour this common inhabitant of the oral cavity. The surface proliferation of *Candida albicans* which is known to occur with the administration of broad spectrum antibiotics, increases the chances of its invading the tissues and thereby causing an infection. This is especially likely to occur in the debilitated patient, in patients using corticosteroids, and if the proliferation is on a surface with already existing disease.

Overgrowth of *Candida albicans* may give rise to numerous clinical features. In the mouth candidiasis may result in a sore mouth (antibiotic stomatitis). Troublesome gastrointestinal symptoms may develop such as diarrhoea and pruritis ani. Rarely, but of serious import, the surface infection caused by *Candida albicans* may be the source of candidal septicaemia.

Tetracyclines may cause terminal renal failure when administered to patients with chronic renal failure. These antibiotics cause a rise in blood urea which is often accompanied by deterioration in renal function. While the normal half-life of tetracycline is in the region of 9 hr., this may be increased to 57–108 hr. in patients with renal failure. Tetracyclines should not, therefore, be given to patients with impaired renal function. One of the tetracyclines, doxycycline, is a possible exception to this general statement as the serum-half life (20–24 hr.) of this preparation is much longer than the other tetracyclines, and it is not significantly changed in patients with chronic renal failure.

Therapeutics

Tetracyclines are not now used so frequently as in the past, possibly because there are more alternatives available. In dentistry tetracyclines have a limited place in treating infections which fail to respond to penicillin, or for those patients hypersensitive to penicillin. Usually, a 5 days' course of tetracyclines is prescribed for dental infections, 250 mg. being taken 6-hourly. Tetracyclines should never be used when a bactericidal effect is required.

A tetracycline mouthbath is sometimes useful in relieving the painful ulcerations of severe recurrent aphthae, the erosions of lichen planus, and especially for oral herpetic ulceration. For this purpose the content of a 250 mg. capsule of tetracycline is added to 15–30 ml. of warm water and this is then held in the mouth for 3 min. before being discarded. The rationale of this treatment is obscure; possibly it is effective in reducing any secondary infection. The procedure is repeated 3 times a day for no longer than 3 days; to continue this form of treatment further invokes the danger of superinfection by *Candida albicans* in susceptible patients.

The use of tetracyclines encourages overgrowth of *Candida albicans* which may be responsible for persistent and troublesome gastrointestinal upsets (e.g. pruritus ani). Such effects are more common than is generally appreciated and it is advocated that 1 nystatin tablet (500,00 units) be swallowed with each dose of tetracycline in the following instances:

(a) when the course of treatment with tetracycline is longer than 5 days;

(b) when the patient has already received a course of tetracyclines recently;

(c) when the patient has had previous untoward experiences with tetracyclines administered alone; and

(d) when the patient is debilitated.

TABLE 1

GROUP	OFFICIAL OR APPROVED NAME	OTHER NAMES	SPECTRUM	DRUG RESISTANCE	ADULT DOSAGE	UNWANTED EFFECTS	COMMENTS
Benzylpenicillin	benzylpenicillin	Penicillin G, Crystapen, Solupen	C+, B+, C—, S. Proteus mirabilis and other proteus often sensitive.		150–600 mg. IM 2–4 times/daily.	An innocuous drug even in high dosages, apart from Hypersensitivity reactions. Hypersensitivity reactions are the most serious hazard—including anaphylactic shock. Procaine penicillin appears to produce a higher incidence of allergic reactions; phenoxymethylpenicillin a low incidence of reactions.	Used for treating severe infections and/or relatively insensitive organisms when high blood levels are required. Rapidly excreted.
	procaine penicillin	Procaine penicillin G, Distaquaine			300–900 mg. IM daily.		
	fortified procaine penicillin (300 mg. procaine penicillin + 60 mg. benzylpenicillin per ml.)	Distaquaine fortified		Many strains of Staphylococcus aureus.	2–3 ml. IM daily.		Effective in all but relatively severe/resistant infections. Lower blood levels maintained for 24 hr.
Acid resistant penicillin	phenoxymethylpenicillin	Penicillin V, Apsin VK, Co-Caps Penicillin V-K, Crystapen V, Distaquaine V-K, Econocil V-K, Econopen V, Ethipen, Stabillin V-K, V-Cil-K, GPV			250 mg. orally 4–6 hourly.	N.B. Cross allergenicity is likely to exist between the penicillins.	Acid resistant. For oral administration. Unsuitable for serious infections because irregular absorption may produce inadequate blood levels.

N.B. Penicillin is the antibiotic of first choice in dentistry. |
Penicillins resistant to penicillinase	methicillin	Celbenin	Penicillinase resistant penicillins reserved for the treatment of resistant Staphylococcal infections.		1 g. IM 4–6 hourly.	Have the same low order of unwanted effects as benzylpenicillin. It has been suggested that methicillin may cause permanent renal damage.	Although active against penicillin sensitive and penicillinase producing strains of Staphylococcus aureus, much less active than benzylpenicillin against other penicillin sensitive species. None of these penicillins is effective against infections due to Gram—bacilli. Reserved for the treatment of serious infections due to resistant Staphylococci.
	cloxacillin	Orbenin		A few strains of Staphylococcus aureus.	500 mg. orally, 6-hourly. 250 mg. IM 4–6 hourly.		
	flucloxacillin	Floxapen			250 mg. orally, or IM, 6-hourly.		
Broad spectrum penicillins	ampicillin	Penbritin	C+, B+, C—, B—,S. Slightly inferior to benzylpenicillin against most Gram + bacteria.	Many strains of Staphylococcus aureus.	250 mg — 1 g. orally, 6-hourly.	Ampicillin produces a higher incidence of skin rashes than other penicillins. The rash is usually of the maculo-papular type and may be unrelated to the usual type of penicillin hypersensitivity. The rash may appear during treatment or days (about 5) after the discontinuation of treatment.	These penicillins are active against Gram + bacteria, but are especially effective against Gram— bacteria. In dentistry these drugs should be reserved for infections caused by identified Gram—organisms. In medicine ampicillin, for example, has been used for a wide variety of infections, especially urinary tract infections.
	amoxycillin	Amoxil			250 mg. orally, 8-hourly.		

GROUP	OFFICIAL OR APPROVED NAME	OTHER NAMES	SPECTRUM	DRUG RESISTANCE	ADULT DOSAGE	UNWANTED EFFECTS	COMMENTS
Carbenicillin	carbenicillin	Pyopen	Pseudomonas infections and infections with Proteus species.	Many strains of Staphylococcus aureus. Strains of Proteus mirabilis which form penicillinase.	20–30 g. daily intravenously, by injection or infusion		This penicillin is of importance because of its activity against Pseudomonas aeruginosa and Proteus species. It is not an antibiotic likely to be used by the dental practitioner.
Cephalosporins	cephaloridine	Ceporin	Similar to ampicillin	A degree of susceptibility to Staphylococcal penicillinase.	500 mg. IM or IV 2–3 times/day.	The incidence of allergic reactions may be lower than that for the penicillins. There is a degree of cross allergenicity between the cephalosporins and the penicillins. Large doses may cause renal damage.	A useful alternative to penicillin when the latter cannot be used, other than because of hypersensitivity. Not, as at first hoped, the answer to Staphylococcal infections, being susceptible to penicillinase. Useful in dentistry in certain cases requiring prophylaxis to prevent the occurrence of bacterial endocarditis. Cephaloridine is to be preferred for IM injection, as cephalothin is painful by that route. Should be used with extreme care in the presence of renal impairment, and may be best avoided.
	cephalothin	Keflin			500 mg. IM or IV 4–6 hourly.		
	cephalexin	Ceporex, Keflex			250–500 mg. orally, 6-hourly.		
Tetracyclines	chlortetracycline	Aureomycin	C+, B+, C−, B−, S, R, V. Often inactive against Proteus species and Pseudomonas aeruginosa.	Slow development of resistance but many Streptococci are resistant and there is an emerging resistance of Pneumococci. Cross resistance between the tetracyclines.	250–500 mg. orally, 6-hourly. 250 mg. orally, 6-hourly but may be doubled in severe infections. 250–500 mg. 6-hourly is the dose range for most preparations; there are exceptions, e.g. Tetrabid. Doses for individual preparations should be checked prior to administration. Preparations are available for injection.	Hypersensitivity reactions are rare. Nausea, vomiting and diarrhoea may occur. Superinfection with resistant strains of Staphylococcus aureus can cause a fatal enterocolitis. Overgrowth of Candida albicans may lead to thrush, glossitis, pruritus ani, etc. Staining of the teeth if administered during the period of calcification of the dental tissues, if given over a long period. May cause terminal renal failure in a stabilized renal failure. *N.B.* **Cross hypersensitivity is likely to exist between the tetracyclines.**	Tetracyclines are useful in dentistry as a second line of defence when penicillin is ineffective, or when the patient is hypersensitive to penicillin. Tetracyclines are contraindicated when a bactericidal drug is required, e.g. prophylaxis against bacterial endocarditis. Whenever possible tetracyclines should be avoided during the period of calcification of the teeth. The least objectionable staining of developing teeth is produced by oxytetracycline. Tetracyclines should be avoided in patients with ulcerative colitis and should be avoided in patients with renal impairment (with the exception of doxycycline).
	oxytetracycline	Berkmycen, Clinimycin, Ethoxytet, Galenomycin, Imperacin, Oxydon, Oxymycin, Stecsolin, Terramycin, Unimycin					
	tetracycline	Achromycin, Clinitetrin, Co-Caps tetracycline, Economycin, Ethitet, Steclin, Sustamycin, Tetrabid, Tetrachel, Tetracyn, Tetrex, Totomycin					

CODE: C+ = Gram + cocci. C− = Gram − cocci. S = Treponema pallidum. B+ = Gram + bacilli. B− = Gram − bacilli. R = Rickettsiae. V = Large viruses, *i.e.* the Psittacosis group.

N.B. Doses of older penicillins were originally expressed in units, but it is now customary to express doses in mg. (or g.), *e.g.* Benzylpenicillin, 250,000 units = 150 mg.; Procaine penicillin, 100,000 units = 100 mg.

Table 1 (*contd.*).

GROUP	OFFICIAL OR APPROVED NAME	OTHER NAMES	SPECTRUM	DRUG RESISTANCE	ADULT DOSAGE	UNWANTED EFFECTS	COMMENTS
Erythromycin group (Macrolides)	erythromycin	Ilotycin, Erythrocin, Erycen, Erythromid, Retcin	C+, B+, C−, S.		250–500 mg. orally, 6-hourly.	Gastro-intestinal upsets (nausea, vomiting, epigastric discomfort, diarrhoea) not uncommon. Hypersensitivity reactions are rare except that erythromycin estolate produces a high incidence of cholestatic hepatitis if given for more than 10 days. In this instance the hepatitis is thought to be due to hypersensitivity.	Similar range of activity to benzylpenicillin. In low concentration it is mainly bacteriostatic, but in higher concentrations it exerts a bactericidal effect. It is another alternative in the treatment of infections when the patient is allergic to penicillin, or when prophylaxis is required. It may be useful in the treatment of infections due to penicillin resistant strains of Staphylococcus aureus, if sensitivity is established.
	erythromycin estolate	Ilosone		Develops rapidly; may occur during treatment.	250 mg. orally, 6-hourly. (For not more than 10 days.)		
Lincomycin	lincomycin	Lincocin, Mycivin	Similar to that of erythromycin.	Some strains of Staphylococcus aureus	500 mg. orally. 3–4 times daily. 600 mg. IM (every 24 hr. in mild to moderate infections; every 12 hr. in severe infections).	Hypersensitivity reactions appear to be rare. Diarrhoea is common with both drugs, possibly less so with clindamycin. Cases of pseudomembranous colitis have been reported following the use of both drugs. *N.B.* **Cross allergenicity is likely to exist between lincomycin and clindamycin.**	Probably best reserved for the treatment of osteomyelitis as they are thought to penetrate well into bone. It is recommended that these drugs be used with extreme caution, and only where no suitable alternative is available, because of the possibility of pseudomembranous colitis. (Pseudomembranous colitis is a serious condition.)
Clindamycin	clindamycin	Dalacin C			150–300 mg. orally, 6-hourly (mild to moderately severe infections), 300–450 mg. orally, 6-hourly (severe infections).		
Anti-fungal antibiotics	nystatin	Nystan, Nystan ointment	Candida albicans. (No antibacterial activity.)	Strains of Candida albicans serially subcultured become resistant. Resistant Candida albicans not yet found clinically.	1 tablet (500,000 units) to be dissolved in the mouth or swallowed, 4 times/day for 1–4 weeks to months. Nystatin ointment applied 4 times/day.	Occasionally produces nausea and vomiting.	It is used locally in the management of candidiasis of the alimentary tract. In treating oral candidiasis (*e.g.* denture stomatitis, angular cheilitis, thrush), 1 nystatin tablet is allowed to dissolve in the mouth, 4 times daily, for a period of from 1–4 weeks or even longer. Nystatin ointment may be applied to the lesions of angular cheilitis and to the fitting surface of the upper denture in the case of denture stomatitis. (Tablets are swallowed to treat intestinal infection and the local treatment of oral infection should be combined with this to help combat the generalized gastrointestinal infection.) Nystatin has an unpleasant taste. Sometimes combined with tetracyclines to prevent overgrowth of Candida albicans.
	amphotericin B	Fungizone (for infusion), Fungilin, Fungilin lozenges, Fungilin ointment	Candida species. Coccidioides immitis. Blastomyces dermatitidis. Cryptococcus neoformans.	Strains of Candida albicans serially subcultured become resistant. Resistant Candida albicans not yet found clini ally.	1 lozenge (10 mg.) to be dissolved in the mouth 4 times/ day for 1–4 weeks. 1–2 tablets (each containing 100 mg.) 4 times/day. Fungilin ointment applied 4 times/day.	Parenterally administered amphotericin B is associated with a large number of unwanted effects, *e.g.*, hypersensitivity reactions, chills, fever, local thrombophlebitis, decreased renal function and rarely irreversible renal failure.	Amphotericin B (Fungizone) is available for injection when it is administered intravenously for the treatment of severe, systemic mycotic disease. Amphotericin B (Fungilin) lozenges and ointment are used for the same purpose as nystatin tablets and ointment, in the treatment of oral candidiasis. Amphotericin tablets are used to combat gut candidiasis. Amphotericin B has not the unpleasant taste of nystatin.

CODE: C+ = Gram + cocci. C− = Gram − cocci. B+ = Gram + bacilli. B− = Gram − bacilli. R = Rickettsiae. V = Large viruses, *i.e.* the Psittacosis group. S = Treponema pallidum.

N.B. Doses of older penicillins were originally expressed in units, but it is now customary to express doses in mg. (or g.), *e.g.* Benzylpenicillin, 250,000 units = 150 mg.; Procaine penicillin, 100,000 units = 100 mg.

ANTI-FUNGAL AGENTS

Fungi are not sensitive to the antibiotics used against bacterial infections, *e.g.* penicillin, tetracyclines, erythromycin. Fortunately, up to now, systemic fungal infections have been rare in Britain, for they are serious diseases and not easy to treat. On the other hand superficial infections by *Candida albicans* are not so uncommon and are usually trivial, but they tend to persist and may be troublesome in susceptible patients. Oral candidiasis (see Chapter 41) may occur as a response to treatment with certain drugs, for example corticosteroids, antibiotics (especially tetracyclines) and immunosuppressive drugs.

A number of anti-fungal agents are now available for local use, but nystatin and amphotericin B have proved particularly useful in dentistry.

Nystatin

Nystatin is effective against *Candida albicans* and some other fungi. It is thought to act by injuring the fungal cell membrane causing a change in its permeability with the loss of potassium ions and other intracellular elements. Bacterial membranes remain unaffected by contact with nystatin.

Absorption and Excretion

Nystatin is not absorbed from the skin or mucous membrane. It is, therefore, used for its local effect in the treatment of candidiasis of the skin or any part of the alimentary tract.

Unwanted Effects

Unwanted effects are exceedingly rare. The occasional patient feels nauseated after oral administration. There have been no reports of hypersensitivity reactions.

Therapeutics

In treating most oral candidal infections one tablet of nystatin (500,000 units) is allowed to dissolve in the mouth, and 4 tablets are prescribed each day for periods varying from 1 week to 4 weeks (*e.g.* denture stomatitis and angular cheilitis, 2–4 weeks, thrush and conditions following drug therapy, 1–2 weeks). In treating candidal leukoplakia the daily regime advocated may have to be continued for many months.

The routine administration of nystatin with tetracyclines has already been discussed. The objection to this measure is that it may induce resistance to the antifungal antibiotic by its widespread use. So far no natural resistance to nystatin has been encountered.

Amphotericin B

Amphotericin B is effective against a number of fungi, including candida species. Its mode of action is thought to be like that of nystatin, and it has no effect on bacteria.

Absorption and Excretion

Amphotericin B is not absorbed from the skin or mucous membranes and is used locally for the treatment of the conditions for which nystatin would be used. Amphotericin B can be used for the treatment of systemic fungal infections, when it is administered intravenously.

Unwanted Effects

Systemic administration is associated with numerous unwanted effects and treatment should only be undertaken in hospital. Some patients develop a fever, some have nausea and vomiting, and it is thought that some undesirable effects on the kidney are almost inevitable, and that a rise in blood urea may occur.

Therapeutics

Amphotericin B is one of the antibiotics effective against systemic fungal infections, and is therefore a valuable weapon in the medical armamentarium. In dentistry amphotericin B is used for the same purposes as nystatin, as a substitute when the patient is unable to accept the unpleasant taste of nystatin. Amphotericin B lozenges (10 mg. in each lozenge) may be used locally in the mouth as an alternative to nystatin tablets. In severe infections, the dose may be doubled. Amphotericin B ointment can be substituted for nystatin ointment and amphotericin B tablets (100 mg. in each tablet) may be substituted for nystatin tablets when the drug is required to be swallowed.

ERYTHROMYCIN GROUP (MACROLIDES)

The group includes erythromycin, oleandomycin and spiramycin, of which the first is of importance to the dental practitioner. Erythromycin has a spectrum of antibacterial activity similar to that of benzylpenicillin. Although it is effective in treating infections due to both benzylpenicillin sensitive and resistant staphylococci, its usefulness in this respect may become more limited because of the development of strains of staphylococci which are also resistant to it. In the absence of known sensitivity it would not be the antibiotic of choice to treat a staphylococcal infection.

Bacterial Resistance

Although cross resistance to other commonly used antibiotics does not occur readily, erythromycin has the disadvantage in that some sensitive organisms (*e.g.* staphylococci) may become resistant to it during prolonged therapy. Bacteria do not produce substances which destroy erythromycin and the resistance which develops is probably due to a mutation. This is not a problem in dental practice where erythromycin is usually employed for only limited periods (its use rarely exceeding 1 week).

Mode of Action

Erythromycin is bacteriostatic in low concentrations, but it also exerts a bactericidal activity in high concentrations depending on the organisms involved. It would appear to act by interfering with protein synthesis within the bacterial cell.

Absorption, Fate and Excretion

Erythromycin base (Erythromycin tablets B.P.) is destroyed by acid gastric juices and so is administered as enteric-coated tablets. Erythromycin estolate (Ilosone), on the other hand, is acid stable and is usually given in the form of capsules. It is absorbed to a greater extent than any other oral preparation of erythromycin and gives peak plasma concentrations within about 2–4 hr. The plasma concentrations provided by erythromycin estolate are also higher and are maintained for a longer time.

Erythromycin is distributed widely throughout the body tissues and 2–5 per cent of it is excreted in its active form in the urine. Although a proportion of the drug is also excreted in the bile, of which some is reabsorbed, the greater part of it seems to be broken down in the body.

Unwanted Effects

All preparations of erythromycin can cause gastrointestinal upsets such as nausea, vomiting, and diarrhoea; epigastric discomfort is not infrequent.

Hypersensitivity reactions are extremely rare with the base, but the estolate form produces a high incidence of cholestatic hepatitis which is thought to be due to hypersensitivity. This condition starts about 10–12 days after the commencement of treatment and is manifested by abdominal pains, jaundice and fever. On stopping the drug the symptoms and signs of liver involvement disappear rapidly, but re-exposure to the preparation may cause an immediate recurrence of the hepatitis.

Therapeutics

Erythromycin is a useful alternative to penicillin when the patient is known to be hypersensitive to the latter. It is administered orally and for most dental infections a 5 days' course will suffice, the dose being 250 mg. 6-hourly. In severe infections the dose can be increased to 500 mg. 6-hourly. Erythromycin base should be used for treating infections, especially if the course is to last more than a week. However, erythromycin is useful as a prophylactic agent in patients with valvular heart defects who, for one reason or another, are unable to have penicillin. In this instance the estolate form is to be preferred, as it probably provides and maintains higher plasma concentrations. Since, under these circumstances it is used only for a period of 3 days, there is little danger of jaundice occurring.

CEPHALOSPORINS
(e.g. Cephaloridine, Cephalothin, Cephalexin)

The cephalosporins are closely related chemically to penicillin. They are active against a range of Gram-positive and Gram-negative cocci and the antibacterial spectrum is similar to that of ampicillin.

Bacterial Resistance

The first of the series to be used in Britain was cephaloridine and originally it was thought to be resistant to β-lactamase produced by staphylococci, but the cephalosporins are now known to be much more susceptible than was at first believed. The cephalosporins cannot be relied upon for treating staphylococcal infections and, in this sense, have proved somewhat disappointing. Furthermore, staphylococci resistant to either methicillin or cloxacillin are likely to be resistant to the cephalosporins.

Mode of Action

Cephalosporins act in the same way as the penicillins by interfering with the biosythesis of the bacterial cell wall in susceptible organisms, thereby exerting a bactericidal effect.

Absorption, Fate and Excretion

Cephaloridine and cephalothin have to be administered parenterally, cephaloridine usually by intramuscular injection and cephalothin by the intravenous route. Of the two injectable cephalosporins, cephaloridine is the one which the dental surgeon is more likely to use. After intramuscular injection maximal blood levels of cephaloridine are reached within 30 min. and therapeutic levels maintained for 6–8 hr. Cephaloridine readily diffuses from the maternal to the fetal circulation and a high proportion of the drug enters the urine through glomerular filtration to be excreted unchanged.

Cephalexin is an acid stable antibiotic and so it may be administered orally. Absorption is quick and peak blood levels are achieved in 1 hr. The drug is excreted unchanged in the urine.

Unwanted Effects

It seems that the incidence of allergic reactions to the cephalosporins is lower than that of the penicillins, possibly in the order of 1–2 per cent. Skin rashes and pruritus are likely to be the most common allergic manifestations.

In penicillin-sensitive patients the use of cephalosporins should be viewed with caution since there is clinical and laboratory evidence of partial cross-allergenicity between the penicillins and the cephalosporins. A study by Thorburn et al. (1966) revealed that patients with a history of penicillin allergy were unusually predisposed to accelerated allergic reactions to cephalothin. These accelerated reactions would seem to suggest that the underlying mechanism is likely to be due to cross allergenicity between the cephalosporins and penicillin, rather than to a generalized and unspecific tendency to drug hypersensitivity.

A serious effect may be on the kidney and Fillastre et al. (1973) report three cases of renal failure following the use of cephalothin and gentamycin. Large doses may cause renal damage and they suggest that the cephalosporins should be used with care in the presence of even minor renal impairment.

Therapeutics

Perhaps the principal use for cephalosporins in dentistry is as a prophylactic in the patient with a valvular heart defect and as an alternative to penicillin when, for some reason other than hypersensitivity, that drug cannot be used. For this purpose cephaloridine would be used and 500 mg. intramuscularly produces satisfactory blood levels for 6–8 hr.

CLINDAMYCIN

Clindamycin is a derivative of lincomycin and both clindamycin and lincomycin have a range of antibacterial activity similar to that of erythromycin. They act on bacterial cells by interfering with protein synthesis and are essentially bacteriostatic.

Clindamycin and lincomycin can be administered orally; clindamycin is rapidly absorbed and, unlike lincomycin, its absorption is not significantly affected by the presence of food in the gut. It produces peak blood levels in about 45 min. which are higher than those achieved with lincomycin. Clindamycin has clear advantages over lincomycin.

It is difficult to evaluate the precise place of clindamycin in dentistry, although it may be useful in the treatment of serious infections such as staphylococcal osteomyelitis. Unfortunately, however useful clindamycin or lincomycin may be, their use in medical and dental practice is likely to be severely restricted because of unwanted effects. Scott *et al.* (1973) reported eight cases of pseudomembranous colitis, in seven of whom the administration of lincomycin preceded the serious illness. Three of these patients died. Wells *et al.* (1974) report similar cases of colitis following the use of clindamycin and suggest that, on present evidence, the use of clindamycin should be restricted to those situations where it is clearly the drug of choice, *e.g.* a potentially life threatening anaerobic infection.

It would seem that clindamycin is a drug which requires further attention and there would appear to be little call for its use in dentistry, or for that of lincomycin.

METRONIDAZOLE

Metronidazole, given orally, is effective in the treatment of trichomonal infections of the genital tract and coincidentally it has been found to be successful in the treatment of acute ulcerative gingivitis. After oral administration it is well absorbed and variable amounts are found in the saliva.

Unwanted Effects

Numerous unwanted effects have been recorded and these are commonly related to the gastrointestinal tract, *e.g.* nausea, vomiting, indigestion, diarrhoea, or constipation. Dizziness and headaches have also been reported, as well as depression. It is not unusual for the patient to complain of a bitter, metallic taste in the mouth. Occasional skin rashes have occurred. Fortunately, the drug is well tolerated and the untoward effects are not often serious. When metronidazole is prescribed, patients should be advised to avoid alcohol as the drug may produce reactions similar to that of disulfiram (Antabuse) when combined with alcohol.

Therapeutics

The efficacy of metronidazole in the treatment of acute ulcerative gingivitis is well established. Metronidazole is perhaps the first choice of drugs for the treatment of this condition, penicillin and other antibiotics being reserved for the more severe cases, *e.g.* patients showing signs of systemic toxicity. Metronidazole is dispensed as a 200 mg. tablet and one tablet is swallowed thrice daily for three days. Discomfort usually decreases after 24 hr. and ulcerations are beginning to heal after 48 hr.

As yet, sensitive organisms have not been found to develop resistance to metronidazole and its use in the treatment of an oral condition does not, therefore, prejudice its efficacy against trichomonal infections.

OTHER ANTIMICROBIAL AGENTS

Many other antimicrobials exist and some are carefully reserved for the treatment of particular infections. For example, streptomycin finds its principal use in the management of tuberculosis, whilst chloramphenicol is the drug of choice in typhoid fever when the seriousness of the complaint over-rides the dangers of its use. Chloramphenicol is a dangerous drug because it can produce irreversible marrow aplasia and it has no place in general dental practice.

Other antibiotics have been used mainly by local application because their parenteral administration is hazardous, *e.g.* polymyxin, bacitracin. Polymyxin, bacitracin and neomycin are contained in Polybactrin aerosol and this is sometimes used by dental surgeons to discourage wound infections. It must always be remembered that the liberal use of many topical antibiotics may encourage the emergence of resistant strains, with the result that the drugs concerned may be found to be ineffective if required systemically at some later date. There is also the risk of encouraging the development of hypersensitivity by local use.

Neomycin sulphate is a member of the streptomycin group which also includes framycetin, kanamycin and paromomycin. It is a bactericidal antibiotic with a wide range of activity on Gram-positive and Gram-negative organisms. It is rarely used parenterally because it may cause renal damage and is liable to produce deafness; the latter may even occur after topical administration. Nevertheless, neomycin alone, or in combination with other drugs, has achieved some popularity in dermatological preparations. Neomycin combined with a steroid (*e.g.* Betnovate-N; betamethasone 17-valerate 0·1 per cent and neomycin sulphate 0·5 per cent) as a cream or ointment is sometimes advocated as being helpful in treating the symptoms of herpes labialis. Various combinations of neomycin with other drugs have been used in dentistry, for example Cicatrin powder (essentially neomycin and zinc bacitracin) on wounds to prevent post-operative infection. However, the topical use of neomycin is not without its dangers and it is a fairly frequent cause of allergic sensitization, usually in the form of skin reactions which are of the delayed type.

Trimethoprim is an antimicrobial agent and has a range of activity similar to that of sulphonamides. It is known that bacteria can be inhibited if they are deprived of certain metabolites which are essential to them, *e.g.* para-aminobenzoic acid. Sulphonamides, by competitive antagonism with para-aminobenzoic acid, prevent the synthesis of bacterial folic acid, whereas trimethoprim acts at a later stage in the bacterial metabolism. When trimethoprim is combined with a sulphonamide, it exerts a bactericidal effect. Trimethoprim is combined with a sulphonamide (sulphamethoxazole) in the preparation Septrin and Bactrim, a tablet containing 80 mg. trimethoprim and 400 mg. sulphamethoxazole. Although trimethoprim is used extensively in medicine, its place in dentistry is not yet established.

Fusidic Acid (Fucidin) is a drug which is effective against staphylococci, although resistant strains do emerge *in vivo*, if rather slowly. Because of this fact it is often used in combined therapy with other antibiotics, *e.g.* erythromycin. Its place in dentistry is not yet established.

Idoxuridine is an anti-viral agent and is useful in the treatment of herpes simplex. Idoxuridine (IDU) is a substance which is incorporated into the DNA of the virus and stops it multiplying. In the amounts used in the local treatment of herpes simplex there does not seem to be any adverse effects on the cells of the host. Juel-Jensen (1973) suggests that for primary and recurrent infections of the skin idoxuridine dissolved in dimethyl sulphoxide (DMSO) is the treatment of choice at the present time. A 5–20 per cent solution of idoxuridine is applied with a brush to the cutaneous lesions four times a day for three days. This causes the vesicles to disappear rapidly and recurrences at the same site become rare.

Idoxuridine in ointment or watery solution will not penetrate the skin and is useless.

PARTICULAR PROPHYLAXIS: THE PREVENTION OF BACTERIAL ENDOCARDITIS

The dental treatment of patients with valvular defects of the heart poses a special problem. Patients with congenital heart defects, with a history of rheumatic fever, or chorea, or those who have undergone cardiac surgery may all be predisposed to bacterial endocarditis. The disease is caused by direct infection from the blood stream, bacteria colonizing the heart valves. Before the era of antibiotics, bacterial endocarditis was almost invariably fatal; even today mortality is about 30 per cent and patients are left with severely damaged hearts in spite of prolonged treatment with antibiotics. Although there is a changing pattern in the disease, as now the older patient is affected rather than the young, rheumatic heart disease is still an important underlying factor in the condition. In the pre-antibiotic era 95 per cent of cases of bacterial endocarditis were caused by *Streptococcus viridans*, an organism found in the mouth, whereas today it is probably less commonly implicated.

Transient bacteraemias follow many dental procedures. In the normal patient such bacteraemias are of little moment, for the bacteria are quickly removed from the bloodstream by the body's defences. However, in the predisposed patient organisms may be implanted on an abnormal heart valve with perpetuation of the bacteraemia from an endocardial focus.

The dental treatment of such patients should be considered as follows:

History

All patients attending for dental treatment should be questioned for any history of heart disease, previous rheumatic fever, or chorea. There is not complete agreement as to which patients should be considered "at risk"; not all would accept that a patient with a history of rheumatic fever, but with no apparent residual heart defects, should be so regarded. Unless a cardiologist is willing to vouchsafe that a particular patient, in spite of having had rheumatic fever, is not "at risk", the dental practitioner should proceed as though that patient were "at risk". However it is important to establish a positive history of rheumatic fever before the patient, on perhaps an indefinite history, is recorded for ever more as having had rheumatic fever.

Treatment Plan

Patients at risk must be encouraged to maintain a high standard of oral care. The teeth must be restored where necessary and periodontal disease prevented. If this state cannot be achieved, either because of indifference on the part of the patient, or because of the inherent quality of the dental tissues, extractions should be contemplated. It must be remembered that diseased tissues may be the source of bacteraemias even in the absence of dental procedures. It must also be emphasized that the edentulous patient is not free from the risk of bacterial endocarditis. Ulcers due to ill fitting dentures may be the cause of a bacteraemia, and such ulcers should receive immediate attention.

All patients concerned should be aware of any risk that dental procedures may involve. If the treatment plan demands many extractions, the patient should be referred to hospital.

The Use of Antimicrobial Agents

In order to prevent the occurrence of bacterial endocarditis in those patients considered to be at risk, antibiotic cover should be provided when certain dental procedures are undertaken, e.g. oral surgery, deep scalings, root canal therapy and any dental treatment likely to cause bleeding. The American Heart Association (1972) states: "Since viridans streptococci are the organisms most commonly implicated in endocarditis following these procedures, prophylaxis is directed specifically against them". A bactericidal agent is required which will kill susceptible organisms before they colonize damaged heart valves; bacteriostatic antibiotics, such as the tetracyclines, are therefore unsuitable. In providing such antibiotic cover a few guiding principles should be observed:

(a) Benzylpenicillin by intramuscular injection is probably the most effective drug for this purpose unless it is contra-indicated (see below);

(b) operative procedures should be undertaken as soon as the antibiotic has provided optimal plasma concentrations and the precise timing will vary with the antibiotic preparation being used. If operative procedures are delayed beyond this time, there is the risk of endocarditis due to the emergence of resistant strains.

(c) some young patients receive small doses of penicillin, on medical advice, as a prophylaxis against the recurrence of rheumatic fever. In these patients penicillin resistant strains of *Streptococcus viridans* will be present in the mouth and when antibiotic cover is required for some dental procedure, an alternative antibiotic should be used, *e.g.* cephaloridine or erythromycin estolate;

(d) when a patient has received penicillin therapy within the previous eight weeks, an alternative antibiotic (e.g. cephaloridine or erythromycin estolate) should be used to provide cover. This is because after penicillin has been discontinued it takes time for the mouth to be recolonized by penicillin sensitive strains; and

(e) if the patient is hypersensitive to penicillin an alternative antibiotic must be used to provide the required cover. As there may be some degree of cross allergenicity between penicillin and the cephalosporins, erythromycin estolate would be a suitable choice.

A few possible regimes are indicated below.

(1) When penicillin is not contra-indicated:

By intramuscular injection, $\frac{1}{2}$ hr. before the operation: benzylpenicillin injection, 600 mg. (1 mega unit) +, 6 hr. later, the oral administration of phenoxymethylpenicillin, 250 mg. 6-hourly for 3 days.

(2) When the patient is hypersensitive to penicillin:

By oral administration, 2 hr. before the operation: erythromycin estolate, 500 mg. +, 6 hr. later, the oral administration of erythromycin estolate, 250 mg. 6-hourly for 3 days.

(3) When penicillin is contra-indicated, other than because of hypersensitivity (see (c) and (d) above):

By intramuscular injection, $\frac{1}{2}$ hr. before the operation: cepahaloridine, 500 mg. +, 6 hr. later, the oral administration of erythromycin estolate, 250 mg 6-hourly for 3 days (an alternative to erythromycin estolate in this instance would be cephalexin, 250 mg. 6-hourly for 3 days).

As the onset of bacterial endocarditis may be insidious, patients should be advised to report any untoward symptoms or signs to their medical practitioner. Endocarditis may develop in spite of prophylaxis, but the present position has been summed up in the *British Medical Journal* (Leader) of 20th October 1973:

"Infective endocarditis presents a complex problem both in temperate and tropical countries. The role of immunological and other factors in the patient is uncertain. When we consider the large number of people at risk who have dental extractions or other procedures without any antibiotic cover, the incidence of the disease must be remarkably small. In two-thirds of patients no precipitating cause is detectable. The host's immunological response is probably more important than the infection, but in our present state of ignorance it remains obligatory to give prophylactic antibiotics for those at risk."

REFERENCES

Anderson, E. S. (1965), "Origin of Transferable Drug-resistance Factors in the Enterobacteriaceae," *Brit. Med. J.*, **2**, 1289.

Anderson, F. M., Datta, N. and Shaw, E. J. (1972), "R Factors in Hospital Infection," *Brit. Med. J.*, **3**, 82.

Chisholm, G. D., Waterworth, P. M., Calnan, J. S. and Garrod, L.P. (1973,) "Concentration of Antibacterial Agents in Interstitial Fluid," *Brit. Med. J.*, **1**, 569.

Davies, J. (1971), "Bacterial Resistance to Aminoglycoside Antibiotics," *J. infec. Dis.*, suppl. Dec.

Dean, A. C. R. and Hinshelwood, C. (1964), "What is Heredity?" *Nature* (*Lond.*), **202**, 1046.

Fillastre, J. P., Laumonier, R., Humbert, G., Dubois, D., Metayer, J., Delpech, A., Leroy, J., and Robert, M. (1973), "Acute Renal Failure Associated with Combined Gentamicin and Cephalothin Therapy," *Brit. med. J.*, **2**, 396.

Gale, E. F. (1973), "Perspectives in Chemotherapy," *Brit. med. J.* **4**, 33.

Garrod, L. P., Lambert, H. P. and O'Grady, F. (1973), *Antibiotics and Chemotherapy*, 4th edition, p. 257. Edinburgh and London: Churchill Livingstone.

Juel-Jensen, B. E. (1973), "Herpes Simplex and Zoster," *Brit. med. J.* **1**, 406.

Lederberg, J. and Lederberg, E. M. (1952), "Replica Plating and Indirect Selection of Bacterial Mutants," *J. Bact.*, **63**, 399.

Lorian, V. (1971), "The Mode of Action of Antibiotics on Gram-Negative Bacilli," *Arch. intern. Med.*, **128**, 623.

O'Grady, F. (1973), *Current Antibiotic Therapy*, p. 7. Edinburgh and London: Churchill Livingstone.

Robertson, M. H. (1973), "Tetracycline Resistant β-Haemolytic Streptococci in South-West Essex: Decline and Fall," *Brit. med. J.*, **4**, 84.

Scott, A. J., Nicholson, G. I. and Kerr, A. R. (1973), "Lincomycin as a Cause of Pseudomembranous Colitis," *Lancet*, **ii**, 1232.

Smith, S. E. and Rawlins, M. D. (1973), *Variability in Human Drug Response*, p. 152. Butterworths.

Thorburn, R., Johnson, J. E. and Cluff, L. E. (1966), "Studies on the Epidemiology of Adverse Drug Reactions," *J. Amer. med. Ass.* **198**, 345.

Wells, R. F., Cohen, L. E. and McNeill, C. J. (1974), "Clindamycin and Pseudomembranous Colitis," *Lancet* (Letter), **i**, 66.

18. GENERAL ASPECTS OF NEOPLASIA

PAMELA J. TARIN AND D. TARIN

AETIOLOGICAL FACTORS

Although the detailed mechanisms which lead to neoplastic change are still unknown, experimental work has shown that several agents can regularly and predictably induce tumours in normal animals. Clinical and epidemiological studies have provided convincing evidence that many of these agents can exert a similar action in man and therefore represent a serious environmental and occupational hazard.

Considerable work is in progress to understand the nature of agents capable of causing neoplasia and the mechanisms by which they do so. Currently, aetiological factors are grouped into four main categories as follows:

(a) chemicals;
(b) viruses;
(c) endocrine secretions; and
(d) radiation.

Genetic constitution is also important as can be seen from the variable responses of different individuals and species to the same carcinogenic agent.

There have recently been great advances in the information available on each of these factors and some of the new findings will now be considered.

Chemical Carcinogenesis

Since the isolation of benzpyrene from coal tar in the 1920s by Kennaway and his group, numerous man-made and naturally occurring chemicals have been shown to be capable of producing cancer. At first it was hoped there might be some chemical properties in common between these substances which would permit the recognition of a particular molecular configuration as being especially associated with carcinogenic activity. This hope was not realized and indeed a vast array of seemingly dissimilar substances have been shown to be capable of producing tumours under one or more circumstances, in various tissues, of many different species. In spite of this, it can still be stated that the majority of highly potent carcinogenic chemicals belong to one of three main groups. The first consists of the polycyclic hydrocarbons, typical examples of which include dimethylbenzanthracene, methylcholanthrene and dibenzanthracene. The second category consists of the aromatic amines, and includes such agents as N-methylaminoazobenzene (MAB), 2-acetaminofluorine and beta-naphthylamine. The third subdivision includes the other carcinogens, amongst which the nitroso compounds such as nitrosourea and the nitrosamines are perhaps the most important. Other significant and naturally occurring substances which should be included in this category are cycasin, a strong liver carcinogen produced by a variety of palm tree, the senecio alkaloids, ethionine and aflatoxin.

It has now been realized, as a result of a lot of work by many different laboratories, that most of these substances do not exert their action in the body in the form in which they are administered. In the course of their metabolism or detoxification extremely active and unstable compounds are formed which either bond very strongly to chemicals within the cell, or donate free radicals to them, thus altering the molecular configuration and the functional properties of the recipients (see review by Ryser, 1971). This process is spoken of as activation and the highly reactive strongly electrophilic compounds formed are termed ultimate or proximate carcinogens. This important generalization explains how carcinogens of totally different structure may act in a similar way.

The site at which the original chemical (or procarcinogen) is activated to form the ultimate carcinogen depends on the metabolic pathway of the substance and the organs in which the enzymes for its conversion reside. The enzymes concerned are usually located in the microsomal fraction and there is some evidence that their production is actually induced by the potentially toxic substances they metabolize. The distribution of such enzymes in the body is variable and accounts for the organ and species specificity of certain carcinogens. For instance the great susceptibility of the liver of some animals to acetylaminofluorene (AAF), azo dyes and ethionine is attributable to its function in the destruction and excretion of foreign substances. In animals, such as guinea-pigs, which cannot hydroxylate AAF, the administration of this substance has no carcinogenic effect, but if the carcinogens are administered in their activated form tumours arise in the animals not previously considered susceptible and are not restricted to the liver.

It is appropriate in this context to mention the related observation that inhibition of activation can prevent carcinogenesis. For instance, it has recently been shown that the administration of 7,8-benzoflavone will inhibit the cellular binding and the carcinogenic action of 7,12-dimethylbenzanthracene (DMBA). Both of these effects are due to the inhibition of an enzyme required for the activation of the procarcinogen (DMBA). It is also known that chloramphenicol and acetanilide inhibit liver carcinogenesis by acetylaminofluorene (AAF). This is because they compete for conjugation in the liver and decrease the formation of the ultimate carcinogen AFF-N-sulphate. Such approaches will probably have important therapeutic consequences in the future.

The intracellular chemicals which are the target of the activated carcinogens have not yet been identified with certainty. However, it has been found that all the major carcinogens so far investigated bind strongly (covalently) to DNA, RNA and protein in varying proportions, depending on the agent in question.

The polycyclic hydrocarbons bind primarily with proteins and DNA and the quantity that attaches to these cellular constituents increases with the potency of the carcinogenic agent. Starch gel electrophoresis of the soluble proteins of mouse skin has revealed a band to which the carcinogenic hydrocarbons bind to a much greater extent than the non-carcinogenic ones. This fraction is absent from fully grown tumours induced by the hydrocarbons but bears an electrophoretic resemblance to the liver protein which binds the carcinogenic aminoazo dyes. In the case of DNA it has been found that its binding to carcinogenic hydrocarbons does not require cell division and it occurs predominantly in the S phase of the cell cycle when DNA synthesis is in progress.

Studies on the aminoazo dyes show that AAF and MAB combine more with protein than with DNA or RNA whereas ethionine reacts more with RNA than with protein or DNA. Thus, although all the carcinogenic chemicals so far examined have tendencies to bind preferentially with tissue DNA, RNA and protein, there are quantitative differences in their affinities for these compounds which make it impossible at present to develop any unified explanation of the chemical basis of carcinogenic action.

Nevertheless, the finding that all carcinogenic chemicals bind to DNA to some extent suggests a mechanism by which they could alter the genome and thereby ensure that the malignant properties that they induce are transmitted to succeeding cell generations. In favour of this possibility is the finding that several ultimate carcinogens are able to elicit mutations in bacteria and bacteriophage. Also supporting it, is the observation that in xeroderma pigmentosum, a genetically transmitted disease in which there is an exceptionally high incidence of skin cancer on exposure to sunlight, many patients display an inability to repair damaged DNA. Conversely, it must be remembered that not all patients with xeroderma pigmentosum possess this defect in DNA repair mechanisms, nor do all genetic mutations lead to the production of cancer. So it is not enough to assume that non-specific alterations in DNA structure will cause cancer. It is therefore necessary to consider whether all the different carcinogens act by producing the same critical mutation. If so, however, it is difficult to explain how different cancers caused by the same mutation can exhibit the marked phenotypic variations seen in nature (see below).

Since the discovery of RNA-primed DNA polymerases, it has become respectable to consider the possibility that the binding of chemical carcinogens to RNA could lead to a heritable neoplastic change in the cell. However, in contrast to the studies on viruses (see below), there is no objective evidence to support this hypothesis in chemical carcinogenesis. Nor is there any factual information on how protein modified by binding with carcinogenic chemicals might produce permanent and heritable changes in cellular behaviour. Nevertheless, it must be conceded that modification of RNA or of membrane proteins by carcinogen binding could be responsible for neoplasia and this cannot be definitely excluded at present.

In an effort to provide a quantitative basis for further study of the interactions between carcinogenic chemicals and cellular constituents Heidelberger and his colleagues (see Heidelberger, 1970 for review) have developed a system for the study of chemical carcinogenesis in vitro. From mouse prostate glands they have derived cell lines which, under their standard culture conditions, ceased to grow after forming confluent monolayers, and do not form tumours on transplantation into the C3H mice from which they were derived. When carcinogenic chemicals are added to the culture medium, the cells continue to grow after a monolayer is attained and, in many foci randomly distributed around the culture dish, pile up on top of each other in an irregular criss-cross orientation. The cells in these foci, but not those in the intervening areas where there is only a monolayer, give rise to tumours when they are transplanted back into intact animals. Since it has also been shown that there is a quantitative relationship between the potency of the carcinogenic hydrocarbons and the number of piled-up colonies seen in the corresponding culture dishes, the method is likely to produce valuable information in future studies.

The three most probable mechanisms of carcinogenic action involved in this system are either:
(a) direct transformation of the cells by the chemical;
(b) selection of pre-existent malignant cells; or
(c) activation of an oncogenic virus in the culture.

Recent studies (see Heidelberger, 1970 for review) involving the exposure of single cells to methylcholanthrene in culture have shown unequivocally that carcinogenesis can be the result of a direct cellular transformation and not necessarily a selection of premalignant cells. This finding must be regarded as an important advance even if it applies only to the mouse prostate-cell culture system studied by Heidelberger's group.

Another significant finding reported by this group is that organ cultures of mouse prostate gland treated with carcinogenic chemicals do not produce tumours on transplantation back into intact animals, even though histological changes in the affected tissue appear to pathologists as being malignant. Treatment of organ cultures from the hydrocarbon experiments with pronase, and the cultivation of the resulting cell suspensions, produces permanent lines which are resistant to the toxicity of the hydrocarbons and develop into malignant transplantable tumours on transfer to C3H mice. The implication is that, whatever the chemical action of the carcinogenic agent within the cell, its effect is enhanced and facilitated by conditions in which cellular arrangement and communication are disturbed (see p. 221).

Viral Carcinogenesis

It is now generally accepted that viruses can cause neoplastic disease in several animal species although this has not yet been established for man (see Allen and Cole, 1972 for review). These viruses can be subdivided into two categories:

(a) DNA tumour viruses, for example polyoma virus, SV 40 virus (Simian vacuolating virus), and the Shope papilloma virus; and

(b) RNA tumour viruses, for example, the Rous sarcoma virus, the Bittner mammary tumour virus, the mouse leukaemia virus of Gross and the mouse sarcoma virus of Harvey. This category of viruses is also known as the oncogenic RNA virus group or simply the oncornaviruses.

The DNA tumour viruses can either bring about a productive infection with cellular lysis, which is accompanied by viral DNA replication and the production of new virions, or be incorporated in the cellular genome with associated "transformation" of the host cells. The use of this term transformation deserves some explanation. It implies only that there has been a permanent and heritable change in the behavioural and growth properties of the cells in culture. Briefly, transformed cells are not subject to contact inhibition of division or movement, and will survive indefinitely in cell culture. There is not necessarily any association between transformation *in vitro* and malignancy *in vivo*. In fact, it has been shown that transformed cells usually need to be passaged *in vitro* before they will proliferate and metastasize on transplantation back into animals.

It has been noted that incorporation of the virus DNA into the cellular genome occurs more readily when host-cell DNA is being synthesized or repaired. This observation is similar to the finding already mentioned, that the binding of carcinogenic hydrocarbons to DNA in tissue cultures occurs predominantly in the S phase of the cell cycle. It is also consistent with the recent observation that when cells are treated with methylcholanthrene (MCA) immediately after plating (*i.e.* when they are multiplying) transformation readily occurs; but if this treatment is delayed until day 8, by which time a monolayer has formed and cell division is contact-inhibited, transformation does not take place. Similarly, when X-rays are used for transformation, cell division must take place soon after for the transformed state to become fixed and stable.

The recent discovery of "conditional" mutants of polyoma virus has provided an opportunity for obtaining further insights into the mechanisms of viral carcinogenesis. For instance, a temperature sensitive form has been found which will only replicate itself, and transform cells, at a lower temperature than that which is optimum for cell culture. Infected cells which are grown at normal body temperature revert to normal morphology and behaviour implying that the continued activity of the viral genome is eqruired to maintain the transformed state and that it is not the product of a single-trigger event. The induction of T antigen synthesis, which in turn induces DNA synthesis, is also temperature-dependent as are alterations of the cell-surface membrane. This information indicates that DNA synthesis and cell-surface characteristics are controlled by adjacent or at least linked genes.

In contrast to the DNA viruses, the oncornaviruses are never cytopathic. In their natural hosts, they simultaneously transform the host cell and replicate themselves. The tumours induced by this group of viruses also have the peculiar characteristic that, after transplantation, their karyotype gradually changes to conform to that of the host rather than that of the donor. This indicates that the enlargement and spread of this type of tumour depends more on infection of adjacent cells than on propagation of neoplastically transformed tissue.

The nucleic acid of oncornaviruses is of course RNA (in single-stranded form) and this is combined with capsid protein and lipid. When visible with the electron microscope, the virus particles may be categorized into three types designated A, B and C. Type C particles are about 100 nm. in diameter and consist of a dense central spherical nucleoid 40 nm. in diameter containing RNA. This is surrounded by a membrane which is separated from the outer envelope by an electron translucent region. The envelope is derived in part from the host cell and resembles the plasma membrane. C particles are commonly seen in animal leukaemias and sarcomas.

Type B particles are similar in appearance to C particles except that their nucleoid is not central and there are regularly spaced projections on the viral surface, demonstrable by negative staining with phosphotungstic acid. Mammary tumour viruses are typical of those with B particle morphology.

Type A particles are considered to be precursors of B particles. They consist of a dense ring resembling a doughnut, located within the cisternae of the endoplasmic reticulum and have been reported in a variety of transplantable murine tumours.

Even in the absence of tumours, or of visible virus particles, it is possible to infer the presence of oncornaviruses in apparently normal cells of various species. In chickens and mice that are free of infectious virus, the group specific antigen of the leukosis virus can be detected and is inherited as a single autosomal dominant trait. In addition, such apparently uninfected chick cells can be made to produce functional oncornavirus components, and it is possible to demonstrate in them the presence of DNA homologous to the RNA of the oncornaviruses. This evidence raises the possibility that oncornaviruses may be very widely, or even ubiquitously, distributed in latent form, and only activated in certain circumstances.

The mechanisms by which RNA viruses produce heritable neoplastic change in the cells they infect have engaged the interest and attention of cancer research workers for some time. The observation that actinomycin D, an inhibitor of RNA transcription from a DNA template, inhibits viral replication suggested that the virus not only replicates but also exerts its effects through an intermediate consisting of DNA. This idea was supported by the later discovery of the requirement for DNA synthesis in the growth of Rous sarcoma and Rous associated viruses. The hypothesis that DNA is synthesized on a template consisting of the viral RNA was confirmed by the subsequent discovery of RNA-directed DNA polymerase (otherwise known as reverse transcriptase). Investigations have now shown that almost all oncornaviruses contain reverse transcriptase whereas most non-oncogenic RNA viruses do not.

These discoveries indicate that mechanisms are available for the transfer of information from extraneous RNA into the genome of the cell. It has recently been proposed that such mechanisms may be important not only in neoplastic conversion of cells by RNA tumour viruses, but also in mediation of the effects of one group of cells on another in normal embryonic development (otherwise known as embryonic induction).

Relevant to this consideration of the mechanism of action of RNA tumour viruses is the recent finding of a temperature-sensitive conditional mutant of the Rous sarcoma virus. It appears, therefore, that in this category of tumour viruses, as with the DNA tumour viruses, the continued action of the viral genome is required for the maintenance of the transformed state.

Since the time it was recognized that viruses can be responsible for causing tumours in animals, clinicians and research workers have sought to establish whether any human tumours are attributable to viral aetiology. As direct experimental methods are obviously not ethically acceptable for obtaining information on this, investigation has depended on epidemiological approaches and attempts to demonstrate viruses or viral antibodies in human tissues and serum. The epidemiological studies have examined the possibility of infective transmission by testing whether certain types of neoplasms emerge in clusters closely grouped in space and time, and have also analysed seasonal and geographic variations in tumour incidence. The most striking evidence obtained by these methods relates to the type of tumour which has come to be known as Burkitt's lymphoma. The incidence of this type of cancer in central Africa was observed by Burkitt to correspond closely to certain climatic zones and to decline rapidly with increasing altitude. The findings seemed most consistent with the interpretation that the disease is transmitted by an arthropod vector carrying an oncogenic virus. The subsequent demonstration of the Epstein-Barr virus in samples from most cases of the disease, lends support to this hypothesis although conclusive proof is still required. Examples of other diseases in which the Epstein-Barr virus has been detected include nasopharyngeal carcinoma and infectious mononucleosis. It has been suggested that the latter condition is the outcome of infection with this virus in individuals who are immune to its oncogenic activity (see p. 227).

Other types of human cancer suspected of being of viral aetiology, on the basis of analogy with comparable tumours in animals, include leukaemias, mammary tumours, and reticuloses such as Hodgkin's disease. There are reports of space time clusters of these neoplastic conditions but the negative studies outnumber the positive. Undoubtedly, with all of them there is evidence for familial aggregation, but this does not necessarily imply viral aetiology. Indeed, in such circumstances it is necessary to be able to show that the disease occurs with equal frequency amongst the genetically unrelated marital partners within the family, before a viral aetiology can be seriously considered. However, it should be mentioned that B and C particles have been identified in a high proportion of tissue specimens from human breast cancers. Similar particles have also been found in milk from human patients with breast cancer more frequently than from controls. Amongst the relatives of patients with mammary cancer, there is also a vastly greater incidence of virus-like particles in the milk than in the relatives of women with no family history of breast cancer. Furthermore, the particles from human milk possessed RNA-dependent DNA polymerase activity similar to that of other oncornaviruses, while milk lacking the particles also lacked the activity. In spite of this, the evidence mainly favours the view that human mammary tumours are closely related to aspects of reproductive life and thus may be primarily hormonal with viruses perhaps acting as promoters (see p. 20 for explanation of tumour promotion).

In contrast to the epidemiological findings, serological work employing fluorescein-labelled antibodies to oncornaviruses has shown that tissues from 49 out of 72 leukaemic patients gave a positive response whereas non-leukaemic tissue did not bind the fluorescent antibody. Similar findings have been reported with human liposarcomas, fibrosarcomas and osteosarcomas. In all of these types of tumours there appears to be a common antigen to which nearly 100 per cent of the patients possess antibodies. Eighty-five per cent of members of the patients' families also have the antibodies but only 20 per cent of normal blood donors, who are regarded as controls in such investigations.

Such findings imply viral aetiology, but as there is no epidemiological evidence in support of this for any of the tumours just mentioned, the findings are difficult to interpret at present.

Endocrine Secretions

There is now ample evidence that endocrine factors can play an important role in the production of tumours. Studies in animals, for instance, have shown that the administration of high doses of oestrogens leads to the production of a high incidence of mammary tumours and a smaller number of other tumours including adenomas of the pituitary, lymphomas of the thymus, carcinomas of the uterus and malignant tumours of the kidney in the hamster. Administration of pituitary growth hormone has been reported to produce lymphosarcoma of the lungs, and tumours of the adrenal cortex and ovaries in rats. A related observation is that androgens inhibit mammary carcinogenesis by oestrogens.

In humans, the dependence of certain mammary tumours on pituitary, ovarian and adrenal hormones, and the success of endocrine therapy of tumours of the prostate provide further evidence of the general importance of endocrine factors in carcinogenesis.

Most of the work on this topic has been concerned with the development of mammary tumours. An important early observation was that ovariectomy in very young animals prevented the subsequent appearance of mammary tumours whereas injections of large doses of oestrogenic hormones into mice of a strain with a high mammary cancer incidence caused a rise in the number of tumours found in females and the development of such tumours even in males. This indicates that the rarity of mammary cancer in the male is due to the fact that male mammary tissue, though potentially responsive, is in an immature condition.

More recently it has been realized that the pituitary hormone prolactin is probably involved in the growth of mammary tumours both in animals and in humans (see Pearson, 1973 for review). The evidence for this conclusion accumulated as follows: it was observed that, in patients whose mammary tumours regressed in response to ovariectomy, administration of oestrogens caused reactivation of tumour growth. In patients who had been hypophysectomized as well as ovariectomized, oestrogens failed to produce such reactivation, suggesting that an intermediate factor released by the pituitary was involved. Studies on carcinogen-induced mammary tumours in mice revealed a similar involvement of a pituitary factor in the reactivation of tumour growth in ovariectomized animals. Further investigation showed that administration of purified prolactin could produce reactivation in animals whose tumours had undergone partial regression after ovariectomy or hypophysectomy.

After development of a radio-immune assay for prolactin it was demonstrated that the administration of oestrogens causes a pronounced increase in plasma prolactin levels. It was also found with this assay that there was good correspondence between plasma prolactin concentration and growth rate of the mammary tumours. The interpretation is that in these mice regression of mammary carcinoma induced by ovariectomy-adrenalectomy is related to a fall in plasma prolactin, and conversely that oestrogen-induced reactivation is related to a rising concentration of this hormone in the blood. Detailed studies of serum prolactin levels in human breast cancer have not yet been reported, but methods for such investigations are being developed.

Radiation Carcinogenesis

Radiation of various types constitutes another factor recognized as capable of causing cancer. Originally, it was observed that radiologists working with X-rays for diagnostic and research purposes frequently developed squamous cell carcinoma on their hands, these being often exposed to the beam in the positioning of patients and other procedures. Later, it was recognized that other forms of ionizing radiations such as rays emitted by radioactive chemicals could also cause cancer. This emerged when it was noted that miners working in pits containing radioactive mineral ores were subject to a high incidence of lung tumours and that women painting the dials of watches with luminous paint were susceptible to developing bone sarcomas. The former group of workers inhaled radioactive dust released by digging and drilling while the latter ingested radioactive material by licking the brushes between strokes to produce a fine point for delicate work.

Following the nuclear explosions in Hiroshima and Nagasaki, it was realized that even single exposures to ionizing radiation of sufficient intensity could induce leukaemia and other malignant diseases in the survivors. Since then, it has also been stated that exposure of a fetus to X-rays in utero as a consequence of investigation of maternal disease carries a greatly increased risk of leukaemia arising in the offspring.

Irradiation with ultra-violet light is also capable of producing skin tumours in humans and animals. This is now known to be the agent responsible for producing solar keratoses and basal-cell carcinomas in some individuals. Although ultra-violet light does not penetrate animal tissues to the same extent as ionizing radiation, it does produce marked scarring and elastosis in the dermis together with hyperplastic and dysplastic changes in the epidermis.

The mechanisms by which various forms of radiation exert a carcinogenic action remain unknown. However, as with the carcinogenic chemicals and viruses, the primary target is currently supposed to be the genome of the parent cells from which the cancer cells are derived. This belief is supported by the observations that exposure of cells to ionizing radiation in vitro results in fracture of chromosomes and other nuclear abnormalities and that radiation exerts a potent mutagenic effect on bacteria and other test organisms such as Drosophila.

The finding, referred to above, that the frequency of transformation in vitro is greater when cells can divide immediately after exposure to X-rays than when they are in confluent monolayers, similarly indicates that the target for the carcinogenic effect of radiation is DNA and that the damage can be repaired if division is deferred.

Defective repair of DNA has been noted in the cells from some patients with xeroderma pigmentosum after exposure to U-V radiation. On the basis of these findings, the marked susceptibility of sufferers from this condition to skin cancer induced by solar radiation is attributed to inability to repair cellular DNA damaged by the ultraviolet rays in sunlight. One difficulty in accepting this interpretation is that not all patients with xeroderma pigmentosum have faulty DNA repair, although they all have the high susceptibility to neoplasia of the skin.

NATURAL HISTORY OF TUMOUR DEVELOPMENT

From this time of conversion of a normal tissue to one with neoplastic potential, to the time a tumour is clinically evident, there is a latent period. The latent period is variable depending on the animal species, the length of exposure to the neoplastic-inducing agent and perhaps even the lifespan of the animal. Studies on industrial disease in man have indicated a latent period of 5–25 years after exposure to a tumour-inducing agent, e.g. aniline dyes, asbestos. Carcinogenic treatment of the back skin of a mouse, however, reveals a latent period of only 14 months. In relation to the two-year lifespan of the mouse, this still represents a long latent period.

With certain agents, continuous exposure to high dosage during the latent period is necessary for tumours to arise. For instance, statistical studies on cigarette smoking have shown that not only do heavy smokers have a high risk of lung cancer but that the risk is reduced when the cigarette smoking is decreased or discontinued. However, constant exposure to a tumour-inducing agent is not always a prerequisite. Depending on the potency of the carcinogenic agent, a transient exposure is sometimes enough to alter the tissue which, after a latent period, becomes neoplastic. Animal experiments suggest that nitrosamines are some of the most potent carcinogens known, requiring in some cases only a single dose to induce tumours.

Tumour induction, in some instances, appears to be a "two stage" mechanism. The sites of tar-induced papillomas on a rabbit's ear were marked with India ink and the tumours allowed to regress. Subsequent treatment with tar, chloroform or punching holes in the ear led to the reappearance of papillomas, many of which arose at the ink-marked sites where previous ones had disappeared. It seems that "latent" tumours, which have been initiated by an agent, can persist and that a change from dormancy to progressive growth may be "promoted" by a further agent. This theory was investigated further.

A single painting of carcinogen at various concentrations was performed on a series of animals. This was the initiating agent whose concentration determined the number of tumours produced. Croton oil was employed as a "promoting" factor and it was found that the speed of production of tumours could be affected by delaying croton oil treatment. By using croton oil treatment prior to painting with a carcinogen virtually no tumours were produced, indicating that the increased tumour yield and reduced latent period observed is not a simple summation effect.

Neoplasia usually manifests as a lump in a tissue or organ. Neoplastic tissues are widely variable in histological appearance, resembling to a greater or lesser degree their tissue of origin. However, most neoplastic tissues have characteristic features in common. All have increased cellularity or increased amount of stroma or both. All possess an increased number of mitotic figures and abnormalities of cellular size, shape and staining properties when compared with normal tissue. There is also a spatial derangement of the cells to one another. The diversity in histological appearance is enormous. Each tumour resembles the normal tissue of origin to a variable degree but there may be changes in cell type from one area of a tumour to another, e.g. squamous carcinoma in areas of adenomatous change in mammary gland. Inflammatory changes may be present, especially if the growth has ulcerated or become necrotic. Lymphocytes may gather at the edge of the growth or be widely distributed within the tumour.

Tumours are designated either benign or malignant. These are rough categories used to indicate the probability of behaviour of a particular tumour. Benign tumours are usually slow growing and may have a capsule of compressed stroma round them. Malignancy in tumours is characterized by invasion of adjacent tissue by tumour cells and the ability to establish metastatic deposits in other organs. However, some tumours are locally invasive and never metastasize (e.g. basal cell carcinoma) and some haemangiomas are more malformations than tumours. Other tumours are so frankly anaplastic and invasive that the tissue of origin is hard to determine.

Invasiveness occurs normally during the growth cycle of the hair follicle, during implantation of the fertilized ovum and during duct development in the pregnant mammary gland. In each instance, the invasiveness is controlled. Studies on the factors controlling normal invasiveness may give clues as to the lack of control in neoplasia.

Once tumours are noticed in humans they are usually at an advanced stage of development. The features of early tumour growth are thus difficult to observe except in those conditions designated "precancerous" in which a proportion can be clinically observed to proceed to tumour formation. Histological studies on precanceroses cannot as yet distinguish which areas of a lesion may become neoplastic or when.

Precancerous changes in human tissue have been studied mainly in skin lesions as these are easily accessible and obvious. Epithelial cells in such premalignant conditions as xeroderma pigmentosum, leukoplakia and actinic keratoses exhibit a certain lack of adhesiveness as compared to normal epithelium. Electron microscopy of epithelial tumours shows more intercellular spaces and a reduction in the number of junctional elements accompanied by some cell degeneration. These features are most marked in malignant tumours, less so in premalignant conditions and much less pronounced in benign tumours. To observe neoplastic changes sequentially, carcinogen-induced tumours in animals have been employed.

The change from normal to neoplastic tissue may not be a simple one-step event but a series of "progressive" changes. For example, studies on mouse mammary tumours have shown that some tumours altered with time, becoming progressively independent of hormonal control. In mice, the usual manifestation of early neoplasia is a macroscopically visible plaque of hyperplastic tissue. This increases in size during pregnancy and regresses during parturition. With successive pregnancies, areas of the plaques "progressed" to carcinomas of various types.

Some carcinomas were, from the outset, independent of hormonal control. Some carcinomas grew during pregnancy and regressed during parturition, but with successive reproductive cycles the tumours grew larger and regressed less until eventually they also became unresponsive to the hormonal stimulus. In a similar way, the mouse mammary tumours varied in their ability to produce milk in late pregnancy.

The development of drug resistance in tumours, immunoresistance, and sarcomatous change after serial transplantation of epithelial tumour tissue are further examples of progressive changes occurring in established neoplastic tissue.

RECENT STUDIES ON PRECANCEROUS CHANGES

Studies of precancerous changes have two main objectives:

(a) to understand how the disease originates; and

(b) to identify features which might prove useful in the early diagnosis of malignancy.

There are, of course, several types of alterations (chemical, structural and functional) in tissues undergoing early neoplasia and here it is proposed to concentrate on some of those which have been the subject of recent study.

Morphological Observations

It is well known, from experimental work and diagnostic experience, that the morphology of tumour cells is very variable and usually differs considerably from that of their normal counterparts. It is important to remember, however, that a tumour is not simply a collection of cancer cells. Consideration of the natural history of tumours shows that they are complex lesions incorporating different tissues of an organ, the histological arrangement of which becomes more disorganized as the disease develops. Thus, it is important to consider not only the tumour cells themselves but also the relationships between different tissues in the developing lesion and between the established lesion and the whole organism.

Recent morphological studies on relationships between different tissues in experimentally-induced skin tumours have shown that there is a sequence of marked ultrastructural changes at the boundary between epithelium and connective tissue prior to and after the development of recognizable tumours (see Tarin, 1972). In the early stages, focal gaps appear in the basal lamina and this is accompanied by accumulation of fragmented basal lamina material in the superficial dermis. The dermal collagen fibres also decrease in size and the acid mucopolysaccharide ground substance between them is increased.

Somewhat later, but still before the appearance of tumours, the fragmented material in the dermis coalesces to form multiple reduplications of the basal lamina focally distributed at the boundary between epithelium and connective tissue. At this time the epidermis is hyperplastic and the cells are irregularly arranged with large intercellular spaces intervening. The dermis is also unusually cellular, most of the new occupants being inflammatory cells among which mast cells predominate. The intervening collagen fibres are still small but otherwise intact.

As soon as small papillomas appear, new ultrastructural features are observed at the dermo-epidermal boundary. These consist of focal disappearance of basal lamina substance, protrusion of bulbous pseudopodia by the basal cells and patchy disintegration of the adjacent connective tissue. Such areas are at first small but later expand to be observed along the entire advancing front of an invading carcinoma and are presumed to be the sites of neoplastic invasion.

Control experiments established that none of these changes is seen in the skin of animals painted with the pure solvent (acetone) in which the carcinogen was dissolved, nor in that of animals treated with irritant chemicals such as benzene or turpentine. Thus it is concluded that the changes are associated with the carcinogenic action of methylcholanthrene and not with its irritative effect. This interpretation is supported by numerous reports of similar features observed in a variety of neoplastic conditions in humans and experimental animals (see Tarin, 1972 for details). Comparative studies on mammary tumours in mice show that the morphological disturbances are similar whether the tumours are of viral, chemical or "spontaneous" aetiology. This suggests that the different carcinogenic agents all act by disturbing similar biological processes in the mammary gland.

It is worthy of note that some of the features described above have been observed in diseases not known to have neoplastic potential (e.g. psoriasis, lichen planus). This means that the individual ultrastructural changes (e.g. fragmentation of the basal lamina, reduplication, pseudopod and vesicle production, connective tissue destruction) are not by themselves characteristic of the carcinogenic process and are therefore probably of limited value for the early diagnosis of cancer. However, this does not invalidate conclusions drawn from the morphological observations since carcinogenesis is the only condition in which they have been seen collectively and in the order described above. Further investigation of the sequence of changes and of their significance may therefore give more insight into the mechanisms of carcinogenesis.

Biochemical Observations

There is good correlation between the ultrastructural observations described above and the results of sequential biochemical studies recently reported by Seilern-Aspang, Mazzucco, Christian and their colleagues (see Mazzuco, 1972 for review).

It was found by this group that painting the skin with carcinogenic chemicals produces a gradual and progressive decrease in its collagen content. In the early stages, cessation of painting resulted in reversal of this trend and a return to normal values without tumour production. Once the collagen content had fallen below a critical value (corresponding to 50 mg. hydroxyproline/mg. dry wt. skin), however, the collagen content did not rise after painting ceased and tumours were formed. The interesting thing about these results is that the collagen content of the skin began to fall long before tumours appeared. Also, despite the fact that the carcinogenic chemical was applied to the epidermis and produced epidermal hyperplasia, biochemical changes which could be directly correlated with the subsequent development or absence of tumours occurred in the adjacent tissue.

Another experiment showed that if one compared groups of mice treated with carcinogens of different potencies, the rate of collagen decrease was greatest in the group treated with the most potent chemical. Comparison of groups of mice of different inbred strains treated with the same chemical shows that the strains with the greatest susceptibility to the carcinogenic agent, in terms of speed of tumour production, manifested the most rapid rate of collagen decrease. In some strains the rate of fall was so constant and reproducible that in any given batch of animals it was possible to predict with reasonable accuracy when the first tumours would arise.

It has been known for a long time that the skin of the mouse varies in its susceptibility to carcinogenic chemicals in different parts of the body. While it is easy to induce carcinomas in the skin of the animal's back, the tail skin is completely refractory to this treatment. The same group of workers established that this was associated with clear differences in the quantity and type of dermal collagen in the two sites. In normal tail skin there was more collagen which possessed a greater degree of intermolecular crosslinking than in back skin. Transplantation of tail skin to the back resulted in a marked fall in its collagen content. This was accompanied by the emergence of the capacity to form tumours in grafts if they were treated with carcinogens.

Since the collagen content of tail skin was found to be low in new born mice and to rise later to normal adult values it was decided to investigate the effects of treating the tail with carcinogenic chemicals in young mice. The result was the production of tumours in tail skin, providing further evidence of a strong association between the formation of epithelial tumours and disturbances in the collagen metabolism of the connective tissue in this organ. There is clearly a great need for similar studies on collagen turnover in human preneoplastic and neoplastic conditions.

Implantation Studies

In certain animals such as mice, rats, dogs and hamsters the introduction of a foreign body such as a plastic film into the subcutaneous tissues results after a long latent period in the development of a sarcoma in relation to the implant. This phenomenon has been used by Brand and Brand and their colleagues to conduct a series of ingenious *in vivo* studies on the mechanisms of tumour formation (see Brand, 1974 for review).

Sequential histological studies show that the process of neoplasia induced by an implant occurs as follows. In the first few days cells accumulate around the implant, macrophages and monocytes being the most common types. After about two weeks, several cells become attached to the surface of the plastic to form a monolayer of macrophages, fibroblasts and smooth muscle cells. Fibroblasts and small blood vessels predominate in the surrounding loose connective tissue which is already forming a thin collagenous investing membrane or capsule. By three months the monolayer of cells on the surface of the implant appears inactive and quiescent and a thick acellular collagenous capsule surrounds it. After this there is little change for several months until sarcomas are detected adjacent to the implants some 14–24 months after their insertion. In this time the monolayer of cells continues to be devoid of any obvious synthetic or mitotic activity.

There seems to be a positive correlation between this quiescent condition, in which the cells on the plastic are surrounded by a thick capsule for months, and the production of tumours because, in species which do not show similar features, tumours do not arise in relation to implanted foreign bodies.

Proceeding now to consider evidence on the mechanisms of foreign-body tumour production, it is clear that the physical qualities of implants can provoke neoplasia quite independently of their chemical composition. This can be shown by converting the plastic film to powdered or finely shredded form prior to implantation. In such experiments, tumours do not arise. Similar results can be obtained with glass, metal and various polymers.

How the physical form of such apparently inert materials causes tumour development is at present not fully understood, but the state of knowledge has been substantially advanced by the following series of experiments performed by Brand and Brand and their co-workers. The information obtained is also pertinent to consideration of the basic processes involved in neoplasia in general.

If the plastic film is removed in the early stages of capsule formation, tumour development does not occur unless the foreign body is replaced by a fresh one. On the other hand, if the film is allowed to remain in position for nine months or longer a tumour sometimes forms in the capsule even if the film is removed. Although this demonstrates that the foreign body needs to stay in place for a long time before the tissues surrounding it become committed to neoplastic behaviour, it can be shown that in the period prior to commitment clones of pre-neoplastic parent cells are already present in the capsule and on the film. The evidence for this was obtained by transferring portions of the film from mice of a strain possessing a marker chromosome (CBA/H-T6) to a syngeneic variety of the same strain which did not possess it (CBA/H)—or *vice versa*. The films were removed from their original carriers many months before tumours would appear and cut into smaller pieces. These were then implanted separately into mice without the marker. It was found that each of the recipients subsequently developed tumours which could be identified as being of donor origin on the basis of the T_6 chromosome. All the tumours from segments of the same film appeared almost simultaneously in the various recipients (*i.e.* had the same latent period), were histologically closely related with regard to sarcoma type and degree of anaplasia, and had identical chromosome constitution as judged by modal chromosome number. Any new chromosome markers which arose were present in all tumours derived from the same film. Furthermore, all the tumours of such a group possessed similar growth characteristics *in vivo* and cell generation times *in vitro*. These findings reveal a homology between tumours arising from the segments of a single film and this is attributed to a common origin from a single clone of pre-neoplastic cells in the original carrier. The same results were obtained when pieces of film/capsule complexes were transplanted but not when portions of capsule alone were used. If the plastic associated with a particular capsule is replaced by pieces of another film the tumours which arise are not homologous. Evidence has recently been obtained to indicate that the cells from which the tumours arise are probably pericytes of the local microvasculature.

Digressing for a moment, it is worth considering the question of the latent period, which is a common feature in the natural history of tumours. It really is very remarkable that the homologous tumours derived from a single film appeared in all recipients at roughly the same time though periods of up to 1–2 years sometimes elapsed after transfer. As Brand has said: "Apparently every member of a pre-neoplastic clone stood under the uniform command of an intracellular timing mechanism" which incidentally was not significantly altered by the different environments into which they were transplanted.

The demonstration of clonal populations of preneoplastic cells implies that they are the progeny of single parent cells, in which the common properties possessed by the clones originally arose. There are indications from other similar transplantation experiments that cells destined to form neoplastic clones migrate from the extracapsular region and multiply to form the clones in the capsule. Most of the progeny probably then settle on the implant surface. Thus is seems likely that direct contact with the implant is not essential for the initiation of neoplastic behaviour. Since the experiment involving the use of the plastic in the form of a powder fails to produce tumours, and one can exclude the action of a chemical agent acting at a distance, it seems reasonable to consider the possibility that cells with pre-neoplastic potential already reside in the tissues. If so, it is necessary to assume that under "normal" conditions their properties put them at a disadvantage in comparison to normal cells and that the introduction of the plastic film then creates some special circumstances which favour their survival and proliferation at the expense of their normal counterparts. Are there any special circumstances created by plastic film and other foreign bodies which might fulfil this role? One of the most obvious properties of such a foreign body is that it functions as a barrier in the tissue. If numerous holes are punched in the film prior to implantation, sarcomas do not arise in the surrounding tissue. Recent studies with Millipore filters have shown that this holds true right down to membranes with nominal pore sizes as small as $0.2\,\mu$. When the pore size is reduced to $0.1\,\mu$ there is a high incidence of tumours in relation to the implants and so there is a sharp cut-off point at which the effect of the pores is eliminated. Histological studies show that the pores of the filters which acted as foreign-body tumour inducers (*i.e.* nominal pore size $0.1\,\mu$) contain no cellular processes. On the other hand, cytoplasmic pro-

cesses or even whole cells can be identified in the pores of those groups of filters (*i.e.* $0.2\,\mu$ nominal pore size or larger) which do not produce tumours. The processes do not appear to reach the centre of the filter and make contact with those from cells on the other side. However, it must be remembered that the spaces in a Millipore filter form an irregular maze and the possibility of contact being made between tenuous processes weaving in and out of the place of section cannot be excluded at present.

Some recent observations made by Saxen, Wartiovaara and their colleagues in Helsinki, on cellular interactions in embryonic development are pertinent to this topic. The metanephrogenic mesenchyme of the kidney needs to be triggered or induced before it can form kidney tubules and the spinal cord is one of the tissues which can do this. Interposition of Millipore filters between the two tissues shows that the effect can be exerted across a barrier with pores of $0.2\,\mu$ or larger diameter but not across one with pores of $0.1\,\mu$ or smaller. Histological studies showed that cytoplasmic processes penetrated the pores of the filters in the former group but did not seem to meet in the middle. Further morphological studies, with Nucleopore membranes which are not sponge-like but are traversed by straight channels like bullet tracks, demonstrated that the filters with larger pores allow processes penetrating from each side to make contact with corresponding ones from the tissue on the other side whereas the filters which prevent induction do not. Since the time required for tubule formation is also closely related to that for contacts to be established between processes there is good reason for believing that intercellular contact is the means for transmitting the inductive signal.

Although this is by no means a universal mechanism of interaction between two different tissues in embryonic organ formation this study shows direct cellular contact to be an important means of cellular communication in some circumstances. The remarkable similarities in the findings in kidney induction and in FB sarcoma production seem to be more than coincidental and suggest that further investigations will reveal that, in the latter, cellular communication across the implant is impaired.

ESTABLISHED TUMOURS

Structural Aspects

Once neoplasms become big enough to be noticed they are already structurally complex and it is extremely difficult to obtain any clues to account for the prevailing impression of disorder which is observed in all tumours or to account for the specific properties of any individual one. There is considerable structural variation, both gross and microscopical, between tumours and this is so not only between those in different sites but also within different parts of the same tumour. Changes, of course, also occur with the passage of time making interpretation still more difficult.

Despite this bewildering diversity, attempts to use the structural features of tumours to assess the prognosis of human disease are meeting with some success. It is not easy to predict the future behaviour of a tumour with reliability on the basis of morphological observations alone, but when this is accompanied by clinical follow-up studies, there is a reasonable possibility of obtaining information which will be useful for therapeutic purposes.

Several grading schemes have been proposed for assessing the severity of malignant disease. These use the presence or absence of features such as pleomorphism, mitotic figures, degree of histological disorder, extent of invasion of adjacent tissues and spread to lymph nodes or distant organs to allocate a particular patient's disease to a category in the scheme. Until recently, such allocation was based on qualitative evaluation of the pattern of features observed in each case. A refinement of this is a new method (see Chapter 19) in which points are awarded, from a standard scale, for each feature observed and the aggregate score is used as a basis for allocation to a place in the grading scheme. This method is intended to reduce the variability attributable to the subjective element in diagnosis.

Because of special anatomical or functional considerations separate grading schemes have to be worked out for neoplasms occurring in different organs and also for some types of malignancy which are diffuse in nature (*e.g.* leukaemia, reticuloses).

The predicted pattern of behaviour of the tumours in each of the categories of a grading scheme has been derived from clinical observation. It must be remembered that observations on the behaviour of the disease are complicated by the effects of therapy. This is to be expected because clinicians cannot merely observe the course of the disease as an academic exercise and do nothing. Because of this inbuilt source of difficulty, continuing long-term studies on large numbers of patients will be required before predictions become really accurate. Nevertheless, such systematic efforts to grade the severity of the disease and correlate it with the effects of treatment are the only way towards attaining the most beneficial results.

Ultrastructure

It was a widely nursed hope that electron microscopy might reveal some fundamental disturbance to which cancerous behaviour could be attributed. In fact electron microscopical observations on established tumours have proved remarkably disappointing from this point of view and it is now quite evident that, like the light microscope, the instrument will have to be used in properly designed investigations in order to reveal useful information.

The ultrastructural features of established tumours are, as one might expect from the histology and the morbid anatomy, extremely variable. Most studies have concentrated on the ultrastructure of the neoplastic cells themselves and the findings are considered in detail in some recent excellent reviews. In essence, however, these investigations have shown that there are no consistent and reliable ultrastructural features which permit the recognition of neoplastic cells; nor are there any intracellular changes which betray how the neoplastic disturbance originates and is perpetuated. The only finding which approached this status was the discovery of round dense bodies in the mitochondria of carcinogen-treated animals. For a short time,

it was thought that this observation might indicate the site of carcinogenic action; but these hopes were destroyed by the realization that they could only be found in epidermis and not other tissues, and that similar changes could be produced by non-specific stimuli such as irritant chemicals or wounding (see Tarin, 1972 for review).

The electron microscope has, however, proved very useful in the study of cancer by revealing changes which cannot be seen with the light microscope in the extracellular tissues and in relationships between cells. Its continuing use in sequential studies of the carcinogenic process is therefore expected to provide information which will contribute to understanding of the basic mechanisms involved.

Behavioural Aspects

Although not all tumours invade and metastasize, these are the most sinister features of tumour behaviour. They not only cause severe destruction but also confer upon the tumour cells the ability to survive excision of the primary lesion. These properties of established malignant tumours have attracted comparatively little direct investigation and remain poorly understood but recent studies have produced information likely to be of therapeutic value.

Invasion

Histological observations show that invasive tumours commonly consist of tightly packed masses of tumour cells which, as they advance into the adjacent tissue, erode and destroy it. The ultimate macroscopical results of this activity vary somewhat depending on the site but often include severe haemorrhage due to the rupture of a large blood vessel, fracture or collapse of bones or the extensive replacement of vital organs such as the liver or the kidney by tumour tissue.

Strauch and his colleagues (see Strauch, 1972 for review) report evidence indicating that many human and animal tumours invade the surrounding tissues by the production of collagenolytic enzymes. Their correlated biochemical and microscopical studies on adjacent slices across the tumour show that the zones with high collagenolytic activity correspond exactly with those displaying morphological features of invasion. In tumours with histological evidence of a radial pattern of invasive growth collagenolytic activity is higher all round the periphery of the tumour than in the centre or in the surrounding tissues, whereas in tumours invading in a single direction collagenolytic activity is increased only in that sector of the periphery where invasion is occurring. Estimations of DNA and nitrogen content in these regions show that the increase in collagenolytic activity is not due simply to an increase in the number of cells but that each cell is putting out more enzyme.

It is also found that malignant tumours, whether of epithelial or mesenchymal origin, all contain high levels of collagenase whereas benign tumours and the normal tissues from which the tumours arise do not.

These observations correlate extremely well with the ultrastructural features of tumour invasion seen in sequential studies of skin carcinogenesis (Tarin, 1972). Here the earliest evidence of penetration of the underlying tissues is seen in papillomas. In these raised lesions the epidermis is thrown into numerous folds within each of which lies a small core of connective tissue. Starting at the centre of the lesion, these small connective tissue enclaves show evidence of disruption, minor at first, but gradually increasing in severity. All amorphous basal lamina-like material eventually disappears and the basal epithelial cells come into direct contact with the connective tissue. From these basal cells large balloon-shaped pseudopodia, devoid of cytoplasmic organelles, extend into the adjacent connective tissue where free-lying vesicular bodies are seen in the immediate vicinity. The latter are believed to derive from the pseudopodia by constriction of the narrow neck and severence of the balloon-like end from the parent cell. Some of the vesicles are intact and contain granular material while others have ruptured with release of their contents. Even more striking, however, is the presence of punctate holes in the connective tissue, often around or next to ruptured vesicles. Collagen fibres next to such holes are fuzzy, frayed and indistinct and the general appearance of the connective tissue is clear evidence that it is undergoing destruction.

In larger papillomas these focal areas of destruction increase and become confluent and the holes in the connective tissue grow and coalesce to form large areas devoid of structural elements. This process, coupled with the advance of the expanding epithelial mass into the space vacated by connective-tissue damage, is the means by which the tumour penetrates into deeper regions.

Similar findings of epithelial pseudopodial projections and dissolution of adjacent connective tissue were reported by Woods and Smith (see Chapter 19) in their studies of the ultrastructural changes in carcinogenesis in the oral mucosa of the hamster.

Confirmation of the release of collagenolytic enzymes and associated ultrastructural evidence of the destruction of the adjacent connective tissue has recently been obtained in studies of basal cell carcinomas and melanomas of human skin. Thus it seems reasonable to conclude that release of collagenolytic enzymes is at least one of the mechanisms by which tumour cells invade the surrounding tissues.

Another, commonly seen in soft parenchymatous organs with less structural collagen content, is the process of infiltration in which tumour cells squeeze between the normal cells of the organ and gradually come to occupy all the available extracellular space within it. Sometimes the tumour cells remain closely grouped as they spread in this manner and at other times they separate from the main tumour mass and infiltrate the surrounding tissues independently. In both situations the observations suggest decreased intercellular adhesion, the derangement being seemingly more severe in the latter where the tumour cells not only fail to adhere to normal cells but to each other as well. Infiltration in such small groups is an indicator of the acquisition of autonomy by the tumour cells and signals the imminence of metastic dissemination.

It is obvious from this account that knowledge of tumour invasion is rudimentary but progressing and it remains to be seen whether further work on the subject will bring means to hand for its control.

Metastasis

Most of knowledge on this important aspect of tumour behaviour has accumulated from clinical observations and post mortem studies. In comparison, little experimental work has been done, perhaps because tumours induced in laboratory animals do not predictably metastasize of their own accord. On the other hand, if animals receive subcutaneous implants of certain transplantable tumours or intravenous inoculations of tumour cells, metastatic deposits are formed, but whether this process is comparable to naturally occurring metastasis is the subject of much debate. Even so, this is so far one of the few means available to study the phenomenon and the results obtained deserve consideration.

The immunological status of the animal seems to affect the formation of metastatic deposits. It has been shown that if mice are treated with antilymphocytic serum prior to implantation of a variety of lymphoma which usually remains localized, metastatic deposits arise in the liver and lungs; also that when mice are thymectomized and/or splenectomized prior to carcinogen treatment, the mammary tumours which arise spread rapidly when transplanted to new hosts. Only the tumours arising late in the course of carcinogen treatment do this; the earlier ones, being presumably too antigenic, were therefore excised to allow the slower ones to develop.

There are also non-immunological systemic factors which affect the growth of metastatic deposits. This has been demonstrated in studies on the Lewis lung tumour. It was found that primary tumours inhibit the growth of secondary deposits and that the secondaries similarly release some inhibitory principle into the blood which eventually retards the growth of the primary. In this work it was also found that removal of the primary resulted in rapid increase in growth of secondary deposits and clearly, if this applies to any other tumours, the implications for the management of human cancer deserve careful consideration.

Therapeutically, little is available at present for the prevention of tumour dissemination. It has been shown, however, that in mice the substance known by the code name ICRF 159 completely prevents metastatic spread from subcutaneous implants of the Lewis lung tumour. Curiously, it does not prevent continued growth of the primary implant, although it does considerably affect its vascular anatomy (Salsbury, Burrage and Hellman, 1970). Although preliminary studies are not producing evidence of regression of secondary deposits in humans treated with this substance, it is not known whether its administration may prevent the spread of early neoplasms. Even if the drug does not prove to be effective in the treatment of human malignancy, further intensive studies of its mode of action in animals are required in the hope that some general principle applicable to other tumours will emerge.

It is a well recognized clinical observation that the distribution of metastatic deposits from a primary tumour tends to be related to its type and location. Thus, for example, secondary deposits from carcinoma of the colon tend to occur preferentially in the liver and lung, while those from carcinoma of the breast favour the lung, the brain and the bones. Some organs, for instance the lung and the liver, commonly contain metastases while others, such as the spleen, thyroid and skeletal muscles, rarely do. The reasons for this "site specificity of metastasis" are at present unknown but most evidence indicates that it is not solely determined by vascular anatomy. There is not sufficient space to consider this evidence in detail here (see Tarin, 1972 for review) but the most remarkable experiment favouring this view should be mentioned. It was shown some 12 years ago that intravascular inoculation of tumour cells with a predilection for forming lung secondaries into animals carrying grafts of lung tissue in the thigh, led to the formation of secondary deposits in the graft. In controls carrying similar thigh grafts from other organs there were no metastatic tumours in the graft. It seems, therefore, that the tumour cells can seek out the organs in which they prefer to establish colonies.

TUMOUR IMMUNOLOGY

The part played by the immune response in either aiding or limiting human tumour growth is not clear. There is, however, a great deal of evidence to suggest that some tumours possess antigens which are capable of stimulating an immune response. In experimental circumstances, virus induced animal tumours provide the clearest evidence for immunological surveillance. Polyoma, SV40 and some adenoviruses are capable of producing tumours in certain species. Wild mice, for instance, carry polyoma virus but rarely get tumours. They have a high antiviral antibody level in the blood. If polyoma virus is administered to a virus-free laboratory strain of mice in the first 24 hr. after birth, tumours subsequently appear. Tumours appear in wild mice only after neonatal thymectomy or after administration of anti-lymphocyte serum. In other words, polyoma virus causes tumours in mice whose cell-mediated immune mechanisms are immature, removed or inhibited. It would seem that the high maternal anti-polyoma antibody level gives passive immunity to the neonatal wild mice until their own immune mechanisms have fully developed. Tumour growth can be prevented in the laboratory mice exposed to polyoma neonatally by administration of either a second viral dose during the latent period or irradiated polyoma-induced tumour cells. These findings suggest that acquisition of immunity against the virus or virus-induced tumour cell antigens leads to obliteration of the virus and the potential neoplastic cells. Another example can be cited here; the Marek disease herpes virus, which produces a highly malignant disease in chicks, can be rendered non-pathogenic by administration of Turkey herpes virus. The latter possesses similar antigens to the Marek disease herpes virus but is not pathogenic in chicks. Antibodies produced under these circumstances are thought to act against virus-induced antigens on malignant cells as Turkey virus production remains unimpaired.

It is necessary to consider the part played by immuno-logical surveillance in chemically-induced experimental tumours. Dimethylbenzanthracene (DMBA) was injected into mice and the injected area of skin was grafted to iso-geneic animals after 5–30 days. These grafts were rejected after a certain time. A second graft taken from the same donor but from a site not injected with DMBA, was given to the same recipient. The second graft was not rejected any quicker than the first, suggesting that DMBA may have caused changes in the antigens of the original skin graft.

More recently, the antigenicity of a variety of chemically-induced tumours in rats has been studied. A wide range of antigenicity was found, some tumours being not detectably antigenic at all. It was suggested that the carcinogenic chemical played an active role in determining the antigens present in a tumour. If immunological surveillance is important in tumour growth, obviously the less antigenic or non-antigenic tumours are favoured under natural conditions. In man, the evidence for involvement of immune mechanisms in tumour formation is slowly accumulating. This involvement was indicated by injecting quantitated suspensions of tumour cells from patients with non-resectable cancer into the subcutaneous tissue of the thigh of these same patients. As a comparison, the patient's tumour cells were injected with some of the patient's leucocytes. The leucocytes were not purified to a single type. This comparatively rough study revealed, however, that localized tumour growth was inhibited in half the patients who had received leucocytes in the inoculum. In these experiments one can deduce that the leucocytes of cancer patients had a specific inhibitory effect on the growth of malignant cells in that individual.

A comprehensive study of malignancy in immuno-deficiency diseases in man was reported by Gatti and Good (1971). Their figures showed that the incidence of malignancy in patients with primary immunodeficiency disease is 10,000 times that of the general age-matched population. Each type of immunodeficiency has a distinctive selection of malignancies associated with it. For instance, deficiencies in the T-cell system in ataxia-telangiectasia and Wiscott-Aldrich syndrome were associated with a high incidence of lympho-reticular neoplasms.

The popularity of organ transplantation in recent years has shown a correlation between immuno-suppressive therapy and an increase in malignant disease in transplant recipients. Early renal transplants were taken from donors dying of metastatic carcinoma and although the organs were macroscopically free of metastases, similar tumours arose in recipients 7–18 months after transplantation. In one case, however, the donor kidney (from a patient with bronchial carcinoma) and its tumour cells were rejected by the recipient on cessation of immuno-suppression. Because of these findings, renal transplants from patients dying of cancer, are no longer employed. Other neoplasms which are thought not to be derived from donor tissue have been reported in renal transplant patients. They are mostly of lymphatic origin.

One reticulum cell sarcoma arose at the site of injection of antilymphocyte globulin which corresponds with experimental findings of a high incidence of reticulum cell sarcoma at the injection site of mice injected with leukaemogenic virus and antilymphocyte serum.

At this stage, there are three questions that could be asked: is the immune response deficient and therefore an aid to spontaneous tumour growth, or does a change occur in the cancer cell allowing it to avoid recognition and destruction, or is the immune response incidental to tumour growth? The possibility of a change occurring in the cancer cell has stimulated lines of research to find tumour-specific antigens.

Chemically induced tumours appear to produce highly specific antigens depending on the carcinogen and the treated tissue. Animal virus-induced tumours stimulate the production of cross-reacting antibodies which attack virus tumour cells in other hosts.

Some interesting results have been obtained from a study of neuroblastomas in children. These tumours are known to grow rapidly and occasionally to undergo spontaneous regression. Lymphocytes taken from patients with neuroblastoma inhibited the colony formation in vitro of their own tumour cells but not their normal cells. Lymphocytes from the mothers and some relatives of these patients were found to inhibit neuroblastoma cell colony formation in vitro from a number of patients. This cross reactivity would be interpreted as virus involvement in animal tumours. No virus has been found associated with neuroblastomas so far.

Cancer-specific antigens promoting cross-reactivity have been reported from melanomas and sarcomas and from carcinoma of colon.

The finding of a "blocking factor" in the sera of neuroblastoma patients indicates that antigen sites on tumour cells become blocked with this antibody-like factor and so prevent reactive lymphocytes (T-cells) from attacking the tumour. Carcino-embryonic antigen and α-fetoproteins have been found associated with certain tumours and also with fetal tissue. The idea has developed that the production of fetal proteins by neoplasms was evidence of dedifferentiation. When fetal tissue was implanted under the kidney capsule in syngeneic and allogeneic mice, the fetal tissue grew poorly. Syngeneic adult tissue transplanted to the same area, however, grew well. Fetal tissue implanted into immunologically "deprived" mice (thymectomized, lethally irradiated and bone marrow reconstituted) grew well also. These experiments indicated that fetal tissue was rejected by an immunological response to fetal antigen. When chemically-induced tumours were transplanted into the normal mice that had rejected the fetal tissue, tumour growth was enhanced. This finding may point to an immunological affinity between fetal and malignant tissues.

Of all human tumours, perhaps Burkitt's lymphoma has the strongest evidence for association with virus. Epstein-Barr virus (EBV) has been isolated in many cases of Burkitt's lymphoma. It is not yet established that EBV is the causative agent but much circumstantial evidence suggests such a role. A humoral factor directed against tumour-associated antigens has been demonstrated on the Burkitt lymphoma cell membrane. The presence of these neoantigens was dependent on infection with EBV. Most patients with Burkitt's lymphoma have high titres of antibodies directed against these viral-induced neoantigens which are not present on the patient's normal cells.

The immunological reaction to tumour cells is thought to be cell-mediated via T-cells and to be of the "delayed hypersensitivity" type. Patients with large tumours have reduced hypersensitivity reactions to BCG vaccination. It is not known whether large tumours impair immune mechanisms or whether a lowered immunity favours tumour growth. However, prior immunization with the patient's own irradiated tumour cells, before chemotherapy, lengthened remission time in patients with small lymphomas. This indicates the importance of the patient's own defence mechanism in chemotherapy.

In conclusion, it could be suggested that tumours escape immunological surveillance either by "blocking factors", by reduced antigenicity or by paralysis of immunocytes by large quantities of antigen.

Conversely, a diminished immunological response would favour spontaneously occurring tumour growth.

SPONTANEOUS REGRESSION OF CANCER

There are many well-documented case histories of tumours and/or metastases that have undergone spontaneous regression. No one knows how frequently latent cancers undergo regression as only clinically evident neoplasia has been documented.

The tumour groups most likely to undergo regression are neuroblastoma, malignant melanoma, choriocarcinoma, hypernephroma. In these instances, the body, by some means, has exercised control over developing tumour cells. Hormonal effects can influence tumour growth as can immune mechanisms. In many of the reported cases there was an accompanying metabolic change, e.g. artificial or natural menopause or an acute febrile episode, but this was not so in all.

POTENTIAL APPROACHES TO TREATMENT

Hyperthermia

It has been known for over 100 years that neoplastic cells are more susceptible to hyperthermia (42°C) than are their normal counterparts but several groups have recently begun re-examining the therapeutic possibilities of this observation (see Dickson and Muckle, 1972 for review). The work of Dickson and Muckle with rabbit XV-2 carcinoma implants in the hind leg showed higher survival rates (up to 50 per cent of the animals being cured) if the heat were locally applied by immersion of the affected limb than if whole-body heating were employed. The significance of this is unknown but it was suggested that whole-body hyperthermia might cause a depression of the immune response.

It has been postulated that survival of animals after local heating may depend in part on the ability of the immune system to destroy metastatic tumours. This hypothesis is supported by the finding that animals challenged by implanting 1×10^6 VX-2 cells into the contra-lateral leg 1–3 months after local hyperthermia of the primary showed no signs of tumour growth. It is believed that stimulation of the immune system by tumour breakdown products, following local heating, accounts for these results.

Studies on the effects of hyperthermia on VX-2 tumour cells in vitro showed that populations of cells actively traversing the cell cycle were much more susceptible than those with a low replication rate. In the former, RNA and protein synthesis were diminished without subsequent recovery and it was considered that the cytopathic effects of hyperthermia are probably due to disturbance of relationships between DNA, RNA and protein.

It is also important to note that temperatures in the region of 39–40°C stimulate growth of tumour cells and that cells surviving hyperthermic shock produce lethal tumours. Thus, in order to avoid facilitation of tumour growth *in vivo*, it is important to ensure that intratumour temperatures reach 42°C for 50 per cent or more of the treatment time and preferably that this should be monitored by thermocouple sensors.

The value of hyperthermic treatment in the management of human cancer is being examined in various centres at present, but there is as yet insufficient evidence to reach firm conclusions on this subject.

Tumour Immunochemotherapy

Cell surface localizing tumour antibodies, whilst incapable of significant destruction of tumour cells, have been used as carriers of cytotoxic drugs leading to their selective concentration in tumour tissue.

Chlorambucil was bound to specific immunoglobulins against mouse EL_4 lymphoma cells and against human melanoma. Intraperitoneal inoculation of EL_4 cells leads to ascites tumour development. Chlorambucil bound to anti EL_4 immune rabbit globulin, injected 2 hr. after tumour inoculation and continued daily for 5 days resulted in survival and for more than 150 days in all mice injected. The survival time was reduced if immunochemotherapy was started more than 72 hr. after tumour cell inoculation.

Similar treatment was given to a patient who had multiple metastases of malignant melanoma. Treatment with localized BCG vaccine, effective to start with, subsequently caused no regression of the metastatic deposits. Serum collected 7 and 16 days after injection with irradiated mela-noma cells showed no anti-melanoma antibody. Intravenous and localized treatment with chlorambucil-bound anti-goat globulin caused regression of all metastatic deposits irrespective of whether these were locally injected or not. The patient's serum acquired high levels of cytoplasmic and cell-surface localizing antibody and lymphocytes from his peripheral blood aggregated round melanoma cells after 12 hr.

This treatment must, of course, be given to a large number of patients before any conclusions as to its efficacy can be drawn. Spontaneous regression despite treatment cannot be ruled out. Preliminary results are, however, encouraging.

REFERENCES

Allen, D. W. and Cole, P. (1972), "Viruses and Human Cancer," *New Engl. J. Med.*, **286**, 70.

Brand, K. G. (1975), "Foreign Body-induced Sarcomas," in *Cancer: a Comprehensive Treatise*, Vol. 1, Ed. F. F. Becker. London: Plenum Publishing Co.

Dickson, J. A. and Muckle, D. S. (1972), "Total Body Hyperthermia Versus Primary Tumour Hyperthermia in the Treatment of the Rabbit VX-2 Carcinoma," *Cancer Res.*, **32**, 1916.

Gatti, R. A. and Good, R. A. (1971), "Occurrence of Malignancy in Immunodeficiency Diseases," *Cancer*, **28**, 89.

Heidelberger, C. (1970), "Studies on the Cellular and Molecular Mechanisms of Hydrocarbon Carcinogenesis," *Eur. J. Cancer*, **6**, 161.

Mazzucco, K. (1972), "The Role of Collagen in Tissue Interactions During Carcinogenesis in Mouse Skin," in *Tissue Interactions in Carcinogenesis* (D. Tarin, Ed.). London: Academic Press.

Pearson, O. H. (1973), "Endocrine Aspects of Breast Cancer," in *Current Research in Oncology* 1972 (C. B. Anfinson, M. Potter and A. N. Schechter, Eds.). New York: Academic Press.

Ryser, H. J. P. (1971), "Chemical Carcinogenesis," *New Eng. J. Med.*, **285**, 721.

Salsbury, A. J., Burrage, K. and Hellmann, K. (1970), "Inhibition of Metastatic Spread by ICRF 159: Selective Deletion of a Malignant Characteristic," *Brit. med. J.*, **4**, 344.

Strauch, L. (1972), "The Role of Collagenases in Tumour Invasion," in *Tissue Interactions in Carcinogenesis* (D. Tarin, Ed.). London: Academic press.

19. NEOPLASIA: ORAL ASPECTS

C. J. SMITH

INTRODUCTION

Many different types of neoplasm can be found in the oral region. These may arise directly from cells in bone, oral mucosa, salivary gland or odontogenic tissues as either benign or malignant lesions; also, metastatic deposits from remote primary malignant neoplasms or local extensions from extra-oral malignant neoplasms sometimes involve oral tissues.

This chapter is concerned primarily with squamous cell carcinoma affecting the oral mucosa, which is one of the most common oral neoplasms. It does not form a large component of the total pool of malignant neoplasms occurring in all sites, but is especially important amongst oral lesions because of its life-threatening characteristics. Attention is also given to conditions which may precede the development of squamous cell carcinoma in human oral mucous membrane and, briefly, to experimental methods for producing squamous cell carcinomas and precancerous states in the oral mucosa of animals. Improvements in prognosis and diagnosis for human oral cancer and precancer are being sought by numerous methods of investigation; some details are given of the current status of this approach. Finally, aetiological factors are considered.

STATISTICS AND EPIDEMIOLOGY

General Considerations

With the increasing number of cancer registration centres set up in recent years, more information is becoming available on the morbidity of various malignant neoplasms. Mortality statistics have, of course, been available over a longer period.

Most reasonably representative studies show that approximately 80–90 per cent of all oral malignant neoplasms are squamous cell carcinomas; those that remain constitute a heterogeneous group comprising sarcomas of bone and soft tissue, adenocarcinomas of salivary gland origin or metastatic from remote glandular sites, malignant lymphomas, malignant melanomas and other extremely rare entities. The number of these latter neoplasms that can be collected together in morbidity and mortality statistics is usually so small that little relevant information can be deduced. Because such a high proportion of malignant neoplasms that affect the oral mucous membrane comprises squamous cell carcinoma, it seems reasonable to assume that statistics collected for all malignant neoplasms in this site can be interpreted as applying, approximately and for comparative purposes, to oral squamous cell carcinoma. Oral cancer is more readily diagnosed clinically and more readily accessible for biopsy than cancer of many other organs; diagnostic errors are therefore expected to be fewer and statistics collected for oral cancer should thus be more reliable than those for many other sites. Use of such statistics concerning oral cancer must, however, be tempered by the understanding that many sources quote figures relating to combined totals for cancer of the lip, oral cavity, and pharynx under the general heading of "malignant neoplasms of the buccal cavity and pharynx". It is important, when extracting information from statistical data on incidence or mortality of oral cancer, that except for the particular point under investigation, like should be compared with like. This applies in particular to the influences of age-structure, sex-composition, geographical region, oral site and time-period (Binnie, Cawson, Hill and Soaper, 1972; Smith, 1973).

Age Distribution

In all populations so far studied, oral cancer predominantly affects the elderly and shows increasing incidence and mortality with each decade. Other malignant oral neoplasms do not necessarily show the same age characteristics.

Geographical distribution

Striking differences are apparent in the oral cancer mortality rates obtained from different countries. In South-East Asia, particularly India and Ceylon, it has long been known that oral cancer has a high prevalence among the malignant neoplasms. Some studies in parts of India have shown that oral cancer accounts for more than half of all known cancers. While this probably reflects some diagnostic shortfall in less accessible sites, for various reasons, recent data from cancer registries confirm the pre-eminence of India in the figures for oral cancer incidence. Within India, as between smaller closely-related countries such as those in Europe, there are marked variations in the oral cancer experience of the populations. France shows a particularly high mortality rate from cancer of the buccal cavity and pharynx, though compared with neighbouring countries most of the excess is related to an increase that affects the male population. This produces a high male/female ratio for oral cancer mortality in the French population of approximately 8:1, whereas in countries such as England and Wales it is approximately 3:1 and in Sweden approximately only 1·3:1. Such variation in the experience of male and female populations probably results from their differing exposure to aetiological agents, though exactly what these are has yet to be established with certainty. There are a few countries or regions in the world where the prevalence of oral cancer, at least for some sites, is greater amongst women than men; in these instances aetiological factors are usually more easily recognizable because of an unusual differential distribution of habits between the sexes.

Temporal Variation

As might be expected, mortality and incidence rates for oral cancer show variation over periods of time. In many countries a gradual decline in oral cancer has been observed over the past few decades. This decline applies to both incidence and mortality figures, so improvements in the latter perhaps bear little relationship to new treatment methods. Suitable correction for any reduction in incidence is therefore necessary if long-term comparisons are being made between the effects of various types of treatment. In certain countries, the rate of decline in oral cancer incidence differs between the sexes, males often showing a sharper fall than females; sometimes in such countries the rate amongst females has remained approximately constant. The reasons for this are obscure, possibly being related to changes in exposure to aetiological agents. Another feature of falling incidence and mortality rates is that different oral sites show a variable involvement in this improvement.

Site Distribution

Statistical studies on oral cancer have long revealed that the different intra-oral sites are affected to a variable degree. Again there is often a large difference between the distribution in males and in females; not only are there differences in the absolute numbers of cancers found in the different oral sites but also the ratio of involvement of one site to another varies between the sexes. Even apparently similar sites may show widely diverging rates of attack by oral cancer; cancer of the lip in males is overwhelmingly found in the lower lip. When a decrease in incidence is observed over the combined sites included in the category of oral cancer, this decrease is not usually equally distributed between the individual sites. Because cancer in some oral sites responds to treatment more readily than in others, the mortality and incidence ratios between different oral sites are not constant; cancer of the lip, for example, makes up a higher percentage of incidence figures than of mortality figures for oral cancer.

CLINICAL MANIFESTATIONS

All too often, patients affected by oral cancer present themselves for diagnosis with the disease in an advanced stage. This is surprising when it is considered that the oral mucosa is a sensitive region which is easily examined by patient, dental surgeon or physician.

Advanced Oral Cancer

At a late stage in the disease there is usually not much doubt about diagnosis, despite variable appearances around the basic forms of either a warty outgrowth or an ulcer. Many late lesions are accompanied not only by extensive spread to important local structures, resulting in such symptoms as tongue immobility, trismus, pathological fracture and disturbance of motor or sensory nerve function, but also by metastatic spread to regional lymph nodes. The involvement of specific nodes depends largely upon the site of the cancer and lymph drainage from the affected area. Metastasis beyond the cervical chain of lymph nodes is relatively infrequent. It should not be forgotten, however, that an enlarged node suspected clinically to harbour a metastatic deposit can sometimes be shown on microscopical examination to be free from tumour; conversely, and of greater significance for the patient, many regional lymph nodes which are believed to be normal on clinical examination contain undetectable cancer cells that will continue to develop even if the primary growth is completely removed. In the exposed conditions of the oral cavity, the ulcerated surfaces readily become infected; this can contribute towards symptoms of pain and enlargement of regional lymph nodes.

"Early" Oral Cancer

The necessity to diagnose oral cancer at earlier stages is unquestionable, but for this to be achieved the potential appearances of early oral cancer need to be appreciated. There is not, however, one particular pattern of manifestation; in any oral site the earliest appearance of cancer may be a localized induration of mucosa covered by a white plaque or fibrinous crust, an erythematous area, small cracks or fissures, a small warty nodule covered by pink or white mucosa, a deeper mass, or an ulcer. More than one of these features may be present even in an early stage. The subsequent rate of growth varies individually and between different sites but ulceration usually develops at some stage, even on the surfaces of exophytic lesions. The ulcers often, though not always, have rolled and everted borders and an indurated base. Early squamous cell carcinoma may or may not be painful. One of the frequent causes of delay in the diagnosis of oral cancer is that the early clinical stages may mimic many other less harmful and more common oral conditions. Attempts have been made to differentiate between early invasive squamous cell carcinoma and non-malignant conditions by *in vivo* staining of tissues with 1 per cent toluidine blue. Despite early claims, however, this technique has not been widely adopted, probably because frequent false positive staining still necessitates a biopsy to provide microscopical confirmation of the nature of any particular lesion. Although apparently not of value in distinguishing malignant neoplasms from simulators of malignancy, the toluidine blue *in vivo* staining technique (or developments along similar lines) might usefully delineate the limits of altered mucosa or disclose previously unsuspected areas. It must be stressed, however, that histopathological examination of an adequate biopsy specimen is the safest and most satisfactory method for establishing the diagnosis whenever malignancy should be suspected.

Lip Cancer

Cancer of the lip accounts for approximately 30 per cent of all carcinoma arising in the oral region among the population of England and Wales; the great majority affect the lower lip. Males are more frequently afflicted than females (in a ratio of 8:1) and the greater numbers amongst males are almost entirely accounted for by increased involvement of the lower lip.

Tongue Cancer

Tongue cancer comprises about 25 per cent of all carcinomas affecting the oral mucosa in the population of England and Wales. Although the disease again affects males more than females, the ratio is only approximately 3:2. The site of tongue cancer is conventionally considered according to the anatomical sub-divisions of the tongue—posterior one-third and anterior two-thirds, with the latter further divided into dorsum, lateral borders and ventral surface. The extent to which cancer is found in any of these sites varies widely between reports, but constant findings are that the dorsum is affected only rarely and the lateral borders most frequently.

Other Sites

For oral sites other than lip and tongue, cancer registry statistics are often amalgamated, either for numerical reasons or because insufficient information regarding location is provided to the registry. Data concerning the relative frequency of lesions in these oral sites are probably less reliable, therefore, than those for tongue and lip. Carcinoma of floor of mouth, gingiva, alveolar mucosa, buccal mucosa, hard and soft palate, and oral mesopharynx, together represent about 45 per cent of the total number of registered oral cancers in England and Wales, with a male to female ratio in the region of 2:1. Largely because of the effects of local aetiological agents (but sometimes for systemic or unknown reasons), the pattern of oral cancer in different populations shows a wide range of both site variability and distribution between the sexes.

Multiple Oral Cancers

Another important aspect which deserves special mention concerns the occurrence of distinctly separate second or multiple primary growths. These appear, either simultaneously or after a variable interval, in the oral mucosa of persons already affected by one oral squamous carcinoma. Among some groups of patients up to 10 per cent might show this capacity for developing oral cancer in multiple sites. The term "field cancerization" has sometimes been applied to this feature. A clear distinction should be drawn between this phenomenon and recurrences in the site of a treated oral carcinoma. Obviously, in a treated patient close surveillance should be maintained of the remainder of the oral mucosa as well as of the site of the original oral cancer.

Prognosis in Relation to Clinical Factors

Once a diagnosis of oral cancer has been established by histopathology, in most instances treatment will be attempted. Arguments concerning particular types of treatment will not be developed here. More often than not it would seem that the choice of different types of surgery, radiotherapy or chemotherapy, alone or in various combinations, is largely a matter of chance for the patient and of personal preference for the clinician determining the treatment plan. There are many reasons for this and it illustrates the fact that no particular method of treatment is supported by results superior in terms of survival or quality of life. Until more information becomes available from properly conducted clinical trials that take into account the many variable factors, such as site and size of lesion and presence of metastases, idiosyncratic approaches to treatment in each case will probably continue.

Although no particular method of treatment is appropriate for all forms of oral cancer, some of the factors that influence the overall success or failure of treatment are better understood. In assessing effectiveness of treatment, one of the most widely used yardsticks is the percentage of patients surviving for a certain number of years, usually expressed in terms of five- or ten-year survival rates. Naturally, when comparisons are being made of survival rates, it is important to make a suitable correction for the ages of the patients. If this is not done, false conclusions may be drawn from survival rates that perhaps do no more than reflect the greater life expectancy of a younger group of patients.

Effect of Site

Of the clinical factors that influence prognosis and treatment, one of the most important is the site of the primary neoplasm. Here, the lip stands out from all other oral sites as showing a completely different pattern of response. Figures in the region of 80–90 per cent are frequently quoted for five-year survival rates in patients with lip cancer. This compares with an overall five-year survival rate of 25–35 per cent when all intra-oral carcinomas are considered as a group. Generally, carcinomas located posteriorly have a poorer prognosis than those found in anterior regions of the mouth.

Effect of Clinical Stage

In addition to site, another important factor with regard to prognosis and survival is the clinical stage of the neoplasm at the time of diagnosis (Binnie *et al.*, 1972). The concept of clinical stage embraces the size of the primary growth and its local extension together with the involvement of regional lymph nodes or more widespread metastases. The TNM classification of the clinical staging of malignant neoplasms takes each of these factors into account. For whatever site, small lesions without evidence of metastasis at the time of diagnosis respond better to treatment than larger lesions or those already accompanied by secondary deposits in regional lymph nodes. Any attempts to compare the relative success of different treatment methods must, therefore, take into account clinical staging as well as site.

For the purposes of cancer registration, it is usual to simplify clinical staging and to classify lesions as either "early" or "late". One of the commonest divisions adopted is to record localized neoplasms up to 4 cm. in diameter as "early", and those which are larger or have evidence of spread as "late". However convenient this might be in clinical terms, there are certain biological inconsistencies inherent in this approach; these mostly revolve around the problem of trying to equate size and spread of neoplasms with the time that they have been present. As it is fairly certain that different carcinomas possess inconstant rates of growth, not least because of variability in cell turnover and cell death, it follows that not all carcinomas of the same age will be the same size (and vice versa). Added to this is the knowledge that individual carcinomas produce metastatic deposits at different stages in their natural history, for reasons as yet unknown. Thus, while it is generally acceptable to consider small localized lesions as being "early" in terms of their duration, it does not necessarily follow that all such lesions have been present for a shorter time than lesions that are larger or show evidence of secondary spread.

As already stated, there is ample evidence that oral cancer survival rates are improved in patients having "early" lesions at the time of diagnosis. Several other features relating to survival rates and clinical staging are also worthy of attention. For example, as has been mentioned earlier, survival rates for patients with lip cancer are far better than for those with intra-oral cancer. Although there might be several contributory causes for this, one important factor must surely be related to the stage of the disease at diagnosis. There is substantial evidence that, in general, patients suffering from lip cancer first seek treatment at an "earlier" stage than do those with intra-oral cancer. This means that lip cancers are first seen by the clinician more frequently as small lesions without metastases than is the case for intra-oral cancers. It might not follow, however, that the lip cancers have been present, on average, for a shorter period of time; indeed, their generally indolent growth pattern suggests that the opposite could be true.

One of the most puzzling features concerning survival rates for patients with intra-oral cancer is why the figures for five- and ten-year survival should be so low. In fact, it appears that only carcinoma of bronchus and of stomach have less favourable survival rates. This is a daunting thought considering how much easier it should be for a small lesion to be noticed in the oral mucosa than almost any other site. More emphasis should be placed on the necessity for advice to be sought earlier when oral lesions do not heal spontaneously or respond quickly to treatment. Also, a high level of awareness needs to be maintained by those responsible for examining the oral mucosa, and more effort should be expended in persuading elderly and edentulous patients in particular of the desirability for occasional oral mucosal examinations.

Surprisingly, men tend to show poorer five-year survival rates for oral cancer than do women. Many studies have confirmed this trend (Smith, 1973), even when the greater natural longevity of women is taken into account. A possible explanation for this phenomenon is that more women than men are diagnosed with their oral cancer in an "early" stage. Whether this represents a greater rate or extent of growth in men than in women, or whether women seek attention more quickly than men, remains an open but interesting question. Moderate improvements in survival figures for oral cancer could probably be simply brought about if men were diagnosed and treated with the disease at the same stages as in women. Further improvement would doubtless follow more frequent diagnosis in the "early" stages for both sexes.

The other major factor often discussed in the context of prognosis and response to treatment is the histological grade of the carcinoma.

Verrucous Carcinoma

The verrucous carcinoma is a distinct clinico-pathological entity separate from the far more common variety of squamous cell carcinoma described above (Shafer, 1972). Because of its special association with certain aetiological factors, there is a wide variation in incidence geographically; in England and Wales, however, it forms a low percentage of oral carcinomas. The most common oral sites for this lesion are the buccal mucosa, especially the commissural region and sulci, and the alveolar mucosa or gingiva. Patients are usually elderly and the average age, particularly in females, is greater than that for patients with the common variety of oral squamous cell carcinoma.

Verrucous carcinoma appears as a warty outgrowth from the oral mucosa which is pink, red, or white depending upon the extent of surface trauma, ulceration and keratinization. Growth is usually slow and tends to spread laterally at first rather than to invade underlying tissues; consequently the lesion might attain a large size before the patient seeks attention. Gradually, however, the underlying tissues, including bone, are invaded and destroyed, though it is rare for metastases to develop.

Survival rates for verrucous carcinoma are better than for the more usual type of oral squamous cell carcinoma, though there is an even greater tendency for the development of multiple primary lesions. As far as treatment is concerned, for once it is possible to give direct guidance. Irradiation of verrucous carcinoma has occasionally been followed by anaplastic changes, rapid growth and metastasis; surgery is therefore the treatment of choice in most instances.

Precancerous Lesions

A premalignant lesion is one in which definite morphological features are seen and which is associated with a greater risk of malignant change than corresponding normal tissue.

Leukoplakia

In the oral mucosa, the best known example of a premalignant lesion is leukoplakia. The reasons for believing leukoplakia to be a premalignant lesion are that (a) it is often found in association with oral cancer; (b) if followed over a period of months or years it may be seen to develop a carcinoma; and (c) it may possess some histological features similar to those seen in squamous cell carcinoma. However, most oral cancers are not preceded by such changes in the mucosa.

Historically, the term "leukoplakia" has signified to some simply any white patch on the oral mucosa but to others has implied the presence of histological features indicating a malignant potential. The varied criteria employed for a diagnosis of leukoplakia, and often the absence of any stated criteria, mean that many previous studies are not comparable with each other. More recently, however, an attempt has been made to standardize the definition of leukoplakia and this is gaining recognition for its usefulness in providing a reference point for several studies. This definition states that oral leukoplakia is a white patch on the oral mucosa which cannot be diagnosed, clinically or histopathologically, as any other recognizable condition. Several features of this definition should be observed. The first is that leukoplakia is now diagnosed on the basis of exclusion of other conditions; the second is that it has a clinical foundation and carries no specific histological connotation, even with regard to the presence of premalignant features; finally, it should be anticipated that some modification of this definition will eventually be desirable. A likely development would be the exclusion of definitely diagnosable conditions through the use of other laboratory tests in addition to histopathology.

Little is known of the prevalence of oral leukoplakia, the few reported studies mostly relating to various Indian populations; in these, up to 5 per cent of the adult population in some regions may be affected by leukoplakia. In India, the aetiological influence of betel-quid chewing is probably of much importance. Aetiological factors of various kinds doubtless also affect the intra-oral site distribution of leukoplakia in different populations as well as the ratio between the sexes. In most studies, males have been affected more than females, the elderly more than other age groups, and the buccal mucosa, commissures, and alveolar ridges more than other sites. Of added interest, the lower regions of oral mucosa are more commonly involved than the upper.

The reported incidence of malignant change in oral leukoplakia has seen a dramatic fall in recent years. Many papers in the older literature quote figures that average out at around 30 per cent of leukoplakias eventually developing oral cancer. More recent studies, however, incorporating a large number of cases and from different population groups, have produced figures in the region of 3–6 per cent. What could be the reasons for this marked change? The most usual explanation offered is that the morbidity of oral cancer has been in decline over the same period and, in particular, there has been a great reduction in the frequency of syphilitic changes in the oral mucosa. In addition, there is probably greater awareness now of the potential significance of oral white lesions, so more oral leukoplakias with benign characteristics and generally less noticeable clinically are included in such studies. It could be argued that even the figures of 3–6 per cent of leukoplakias undergoing malignant change represent an overestimate because many of the cancers have occurred within a short time of the original biopsy and diagnosis of leukoplakia. In some of these instances the first biopsy may have simply missed the site of an already existing small oral cancer which only became evident over the succeeding months. Thus, such leukoplakias should not truly be classified as having demonstrated a malignant transformation but only as having been associated with an oral cancer. This is an important consideration in practical clinical terms and in studies where an attempt is being made to understand the likely behaviour of oral leukoplakias. There is a broad spectrum of clinical appearances; individual leukoplakias cover a variable area of oral mucosa, have a regular or irregular shape, possess a distinct or indistinct margin, are raised, flat, fissured, nodular or smooth, and show any of a range of colours from white to grey or yellow. Opaque or translucent lesions may be seen and the texture of affected mucosa is also variable. Some workers choose to subdivide oral leukoplakias into separate clinical types according to their appearances, though not every lesion can by any means be conveniently slotted into such categories. Of these separate groupings, the most commonly employed are the "homogeneous" and the "speckled" types. The latter, in which whitish raised nodules are distributed on an erythematous background, has special significance because malignant change occurs more commonly in this group than in others. A greater proportion of the "speckled" leukoplakias exhibit epithelial dysplasia and the presence of Candida organisms than do other leukoplakias.

Erythroplakia

A lesion of different appearance, comprising a well-defined bright red patch with irregular margins and often a granular or velvety surface, can also be classified amongst the oral precancerous lesions. This is called "erythroplakia", (sometimes "erythroplasia"), a term that should be used in the same manner as leukoplakia; diagnosable lesions that appear as reddened areas of oral mucosa should be excluded and the remainder can be considered in the category of erythroplakia. Erythroplakia is less common than leukoplakia, tends to affect the posterior parts of the mouth rather than the anterior, and has a greater propensity for malignant change than leukoplakia. Carcinoma *in situ* of the oral mucosa often appears clinically as an erythroplakia. Difficulty in classification sometimes arises because patches of erythroplakia are interspersed with those of leukoplakia, or small white flecks and nodules may be scattered over an erythroplakic patch. In these circumstances, the soundest policy for treatment is to regard the lesion in the category of erythroplakia.

Prognosis in Relation to Clinical Factors

The main clinical factors of influence in treatment are, as for oral cancer, the site and size of the affected area. The most favoured method of treatment has been surgery, with or without grafting depending upon the size of the mucosal area removed. More recently cryosurgery, chemotherapy with cytotoxic drugs, radiotherapy using local applicators to the mucosal surfaces, and large doses of vitamin A, have all been employed. However, no properly conducted clinical trials have produced firm guidelines for the most appropriate form of treatment for different types of oral premalignant lesion. The factor most commonly taken into account when determining the necessity and extent of any treatment, is the presence and degree of epithelial dysplasia as revealed by a biopsy. Often, an excision biopsy can be performed and treatment is carried out along with diagnosis. If possible aetiological factors can be recognized, then one aspect of treatment is to eliminate these where feasible; sometimes, the removal of aetiological factors is the only treatment necessary. In any event, it is wise to keep regular surveillance of these lesions, sites at which they have been treated, or adjacent apparently normal mucosa.

Precancerous Conditions

There is a subtle difference between a premalignant lesion and a premalignant condition. The latter is any generalized condition that might predispose to the development of cancer in a particular site and does not necessarily imply the existence of any observable change in that site beforehand. Examples of possible premalignant conditions related to oral cancer are sideropenic dysphagia (Patterson-Kelly syndrome, Plummer-Vinson syndrome) and oral submucous fibrosis.

Sideropenic Dysphagia

The syndrome comprising dysphagia, superficial glossitis, and anaemia (sideropenic dysphagia), is associated with an increased susceptibility to carcinoma at the junction between pharyngeal and oesophageal mucosa. There is probably also an accompanying increase in the risk of carcinoma developing in the oral mucosa. The condition appears to have an unusually high incidence amongst Swedish women and this has been suggested as an explanation for the comparatively high mortality and incidence rates for oropharyngeal cancer in Sweden.

Oral Submucous Fibrosis

Submucous fibrosis is discussed in Chapter 39. The main reasons for suspecting an association with oral cancer are that submucous fibrosis has been observed to be more common in oral cancer patients than amongst a control group, and that epithelial dysplasia is more often found in biopsies from submucous fibrosis lesions than from normal controls. Follow-up studies of large numbers of patients with oral submucous fibrosis and of properly matched control groups are required, however, before a close relationship with oral cancer development can be definitely confirmed.

HISTOLOGICAL APPEARANCES OF ORAL CANCER AND PRECANCEROUS LESIONS

Squamous Cell Carcinoma

Squamous cell carcinoma arising from the oral mucosa shows microscopical appearances similar to those in other sites; the features have been described in detail by Lucas (1972). Many oral squamous cell carcinomas are well-differentiated, resembling normal stratified squamous epithelium and producing keratin, while in a lesser proportion there is poor differentiation; considerable variation in these features may be seen within a single lesion. Some authorities hold the view that the more differentiated carcinomas are associated with longer survival and better response to therapy. However, the clinical stage of the neoplasm is a more reliable indicator of future behaviour than any histological grading system so far tested. Unfortunately, many of the studies on grading of oral squamous cell carcinoma have neglected to correlate this feature with all-important information concerning exact site, size of lesion and metastatic spread.

Verrucous Carcinoma

Microscopically, the verrucous carcinoma is a type of squamous cell carcinoma, for it arises from squamous epithelium. It is distinct enough from other squamous cell carcinomas to be considered a separate entity (Shafer, 1972). This distinction is not made solely on histopathological grounds, because clinical appearance and behaviour must also be taken into account. The papillary pattern seen clinically is reproduced microscopically; broad and deep invaginations of surface epithelium extend into underlying connective tissue and separate the slender connective tissue papillae which are covered by hyperplastic stratified squamous epithelium. A thick layer of parakeratinized cells usually covers the surface and characteristically packs the deep clefts separating individual nodules or papillae. Active infiltration of underlying connective tissue by columns or islands of malignant cells is seen but rarely, then sometimes being confused with pseudo-epitheliomatous hyperplasia; there are usually few cytological features characteristic of the more usual squamous cell carcinomas. Both these factors combine to produce occasional diagnostic problems, especially when a biopsy is taken from superficial tissue; simulation of benign papillomatous conditions can easily occur. Despite the lack of obvious microscopical features associated with malignancy, there is no doubt about the inexorable spread and destructive capacity of oral verrucous carcinoma. When verrucous carcinomas have been irradiated, some have subsequently shown histopathological alteration to an anaplastic type of carcinoma. A change in behaviour accompanies this alteration and the affected lesions show rapid invasion with more obvious malignant properties. Most authorities today agree that the category of oral verrucous carcinoma also includes the lesion hitherto known as oral florid papillomatosis.

Perhaps associated with its well-differentiated appearance, the oral verrucous carcinoma has a better prognosis than other oral carcinomas, with the possible exception of squamous carcinoma of the lip.

Leukoplakia

As explained previously the current concept of the diagnostic category "leukoplakia" is based on clinical rather than histological criteria. The range of different histological appearances within the whole of this clinically-defined group is broad. Fundamentally, especially when considering them in the context of premalignancy, leukoplakias can be divided into two groups according to whether or not they possess features suggestive of malignant potential. Thus, in simple terms, one group shows

normal cytological features throughout the thickness of epithelium but the other shows atypical cytological features (atypia). Depending upon the number and severity of these atypical epithelial features (some workers use the rule-of-thumb that at least two must be present), lesions are said to show slight, moderate, or severe epithelial dysplasia. The histological and cytological features currently considered of importance in the diagnosis of epithelial dysplasia are as follows:

(a) irregular epithelial stratification;
(b) hyperplasia of the basal cell layer;
(c) drop-shaped rete-processes;
(d) keratinization of single cells or groups of cells in the prickle-cell layer;
(e) loss of intercellular adherence;
(f) an increase in the number of mitotic figures, amongst which the occasional abnormal mitosis may be found;
(g) increased nuclear-cytoplasmic ratio;
(h) loss of polarity of the basal cells;
(i) cellular pleomorphism;
(j) nuclear hyperchromatism; and
(k) enlarged nucleoli.

No invasion of underlying connective tissue is present. When atypical features extend throughout the entire epithelial thickness, or almost its entire thickness, a diagnosis of carcinoma *in situ* can be applied. These are often red lesions because they lack a keratinized surface and usually have thinner epithelium than is seen in normal mucosa. Leukoplakias, on the other hand, possess a keratinized layer of variable thickness which is often not uniform in a single lesion; they exhibit orthokeratosis, parakeratosis, or a mixture of both types of keratin.

Amongst the whole range of histological appearances seen in leukoplakia there is a wide variation in epithelial thickness. Atrophy or hyperplasia may be observed in extreme forms, or any intermediate thickness, and frequently the thickness of epithelium varies within a single lesion. Some believe that epithelial atrophy is an important factor in the assessment of premalignancy and that lesions with atrophic epithelium are more likely to develop into invasive carcinoma. Support is provided for this view by the evidence that leukoplakias clinically exhibiting erythematous areas (*i.e.* the "speckled" type) show regions of epithelial atrophy as well as a greater tendency for malignant change.

The presence of inflammatory cells in the connective tissue beneath leukoplakic epithelium is another variable feature. Some leukoplakias, usually those without epithelial dysplasia, show few if any inflammatory cells beneath the epithelium. Conversely, many of those most severely affected by epithelial dysplasia are accompanied by a heavy infiltrate of lymphocytes and plasma cells. Occasionally, however, heavy infiltrates occur beneath comparatively normal but hyperkeratotic epithelium and some lesions exhibiting marked epithelial dysplasia have only a slight accompanying inflammatory reaction. When Candida organisms are present in the surface keratotic layer to any extent, polymorphonuclear leucocytes are found in the connective tissue, especially within the capillaries of papillae, and plasma cells appear to be more prevalent than they are beneath other leukoplakias. Although the attention of some workers is turning towards the possible significance of this inflammatory infiltrate, no definite results have so far emerged. It has been suggested that an increase in number of plasma cells might accompany the transformation from epithelial dysplasia to carcinoma; some support is provided for this view by the finding that Russell bodies are present more often beneath leukoplakias that subsequently develop malignancy.

Significance of Epithelial Dysplasia

The most important unsolved problem is how to estimate the role played by epithelial dysplasia in the development of invasive carcinoma. The cytological features of epithelial dysplasia can often be seen in lesions which do not otherwise possess premalignant characteristics. Usually these are inflammatory lesions, and lichen planus not uncommonly provides an example of epithelial dysplasia. As the cellular atypia does not seem to be of great importance in many of these examples, though even this has yet to be shown conclusively, some doubt has been expressed as to its predictive value in so-called premalignant lesions. More evidence is clearly required, particularly with regard to the significance of each component of dysplasia.

A few attempts have recently been made to assess the importance of various cytological features in the epithelium of oral leukoplakias. In one study, many individual cytological and histological characteristics were classified for each of a large number of lesions falling into the leukoplakia category (Kramer, Lucas, El-Labban and Lister, 1970). The leukoplakias were divided into two groups, those that had been followed by the development of a carcinoma in the years succeeding original biopsy and those that had not. A computer-aided discriminant analysis was performed to select features in leukoplakia biopsies that helped to separate those cases that did not develop carcinoma from those that did. The results of this study suggest that the most important features are:

(a) abnormal mitoses in the spinous layer;
(b) disturbed polarity of epithelial cells;
(c) abnormal mitoses in the basal layer;
(d) nuclear hyperchromatism in epithelial cells;
(e) Russell bodies in the lamina propria;
(f) enlarged nucleoli in the spinous layer;
(g) epithelial cell pleomorphism; and
(h) intraepithelial keratinization.

Another study has been based on an attempt to provide a slightly more objective appraisal of cellular features than is usual. In this method, sections of leukoplakias are evaluated against photographic standards for each individual characteristic of epithelial dysplasia. This work has confirmed a fairly high level of intra- and inter-observer variation in assessment of different cellular features. Consequently, methods relying upon a subjective appraisal of cytological characteristics are in doubt and

more objective, quantitative and reproducible methods should be sought for the evaluation of epithelial dysplasia.

Any discussion on the diagnosis of epithelial dysplasia in precancerous lesions must take into account results obtained from the few longitudinal studies of oral leukoplakia so far reported. Despite the large number of leukoplakias followed, only a small proportion have developed carcinoma. When the original biopsies from leukoplakias which showed subsequent malignancy were retrospectively assessed for atypical features, surprisingly few showed epithelial dysplasia. Some absence of dysplasia could doubtless be accounted for by poor (or unlucky!) selection of biopsy sites or sections for examination; however, these factors will continue to be a problem and important questions arise concerning the wisdom of reliance solely upon epithelial dysplasia for prognosis.

In the treatment of oral leukoplakia, it would seem wise on the basis of present knowledge to remove completely, where possible and otherwise desirable, any lesion exhibiting severe dysplasia. Those which show moderate or slight dysplasia should be watched carefully for any change in clinical appearance as a possible indication for a further biopsy. From the foregoing it should be obvious that there is a need for biopsy of any white lesion found on the oral mucosa.

Candidal Leukoplakia

The tendency to malignant transformation of the speckled type of leukoplakia has already been referred to. Speckled leukoplakias are also more commonly associated with chronic infection by Candida albicans. On histological examination, hyphae, and occasionally spores, are seen in the superficial layers of a parakeratotic lesion. Epithelial hyperplasia is often a feature but atrophic areas are frequently interspersed; usually, polymorphonuclear leucocytes infiltrate superficial layers and may form microabscesses. It is more common to find epithelial dysplasia in this type of leukoplakia than those not infested with Candida, but this property usually resolves following successful treatment of the infection. This might suggest that the type of dysplasia seen is not of premalignant significance.

The question that naturally arises is whether or not Candida affects the predisposition to malignant change in these lesions. Two main suggestions have been put forward to explain the role of Candida organisms in leukoplakias. One of these proposes that the fungal hyphae play a direct part in stimulating epithelial dysplasia and development of carcinoma; the other requires less direct involvement, implying that immunological changes occur in leukoplakias likely to undergo malignant transformation and these coincidentally create more suitable conditions for Candidal infection. At the moment it is not possible to resolve these problems. (See also Chapters 10 and 41).

Oral Submucous Fibrosis

In this condition abnormal deposition of fibrous tissue is seen beneath oral epithelium; sometimes the fibrous tissue infiltrates underlying muscle. Both epithelial hyperplasia and epithelial atrophy have been described in association with the fibrosis, and epithelial dysplasia of currently indeterminate significance may also be seen.

Exfoliative Cytology

Brief reference should be made to the use of exfoliative cytology as a diagnostic aid. This technique, which involves removal of superficial cells from a mucosal lesion and their microscopical examination following suitable staining, has achieved much prominence in the diagnosis of carcinoma *in situ* of the uterine cervix. As already explained, however, carcinoma *in situ* is only rarely found in the oral mucosa and the great majority of oral pre-malignant lesions have a keratotic surface; this makes the retrieval of recognisably affected cells from the oral surface far less certain. Poor results obtained from the few satisfactory studies on exfoliative cytology in the diagnosis of epithelial dysplasia in oral leukoplakias can be explained on this basis. In fact, less than half the lesions with epithelial dysplasia are likely to be detected by exfoliative cytology alone (Dabelsteen, Roed-Petersen, Smith and Pindborg, 1971). Oral cancers, too, tend to have keratotic surfaces or to be covered with a fibrinous slough and debris. It is not surprising, therefore, that exfoliative cytology appears to be effective in detecting malignant cells in up to only 80 per cent of oral cancers. This is not acceptable for individual diagnosis or screening purposes because at least one out of every five oral cancers would produce a false negative smear. Exfoliative cytology is not necessarily valueless in the diagnosis of oral cancer and precancerous lesions, however, for it may be useful where biopsy is not easily performed, not a wise procedure medically, or not permitted by the patient.

OTHER METHODS FOR THE STUDY OF ORAL CANCER AND PRECANCEROUS LESIONS

Experimental Oral Carcinogenesis

Apart from a few minor studies, little success was achieved in experimental oral carcinogenesis until it was discovered that the hamster cheek pouch mucosa is particularly susceptible to chemical carcinogens. Many experiments have since been reported using this model and some will be mentioned briefly below. Although the end result is the production of squamous cell carcinomas that are closely similar to their human oral counterparts, several factors make the model far from ideal. Amongst these should be mentioned the almost complete trans-formation of "premalignant" lesions to malignant neo-plasms, the generally exophytic character of resultant tumours, the immunologically privileged status of the hamster cheek pouch and, in common with many other experimental models of carcinogenesis, an extreme scarcity of metastatic spread. A few workers have used alternative sites in the hamster, such as tongue mucosa, in an attempt to overcome some of these difficulties whereas others have tried to produce oral cancer in different animals,

usually without success. There may be some important lessons to be learnt, however, from a study of the reasons why some animals' oral mucosa is refractory to carcinogens or why most experimental oral carcinomas do not metas-tasize. Occasional reports have appeared relating to the testing of suspected aetiological agents for human oral cancer against the oral mucosa of experimental animals. These have occasionally produced interesting results though there is always a problem in extrapolating such observations to the human situation.

Electron Microscopy

Electron microscopical investigations of cancer have so far been a disappointment. The main reason for this is that, although numerous observations have been made of various parts of the cell, none has proved to be unique to the cancer cell or its precursors. However, in common with premalignant and malignant lesions in other epithelial sites, human and experimental oral cancer and precancer reveal some interesting properties. In early stages of experimental carcinogenesis and in certain human oral premalignant lesions, the basal plasma membrane sends pseudopodia-like structures into underlying connective tissue. These pass through gaps in the lamina densa and enter areas where collagen destruction is evident. There is doubt, however, about whether the collagen damage arises first and allows or encourages epithelial penetration, or whether the epithelial pseudopodia are active in producing such damage. This process continues until, in the fully malignant state, little lamina densa remains, the malignant epithelial cells have an extremely convoluted surface, and connective tissue destruction is widespread. The pseudo-podial extensions through damaged lamina densa are not confined to premalignancy, though, also being seen during wound healing, vesicle formation and in a few other circumstances. However, in the premalignant states they are apparently uncontrolled and may be indicative of early invasion, whereas in other situations once their function is complete or the stimulus removed they disappear.

As well as changes at the junction between epithelium and connective tissue, electron microscopy reveals loss of adhesion between malignant epithelial cells and increased irregularity of the plasma membrane. These have their counterparts under the light microscope, appearing as loss of intercellular adherence and increased cellular pleo-morphism. There is current interest in the significance and extent of alterations in the attachment apparatus between cells during oral carcinogenesis, in the ultrastructural alterations accompanying Candida invasion, and in various features of the cell membrane. The coating on the surface of epithelial cells contains several important com-ponents, including various antigens; both histochemical and immunological techniques are being combined with electron microscopy to determine more of their characteris-tics. An ultrastructural study of oral submucous fibrosis has revealed that the affected connective tissue contains an excessive number of fine collagen fibrils and of interfibrillar matrix. In common with the other ultrastructural features of oral cancer and precancerous lesions, the significance of this is still obscure. Advances beyond the compilation of purely descriptive records await correlation with follow-up information of the clinical states.

Histochemistry

Histochemical studies, like electron microscopy, have failed to disclose clear differences between oral carcinoma and non-malignant conditions.

Nevertheless, some interesting features have emerged. For example, lactate dehydrogenase activity appears to be increased in both oral cancer and in certain leukoplakias. Other studies showed changes in the state of lysosomal enzymes both during experimental oral carcinogenesis and in human oral cancer and precancerous lesions. There could be a correlation between altered lysosomal enzyme activity, changes observed by histochemical methods in juxta-epithelial connective tissue, and the electron microscopical observations referred to above (Smith, 1972). Extra-lysosomal acid phosphatase in intercellular spaces has been described in human oral leukoplakias and is perhaps associated with increased keratinization. Combining histochemical methods with electron microscopy should help to clarify the nature of alterations that accompany oral malignancy. In common with many other methods, histochemistry awaits more complete exploitation both in the range of techniques and in their application to lesions with well-defined properties.

Cell Turnover Studies

Investigations of cell kinetics in human oral cancer have produced variable and complex results that defy a uniform interpretation. Experimental carcinogenesis in hamster cheek pouch has been studied with more success. The main conclusions are that cell cycle time, including each component phase, is progressively reduced as carcinoma ensues; also, suprabasal progenitor cells appear with increasing frequency during carcinogenesis.

In human oral leukoplakias cell turnover and mitotic rate are both increased. Mitotic values are higher in leukoplakia lesions that exhibit epithelial dysplasia than in those that do not.

Immunological Methods and Prognosis of Cancer

As far as oral malignancy is concerned, two particular areas of investigation have attracted attention. One relates to the presence of blood group antigens on the surface of oral epithelial cells. These can be examined by fluorescence or peroxidase techniques, and are markedly reduced, or sometimes completely absent, in sites of oral cancer. Areas of epithelial dysplasia usually show reduced staining of blood group antigens, but to less extent than in carcinoma.

The second approach has been based upon the expectation that cell-mediated immune mechanisms might be involved in oral premalignancy and its transformation. Both the lymphocyte transformation test and leucocyte migration test have produced results suggesting an association of cell-mediated immunity with oral leukoplakia. Whether this is of predictive value, however, awaits the outcome of further studies.

Defects of cell-mediated immunity have been reported in patients suffering from iron-deficiency anaemia. Should this be confirmed, it raises the prospect that such a mechanism might explain the possible association between iron-deficiency anaemia and conditions such as oral cancer and chronic hyperplastic candidiasis.

Administration of anti-lymphocytic serum to hamsters during cheek pouch carcinogenesis has the effect of both depressing the cell-mediated immune system and causing earlier formation of malignant tumours which grow in greater profusion. This provides yet another illustration of a possible involvement of cell-mediated immune mechanisms in oral malignancy.

AETIOLOGICAL FACTORS

Oral Cancer

No single cause has been found for all oral cancers though several factors have been implicated; often, these are related particularly to a defined population group and one or two sites (Smith, 1973). Recognition of aetiological agents encourages the view that prevention is possible, at least to some extent, and one looks forward to the time when active preventive measures can be instituted that will lead to significant reductions in the morbidity and mortality from oral cancer. For some oral cancers no recognizable aetiological factors can be found.

Sunlight

This is an important aetiological factor for cancer of the lip.

Pipe Smoking

In the past this was thought to be a significant contributor to cancer of the lip. More recently, however, although some studies have confirmed previous suspicions, others have failed to demonstrate a relationship.

Cigarette Smoking

For oral sites, excluding the lip, there appears to be a direct correlation even though it is not particularly marked. One puzzling feature, therefore, is that one might not expect to find a declining incidence of oral cancer among a population where cigarette consumption is on the increase. As this is contrary to experience in many countries, it probably indicates that different aetiological factors have been reduced more drastically.

Other Smoking Habits

Cigar smoking appears to be associated with cancer of the buccal mucosa, the habit of reverse smoking (under some conditions) with cancer of the palatal mucosa, and "bidi" smoking in India with oropharyngeal cancer.

Tobacco Chewing

There is substantial evidence in support of the long-suspected association between betel quid chewing and oral cancer in South-East Asia. What is more in doubt, however, is the identity of the harmful ingredient. Some evidence points to the lime content, other evidence to the tobacco, and yet a third view implies that both act in concert. Animal experiments have shown that oral mucosa exposed to lime or tobacco undergoes changes, at the light and electron microscopical levels, similar to those seen in human oral premalignant lesions.

Oral verrucous carcinoma in Papua-New Guinea is possibly induced by the application of slaked lime to the oral mucosa, though the action of tobacco in addition cannot be entirely excluded. In parts of the U.S.A. where verrucous carcinoma is more common than usual, both "snuff-dipping" and tobacco-chewing habits are widely practised among the affected individuals.

Alcohol

Various studies have investigated the role of alcohol in the aetiology of oral cancer. Most have demonstrated a positive relationship of some form and have included the direct influence of heavy drinking or the indirect effect of liver cirrhosis. Cancer of the tongue and floor of mouth show a particularly positive association. Conversely, population groups which abstain from alcohol reveal a reduced mortality rate from oral cancer. All investigations into drinking habits, however, are hampered by two complicating factors. One is that heavy drinkers are usually heavy smokers and it is difficult therefore to exclude the effects of smoking. The other factor is the difficulty in obtaining a truthful history about drinking habits. Animal studies have provided some evidence that liver cirrhosis is a predisposing factor to the development of oral cancer.

Syphilis

Through comparison of registration details for persons suffering from syphilis and those suffering from various forms of cancer, it has been possible to determine a direct association between syphilis and cancer of the tongue; other parts of the mouth and lips did not show such an association. From other investigations, the association is more accurately defined as one with cancer of the anterior two-thirds of the tongue and not of the posterior one-third. When correction is made for alcohol and tobacco consumption, the relationship is still present.

What is not known, however, is whether the involvement of syphilis in the aetiology of oral cancer is direct, through the presence of the infection, or indirect, perhaps through the methods of treatment. The suggestion has been made that there is a connection between the declining rates of oral cancer incidence in some countries and the changing pattern of treatment of syphilis, with arsenicals and heavy metal compounds no longer in common use. There is no direct evidence in support of this view and the possibility that long-term effects of the disease are implicated cannot be ignored.

Dental Factors

Although poor oral hygiene, jagged restorations or teeth, and ill-fitting dentures have often been accused of being aetiological factors in oral cancer development, there is little or no direct evidence of such an association.

On the other hand, it is difficult to see how convincing evidence could ever be obtained with the difficulties involved in obtaining accurate dental histories retrospectively. By the time investigations are made amongst persons who already have oral cancer, it is hardly surprising that a deterioration in their oral hygiene can be found. Also, in many mouths, it is not difficult to find traumatic factors if they are sought. Loss of teeth is a frequent accompaniment of treatment for oral cancer; it is likely, therefore, that an association would be found at this stage between oral cancer and the edentulous state. This would not imply, however, a previously poor dental condition. There is no direct evidence to support the hypothesis that declining rates of oral cancer incidence are a result of improvements in the standard of dental health.

Oral Precancerous Lesions

For the most part, aetiological factors for oral cancer are also involved in the aetiology of oral precancerous lesions. The available evidence relates mostly to leukoplakia. The possible role of Candida infection has been discussed in previous sections but additional information concerning other factors is provided by Pindborg (1971) and, in brief, below.

Tobacco Habits

These would appear to be the most common of the aetiological factors that can be implicated for leukoplakias, though the type of habit varies geographically and the leukoplakias are preferentially distributed in different oral sites accordingly. Cheroot smoking apparently has a positive correlation with floor of mouth leukoplakia in Danish females, snuff-induced leukoplakias are found in sites that correspond to where the snuff is habitually placed, hookli pipe-smoking is associated with leukoplakia of labial mucosa, reverse smoking induces leukoplakia in the mucosa of the hard palate, and bidi-smoking particularly encourages development of lesions on buccal mucosa. Chewing habits, similar to those involved in the production of oral cancer, are equally important in the consideration of aetiological factors for leukoplakia.

Other Factors

Local trauma probably plays a large part in the development of oral leukoplakias and its removal is often accompanied by resolution to a normal mucosa. Some workers have suggested that vitamin A deficiency might be associated with oral leukoplakia, especially as large doses of vitamin A can be followed by reduction or disappearance of the lesions. Although finding some initial favour as a method for treating oral leukoplakias, vitamin A supplementation has largely been abandoned because the doses required could not be sustained and the lesions recurred when therapeutic levels of vitamin A were reduced.

Heavy consumption of chillies has been suggested as an aetiological factor in the production of oral submucous fibrosis. However, there is no convincing evidence that this view can be supported either from population studies or work on experimental animals.

REFERENCES

Binnie, W. H., Cawson, R. A., Hill, G. B. and Soaper, A. E. (1972), "Oral Cancer in England and Wales: A National Study of Morbidity, Mortality, Curability and Related Factors." London: H.M.S.O.

Dabelsteen, E., Roed-Petersen, B., Smith, C. J. and Pindborg, J. J. (1971), "The Limitations of Exfoliative Cytology for the Detection of Epithelial Atypia in Oral Leukoplakias," *Brit. J. Cancer*, **25**, 21.

Kramer, I. R. H., Lucas, R. B., El-Labban, N. and Lister, L. (1970), "The Use of Discriminant Analysis for Examining the Histological Features of Oral Keratoses and Lichen Planus," *Brit. J. Cancer*, **24**, 673.

Lucas, R. B. (1972), *Pathology of Tumours of the Oral Tissues*, 2nd edition. London: Churchill Livingstone.

Pindborg, J. J. (1971), "Oral Leukoplakia," *Aust. J. Dent.*, **16**, 83.

Pindborg, J. J. (1972), "Is Submucous Fibrosis a Precancerous Condition in the Oral Cavity?" *Int. dent. J.*, **22**, 474.

Shafer, W. G. (1972), "Verrucous Carcinoma," *Int. dent. J.*, **22**, 451.

Smith, C. J. (1972), "Variations in Histochemical Properties of Hydrolytic Enzymes in Oral Precancerous Conditions," *J. dent. Res.*, **51**, 308.

Smith, C. J. (1973), "Global Epidemiology and Aetiology of Oral Cancer," *Int. dent. J.*, **23**, 82.

20. ODONTOGENIC TUMOURS AND TUMOUR-LIKE LESIONS

R. B. LUCAS and J. J. PINDBORG

Classification and nomenclature

Benign and malignant tumours

Behaviour of odontogenic tumours

    Malignant tumours
    Locally invasive tumours
    Benign tumours and hamartomas

Odontogenesis and oncogenesis

    Epithelial tumours
    Tumours with epithelial and mesenchymal elements

Appendix

The general aspects of neoplasia have been discussed in Chapter 18. This section is concerned particularly with the odontogenic neoplasms.

CLASSIFICATION AND NOMENCLATURE

That the terminology and designations used in scientific discussions should have agreed and stable meanings would seem both obvious and necessary. Yet pathological, including tumour, nomenclature has been most inconsistent, not only as between different languages but even in the same ones. The World Health Organization defines the problem in the introductory paragraph to its series of monographs on the histological classification of tumours:

"Among the prerequisites for comparative studies of cancer are international agreement on histological criteria for the classification of cancer types and a standardized nomenclature. At present, pathologists use different terms for the same pathological entity, and furthermore the same term is sometimes applied to lesions of different types. An internationally agreed classification of tumours, acceptable alike to physicians, surgeons, radiologists, pathologists and statisticians, would enable cancer workers in all parts of the world to compare their findings and would facilitate collaboration among them."

WHO not only recognized the problem but itself set about finding a remedy, by setting up international reference and collaborating centres for the study of tumours of various tissues and sites and by publishing the agreed classifications and descriptions that resulted from the work of these centres. Recently, "Histological Typing of Odontogenic Tumours, Jaw Cysts and Allied Lesions" has been published (Pindborg, Kramer and Torloni, 1971); this classification, which is the result of a five year international collaborative effort, is appended to this chapter and the nomenclature set out there is used throughout this section.

As well as agreeing on nomenclature, it would clearly be helpful to discussion if agreement could be reached upon definitions for terms and concepts. But when an attempt is made to define even such a basic term as that which constitutes the subject of this chapter, it is found that a precise definition still eludes us today as it did Virchow a century ago, when he said that no man, even under dire compulsion, could say exactly what a tumour is. However carefully a definition may be formulated, exceptions can always be found, often with regard to common neoplasms and not, as might be thought, mainly in connection with the rarities and curiosities. Indeed, the oral region provides good examples. It is, for instance, generally accepted that neoplasms are lesions characterized by progressive growth, but exceptions to this rule are found amongst the salivary gland tumours. Thus, pleomorphic adenomas may grow to a certain size and then remain stationary for many years, sometimes even for the rest of the patient's life. Subcutaneous lipomas are another example, since these tumours can frequently remain dormant for long periods. Similarly, exceptions to all other features generally accepted as criteria of neoplasia could be cited without difficulty.

The foregoing remarks are not intended to convey the impression that formal definitions of neoplasia are of little practical value. On the contrary, by stressing the important features of many common neoplasms, such as persistent and progressive growth, "autonomy", incoordinated proliferation and the like, they give a good idea, although not a strict scientific definition, of what neoplasms are like and what they may do to the host who harbours one. Although knowledge of the behaviour and the response to available treatments of most tumours is reasonably comprehensive and the terminology used is adequate for the everyday purposes of diagnosis and treatment, the point has not been reached where the subject can be discussed in terms of rigorous scientific exactitude. This applies no less to tumours of the odontogenic tissues than to any others elsewhere in the body.

BENIGN AND MALIGNANT TUMOURS

The difficulties encountered in the precise definition of neoplasms in general extend also to the distinction between benign and malignant tumours. The concepts "benign" and "malignant" are of course readily comprehensible, and every textbook of pathology lists the essential features typifying each group, but just as anomalies, exceptions and contradictions prevent the formulation of a precise definition of neoplasms as such, so they also prevent rigorous definition of these groups. In practice, this lack of precision is recognized and has to be accepted. It is known, for example, that certain tumours are almost always benign and others are nearly always malignant, but it is also known that a tumour of the benign group may show evidence of malignancy and that a tumour of the malignant group may not in fact behave in such a way. And also, in addition to tumours that usually pursue a predictable course but occasionally behave in an unexpected manner, there are numerous types of tumours whose behaviour is always unpredictable. Moreover, the prognosis in a given case may depend as much or even more on the anatomical situation of a tumour as on its histological constitution. This is a familiar situation in the oral region—the outlook for a patient with, for example, carcinoma of the floor of the mouth is much less favourable than for a patient with a lip tumour because, at least in part, of the technical difficulty of eradicating a tumour in the former situation and the ease of doing so in the latter, although histologically the two tumours might be identical.

Because of these and other considerations it is not possible to establish precise definitions distinguishing innocence and malignancy in tumours, and this is recognized by many systematists when they speak of these attributes being the extremes of a range of spectrum, with all gradations between. As Willis (1967) puts it, when the clinician asks the pathologist about a tumour he has removed, "Is it innocent or malignant?" the pathologist should encourage him to ask rather, "*How* innocent or malignant is this tumour?". Such a question is of course as applicable to many of the tumours that can occur in the oral tissues as to those in other parts of the body. However, in the case of the odontogenic tumours, the problem is not so troublesome since many of these neoplasms are benign and only rarely depart from such behaviour, although some difficulties do exist, as will be seen. Because perhaps of this general pattern of behaviour, there are frequently instances in the literature on odontogenic tumours of a certain looseness in the use of terminology. For example, lesions may be referred to as benign, when the meaning intended is that they do not metastasize. Or again, if a lesion is judged not to be malignant, it may be referred to as hamartomatous, when it might be more appropriately termed a benign tumour. Clearly, then, some additional concepts are desirable and one such is that of local malignancy. This term is used for tumours that cannot be classified without qualification as malignant since they rarely, if ever, metastasize. At the same time, they cannot be termed benign since they infiltrate and destroy tissue. The classic example of a neoplasm of this type is the basal cell carcinoma or rodent ulcer, which if left untreated relentlessly invades the adjacent tissues and in the course of time destroys great areas. However, it rarely metastasizes, and death is ultimately due to the local destructive effects of the lesion itself, or to complications directly connected therewith.

It should be noted that the invasion and destruction of tissue is the essential feature of the locally malignant neoplasm. This point is made because some benign neoplasms can also produce serious or fatal results for their host. Highly differentiated and completely circumscribed tumours can still be lethal if they should interfere with a vital structure, for example, compression of the trachea by a benign mediastinal tumour. In such cases there is no question of infiltration and tissue destruction, the fatal effects of the tumour being incidental, as it were, due to its anatomical position and not to any inherent lethal properties. On the other hand, a benign tumour may be poorly demarcated from surrounding tissues and may even intermingle with them. The tortuous and dilated lymph channels of cystic hygroma, for example, extend irregularly into the adjacent normal tissue, and similarly some of the lesions in neurofibromatosis may be closely intermingled with normal tissue. However, the element of progressive infiltration and tissue destruction is absent in such lesions and any ill-effects they may produce are due to other reasons.

In addition to the terms and concepts already mentioned, it is necessary to consider the class of lesions designated as hamartomas. Here again, there are difficulties with precise definitions, but Albrecht's original description is still generally valid. He used the term hamartoma to describe those tumour-like masses that are composed of a mixture of tissues normal to the part in which they are occurring and that are due to an anomaly in tissue development. Although these lesions resemble neoplasms in many ways, such as in clinical presentation and microscopic appearance, they are not true neoplasms; their growth potential is limited, and growth ceases when the host has reached full maturity. Many hamartomas conform closely to this general description. The haemangiomas of infants and children are familiar examples, these masses of excess tissue being tumour-like in clinical appearance and microscopic structure, and they may even appear to be invading adjacent normal tissues. Furthermore, they may grow rapidly and even alarmingly, but in time the growth rate diminishes and finally ceases. Some lesions may diminish in size and may even regress completely. In other cases, however, there are divergences from what is accepted as the characteristic pattern of behaviour of hamartomas. For example, in neurofibromatosis the lesions generally cease growing in adult life; in some cases, however, they continue to enlarge slowly but indefinitely. Then again, although hamartomas are by definition non-neoplastic, some are rather prone to undergo neoplastic change. Neurofibromatosis is once more an example; there is a marked predisposition for the hamartomatous tissue to become sarcomatous.

Hamartomas must be distinguished from embryonic tumours, which are true neoplasms arising during embryonic, fetal or early post-natal development from a particular organ rudiment or tissue while this is still immature (Willis, 1958). In many cases, of course, such tumours will appear during early life. In some tissues and organs, however, post-natal development goes on for a long time, as in the case of the teeth, and full maturity is not attained until adult life. Tumours occurring in tissues that are still developing can thus appear in childhood, adolescence and even adult life, and although of post-natal origin can be considered as embryonic tumours. These tumours, as Willis points out, are therefore both malformations and neoplasms and often the latter attribute is only too obvious, as in the case of some of the tumours of infancy and childhood, such as neuroblastoma, retinoblastoma and nephroblastoma.

Most, if not all, of the odontogenic tumours come into the category of embryonic tumours. The evidence is largely inferential, but nevertheless it is strong. Most of the tumours occur in children, adolescents and young adults. Even when they occur in older people they may well have been present for a long period without having been noticed. Many of the tumours are associated with anomalies of dental development such as unerupted teeth, and microscopically all of them display undoubted affinities with developing dental tissues. Although some tumours may arise from the odontogenic tissues while they are actually in the process of developing, it is likely that others originate in those vestiges of the odontogenic apparatus that remain in the jaws after dental development has been completed. There is thus an alternative explanation for the occurrence of apparently embryonic tumours in later adult life or indeed in old age, other than their persistence in a dormant or slowly progressive state since the period of odontogenesis. They may, instead, develop from the odontogenic residues and this seems to be a likely origin in many cases.

Embryonic tumours in general are much less common than are tumours of adult tissues; clearly, developing tissues have a limited life as such, so that the tumorigenic mechanisms operating in the case of embryonic tumours must be of a different order from those concerned in the tumours of adult tissues. Odontogenic tumours are like other embryonic tumours in their relative infrequency; here again, for those that arise during active dental development there is a limited period for their onset. For those that arise from odontogenic residues it could be speculated that, although these residues remain in the jaws permanently, they are not exposed in the same way and to the same degree at least, to the carcinogenic agents that must undoubtedly be brought into contact with the oral mucosa (and other body surfaces in contact with the external environment) throughout life.

In one respect odontogenic tumours are unlike many other embryonic neoplasms. The rapid growth, proneness to metastasize and poor prognosis of tumours like neuroblastoma are regrettably familiar features of these neoplasms. Fortunately, the majority of odontogenic tumours behave differently, either being benign or having local invasive properties only. Indeed, the status of some odontogenic tumours is still not certain—whether they are benign or hamartomatous, a matter to be discussed later.

Teratomas are neoplasms composed of more than one tissue not normally present in the part in which the tumour occurs. They differ from simple malformations in showing the neoplastic quality of progressive growth, and from embryonic tumours in that the latter are neoplasms of the tissues proper to the part in which they arise.

BEHAVIOUR OF ODONTOGENIC TUMOURS

Although the odontogenic tumours are, on the whole, of less unpredictable behaviour than are many other tumours elsewhere in the body, there is still a great deal to be learned about their precise nature.

Malignant Tumours

Only a few odontogenic tumours come into this category.

Intra-alveolar Carcinoma is a rare tumour and although it has been recognized for some considerable time, few cases have been recorded. In recent years, however, more attention has been given to this group of tumours and probably in future an increasing number of cases will be reported (Shear, 1969). These tumours are squamous cell carcinomas, showing the usual microscopic features and behaviour of such growths although there is often a tendency for an ameloblastoma-like pattern to be developed. The intraosseous situation of these neoplasms, well away from the mucosal epithelium that is the source of the common squamous cell carcinoma of the mouth, indicates that they originate in odontogenic epithelial rests.

Squamous Cell Carcinoma Arising in Odontogenic Cysts constitutes another category of malignant odontogenic tumour. These tumours are not common and many of the reports, like those of malignant ameloblastomas, do not withstand critical examination. Nevertheless, several acceptable reports have been published and there is evidence that the primordial cyst (keratocyst) is much more likely to undergo malignant change, uncommon though this is, than the other varieties of odontogenic cysts (Toller, 1972). Precancerous changes such as dysplasia and carcinoma *in situ* have been reported in primordial cysts.

Connective tissue malignancy in the odontogenic series is even less common than epithelial malignancy. It is not certain whether or not there occurs a pure **fibrosarcoma** of odontogenic origin, although theoretically there is no reason why this should not be the case, the tumour being the malignant counterpart of the benign odontogenic fibroma or myxoma. Intraosseous fibrosarcoma does occur in the jaws but is a rare tumour, and in the cases so far reported it would be no more than conjecture to characterize any of these neoplasms as odontogenic.

Ameloblastic Fibrosarcoma is in rather a different category as this is clearly an odontogenic tumour, being the counterpart of the ameloblastic fibroma. The latter is itself a rare tumour although its clinical and pathological attributes are well known. Ameloblastic fibrosarcoma is correspondingly even rarer and less than 20 cases have been reported so far (Leider *et al.*, 1972). They have occurred most frequently in young adults, in the mandible more often than in the maxilla. The diagnosis of sarcoma has depended on the histological features, together with the clinical behaviour. Microscopically, the epithelial element of these tumours has appeared identical to that in ameloblastic fibroma, but the fibroblastic component has shown the usual cytological features of malignancy such as pleomorphism, excessive mitotic activity and abnormal mitoses. Clinically, the tumours have behaved like fibrosarcomas of low-grade malignancy. It may be that this tumour is a lesion of local invasiveness only.

Locally Invasive Tumours

A number of odontogenic tumours are locally invasive. Tumours of this type are not encapsulated or circumscribed and although they may not grow particularly rapidly, they do extend through and replace adjacent tissues, rather than pushing them aside as occurs with the purely expansile growth of circumscribed and encapsulated benign neoplasms. From the point of view of treatment, it is possible to obtain a satisfactory result by simple enucleation in the case of circumscribed tumours, whereas locally invasive tumours require a resection that will remove the tumour together with surrounding tissue sufficient to reach beyond the limits of tumour permeation. If this can be done, then an equally satisfactory result is obtained. If removal of the tumour is incomplete there will of course be recurrence. This was not infrequently the case with the old treatment of curettage for ameloblastoma; the patient who has had several such operations with subsequent recurrence over a period of years is still familiar to clinicians, since old patients treated in the past by the now outmoded methods still present for definitive treatment.

Even apparently completely circumscribed or encapsulated tumours may not be without risk of recurrence if treated conservatively, for example, pleomorphic adenoma. For this reason surgeons often prefer to resect tumours rather than enucleate them or use other conservative

procedures, since this will be satisfactory both for tumours that are known to be locally invasive and for those that are circumscribed and encapsulated, but might still recur.

One result of the understandable desire of surgeons to err on the side of safety—if indeed there is any error—is that little is known of the full life history of a number of odontogenic tumours, and what the pattern of growth would be, uninfluenced by treatment, or whether more conservative measures than are now generally practised would perhaps be effective. This is particularly so for those lesions that have been recognized as entities mainly in recent years and have thus been treated by modern methods.

Evidence is now accumulating that invasive tumours, both epithelial and mesenchymal, contain high levels of collagenolytic substances and that collagenolytic activity is most pronounced in areas where invasion is actively occurring. Such substances have recently been demonstrated in various odontogenic cysts and in **ameloblastoma,** and it may well be that the ability of such lesions to cause bone resorption depends in part at least on the production of collagenolytic or osteolytic substances. But, in addition, perhaps it might be speculated that the invasiveness of ameloblastoma is of a different nature from that of other locally invasive or malignant tumours. The epithelial component of the odontogenic apparatus is endowed with properties that enable it to penetrate mesenchyme in the process of odontogenesis. This is of course a perfectly normal and indeed essential element in dental development, and this invasiveness of the epithelium, if it may be so termed, is also seen in organogenesis in other tissues that have a comparable mode of development, for example the hair follicles. It is generally considered that many ameloblastomas originate in rests of odontogenic epithelium, and thus may have properties that were normal to that epithelium. If such were the case the local invasiveness of ameloblastoma would represent the altered activity of a normal property. This might well be a different sort of invasiveness from that seen in many other invasive tumours.

The question of frank malignancy has also arisen in connection with ameloblastoma. Numerous cases have been reported in which metastases were considered to have occurred; these are fully analysed in the literature by a number of authors and need not be discussed in detail here. Suffice it to say that when the unacceptable cases have been rejected, because of inadequate documentation, absence of photomicrographs, or inconclusive nature of those presented, or for other relevant reasons, only a few remain in which it can be accepted that metastatic deposits have genuinely occurred (Ikemura *et al.*, 1972). In these cases the metastases have generally occurred in the lungs and there has usually been a long history with several or many operations on the jaw tumour. This suggests that when pulmonary metastases do occur, spread is likely to have been by inhalation and not by the haematogenous route. Inhalation metastases of this type are probably implantation deposits of fragments of tumour mechanically dislodged from the primary growth in the course of operative intervention. They are therefore in a different category from the secondary deposits that occur in most of the common metastasizing tumours, where the dissemination of tumour cells from the primary growth occurs by way of the blood stream or lymphatics, and for reasons still largely unknown. However, there are exceptional cases of ameloblastoma in which the metastases have been blood-borne. On the whole, it is reasonable to conclude that the ameloblastoma, like the basal cell carcinoma, is a locally invasive non-metastasizing tumour, but that, exceptionally, metastases have occurred.

Some examples of ameloblastoma have been described as malignant, not because of metastasis but because the microscopic appearance has provided cytological evidence of malignancy, or because the tumour has progressed unusually rapidly, or because both of these features were present. Apart from rare cases in which squamous cell carcinoma has occurred together with, or developed in, ameloblastoma, considerable reserve should be exercised in regard to such cases, since the histological identity of these tumours is frequently not above suspicion. Moreover, since local invasiveness is in any case a characteristic feature of ameloblastoma, it is not justifiable to designate a particular tumour as malignant simply because it exhibits this feature to a more pronounced degree than is usual. The diagnosis of malignancy should depend on evidence of metastasis as well as invasiveness. It is not sufficient to say that a tumour is malignant because it looks malignant under the microscope. It must be shown to behave malignantly, or at least it must be known that tumours showing such a microscopic appearance do in fact so behave, in most cases. This is an aspect of the pathology of ameloblastoma for which little objective evidence has as yet been put forward.

The **calcifying epithelial odontogenic tumour** is another neoplasm that is considered to be locally invasive. Although some of the reported tumours have seemed to be well circumscribed, these growths are not encapsulated and they would certainly appear histologically to comply with general concepts of local invasiveness. Some tumours have recurred after treatment, but others appear to have been permanently cured (Krolls and Pindborg, 1974). These different therapeutic results are probably due to completeness or otherwise of excision; no data are available with regard to long term behaviour, uninfluenced by treatment. A point that should be mentioned is the cellular pleomorphism frequently seen in this tumour. Sometimes it is pronounced, and giant cells with large irregular nuclei may be conspicuous (fig. 1). Such features might suggest frank malignancy to the inexperienced observer, but these tumours do not metastasize.

Tumours of the odontogenic **fibroma-fibromyxoma-myxoma group** are of variable behaviour (Harrison and Eggleston, 1973). Those in which collagen is a major component tend to be circumscribed, but those that are largely myxomatous are unencapsulated and frequently extend through bone and into soft tissues and the margin of the growth is ill-defined. These tumours therefore have to be treated as locally invasive and resected with an ample margin of surrounding tissue. Adequately done this effects a cure, which of course is the overriding aim, but

from the theoretical point of view it is still not known whether this is a truly locally malignant neoplasm, in the sense that its cells infiltrate and destroy adjacent tissues, or whether the penetration of surrounding tissues is not due mainly to the physical characteristics of the neoplasm. The diffluent myxomatous material may readily penetrate and percolate through tissue spaces even in the absence of some inherently invasive quality of the neoplasm, such as might be supposed to be possessed by locally invasive tumours like basal cell carcinomas or indeed by invasive tumours in general.

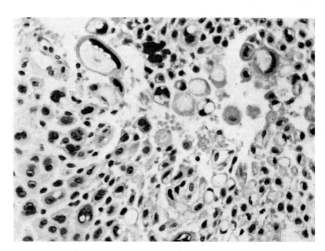

Fig. 1. Nuclear pleomorphism in a calcifying epithelial odontogenic tumour. × 260. Courtesy of Dr. F. V. Howell, La Jolla, California.

Benign Tumours and Hamartomas

These two categories are best considered together since there is not infrequently some difficulty in deciding which is the appropriate designation for certain lesions.

The **adenomatoid odontogenic tumour** is a case in point. This lesion generally occurs in adolescents and young adults, often in association with an unerupted tooth. In a recent compilation and analysis of over 100 published cases it was shown that recurrence was extremely rare, despite the fact that many tumours appeared clinically to be cysts and therefore received conservative treatment (Giansanti et al., 1970). Indeed, in some cases in which there had been no recurrence, it was known that removal of the lesion had probably been incomplete. On the other hand, although the rate of growth of many lesions appears to be slow, it does seem to be progressive, at least in those cases followed sufficiently long for this to be assessed. Thus, while there are some features in favour of regarding this lesion as a hamartoma, there are others suggesting that it is a benign tumour. One piece of evidence that could help is as yet lacking; knowledge of the natural history of the lesion in the absence of treatment. Thus, if it were to transpire that the majority of lesions cease to grow or even regress after a period, this would be in favour of their hamartomatous nature, but it must be recognized that some hamartomatous lesions can continue to grow slowly over a long period and some benign tumours may cease to grow and remain quiescent, as has already been mentioned. The dividing lines between the various classes of tumours and allied lesions are thus indefinite, and for lesions that happen to come into the borderlands, this situation can only be accepted and further knowledge awaited.

The **calcifying odontogenic cyst** is another lesion that, like the adenomatoid odontogenic tumour, fortunately presents few problems in terms of practical management but again poses questions of basic importance. Although many of the lesions are indeed cystic, a number are not. The designation is therefore inappropriate, both factually and also because it implies that the lesion is not neoplastic. This, however, is not known. Certainly the lesion is benign. Many cases have now been reported and few have recurred after conservative treatment.

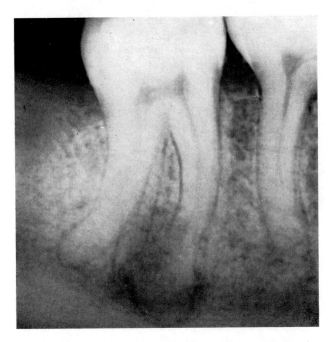

Fig. 2. Benign cementoblastoma. An early lesion involving the mandibular right second molar tooth and resembling apical osteitis.

Ameloblastic fibroma appears to be a benign tumour. A recent analysis of 24 cases—a relatively large number for this rather rare growth—has shown that most tumours appeared to be circumscribed, but there was a recurrence rate of over 40 per cent (Trodahl, 1972). This was probably due to unduly conservative treatment in some cases, but in most it was thought that the primary excision had been complete, although there was no proof that this in fact was so. These findings contrast strikingly with those noted for the adenomatoid odontogenic tumour, with its negligible recurrence rate. However, the ameloblastic fibroma is generally considerably larger and more of a centrally situated lesion than is the adenomatoid odontogenic tumour, and may well be more difficult to remove completely. It seems reasonable to consider this tumour benign although, like the other benign tumours, it will recur if incompletely removed.

Lesions that come under the general heading of **cementoma** pose no problems of behaviour since they are all uniformly benign. They do, however, have many features of interest and importance with regard to histogenesis and classification. At present, they are considered to constitute four groups. The **benign cementoblastoma** is the entity formerly designated as "true cementoma". It is always attached to the roots of a tooth. Radiographically, it is essentially a sclerotic lesion which appears to be attached to or overlying the apical third of the root and surrounded by a radiolucent zone of uniform width. In the early stages of development the benign cementoblastoma may resemble apical osteitis (fig. 2). Histologically, the neoplasm is characterized by the formation of sheets of cementum-like tissue that may contain a large number of reversal lines (fig. 3). The peripheral and more active growth areas may be unmineralized. The cementum-forming cells, which are unusually large and occasionally pleomorphic, become entrapped in the hard tissue which they have formed.

There may be histological variants of this tumour. While in some cases the cementum is strongly basophilic, with many deeply staining reversal lines somewhat reminiscent of osteitis deformans, in others it is uniformly eosinophilic. Some tumours may be indistinguishable histologically from osteoid osteoma or benign osteoblastoma.

The **cementifying fibroma** and **periapical cemental dysplasia** are histologically identical. They differ in that periapical cemental dysplasia occurs in the mandibular incisor region in post-menopausal women whereas the cementifying fibroma has no sex predilection and occurs mostly in the mandibular premolar and molar region.

The so-called **gigantiform cementoma** appears to be seen most often in middle-aged Negro females. Only a few cases have been reported.

The **odontomes,** complex and compound, have been well known and fully recognized for many years and their natural history is fully documented. They are developmental malformations of the odontogenic tissues that occur in children and display their period of active growth during this stage of life. When adult life is reached, they cease to grow and become quiescent. They conform in all respects to categorization as hamartomas. There are many interesting questions with regard to their composition and origin, and some of these are considered in the next section.

A lesion that has been designated as a hamartoma, the **gingival epithelial hamartoma,** has recently been described. Some of the queries raised about the hamartomatous versus neoplastic status of some other lesions also apply here. The status of this interesting gingival lesion cannot be taken for granted as yet, and more cases must be studied.

ODONTOGENESIS AND ONCOGENESIS

This discussion of odontogenesis and oncogenesis mainly concerns the changes that occur in odontogenic tumours from the time of their appearance onwards, rather than the problems of tumour induction.

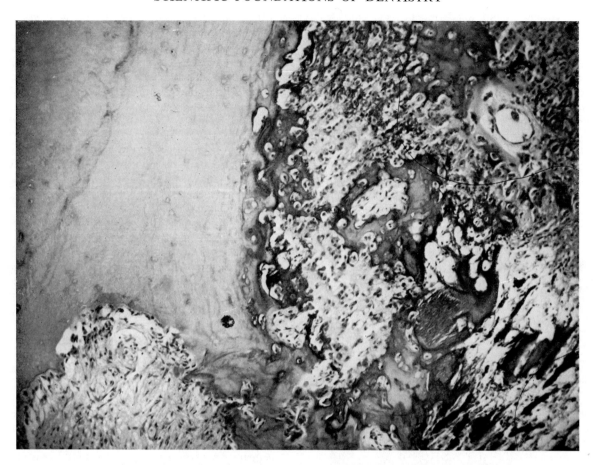

FIG. 3. Benign cementoblastoma, showing the basophilic tumour tissue continuous with osteocementum at the tooth root. × 90.

Practically all microscopists who have studied odontogenic tumours and commented on their histogenesis have noted how close a parallel may be drawn between the different stages of normal odontogenesis and the various odontogenic tumours. Undoubtedly, some fundamental considerations underlying the origin and development of these tumours will be illuminated as a result of the intensive and detailed investigations into normal development now being carried out and, conversely, studies of oncogenesis may well contribute to our knowledge of the normal. However, a certain amount of reserve is necessary. Because of the remarkable structural similarities of many odontogenic tumours to the developing dental tissues, it is tempting to construct classifications placing tumours in order of differentiation corresponding to different stages of odontogenesis, to ascribe their origin to elements of the odontogenic apparatus at various stages of development, or to try to correlate their biological activity with these features. It is essential to keep an open mind about all these matters since so much in fundamental knowledge is still lacking.

Another point that must be made concerns the range and identity of odontogenic tumours. Although textbooks and other formal accounts categorize the odontogenic tumours in a number of well-defined types—as indeed they must do both for the sake of clarity and because the majority of

tumours do in fact fall into such classes—there are also neoplasms that are difficult to classify or that otherwise pose problems in diagnosis or nomenclature. Some such tumours, although almost certainly of odontogenic origin, appear not to correspond with any of the accepted diagnostic categories. Others have more familiar features but show characteristics of more than one of the currently accepted tumour types. It must therefore be expected that current ideas on the histogenesis of odontogenic tumours, although certainly not rigid at the moment, as most authorities would agree, will undergo continuous modifications and evolution for some time to come.

With regard to normal odontogenesis, it is to be noted that a number of other tissues or organs develop in a fashion similar to the teeth, and some of the neoplasms of these tissues are again in some ways comparable to odontogenic neoplasms. The mammary, salivary, lacrimal and other glands, and the hair follicles, are all primarily derivatives of epithelium, as is the enamel organ. And, as in the teeth, interaction between epithelium and mesenchyme is an essential element in the development of these structures. It is in the teeth, however, that these interactions are most prominent, and this is reflected in odontogenic neoplasms.

Although a great deal of experimental work has been done in recent years on the normal development of most organs and tissues, including the teeth, and much has been learned, particularly about the way developing tissues interact with each other, knowledge is still at an early stage. So far as the odontogenic neoplasms are concerned, it could be rewarding to investigate these lesions in ways that have been applied to normal tissues, particularly with regard to tissue culture and transplantation experiments, but the experimental material and the nature of the experiments themselves, is extremely limited because of the relatively infrequent appearance of neoplasms in man. However, a start has been made in producing tumours in experimental animals, for example by infection with polyoma virus, and no doubt this and further methods will be exploited in the future. For the moment then, it must be accepted that little experimental work has been done on odontogenic tumours, and much of what is said about the possible implications of normal odontogenesis for onco-genesis can only be speculative.

A basic finding in developmental research is the great importance of mesenchyme for epithelial development. However, not only does mesenchyme influence epithelium to develop in certain directions, but epithelium also reacts on the mesenchyme. This interaction in odontogenesis is well recognized; its importance in other tissues also has now been established. In dental development, it has been shown that the dental papilla controls the shape of the developing tooth. Moreover, if dental papilla is added to explants of various types of epithelium, including integu-mental epithelium, tooth formation can be induced. In the case of other specialized derivatives of integument in various species, such as hairs, scales and feathers, there is also evidence that the dermal component can control the development of these structures. Not all epithelia will produce any of these structures if the corresponding dermal component be added. The epithelium has to be competent to respond, but this competence tends to be rather wider than might be thought, as suggested by the integumentary response to dental mesoderm. Epithelial cells, like all other somatic cells, possess genetic inform-ation for the development of a range of structures; the dermal element in each site—jaws, skin, feather tracts—has the specific inductive information for the adnexal structure appropriate to it.

Epithelial Tumours

On the basis of experimental results, it is possible to speculate on the histogenesis of those odontogenic tumours that may arise from surface epithelium. Some ameloblastomas may arise in this way and it is also possible that other usually intraosseous tumours may on occasion do so. An appreciable proportion of the reported cases of calcifying odontogenic cyst have been extraosseous lesions situated in the gingiva. Some calcifying epithelial odontogenic tumours have also been extraosseous and a small number of adenomatoid odontogenic tumours have been similarly situated. Naturally, the submucosal situ-ation alone of these tumours is not sufficient evidence to indicate origin from the overlying epithelium and indeed, except in the case of ameloblastoma, there is no objective

evidence that such might be the case. A small number of ameloblastomas have, however, appeared to arise from this epithelium; although the evidence in these cases may not be conclusive, at least the possibility is reasonable. If these extraosseous tumours do not develop from the surface epithelium, then they must do so from more deeply situated epithelium, in effect, the remnants of the dental formative epithelium.

The concept that odontogenic tumours should develop from epithelial rests is entirely logical, but when tumours arising from the surface epithelium are considered the question arises as to why some should appear as ordinary tumours of squamous epithelium, such as papillomas or squamous cell carcinomas, while others are of odontogenic type. As already noted, it seems likely that the carcinogenic stimuli leading to the development of embryonic tumours are different from those that produce post-embryonic neoplasms. It may be that a stimulus from the external environment leads to proliferation along the paths leading to squamous cell carcinoma, whereas a stimulus to the epithelium from the dermis leads to proliferation along the odontogenic pathway. Experimentally, it has been shown that in grafts of mouse enamel organ and dermis from the plantar surface of the foot, the epithelium forms strands that permeate the connective tissue in a manner and pattern thought reminiscent of ameloblastoma (Kollar, 1972). It has been suggested from such experiments that neoplasia need not imply a defect in the epithelium itself, but that some alteration in the stroma might elicit neo-plastic responses in epithelium. The role of the mesen-chyme seems not to be simply nutritive, but also inductive.

The odontogenic tumours that consist principally of epithelium are ameloblastoma, adenomatoid odontogenic tumour, calcifying epithelial odontogenic tumour and calcifying odontogenic cyst. Although ameloblastoma is usually regarded as a purely epithelial growth, there is now some evidence at the ultra-structural level (fig. 4) of inductive changes (Mincer and McGinnis, 1972). The adenomatoid odontogenic tumour is also in most cases purely epithelial, apart from the amorphous calcified deposits that are not infrequently present. However, dentine has been noted in some tumours.

In ameloblastoma, a marked resemblance to phases of dental development can occur and histochemical and ultrastructural studies have confirmed the similarity of the tumour cells to those of normal dental lamina and enamel organ. An appreciable number of tumours arises in connection with unerupted teeth and in such cases the point of origin can hardly be in doubt, since tumour epithelium is found lining the dental follicle in place of normal follicular epithelium. Cases of this type have been widely reported in the literature, frequently with the conclusion, explicit or implicit, that the tumour has developed in what was previously a non-neoplastic denti-gerous cyst. It should be noted, however, that the number of cases in which such a change has been convincingly demonstrated is small. In the majority, it is much more likely that the error in development that led to the develop-ment of the tumour took place when tooth development was nearly complete, at which stage the changes that lead

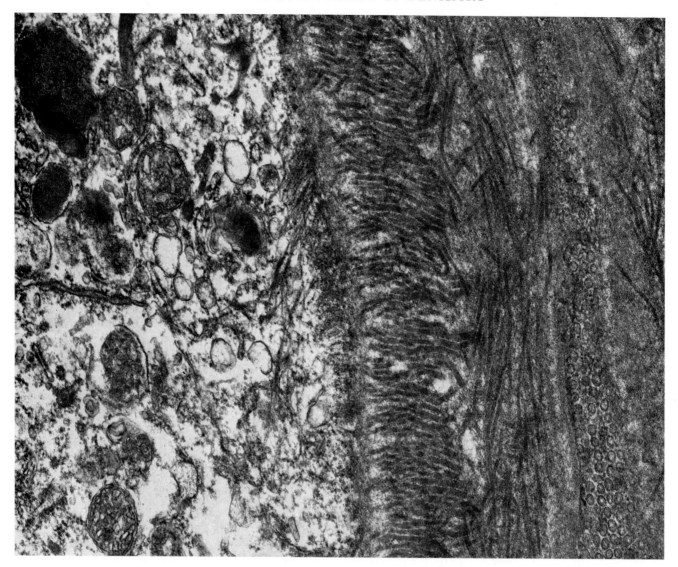

FIG. 4. Ameloblastoma. Light microscopy showed zones of juxtaepithelial hyalinization in this tumour; this electron-micrograph is from such a zone and shows a band of collagen corresponding to it. From Mincer and McGinnis (1972).

to dentigerous cyst formation also occur. It may well be that disturbance of development at this stage can proceed in different directions—to tumour formation or to non-neoplastic cyst formation.

Other ameloblastomas appear to develop independently of the teeth, or perhaps they may appear in place of missing teeth. It is generally considered that such tumours arise from remnants of odontogenic epithelium, and the similarities between dental formative epithelium and ameloblastoma have already been mentioned. Another possible point of origin for ameloblastoma is the basal layer of the mucous membrane. The arguments for and against these various possibilities are fully covered in standard textbooks and in the literature and need not be pursued further here. The point of importance for the purposes of the present discussion is that the ameloblastoma is an embryonic tumour arising as the result of a disturbance in the course of odontogenesis. The nature of

this disturbance is not yet known, but it seems to operate wholly or almost wholly, as a stimulus to growth. The epithelium, now endowed with the properties of progressive and invasive growth, does not have the capability of inducing mesenchymal change.

Like ameloblastoma, the adenomatoid odontogenic tumour appears usually to be a wholly epithelial growth, although on occasion dentine may be present. Again, like the ameloblastoma, the tumour often occurs in association with unerupted teeth and often the clinical diagnosis is dentigerous cyst. Thus the abnormality in odontogenesis appears to become manifest at more or less the same stage as occurs in ameloblastoma, although obviously the results are different, both in terms of histological structure of the abnormal growth that results, and in behaviour. With regard to structure, both morphologically and histochemically, the similarity of the cells lining the tubular structures in the adenomatoid odontogenic tumour to the preameloblastic stage in normal odontogenesis has been noted by a number of workers. The difference in behaviour between ameloblastoma and the adenomatoid odontogenic tumour has already been noted.

The calcifying odontogenic cyst is also an essentially epithelial lesion, in which the cells most closely resemble those of the reduced enamel epithelium. Although in its typical form it is purely epithelial, in some cases immature dentine may be deposited in proximity to the epithelium. In an analysis of the 52 cases that have been published to date, Fejerskov and Krogh (1972) found 7 cases where the lesion was associated with an odontoma; they propose the term, calcifying ghost cell odontogenic tumour. Praetorius (1973) distinguishes between four different odontogenic tumours which may be associated with a calcifying odontogenic cyst:

(a) an ameloblastoma-like tumour with formation of dentinoid;

(b) odontoameloblastoma;

(c) ameloblastic fibro-odontoma; and

(d) complex odontoma.

The characteristic ghost cells of the lesion are of particular interest. They are anuclear, or if nuclei are present, these are pyknotic. The only organelles found in an electron microscopical study were thick electron-dense fibrils of uniform size, sharply defined against large empty spaces. Small needle-like crystalloid structures were seen in most cells, indicating early dystrophic calcification. So far, no agreement has been reached as to the nature of the ghost cells.

Apart from the element of inductive change, the four lesions just dealt with all appear to result from some error in odontogenesis that causes epithelial proliferation. This proliferation produces structures that resemble aspects of the normal epithelial component of odontogenic tissues. The precise appearances produced—in other words, the particular type of neoplasm—may depend on either the site of origin or the time of origin, but as yet there is little factual knowledge in this respect.

Tumours with Both Epithelial and Mesenchymal Elements

Odontogenic tumours that consist of both epithelium and mesenchymal elements may or may not show inductive changes. Ameloblastic fibroma, for example, generally does not show such changes, but they are prominent in ameloblastic fibro-odontoma and odontoameloblastoma, and the complex and compound odontomes are familiar end results of inductive activity. It is in this range of tumours, if they may be placed in a range for purposes of discussion, that many debatable lesions are found, since there are all degrees of epithelial-mesenchymal interaction to be observed within this series. Thus, in the usual types of ameloblastic fibroma, there is no evidence of inductive change or at the most there is some hyalinization of the mesenchyme around the epithelial follicles or strands. Rarely, however, hyalinization may be pronounced (fig. 5)

and the epithelium itself may show changes where it is in contact with the hyaline tissue.

In the **ameloblastic fibro-odontoma** the general appearances are those of ameloblastic fibroma but in addition, dentine and enamel are present. The question therefore arises as to whether this lesion might not represent a stage in the development of a complex odontome. That is to say, might it be envisaged that the earliest lesion is the ameloblastic fibroma, that this lesion may go on to the formation of dentine and enamel (ameloblastic fibro-odontoma) with final maturation and more or less disappearance of the epithelium (complex odontome)? The possibility of such a mode of progression was suggested many years ago, but subsequent experience has not added support to this view.

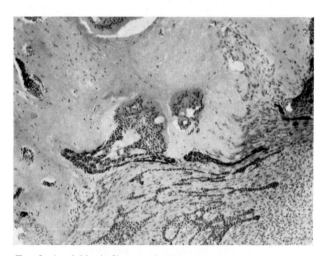

Fig. 5. Ameloblastic fibroma, showing appearance of hyalinization of the mesenchymal component. × 70.

Thus, a recent analysis of the cases of ameloblastic fibroma and ameloblastic fibro-odontoma reported in the literature showed that these tumours occurred in the same general age group (Eversole *et al.*, 1971). Were progression the general course for these lesions, complex odontomes would occur at a distinctly later age than the other lesions. The same analysis also showed that complex odontomes occurred twice as often in females as in males, whereas the other tumours occurred two or three times more frequently in males. Clearly, the sex ratios would have to be equal were progression to represent the usual course of events. While the available evidence thus suggests that the various odontogenic tumours are indeed separate entities and not merely stages in progression or differentiation, it is still possible that some examples may be transitional forms. This possibility can pose diagnostic problems for the pathologist.

Other lesions in the general group of epithelial and mesenchymal tumours are dentinoma and odontoameloblastoma. **Dentinoma** is rare and its status is somewhat equivocal. Some lesions described as dentinoma resemble ameloblastic fibroma in which there is also present an irregular or poorly formed type of dentine, but in which no enamel is seen. In other lesions no epithelium is present; this is assumed to have atrophied and disappeared after fulfilling its formative role, as occurs in normal odontogenesis.

Odonto-ameloblastoma is a rare tumour in which there is an epithelial component resembling ameloblastoma (rather than the epithelium of ameloblastic fibroma) and enamel and dentine are also present.

It is evident from the foregoing remarks that the epithelial-mesenchymal tumours can show a varied range of appearances, and indeed they provide some of the most interesting problems in odontogenesis and oncogenesis. Recent investigations of normal development have indicated the presence of an electron-dense membrane between the preameloblasts and the adjacent mesenchyme just before differentiation of the latter, and when odontoblasts appear desmosomes can be demonstrated between them and the preameloblasts. There is evidence to indicate that if this membrane is unusually thick mesenchymal differentiation may be retarded, and also that the membrane may have to break down for normal differentiation to proceed. It may well be that in tumour formation there are abnormalities in the mechanisms of interaction between epithelium and mesenchyme, just as the epithelium and the mesenchyme themselves are abnormal in their neoplastic growth characteristics. Investigation of the interface between the two tissues seems a promising field from which to learn something of the reasons why induction does not occur in some tumours whereas it does in others.

APPENDIX

W.H.O. Classification of Tumours Related to the Odontogenic Apparatus

A. Benign

1. Ameloblastoma
2. Calcifying epithelial odontogenic tumour
3. Ameloblastic fibroma
4. Adenomatoid odontogenic tumour (adeno-ameloblastoma)
5. Calcifying odontogenic cyst
6. Dentinoma
7. Ameloblastic fibro-odontoma
8. Odonto-ameloblastoma
9. Complex odontoma
10. Compound odontoma
11. Fibroma (odontogenic fibroma)
12. Myxoma (myxofibroma)
13. Cementomas
    (a) Benign cementoblastoma (true cementoma)
    (b) Cementifying fibroma
    (c) Periapical cemental dysplasia (periapical fibrous dysplasia)
    (d) Gigantiform cementoma (familial multiple cementomas)
14. Melanotic neuro-ectodermal tumour of infancy (melanotic progonoma, melano-ameloblastoma)

B. Malignant

1. Odontogenic carcinomas
    (a) Malignant ameloblastoma
    (b) Primary intra-osseous carcinoma
    (c) Other carcinomas arising from odontogenic epithelium, including those arising from odontogenic cysts
2. Odontogenic sarcomas
    (a) Ameloblastic fibrosarcoma (ameloblastic sarcoma)
    (b) Ameloblastic odontosarcoma

REFERENCES

Fejerskov, O. and Krogh, J. (1972), "The Calcifying Ghost Cell Odontogenic Tumor—or the Calcifying Odontogenic Cyst," *J. Oral Path.*, **1**, 273.

Giansanti, J. S., Someren, A. and Waldron, C. S. (1970), "Odontogenic Adenomatoid Tumor (Adenoameloblastoma). Survey of 111 Cases," *Oral Surg.*, **30**, 69.

Harrison, J. D. and Eggleston, D. J. (1973), "Odontogenic Myxoma of the Maxilla; A Case Report and Some Interesting Histological Findings," *Brit. J. Oral Surg.*, **11**, 43.

Ikemura, K., Tashiro, H., Fujino, H., Ohbu, D. and Nakajima, K. (1972), "Ameloblastoma of the Mandible with Metastasis to the Lungs and Lymph Nodes," *Cancer*, **29**, 930.

Kollar, E. J. (1972), "Histogenesis of Dermal-epidermal Interactions," in *Developmental Aspects of Oral Biology*, (H. C. Slavkin and L. A. Bavetta, Eds.). New York and London: Academic Press.

Krolls, S. O. and Pindborg, J. J. (1974), "Calcifying Epithelial Odontogenic Tumor. A Survey of 23 Cases and Discussion of Histomorphologic Variations," *Arch. Path.*, **98**, 206.

Leider, A. S., Nelson, J. F. and Trodahl, J. N. (1972), "Ameloblastic Fibrosarcoma of the Jaws," *Oral Surg.*, **33**, 559.

Mincer, H. H. and McGinnis, J. P. (1972), "Ultrastructure of Three Histological Variants of the Ameloblastoma," *Cancer*, **30**, 1036.

Pindborg, J. J., Kramer, I. R. H. and Torloni, H. (1971), "Histological Typing of Odontogenic Tumours, Jaw Cysts and Allied Lesions." International Classification of Tumours No. 5. World Health Organization, Geneva.

Praetorius, F. (1973), "Calcifying Odontogenic Cyst. Range, Variations and Neoplastic Potential." Paper given at the Annual Meeting 1973 of the American Academy of Oral Pathology.

Shear, M. (1969), "Primary Intra-alveolar Epidermoid Carcinoma of the Jaw," *J. Path.*, **97**, 645.

Toller, P. A. (1972), "Newer Concepts of Odontogenic Cysts," *Int. J. Oral Surg.*, **1**, 3.

Trodahl, J. N. (1972), "Ameloblastic Fibroma. A Survey of Cases from the Armed Forces Institute of Pathology," *Oral Surg.*, **33**, 547.

Willis, R. A. (1958), *The Borderland of Embryology and Pathology*. London: Butterworth and Co. (Publishers) Ltd.

Willis, R. A. (1967), *Pathology of Tumours*, 4th edition. London: Butterworth and Co. (Publishers) Ltd.

21. CYSTS

M. SHEAR

A cyst is a pathological cavity containing fluid or semi-fluid material. It is usually, but not always, lined by epithelium. Numerous classifications have been published of cysts of the jaws. Most of these are perfectly satisfactory and the reader is advised to use any classification which he finds valuable as an aid to memory and understanding. The classification used in this chapter is modified from the one recommended by the World Health Organization for the Histological Typing of Odontogenic Tumours, Jaw Cysts and Allied Lesions (Pindborg, Kramer and Torloni, 1971).

CLASSIFICATION

I. CYSTS OF THE JAWS
A. EPITHELIAL

1. *DEVELOPMENTAL*
   (a) *Odontogenic*
       (i) Primordial cyst (keratocyst)
       (ii) Gingival cyst of infants
       (iii) Gingival cyst of adults and lateral periodontal cyst
       (iv) Dentigerous (follicular) cyst
       (v) Eruption cyst

   (b) *Non-odontogenic*
       (i) Nasopalatine duct (incisive canal) cyst
       *(ii) Median palatine, median alveolar and median mandibular cysts
       *(iii) Globulomaxillary cyst
       (iv) Nasolabial (naso-alveolar) cyst

2. *INFLAMMATORY*
   Radicular cyst
3. Surgical ciliated cyst of maxilla

B. NON-EPITHELIAL
1. Solitary bone cyst (traumatic; haemorrhagic; simple bone cyst)
2. Aneurysmal bone cyst

II. CYSTS OF THE SOFT TISSUES OF THE MOUTH, FACE AND NECK
1. Anterior median lingual cyst
2. Dermoid and epidermoid cysts of the floor of mouth
3. Thyroglossal duct cyst
4. Branchial cleft (lymphoepithelial) cyst
5. Oral cysts with gastric or intestinal epithelium
6. Mucous extravasation cyst, mucous retention cyst, ranula

PRIMORDIAL CYST (ODONTOGENIC KERATOCYST)

There has been a great deal of interest in these cysts since the realization that they may grow to a large size before they become clinically apparent and that, unlike other jaw cysts, they have a particular tendency to recur following surgical treatment.

The term, odontogenic keratocyst, was introduced originally to describe any jaw cyst in which keratin was formed to a large extent and some dentigerous, radicular and residual cysts were therefore included under this heading. Although other cyst linings may occasionally become keratinized by metaplasia, these linings are distinctly different from the characteristic lining epithelium of the primordial cyst. While primordial cyst linings do keratinize, they have other features which

---

* These cysts, previously regarded as developmental non-odontogenic cysts, are of debatable origin.

---

distinguish them and it is these which are probably responsible for their biological behaviour rather than the presence of keratin. A number of studies such as that by Browne (1969) have shown moreover that the primordial cyst occurs at a significantly earlier age than, and has a significantly different site distribution from dentigerous and radicular cysts. This suggests that it is not a dentigerous or radicular cyst in which keratinization has occurred. This cyst therefore should be regarded as a distinct entity of developmental origin and the term "primordial cyst" is preferable to the non-specific histological term "keratocyst."

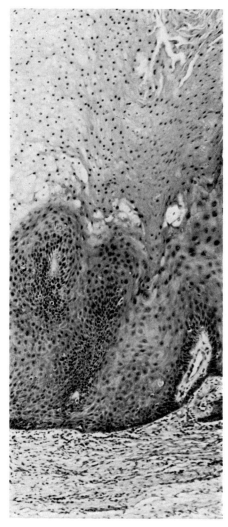

Fig. 1. Parakeratinized stratified squamous epithelium lining a radicular cyst. H. and E. × 100.

Clinical Features

Primordial cysts represent approximately 11 per cent of all jaw cysts. They occur over a wide age range and cases have been recorded as early as the first and as late as the ninth decade. There is a pronounced peak incidence in the second and third decades. They are generally found more frequently in males than in females. About 75–80 per cent of primordial cysts involve the mandible and most of these occur in the angle, extending for varying distances into the ascending ramus and forward into the body.

Patients with primordial cysts may complain of pain, swelling, or discharge but many are remarkably free of symptoms until the cysts have reached a large size or are discovered fortuitously during dental examination when radiographs are taken. Only about 60 per cent of cases produce expansion of bone. Some 10 per cent of patients with primordial cysts develop more than one.

A particular feature of primordial cysts is their tendency to recur after surgical treatment. The recurrence rates in different reported series have varied from 11 to 62 per cent. Probable reasons for this are the presence of satellite cysts and the fact that their thin fragile linings are difficult to enucleate and may be retained during some surgical procedures.

There is not much information about the rate of growth of primordial cysts, but although their rate of enlargement may not be greater than that of other jaw cysts, it seems clear that their growth is more unremitting and there is evidence that their epithelial linings exhibit greater mitotic activity than the epithelial linings of other jaw cysts (Main, 1970). It has also been shown (Toller, 1970b) that primordial cyst fluids have a significantly higher osmolality than corresponding serum, and this may also play a part in the expansive growth in size of the primordial as well as other jaw cysts.

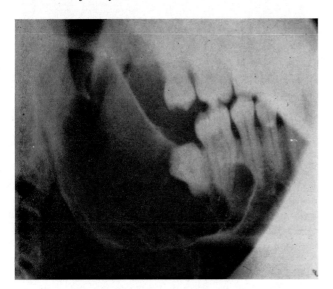

Fig. 2. Radiograph of extensive primordial cyst with scalloped margins.

Radiological Features

Most primordial cysts are well demarcated, with a distinct sclerotic margin. The majority are unilocular radiolucencies and most of these have a smooth periphery. Almost all the maxillary lesions are of this variety and tend to be small as they make their clinical appearance earlier than the mandibular lesions. Some of the unilocular lesions have scalloped margins and these may be interpreted as multilocular (fig. 2). True multilocular lesions are not uncommon, particularly in the mandible, and this variety is particularly liable to be misdiagnosed as ameloblastoma. Primordial cysts may impede the eruption of related teeth and this results in a "dentigerous" appearance radiologically. These lesions are frequently incorrectly diagnosed as dentigerous cysts and this has given rise to two misconceptions. One is that many dentigerous cysts have keratinized epithelial linings similar to those found in primordial cysts; and secondly that dentigerous cysts may have an extra-follicular origin.

Pathogenesis

Evidence derived mainly from the histological examination of primordial cysts from patients with the basal cell carcinoma syndrome, suggests that the cysts may arise directly from the dental lamina. Satellite microcysts in the walls of the main cysts are often seen apparently arising directly from the remnants of the dental lamina (fig. 3). The stimulus for this phenomenon is not known, but as the basal cell carcinoma syndrome is transmitted genetically as an autosomal dominant, and the occurrence of multiple primordial cysts in patients with the syndrome is a common finding, it is possible that there is a predisposition in some individuals to form primordial cysts and it may be for this reason that they are so frequently multiple. However, no one has yet shown a familial tendency to develop primordial cysts in the absence of other features of the syndrome and although the possibility that their occurrence may be genetically determined cannot be excluded, it must be regarded at present as speculative.

Histopathology

Unless the cyst is very small, the linings of primordial cysts are rarely received intact in the laboratory. They are invariably thin-walled, collapsed and folded.

The histological features are characteristic and are illustrated in fig. 4. There is a regular cyst lining of keratinized stratified squamous epithelium which is usually about five to eight cell layers thick and without rete ridges. The form of keratinization is predominantly parakeratotic but is sometimes also orthokeratotic and both varieties may be found in different parts of the same cyst. There is a well-defined basal layer consisting usually of columnar and occasionally cuboidal cells. The nuclei frequently tend to be orientated away from the basement membrane and in the majority of cases are intensely basophilic. Desquamated keratin is present in many of the cyst cavities. Mitotic figures are found in the basal layer but more frequently in the suprabasal layers. Features of epithelial atypia are seen occasionally and some workers, while stressing that malignant transformation in jaw cysts is extremely rare, make the point that keratinizing cysts appear to have a greater tendency to such change than others. The fibrous wall of the primordial cyst is usually thin with relatively few cells widely separated by a stroma that is often rich in mucopolysaccharide and resembles embryonic mesenchyme. Inflammatory cells are infrequent but there may be a mild infiltration of lymphocytes and monocytes. If the cyst wall is heavily inflamed, the adjacent epithelium may lose its keratinized surface, thicken, and develop rete processes.

Estimation of the soluble protein level in aspirated cyst fluid may be a valuable aid in the pre-operative diagnosis of primordial cysts. Toller (1970a) believes that a protein level of less than 4·0 g./100 ml. indicates a diagnosis of primordial cyst whereas a value of over 5·0 g./100 ml. will suggest a radicular, dentigerous or fissural cyst, or even an ameloblastoma.

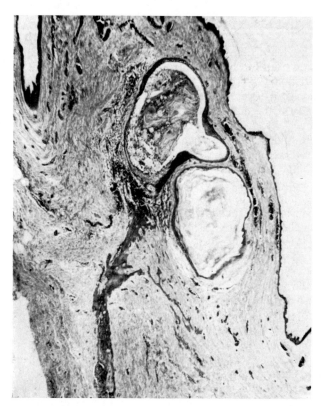

FIG. 3. Satellite microcysts in the wall of a primordial cyst, apparently arising directly from the dental lamina. H. and E. × 80. (Previously published in the *British Dental Journal*, **123**, 321, 1967, and reproduced with kind permission of the Editor.)

It has also been shown that a pre-operative diagnosis of primordial cyst might be made by aspirating cyst fluid and demonstrating keratinized squames in a stained film.

Treatment

In view of the now well-known tendency for the primordial cyst to recur, its treatment has given rise to much discussion amongst oral surgeons. Bramley (1971) has suggested an approach depending on which of the three radiological types is dealt with. Provided that there is adequate access, the unilocular type should be enucleated by an intra-oral approach. If access is difficult a two-stage treatment should be carried out, the first stage being decompression and the second complete enucleation of the reduced area. Great care must be taken during enucleation to ensure that all fragments of the extremely thin lining are removed. The unilocular lesion with scalloped margins is excised in a block of mandible if the lesion is not too large,

leaving continuity of the jaw. If too large for this procedure, careful enucleation is done by whichever route gives best access, followed by a careful watch for recurrence. Any recurrence will be small if detected early and can then be excised with the surrounding bone. Neither enucleation

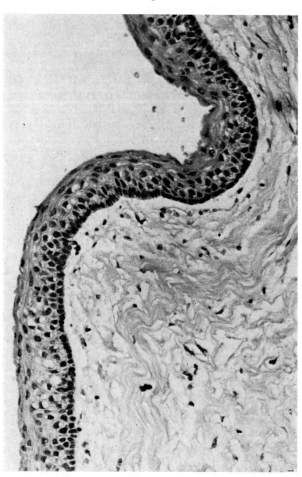

FIG. 4. Characteristic histological features of a primordial cyst. H. and E. × 200.

nor the two-stage procedure is suitable for multilocular lesions. If the lesion is small then block excision leaving continuity of the mandible is indicated; if large, the lesion must be excised and immediate bone grafts placed.

GINGIVAL CYST OF INFANTS

The incidence of gingival cysts is high in new-born infants but they are extremely rare over three months of age. They occur as white or cream-coloured nodules along the alveolar ridges (fig. 5) and may be single or multiple. They arise from epithelial remnants of the dental lamina which has the capacity, at an early stage in development, to proliferate, keratinize, and to form small cysts. This capacity to proliferate is of limited potential, unlike that of the dental lamina in the formation and growth of primordial cysts. Very few become clinical problems. Some probably open on the surface, leaving clefts; others may be involved by developing teeth and some degenerate and disappear, the keratin and debris being digested by giant cells.

Histologically, they have a thin lining of stratified squamous epithelium with a keratotic surface. The basal cells are flat, unlike those in the primordial cyst.

The mid-palatal raphe cysts of infants have a similar clinical and histological appearance but they arise from epithelial inclusions at the line of fusion of the palatal folds and the nasal processes.

many lateral periodontal cysts are discovered on routine radiological examination in the absence of any clinical symptoms and signs. These seem likely to have arisen within the alveolar bone and eroded outwards. One must conclude therefore that the gingival cyst of adults and the lateral periodontal cyst are distinct entities which have different pathogeneses.

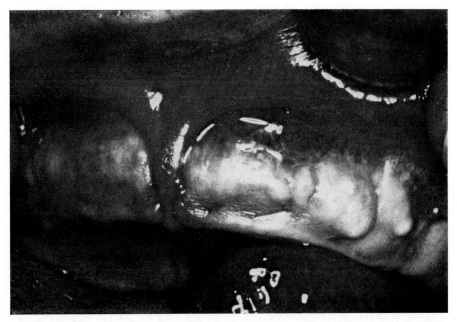

FIG. 5. Gingival cysts in an infant. (Reproduced from the *British Dental Journal*, **132**, 457, 1972, Fig. 1, with kind permission of the author, Mr. I. D. F. Saunders, and the Editor.)

There is no indication for any treatment of gingival or mid-palatal raphe cysts in infants.

GINGIVAL CYST OF ADULTS AND THE LATERAL PERIODONTAL CYST

There is a great deal of confusion about the relationship between the gingival cyst of adults and the lateral periodontal cyst. Some workers believe that they should be grouped together as gingival cysts. They consider that both arise from extraosseous odontogenic epithelium and that when radiolucencies are present they are the result of cup-shaped depressions on the periosteal surfaces of the cortical plates produced by enlargement of the gingival cysts.

Only those lesions which do not communicate with the tooth should, however, be classified as gingival cysts. Where there is resorption of adjacent alveolar bone with direct communication with the tooth, the lesions should be termed lateral periodontal cysts, since it is impossible to determine from where they arose. Gingival cysts do occur without bone involvement or may produce a cup-shaped depression on the periosteal surface. There may be a gingival swelling but they usually go unnoticed and most of the reported examples have been detected in the course of histological examination of gingival biopsies. It is difficult to imagine that cysts originating in the gingival soft tissues could enlarge sufficiently to produce a radiologically-evident bone erosion without any gingival swelling. Yet

Clinical Features

When a gingival cyst is present in an adult, there may be a history of a slowly enlarging swelling which may or may not be painful. They are well circumscribed, up to 1 cm. diameter. The lesions are soft and fluctuant and the adjacent teeth are usually vital.

Radiographs of lateral periodontal cysts show a well-defined round or ovoid radiolucent area with a sclerotic margin somewhere between the apex and the cervical margin of the tooth.

Pathogenesis

The most likely origin of the gingival cyst in adults is from odontogenic epithelial cell rests which are frequently discernible in histological sections of adult human gingivae. The stimulus for proliferation of these rests is unknown. There is no evidence of an inflammatory stimulus and proliferation with subsequent cyst formation probably occurs spontaneously.

As the lateral periodontal cyst is lined by narrow non-keratinized epithelium which resembles reduced enamel epithelium, the proposal that it arises initially as a dentigerous cyst developing by expansion of the follicle along the lateral surface of the crown, is an attractive one. If tooth eruption is normal, the expanded follicle may finally come to lie on the lateral aspect of the root (fig. 6).

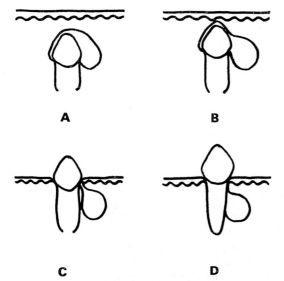

Fig. 6. Diagram illustrating the possible pathogenesis of a lateral periodontal cyst. At A there is expansion of the follicle on the lateral surface of the crown of an unerupted tooth. At this stage a radiograph would show a lateral dentigerous cyst. At B-D the tooth erupts leaving the expanded follicle behind.

Histopathology

Gingival cysts in the adult have a variable histological pattern. They are usually small. Some have an extremely thin lining of one or two layers of flat cells with pyknotic nuclei. In others, the epithelial lining may be of a rather thicker stratified squamous nature. A parakeratinized layer may be found on the surface of the epithelium and there may be desquamated cells in the cyst cavity.

The classical lateral periodontal cyst, as distinct from the primordial cyst in a lateral periodontal position, is lined by a thin, non-keratinizing layer of squamous or cuboidal epithelium, usually ranging from one to five layers thick, which resembles reduced enamel epithelium.

Treatment

When it is a clinical problem, the gingival cyst can be removed sugically. The lateral periodontal cyst can also be removed by enucleation. There is no tendency for recurrence.

DENTIGEROUS CYST

A dentigerous cyst is one which encloses the crown of an unerupted tooth and is attached to the neck. It is important that this definition is applied strictly and that the diagnosis of dentigerous cyst is not made on radiographic evidence alone, otherwise primordial cysts of the envelopmental variety and unilocular ameloblastomas involving unerupted teeth are liable to be misdiagnosed as dentigerous cysts.

Clinical Features

Dentigerous cysts represent about 14 per cent of all jaw cysts. The majority occur during the second, third and fourth decades. About 60 per cent of cases occur in males and data from the author's material suggest that they are more common among caucasoids than among negroids. A substantial majority of dentigerous cysts involve the mandibular third molar. The maxillary permanent canine

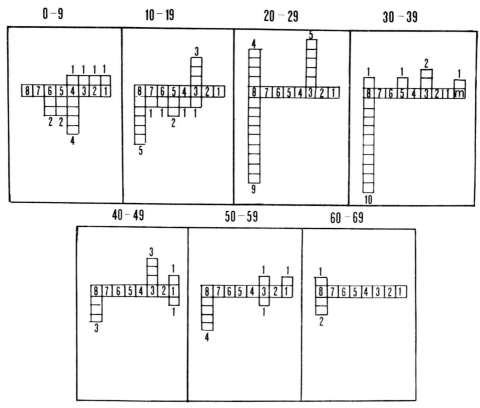

Fig. 7. Diagram illustrating which teeth are involved by dentigerous cysts in different decades.

is next in order of frequency of involvement, followed by the maxillary third molar and the mandibular premolars (fig. 7).

Like primordial cysts, dentigerous cysts may grow to a large size before they are diagnosed. Most of them are discovered on radiographs when these are taken because a tooth has failed to erupt, or a tooth is out of alignment. Many patients first become aware of the cysts because of slowly enlarging swellings and this is the common mode of occurrence in edentulous patients in whose jaws unerupted teeth have inadvertently been retained.

Radiological Features

Radiographs show unilocular radiolucent areas associated with the crowns of unerupted teeth. The cysts have well-defined sclerotic margins unless they become infected. The most common relationship of the cyst to the unerupted crown is central or coronal, where the crown is enveloped symmetrically. Expansion of the follicle may however also produce either a lateral or circumferential relationship between the cyst and the involved tooth.

Pathogenesis

The risk of a dentigerous cyst forming in relation to an unerupted tooth has been calculated at only about 1 per cent. It is clear therefore that there must be a factor or factors as yet unidentified, other than the mere failure to erupt, which is responsible for the formation of the cyst. The histological features of dentigerous cysts provide evidence that they arise by accumulation of fluid between the reduced enamel epithelium and the enamel. It has been suggested that the pressure exerted by a potentially erupting tooth on an impacted follicle obstructs the venous outflow and thereby induces rapid transudation of serum across the capillary walls. The increased hydrostatic pressure of this pooling fluid separates the follicle from the crown, with or without reduced enamel epithelium. In the presence of an inflammatory process in part of the cyst wall, exudation will play some part in its expansion. Furthermore, the passage of desquamated epithelial cells and inflammatory cells into the cyst cavity will probably contribute to the increase in intracystic osmotic tension and thereby probably to further expansion of the cyst.

Histopathology

Pathologists should do a careful dissection of the gross specimen to determine that the cyst surrounding the crown is indeed a dilated follicle and that it attaches at the amelocemental junction. Histological examination usually shows a thin fibrous cyst wall lined by epithelium which is in fact reduced enamel epithelium and consists of two to five layers of flat or low cuboidal cells (fig. 8). Characteristically, the epithelial lining is not keratinized and most that have been described as keratinized have usually been primordial. Rarely, a true dentigerous cyst lining may form keratin. Sometimes, the superficial layer of the epithelial lining is low columnar and retains some of the morphology of the ameloblast layer which, of course, it

originally was. In some cysts part of the epithelial lining may contain metaplastic mucus-secreting cells or ciliated cells. Occasional bud-like thickenings of the epithelium may be seen in the absence of inflammation and sometimes there may be budding of the basal cells into the fibrous capsule.

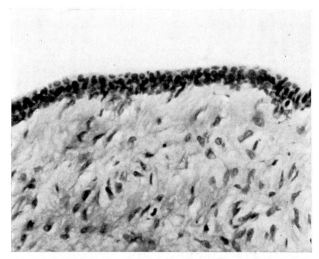

FIG. 8. Histological features of a dentigerous cyst. H. and E. × 220.

The Dentigerous Cyst as a Potential Ameloblastoma

A number of workers have claimed that many ameloblastomata arise in dentigerous cysts, but the author has seen no evidence to support such a contention. Indeed, the fact that dentigerous cysts are rare in South African negroids compared with caucasoids, whereas ameloblastoma is five times more common in negroids, provides contrary evidence. While an ameloblastoma, being of odontogenic epithelial origin, may of course theoretically arise from dentigerous cyst lining as well as from any other odontogenic epithelium, the belief that it commonly arises in this situation and that the dentigerous cyst should therefore be regarded as pre-ameloblastomatous, should be viewed with caution. A possible reason for this confusion is that an ameloblastoma, like a primordial cyst, may involve an unerupted tooth, particularly a third molar at the angle of the mandible, and this may be incorrectly interpreted as a dentigerous cyst on radiographs. When subsequently the lesion is removed and diagnosed histologically as an ameloblastoma, the erroneous conclusion may be reached that the ameloblastoma developed from a dentigerous cyst.

Treatment

When the dentigerous cyst has developed around a mandibular third molar, the treatment is usually careful enucleation together with the involved tooth. In children, when the involved tooth and possibly adjacent teeth are prevented from assuming their normal position in the arch, marsupialization is recommended. This procedure usually results in the involved teeth erupting into functional occlusion as the cyst cavity fills with new bone.

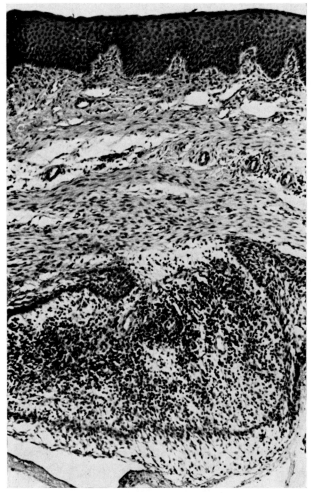

FIG. 9. Eruption cyst. The surface epithelium is at the top and the cyst epithelium at the bottom of the photomicrograph. H. and E. × 100.

ERUPTION CYST

An eruption cyst is in fact a dentigerous cyst occurring in the soft tissues. Whereas the dentigerous cyst develops around the crown of an unerupted tooth lying in bone, the eruption cyst occurs when a tooth is impeded in its eruption only by soft tissues.

Clinical Features

Eruption cysts are not commonly seen in pathology departments but it is possible that they occur more frequently clinically and that as some open spontaneously they are not excised and are therefore not submitted for histological examination.

The eruption cyst produces a smooth swelling over the erupting tooth. The swelling may be either the colour of normal gingiva or blue. It is soft and fluctuant.

Histopathology

As most eruption cysts are treated by marsupialization the pathologist usually receives only part of the cyst wall. The superficial aspect is covered by gingival epithelium.

This is separated from the cyst by a strip of dense connective tissue of varying thickness that usually shows a chronic inflammatory cell infiltrate, mild superficially, but more intense closer to the epithelial lining of the cyst. In non-inflamed areas the epithelial lining of the cyst is characteristically of reduced enamel epithelial origin consisting in the main of two to five cell layers of squamous or low cuboidal epithelium. Invariably, the epithelial lining is intensely inflamed and the cells are separated by fluid (fig. 9).

Treatment

As previously mentioned eruption cysts are usually treated by marsupialization. The dome of the cyst is excised exposing the crown of the tooth, which is thus allowed to erupt.

NASOPALATINE DUCT (INCISIVE CANAL) CYST

The nasopalatine duct cyst may occur within the nasopalatine canal or in the soft tissues of the palate at the opening of the canal where it is called cyst of the palatine papilla.

Clinical Features

Nasopalatine duct cysts form approximately 12 per cent of all jaw cysts. They practically never occur in the first decade, are extremely rare during the second and third decades, and most are found in the fourth, fifth and sixth decades. In the author's material, 79 per cent occurred in males.

The most common symptom is swelling, usually in the anterior region of the midline of the palate. Swelling also occurs in the midline of the labial aspect of the alveolar ridge and in some cases "through and through" fluctuation may be elicited between the labial and palatal swellings. It is when midline swellings of the palate occur further posteriorly, that diagnoses of median palatine cysts tend to be made. Other symptoms are pain and discharge although, in general, symptoms are not severe and patients often disregard them for many years. The cyst is sometimes discovered fortuitously by the dentist during routine radiological examination. In establishing the diagnosis of nasopalatine duct cyst it is important to attempt to exclude the possibility of a periapical lesion by testing the pulp vitality of the anterior teeth.

Radiological Features

The nasopalatine duct cyst occurs in the incisive canal and it may be difficult to decide whether a radiolucency in that area is a cyst or a large incisive fossa. In general, a radiograph of the fossa which shows a shadow less than 6 mm. wide, may be considered within normal limits provided the patient has no other symptoms. However, a radiolucency slightly larger than this is not an indication for immediate surgical intervention and in the absence of any symptoms the patient may be referred for further examination six months later.

Nasopalatine duct cysts occur in the midline of the palate above or between the roots of the central incisor teeth. In the latter case the incisor roots may diverge. Some cysts may appear heart-shaped either because they become notched by the nasal septum during their expansion or because the nasal spine is superimposed on the radiolucent area, or if there are bilateral cysts. Very large cysts extend posteriorly and superiorly and it is these which give rise to the diagnosis of median palatine cyst. If on a dental radiograph the radiolucent area appears to be related to the apex of an incisor tooth, an occlusal view will usually demonstrate that the cyst and the apex are separated. In addition to the demonstration of pulp vitality it may also be possible to see an intact lamina dura around the tooth apices.

Pathogenesis

Nasopalatine duct cysts are thought to arise from the nasopalatine ducts in the incisive canal but the aetiological factors associated with their formation and their pathogenesis are largely speculative. It has been suggested that trauma or bacterial infection could stimulate the nasopalatine duct remnants to proliferate. There is, however, very little evidence to support such an hypothesis. It has also been postulated that nasopalatine duct cysts, like primordial cysts, develop spontaneously. Although there is no proof for such a theory, the concept is in accord with some of the facts. Firstly there is the observation that small cystic dilatations of portions of the nasopalatine ducts are occasionally seen in fetal material. Secondly, the cysts occur very rarely in relation to the frequency of trauma in the nasopalatine area.

Fluid accumulation is likely to be responsible for their enlargement but what leads to the initial collection of fluid in the cavity is uncertain. Osmotic attraction of serum through normal capillary walls may occur and in the absence of drainage of this fluid, the hydrostatic pressure would increase. Osmotically active particles are supplied by the breakdown of cells shed into the cyst cavity. The mechanism which might initially trigger the spontaneous development of nasopalatine duct cysts, if this is indeed what happens, is yet to be identified. It seems possible that the occurrence of these cysts, as with other jaw cysts, may have some genetic determinant.

Histopathology

The epithelial linings of nasopalatine duct cysts are extremely variable. Stratified squamous, pseudostratified columnar, cuboidal, columnar, or primitive flat epithelium may be seen, individually or in combination. Mucous cells may be found in pseudostratified columnar epithelial linings, and cilia, although most frequently seen on the surface of pseudostratified columnar epithelia, may also be present in association with columnar and, rarely, with cuboidal epithelium. Although it is frequently stated that cysts lined by respiratory epithelium originate from nasopalatine duct adjacent to the nasal cavity, whereas those lined by stratified squamous epithelium develop from

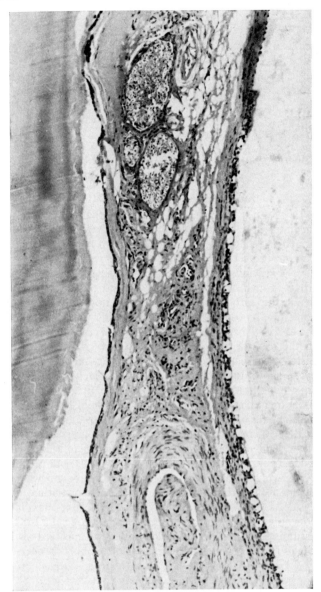

FIG. 10. Bilateral nasopalatine duct cyst. A neurovascular bundle is present in the intervening wall. H. and E. × 100.

the lower portion of the duct, this should not be regarded as a rule. For one thing, cysts of the palatine papilla may be lined by pseudostratified ciliated columnar epithelium and for another, it is rare to find a nasopalatine duct cyst lined entirely by one variety of epithelium.

A valuable diagnostic feature of nasopalatine duct cysts is the presence of nerves and muscular-walled blood vessels in the fibrous capsule (fig. 10). The explanation for this phenomenon is that the long sphenopalatine nerve and vessels which pass through the incisive canal are either included in the cyst wall or are removed with the cyst in the course of surgical enucleation.

Small foci of mucous gland elements are sometimes found in the fibrous cyst walls. It has been suggested that their presence in a cyst wall is strong evidence in favour of the diagnosis of nasopalatine duct cyst but they have been seen in an undoubted nasolabial cyst.

As far as evidence of inflammation is concerned, approximately one quarter of the author's cases were relatively free of inflammatory cell infiltrate. In about one-half there was a mild chronic inflammatory cell infiltrate and the remainder could be regarded as showing moderate to severe inflammation.

Treatment

Nasopalatine duct cysts are treated by surgical enucleation.

THE SO-CALLED MEDIAN CYSTS

In recent years, the existence of separate entities of median palatine and median alveolar cyst have been questioned and they have been excluded from the World Health Organization classification (Pindborg, Kramer and Torloni, 1971). Previously it was thought that such cysts developed from epithelium entrapped in the process of fusion of embryonic processes, whereas it is now felt that they constitute a posterior extension of an incisive canal cyst in the case of a median palatine cyst and an anterior extension in the case of a median alveolar cyst. Examination of histological sections of cases diagnosed as median palatine cysts, shows that some are lined exclusively by stratified squamous epithelium while others are lined in part by pseudostratified ciliated columnar, cuboidal, or columnar epithelium. Some contain neurovascular bundles in the wall and some contain large muscular blood vessels. Some show remnants of nasopalatine ducts in their walls. This evidence indicates that should a median posterior palatine cyst in fact exist as an entity, there can be no way of distinguishing it histologically from a nasopalatine duct cyst. As far as the median alveolar cyst of the maxilla is concerned, there appears to be no embryological basis for assuming that it develops from epithelium enclaved at the site of fusion between the right and left globular processes.

Median Mandibular Cyst

Occasionally a cyst occurs in the midline of the mandible producing a well-defined round or ovoid or irregular radiolucent area, which may separate the roots of the lower incisor teeth. In some reported cases, the associated teeth have been non-vital and in others they have all been vital. The presence of a cyst in the midline of the mandible, associated with vital teeth, has tempted some workers to postulate its origin from epithelial inclusions trapped in the area during embryonic development. This concept is however not tenable, as the mandible forms in the mandibular process which forms as a single unit. No fusion takes place between ectodermal processes and there is no possibility of epithelial entrapment.

Those cysts associated with non-vital teeth are likely to be radicular and when these are lined by ciliated pseudostratified columnar epithelium, it is probably the result of secretory metaplasia which occurs not infrequently in radicular cysts. When associated with vital teeth, these cysts may be either primordial, lateral periodontal or solitary bone cysts.

GLOBULOMAXILLARY CYST

The globulomaxillary cyst has traditionally been described as a fissural cyst found within the bone between the maxillary lateral incisor and canine teeth. Radiologically it is a well-defined radiolucency which frequently causes the roots of the adjacent teeth to diverge. While there can be no doubt that cysts occasionally occur in this region and that the pulps of adjacent teeth may give positive vitality responses, there is now a considerable body of opinion against the idea that they are fissural cysts.

It was believed for many years that they arose from non-odontogenic epithelium included at the site of fusion of the globular process of the medial (fronto-nasal) process, and the maxillary process. Embryologists have pointed out however that the surface bulges seen in the naso-maxillary complex of the embryo and which are called "facial processes", are not in fact prolongations with free ends which meet in the nasal region. Other than at the median palatal raphe there is no ectoderm to ectoderm contact which requires dissolution of the ectodermal surfaces prior to fusion, and there is therefore no possibility of enclavement of ectodermal residues. The facial processes are in fact merely elevations or ridges which correspond to centres of growth in the underlying mesenchyme. These are covered by a continuous sheet of folded epithelium. As these growth centres proliferate and develop, the surface furrows between them become more shallow and eventually smooth out.

Critical analysis of clinical, radiological and histological features of cysts in the "globulomaxillary" area has shown that a number of them have the features of primordial cysts and some of them fulfil the criteria for the diagnosis of lateral periodontal cyst. In others, the adjacent teeth are non-vital and the cysts are probably radicular.

The available evidence, then, would appear to indicate that the globulomaxillary cyst is not in fact a discrete entity.

NASOLABIAL (NASO-ALVEOLAR) CYST

The nasolabial cyst occurs outside the bone in the nasolabial folds just below the alae nasi. It is traditionally regarded as a jaw cyst although strictly speaking it should be classified as a soft tissue cyst.

Clinical Features

Nasolabial cysts are rare lesions. They have a wide age distribution. Most cases occur in the third to the sixth decades, with a peak in the fourth decade, and about 80 per cent are found in women (Roed-Petersen, 1969).

The most frequent symptom is swelling and often this is the only complaint. Sometimes the patients complain of pain and difficulty in nasal breathing. The cysts grow slowly, producing a swelling of the lip. They fill up the naso-labial fold and may lift the alae nasi. Intra-orally they form a bulge in the labial sulcus.

Radiological Features

There is a localized increased radiolucency of the alveolar process above the apices of the incisor teeth resulting from a depression on the labial surface of the maxilla. This may be detectable in a tangential view. The cyst may be aspirated and a radio-opaque liquid introduced after which it may be examined in tangential and postero-anterior views of the jaw or in vertex occlusal views.

Pathogenesis

The pathogenesis of the nasolabial cyst is unresolved. The traditional concept is that the nasolabial cyst is the soft tissue equivalent of the globulomaxillary cyst. However, as mentioned in the section on the globulo-maxillary cyst, this concept is not tenable on embryological grounds.

The location of nasolabial cysts is such that they could conceivably develop from remnants of the embryonic nasolacrimal rod or duct. The mature nasolacrimal duct is lined by pseudostratified columnar epithelium and this is the type of epithelium usually found lining nasolabial cysts. A developmental origin is supported by the frequent occurrence of bilateral examples.

Histopathology

Nasolabial cysts are lined by pseudostratified columnar epithelium, usually alone, but sometimes associated with stratified squamous epithelium or cuboidal epithelium. Goblet cells and ciliated cells may also be present.

Treatment

Nasolabial cysts are treated by surgical excision through an intra-oral approach.

RADICULAR CYST

A radicular cyst is one which arises from the epithelial residues in the periodontal ligament as a result of inflammation. The inflammation usually follows the death of the dental pulp and cysts arising in this way are found most commonly at the apices of the involved teeth. They may however also be found on the lateral aspects of the roots in relation to lateral accessory root canals. Less commonly, inflammatory cysts may occur towards the cervical margin of the lateral aspects of the root as a consequence of an inflammatory process in a periodontal pocket. This latter lesion is perhaps best referred to as an inflammatory periodontal cyst or an inflammatory collateral cyst to distinguish it from radicular cysts resulting from pulp death, and from the lateral periodontal cyst which is of developmental origin. Radicular cysts may remain behind in the jaws after removal of the offending tooth and are then referred to as residual cysts.

Clinical Features

Radicular and residual cysts are by far the most common cystic lesions in the jaws, comprising 58 per cent of jaw cysts in the author's material. They have a wide age distribution but few cases are seen in the first decade. Thereafter there is a fairly steep rise with a peak incidence in the third and fourth decades. Large numbers of cases are still seen in the fifth decade, after which there is a gradual decline. The low incidence in the first decade has been shown in a number of studies and indicates that although dental caries is frequently found in children during this period, radicular cysts are not commonly found associated with deciduous teeth. There is a higher incidence of radicular cysts in males than in females, a ratio of 1·7:1. The lower incidence in females may be because they are less likely than males to neglect their teeth, particularly the maxillary incisors which is the area where many radicular cysts occur. Males, moreover, are more likely to sustain trauma to maxillary anterior teeth.

They occur in all tooth-bearing areas of the jaws although about 60 per cent are found in the maxilla and 40 per cent in the mandible. There is a particularly high incidence in the maxillary anterior region (approximately 37 per cent of the total). There are a number of possible reasons for this high incidence. Maxillary incisors have in the past, perhaps more frequently than other teeth, had silicate restorations placed in them with consequent high risk to their pulps. Then there is the high incidence of palatal invaginations in the maxillary lateral incisors and the frequency with which pulp death supervenes in these teeth; and thirdly, maxillary anterior teeth are probably more prone than others to traumatic injuries which lead to pulp death.

Many radicular cysts are symptomless and are discovered when periapical radiographs are taken of teeth with non-vital pulps. Often, however, there is a slowly enlarging swelling. When the cyst has completely eroded the overlying bone fluctuation can be elicited. Pain and infection are other clinical features of some radicular cysts. A *sine qua non* for the diagnosis of a radicular cyst is the related presence of a tooth with a non-vital pulp. Occasionally a sinus may lead from the cyst cavity to the oral mucosa.

Radiological Features

It is difficult to distinguish a small radicular cyst radiologically from a periapical granuloma or a chronic abscess. Larger radiolucent lesions associated with roots of teeth, particularly if they are more than 1 cm. in diameter, are more likely to be cystic. The lesions are usually round or ovoid radiolucencies surrounded by a narrow radio-paque margin which may extend from the lamina dura of the involved tooth. A radicular cyst on the lateral margin of a root in association with an accessory root canal must be differentiated from a lateral periodontal cyst.

Pathogenesis

It is convenient to consider the pathogenesis of radicular cysts in three phases: the phase of initiation, the phase of cyst formation and the phase of enlargement. The precise mechanisms involved in all phases are controversial. It is generally agreed that the epithelial linings of these cysts are derived from the epithelial cell rests of Malassez in the periodontal ligament. There is also no doubt that these cells may proliferate and when they do so, either *in vivo* or in tissue culture experiments, there are consistent morphological and histochemical changes. Precisely how these epithelial cells are stimulated to proliferate is not clear. There is some evidence that decreased oxygen and increased carbon dioxide tension, and a local reduction in pH produced in the course of a chronic inflammation, may be critical factors.

The next phase in the pathogenesis of the radicular cyst is the process by which a cavity comes to be lined by proliferating odontogenic epithelium. Two possibilities are generally recognized and it seems likely that both are feasible and each may operate independently of the other. The first concept proposes that the epithelium proliferates and covers the bare connective tissue surface of an abscess cavity. The other suggests that a cyst cavity forms within a proliferating epithelial mass in an apical granuloma by degeneration and death of cells in the centre (fig. 11). There is histological evidence for the latter hypothesis. The proliferating epithelial masses show considerable inter-cellular oedema. These intercellular accumulations of fluid coalesce to form microcysts containing epithelial and inflammatory cells. The demonstration of high levels of acid phosphatase activity in the central cells of apical granulomas, and in the exfoliating epithelial cells of radicular cysts, suggests that these cells are undergoing autolysis. Moreover, ultrastructural examination of epithelial islands in experimentally induced granulomas shows evidence of death in the central cells. Microcysts may increase in size by coalescence with adjacent micro-cysts and, once established, the cyst increases in size by accumulation of fluid within its cavity.

The third phase in the pathogenesis of radicular cysts is also controversial but Toller's experimental work provides evidence for the hypothesis that most cysts increase in size as a result of osmosis. Lytic products of the epithelial and inflammatory cells in the cyst cavity provide the greater number of smaller molecules which raise the osmotic pressure of the cyst fluid. The absence of lymphatic drainage promotes this osmotic imbalance.

There do not appear to be data on the rate of radicular cyst growth although it has been estimated at approximately 5 mm. in diameter annually. They tend to expand progressively and, if untreated, may grow to a large size. Epithelial proliferation continues as long as there is an inflammatory stimulus, but probably plays little if any part in the growth of the cyst. When the stimulus to epithelial proliferation ceases, the epithelium is able to differentiate to a certain extent although keratinization is rare.

Histopathology

Radicular cysts are lined completely or in part by stratified squamous epithelium ranging in thickness from 1–50 cell layers. Most linings are between 6 and 20 layers thick. The epithelial linings may be proliferating and may show arcading with an intense associated inflammatory process, or may be quiescent and fairly regular. Keratinized and parakeratinized linings are rarely seen in radicular cysts. When they do occur they are different morphologically from those seen in primordial cysts (fig. 1).

Mucous and ciliated cells are frequently found in the epithelial linings and probably result from metaplasia. They are found in cysts of both the maxilla and mandible.

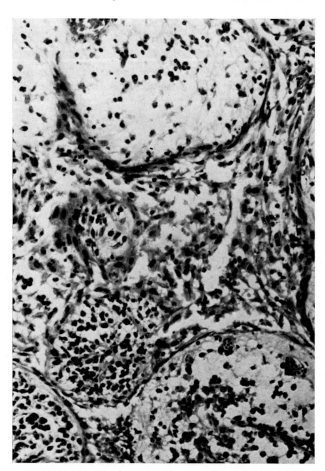

FIG. 11. Proliferating epithelium in an apical granuloma showing degeneration and death of cells in the centre with the formation of a microscopic cavity. H. and E. × 180.

In approximately 10 per cent of radicular cysts, hyaline bodies are found in the epithelial linings but only rarely in the fibrous capsule. These bodies measure up to about 0·1 mm. and are linear, straight or curved, or of hair-pin shape and sometimes they are concentrically laminated. They are brittle and frequently fracture. Circular or polycyclic bodies are also seen with a clear outer layer surrounding a central granular body. The bodies contain cystine and have other histochemical similarities to keratin although the correspondence is not complete. It has also been postulated that the hyaline bodies are derived from thrombi in venules of the connective tissue rendered varicose and strangled by epithelial cuffs which encircle them, and that they react histochemically as haematogenous. If they are haematogenous then the presence of disulphide groups in erythrocytes would account for the reactions which have been attributed to keratin. However, it is surprising that structures of haemic origin do not occur in other situations and they do not seem to have been described other than in jaw cysts. The author has not seen them in nasopalatine duct cysts.

Deposits of cholesterol crystals are found in many radicular cysts but by no means in all. The cholesterol crystals are first deposited in the fibrous cyst walls where they evoke a foreign body giant cell reaction. As a result a mass of granulation tissue containing the cholesterol fungates into the cyst cavity and appears macroscopically and microscopically as a "mural nodule" producing ulceration as it enlarges. Once the entire mass has passed into the cavity the epithelial breach presumably heals and the cholesterol crystals lie free in the cyst fluid.

Carcinomatous Change

A number of well-documented cases have been reported which indicate that squamous carcinoma may arise from the epithelial lining of radicular and other odontogenic cysts. Other reported cases are however dubious in that the possibility of secondary cystic change in a carcinoma cannot be excluded. Nevertheless, in relation to the large numbers of cysts which do occur, the incidence of neoplastic change is exceptionally rare. There is no evidence whatsoever that radicular cyst epithelium is at particular risk and there is therefore no justification for regarding these cysts as precancerous.

Treatment

There are two forms of surgical treatment for radicular cysts: enucleation and marsupialization. The non-vital tooth responsible for the cyst should be extracted or root-filled with an apicectomy.

SURGICAL CILIATED CYST OF THE MAXILLA

These cysts may develop in patients whose maxillary sinuses have been opened surgically during a Caldwell-Luc operation. They do not seem to be common, possibly because they are not diagnosed. The cysts are probably derived from the epithelial lining of the maxillary sinus which is trapped in the wound during closure of the Caldwell-Luc incision, and subsequently begins to proliferate. Patients usually complain of a poorly localized pain or discomfort in the maxilla. Radiographs reveal a well-defined radiolucent area closely related to the maxillary sinus. Histologically, they are lined by pseudostratified ciliated columnar epithelium with squamous metaplasia in inflamed areas.

SOLITARY BONE CYST (TRAUMATIC; HAEMORRHAGIC; SIMPLE BONE CYST)

The solitary bone cyst of the jaw is probably the same lesion as the solitary or unicameral bone cyst which is most frequently located in the metaphyses at the upper end of the humerus and the femur in children and adolescents.

Clinical Features

The solitary bone cyst occurs in young individuals. There is a prominent peak incidence in the second decade and it is rare to find a case in a patient more than 40 years old. There is no definite sex predilection. Solitary bone cysts occur almost exclusively in the mandible and approximately one-quarter of these are located in the anterior part (Howe, 1965).

Most cases are diagnosed fortuitously and almost all are chance radiographic findings. About a quarter of the patients, however, complain of swelling. Pain is an unusual feature. In many instances there is a history of significant trauma to the area and the time lag between injury and diagnosis varies from 1 month to 20 years.

Radiological Features

There is a radiolucent area with an irregular but definite edge and slight cortication (fig. 12). The majority of cases show some degree of marginal condensation but neither as

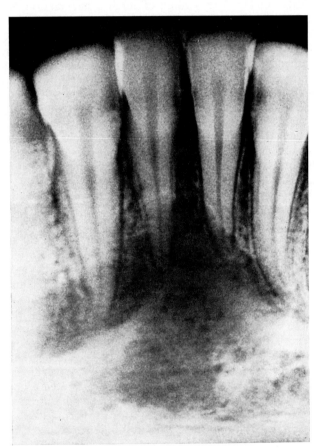

FIG. 12. Radiograph of a solitary bone cyst in the symphyseal region of the mandible.

sharp nor as opaque as in radicular cysts. In about three-quarters of cases, usually in the posterior mandible, the cyst envelops the roots of erupted teeth. Scalloping is a prominent feature and occurs both between teeth and away from teeth.

Pathogenesis

The pathogenesis of the solitary bone cyst is not known but there are a number of theories. The most favoured concept (Howe, 1965) appears to be that trauma or some other stimulus leads to rupture of a thin-walled sinusoid and produces intramedullary haemorrhage. A haematoma forms, and when it breaks down the products of haemolysis produce a local rise in osmotic pressure. This in turn leads to transudation into the cyst fluid. In the presence of intact cortical bone there is increased intraosseous pressure which leads to resorption of bone by osteoclastic activity and sometimes to swelling by concurrent periosteal bone deposition. As transudation into the cyst occurs, the fluid is diluted so that intracystic pressure drops, but further bleeding may be responsible for progression of the lesion. Once no more bleeding occurs there will be gradual absorption of the serous fluid in the cavity until it is empty. The fact that they are practically never found in patients over 30 years suggests that they are self-limiting and undergo spontaneous regression. When the space is filled with blood as a result of surgical intervention, the defect heals and it has been suggested that a spontaneous haemorrhage into an empty cyst cavity may do the same.

This however, is the main problem in accepting the pathogenesis described above. Essentially it proposes that on the one hand, intrabony haemorrhages are responsible for initiating and then maintaining the process, whereas on the other hand haemorrhage into the cyst cavity in the course of treatment leads to ready repair, and spontaneous haemorrhage is postulated as the reason for resolution without treatment. While this does not invalidate the hypothesis, it does mean that further information is necessary in order to clarify the pathogenesis.

Histopathology

When the cyst cavities are opened about 30 per cent are found to be empty. In the other cases blood, serosanguinous or serous fluid may be present. In most cases, no visible lining is present and in the remainder either a thin membrane, granulation tissue, or blood clot may be found. When lining is present, it consists of a loose vascular fibrous tissue membrane of variable thickness, with no epithelial lining, although fragments of fibrin with enmeshed red cells may be seen. Haemorrhage and haemosiderin pigment are usually present, and scattered small multinucleate giant cells are often found. Some cyst walls, possibly cases of longer standing, are more densely fibrous. The adjacent bone, when included in the specimen, shows osteoclastic resorption on its inner surface.

Treatment

Surgical treatment is usually recommended because when the cavity is opened and haemorrhage encouraged, rapid obliteration of the lesion results. However, many cases of solitary bone cyst appear to heal spontaneously, so that the need for surgical intervention may well be questioned provided that an accurate diagnosis can be established on clinical and radiological grounds, and that the patient is able to attend for follow-up radiographs at yearly intervals.

ANEURYSMAL BONE CYST

The aneurysmal bone cyst is an uncommon lesion which has been found in most bones of the skeleton, although most occur in the long bones and in the spine. The term "aneurysmal bone cyst" was originally suggested to describe the characteristic "blow-out" of the bone seen in radiographs of the lesions.

Clinical Features

Most aneurysmal bone cysts of the jaws occur in children and adolescents, an age distribution similar to that for aneurysmal cysts in other bones. There does not appear to be any sex predilection. They usually occur in the mandible and most of these are in the posterior part of the body or involve the angle or ascending ramus. The result is a firm, usually painful swelling.

Radiological Features

The aneurysmal bone cyst produces a radiolucent area which expands the bone and may balloon the cortex. It is usually unilocular but some have been described as having faintly discernible septation. Some are described as multilocular or honeycomb-like.

Pathogenesis

The pathogenesis is not known but there is evidence which suggests that at least some cases develop in pre-existing lesions. Cases have been described in bones outside the jaws in which aneurysmal bone cysts have occurred in association with areas which have the appearance of fibrous dysplasia or with features of chondromyxoid fibroma. Jaw cases have been seen in association with areas indistinguishable from ossifying fibroma and giant cell granuloma.

At operation, a thin shell of bone covers the cyst. When this is removed dark venous blood wells up. The cyst contains variable amounts of friable vascular tissue which subdivides the cavity into a number of blood-filled locules. Areas of more solid tissue may also be present.

Histopathology

The lesions consist of many capillaries and blood-filled spaces of varying size, separated by delicate loose-textured fibrous tissue containing small multinucleate cells and scattered trabeculae of osteoid and woven bone. In some of the solid areas, sheets of vascular tissue containing large numbers of multinucleate giant cells resemble giant cell granuloma of the jaws. Other solid areas may have the appearance of fibrous dysplasia, ossifying fibroma, and possibly other jaw lesions, and this gives credence to the view that the aneurysmal bone cyst may constitute secondary change in a pre-existing lesion.

Treatment

The aneurysmal bone cyst is a benign condition but may recur after incomplete curettage. Where possible, excision is advisable provided that this does not interfere with function. Failing this, thorough curettage and bone grafting, repeated if necessary, should be done.

REFERENCES

Bramley, P. A. (1971), "Treatment of Cysts of the Jaws," *Proc. roy. Soc. Med.*, **64**, 547.

Browne, R. M. (1969), "The Pathogenesis of the Odontogenic Keratocyst," *Fourth Proceedings of the International Academy of Oral Pathology*, p. 28.

Howe, G. L. (1965), " 'Haemorrhagic Cysts' of the Mandible," *Brit. J. Oral Surg.*, **3**, 55.

Main, D. M. G. (1970), "Epithelial Jaw Cysts: A Clinicopathological Reappraisal," *Brit. J. Oral Surg.*, **8**, 114.

Pindborg, J. J., Kramer, I. R. H. and Torloni, H. (1971), *Histological Typing of Odontogenic Tumours, Jaw Cysts and Allied Lesions*. Geneva: World Health Organization.

Roed-Petersen, B. (1969), "Nasolabial Cysts," *Brit. J. Oral Surg.*, **7**, 84.

Toller, P. A. (1970a), "Protein Substances in Odontogenic Cyst Fluids," *Brit. dent. J.*, **128**, 317.

Toller, P. A. (1970b), "The Osmolality of Fluids from Cysts of Jaws," *Brit. dent. J.*, **129**, 275.

22. THE NATURE OF PAIN

D. J. ANDERSON

INTRODUCTION

The object of this section is to make as many generalizations as seem useful on the subject of pain and then to discuss pain from the teeth in an attempt to discover whether the generalizations are helpful towards an understanding of this particular problem. Of all the sensations experienced by man, pain is accompanied by the most widespread reactions and can sometimes be said truly to involve the whole being. The experience of pain is a subjective, private sensation which can be described only imperfectly to others. Whereas it is possible to share other sensations by, for example, looking, listening, tasting or touching, with reasonable certainty of the same experience as another person, this is not possible with pain. What is described as moderately painful by one person, may be unbearable to another or reported as uncomfortable by a third. It is necessary to rely on verbal descriptions, or observations upon a person actually in pain and to judge from the descriptions, or the reactions, the severity of the painful sensation. Even were the stimulus of the same intensity and the neurological responses identical, descriptions of sensations can be very unreliable, since they depend on the ability of the sufferer to put his feelings into words, the choice of which is influenced by intelligence, education, race, social class and previous experience of the sensation. Their inability to give verbal expression to sensation makes the management of pain a particularly difficult problem in infants and young children.

PERCEPTION OF PAIN

Aside from problems of communication there are, between the application of a stimulus and the onset of a sensation, many points at which the sensory input can be influenced with effects on the ultimate sensory experience. One of the difficulties in the study of pain is the separation of what a person judges to be painful (the pain perception threshold) from what he can tolerate without taking avoiding action and showing signs of distress. Everyone is aware from his own experience, and that of others, that a painful stimulus can be tolerable on one occasion and unbearable on another. Pain at night seems totally to involve body and mind, when there is little else to occupy the attention, yet severe injury during a game may go unnoticed. The classical example is of the soldier who scarcely notices injury suffered in battle but afterwards finds the injection of drugs extremely unpleasant. There are many examples in the context of dentistry; the simplest is in the injection of local anaesthetics. In some patients, penetration of the oral mucosa is not noticed, in others it cannot be tolerated without the preliminary application of a surface anaesthetic. It is inconceivable that this can be due in more than the smallest part to differences in the physical damage presumed to be the stimulus; in other words the afferent input in the different patients is likely to be almost the same; what differs is the response that this evokes in the central nervous system.

In carefully controlled laboratory experiments the variability of pain thresholds can be reduced to a minimum (see fig. 1); however, it must be emphasized that even in trained subjects protected from outside influences, pain thresholds can be affected by suggestion and by other afferent inputs, and furthermore, what is being measured is not the whole pain experience. Pain as a mind and body experience has much in common with pleasure and for centuries Aristotle's view was accepted that pain and pleasure were opposites. There is much to recommend this idea; pain, like pleasure, seems to affect the whole being and its character is difficult to explain to other people. The intensity of pain or pleasure evoked from time to time in one person or among different people varies according to factors such as age, sex or mood. The obvious difference is that a variety of receptor mechanisms can be instrumental in arousing feelings of pleasure; it now seems that a particular group of receptors, stimulated by events which cause actual tissue damage or threaten to

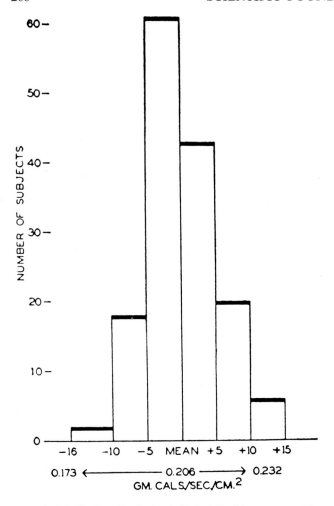

Fig. 1. Distribution of pain thresholds in 150 subjects, measured by thermal radiation applied to the forehead. In this group the mean value for stimulus intensity is about 0·21 gm. cals/sec/cm.² and all the subjects fall within ± 15% of the mean. From Wolff and Wolf (1958). Pain 2nd. Ed. Oxford, Blackwell.

these subjects the latency between the application of a stimulus and the withdrawal response is shorter than the latency between stimulation and the onset of pain in an intact individual. Even allowing for the possibility of shorter reflex latencies in subjects after spinal transection, these findings are not consistent with the view that withdrawal from injury is a consequence of the sensation of pain. The question as to whether the same receptor mechanism serves both pain and the withdrawal responses associated with it has been investigated in a human subject who had suffered spinal transection. The stimulus intensity necessary to cause pricking pain was not significantly different from that which evoked a flexion withdrawal response, and this adds further support to the view that the peripheral mechanisms for protection and for pain are the same.

If pain is not an essential part of immediate protective responses, what then are its functions? There are those who hold the view that it is a rather pointless addition to the many other unpleasant aspects of life, and point out that it frequently comes too late to give a warning of disease and that it causes needless suffering, especially in the terminal stages of disease, when its value is nil. Furthermore, as mentioned already, the severity of the pain rarely relates closely or usefully to the severity of the injury or disease.

On the other hand, survival of children congenitally incapable of feeling pain is less likely than in normal children; however, the longer they survive, the more skilled they become in using other evidence to detect injury, just as is possible in adjusting to other sensory loss. If pain depends on specific receptors and afferent pathways, one would expect some evidence of structural abnormalities in these children, but none has been reported. On the other hand if pain is the result of a discharge of an appropriate pattern of impulses from other receptors, one would expect other sensory loss in addition to pain. A slight impairment of temperature sensation has been noted in children showing hereditary insensitivity to pain.

do so, are responsible for the sensation of pain. Whether actual or potential damage is considered necessary to evoke pain, depends on the resolving power of methods used to detect tissue damage. The absence of damage at a gross level does not mean that there has not been damage of one or two cells, which given a suitable degree of sensitivity or proximity of the receptor mechanism could cause an impulse discharge and evoke a sensation.

PROTECTIVE RESPONSES

Since injurious stimuli are frequently associated with a pattern of responses which seem to minimize the damage or protect the organism, it is often said that the sensation of pain is responsible for the protective responses. This is not so. It can shown in animals or in human subjects after transection of the spinal cord that protective reflexes can be elicited by injury to the skin supplied by nerves at a segmental level below the spinal cord section, although the subject feels no pain in that region. Furthermore, in

EARLY THEORIES

In attempting to understand the problems of pain, it is worth going over paths taken by biologists in the past and, in particular, the writings of Johannes Müller (1842) who, though quoted often, seems to have been frequently misinterpreted. Müller introduced the idea of "the nerve of each sense having its own peculiar quality or energy". It does not seem that in using the phrase "peculiar quality or energy" Müller meant specificity as commonly understood today. Although he also wrote "the nerves of the senses have a specific irritability for certain influences, for many stimuli which exert a violent action upon one organ or sense have little or no effect on another", he went on to point out that electrical, chemical and mechanical stimuli can excite all nerves but produce different sensations; and concluded that "the hypothesis of specific irritability of the nerves of the senses for certain stimuli, is therefore insufficient and we are compelled to ascribe with Aristotle, peculiar energies to each nerve, energies which are vital qualities of the nerve just as contractility is a vital property of muscle". It is clear that Müller was in doubt as to what the "peculiar energies" consisted of, or where they might reside, for he wrote: "It is not known whether the essential cause of the peculiar 'energy' of each nerve of sense is seated in the nerve itself, or in the parts of the brain and spinal cord with which it is connected."

As far as can be gathered without recourse to the original writings, but to translations thereof, it is doubtful as to whether Müller or Helmholtz was responsible for the introduction of the idea of modalities as we understand it. Müller wrote: "Sensation is a property common to all senses, but the kind or 'modus' of sensation is different in each, thus we have sensations of sound, of taste, of smell and of feeling or touch." This seems to be as close as Müller approached to the concept of sensory modalities. Helmholtz (1860), in discussing the five senses said: "The qualities of the sensations cannot be compared with each other unless they belong to the same group. For example, we can compare two different sensations of the sense of sight as to intensity and colour, but we cannot compare either of them with a sound or smell, . . . the only sensations that can be produced by stimulation of a single sensory nerve fibre are such as belong in the group of qualities of a single definite sense."

Certainly Müller did not recognize separate components in somaesthetic sensation, e.g. sensation deriving from the surface of the body; for him there were five senses of which touch encompassed all the components of the somaesthetic system which we now regard as separate modalities. He seemed certain that the identity of the five senses was maintained; "even in the most excited condition the sensation preserves its specific character" and "it is an admitted fact that the sensations of light, sound, taste and odours can be experienced only in their respective nerves". However, he was in doubt about pain, which he considered to be a component of common sensation, for he said "it is a question whether the sensation of pain may not be felt in the nerves of the higher senses—whether, for example, violent irritation of the optic nerve may not give rise to the sensation of pain". However, he did not give any support to the idea that pain arises by overstimulation of optic nerve fibres and suggested that to explain pain experience when the optic nerve is violently stimulated "there are filaments of the nerves of common sensation [in which he included pain] distributed in the nerves of other organs of sense".

From the extracts quoted already, it is clear that as far as the so-called special senses are concerned, Müller's law of specific or peculiar nerve energies remains undisturbed by information obtained since the nineteenth century. His view of somaesthetic sensation which he called feeling or touch and in which he included itching, pleasure, pain, heat, cold and "those excited by the act of touch in its more limited sense" is no longer acceptable. Since all these sensations, which are aroused when the body surface is stimulated, were in Müller's view subdivisions of a single mode they must have been regarded as qualities, not separate modalities. It therefore seems that while Müller did not believe that pain could be evoked by overstim-

ulation of the other sensory modalities which we now call special senses, he did believe that on the body surface pain was a quality of the feeling or touch modality and presumably therefore could be aroused by excessive stimulation of the receptor mechanisms of this modality and had no specific receptors or afferent pathways.

PAIN RECEPTORS

In fact debate on this point has continued since Müller's time and it is only recently that the evidence for pain as a separate modality has increased substantially. If any one of the qualities of somaesthetic sensation can be evoked from a point on the body surface, then in a unitary system it ought to be possible to evoke all. This is not possible however, and the discovery in the skin of a punctate distribution of discrete sensory areas and complex structures surrounding nerve endings led von Frey (see Sherrington, 1900) to propose the existence of four sensory modalities in the skin; touch, warmth, cold and pain. This proposition carried with it the assumption that Müller's doctrine of specific nerve energies applied to all of these modalities and furthermore, that each modality was served by anatomically specialized receptor mechanisms. The question of anatomical specialization will not be dealt with here; suffice to say that it is now generally accepted that while certain structures such as Pacinian corpuscles impart special characteristics to the nerve ending with which they are associated, such as threshold and directional sensitivity, they are probably not responsible for the specificity of nerve endings. Furthermore, even von Frey had doubts as to whether the number of end organs in the skin was sufficient to account for all the points from which the sensation of cold could be evoked. Whatever the claims regarding anatomically specialized endings associated with other sensations in the skin, no one has ever claimed, given that pain is a separate modality, that it is served by a recognizable anatomically specialized receptor mechanism. All the evidence points to bare nerve terminals. Their involvement in the sensation of pain and support for the concept of pain as a separate modality was based for a long time on the observation that the "central cornea appears to be endowed with pain sensation only. It is found to possess histologically only one form of nerve endings, namely, free nerve filaments" (Sherrington, 1900). However, from the cornea and, indeed, other structures served by bare nerve endings, it is known to be possible to evoke sensations other than pain. This observation is further evidence against the anatomical basis of specificity and in addition it can be used against the hypothesis that pain is a separate modality. While the former no longer has any supporters, the question of pain as a separate modality still remains. In answering this question it would be helpful to know if there are any parts of the body (a) from which pain but no other sensation can be evoked, or (b) from which other sensations can be evoked but not pain. Regarding (a) the dental pulp, which was previously linked with the cornea as endowed only with pain receptor mechanisms, now remains alone. Whether its unique position is real or simply inadequately investigated is in doubt; certainly it would not be a popular structure on which to study a sensation from which most people shrink. Regarding (b) it was said many years ago that the mouth is poorly supplied with pain endings and that there are parts of the inner lining of the cheek from which pain cannot be aroused; the glans penis is insensitive to touch but sensations of warmth and pain can be aroused from it. This kind of evidence runs against the view that pain is the result of overstimulation of other receptor mechanisms and is merely a quality difference as, for example, red is from orange. The fact that in everyday experience pure pain is never experienced, but follows as an unpleasant extension of other sensations—temperature, touch and pressure, is not incompatible with the separate modality hypothesis. Reference was made earlier to the possible connection between tissue damage and the

end-organ is an apparatus amenable to some particular physical agent and at the same time rendered less amenable to, *i.e.* is shielded from, other excitants. It lowers the value of the limen (the threshold) of one particular kind of stimulus; it heightens the value of the limen of stimuli of other kinds." A nociceptor could not conform with this definition if it were a mechanoreceptor or thermoreceptor which responded to normal mechanical or thermal stimuli with a progressively increasing response to stimulus intensities ranging from harmless to noxious. Were this so, the organism would have difficulty in distinguishing reliably between innocuous and injurious stimuli and its protective responses might on some occasions fail to spring into action and on others be subject to false alerts. Since tissue damage results from severe mechanical stimulation or extremes of temperature, a nociceptor must,

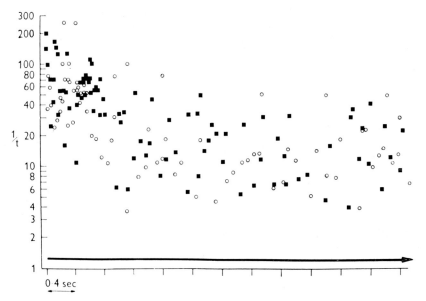

FIG. 2. Impulse discharge pattern by innocuous but firm pressure (filled squares) and noxious pressure (open circles) from a receptor in primate glabrous skin. Ordinate: instantanous frequency (1/t). Abscissa: time, with stimulus constant. From Burgess and Perl (1973).

sensation of pain and it is difficult to see how tissue damage can occur without the application of stimuli which, at any rate initially, stimulate touch, pressure, or temperature receptors. As far as can be judged macroscopically, injury seems to be what Sherrington called the "adequate stimulus" and he described stimuli which caused tissue damage as noxious; from this the term "nociceptor", meaning receptor responding to injury, was derived.

The great difficulty which faces investigators of somaesthetic mechanisms is to fit receptors into modality categories, since the anatomical basis which was fundamental to von Frey's proposition has been shown not to exist. The question to be answered is whether there are any receptors which could by their performance qualify for the title of nociceptor as defined by Sherrington, while satisfying also his classical definition of a receptor. Pain as a separate modality must depend on a physiologically unique receptor mechanism in Sherrington's terms "The sensorial

if it is to make discrimination possible, be a high-threshold receptor, unresponsive to stimulus intensities which evoke normal sensations of touch, pressure and temperature.

Figure 2 illustrates the inability of low-threshold mechanoreceptors, which respond to mild stimulation, to function as nociceptors. It can be seen that impulse frequencies have much the same distribution whether the stimuli are noxious or not. Clearly, "overstimulation" of receptors of this type would not provide the animal with suitable information on which to base a reliable decision as to the nature of the stimulus. Iggo (1972) reported that low-threshold mechanoreceptors of the type illustrated in fig. 2 can be driven to maximal activity by innocuous stimuli and cannot increase their response if the stimuli are intensified to noxious levels. Similar observations were made many years ago when mechanoreceptors in the frog's skin were found to fire maximally when the skin was subjected to puffs of air which could not possibly have been noxious.

Recent work has established the existence and characteristics of receptors which satisfy criteria for nociception. Investigators have found mechanoreceptors serving the skin in cats, which had conduction velocities mainly in the 10–20 m./sec. range (A delta group) and which showed high thresholds. They appeared to supply 20 or more spots on the skin and the spots supplied by one nerve fibre were distributed over an area of several square centimetres. The punctate distribution and the rather rapid adaptation rates are consistent with the idea that these might be involved in pricking pain. These high threshold mechanoreceptors are not excited by heat or chemical changes at damaging levels. However, C fibre receptors have been found which are not only high threshold mechanoreceptors but respond also to damaging heat and noxious chemicals. Because of their ability to respond to

maintaining a fairly steady impulse frequency after the stimulus has ceased to move. The polymodal receptors show interesting responses to prolonged heating. Not only do they continue to fire during maintained heating—in bursts of impulses rather than a steady frequency, but the threshold may actually fall by 2–8°C. Alternatively if they are repeatedly stimulated at the same temperature the impulse discharge increases (Burgess and Perl, 1973).

This finding is of particular interest in attempting to correlate the behaviour of receptors with sensory experience in man. Greene and Hardy (1962) found that with repeated or long maintained thermal stimulation of the skin, the minimum temperature necessary to evoke pain fell during a 12 min. period. Also, with a steady level of heat flux for 50 min., the subject changed his description of the sensation from warm to hot and after 30 min., to painful. At this

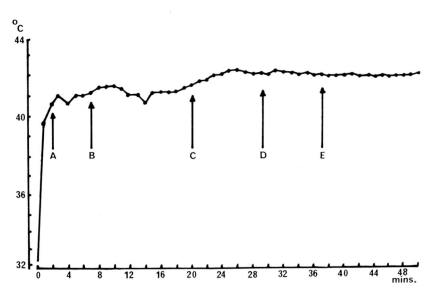

FIG. 3. Record of skin temperature during exposure to constant thermal radiation for 50 minutes. The reports of the subject were at A, warm; at B, hot; at C, very hot; at D, pain. From E onwards the subject reported continuous pain. Redrawn from Greene and Hardy (1962).

injury inflicted in several ways these are called polymodal.

It has also been shown that the cat skin contains thermoreceptors which do not fire until the skin temperature reaches 44°C, well beyond the point at which sensitive "warm" fibres would have ceased to fire. These high threshold thermoreceptors go on firing with increasing frequency up to about 60–65°C.

Adaptation

An important feature of the behaviour of receptors, and one of particular interest when considering human experience of pain, is the phenomenon of adaptation. All receptors, nociceptors included, show a decline in the frequency of impulse discharge during maintained stimulation. In the mechanical nociceptor group there are in the high threshold range, receptors which are rapid adaptors, responding only to moving stimuli. In the more sensitive group there are slowly adapting receptors capable of

point the skin temperature was 42.2°C, well below the usual pain threshold of 45°C (fig. 3). This is an example of the phenomenon of hyperalgesia which will be referred to again. The rather precise categorization of nociceptors which has been achieved in neurophysiological terms has not yet been matched histologically but it is inconceivable that physiological specificity is not associated with some structural specialization. The profuse innervation of the skin and the great difficulties of single unit analysis of pain in human subjects are responsible for the failure to identify these receptors anatomically.

Chemical Stimulation of Pain Receptors

If the adequate stimulus is tissue damage it is reasonable to suppose that direct excitation of the nerve endings would be by chemical means and it seems plausible to suggest that nociception, so essential for the survival of unicellular protozoa and multicellular organisms, is a descendant of the primitive chemical sense. The normal skin provides protection against stimulation, and chemical sensitivity is restricted to olfactory and gustatory receptor areas and to mucous membranes such as those of the eye, nose and mouth. However, if the epidermis is removed, for example, after the formation of a blister during which the outer layers of the epidermis separate off, exposing the stratum basale, many chemical agents can reach nerve endings and cause pain. The skin blister preparation has been used extensively to study the chemical basis of pain (Keele and Armstrong, 1964). Nearly fifty years ago Lewis first demonstrated the role of histamine in the vascular responses to various stimuli applied to the skin and he later (1942) reported that in addition to producing the so-called triple response, histamine also caused itch when pricked into the skin. In the blister base preparation it sometimes causes pain as well as itch and others found that intradermal injection caused pain, but only when high concentrations were injected. However, this effect is greatly potentiated by acetylcholine, and it has been found that the nettle sting contains a mixture of acetycholine and histamine. The presence of histamine in many tissues, particularly the skin, makes it an obvious candidate for the role of an endogenous pain-producing agent; however, others have been discovered. Obviously if cell damage occurs, potassium, the chief intracellular ion, will be released and it has indeed been found that by intramuscular injection, intradermal injection, and by application to the exposed blister base, potassium chloride causes pain. The potassium concentration in inflammatory exudates is near threshold levels for pain production and so it may be a contributory factor. More recently many other substances more effective than histamine and potassium salts have been discovered. These include 5-hydroxytryptamine (serotonin) released from blood platelets, which is effective in the blister base preparation in concentrations as low as 10^{-8} g./ml. It was also discovered that blister fluid and plasma can cause pain if collected in a glass vessel and applied to the base of the original or another blister. The active agent is bradykinin and other so-called plasma kinins increase capillary permeability and cause oedema. Keele and Armstrong (1964) have also looked at the effect of acetylcholine on the blister base and found that it caused pain which the subjects could grade in severity, and their estimates of severity corresponded well with the concentrations over the range 1×10^{-5} g./ml. to 5×10^{-5} g./ml. The blister area was completely refractory to further stimulation for 1 min. after washing off the solution and recovery to full sensitivity took 9 min.

From all these studies it is clear that there are many products of cell damage which could cause pain. Further evidence for the production within the skin of chemical agents capable of causing pain was obtained in man by perfusion of the skin under a "triple response" reaction and the demonstration by means of bio-assay that the perfusate contained a bradykinin-like substance, the concentration of which rose and fell with the development and decline of the "flare".

The sensitivity of polymodal nociceptors (see above) to bradykinin and various other chemicals likely to act as intermediaries in pain production has been investigated and it appears that bradykinin excites them only weakly and histamine is even less effective. However in very low concentration acetylcholine evokes a vigorous discharge, and potassium in twice to four times the concentration in extracellular fluid is also very potent. It was found that these agents did not excite mechanical nociceptors (Burgess and Perl, 1973).

TYPES OF PAIN

It is an old observation that the sensation of pain can be divided into two components; an immediate sharp pain of short duration, followed after a time lapse of 0·9–2·5 sec. (in experimental studies) by a more intense burning pain, described as radiating from the point stimulated and swelling rapidly to a maximum, then fading gradually. A number of pieces of evidence point to the conclusion that this phenomenon depends on a double afferent pathway; the A delta fibres giving rise to the short latency sharp component and the C fibres to the long latency burning component. For example, pressure or hypoxia first block conduction in the myelinated fibres and the fast component disappears leaving the slow burning component, sometimes in a more unpleasant form. Local anaesthetics block C fibres before A fibres and abolish the second pain before the first. More light on the double pain phenomenon has been shed by one of the few electrophysiological studies on pain in man. In these experiments a nerve bundle in the leg was exposed under general anaesthesia and after the subjects had recovered from the anaesthetic, the nerve bundle was stimulated electrically and the compound action potential recorded. Using the fact that the threshold stimulus intensity is lower the greater the fibre diameter, it was possible by progressively increasing the stimulus intensity to excite first the A group and then with large voltages to bring in the C fibres. The subjects began to report pain only when the stimulus voltage rose to between 0·25 and 7·0 V. and the tapping or thumping sensations previously experienced were described as sharper. At that stimulus intensity the A delta fibres were firing, and with repetitive stimulation the sensation was in most cases too uncomfortable for the patients to bear. At much higher voltages the C wave appeared on the record and all the subjects described the sensation in response to a single stimulus as unbearable and with repetitive stimulation refused to continue the experiment. At that stage, of course, the A fibres were also firing but in later experiments it was possible to block conduction in these fibres. When this was done, leaving only the C fibres capable of conduction it was found that a single stimulus was not painful but repetitive stimulation at 3 or more/sec. was always unbearably painful. From the onset of stimulation there was a delay of between 2–4 sec. before pain was felt.

FACTORS MODIFYING THE PAIN THRESHOLD

Before discussing the problem of pain from teeth there remains one aspect of the receptor mechanism to be discussed in general terms. Reference has been made already to the considerable differences from time to time in the same individual and between individuals in the sensation of pain evoked by stimuli which do not differ greatly in intensity. The question arises as to the level at which filtering or amplifying mechanisms exist. It is not intended in this section to deal with the pathways taken by impulses from nociceptors after the spinal cord has been entered but simply to illustrate the general principles by which input to the central nervous system can be modified.

The first point at which input from the periphery can be influenced is actually at the receptor, where changes can be produced by various mechanisms, some of which are accessible to central nervous control. Recalling the observations that injury in battle or other occasions of stress may

extensive than normal. It has also been shown that suggestion under hypnosis can influence the tissue response to injury. Here then are examples of the way that higher nervous control can influence the input from nociceptors to the central nervous system, but although this effect is at a receptor level it is an indirect effect, via local vascular mechanisms.

Later, Lewis obtained evidence for a more local action when he investigated the tenderness which some people experience in the skin near an area of injury. He found this, for example, in the skin of the face over the maxillary antrum and upper teeth after a period of electrical stimulation of the antral mucosa and teeth. He postulated that impulses from nociceptors spread to other terminals in the distribution of a nerve in areas of skin not being stimulated

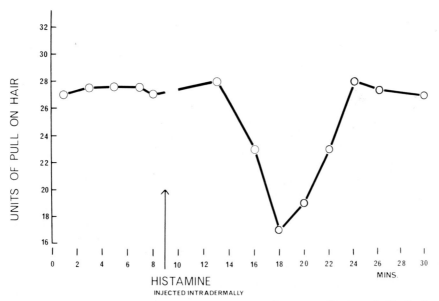

FIG. 4. Pain threshold, measured in units of pull on a hair, in an area of hyperaemia (the flare) produced by intradermal injection of histamine. From Bilisoly, Goodell and Wolff (1954).

be unnoticed poses the question as to whether sympathetic nervous activity could affect receptor thresholds. There is no evidence to show that sympathetic nerves can directly affect nociceptors, although a threshold-lowering effect has been demonstrated on mechanoreceptors in frog skin. In this isolated preparation indirect influences via changes in blood flow could not have occurred.

Many years ago Lewis performed many simple and elegant experiments on local vascular changes associated with injury (the "triple response") and postulated that impulses from the injured skin travelling in a central direction also passed antidromically along branches supplying local arterioles to cause vasodilation. He demonstrated that in an area of inflammation the pain threshold was apparently lowered and because this hyperalgesia was associated with redness, he called it erythralgia. Others since Lewis have extended his observations (see fig. 4). For example, it has been shown that in skin exhibiting reflex vasodilation during heating, the pain threshold is lowered and the triple response to noxious stimulation is more

and that these terminals were somehow raised to a hyper-excitable level. More recently it has been shown that antidromic stimulation of nerves can cause the liberation of chemical agents which cause vasodilation and would presumably result in a lowered pain threshold.

The next point at which nociceptor input might be modified is at segmental level in the spinal cord. Mechanisms at this level or higher are required to account for the common observation that with the same stimulus, and when the condition of tissues seems to be similar, pain thresholds differ markedly. The fact that experience and training can narrow the variability of pain thresholds in subjects tested in carefully regulated laboratory conditions bears witness to the influence of the central nervous system. Part of this effect can be attributed to the fact that at every moment of life the brain and spinal cord are being bombarded by information from countless receptors and when this is controlled and reduced in laboratory conditions, attention can be focused more reliably on a test stimulus. However, even in these circumstances there is evidence that stimulus intensities considered to be painful (the pain perception threshold) differ in people of differing cultural background or race and can be influenced by other sensory inputs, especially from other nociceptors, by past experience, by the psychological state of the subject and by suggestion during hypnosis.

There are many examples of conditions pertinent to dentistry in which pain thresholds can be influenced: two will be cited. One well known example is counter-irritation or hyperstimulation analgesia. The application of irritating chemicals or heat or cold close to a painful area can reduce the intensity of pain. The proximity of the counter-irritation and the painful area might suggest that there is some interaction peripherally; however, while this may be so in some instances, it is not always a requirement for the success of counter-irritation. It has been shown, for example, that the pain threshold to electrical stimulation of the teeth is raised by applying ethyl chloride to the skin over the tibia for about 20 sec., producing in that region pain of burning or aching character. The remarkable result is that pain thresholds are raised for a period of 2 hr. afterwards, the pain from the leg presumably having disappeared long since.

The technique of audio-analgesia, practised in the past by the itinerant surgeon with a brass band, or more recently by using "white noise" for dental operations, is considered to achieve true analgesia, i.e. it raises the pain perception threshold, in some instances. However, there is evidence that its effect is more likely to depend on suggestion and distraction since no evidence was found that sensitivity of teeth was lowered.

REFERRED PAIN

This is a suitable point at which to discuss "referred pain". When deep structures such as viscera, the maxillary air sinus and, surprisingly, the teeth are injured or diseased, the patient may have difficulty in localizing the origin of the sensation and is generally much less precise in his description of the pain than when it originates from superficial areas. Furthermore, the patient often reports that the pain seems to be located in an area superficial to and often remote from the injured or diseased organ; for example, anginal pain is often referred to the left arm. Pain from teeth may be referred to the opposing arch or to the ear or the maxillary sinus and from the latter two structures to the teeth. In every case the area of reference has the same segmental innervation and reference does not occur across the midline except from the gut which has bilateral innervation. Difficulty in localizing the origin of pain from deep structures may be due simply to lack of information from sparsely innervated structures and reference has been attributed to the fact that the predominant sources of information throughout life are superficial structures and the brain has learned to expect that all the information comes from these areas. It might be supposed, if this explanation is correct, that anaesthetizing the area of reference would not abolish the referred pain. Unfortunately the results of this type of experiment are equivocal and leave us with the mechanism unexplained.

Whatever the answer may be, it is certain that the phenomenon depends on mechanisms at a spinal or higher level and not at the level of the receptor terminals.

Phantom Limb

The condition of phantom limb provides further evidence for the influence of central mechanisms on the experience of pain. Phantom limb pain may occur in as many as a third of patients who have suffered amputation. There is ample evidence to show that, although sensory input from the stump and other areas called "trigger zones" can start and modify phantom limb pain, they are not the principal cause and indeed section of the dorsal roots often fails to remedy the condition.

Aerodontalgia

The phenomenon of aerodontalgia appears to have characteristics in common both with phantom limb and referred pain and so for this reason and for its interest to dentistry it is worth attention. Aerodontalgia is dental pain which people sometimes experience when exposed to changes in barometric pressure such as during unpressurized high flying. It has been shown to be pain referred to the teeth from an infected maxillary sinus. Furthermore, in a remarkable study (Hutchins and Reynolds, 1947) which ought to have stimulated great interest, it was found that the pain was generally referred to teeth or a tooth which had previously been subjected to painful trauma, disease, or dental treatment without anaesthesia, but which was symptomless at the time of aerodontalgia. Reference of pain was also reported even to areas from which teeth had been extracted. In their approach to this problem, the experimenters performed dental treatment without anaesthesia (or under nitrous oxide anaesthesia for extractions) and then tested for referred pain several weeks later by pricking the nasal epithelium in the region of the ostium of the maxillary antrum. The dental treatment was bilateral and so the subjects were their own controls in the next step of the experiment which was to produce block anaesthesia by injecting local anaesthetic on one side of the mouth. After a further 10–16 days both sides were tested again and on the control side 13 of the 14 subjects still reported pain on stimulation of the maxillary ostium while no referred pain was produced on the side which had been anaesthetized previously. The similarity between this phenomenon and phantom limb is in the long duration effect of the original traumatic experience and the fact that in some cases injection of local anaesthetic may stop the pain even after the anaesthetic effect has worn off. There are many differences of course; phantom limb pain is often extremely severe, arises spontaneously, and sometimes from distant trigger zones.

In these brief references to pain thresholds, referred pain, phantom limb and aerodontalgia, there is enough evidence to show that the central nervous system can indirectly and possibly directly set the sensitivity level of nociceptors; it can sift, reject, or amplify information it receives from receptors and it uses previous experience in the interpretation of data.

THE GATE CONTROL THEORY

One of the most dramatic aspects of the nervous system is the enormous quantity of information that continuously pours in from receptors all over the body, and it can be assumed that the input is greater than the maximum number of impulses the spinal cord can deal with. There is no evidence of direct inhibitory action at a receptor level (see above) and control of what can be called surplus inflow seems to be at spinal cord level and above. Inhibitory mechanisms have been shown to operate at axonal terminals of afferent fibres, controlling the amount of chemical transmitter released at their terminals, and thereby influencing the excitation of the next neurone in the conducting chain from the periphery to the brain. Evidence obtained during the past 10–15 years indicates that the part of the dorsal horn of spinal grey matter known as the substantia gelatinosa may have a key role in determining how much information reaches the antero-lateral pathways which are essential for pain. The substantia gelatinosa has been described as the site of a "gate control" mechanism by which supraspinal descending pathways can influence spinal afferent conduction. The "Gate Control Theory" of Melzack and Wall proposes in addition, that spinal cord transmission cells are subjected to modulating influences in the substantia gelatinosa from large and small diameter fibres coming in from the periphery. Large diameter fibre input, according to this theory tends to close the gate, small diameter fibre input (such as A delta and C) tends to open the gate. This theory provides neat explanations for many of the puzzling features of pain such as phantom limb, referred pain and counter-irritation: it is however, by no means universally accepted.

PAIN FROM THE TEETH

Turning now to the problem of pain from teeth, the first and oldest question concerns the nature of the receptor mechanism. Recalling the characteristics of pain from other parts of the body it may be that a description of dental pain would be useful in providing clues about the receptors. One of the difficulties, however, in using information of this kind is that stimuli applied to dental enamel must penetrate this tissue to reach dentine or pulp, or in some way excite receptor mechanisms in the periodontal ligament to evoke pain, for there is no receptor mechanism in enamel. This means, provided the enamel is intact, that chemical stimuli cannot evoke pain, and other stimuli are likely to be somewhat modified in their passage to the receptor mechanisms wherever these may be. Even the results of electrical stimulation must be looked at with caution because it has been shown in animals that with monopolar stimulation the difference between the stimulus intensity which will excite "intradental" mechanisms and that which excites periodontal receptors is not large.

Pain can be evoked from sound intact teeth by tempera-ture change, by pressure, and by electrical stimulation. There is no evidence that sensations other than pain can be aroused although of course the quality differs with different stimuli. Subjects involved in experiments will often use previous experience of pain from known stimuli in describing the sensations evoked when they are kept in ignorance of the nature of the test stimulus. It is well established however, that bright sharp pain can occur in response to electrical stimulation or to pressure applied to the enamel. It would therefore be reasonable to expect to see A delta fibres in either the periodontal ligament or the pulp or in both sites. Again, since pain considered to be the result of C fibre activity can also be evoked from the teeth, these fibres would also be expected to be present. Light microscopical studies have shown fibres in the 5–6 μm. range and various authors have reported conduction velocities in the range 11–83 m./sec. Figures of 11–17 m./sec. have been obtained for pulpal fibres, whilst for periodontal fibres conduction velocities between 24 and 60 m./sec. have been found in the cat. With longer lengths of nerve in the dog and therefore more reliable measurements, the range has been extended to between 28 and 83 m./sec. with most of the units conducting at about 50 m./sec. While electronmicroscopic evidence is available from many sources for the presence of unmyelinated fibres in the dental pulp, there are hardly any data for conduction velocities in the C fibre range except for one study which found a range of 0·8–38 m./sec. and only one fibre in the C range.

Sensitivity of Dentine

Since enamel is completely insensitive it might be considered that dental pain could be studied more sucessfully by removing the enamel and testing the dentine direct, by analogy with skin after removal of the epidermis by blister formation and testing the exposed blister base. Other possibilities are to test the dental pulp exposed by trauma or disease. However, the dental pulp does not offer a particularly exciting challenge since we know that it contains nervous elements and presumably the mechanism of excitation is no different from that in other parts of the body. Furthermore, there would be few volunteers for that kind of experiment. Exposed dentine at the neck of the tooth is another possibility, but here, as with pathologically exposed pulps, or indeed carious dentine one would be faced with unknown variables.

It is well established that under carious dentine or even when only the enamel is affected by caries, the pulp may be hyperaemic. It therefore follows that since the overwhelming mass of clinical evidence and common experience which has been responsible for the general view that dentine is exceptionally sensitive, comes from observations and experience of carious teeth, it may be as far from the true picture as would have been obtained by studies of skin sensitivity were these made on hyperaemic skin. Such a criticism can of course be aimed at the work on the blister-base preparation and the only answer to it is that the pain threshold to acetylcholine in the blister base preparation is about the same concentration as excites C fibre endings when injected close arterially in normal cat's skin (Keele and Armstrong, 1964).

Contrary to the common view of dentine, studies on near normal dentine in teeth only slightly affected by caries as indicated by a probe sticking in an occlusal fissure, have consistently demonstrated how insensitive is this tissue. When heat production is kept down by using a slow-running bur with a coolant, cutting the dentine only rarely caused pain and stimuli applied subsequently were also rather infrequently successful. However, the procedure of filling the cavity in dentine with gutta percha for a week results in enhanced sensitivity as might be expected, in view of the hyperaemia known to occur in the pulps of teeth treated this way.

The author's early experiments in this field were stimulated by the work of Keele and associates (Keele and Armstrong, 1964), and by analogy with the blister base preparation in skin, it was thought that removal of the enamel would leave the nervous elements (if there were any) in the dentine accessible to stimulation by various chemicals found effective on nerve endings in the dermis. This was not so, and it became apparent that whether through inaccessibility or insensitivity, intradental nerves could not be excited by acetylcholine, potassium chloride, and other substances applied to dentine although it was possible to evoke acute pain when these substances were applied directly to the freshly exposed dental pulp. Greater success in evoking pain from dentine was achieved by applying solutions which exerted a high osmotic pressure and such was the relationship between the osmotic pressure of a wide range of different solutions and the production of pain that it was found appropriate to express pain thresholds in terms of osmotic pressure. It was also found that repeated application of these solutions depressed sensitivity, but only in the dentine being stimulated, not in the tooth as a whole.

Evidence of this type was obtained by other investigators, who also showed that when dentine was subjected to pressure changes or to drying there was displacement of odontoblast nuclei into the dentinal tubules. The accepted clinical belief that local anaesthetics do not block pain when applied to dentine has been supported by experiments; it has also been found that protein precipitants were ineffective.

Hydrodynamic Hypothesis

Taken as a whole this evidence strongly suggested the intervention of a physical rather than a nervous transduction mechanism between the stimulus applied to the surface of the dentine and the nervous response arising at a deeper level in the tooth, either in the dentine or in the pulp. Until recently the hydrodynamic hypothesis (Brännström and Åström, 1964) seemed to provide an adequate explanation for the facts available at that time. According to this hypothesis stimuli cause pain when applied to dentine, by some means involving displacement of the contents of the dentine tubules, which excites mechanoreceptors in the dental pulp. More recently it has been suggested that different mechanisms are involved depending on whether the stimulus causes inward or outward movement of fluid.

Fluid movement *in vitro* has been measured by several investigators. From the most recent however, doubts as to the validity of the hydrodynamic hypothesis arose, because whereas a good correlation between osmotic pressure and pain-producing power had been established earlier and the link had been assumed to be fluid movement, the new studies showed that, at any rate in freshly extracted teeth, fluid movement did not match osmotic pressure in all cases. The results of human experiments and recent experiments *in vitro* on fluid movement are consistent with the hydrodynamic hypothesis for calcium chloride, dextrose and sugar syrup. However, with urea, sodium chloride and ammonium chloride solutions there was disagreement because they caused less fluid movement than other solutions of similar osmotic pressure and similar pain producing effect.

Electrophysiological studies of the response of dentine to stimulation, using the standard technique of dissecting small filaments from dental nerves which were first attempted in 1939 have through the years provided rather disappointing results. When a technique was described of direct recording from dentine it seemed that a solution to the problem of the site and nature of the intradental receptor mechanism was near (Scott, Schroff and Gabel, 1953). However there were difficulties. Firstly, the structure of dentine permits the recording through a layer of dentine of electrical activity in the underlying pulp cavity, and so it does not necessarily follow that electrical activity recorded from the surface of the dentine has its origin in dentine. Secondly, thorough study of the technique showed that it was capable of recording electrical changes which were not of biological origin. Since then an electrode was devised with which non-biological artefacts were eliminated, and on occasions impulses have been recorded simultaneously from the dentine surface and from a filament dissected from the inferior dental nerve (Horiuchi and Matthews, in Emmelin and Zotterman, 1972).

Several facts have emerged from these studies which raise more questions about sensory mechanisms. Before considering them it is important to be reminded that attempts are being made to correlate studies on pain using various solutions applied to dentine in man, electrophysiological studies on animals, and measurements of fluid movement in extracted human teeth. The reader should be aware of the pitfalls of such an exercise.

In human studies, if pain was evoked by the application of solutions to dentine the latency was short, and sometimes the response was instantaneous and vigorous. The latency of the neural response in cats was never less than five minutes when solutions were applied to outer dentine, but was reduced as the pulp was approached. It is possible, as mentioned earlier, that in human experiments the dental pulp was hyperaemic. Furthermore most of the painful responses in human subjects were obtained not from the freshly exposed dentine, which we found both during cutting and testing to be unexpectedly insensitive, but from dentine in cavities filled for a week with gutta percha, below which the pulp was almost certainly hyper-aemic. In the animal experiments there was no doubt that the teeth were non-carious.

Comparing the animal results with those obtained on fluid flow *in vitro*, it was surprising that 2·5 mol./l. NH_4Cl caused a vastly greater impulse discharge than 4 mol./l. dextrose although the dextrose had an osmotic pressure about twice that of the NH_4Cl and would be expected to produce a greater fluid flow. In fact in some flow measurements 4 mol./l. dextrose produced eight times the fluid movement achieved by an iso-osmotic solution of NH_4Cl

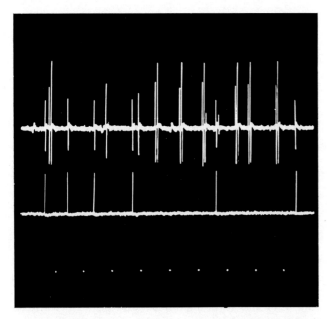

FIG. 5. Simultaneous recordings in the cat from the surface of dentine (upper record) and a single fibre dissected from the inferior dental nerve (centre record). The discharge was evoked by the application of 2·5 mol/l NaCl to dentine under the electrode at the tip of the crown. Note that the potentials in the centre recording are separated by the same intervals as a group of constant amplitude potentials in the top recording. *Calibrations*—Upper record: 1 cm. = 50 μV. Centre record: 1 cm. = 0·25 mV. Lower record: time intervals 0·1 sec. (From Horiuchi and Matthews, 1972, in *Oral Physiology*, pp. 291–302. Eds. Emmelin, N. and Zotterman, Y., Oxford, Pergamon.)

(Horiuchi and Matthews, *op. cit.*). These findings do not support the hydrodynamic hypothesis, and the problem has not yet been resolved. However, experiments are in progress to test the hydrodynamic hypothesis and preliminary results have been reported. The first objective was to look specifically at the effect of 4 mol./l. NH_4Cl and 4 mol./l. dextrose which have an osmotic pressure of about 240 atmospheres. This value had of course been within the range of osmotic pressures previously investigated but these two solutions had not been used in 4 mol./l. concentrations in the previous series. Whereas this concentration of dextrose achieved a much greater fluid movement *in vitro* than NH_4Cl and therefore would be expected according to the hydrodynamic hypothesis to produce more reports of pain, the neural response animal to dextrose was less than to HN_4Cl. First results (Anderson, Matthews and Yemm, 1973) indicate that the two solutions have much the same effect in man, producing

pain in about 50 per cent of tests. This is in line with previous findings, but is not what would have been expected according to the hydrodynamic hypothesis or from animal experiments.

Neurohistology

How does this work relate to histological findings? When the first descriptions were published of what appeared to be unmyelinated nerve fibres in the inner dentine and the specialized junction between these elements and the odontoblast processes, it was tempting to regard this as a functional relationship akin to that of a receptor organ and nerve terminal (R. M. Frank in Symons, 1968). While some investigators claim to have found that two months after the inferior dental nerve resection, fibres could still be seen in dentine, there are conflicting reports and conflicting interpretations of electronmicroscopic appearances. Others have found that resection of the inferior dental nerve in mice resulted in the disappearance of intradentinal nerves. Electron microscopy of dentine and of nerve fibres is notoriously difficult, and final judgements are impossible while experienced workers disagree, expecially when the point at issue depends on seeing or not seeing nerve fibres which are known to be only sparsely distributed in dentine. Furthermore, whatever the outcome, there remains the clinical and experimental evidence from man that the outer part of the dentine is sensitive, yet there is no evidence that nerve fibres penetrate further than the inner third of the dentine. Indeed, it has been shown that the outer region of the dentinal tubules does not contain any cellular material, so presumably the odontoblast process does not extend throughout the entire length of the tubule.

It can be said, in conclusion, that substantial progress has been made in recent years. It is common experience in research that as the answer to one question is approached, others spring up and the horizon seems constantly on the move. That nerve fibres enter the dentine from the pulp and that electrical activity of indisputably biological origin can be recorded from the surface of dentine there is no doubt, and these are advances made during the last decade or so. The function of the nerves remains to be established. If there is indeed a functional relationship between the nerve fibre and the odontoblast, and together they provide the anatomical basis of a dentinal receptor mechanism, then the odontoblast will have been shown to be a unique cell capable on the one hand of taking part in histogenesis and on the other of nociception.

REFERENCES

Bilisoly, F. N., Goodell, H. and Wolff, H. G. (1954), "Vasodilatation, Lowered Pain Threshold and Increased Tissue Vulnerability," *Arch. intern. Med.* **94**, 759.

Brännström, M. and Åström, A. (1964), "A Study on the Mechanism of Pain Elicited from the Dentine". *J. Dent. Res.*, **43**, 619.

Burgess, P. R. and Perl, E. R. (1973), "Cutaneous Mechanoreceptors and Nociceptors" in *Handbook of Sensory Physiology*, vol 2, *Somato-sensory System*, p. 67 (A. Iggo, Ed.). Berlin: Springer-Verlag.

Greene, L. C. and Hardy, J. D. (1962), "Adaptation to Thermal Pain in the Skin," *J. appl. Physiol.* **17**, 693.

Hutchins, H. C. and Reynolds, O. E. (1947), "Experimental Investigation of the Referred Pain of Aerodontalgia". *J. Dent. Res.*, **26**, 3.

Iggo, A. (1972), "The Case for 'Pain' Receptors," in *Pain, Basic Principles, Pharmacology, Therapy*, p. 60 (R. Janzen, W. D. Keidel, A. Herz and C. Steichele, Eds. London: Churchill Livingstone.

Keele, C. A. and Armstrong, D. (1964), *Substances Producing Pain and Itch*. London: Arnold.

Scott, D. Jr., Schroff, F. R. and Gabel, A. B. (1953), "Response Pattern of Sensory Endings in the Tooth of the Cat". *Fed. Proc.*, **12**, 129.

Sherrington, C. S. (1900), "Cutaneous Sensation," in *Textbook of Physiology*, pp. 988 and 995 (E. A. Schafer, Ed.). Edinburgh and London: Pentland.

Wolff, H. G. and Wolf, S. (1958), *Pain*. 2nd ed. Blackwell, Oxford. p. 15.

FURTHER READING

Anderson, D. J., Hannam, A. G. and Matthews, B. (1970), "Sensory Mechanisms in Mammalian Teeth and Their Supporting Structures," *Physiol. Rev.*, **50**, 171.

Emmelin, N. and Zotterman, Y. (1972), *Oral Physiology* (Wenner-Gren Symposium, 1972). Oxford: Pergamon.

Melzack, R. (1973), *The Puzzle of Pain*. Harmondsworth, England: Penguin Books.

Perl, E. R. (1971), "Is Pain a Specific Sensation?," *J. psychiat. Res.* **8**, 273.

Symons, N. B. B. (1968), *Dentine and Pulp, Their Structure and Reactions*. London: Livingstone.

23. NEUROLOGICAL ASPECTS OF THE DIAGNOSIS AND TREATMENT OF FACIAL PAIN

B. D. WYKE

"There's no art
To find the mind's construction in the face."
(William Shakespeare, *Macbeth*, IV, 7)

The experience of pain

Special significance of facial pain

Peripheral facial pain systems

Nociceptive receptors in facial tissues
Nociceptive afferent pathways from facial tissues

Central facial pain projection systems

Perceptual component
Afferent component
Memory component
Visceral-hormonal reflex component

Awareness of facial pain

Peripheral modulation
Central modulation
    Within the caudal spinal nucleus
    Within the thalamic relay nuclei
    Within the cerebral cortex

Clinical varieties of facial pain

Primary
Secondary
Referred
Ictal

No matter where it is felt in the body, and no matter from what cause, pain—which is the commonest of all clinical symptoms encountered in medical and dental practice—represents a disturbance of neurological function;

and as such, its diagnosis and treatment should (ideally) be founded upon precise understanding of the neurological mechanisms involved in its production. Unfortunately—because the necessary anatomical and physiological data are seldom available in sufficient detail—this is rarely possible in practice, and the clinician confronted by a patient in pain must perforce adopt a pragmatic approach to relief of this distressing symptom. This is particularly so in the case of facial pain, the complexities of which are compounded by the fact that as a practical clinical problem it engages the disparate interests of oral and dental surgeons, otorhinolaryngologists and psychiatrists as well as those of neurological physicians and surgeons.

For these reasons, this Chapter attempts to draw together some of the threads of data from each of these disciplines, as well as from modern neuro-anatomical, neurophysiological and neuropharmacological studies, into a systematized pattern that may serve as an operational basis for a more ordered approach to the problem presented by patients suffering from facial pain—which, for the purposes of this discussion, is taken to refer to pain experienced in the extra-oral, extra-nasal and extra-orbital tissues covering the anterior and antero-lateral aspects of the skull and mandible. Information concerning earlier studies in this field relevant to the interests of dental and oral surgeons is contained in previous communications by the writer over the last twenty-five years and in several special monographs, so this account concentrates on certain recent fundamental developments in neurological science that may contribute to improved understanding of the clinical problems of facial pain.

THE EXPERIENCE OF PAIN

As a phenomenon of human experience, pain is not (as has often been asserted) a perceptual sensation in the sense that vision, hearing, smell, taste, touch or kinaesthesis are, but is an abnormal emotional state that is called into being usually by the development of chemical and/or structural changes in various tissues of the body that give rise to activity in afferent systems within the neuraxis that normally are relatively quiescent. In other words, pain is an abnormal affective state that is aroused by unusual patterns of activity in specific afferent systems, and which is coloured (see p. 287) by the variety of somatic and visceral reflex responses and hormonal changes that are simultaneously evoked by such activity. In spite of a recent re-affirmation to the contrary, pain is not merely an unpleasant subjective experience provoked by perception of particularly intense stimulation of any morphological variety of sensory receptor, but is a specific emotional disorder that is provoked by abnormal activation of an anatomically discrete peripheral afferent system that is, for the most part, distinct from those afferent systems whose activity evokes the primary perceptual experiences of normal everyday life. Thus it is not so much the nature or intensity of a tissue disturbance that determines whether or not it will be painful, as the extent to which the afferent activity that it evokes is channelled into those central pathways (see p. 284) whose cerebral connexions are such that they evoke the experience of pain when appropriately activated.

The affective state of pain—no matter how bizarre its clinical presentation may be—is therefore always indicative of pathological change (either structural or chemical, or both) somewhere in the body, unless the complainant is to be regarded as hysterical or as a malingerer. This affective state also differs from all other affective states of human experience in that it is always invested with a local habitation in the sufferer's body: for unlike elation or sorrow (for example), pain is always felt in some particular part of the body with varying degrees of precision—even though that part be no longer present, as with the "phantom pain" that may follow amputation of a limb or a breast. Furthermore, although the experience of pain is regarded by most individuals as highly unpleasant and undesirable, and therefore as something to be got rid of as soon as possible, this is not always the case—thus in some cultures and in certain religious sects it is regarded as morally elevating, or as a means of expiating feelings of guilt attached to some transgression of ethical or social principles; whilst some psychiatrically disturbed individuals (i.e. hypochondriacs and masochists) may derive emotional satisfaction from the experience, often to the point of resisting therapeutic attempts to relieve them of it. Yet other individuals (who are very few in number) lack the capacity to experience pain that is possessed by most of the human race.

The Special Significance of Facial Pain

Neurologists and otolaryngologists especially are familiar with the fact that the emotional disturbance engendered by pain in the face is generally far more intense than that associated with the occurrence of pain in any other part of the body (except the genitalia). This special emotional significance of facial pain arises from the considerable psychological and sociological importance of the face which, in most sophisticated communities, is the only part of the body (except the hands) that is regularly presented directly to the inspection of society. As every actor knows, it is with the face that most of the external expression of an individual's internal emotional life is conveyed to his fellows; and in women especially, the attractiveness and expressiveness of the face play a major rôle in intersexual relations—so much so, in fact, that in some cultures women are required to veil their faces from the public gaze of males.

For these reasons—which are more cogent in women than in men—the occurrence of pain in the face is charged with particularly intense emotional overtones whose existence cannot be ignored by those responsible for the management of patients thus afflicted. This socio-psychological significance of facial pain is only too clearly and piteously exemplified by those patients (more often women than men) who—suffering from chronic pain in the face, or repeated acute episodes of facial pain—become social recluses; and such patients may even be driven to the point of attempting suicide as a result of their distressing social isolation.

At the outset of this account, then, it may be said that some of the complexities inherent in the clinical management of facial pain may be resolved by realizing that one is dealing with an affective disorder that is of a special nature and peculiar intensity. This disorder is generally evoked when specific receptor endings (see below) in or related to the facial tissues are irritated by the local development of chemical or structural abnormalities (see pp. 280–1), or when irritation of receptors in tissues located outside the face leads to reference of pain to the facial territory (see p. 296); but it may also present without overt evidence of such irritation as the clamant signal of a basic psychiatric disorder, or as an epileptic manifestation (see p. 297).

PERIPHERAL FACIAL PAIN SYSTEMS

With the foregoing considerations as background, the structural and functional features of the neurological systems whose activity gives rise to facial pain may now be reviewed, commencing with those that lie peripheral to the neuraxis.

Nociceptive Receptors in Facial Tissues

In spite of prolonged argument ever since 1895, there is now no doubt that most tissues of the body are equipped with a specific system of receptor nerve endings that are particularly sensitive to tissue damage, and which as such can be categorized as nociceptive receptors. In the facial tissues (as elsewhere) this system is represented by plexiform and freely-ending arrangements of unmyelinated nerve fibres that are distributed throughout the skin (fig. 1) and subcutaneous tissues, adipose tissue, fasciae, periosteum, the

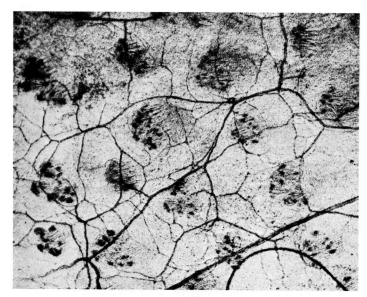

Fig. 1. The nociceptive system of plexiform unmyelinated nerve fibres in human skin. Corpuscular receptor end organs are distributed in the interstices of the network. Methylene blue preparation of biopsy specimen. × 100. From Weddel (1941).

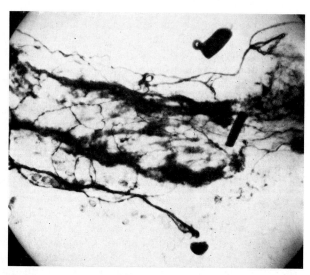

Fig. 2. The perivascular nociceptive system of plexiform unmyelinated nerve fibres in the adventitial sheath of a small subcutaneous blood vessel. Teased gold chloride preparation. × 225. From Wyke (1968).

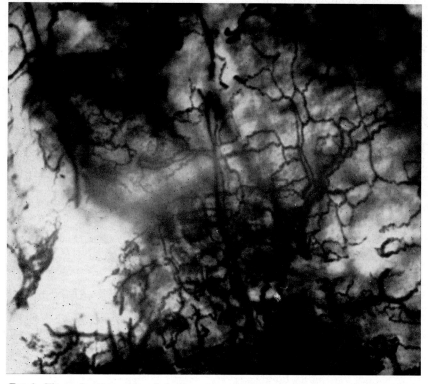

Fig. 3. The nociceptive system of plexiform unmyelinated nerve fibres ramifying through the superficial layers of the fibrous capsule of the temporomandibular joint. Teased gold chloride preparation of posterior joint capsule (external surface above and to right, synovial surface below and to left). × 250.

adventitia of the blood vessels (fig. 2) and the fibrous capsules and ligaments of the temporomandibular joints (fig. 3)—although not in the articular cartilage, synovial tissue or menisci in these joints (see p. 293).

In normal circumstances this receptor system is relatively (although not entirely) inactive: but its afferent activity is markedly enhanced when the unmyelinated nerve fibres comprising it are excited by the application of mechanical forces to the containing tissue that sufficiently deform or damage it (as with pressure, distension, abrasion, contusion or laceration), or by their exposure to the presence in the surrounding tissue fluid of irritating chemical substances (such as potassium ions, lactic acid, bradykinin and other kinins, 5-hydroxytryptamine and histamine) that are released from damaged, necrosing, inflamed or metabolically abnormal (and particularly, ischaemic) tissues. When the frequency of the afferent discharges evoked from the receptor endings in the skin by these stimuli (particularly the chemical agents) is relatively low, the sensory experience thereby provoked is that of itching, whilst higher-frequency discharges give rise to the emotional disorder of pain: thus it is that constant scratching of pruritic cutaneous lesions (which progressively increases the amount of locally damaged tissue) eventually renders them painful, after initially suppressing the itch on account of coincident stimulation of mechanoreceptors (see p. 287) located in the affected tissue.

Nociceptive Afferent Pathways from Facial Tissues

Afferent impulses from the nociceptive receptor systems in the facial tissues are transmitted into the central nervous system through small-diameter nerve fibres that traverse the related cranial and upper cervical nerves from their peripheral branches (see below)—although the ratio of the number of such fibres to that of the larger myelinated afferent fibres is less in these nerves than it is in most of the nerves of spinal origin. Most of these nociceptive afferent fibres are unmyelinated and less than 2 μ in diameter, but some are small myelinated fibres 2–5 μ in diameter—thus all the facial nociceptive afferents belong to the Group III range of nerve fibre diameters, upon which fact depends (*inter alia*) their differential sensitivity to local anaesthetic blockade, their slow conduction velocity and their low sensitivity to direct stimulation of the nerve trunks containing them. All such small diameter fibres are not exclusively activated by nociceptive stimulation, however, for afferent impulses can be evoked in fibres in the Group III diameter range (including in some unmyelinated fibres) by non-traumatic stimulation of peripheral tissues—but it may be that in man the nociceptive afferent fibres are different fibres from those in this same diameter range that respond to innocuous peripheral stimuli (such as tickling, for instance).

Neurosurgical experience extending over seventy years has amply demonstrated the topography of the peripheral distribution of the nociceptive afferent fibres in the nerves supplying the superficial tissues of the face, which is illustrated in fig. 4. The clinician's attention is particularly directed to the precise boundaries of the regions innervated from the ophthalmic, maxillary and mandibular branches of the trigeminal nerve (between which there is little overlap), and to the fact that the latter branch does not supply the tissues overlying the postero-lateral and inferior portions of the mandible—which tissues are innervated from the dorsal roots of the second and third cervical nerves. It should also be noted that the concha of the ear receives an additional innervation from the glossopharyngeal and vagus nerves, and that the latter (vagus) nerve contributes to the innervation of the posterior wall of the external auditory meatus. Some afferent fibres from the concha of the ear, as well as many from the blood vessels

in the face, also travel in the facial nerve (15 per cent of whose fibres are facial afferents) to enter its nervus intermedius root (their cell bodies being located in the geniculate ganglion). Details of the disposition of individual peripheral branches of the nerves supplying the face may be found in specialized neuro-anatomical works.

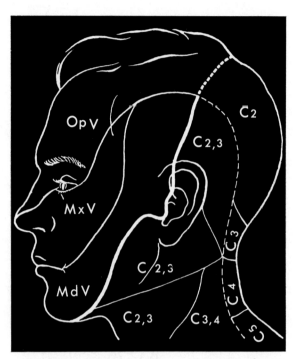

FIG. 4. The cranio-facial dermatomes. The diagram depicts the sectors of the face and head innervated from the ophthalmic (Op V), maxillary (Mx V) and mandibular (Md V) branches of the trigeminal nerve, and from the dorsal roots of the upper cervical nerves. (From Wyke (1968), redrawn and modified from Haymaker, W., and Woodhall, B. (1945), *Peripheral Nerve Injuries*. Philadelphia: Saunders.)

Irrespective of whether they enter the lower brain stem by way of the trigeminal (sensory root), facial (intermedius root), glossopharyngeal, vagus or upper cervical nerves, the afferent fibres from the nociceptive receptor systems in the facial tissues terminate by synapsing on cells located in the ipsilateral spinal nucleus of the fifth nerve (see p. 283), after traversing the spinal tract of the fifth nerve (fig. 5). The cell bodies of these small diameter afferent fibres are located respectively in the trigeminal ganglion, geniculate ganglion, jugular ganglion, ganglion nodosum and in the dorsal root ganglia of the second and third cervical nerves: in the trigeminal ganglion the cell bodies of fibres innervating the peri-oral tissues lie ventral to those innervating more peripheral regions of the face.

As the sensory root of the trigeminal nerve enters the pons, most of the myelinated fibres within it divide into an ascending and a descending branch. These latter branches turn caudally into the medulla oblongata along with the unmyelinated trigeminal afferents as the superficially located spinal tract of the fifth nerve (fig. 5), which is also joined (in the medulla) by small diameter afferents from the facial, glossopharyngeal and vagus nerves and in the

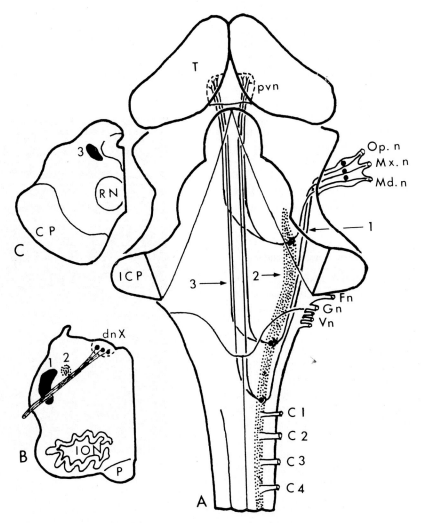

Fig. 5. Diagram illustrating the central projections of the nociceptive afferents from the oro-facial tissues within the lower brain stem—in longitudinal section (A), and in transverse sections of the medulla oblongata (B) and mesencephalon (C). Projections from the facial (Fn), glossopharyngeal (Gn), vagus (Vn) and cervical (C) nerves are omitted. (From Wyke (1968).)

Op.n.	ophthalmic branch of trigeminal nerve
Mx.n.	maxillary branch of trigeminal nerve
Md.n.	mandibular branch of trigeminal nerve
1	spinal tract of trigeminal nerve
2	spinal nucleus of trigeminal nerve
3	bulbothalamic tracts
pvn	posterior ventral nucleus of thalamus (T)
ICP	inferior cerebellar peduncle
P	medullary pyramid
ION	inferior olivary nucleus
dnX	dorsal vagal nucleus
RN	red nucleus
CP	cerebral peduncle

upper cervical spinal cord by similar afferents in the cervical nerves. Most of the fibres in the spinal tract are therefore thin and hence slowly-conducting, 90 per cent being less than 4 μ in diameter—although the thinnest fibres extend more caudally than the thicker fibres; and in spite of its name, it contains facial nociceptive afferents of non-trigeminal as well as of trigeminal origin. Within the tract—which extends caudally throughout the medulla oblongata into the dorso-lateral regions of the upper cervical spinal cord as far as the third cervical segment—

the fibres of trigeminal origin are somatotopically orientated (see fig. 5) in the dorso-ventral plane, those derived from the mandibular division lying dorsal to those of maxillary origin, with the fibres from the ophthalmic division being most ventrally located: furthermore, the cutaneous afferents are more superficially (i.e. laterally) placed in the tract than are the afferents from the deeper facial and oral tissues, whilst the afferents of non-trigeminal (that is, of nervus intermedius, glossopharyngeal and vagal) origin lie dorsal and caudal to the fibres of trigeminal origin. The

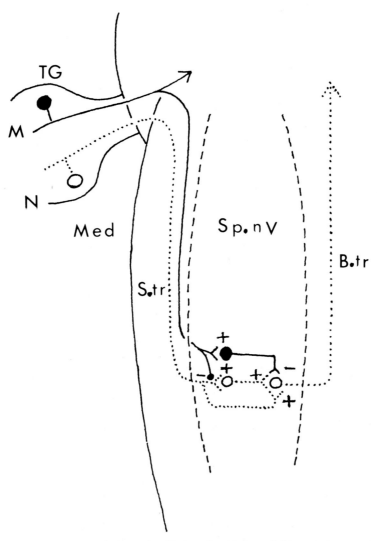

FIG. 6. Diagram illustrating a simplified version of the probable synaptic arrangements within the spinal nucleus of the trigeminal nerve. Description in text (plus signs indicate facilitatory synapses: minus signs indicate inhibitory synapses).

TG	trigeminal ganglion
N	oro-facial nociceptive afferents
M	ore-facial mechanoreceptor afferents
Med	medulla oblongata
S.tr	spinal tract of trigeminal
Sp.nV	spinal nucleus of trigeminal nerve
B.tr	bulbothalamic tract

more caudal parts of the tract are also joined by the afferents from the dorsal roots of the upper cervical nerves. Finally, it should be noted that only about 50 per cent of the smaller fibres in the spinal tract are central processes of afferents from the oro-facial tissues, for many of them are internuncial projections linking one part of the trigeminal nuclear complex with another.

On cytoarchitectonic grounds, the spinal nucleus of the fifth nerve—which lies immediately medial to the spinal tract (see fig. 5), and on whose cells the tract fibres establish terminal synaptic relations (fig. 6)—is subdivided rostrocaudally into a nucleus oralis, nucleus interpolaris and nucleus caudalis, the latter portion being the principal (although not the exclusive) site of synaptic projections from the nociceptive receptor systems in the oro-facial

tissues. Contrary to earlier views, the projections from the different regions of the face are not somatotopically distributed in a rostro-caudal direction within the spinal nucleus: instead, the nucleus contains a series of overlapping receptive fields whose individual vertical dimensions vary with different regions of the facial tissues. As is the case with nociceptive afferents in the dorsal horns of the spinal grey matter, however, most of the facial nociceptive afferents do not relay exclusively on to projection neurones within the spinal nucleus—which represent only 30–40 per cent of the cells in the nucleus caudalis (see p. 284)—but instead terminate additionally (fig. 6) on more numerous interneurones whose activity is also influenced by mechanoreceptor afferents from the oro-facial tissues: these interneurones (which appear to be the rostral homologue of the cells of the substantia gelatinosa Rolandi in the dorsal horns of the spinal grey matter) then relay to the projection cells, where they terminate presynaptically (in axo-axonic synapses) on the terminals of the collaterals of the myelinated and unmyelinated afferent fibres that do reach the projection neurones directly. These anatomical details (see fig. 6) are not merely of academic interest, for they suggest—because of their resemblance to the mode of termination of the dorsal root afferents in the spinal cord (see also p. 287)—that the centripetal projection into the central nervous system of afferent impulses from the peripheral nociceptive systems in the facial tissues is not an inevitable, direct on-line process, but is instead modulated (at the synapses within the spinal nucleus of the fifth nerve) by concurrent inputs from other (principally mechano-sensitive) oro-facial receptor systems delivered to the spinal nuclear synaptic systems by way of the collateral branches of the larger myelinated (i.e. mechanoreceptor) afferents (see also p. 287) entering the lower brain stem through the roots of the related cranial and upper cervical nerves, as well as by central mechanisms (see p. 288). This matter is considered further, in relation to its clinical implications, at p. 287.

CENTRAL FACIAL PAIN PROJECTION SYSTEMS

The activity that is eventually generated in the projection neurones of the spinal nucleus of the fifth nerve (which represent only about 40 per cent of the total number of cells in the nucleus caudalis) by the afferent systems just described is propagated rostrally in the brain stem in fibres of the bulbothalamic tracts (see figs. 5 and 7), which represent the axons of the spinal nuclear projection neurones. These fibres leave the nucleus on its medial aspect and turn rostrally in the medulla oblongata in two bundles: those derived from the rostral (oral and interpolar) regions of the spinal nucleus ascend mainly in the contralateral medial bulbothalamic tract that lies dorsal to the medial lemniscus, whereas those from the nucleus caudalis on each side ascend bilaterally and lie more laterally in the medulla (as the lateral bulbothalamic tract—see fig. 5B), just medial to the spinothalamic tracts—and surgical experience indicates that it is this latter bilateral tract system that is particularly involved in the production of facial pain. The bilaterality of this caudally-derived central facial projection system is also evidenced by the fact that performance of the operation of hemispherectomy (removal of one cerebral hemisphere) results in no difference in the pain sensitivity of the two sides of the face.

The fibres of the lateral bulbothalamic tract ascend from the medulla into the mesencephalon, where they lie (fig. 5C) just beneath the dorso-lateral surface, ventro-medial to the more superficially placed spinothalamic tract. Thereafter they proceed to the thalamus, within which they terminate by synapsing with cells located in the medial part of the posteroventral nucleus and in some of the intralaminar nuclei, and in the magnocellular portion of the medial geniculate body. Not all of the projection fibres from the caudal part of the spinal nucleus of the fifth nerve follow

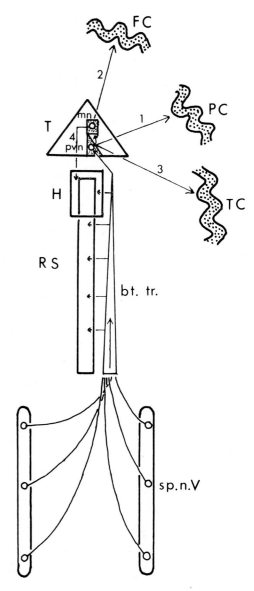

Fig. 7. Diagram depicting the reticular (RS), cortical (1,2,3) and hypothalamic dispersal of nociceptive afferent activity of oro-facial origin described in the text. (From Wyke (1968).)

sp.n.V	spinal nucleus of trigeminal nerve
bt.tr.	bulbothalamic tract
RS	brain stem reticular system
T	thalamus
pvn	posterior ventral nucleus of thalamus
mn	medical nucleus of thalamus
H	hypothalamus
FC	frontal cortex
PC	paracentral cortex
TC	temporal cortex

this course to the thalamus, however, for many of them terminate (see fig. 7) on cells in the longitudinal recticular system of the lower brain stem. Activity reaching the reticular cells by this route is then propagated further rostrally through a series of intermediate relays within the mesencephalic portion of the reticular system to the centre-median and intralaminar nuclear systems in the thalamus.

The above observations suggest that activity originating in nociceptive receptor systems located in the facial tissues may be propagated from the nucleus caudalis to the thalamus through two parallel pathways—one being a paucisynaptic system that terminates mainly in the medial posteroventral nuclear complex of the thalamus, and the other a multisynaptic system that terminates mainly in the centre-median and intralaminar thalamic nuclei; and it is tempting to equate the initial acute pain that rapidly follows peripheral nociceptive stimulation (so-called "fast" pain) with transmission through the former pathway, and the duller, more persisting aching pain that develops later (so-called "slow" pain) with transmission through the latter. However, it should be noted that there are no cells in any of the above-mentioned thalamic sites that respond uniquely to peripheral noxious stimulation (all of them being affected by both noxious and innocuous stimuli)—even though surgical lesions placed stereotactically in certain of these sites may sometimes result in temporary clinical relief of pain, and their direct electrical stimulation in animals and human subjects produces behavioural responses indicative of the experience of pain. In the light of present knowledge, then, it seems that evocation of the experience of facial pain is contingent upon production, in the cells of several of the thalamic nuclei, of a critical degree of activity—and that this is not merely a function of the discharge frequency of the nociceptive receptor systems in the facial tissues, but depends also upon the extent to which the centripetal transsynaptic flow of such activity is modulated (in the nucleus caudalis and in the thalamic nuclei) by coincident inputs from peripheral mechano-receptor afferent systems and by the activity of central projection systems to these synaptic sites (see pp. 287, 290).

Once an adequate degree of activity has been generated in the thalamic nuclei mentioned above by the inputs ascending to them from the spinal nucleus, it is dispersed therefrom (figs. 7, 8, 10) in four directions; and each member of this quadruple intracerebral projection system provides a specific component to the patient's experience of pain in the face, as follows:

1. The Perceptual Component

First (see figs. 7, 8 and 9), impulses reaching the postero-ventral nucleus of the thalamus (whether of nociceptive or mechanoreceptor origin) are projected therefrom (in the

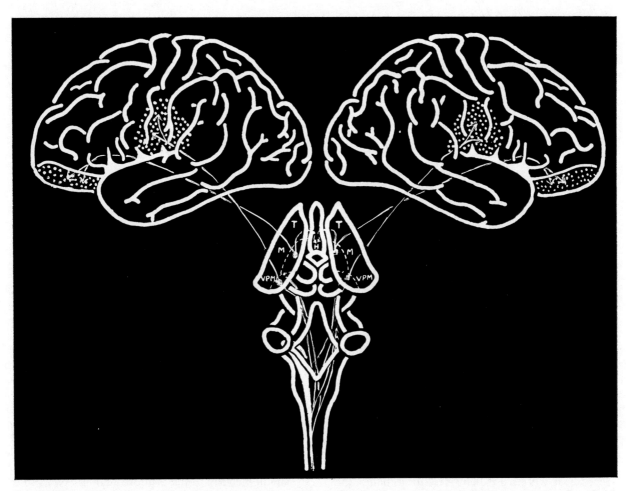

FIG. 8. Diagram illustrating the bilateral thalamo-cortical projections subserving the perceptual and affective components of oro-facial painful experience described in the text. The former passes from the medial portion of the posterior ventral nucleus (VPM) of the thalamus (T) to the inferior paracentral cortex (see also fig. 9): the latter from the medial thalamic nucleus (M) to the orbito-frontal cortex. (From Wyke (1958b).)

thalamo-cortical radiation traversing the posterior limb of the internal capsule) to the inferior paracentral and parietal regions of the cerebral cortex—and because of the bilaterality of the bulbothalamic projection system described at p. 284, both sides of the face relay to this cortical sector in each cerebral hemisphere. Activation of this somatotopically organized (see fig. 9) thalamo-cortical projection system leads to the patient's recognition (with varying degrees of accuracy) of the peripheral anatomical location of the painful stimulus, and of its physical nature

other modalities of oro-facial sensory experience). Furthermore, traumatic, infarctive or neoplastic lesions in the paracentral regions of the cerebral cortex do not impair a patient's awareness of the unpleasant nature of peripheral painful stimulation, although they seriously impair his capacity to recognize its anatomical location.

2. The Affective Component

A second set of projections passes from certain of the thalamic nuclei to the cortex of the frontal lobes in the

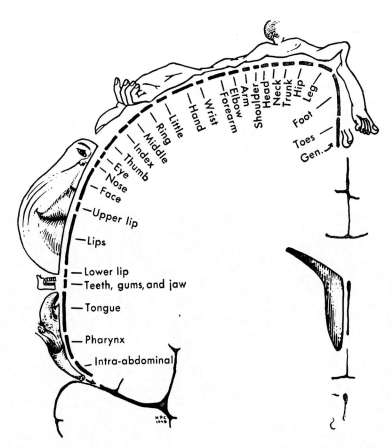

FIG. 9. Cortical homunculus illustrating the somatotopic organization of the oro-facial projection system from the thalamus to the paracentral cortex. From Penfield and Rasmussen (1950).

(i.e. whether pricking, pressing, bursting, stabbing, throbbing or burning)—which latter information is provided mainly by coincident stimulation of the non-nociceptive receptor systems located in the affected tissues.

Arrival of impulses in the inferior paracentral regions of the cerebral cortex may thus be said to provide the perceptual component of the patient's painful experience—that is to say, his knowledge of where in his face the painful site is located and of what nature the causative stimulus is. Activation of this particular thalamo-cortical projection system does not, however, of itself give rise to the emotional disturbance (see p. 279) that patients describe as pain; nor does direct electrical stimulation of the inferior paracentral regions of the cerebral cortex in unanaesthetized patients evoke the experience of pain in the face (although it evokes

thalamo-frontal radiation—of which the inferior portion, passing from the dorsomedial nucleus of the thalamus to the orbital cortex of the ipsilateral frontal lobe (figs. 7 and 8), is of major significance in relation to pain. Within the thalamus, intrathalamic connexions link the various relay nuclei in which the bulbothalamic tracts terminate (see p. 284) to the dorsomedial nucleus, whose efferent fibres ascend through the anterior limb of the internal capsule to (inter alia) the orbitofrontal cortex, which is part of the limbic system. Impulses reaching the thalamic nuclei from the spinal nucleus of the fifth nerve are thus propagated simultaneously to the orbitofrontal as well as to the paracentral regions of the cerebral cortex (see figs. 7 and 8); and it seems that it is activation of this former thalamocortical projection system that gives rise to the specifically unpleasant emotional state that patients complain of as pain (see p. 279)—in short, it is by its evocation of an adequate degree of activity in the orbitofrontal projection system that a peripheral tissue disturbance "hurts".

This proposal receives support from neurosurgical observations on the effects of selective interruption of the orbitofrontal thalamic projection system in patients afflicted with intractable pain. This system may be interrupted at its distal end by the operation of orbito-frontal leucotomy, or at its origin in the medial thalamic nuclei by the operation of stereotactic thalamotomy; in either instance the procedure (when successful) relieves the emotional distress of which the patient complains (and thus his need for powerful analgesic drugs) without removing his perceptual awareness of a bodily abnormality. In short, after such operations the patient is still aware that something is wrong with some part of his body but no longer complains that it hurts him, because the surgical procedure has specifically dissected out the principal central neurological system whose abnormal activity is responsible for the affective disorder (see p. 279) that patients describe as pain.

3. The Memory Component

A third cortical projection system links certain of the thalamic nuclei on each side (fig. 7) to the cortex of the related temporal lobe, in the ventro-medial parts of which the recent and long-term memory storage systems are located. This thalamo-cortical projection system is also activated, along with the other two already mentioned, by the arrival within the thalamus of afferent impulses in the bulbothalamic tracts; and in this way a subject builds up his memory of past oro-facial painful experiences. Clinical and personal experience (as well as experimental studies) suggests, however, that long-term memory retention of painful experiences depends not so much upon the intensity of an individual painful episode as upon the length of time it lasts or the frequency with which it is repeated.

4. The Visceral-hormonal Reflex Component

A fourth (non-cortical) projection system passes from the thalamic nuclei to the subjacent hypothalamic nuclei located in the ventral diencephalon, which also receive afferent inputs (*inter alia*) from cells in the reticular system and from various parts of the limbic system. As it is the activity of cells in various nuclear sub-groups of the hypothalamus that controls the efferent activity in the sympathetic and parasympathetic outflows, and as some of these cells also synthesize the hypophysoportal hormones that control the secretory activity of the anterior lobe of the pituitary gland (as well as the antidiuretic and oxytocic hormones), it will be apparent that these subcortical projections to the hypothalamus provide a means whereby afferent activity in the bulbothalamic tract system may evoke the complex of visceral reflex effects (*e.g.* on the pupil, and on the cardiovascular and gastro-intestinal systems) and hormonal changes that are associated with the experience of pain.

AWARENESS OF FACIAL PAIN

The quadripartite dispersal within the brain of activity of nociceptive origin that has been described indicates that each thalamic projection system provides a specific component to the global experience of pain. But all clinicians are aware (contrary to some early experimental claims based on studies of so-called "pain thresholds") that individual patients vary in the intensity of their experience of chronic pain from time to time in the course of the day; that different patients with apparently comparable pathological lesions giving rise to pain report (and manifest) widely differing degrees of suffering; and that the intensity of pain suffered varies widely with emotional state, with the extent to which the patient's attention may be occupied by concentration on daily tasks, and in response to suggestion.

Nevertheless, these everyday aspects of painful experience have always been ignored in the traditional view of pain as a sensory modality inevitably evoked by activity in a direct on-line projection system from peripheral pain receptors into the brain (see p. 284): furthermore, nowhere within the fourfold intracerebral projection system outlined above is there any neurological mechanism capable of explaining these seeming vagaries in a patient's awareness of pain. Fortunately, however, a series of neuro-anatomical, neurophysiological and neuropharmacological studies in the last decade has thrown considerable light on these clinically important matters by revealing that the experience of pain may be modulated in its intensity by concurrent activity in peripheral and in central neurological systems that play upon the nociceptive afferent systems at various synaptic stages in their course within the neuraxis.

Peripheral Modulation of Awareness of Pain

All human beings (and many animals) are instinctively aware that rubbing or pressing on a painful tissue may temporarily abort the pain. Massage, vibration and compression of tissues—all of which may be employed for analgesic purposes—are procedures that stimulate the rapidly- and slowly-adapting mechanoreceptors located therein; and there is now substantial evidence to show that the excitability of the synapses at which small-diameter nociceptive afferents relay as they enter the central nervous system is modulated by on-going afferent activity reaching the same synapses from collateral branches of the larger-diameter myelinated afferents innervating mechano-receptors located in the same or related regions of tissue (see fig. 6). Such collaterals of mechanoreceptor afferents subtend facilitatory synapses on interneurones as they enter the neuraxis (which, in the case of the dorsal horns in the spinal grey matter, are the cells of the substantia gelatinosa located in lamina II), whose axons in turn relay presyn-aptically (fig. 6), in inhibitory axo-axonic synapses, on the terminals of the nociceptive afferents subtended on the central projection neurones that transmit activity into the brain. Thus it is clear that centripetal transmission of activity originating in peripheral nociceptive systems is not merely a function of the intensity of their stimulation, but is continuously determined by the frequency of concurrent afferent discharges from related mechanoreceptors—whose activity normally suppresses the onward flow of nociceptive impulses at their first synaptic relay in the neuraxis.

As already indicated at pp. 283–4, similar neuro-anatomical arrangements (see fig. 6) have been shown to exist in the spinal nucleus of the fifth nerve; and neuro-physiological studies have revealed that comparable presynaptic inhibitory modulation of the centripetal flow of nociceptive impulses through this nucleus is effected from mechanoreceptors in the oro-facial tissues via internuncial neurones in the nucleus that are homologous (see p. 283) to

lost until (and if) they regenerate; and selective alterations of function in trigeminal ganglion cells related to facial and oral mechanoreceptor afferents have been implicated in the mechanisms of production of trigeminal neuralgia (see also p. 295). Furthermore, as increasing age in late adult life is associated with progressive degeneration of the larger-diameter (mechanoreceptor) myelinated afferent fibres in peripheral nerves throughout the body, the consequent loss of their central synaptic inhibitory effects may go some way towards explaining the diminishing pain tolerance that characterizes middle-aged and elderly patients, and the greater incidence of trigeminal neuralgia in older than in younger subjects.

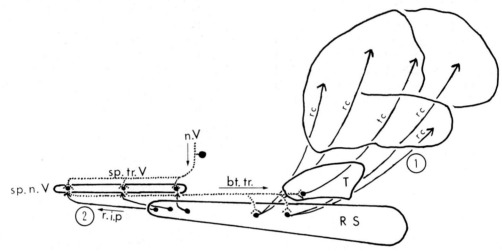

FIG. 10. Diagram illustrating the rostral (1) and caudal (2) reticular projection systems involved in the modulation of awareness of oro-facial pain described in the text. (From Wyke (1968).)

n.V	sensory root of trigeminal nerve
sp.tr.V	spinal root of trigeminal nerve
sp.n.V	spinal nucleus of trigeminal nerve
bt.tr.	bulbothalamic tract
T	thalamus
tc	thalamo-cortical projections
RS	brain stem reticular system
rc	reticulo-cortical projection system
r.i.p.	caudal inhibitory reticular projection to spinal nucleus

the cells of the substantia gelatinosa in the spinal cord. It should also be noted that whilst mechanoreceptor afferent activity generally inhibits the onward flow of concurrent impulses of nociceptive origin, in certain circumstances (which influence the precise frequency of mechanoreceptor afferent discharge) it may facilitate synaptic transmission from nociceptive inputs.

While much still remains to be done in developing the applications of these experimental data to the various facial pain syndromes encountered in clinical practice (see p. 290 and Table 1), realization of the biphasic (inhibitory and facilitatory) modulating influence of peripheral mechanoreceptor activity upon centripetal transmission of oro-facial nociceptive receptor activity has already proved helpful. Thus, it has been suggested that the extreme cutaneous hyperalgesia that characterizes post-herpetic neuralgia is the result of selective viral damage to the parent nerve cells of mechanoreceptor afferents, whose normal central synaptic inhibitory effects are therefore

Central Modulation of Awareness of Pain

In addition to the modulating influence of peripheral mechanoreceptor inputs that has just been described, awareness of facial pain is further modulated within the brain by three central projection systems that influence the sequential centripetal propagation of impulses of nociceptive origin through the synapses in the spinal nucleus of the fifth nerve, in the thalamic nuclei and in the cerebral cortex itself.

(1). **Within the caudal spinal nucleus,** onward propagation of impulses is influenced through projections that reach it from the nearby medullary portion of the brain stem reticular system, and from the paracentral regions of the cerebral cortex.

Axons pass from large neurones in the caudal reticular system (fig. 10) to synapse with the interneurones in the nucleus caudalis (see p. 283 and fig. 6) that exert presynaptic inhibitory effects on the facial nociceptive afferent terminals, which interneurones they stimulate. As this centrifugal reticular projection system is continuously active throughout life, it will be clear that it normally restricts the onward flow into the brain of impulses from the peripheral nociceptive systems located in the oro-facial tissues, thereby reinforcing the similar effect of inputs from the mechanoreceptors in the same tissues (described on p. 287) and so suppressing awareness of nociceptive stimulation in the facial tissues.

The normal inhibitory effect of this reticular cascade system is augmented when a subject's attention is diverted away from his oro-facial tissues; when sleep supervenes; when hypnosis is induced; when hysterical anaesthesia develops; or when the blood concentration of catecholamines becomes very high (as in states of great emotional tension). These facts may explain (inter alia) why distraction diminishes awareness of facial pain, why hypnotic suggestion is often effective in producing degrees of analgesia adequate for oro-facial surgery, and why soldiers in battle (with consequent high blood concentrations of catecholamines) may sustain severe facial injuries without complaining of pain. It is also relevant for the clinician to note that numbers of drugs (if administered in appropriate doses) may selectively stimulate the reticular neurones that operate this inhibitory system, and thereby reduce a patient's awareness of facial pain without diminishing his general state of alertness. Examples of such drugs are methylamphetamine, chlorpromazine (Largactil), diazepam (Valium), morphine and its analogues, carbamazepine (Tegretol) and diphenylhydantoinate (Phenytoin; Epanutin; Dilantin); and it is partly for this reason that chlorpromazine and diazepam are such useful premedicating agents preparatory to oro-facial surgery, and that carbamazepine and diphenylhydantoinate often effectively depress a patient's awareness of the attacks of facial pain in trigeminal neuralgia (see p. 295)—which latter effect is exerted more powerfully by carbamazepine than by diphenylhydantoinate.

Conversely, a reduction in the centrifugal inhibitory effect of the caudal reticular system enhances the intensity of on-going painful experiences, and also increases the probability that a particular peripheral stimulus (whether mechanical or chemical) operating in the facial tissues will evoke an attack of pain—examplified, for instance, by the provocation of attacks of trigeminal neuralgia by relatively gentle mechanical stimulation of "trigger zones" in the oro-facial territory (see also p. 295). Such a situation arises with exposure to sudden, intense painful stimuli that canalize attention on the oro-facial tissues; with specific direction of the patient's attention to those tissues in the absence of distracting stimuli; and following the administration of small doses of barbiturates or ethyl ether. It is for this latter reason that patients suffering from chronic facial pain, or from repeated attacks of paroxysmal facial pain, should never be given barbiturates (such as quinalbarbitone (Seconal), pentobarbitone (Nembutal) or phenobarbitone (Luminal)) for soporific or sedative purposes—for then the facial pain will be intensified to the point where it becomes excruciating. For the same reason, anaesthesia should never be induced in patients with facial pain (due to facial injuries, for example) by slow intravenous injection of thiopentone (Pentothal)—instead, the previously calculated dose of thiopentone should be injected as a single bolus as quickly as possible.

In addition to the modulating influence of this reticular projection system, which may in turn be influenced through projections from several sectors of the cerebral cortex to reticular neurones, there is also evidence that more direct projections from the paracentral regions of the cerebral cortex (especially in the contralateral hemisphere) may exert inhibitory effects on transmission through the synaptic systems in the spinal nucleus of the trigeminal nerve. Whilst this latter effect (which is mainly presynaptic) is exerted more powerfully on synaptic transmission of mechanoreceptor afferent activity through the rostral portions of the trigeminal nuclear system, it also operates on facial nociceptive relays through the caudal portion of the spinal nucleus and thus modifies awareness of facial pain. Clearly, then, the regions of cerebral cortex to which the "perceptual" projections (see p. 285) of the facial afferent system are directed exert a negative feed-back influence on the centripetal transmission of activity within this system—which process may assist in "sharpening" the subjective localization of the evocative stimulus within the oro-facial tissues.

(2). Within the thalamic relay nuclei, additional modulation of the centripetal propagation of bulbothalamic tract activity is effected through projections to the thalamic relay nuclei from the cerebral cortex. These corticothalamic projections arise mainly from neurones in the inferior paracentral regions of the cerebral cortex and descend through the internal capsule to synapse with the thalamic neurones (see p. 284) on which the ascending bulbothalamic fibres relay, on which neurones they exert long-lasting postsynaptic inhibitory effects. Similar (as well as presynaptic) inhibitory effects on thalamic synaptic transmission of afferent activity may also be exerted from more widely dispersed cortical neurones in the frontal, parietal and temporal regions and from other parts of the limbic system.

It seems, therefore, that neurones in each of the cortical regions to which centripetal bulbothalamic activity is projected to evoke the perceptual, emotional and memory aspects of facial painful experiences (see pp. 285-7) exert a retrograde inhibitory (negative feed-back) influence on the thalamic sites through which such activity is relayed to the cerebral cortex, and thereby "damp down" awareness of facial pain. However, the precise circumstances in which these corticofugal inhibitory projections to the thalamic relay nuclei operate is still unknown—although loss of their normal inhibitory influence because of interruption of their pathways by internal capsular or parathalamic lesions (such as may occur in patients with cerebral vascular disease, or following intracerebral stereotaxic surgery) may have something to do with the production of the syndrome of so-called "thalamic pain".

(3). Within the cerebral cortex, the excitability of the neurones on which the thalamocortical projections (see p. 285) terminate is continuously modulated by ascending activity that reaches them (see fig. 10) from neurones located in the rostral portions of the brain stem reticular system, via the reticulocortical projection system. The influence of this continuously-active system on cortical neurones is generally facilitatory, so that the excitability of cortical neurones at any moment is a function of the prevailing frequency of reticulocortical discharge—and for this reason this system was originally designated as the 'reticular activating system'. More recent study, however, has led to some modification of the original anatomical implications of this term—although the functional concept of cortical activation provided from neurones located in the rostral brain stem has been thoroughly validated, both in experimental and in clinical contexts.

It now seems that this cortical activating system is derived from rostral reticular and "non-specific" thalamic (for example, intralaminar—see p. 284) neurones, and functions as a driving (or "alerting") mechanism for the synaptic systems within the cortical mantle, to which it normally contributes an unceasing but varying stream of facilitatory impulses. Thus an individual's prevailing global awareness of his environment, and the intensity of all his sensory and emotional experiences (including pain), is continuously conditioned by the degree of activity prevailing in this system. As afferent activity from nociceptive systems in the oro-facial tissues is channelled into the brain stem reticular system (see p. 284) and into the intralaminar thalamic nuclei (see p. 284), and thereby influences cortical activation, it will be clear that the state of excitability obtaining in the cells of the reticular system and intralaminar thalamic nuclei at the time when impulses are delivered thereto from the spinal nucleus of the fifth nerve will, from moment to moment, influence the intensity of a patient's painful oro-facial experiences. In this connexion, it is relevant to note that nociceptive stimulation in the peripheral distribution of the trigeminal nerve has been shown to be a particularly potent means of evoking augmented activity in the reticular system and in its cortical activating projections.

Experimental and clinical studies extending over the last fifteen years have shown that many afferent, metabolic, hormonal and pharmacological influences, too numerous to describe in detail here, may produce moment-to-moment fluctuations in the excitability of reticular and other cortical-activating neurones—and thus in the intensity of awareness of pain. Thus, cortical activation is enhanced (and pain is therefore intensified) in states of moderate anxiety; by a moderate increase in the blood concentration of catecholamines; by moderate degrees of hypercarbia; and by the intake or administration of moderate amounts of alcohol, caffeine (in the form of tea or coffee), dextro-amphetamine (*Benzedrine*), cannabis indica (marijuana) and lysergic acid diethylamide (LSD-50). Conversely cortical activation is reduced (and pain is diminished) by emotional tranquillity (induced by suggestion, for instance); by the onset of sleep; by hypocarbia (induced by hyperventilation, for instance); by the intake or administration of large amounts of alcohol; and by the administration of agents such as meperidine (*Pethidine*) and the volatile and non-volatile general anaesthetic agents.

As the rostral cortical activating system projects (*inter alia*) to the orbito-frontal, inferior paracentral and temporal sectors of the cerebral cortex (fig. 10), it follows that

should afferent impulses from facial nociceptive receptors be delivered into the brain stem at a time when reticular excitability is augmented for any of the reasons mentioned above, then the facial pain will be felt to be intense, it will be relatively well localized within the facial tissues and it will be likely to be remembered vividly: on the other hand, should the same afferent input enter the brain stem when reticular excitability is diminished the pain will be felt to be less severe, it will be poorly localized, and memory of the experience will be poor and of short duration. In this way, then, the intensity of the emotional experience of facial pain, the precision of its perceptual localization within the face and the vividness with which it is remembered are all conditioned by the degree of activity prevailing in the rostral activating projections to the orbito-frontal, inferior paracentral, and temporal regions of the cerebral cortex respectively—and thus are not solely determined by the intensity of the peripheral nociceptive stimulus (whether it be mechanical or chemical). It is hardly surprising, then, that individual pain tolerance is a widely varying parameter, and that it does not necessarily correlate with the relatively constant pain threshold (see p. 279).

CLINICAL VARIETIES OF FACIAL PAIN

In the light of the foregoing observations, it is convenient —and apposite for diagnostic and therapeutic purposes— to classify facial pain into four main categories in terms of the neurological mechanisms whose disordered activity may give rise to the experience of pain in the oro-facial tissues. These groups, and their various subdivisions, are summarized in Table 1 and will now be discussed *seriatim*.

TABLE 1

CLINICAL CATEGORIES OF FACIAL PAIN

I. **Primary**
　(1) Dental and periodontal
　(2) Cutaneous, mucosal (oral cavity and sinuses), periosteal and fascial
　(3) Vascular (superficial and deep)
　(4) Articular (temporomandibular)

II. **Secondary**
　(1) Peripheral (cranial)
　(2) Peripheral (cervical)
　(3) Central

III. **Referred**
　(1) From teeth
　(2) From nose and paranasal sinuses
　(3) From heart

IV. **Ictal**
　(1) Sensory epilepsy

Primary Facial Pain

Primary facial pain is defined as pain experienced in the oro-facial tissues as a result of direct mechanical and/or chemical irritation of one or more of the nociceptive receptor systems located therein (see p. 279)—in other words, the pain is felt in tissues where the lesion is located.

Within this category, further subdivision is possible in terms of the particular tissues containing the irritated nociceptive nerve endings.

Dental and Periodontal Pain

In clinical practice this is the commonest of all varieties of oro-facial pain, and its differential diagnosis and treatment are certainly the province of the dental and oral surgeon. It is not discussed here, however, as it does not fall within the purview of this Chapter (being dealt with elsewhere in this volume): but physicians and surgeons generally should remember to include a careful examination of the teeth and their related tissues in any investigation of pain in the face.

Cutaneous, Mucosal, Periosteal and Fascial Pain

The skin covering the face, the mucous membrane lining the nose, paranasal sinuses and mouth, the periosteum covering the facial skeleton, and the fascial sheaths of the muscles and salivary glands are all provided with the plexiform system of nociceptive nerve endings described at p. 279 and illustrated in fig. 1. Direct irritation of this system in the facial skin by trauma (involving contusion, laceration or burning) or infection (as with abscesses or cellulitis); in the mucosa by infective lesions (as sinusitis or nasal infections); in the periosteum (as a result of facial fractures or osteomyelitis); or as a result of involvement of any of these tissues by ulcers or neoplasms, will lead to facial pain. In like manner, irritation of the nociceptive plexiform system in the parotid fascia in the presence of acute parotitis or of malignant neoplasms of the parotid gland may lead to primary facial pain, as may distension of this (or more often, of the submandibular) gland resulting from sialolithiasis.

Clearly, the management of any of these varieties of facial pain involves direct treatment of the painful lesion where possible—if necessary by surgery or with antibiotics, or a combination of both; or with radiotherapy, in the case of appropriate neoplasms. But temporary relief of the pain for periods of varying duration may be obtained by infiltration of the appropriate afferent nerves supplying the affected regions of the face (see fig. 4) with local anaesthetic agents or with alcohol, or by the administration of analgesic agents such as acetylsalicylic acid (*Aspirin*), meperidine (*Pethidine*), codeine or morphine. In the presence of intractable lesions, more prolonged relief may be afforded by surgical division of the related cranial nerve branches (peripheral neurectomy), or of their central projections in the sensory root (rhizotomy) or spinal tract of the fifth nerve (tractotomy), or by the performance of orbitofrontal leucotomy or thalamotomy (see p. 287).

Vascular Facial Pain

Facial pain of vascular origin (Table 1) is far more common in clinical practice than is generally realized (either by doctors or dentists), and arises from mechanical or chemical irritation of the plexiform system of unmyelinated nerve fibres that is embedded in the adventitial sheaths of the blood vessels supplying the superficial facial tissues and the deeper mandibular musculature (see p. 280 and fig. 2). For clinical purposes, these two groups of vascular nociceptive receptors can be treated separately, in terms of their respective contributions to superficial or deep vascular facial pain.

Superficial Vascular Facial Pain. This is evoked by irritation of the receptor system related to the superficial blood vessels (mainly branches of the supra-orbital, facial or superficial temporal arteries) that supply the skin and

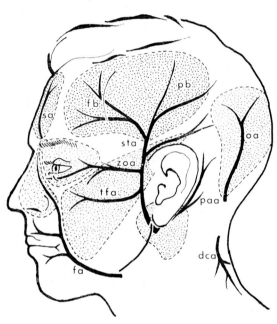

FIG. 11. The principal sectors of pain distribution in the face and head in patients suffering from superficial vascular pain (see text), in relation to the superficial arterial system of the head. (From Wyke (1968).)

sa	supra-orbital artery
fa	facial artery
sta	superficial temporal artery
fb	frontal branches
pb	parietal branches
zoa	zygomatico-orbital artery
tfa	transverse facial artery
paa	posterior auricular artery
oa	occipital artery
dca	descending cervical artery

subcutaneous tissues of the face (fig. 11). Such irritation occurs in patients with primary vascular disease (as in arteriosclerosis, periarteritis nodosa and temporal arteritis, for example), but more often results from episodic excessive dilatation of these blood vessels (as in facial migraine—see below).

Whilst the former varieties of superficial vascular facial pain (namely, those associated with vascular pathology) are readily recognized by the competent physician or surgeon, the clinical syndrome of facial migraine often goes unrecognized for what it really is—largely because the anatomical distribution of the pain outlined in his own face by the patient does not have a dermatomal distribution (see fig. 4), but instead is distributed in the vascular territory of one or more of the branches of the superficial facial arterial system (as indicated in fig. 11). For this reason, patients with this complaint may be labelled as "hysterical", or have their condition designated by an enormous variety of names by clinicians working in different fields—twenty representative examples of which, culled from the literature, are listed in Table 2.

TABLE 2

SOME DESIGNATIONS OF SUPERFICIAL VASCULAR FACIAL PAIN*

Psychogenic facial pain	Autonomic faciocephalgia
Hysterical facial neuralgia	Sympatheticalgia
Atypical facial neuralgia	Sphenopalatine neuralgia
Idiopathic facial neuralgia	Petrosal neuralgia
Facial causalgia	Vidian neuralgia
Facial migraine	Ciliary neuralgia
Migraine variant	Charlin's syndrome
Cluster headache	Sluder's syndrome
Periodic migrainous neuralgia	Horton's syndrome
Histaminic cephalgia	Anaesthesia dolorosa

* After Kabler (1965) and Wyke (1968).

This variety of vascular facial pain can be recognized diagnostically, however, by the fact that it often wakes the patient up from sleep (when the facial blood vessels are widely dilated); that it may occur in other situations (such as physical exercise or exposure to radiant heat) that lead to dilatation of the facial vasculature; that it is provoked in situations that increase vascular pressures in the face (as by bending the head downwards, or prolonged bouts of coughing); and by the fact that one or more of the superficial facial arteries is often tender to pressure. Furthermore, patients often discover for themselves that attacks of this variety of facial pain (like some forms of cranial migraine) may be provoked by eating certain tyramine-containing foodstuffs (such as cheese or chocolate), by the ingestion of alcohol, or (in women) by taking oestrogen-containing oral contraceptive agents. Attacks of such pain are also often accompanied by other evidences of vasodilatation in the oro-facial region—such as unilateral nasal obstruction and/or watery rhinorrhoea, unilateral conjunctival injection, lachrymation, salivation, or erythema in the affected region of the face. These diagnostic features are further reinforced by demonstration that an attack of facial pain may be aborted by digital compression of the ipsilateral common carotid artery, or by administration (preferably in aerosol or inhalant nasal spray form) of a directly-acting vasoconstrictor drug such as ergotamine tartrate.

If correctly diagnosed, this condition of facial migraine may be treated (if attacks of pain are infrequent) by use of a nasal inhalant preparation of ergotamine tartrate at the onset of an attack; or if attacks are frequent, they may be warded off by daily oral administration (in maintenance doses of 6–12 mg. per day) of methysergide maleate (*Deseril; Sansert*), or of clonidine hydrochloride (*Dixarit*) in daily divided doses totalling 50–150 μg. Such medication should be carried out only by an experienced physician, however, because of a variety of side-effects that may be produced by these drugs—most serious of which, in the case of methysergide, is retroperitoneal fibrosis that may lead to ureteric obstruction.

The potent therapeutic effect of methysergide is of particular interest in relation to the possible mechanism of production of paroxysmal superficial vascular facial pain (*i.e.* facial migraine), in view of the fact that this drug is ineffective in aborting an attack of such pain once it has begun (in contrast to the immediate effect of the direct vasoconstrictive ergotamine derivatives), although it is highly effective as a prophylactic agent when taken regularly in daily maintenance doses. Methysergide is a powerful antagonist of the arterial vasoconstrictor effect of 5-hydroxtryptamine; and it has been shown (in patients with cranial vascular migraine) that attacks of headache are preceded for several days by a gradual rise and are then precipitated by an abrupt fall (of between 45 and 60 per cent) in the plasma concentration of 5-hydroxytryptamine —and that it is this latter fall that results in the marked dilatation of the scalp blood vessels that produces the headache. The clinical histories and physical appearance of patients afflicted with facial migraine suggest that a similar chemical mechanism may be involved in the sudden dilatation of the facial blood vessels that gives rise to their pain (and in the increasing pallor in the affected region of the face that heralds the onset of pain by two or three days); and it is probable that the protective effect of methysergide (which itself has no direct action on blood vessels) results in its antagonism of the action of 5-hydroxytryptamine on the smooth musculature of sensitized regions of the facial vasculature—thereby preventing abrupt (and painful) changes in their diameter.

It is also relevant at this point to reiterate (as already noted at p. 281) that many of the afferent nerve fibres from the nociceptive receptor system in the walls of the superficial facial blood vessels (see fig. 2) project to the caudal end of the spinal nucleus of the fifth nerve by way of the nervus intermedius root of the facial nerve—which they reach by traversing the nerve of the pterygoid canal, the sphenopalatine ganglion, the greater superficial petrosal nerve and the geniculate ganglion. This may explain why pain sensitivity persists in the subcutaneous tissues of the face in the presence of complete skin surface analgesia resulting from trigeminal nerve block or section; why patients with facial migraine who are mistakenly diagnosed as suffering from trigeminal neuralgia and subjected in consequence to alcohol injection or section of the trigeminal nerve continue to have attacks of pain in superficially analgesic regions of the face (the so-called syndrome of "anaesthesia dolorosa"); and why some surgeons have claimed that this type of facial pain (to which they attach various of the names listed in Table 2) may sometimes be relieved by sphenopalatine ganglionectomy, or division of the Vidian or petrosal nerves—which surgical procedures should not, of course, be carried out on patients who are in fact suffering from facial migraine.

Deep Vascular Facial Pain. The deep variety of vascular facial pain is so designated because it arises from irritation of the perivascular nerve plexuses in the adventitia of the blood vessels (see p. 280) ramifying within the mandibular muscles, usually (as with muscles elsewhere) as a result of their exposure to abnormal concentrations of muscle metabolites (see also p. 281) in the surrounding tissue fluid. As with the afferents from superficial facial blood vessels (see p. 292), many of those derived from the nociceptive receptor system related to the intramuscular blood vessels enter the brain stem through the nervus intermedius branch of the facial nerve. Such pain is always clearly distinguished by patients from pain of cutaneous or superficial vascular origin because it feels "deep" in the face or jaws and because it has a dull, aching quality that is all its own: it may be localized in a single muscle or part of a muscle or be diffused through a number of muscles, and the affected musculature is tender to pressure and hurts on attempted movement while the pain is present and for varying periods (which may last several hours) after it has gone.

This type of facial pain is also very common in clinical practice, and is encountered most often as a result of localized mandibular muscle spasm engendered reflexly by irritating (and especially inflammatory) lesions located in various parts of the oro-facial territory—especially the teeth and periodontal tissues, the paranasal sinuses, the external auditory meatus and the temporomandibular joints. It is also a frequent cause of the facial pain (usually bilateral) that is experienced by persistently anxious patients and by patients with persisting bruxism and with trismus. Figure. 12 indicates the characteristic distribution of this type of pain (and deep tenderness) when produced by temporalis [A] and masseter [B] muscle spasm—pterygoid spasm leads to pain felt deep in the throat below the ear and behind the angle of the mandible.

In many of the circumstances mentioned the more intense pain is often experienced (misleadingly) by the patient in the affected muscles, and not in the site of primary pathological change; for the persisting muscle spasm is a self-reinforcing process, due to the increasing accumulation of irritant metabolites in the tissue fluid of the hyperactive muscles that leads reflexly to further spasm and limitation of movement, and gradual intensification of the myalgic pain. For diagnostic purposes, however, the muscular origin of the pain is readily disclosed (if need be) by electromyographic demonstration of excessive motor unit activity in the muscles located in the painful regions of the face: whilst confirmation of its reflex origin is readily provided by the immediate abolition of this excess motor unit activity (and slower disappearance of the pain) that is produced by local anaesthetic blockade of the afferent nerve fibres that innervate the site of primary abnormality.

In dealing with this particular variety of primary facial pain, then, it is clear that treatment must be directed at removing or correcting the underlying cause of the reflex muscle spasm (wherever and whatever it may be), and not at the muscles themselves—even though these may be the

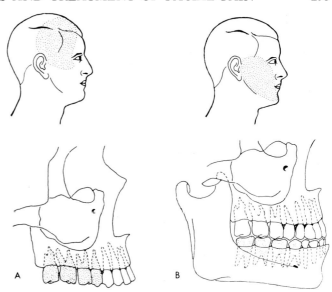

FIG. 12. The common areas of distribution of pain and tenderness in patients suffering from deep vascular facial pain (see text). (From Wyke (1968).) A. Pain distribution associated with reflex temporalis muscle spasm resulting from irritation of receptors or afferent nerve fibres related to the posterior maxillary teeth. B. Pain distribution associated with reflex masseter muscle spasm resulting from irritation of receptors or afferent nerve fibres related to the posterior mandibular teeth.

site of the pain of which the patient complains on presentation.

Temporomandibular Articular Pain

The temporomandibular joint tissues make a substantial contribution to the production of facial pain—not only because abnormal activity of the various receptor systems located therein may lead to painful reflex spasm in some part of the mandibular musculature (as described above), but also because mechanical or chemical irritation of the nociceptive receptor system related to the joint tissues themselves (see below) may lead directly to primary articular pain (Table 1).

As perusal of the literature will readily indicate, the subject of tempromandibular joint pain has long been in a state of extreme confusion from a clinical point of view—but some of this confusion can fortunately now be resolved in the light of neuro-anatomical, neurophysiological and clinical neurological studies of this joint system that have been made in the last decade. These studies indicate that the nociceptive system of each temporomandibular joint consists of a dense plexus of unmyelinated nerve fibres that weaves (with regionally varying density) throughout the fibrous capsule of the joint (fig. 3) and the related fat pads: this plexus is most dense in the posterior portion of the fibrous capsule and in the small para-articular fat pad (fig. 13) related thereto. As in all other synovial joints in the body, no nerve endings of this (or any other) variety are present in the articular cartilages, menisci or synovial tissue in the temporomandibular joints (in spite of frequent claims to the contrary)—which tissues, therefore, can never serve as a source of primary articular pain. The small diameter afferent fibres from this nociceptive system enter the regionally-related articular branches of the auriculo-temporal, masseteric, deep temporal (and sometimes the lateral pterygoid) nerves, whence they pass into the sensory root and spinal tract of the trigeminal nerve (their cell bodies lying in the trigeminal ganglion).

One of the many myths that still continues to plague clinical discussion of temporomandibular joint pain is the so-called Costen's syndrome; but in order to avoid needless

its fibrous capsule, or in the related posterior articular fat pad. A common cause of such primary articular pain is the creation of abnormal mechanical stresses in the fibrous capsules of one or both temporomandibular joints as the result of some form of malocclusion—occurring either in patients with natural teeth, or (more often) in patients provided with dental prostheses. Less common causes of such primary articular pain are traumatic lesions of the

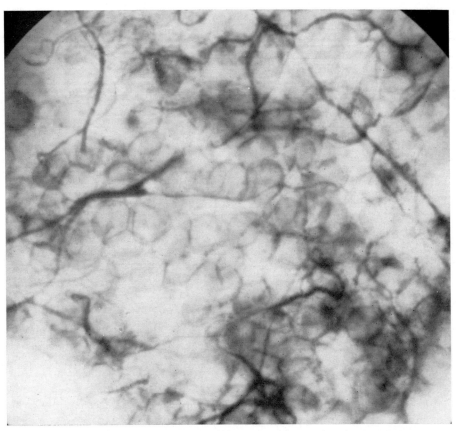

Fig. 13. The nociceptive system of plexiform unmyelinated nerve fibres distributed through the posterior articular fat pad related to the temporomandibular joint. The attachment of the fat pad to the posterior capsule of the joint lies to the left. Teased gold chloride preparation. × 400.

waste of space, and in the hope that this matter may finally be disposed of once and for all, it can be stated now that the morphological studies just described are totally incompatible with the purported aetiological implications of Costen's hypotheses. It should also be clear from the foregoing data that neither surgical removal of the meniscus from the temporomandibular joint (meniscectomy) nor excision of its synovial tissue (synovectomy) are procedures that can be claimed as extirpating tissues that are the primary source of articular pain—for neither tissue contains nociceptive nerve endings: the joint menisci are only causally involved in the production of articular pain when they are displaced against the sensitive fibrous capsular tissues that surround the joint.

Pain experienced in the region of the temporomandibular joint (including the external auditory meatus) only arises primarily from the articular tissues if there be mechanical or chemical irritation of the nociceptive receptor system in

fibrous capsule (with or without joint dislocation)—produced directly by injuries (accidental or surgical) to the joint region, or indirectly by forces transmitted to the joint tissues from a blow on the chin (as in boxing, for example)—or the development (more rarely) of acute or chronic inflammatory changes in the joint capsule (as may occur in patients afflicted with osteo-arthritis, rheumatoid arthritis or Reiter's syndrome, for instance).

Attention should also be drawn here to a common (but often unrecognized) primary articular facial pain syndrome that occurs particularly (but not exclusively) in young women in late adolescence or young adult life. This type of pain, which is usually (but not always) bilateral, develops in the temporomandibular joint region and external auditory meatus: it is felt in the morning on waking after an evening spent in prolonged periods of intra-oral osculation, and is accompanied by severe limitation of jaw opening. When this common form of sexual play is performed clumsily for long periods, the fat pad behind the condylar head of the mandible (usually in the female partner) is subjected to severe and prolonged compression that irritates the dense plexus of unmyelinated nerve fibres within it (see p. 293 and fig. 13)—thereby producing the characteristic pre-auricular and meatal pain and local tenderness. Diagnosis of this syndrome is established by a history of the morning onset (and subsequent persistence) of intense pre-auricular pain and limitation of jaw movement following upon an evening spent in sexual play, and by the presence of an extremely tender spot just in front of the tragus of the ear; and it may be confirmed by the fact that infiltration of the posterior articular fat pad with 0·5 ml. of Lignocaine hydrochloride solution abolishes the pain for about 45 min. The practical importance of recognizing this syndrome as a cause of primary facial pain lies in the fact that young women thus afflicted will not then be regarded as hysterical, or (conversely) be subjected to unnecessary and sometimes disfiguring surgical operations on the lateral aspect of the face. Instead, all that is required in the way of treatment is the administration (for two or three days) of mild analgesics such as acetylsalicylic acid or codeine—supplemented by direct infiltration of the fat pad with a long-acting local analgesic agent, if necessary in the acute stage—followed, perhaps, by some appropriate advice (for prophylactic purposes) on less traumatic techniques of osculation.

Secondary Facial Pain

Secondary facial pain (Table 1) embraces those varieties of pain that are experienced in the face although the causative lesion is located outside the facial tissues themselves, somewhere along the pathways (see pp. 281, 284) pursued by the small diameter afferent nerve fibres that link the various nociceptive receptor systems in the oro-facial tissues (described on p. 279) with the spinal nuclei of the fifth nerve on either side of the medulla oblongata and upper cervical spinal cord (see p. 283). Depending on whether the irritative lesion involves the extracranial and extraspinal branches of the sensory nerves to the oro-facial tissues, or their intracranial roots and centripetal extensions into the spinal tract of the fifth nerve, a peripheral and a central type of secondary facial pain may be differentiated.

Peripheral Secondary Facial Pain

The most familiar example of peripheral secondary facial pain (Table 1) is probably provided by the trigeminal neuralgias—and especially *tic douloureux*. Long clinical experience (extending over almost three-quarters of a century) of the palliative effects of alcohol injection into, or surgical operations on, the peripheral branches of the trigeminal nerve, the trigeminal ganglion, or the sensory root and spinal tract of the trigeminal nerve in this latter condition has convinced most neurologists and neuro-surgeons that the cause of *tic douloureux* lies in some disturbance of function in the peripheral neurones of the trigeminal system. Reference has already been made (on pp. 288 and 289) to the fact that this may involve loss of the presynaptic inhibitory effects on nociceptive relays through the spinal nucleus of the fifth nerve that are normally exerted by myelinated mechanoreceptor afferents from the oro-facial tissues; and in recent years, light and electron microscopic studies of biopsy material from patients afflicted with this distressing complaint have demonstrated degenerative changes in such myelinated afferent fibres within the trigeminal system. This would seem to settle the matter—were it not for some pertinent neuropharmacological data that require mention at this point.

These data arise from the clinical observation that considerable relief may be afforded to a high proportion of patients suffering from *tic douloureux* by administration of diphenylhydantoinate (*Phenytoin; Epanutin; Dilantin*) in divided daily doses totalling 300–400 mg., and of carbamazepine (*Tegretol*) in daily doses totalling 400–600 mg.—the latter drug (which is chemically related to imipramine) being the more effective. Basically, these two drugs are rostral reticular system depressants that act (for this reason) as anti-ictal agents—in respect of which latter action, however, diphenylhydantoinate is the more powerful: but although diphenylhydantoinate also possesses a peripheral local analgesic action, its effect in trigeminal neuralgia seems to depend (as does that of carbamazepine) upon an additional central action on caudal reticular neurones. Thus, experimental studies have shown that diphenyl-hydantoinate and carbamazepine both reduce the synaptic excitability of projection neurones in the spinal nucleus of the fifth nerve, probably by enhancing activity in the presynaptic inhibitory projections thereto from neurones in the caudal portion of the brain stem reticular system (see p. 289), and that carbamazepine additionally depresses synaptic transmission through the thalamic nuclei. Whilst there is now little doubt, then, that *tic douloureux* arises as a result of loss of the normal degree of presynaptic inhibitory activity that restricts the flow of nociceptive afferent discharges through the spinal nucleus of the fifth nerve, it seems that this situation may arise from disturbance of function in either the peripheral or the central neurological systems that are responsible for such inhibition; and similar considerations may apply to paroxysmal glossopharyngeal neuralgia and to facial postherpetic neuralgia.

Other varieties of trigeminal neuralgia that represent peripheral secondary facial pain require mention at this point, for in some instances their differential diagnosis from *tic douloureux* may require considerable clinical expertise. Thus, supra-orbital or maxillary neuralgia may result from irritation of the peripheral branches of the divisions of the fifth nerve related to the frontal, ethmoidal, sphenoidal and maxillary sinuses as a result of sinusitis or of malignant neoplasms developing in these sinuses; or pain may be felt anywhere in the face because of irritative involvement of these (or other) trigeminal nerve branches in fractures of the facial skeleton. For these reasons, careful radiological examination of the paranasal sinuses and facial skeleton is an essential part of the investigation of patients suspected of having secondary facial pain.

A less familiar (although in fact more common) variety of peripheral secondary facial pain than those mentioned above is that experienced in the inferior facial dermatomes innervated (fig. 4) from the dorsal roots of the second and third cervical nerves (Table 1), as a result of their irritation at or near the upper cervical intervertebral foramina. This usually arises (in older patients) as a result of upper cervical osteo-arthritis or spondylitis, or (in younger patients) as a sequel (delayed sometimes for several months) to accidental whiplash injuries involving the apophyseal joints of the upper cervical spine: it also occurs (less often) in the presence of degenerative conditions affecting the cervical intervertebral discs, should the upper cervical dorsal nerve roots be squeezed and irritated in the intervertebral foramina as the vertical height of the cervical spine decreases. The pain experienced in these circumstances is always felt in the postero-inferior region of the face around the mandibular angle—but in different patients may extend into the regions beneath the ear or beneath the ramus of the mandible, or into the post-auricular, mastoid and/or occipital regions (see fig. 4). The pain may be bilateral, but often is unilateral; and as it sometimes may be episodic, patients may be diagnosed (and often are, in a surprising number of instances) as suffering from "atypical" trigeminal neuralgia—in spite of the fact that the mandibular nerve does not innervate the affected regions of the face. When patients complain of pain in any of the facial regions just mentioned, their examination should include a careful radiological study (in oblique, as well as in anterior and lateral projections) of the upper cervical spine; treatment of this type of facial pain requires immobilization and support of the neck in a cervical collar, manipulation, traction or (occasionally) surgery—depending upon the causal pathology.

Central Secondary Facial Pain

Varieties of facial pain symptomatically identical to those just described may be produced by irritative lesions that impinge on the more proximal parts of the nociceptive afferents from the facial tissues in the intracranial portions of the trigeminal, facial, and glossopharyngeal nerves and their intracerebral extensions into the spinal tract of the fifth nerve, and these comprise (Table 1) the central type of secondary facial pain.

This situation is exemplified by the facial pain (often preceded by facial paraesthesiae) that is associated with intracranial tumours—for instance, gliomas, meningiomas or neuromas—or intracavernous carotid aneurysms that involve or press on the trigeminal ganglion; or intracranially extending nasopharyngeal carcinomas. Other examples are provided by the facial pain resulting from neoplasms, aneurysms or other space-occupying lesions located within the posterior cranial fossa or upper vertebral column (for example, syringomyelia and syringobulbia) that impinge on and thus irritate the nociceptive afferent fibres in the roots of the trigeminal, facial, glossopharyngeal or vagus nerves or in the spinal tract of the fifth nerve in the medulla oblongata and upper cervical spinal cord—of which the classic instance is the neuroma of the eighth nerve.

It should also be emphasized here that comparable types of secondary facial pain (which may sometimes be clinically indistinguishable from *tic douloureux*) are frequently encountered in patients with disseminated (multiple) sclerosis—in whom it may be the initial presenting symptom—as a result of the irritation of fibres in the spinal tract of the fifth nerve by the development of glial plaques in the lateral region of the medulla oblongata and upper cervical spinal cord. Vascular insufficiency states involving the lower brain stem, particularly that part of it supplied by the posterior inferior cerebellar artery, may likewise give rise to episodic hypoxic irritation of the fibres of the spinal tract of the fifth nerve and the neurones in the caudal part of the spinal nucleus to produce paraesthesiae and pain in the ipsilateral face—as in patients with cerebral arteriosclerosis, for instance.

Referred Facial Pain

As indicated in Table 1, pain may be referred to the face from three main sets of tissues, namely, the teeth, the nose and paranasal sinuses, and the heart. Such pain is designated as referred because it is felt in some portion of the face even though neither the nociceptive receptor system in that part of the face nor the related afferent nerve fibres are involved in any pathological process—which instead involves non-facial tissues whose nociceptive afferent innervation is embryologically related to the segmental innervation of the face. For this latter developmental reason, afferent projections from nociceptive receptor systems in the teeth, nose, sinuses and heart converge synaptically on neurones in the caudal spinal trigeminal nucleus (see p. 281) or posteroventral thalamic nuclei (see p. 284) to which afferents from facial tissue receptor systems also project; and when the former input system is activated by peripheral mechanical or chemical irritation, the perceptual thalamo-cortical projection system (see p. 285) interprets the situation as if the input were really being derived from receptors in the related part of the face—in which the pain is felt to be deeply located, in which the tissues may be tender to pressure or pricking, and in which local anaesthetic infiltration may abolish the pain.

Thus, pain from disease affecting particular groups of maxillary or mandibular teeth may be referred to specific, relatively small regions of the ipsilateral face and nose, or else be referred diffusely to large areas of the face innervated by the ipsilateral maxillary or mandibular nerves —and in these circumstances the patient may complain only of his facial pain and make no initial reference to toothache. On the other hand, some of the characteristic sites in the face (and jaws) to which pain is referred from irritative lesions of the mucosa lining the nose and paranasal sinuses are indicated in fig. 14—thus, pain felt in the malar and pre-auricular regions may be referred from a lesion affecting the ipsilateral middle turbinate or the region of the antral ostium, whilst ethmoidal lesions give rise to pain felt in these same regions of the face together with the upper molar teeth; and inferior turbinate and intra-antral mucosal lesions produce pain referred to the

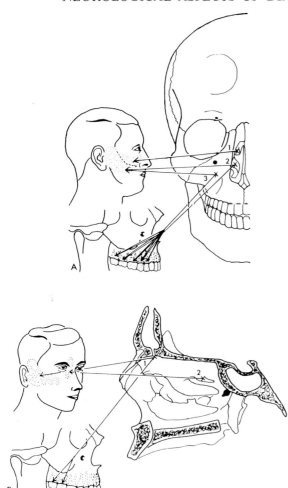

FIG. 14. Common sites of pain referred to the oro-facial region from irritative lesions of the nose and paranasal sinuses. (From Wyke (1968).) A. Sites of reference from lesions involving the middle turbinate (1), the inferior turbinate and aditus of the maxillary sinus (2) and the mucosal lining of the maxillary antrum (3). B. Sites of reference from lesions involving the ethmoid sinus (1) and the superior turbinate (2).

ipsilateral cheek and most of the ipsilateral maxillary teeth.

Finally, it should be noted that patients with coronary vascular insufficiency often experience pain in the postero-inferior regions of the face that are innervated (see fig. 4) from the branches of the upper cervical dorsal nerve roots on the left side. Whilst there is little difficulty in recognizing such pain for what it is when it is provoked by exercise or emotional tension and accompanied by pain in the chest or down the inside of the left arm and by dyspnoea, it should be emphasized that left-sided inferior facial (and neck) pain may occasionally be the only manifestation of coronary insufficiency—until an electrocardiogram is taken. Electrocardiography should always be carried out, therefore, in any patient who has episodic pain in the postero-inferior region of the left side of the face in the absence of evidence of disease affecting his upper cervical spine.

Ictal Facial Pain

Ictal facial pain is the least common of all varieties of facial pain (Table 1), and for this reason usually goes unrecognized in general clinical practice. It is in fact an unusual manifestation of sensory epilepsy and results from paroxysmal discharges generated within the reticular system of the brain stem that are projected to sectors of the cerebral cortex (see pp. 289–90) to which the nociceptive afferents from the face also project. As a result, when the epileptogenic disturbance in the brain fires off, the patient develops an attack of pain in the face that may be unilateral and regionally localized in some part of the face at first, but which gradually intensifies in severity and expands over the face (often becoming bilateral) as the seizure discharge develops. The pain is felt to be deep in the facial tissues, and is often preceded (in the initially affected region of the face) by feelings of numbness, tightness or tingling. When the pain commences, it is usually described as being "throbbing" or "bursting"; but it then develops a "burning" quality as the attack develops. The incrementing phase of the attack may be spread over varying periods up to 2 min. in duration; and once developed, the pain may last for 15–20 min., after which it subsides gradually (the affected regions of the face often feeling "numb" or "cold" for up to 2 hr. thereafter).

In some patients, such episodes of facial pain may be heralded or accompanied by other clinical evidences (see Table 3) of ictal sensory or motor disturbance—such as transient dysphasia, feelings of unreality, mental confusion, sensations of abdominal cramp or distension, an urgent desire to micturate, facial and/or limb paraesthesiae, blurring of vision, or unilateral or bilateral twitching of the facial and/or mandibular musculature—or may (rarely) terminate in a generalized convulsion. In other patients, however, such additional manifestations of ictal dysfunction may be entirely lacking—which renders diagnosis extremely difficult. Further features which assist recognition of this syndrome, however, are the patient's recognition of the fact that attacks of pain are particularly associated with periods of severe emotional tension or states of drowsiness (often occurring as he is falling off to sleep at night or as he is awakening in the morning)—which characterize most varieties of ictal disturbance. Most patients with ictal facial pain develop the disorder in adult life as a late manifestation of a genetic epileptogenic predisposition—but a few cases have been reported, and one has been seen by the writer, in which the disorder has developed as a manifestation of post-traumatic epilepsy. The principal clinical features of the syndrome of ictal facial pain are summarized for convenience in Table 3.

Recognition of this type of facial pain is facilitated by performance of electroencephalography. Patients afflicted with this disorder may show evidence of bilateral paroxysmal activity (at 4–6 Hz., or consisting of a mixture of fast and slow waves) in the resting record at times when they are not complaining of pain—as do many patients with a variety of ictal disorders; but, on the other hand, such a record may be entirely normal. More significant,

TABLE 3

THE SYNDROME OF ICTAL FACIAL PAIN*

Sex incidence	Usually female (10 of 11 cases)
Age at onset of pain	40–60 years
Location of pain	Deep and expanding (often becoming bilateral)
Duration of pain	Up to 20 min.
Quality of pain	Throbbing or bursting, then burning
Associated subjective ictal phenomena (usual)	Dysphasia Feelings of unreality ("like a dream") Confusion and disorientation Tinnitus Blurring of vision Abdominal cramp or distension Desire to micturate Paraesthesiae in face and/or limbs
Associated overt ictal phenomena (sometimes)	Dysphasia or dysarthria Twitching of facial muscles Twitching of mandibular muscles Generalized convulsions
Previous personal history of epilepsy	Occasional (3 of 11 cases)
Ictal phenomena in relatives	Usual (8 of 11 cases)
Attacks precipitated or potentiated by	Emotional tension Drowsiness Hyperventilation Barbiturate sedation
EEG correlates of attacks	Paroxysmal slow (or fast and slow) waves, bilaterally.
Attacks relieved by	Diphenylhydantoinate Carbamazepine
Attacks unrelieved by	Phenobarbitone Chlorpromazine Valium Trigeminal nerve injection or section

* Data based on a personal series of 11 cases.

however, is a demonstration that voluntary hyperventilation provokes an attack of facial pain that is accompanied by potentiation (or emergence) of paroxysmal discharges in the electroencephalogram—a phenomenon that occurs in some (but not all) patients suffering from ictal facial pain. It should be noted that this type of electroencephalographic response is in marked contrast to that associated with attacks of other varieties of facial pain—which involves desynchronization of normal activity into low-voltage discharges at a mixture of fast frequencies.

Once diagnosed, ictal facial pain usually responds satisfactorily to treatment with the anti-ictal agents diphenylhydantoinate (*Phenytoin; Dilantin; Epanutin*) or carbamazepine (*Tegretol*), administered in divided daily doses commensurate with the patient's age, body size, and severity and frequency of symptoms. It should be noted, however, that patients suffering from ictal facial pain are often told (if they are not regarded as "hysterical") that they have some "atypical" variety of trigeminal neuralgia (in spite of the totally uncharacteristic features of their clinical history), and this diagnosis may then be regarded as being "confirmed" by a satisfactory therapeutic response to administration of carbamazepine (*Tegretol*) (see p. 295); or worse, they may be subjected to alcohol injection or surgical division of one of their trigeminal nerves—which leaves them with continuing attacks of pain felt deeply in regions of the face that now are superficially analgesic, and thus creates a state of so-called "anaesthesia dolorosa" (see also p. 292).

FURTHER READING*

Alling, C. A. (Ed.) (1968), *Facial Pain.* Philadelphia: Lea and Febiger.
Beecher, H. K. (1968), "The Measurement of Pain in Man", in *Pain*, pp. 207–208 (A. Soulairac, J. Cahn and J. Charpentier, Eds.). New York: Academic Press.
Bosma, J. F. (Ed.) (1967), *Symposium on Oral Sensation and Perception.* Springfield, Illinois: Thomas.
Brodal, A. (1969), *Neurological Anatomy in Relation to Clinical Medicine*, 2nd edition. London: Oxford University Press.
Dubner, R. and Kawamura, Y. (Eds.) (1971), *Oral-Facial Sensory and Motor Mechanisms.* New York: Appleton-Century-Crofts.
Eccles, J. C. (1964), *The Physiology of Synapses.* Berlin: Springer.
Hall, I. S. and Colman, B. H. (1971), *Diseases of the Nose, Throat and Ear.* Edinburgh: Livingstone.
Harris, W. (1937), *The Facial Neuralgias.* London: Oxford University Press.
Hassler, R. and Walker, A. E. (Eds.) (1970), *Trigeminal Neuralgia: Pathogenesis and Pathophysiology.* Stuttgart: Thieme.
Janzen, R., Keidel, W. D., Herz, A. and Steichele, C. (Eds.) (1972), *Pain: Basic Principles, Pharmacology, Therapy.* Stuttgart: Thieme.
Kenshalo, D. R. (Ed.) (1968), *The Skin Senses.* Springfield, Illinois: Thomas.
Klineberg, I. J., Greenfield, B. E. and Wyke, B. D. (1971), "Afferent Discharges from Temporomandibular Articular Mechanoreceptors: An Experimental Analysis of Their Behavioural Characteristics", *Arch. oral Biol.*, **16**, 1462.
Klineberg, I. J. and Wyke, B. D. (1973), "Articular Reflex Control of Mastication", in *Oral Surgery. IV*, pp. 252–258 (Lester W. Kay, Ed.). Copenhagen: Munksgaard.
Knighton, R. S. and Dumke, P. R. (Eds.) (1966), *Pain: An International Symposium.* Boston: Little, Brown.
Lance, J. W. (1969), *The Mechanism and Management of Headache.* London: Butterworths.
Merskey, H. and Spear, F. G. (1967), *Pain: Psychological and Psychiatric Aspects.* London: Baillière, Tindall and Cassell.
Ostfeld, A. M. (1962), *The Common Headache Syndromes.* Springfield, Illinois: Thomas.
Noordenbos, W. (1959), *Pain. Problems Pertaining to the Transmission of Nerve Impulses Which Give Rise to Pain.* Amsterdam and London: Elsevier.
Rasmussen, P. (1965), *Facial Pain.* Copenhagen: Munksgaard.
de Reuck, A. V. S. and Knight, J. (Eds.) (1966), *Touch, Heat and Pain.* London: Churchill.
Schwartz, L. L. and Chayes, C. M. (Eds.) (1968), *Facial Pain and Mandibular Dysfunction.* Philadelphia: Saunders.
Sternbach, R. A. (1968), *Pain. A Psychophysiological Analysis.* New York: Academic Press.

* Detailed references, omitted in accordance with editorial policy (see Preface), may be found in the monograph *Neurology of Facial Pain* by B. D. Wyke, to be published by Heinemann.

White, J. C. and Sweet, W. H. (1969), *Pain and the Neurosurgeon. A Forty Year's Experience.* Springfield, Illinois: Thomas.

Wolff, H. G. (1963), *Headache and Other Head Pain*, 2nd edition. London: Oxford University Press.

Wolstenholme, G. E. W. and O'Connor, M. (Eds.) (1959), *Pain and Itch. Nervous Mechanisms.* London: Churchill.

Wyke, B. D. (1958), "The Surgical Physiology of Facial Pain", *Brit. dent. J.*, **104**, 153.

Wyke, B. D. (1960), *Neurological Aspects of Hypnosis.* London: Dental and Medical Society for the Study of Hypnosis.

Wyke, B. D. (1968), "The Neurology of Facial Pain", *Brit. J. hosp. Med.*, **1**, 46.

Wyke, B. D. (1969), *Principles of General Neurology. An Introduction to the Basic Principles of Medical and Surgical Neurology.* Amsterdam and London: Elsevier.

Wyke, B. D., Greenfield, B. E. and Klineberg, I. J. (1972), "Mechanoreceptor Reflex Innervation of the Temporomandibular Joint", in *Morphology of the Maxillo-Mandibular Apparatus*, pp. 138–146 (G.-H. Schumacher, Ed.). Leipzig: Thieme.

24. THE PHARMACOLOGY OF LOCAL ANAESTHETIC DRUGS

FELICITY REYNOLDS

Chemical structure

Mode of Action
  Nerve conduction
  Active form of the molecule
  Action on cell membrane
  Possible mechanisms

Duration of action

Pharmacological effects
  Local
  Systemic

Hypersensitivity

Vasoconstrictors
  Uses and dangers
  Adrenaline
  Noradrenaline
  Levonordefrin
  Felypressin

Assessment
  Laboratory investigations
  Clinical trials

Individual local anaesthetics
  Procaine
  Amethocaine
  Lignocaine
  Mepivacaine
  Prilocaine

A local anaesthetic drug is one which reversibly blocks conduction in nerve fibres, when applied locally. This it does by an action upon the axonal membrane, preventing its depolarization. Complete conduction blockade can only be produced by direct application of the drug; a sufficient concentration cannot be achieved clinically by systemic as opposed to local administration.

CHEMISTRY AND STRUCTURE-ACTIVITY RELATIONSHIPS

The local anaesthetics in current use are all weak bases with the following general formula:

Aromatic group—intermediate chain—2° or 3° amine

Individual formulae of drugs that are or have been widely used in dentistry are shown in fig. 1.

Since in the first local anaesthetic, cocaine, the intermediate chain and aromatic residue consisted of an ester of benzoic acid, early synthetic substitutes, for example procaine and amethocaine, tended to imitate this structure.

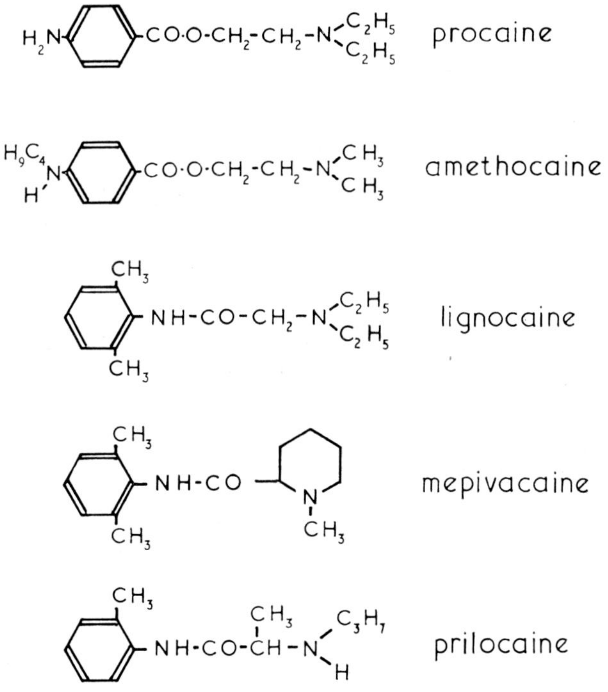

FIG. 1. Formulae of some local anaesthetic drugs.

Procaine is an ester of *p*-aminobenzoic acid. However, such a structure has a number of disadvantages: an ester is unstable in solution, it may hydrolyse, and it cannot be autoclaved. Moreover, it may be highly antigenic (see later under Hypersensitivity). In all local anaesthetics synthesized since the advent of lignocaine in the 1940s the intermediate chain has taken the form of an amide linkage, a more chemically stable structure.

All agents referred to in this chapter are tertiary amines, with the exception of prilocaine, a secondary amine. The tertiary amine in mepivacaine has been incorporated into a piperidine ring.

The importance of the amine group is that it confers on the molecule the property of a weak base, or proton acceptor. Thus, in acid solution, it acquires one proton (H$^+$) and becomes a cation:

$$R_1 \diagdown \quad \diagup R_2 \qquad\qquad R_1 \diagdown \quad \diagup R_2$$
$$N \quad + \ HCl \rightleftharpoons \quad N^+ \qquad Cl^-$$
$$R_3 \diagup \qquad\qquad\qquad R_3 \diagup \quad \diagdown H$$
$$\text{base} \qquad\qquad\qquad\qquad \text{cation}$$

The cationic form of the molecule is of course compulsively water-soluble, but the non-ionized form, the base, tends to be lipid-soluble and thus can penetrate lipid membranes and tissue barriers.

The proportion of the two forms of the molecule present in solution depends not only on the pH of the environment, but also on an inherent property of the molecule, termed the pK$_a$ (negative logarithm$_{10}$ of the dissociation constant of the acid) and thus can be calculated from the Henderson-Hasselbalch equation:

$$pH = pK_a - \log \frac{[\text{cation}]}{[\text{base}]}$$

At a pH of 7·4, that of the extracellular fluid, lignocaine, with a pK$_a$ of 7·86 is thus approximately 75 per cent ionized, whereas procaine with a pK$_a$ of the order of 9, is 97·5 per cent ionized. At physiological pH, therefore, and with equal total concentrations, the concentration of lignocaine base is ten times that of procaine base. This can account for the greatly enhanced penetrative powers of lignocaine over procaine.

A local anaesthetic for injection is presented as the salt, usually the hydrochloride. The pH of the resulting solution is less than 7 as the salt is derived from a strong acid and a weak base.

Potency. A certain minimum concentration of the basic form of the molecule must be present in tissues *in vivo* in order to penetrate to the site of action and achieve nerve blockade. This minimum concentration, or threshold anaesthetic concentration, gives a measure of the potency; it depends upon the molecular configuration of the drug and is related to its lipid solubility. In one homologous series these factors can be altered, for example, by changing the number of carbon atoms in the alkyl radicals attached to the amine nitrogen. In the mepivacaine series, for instance, if the chain length is increased from methyl, an increased potency is achieved but with increased tissue irritancy and reduced aqueous solubility. The optimum is reached with C$_4$, bupivacaine, a potent drug of long duration which is used extensively for epidural analgesia.

MODE OF ACTION

Nerve Conduction

A nerve fibre consists of a central semi-fluid core, the axoplasm, enclosed in a tube, the cell membrane. The cell membrane is believed to be built up of a bimolecular lipid palisade, bounded inside and out by a monomolecular protein layer. Each fibre of a peripheral nerve is enclosed in a tube of neurilemma, from which it is separated by the myelin sheath, except at the nodes of Ranvier. The myelin sheath, an insulating layer, is absent—or nearly so—in nonmedullated nerves. Nerve fibres so encased are collected in bundles within the endoneurium. The perineurium surrounds a collection of bundles, and the epineurium encloses a whole nerve. There is therefore a substantial barrier between a local anaesthetic placed in the surrounding tissues and its site of action at the nerve cell membrane.

During nerve conduction, changes occur in the cell membrane. In the **resting state** there is a potential difference across the cell membrane, with the inside negative, due to a higher concentration of sodium ions outside than in. The cell membrane is relatively impermeable to sodium ions which, being heavily hydrated, are larger than the pores in the lipid layer of the cell membrane. Potassium ions therefore tend to be held within the cell by an electrical gradient created by the sodium pump.

Depolarization phase. When a nerve is stimulated, partial depolarization of the membrane is accompanied by a release of calcium ions and leads to a large transient increase in permeability to sodium ions which therefore enter the fibre, resulting in massive depolarization. This is termed the depolarization phase. Thus, the threshold required to produce the action potential is exceeded, with consequent propagation of the nerve impulse. The increase in permeability to sodium ions is thought to be due to an altered configuration of the lipid layer of the cell membrane, increasing its pore size.

During the **neutralization phase,** potassium ions pass out of the fibre to restore electrical neutrality.

In the **restoration phase** sodium ions return to the outside and potassium ions re-enter the fibre.

In myelinated nerves these changes take place only at the nodes of Ranvier, giving rise to saltatory conduction of the nerve impulse.

The Active Form of the Local Anaesthetic Molecule

The primary action of a local anaesthetic is on the cell membrane. Thus, in order to act, the local anaesthetic must first penetrate the surrounding tissues and the nerve sheath. Only the uncharged form, therefore, can gain access to the cell membrane.

According to the evidence of Ritchie, Ritchie and Greengard (1965), however, the cation is probably the active form of the molecule. This was demonstrated in the following way. Intact and desheathed nerves were suspended in bath fluids of different pH values and different concentrations of lignocaine were added. By measuring the action potential produced by stimulation of the nerve, the investigators were able to find the minimum concentration of lignocaine necessary to produce conduction block in different pH conditions. It was shown that while a high pH favoured block by lignocaine of an intact nerve, in a desheathed preparation the optimum pH for the action of lignocaine was neutral. Thus, where little or no penetration was required the lowest effective concentration was one which contained a predominance of the cationic form of the drug.

The Action of Local Anaesthetics on the Cell Membrane

The action of local anaesthetics has been termed membrane stabilization, or more correctly electrical stabilization (Seeman, 1972): the resting potential is unaltered but response to stimulation is inhibited.

Initially the threshold for electrical excitation is increased, the rate of rise of the action potential reduced and conduction of the impulse slowed; eventually, nerve conduction is completely blocked. This stabilizing action is secondary to inhibition of the transient increase in permeability to sodium ions that normally occurs in response to stimulation.

The production of nerve conduction blockade is associated with a concentration of local anaesthetic of about 0·04 mole/kg. dry membrane (Seeman, 1972). This figure is clearly of the same order as that historically associated with the production of general anaesthesia, that is about 0·05 mole/l. olive oil, according to the Meyer-Overton rule. However, this latter figure is far from constant, and the more constant factor may be the volume occupation of the membrane by the anaesthetic, since large molecules cause greater membrane perturbation than small molecules. The volume occupation for local anaesthetics is 10–20 times that for general anaesthetics. Under conditions of local anaesthesia there is about a 3·5 per cent expansion of membrane volume; the actual volume of the anaesthetic occupying the membrane, however, is only about 0·3 per cent or less. The equivalent figures for general anaesthesia are a volume expansion of the membrane of 0·6 per cent compared with the volume of the anaesthetic of about 0·02 per cent (see Chapter 25).

Possible Mechanisms. The fact that high atmospheric pressure can reverse general and local anaesthesia suggests that this membrane expansion is the cause of nerve conduction block.

However, the volume occupied by the anaesthetic can only account for about 10 per cent of this membrane expansion (see above). A number of other mechanisms may be involved (Seeman, 1972):

(a) disordering of the lipid component of membrane;
(b) formation of ice crystals in the membrane;
(c) distortion of membrane proteins; and
(d) displacement of membrane-bound Ca^{++}. Calcium is known to condense lipid monolayers. Local anaesthetics displace membrane-bound Ca^{++} whereas general anaesthetics increase it. This could account for the greater membrane expansion by the former.

DURATION OF ACTION

It is possible to increase the duration of action of a local anaesthetic to a certain extent by increasing the concentration and dose. Prolongation by the addition of vasoconstrictors is discussed later. Certain properties of the drug itself also influence its duration.

The more lipid soluble, potent local anaesthetics are likely to be longer acting. A high pK_a tends to reduce the concentration of base present in the tissues, increase the water solubility of the molecule and therefore to accelerate its removal from the site of action. The production of local vasodilatation by the local anaesthetic drug itself also accelerates its removal and so shortens its action. Dextro-isomers of prilocaine and mepivacaine are longer-acting than the laevo-isomers, probably because they are more powerful vasoconstrictors. A high tissue irritancy depresses absorption possibly because local oedema compresses capillaries. This is of little importance at clinical concentrations.

Rapid biotransformation cannot reduce the duration of action of amide local anaesthetics, which are metabolized in the liver only after removal from the site of action. Theoretically there might be some curtailment of action by pseudocholinesterase injected into vascular areas.

A further discussion of duration of action, including the relationship between dental and soft-tissue anaesthesia, will be found in the section on vasoconstrictors.

PHARMACOLOGICAL EFFECTS

The effects of local anaesthetics may be local or general (systemic). The local effects, occurring only at high concentrations of the drug, are due to its primary action of blocking nerve conduction and are seen in the area of supply of the nerves affected by the block. All types of nerve fibres are affected, but small fibres are more readily blocked than large fibres, and non-myelinated more readily than myelinated. Thus pain and temperature are the most sensitive modalities, and somatic motor power the least. Vasomotor tone may be affected locally in two ways: firstly by blockade of sympathetic vasoconstrictor fibres, producing vasodilatation in the area of supply; secondly, by a direct action of the drug on the smooth muscle of blood vessels at the site of injection. Here local anaesthetics may be divided into pre- and post-lignocaine categories. With the exception of cocaine (which produces marked vasoconstriction since it inhibits noradrenaline uptake and so potentiates its action) all pre-lignocaine drugs, such as procaine, produce vasodilatation. Lignocaine may be neutral or mildly vasodilator, while mepivacaine and prilocaine tend to produce vasoconstriction.

Systemic effects occur with absorption from the site of local administration or as a consequence of systemic administration. They are seen at lower ambient concentrations than the local effects. Nevertheless, the dose required to produce systemic effects is several times that customarily used in dentistry, while systemic toxicity would be expected with a dose about ten times that used in dentistry, even if the entire dose is given accidentally intravenously. Unwanted effects of dental local anaesthesia are generally due to the addition of vasoconstrictor drugs, or to hypersensitivity, which will be dealt with in later sections. Systemic pharmacological effects of local anaesthetics will be discussed here, only briefly.

Cardiovascular System

Local anaesthetics have a stabilizing effect on the cell membrane of cardiac tissue. They tend to depress automaticity in abnormal or damaged fibres and thereby suppress cardiac arrhythmias. Procaine has quinidine-like effects and may slow the rate of rise of the action potential and increase the effective refractory period of cardiac cells. In large doses it may slow conduction in Purkinje tissue and effectively depress myocardial contractility, as does quinidine. Lignocaine, on the other hand, even in large clinical doses does not depress myocardial contractility. It is used as an anti-arrhythmic in a dose of 1–2 mg./kg. by intravenous bolus, followed by a slow infusion.

Local anaesthetics cannot be expected to have a direct effect on smooth muscle in vessel walls via the systemic circulation. Circulatory collapse after local anaesthesia in dentistry therefore cannot be a direct effect of the local anaesthetic drug. It may be due most commonly to a faint, or more rarely and disastrously to an arrhythmia caused by a catecholamine vasoconstrictor, or to anaphylactic shock. The latter is very unusual in relation to amide local anaesthetics (see later).

Central Nervous System

Synthetic local anaesthetics primarily cause sedation, and in massive doses, or in large doses given intravenously, may cause restlessness, pins and needles, tremors, twitching and occasionally convulsions. Intravenous doses cause only relatively transient effects. Respiratory and circulatory collapse, which may accompany massive overdose, occur because of medullary depression rather than as a peripheral effect.

HYPERSENSITIVITY

Hypersensitivity implies an abnormal antigen-antibody response, and not an exaggerated normal response, correctly termed **supersensitivity.** The term has even been misused to describe adverse reactions due to accidental intravenous injection and frank overdose, while the lay public frequently claim "sensitivity" to the local anaesthetic when they have suffered a classical faint or a typical adrenaline reaction. It appears that dentists encounter true hypersensitivity to modern local anaesthetics, though rarely, more frequently than do anaesthetists, probably because of the much larger number of patients given dental anaesthesia.

The occurrence of hypersensitivity theoretically requires previous sensitization to the antigen, though such a history cannot always be obtained. An antigen is typically a foreign protein; thus, a local anaesthetic must act as a hapten. Hypersensitivity to a local anaesthetic is more frequent in atopic individuals and may be manifested as local oedema initially, as generalized urticaria, or as angioneurotic oedema with or without lymphadenopathy. Dermatitis may be encountered as a delayed reaction to skin applications and as contact dermatitis in dentists. Anaphylaxis, an acquired, immediate reaction to injection, appears less common than atopic reactions.

Hypersensitivity to procaine and other ester derivatives of benzoic acid is not uncommon. There is likely to be cross sensitivity within the ester group of drugs and with p-aminobenzoic acid, widely used as a sunscreen, and p-hydroxybenzoic acid and its derivatives (paraben, methylparaben) which are preservatives and may be incorporated into amide local anaesthetic preparations. All these benzoic acid esters are relatively highly antigenic whereas the amide local anaesthetics are not, though true hypersensitivity to lignocaine has been reported (Waldman and Binkley, 1967; Eyre and Nally, 1971; Walker, 1971).

Testing for hypersensitivity in suspected cases can avoid suffering and danger if carried out correctly. Patch testing is ineffective for local anaesthetics, which do not penetrate intact skin. Intradermal and scratch testing may also give false negative results, since local anaesthetics must act as haptens, or a metabolite may be the antigen in delayed reactions. Moreover, intradermal testing may give rise to extensive and painful cutaneous reactions. Nasal testing has been advocated (Eyre and Nally, 1971) but this too can be dangerous and, moreover, may give false negative results for the same reason as intradermal testing. There is no doubt that *in vitro* testing is free from danger to the patient and also more reliable than other methods; the lymphocyte transformation test (see Chapter 14) and histamine release from sensitized lung tissue have both been advocated for detecting circulating antibody to local anaesthetics.

VASOCONSTRICTORS

The addition of a vasoconstrictor to a local anaesthetic preparation delays its removal from the site of action and so prolongs and enhances its effect. Such an addition is especially valuable in dentistry because of the high vascularity of oral mucosa, and because some local anaesthetics such as procaine have a vasodilator action and high pK_a. Even lignocaine without a vasoconstrictor may produce successful anaesthesia in dentistry in fewer than 50 per cent of cases (see Table 1). The incidence of successful blockade without vasoconstrictor is higher with the newer drugs of lower pK_a and mild vasoconstrictor properties such as mepivacaine and prilocaine. However, the duration of dental anaesthesia is usually unacceptably short, though both efficacy and duration can be increased to a certain extent by increasing the concentration of the latter two drugs.

The addition of a vasoconstrictor, however, is not without disadvantages. The first, and one most prominent in the lay mind, is the increased duration of soft tissue anaesthesia, lasting more than four hours with some preparations (see Table 1). In some circumstances, by reducing the concentration of vasoconstrictor, substantial reduction in duration of soft tissue anaesthesia can be obtained while maintaining a satisfactory degree of operative analgesia. There may,

TABLE 1

THE DURATION OF ACTION AND INCIDENCE OF SUCCESSFUL ANALGESIA OF SOME DENTAL LOCAL ANAESTHETIC PREPARATIONS

Local Anaesthetic	Vasoconstrictor	Author	Mean Duration of Anaesthesia, min.		Ratio STA/DA	Incidence %
			Dental (DA)	Soft Tissue (STA)		
Lignocaine 2%	adrenaline 12·5 µg./ml.	1	63·3	192·8	3·0	97
		2 infiltration	31	172	5·5	80
		regional	34	188	5·5	86
	adrenaline 10 µg./ml.	3		199·5		90
	adrenaline 5 µg./ml.	1	35·0	155·1	4·4	97
	0	1	6·3	59·9	9·5	38
		4	19·5	105	5·4	48
Mepivacaine 2%	adrenaline 12·5 µg./ml.	1	45·1	171·7	3·8	93
		2 infiltration	32	116	3·6	90
		regional	40	188	4·7	76
	adrenaline 10 µg./ml.	1	35·6	145·0	4·1	93
	adrenaline 5 µg./ml.	1	35·1	155·0	4·4	94
	0	1	13·1	82·1	6·3	83
		3		115·7		75
		4	19·5	105	5·4	83
	levonordefrin 50 µg./ml.	3		244·6		92
Mepivacaine 3%	0	1	17·2	102·6	5·9	91
		2 infiltration	20	102	5·1	84
		regional	33	156	4·7	84
		3		148·6		85
Prilocaine 3%	felypressin 0·4 i.u./ml.	5	18·6	139·4	7·5	
	felypressin 0·03 i.u./ml.		37·4	247·7	6·6	
	0		14·9	132·8	8·9	

Authors

1. Berling, C. (1958), "Carbocaine in Local Anaesthesia in the Oral Cavity," *Sartryck ur Odontologisk Revy*, **9**, 254.
2. Mumford, J. M. and Geddes, I. C. (1961), "Trial of Carbocaine in Conservative Dentistry," *Brit. dent. J.*, **110**, 92.
3. Dobbs, E. C. and Ross, N. (1961), "A New Local Anesthetic, Carbocaine," *N.Y. St. dent. J.*, **27**, 453.
4. Mumford, J. M. and Gray, T. C. (1957), "Dental Trial of Carbocaine—a New Local Anaesthetic," *Brit. J. Anaesth.*, **29**, 210.
5. Goldman, V., Killey, H. C. and Wright, C. (1966), "Effects of Local Analgesic Agents and Vasoconstrictors on Rabbits' Ears," *Acta Anaesth. scand.*, suppl. 23, 353. Quoting a personal communication from Berling (1965).

however, be negligible reduction in the period of soft-tissue anaesthesia after mandibular block with plain solutions. The work of Berling (see Table 1) suggests that while the addition of adrenaline substantially increases the duration of soft-tissue anaesthesia, it increases the duration of dental anaesthesia even more, and that the ratio of soft tissue to dental anaesthesia duration increases as the concentration of vasoconstrictor decreases. Thus despite recent additions

to the local anaesthetic field, it appears that for anything but the shortest procedures (or the most rapid workers) some sort of vasoconstrictor is needed, if repeated injections are to be avoided.

Here, however, the second and more disastrous, if less frequent, disadvantage of vasoconstrictors must be considered. While there is no doubt that vasoconstrictors reduce the danger of systemic intoxication (such as may be due to big doses of local anaesthetics used by anaesthetists) by reducing absorption, there is no such requirement in dentistry (see Pharmacological Effects, p. 301). The danger in this field lies rather in accidental intravenous injection. Here the dose of local anaesthetic is negligible but the nature and dose of the vasoconstrictor is highly significant. It is to the latter drug that accidental intravenous injection owes its danger.

Accidental intravenous injection is more common in dentistry than in other forms of local anaesthesia both because of the vascularity of the area and because of the less frequent use of aspiration prior to injection. The incidence of aspiration of blood depends on the technique and type of injection; Goldman and Gray (1963) report an incidence of 7 per cent for infiltration, 10·5 per cent for mandibular block, 13 per cent for maxillary block and 15 per cent when infiltration and nerve block are combined, while it may be as high as 50 per cent with certain techniques using a fine needle (Cowan, 1972). There is thus a strong indication in all cases for using as aspiration technique, in order to detect when the needle tip is intravascular, and so to avoid both intravenous injection and failed blockade.

The danger to the patient, should intravenous injection occur, varies with the nature and concentration of the vasoconstrictor, and with the possibility of drug interactions (*vide infra*).

Adrenaline

Adrenaline is the longest established and most widely used vasoconstrictor in local anaesthesia. While it is commonly used by anaesthetists in concentrations of 5 µg./ml. (1:200,000) or less for epidural analgesia, 4 µg./ml. may lead to a low success rate in dental anaesthesia (Cardwell and Cawson, 1969). With prilocaine, though the success rate may be higher, the duration of action is often inadequate (Goldman and Evers, 1969).

As 2 per cent lignocaine with adrenaline 12·5 µg./ml. (1:80,000) has such a high success rate in skilled hands as well as a more than adequate duration, there can be no indication for the inclusion of such high concentrations of adrenaline as 20 µg./ml. (1:50,000).

Cardiovascular Effects

Adrenaline acts on both α and β receptors, the β stimulant properties increasing heart rate and stroke volume and the tendency to arrhythmias, while causing peripheral vasodilatation which tends to counteract α vasoconstriction. The net effect on blood pressure in man is thus usually increased pulse pressure without an increase in mean arterial blood pressure. Clinically, therefore, adrenaline, entering the systemic circulation rapidly, may cause palpitations, anxiety and sweating, accompanied by a precipitate rise in pulse rate. These changes are likely to be short-lived since adrenaline is rapidly inactivated by neuronal uptake. Fainting, which may accompany such changes, is not directly caused by adrenaline. The incidence of such side effects is relatively low in skilled hands using a concentration of adrenaline of 12·5 µg./ml. or less (Goldman and Evers, 1969). However, adrenaline is contra-indicated in all

patients with coronary artery disease and thyrotoxicosis and in those taking antihypertensive or tricyclic antidepressant drugs, which markedly potentiate its actions (Boakes *et al.*, 1973).

Local Effects

It has been found experimentally that when adrenaline and noradrenaline are given intradermally the pale zone they induce may become cyanotic. This is thought to be due to a local increase in oxygen consumption (Klingenström and Westermark, 1964), and may be the cause of pain, oedema and subsequent necrosis sometimes associated clinically with local anaesthesia.

Noradrenaline

Noradrenaline is less widely used than adrenaline in local anaesthetic preparations. Its effect on peripheral β receptors is weak compared to that of adrenaline, and it is also a slightly less potent α receptor stimulant and prolongs local anaesthesia less. It is used in concentrations of 20 or 40 µg./ml. (1:50,000 or 1:25,000). In such concentrations it may cause a marked and dangerous rise in both systolic and diastolic pressure, associated with severe headache and

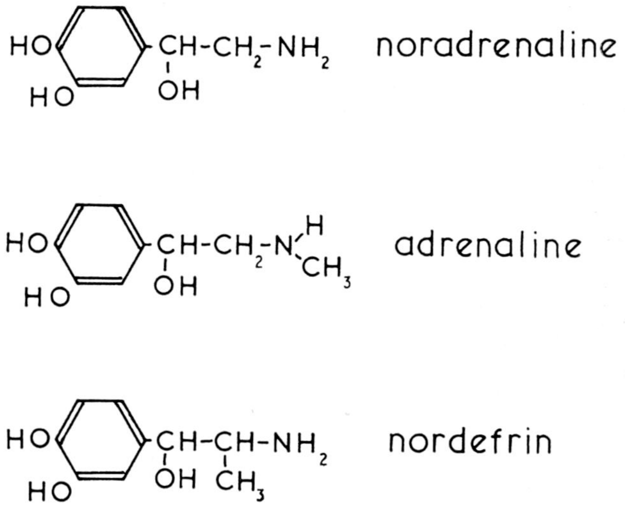

FIG. 2. Formulae of catecholamine vasoconstrictors.

a danger of cerebrovascular accident. Preparations containing 40 µg./ml. (Xylestesin, now no longer available as such, and Hostacaine-with-noradrenaline) were the subject of 12 cases of adverse drug reactions reported to the Committee on Safety of Medicines between 1964 and 1972. Of these, three cases involved a period of unconsciousness and there was one death associated with subarachnoid haemorrhage. Noradrenaline is contraindicated in all those patients in whom adrenaline is contraindicated and in hypertension. Tricyclic antidepressant drugs cause a four- to eight-fold potentiation of its pressor effects (Boakes *et al.*, 1973). Noradrenaline is associated with local effects similar to those of adrenaline, which may be severe with high concentrations. There may, moreover, be reactive hyperaemia and consequently an increased risk of reactionary haemorrhage.

There can thus be no indication for the use of noradrenaline in place of adrenaline in this field.

Levonordefrin

Nordefrin is α-methyl noradrenaline or isoadrenaline (see fig. 2). Cobefrin is a trade name. The **laevo-**isomer is the more potent vasoconstrictor. It is not marketed in Britain but has been used in the United States of America and Scandinavia, principally with mepivacaine.

It has an action similar to that of noradrenaline, being an α receptor stimulant, but it is much less potent and is used in a concentration of 50 μg./ml. (1:20,000). In this concentration it is probably as likely as noradrenaline 10 μg./ml. to produce a rise in blood pressure which may be more sustained since it is less rapidly inactivated by tissue uptake. Some poorly controlled trials report "fewer side effects" referable to the vasoconstrictor using mepivacaine 2 per cent with levonordefrin 50 μg./ml. than using lignocaine 2 per cent with adrenaline 10 μg./ml. It may be associated with an undesirably long duration of soft-tissue anaesthesia (see Table 1).

Felypressin

Felypressin (Octapressin) is a synthetic polypeptide related to vasopressin. It is at present marketed with prilocaine in the United Kingdom as Citanest Octapressin which is prilocaine 3 per cent with felypressin 0·03 i.u. This concentration of felypressin gives a longer duration of dental anaesthesia than does 0·4 i.u./ml., though it may cause an excessively long period of soft-tissue anaesthesia (Table 1). It prolongs the action of prilocaine better than does adrenaline, 3·3 μg./ml., (Goldman and Evers, 1969) and better than it does the action of lignocaine. Experimentally it does not increase the intravenous toxicity of local anaesthetics as does adrenaline (Åkerman, 1969) and clinically it is less likely to produce systemic cardiovascular side effects. It is therefore advocated as the most suitable vasoconstrictor for use in patients with cardiovascular disease or taking tricyclic antidepressant drugs.

It is less likely to produce local cyanosis on intradermal testing than are catecholamines (Klingenström and Westermark, 1964) and therefore there is less potential risk of local tissue damage.

ASSESSMENT

Most local anaesthetics are fairly satisfactory drugs and improvements gained in the manufacture of new drugs are likely to be only marginal. Therefore, careful assessment of a new drug is mandatory before it can be adopted in preference to a well-tried agent.

Local anaesthetics lend themselves to fairly accurate assessment as their effects can be measured objectively more easily than those of systemic analgesics. However, multifarious methods of testing have led to conflicting reports of efficacy.

Before the first clinical trials of a new drug take place, extensive preliminary investigations in both animals and man will have established a number of facts. It behoves the clinician about to embark on a clinical study to acquaint himself with the relevant literature.

Laboratory Investigations in Animals and Man

Animal studies can be used to make a rough assessment of latency, potency, local tissue irritancy and duration of action. Inhibition of the corneal reflex in the rabbit is used to measure surface anaesthetic activity. Inhibition of reaction to pinprick after intracutaneous injection in the guinea-pig can test infiltration anaesthesia. Conduction anaesthesia may be tested by sciatic nerve block in guinea-pig or frog, or by mouse tail root infiltration measuring inhibition of the pain reflexes. In man a series of intradermal injections of different concentrations of the new drug, together with a standard drug and a blank (physiological saline) can be given in the forearm. A quantitative assessment of analgesia to pinprick can be made by counting the number of standard, regularly interspersed pinpricks felt as sharp out of a total of, say, five per intradermal weal. This can give a crude estimate of potency and duration of action.

Clinical Trials

Drugs Used. It is generally considered desirable to use a new drug initially in a short series of cases without the use of a control or double-blind technique: a "clinical impression" trial. In this way, approximate potency may be confirmed and the most suitable concentration or range of concentrations established for use in a well-controlled double-blind trial. In this trial, the agent should be compared with a standard drug such as lignocaine, plain solutions should be included where suitable and the same vasoconstrictor, in the same concentration or range of concentrations, should be added to both local anaesthetics. If a vasoconstrictor is to be tested, it should be compared with plain solutions and with adrenaline, and comparable ranges of concentrations of each vasoconstrictor added to the same local anaesthetic or series of local anaesthetics. Only thus will it be possible to draw conclusions about any single new agent. Undue use of plain solutions that are already known to be ineffective must, of course, be avoided on ethical grounds.

Selection of Patients. As few patients as possible should be eliminated from the trial, and these should be specified beforehand; for example, some may be disqualified if catecholamines are to be included. The age, sex and concurrent diseases or medication should be noted. Males and females have been observed to react differently to infiltration anaesthesia. The type of procedure should be specified.

Technique of Administration. A double-blind trial must be used, with coded ampoules and random allocation of patients. Further details concerning methods in general are covered in Chapter 58.

A single administrator reduces the number of patients necessary, but a large-scale field trial is often considered desirable, in which case careful randomization, and standardization of the technique of administration are necessary. The type of anaesthesia, *i.e.* nerve block or infiltration, should be specified in each case, since each may yield different results (see Table 1). It is simpler statistically if the initial volume injected is kept constant for each type of blockade.

Assessment. (1) **Incidence** of successful anaesthesia. If analgesia is inadequate beyond 10 min. after the injection, this may be recorded as a failure.

(2) **Onset.** With modern drugs, onset is generally so rapid as to make differences between preparations clinically unimportant. To record the time of onset for conservative dentistry accurately it may be necessary to remove the enamel and produce pain before giving the injection, and then to stimulate the tooth at short intervals thereafter. This is not essential to validate a clinical trial.

(3) **Duration of dental anaesthesia.** This is generally recorded as the time at which a further injection becomes necessary, or the duration of the procedure (minimum duration). Since many procedures may be shorter than the duration of analgesia this can be inaccurate, but may be sufficient in a large-scale trial. Electrical stimulation of the teeth is more laborious but can give more accurate results.

(4) **Duration of soft-tissue anaesthesia.** Every patient must be given a stamped addressed postcard, on which he is asked to state the time at which normal sensation returns to his mouth, tongue and lips. The meaning and importance of this must be carefully explained to him.

(5) **Side effects.** Ideally, changes in pulse and blood pressure should be measured, though these may be more accurately assessed in a separate trial by continuous recording, on a smaller number of patients. Symptoms such as sweating, palpitations and faintness, and obvious signs such as pallor and syncope should be noted. If direct questioning is used some unlikely symptom should be sought, to detect indiscriminate positive responses. Post-operative symptoms such as local pain, swelling, bleeding, ulceration and jaw stiffness, and those related to hypersensitivity should be included on the postcard.

An estimate of blood loss may be made at the time of operation where appropriate.

Careful recording of what may appear an excessive number of data is essential to useful statistical evaluation of the results, and can enable meaningful comparisons to be made between different but similarly constructed clinical trials.

INDIVIDUAL LOCAL ANAESTHETICS

The number of local anaesthetics that have been marketed is legion, but only those that have been widely used in dentistry are described here. They are presented in chronological order. Their individual formulae are given in fig. 1. BP names are used; popular trade names and USP names are given in parenthesis.

Procaine

(Novocaine)

Procaine was synthesized in 1905, as a less toxic substitute for cocaine. Though now largely superseded, it enjoyed a long period of use.

Physico-chemical Properties. Procaine is an ester; solutions of the hydrochloride are unstable and cannot be autoclaved. It is poorly lipid-soluble; it has a pK_a of about 9·0 and is therefore highly ionized at physiological pH.

Local Anaesthetic Properties. It has a slow onset, a short duration of action and extremely poor penetrative powers. Even with a vasoconstrictor, it produces a relatively low incidence of successful dental anaesthesia. These properties stem from its vasodilator activity and highly ionized state. It is inactive as a surface anaesthetic.

Fate. It is rapidly hydrolysed by the enzyme pseudocholinesterase in the plasma and the liver to *p*-aminobenzoic acid and diethylaminoethanol.

Complications. It is more likely to be associated with hypersensitivity reactions than are amide local anaesthetics (*vide supra* under Hypersensitivity).

Preparations. Numerous dental preparations are available, including a 3 per cent solution with adrenaline 20 μg./ml. (1:50,000) as Novutox, a 1 per cent solution with butanilicaine 2 per cent (a little-used local anaesthetic) as Hostacain and with, in addition, noradrenaline 40μg./ml. as Hostacain-with-noradrenaline. These preparations might be considered to contain dangerously high concentrations of vasoconstrictor.

Indications. The only current indication for using procaine would appear to be in patients found to be hypersensitive to all amide local anaesthetics, but not to procaine.

Amethocaine

(Tetracaine, USP; Decicaine; Pontocaine)

Amethocaine is a homologue of procaine. It is highly lipid-soluble and has a pK_a of 8·39. It is potent and long-acting and a highly effective surface anaesthetic. It is extremely effective in solution applied as a spray or on cotton wool pledgets to the mucous membrane before injections or to the gum margins before scaling. It has been recommended in 0·5–2 per cent solutions or as a 10 per cent paste for surface application, but care should be exercised with higher concentrations since amethocaine is rapidly absorbed from mucous surfaces and the maximum safe dose is only 1 mg./kg. or less for the solution.

Indications. Amethocaine is indicated when a long-acting surface application is required.

Lignocaine

(Lidocaine, USP; Xylocaine)

Lignocaine was introduced into clinical practice in the 1940s, has wide applications and has been popular ever since.

Physico-chemical Properties. Lignocaine is an amide derivative of xylidine; solutions of the hydrochloride are extremely stable and can be autoclaved repeatedly. It is of intermediate lipid solubility; it has a pK_a of 7·86.

Local Anaesthetic Properties. It has a rapid onset of action, good powers of penetration, and only slight vasodilator activity. Nevertheless, for dental anaesthesia, the incidence of successful anaesthesia and the duration of action may both be inadequate without the addition of a vasoconstrictor (Table 1). It is active as a surface anaesthetic applied to mucous membranes.

Complications. Hypersensitivity is rare but has been reported (*vide supra*). The maximum safe dose of lignocaine by direct intravenous injection is about 2 mg./kg., so that the possibility of systemic toxicity is negligible. Most complications associated with the use of lignocaine in dentistry are due to the incorporation of high concentrations of adrenaline.

Preparations. Lignocaine 2 per cent with adrenaline 12·5 μg./ml. is the most widely used, though lower concentrations of adrenaline may be sufficient (Table 1). Plain solutions and solutions with noradrenaline 20 μg./ml. (Fastocaine) are also obtainable as dental preparations. The indications for noradrenaline are doubtful, and still more so such high concentrations of vasoconstrictors as are to be found in Xylestesin S for example, which contains adrenaline 20 μg./ml. and noradrenaline 20 μg./ml., thereby subjecting the recipient to the risk of both dangerous arrhythmias and hypertension.

Lignocaine is also available as a 5 per cent paste with or without amethocaine.

Indications. Lignocaine with adrenaline is indicated for painful procedures likely to last more than 15 min., in patients for whom adrenaline is not contra-indicated (*vide supra* under Vasoconstrictors). Plain solutions have too low an incidence of success for most purposes.

Mepivacaine
(Carbocaine)

Mepivacaine, like lignocaine, is an amide derivative of Xylidine, and is stable in solution. It has a pK$_a$ of 7·8, and its lipid solubility is of the same order as that of lignocaine.

It has been used in dentistry in a 2 per cent and a 3 per cent solution. It has superior penetrative powers and mild vasoconstrictor activity, and when used in a 3 per cent solution without vasoconstrictor it has a much higher success rate than does lignocaine (see Table 1). When used with adrenaline, it is indistinguishable from lignocaine in terms of success rate, duration of action and complications. In the U.S.A. and Scandinavia it has also been used with levonordefrin, which is said to be associated with few side effects, but the duration of soft-tissue anaesthesia is excessively long.

Indications. Mepivacaine 3 per cent is probably the best preparation for procedures of short duration.

Prilocaine
(Citanest)

Prilocaine is an amide derivative of *o*-toluidine, and is stable in solution. Its pK$_a$ is about 7·8, and is slightly less lipid soluble than lignocaine. Prilocaine has a rapid onset of action, good penetrative powers and some vasoconstrictor activity. In dentistry it has a moderately high success rate when used without a vasoconstrictor, but a short duration of action, especially for infiltration anaesthesia. It has been used as a 3 per cent solution plain and with adrenaline 3·3 μg./ml. (1:300,000) or with felypressin 0·03 i.u./ml., as a 4 per cent plain solution and as a 2 per cent solution with adrenaline 5 μg./ml. (1:200,000). Goldman and Gray (1963) found the solutions with adrenaline to be similar in activity to lignocaine 2 per cent adrenaline 12·5 μg./ml., though the action of prilocaine with adrenaline may be of insufficient duration for dental anaesthesia (Goldman and Evers, 1969). With felypressin the duration is longer, but the duration of soft-tissue anaesthesia may be unduly prolonged (see Table 1).

Prilocaine, being a secondary amine, is rapidly metabolized in the liver and the metabolite *o*-toluidine produces methaemoglobinaemia in large doses. This is of no significance in dentistry.

Indications. Prilocaine with felypressin (Citanest Octapressin) in indicated for long procedures in patients for whom catecholamines are contraindicated.

REFERENCES

Åkerman, B. (1969), "Effects of Felypressin (Octapressin) on the Acute Toxicity of Local Anaesthetics," *Acta pharmacol. (Kbh.)*, **27**, 318.

Boakes, A. J. Laurence, D. R., Teoh, P. C., Barar, F. S. K., Benedikter, L. T. and Prichard, B. N. C. (1973), "Interactions Between Sympathomimetic Amines and Antidepressant Agents in Man," *Brit. med. J.*, **1**, 311.

Cardwell, J. E. and Cawson, R. A. (1969), "A Trial of Lignocaine with 1:250,000 Adrenaline," *Brit. J. Oral Surg.*, **7**, 7.

Cowan, A. (1972), "A New Aspirating Syringe," *Brit. dent. J.*, **133**, 547.

Eyre, J. and Nally, F. F. (1971), "Nasal Test for Hypersensitivity—Including a Positive Reaction to Lignocaine," *Lancet*, **2**, 264.

Goldman, V. and Evers, H. (1969), "Prilocaine-Felypressin: a New Combination for Dental Analgesia," *Dent. Practit.*, **19**, 225.

Goldman, V. and Gray, W. (1963), "A Clinical Trial of a New Local Analgesic Agent," *Brit. dent. J.*, **115**, 59.

Klingenström, P. and Westermark, L. (1964), "Local Tissue-oxygen Tension After Adrenaline, Noradrenaline and Octapressin ® in Local Anaesthesia," *Acta anaesth. scand.*, **8**, 261.

Ritchie, J. M., Ritchie, B. and Greengard, P. (1965), "The Effect of the Nerve Sheath on the Action of Local Anesthetics," *J. Pharmacol.*, **150**, 160.

Seeman, P. (1972), "The Membrane Actions of Anesthetics and Tranquilizers," *Pharmacol. Rev.*, **24**, 583.

Waldman, H. B. and Binkley, G. (1967), "Lignocaine Hypersensitivity: Report of Case," *J. Amer. dent. Ass.*, **74**, 747.

Walker, R. T. (1971), "Hypersensitivity Reaction to Local Anaesthetic," *Brit. dent. J.*, **130**, 2.

25. GENERAL ANAESTHESIA

J. G. WHITWAM

INTRODUCTION

Modern dental anaesthesia may be said to have started in 1800 with the observation by Davy that nitrous oxide alleviated "toothache".

Once sleep is induced, a subject, while probably unaware of pain, may still show reflex somatic and autonomic responses to surgical stimulation which are exhibited as musculo-skeletal movement, usually associated with changes in respiration, and cardiovascular changes, for example in heart rate and blood pressure. Unless the afferent pathway from the site of surgical stimulation or the efferent neuromuscular pathways are blocked with local anaesthetic or muscle relaxants respectively, in order to provide optimum surgical conditions, anaesthesia must be deep enough to prevent reflex muscle movement. An adequate level of anaesthesia is associated with changes in cardiorespiratory function and also depression of the reflexes which normally maintain the airway. There may be inadequate ventilation, respiratory obstruction, a fall in blood pressure or a combination of factors which cause failure of oxygen delivery to the heart and brain, leading to cardiac arrest and death. The possibility of this complication occurring is increased during dental surgery by the competition between operator and anaesthetist for the airway, and often by the use of the sitting position.

EFFECT OF ANAESTHETICS ON THE CENTRAL NERVOUS SYSTEM (CNS)

The basic unit of the nervous system is the neurone which has been described as having input (cell body and dendrites), integrative (axon hillock), conductile (axon) and output (secretory terminal) segments. Nerve cells are linked by their axons to either the dendrites and cell bodies or to the axons of other cells by means of synapses. Electrical impulses (action potentials) arriving at presynaptic terminals release transmitter substances which can cross the synaptic cleft and cause either depolarization (excitation) or hyperpolarization (inhibition) of the membrane of the post-synaptic cell.

Anaesthetics act at synapses to impair conduction and exert profound effects on complex multisynaptic pathways, causing a breakdown of the normal interrelationships of activity within the brain, which is associated with and presumably causes the anaesthetic state. It has been suggested that barbiturates reduce the amount of transmitter released at presynaptic terminals. Inhalational agents (*e.g.* halothane, chloroform, ether) are thought to act by increasing the threshold of post-synaptic cells to excitation. However, Richards (1973) has suggested that in the cerebral cortex halothane reduces excitatory synaptic transmission not by an increase in the electrical threshold of post-synaptic cells, but by interference with the process of chemical transmission, either by reducing the output of transmitter from presynaptic terminals or by reducing the sensitivity of the post-synaptic membrane to the transmitter substance.

Drugs used to induce anaesthesia are usually administered through the lungs or intravenously. In children the intramuscular injection of methohexitone may sometimes be preferred.

INHALATIONAL AGENTS

A mixture of nitrous oxide and oxygen provides an inhalational background for most anaesthetic techniques. Because of changes in lung function caused by anaesthesia it is advisable to administer an inspired oxygen concentration greater than that in air, *e.g.* in the range of 30–40 per cent.

Nitrous oxide has analgesic properties but does not induce full surgical anaesthesia. It is used either in conjunction with intravenous drugs or as a vehicle for the vaporization and administration of other inhalational agents which are liquid at room temperature (*e.g.* halothane, trichlorethylene, methoxyflurane).

Storage of Oxygen and Nitrous Oxide. Oxygen is pumped into cylinders to a pressure of 13700 kPa for storage and delivery.

At normal ambient temperatures nitrous oxide is below its critical temperature (*i.e.* the temperature below which it can be liquefied by pressure, 36·5°C) and full cylinders contain liquid nitrous oxide with a relatively small amount of vapour (*i.e.* nitrous oxide gas below 36·5°C). At 20°C, the cylinder pressure gauge will indicate a steady pressure of 5065 kPa as long as any liquid nitrous oxide remains in the cylinder; once it has all evaporated, the pressure falls steadily until the cylinder is empty. Hence unlike oxygen, where there is a progressive reduction in pressure as gas is withdrawn, the pressure dial on a nitrous oxide cylinder gives little indication of the amount remaining. Because liquids are virtually incompressible nitrous oxide cylinders are not filled to the point where they contain only liquid, since a small increase in ambient temperature would cause a dangerous rise in pressure in the cylinder. The degree of filling is expressed as the Filling Ratio:

$$\text{Filling ratio} = \frac{\text{Weight of nitrous oxide (liquid + gas in cylinder)}}{\text{Weight of water required to fill cylinder completely}}$$

This is normally 0·75 when nine-tenths of the nitrous oxide is liquid.

By knowing the tare weight, *i.e.* the weight of the container (in this case the empty cylinder), it is possible by weighing a cylinder to assess the amount of nitrous oxide remaining.

Pre-mixed Nitrous Oxide—Oxygen Mixtures. When oxygen is bubbled through liquid nitrous oxide, some of the oxygen dissolves in the nitrous oxide. The gas bubbles also carry nitrous oxide into the gaseous phase and the process can be continued until all the liquid nitrous oxide disappears. The addition of oxygen in this way lowers the critical temperature of the nitrous oxide.

Entonox is the term used for a gas introduced by the British Oxygen Company which contains 50 per cent nitrous oxide and 50 per cent oxygen. If the temperature falls below −7°C (as may occur in winter in temperate climates) liquid nitrous oxide will reform. If this occurs, the first gas to be delivered will contain a relatively high concentration of oxygen. As usage continues the nitrous oxide will evaporate and since the cylinder has already given up most of its oxygen a gas mixture deficient in oxygen will be delivered.

Reducing Valves. Before delivery to the patient nitrous oxide and oxygen are passed through reducing valves. The final pressure varies between 101 kPa (1 atm.) and 405 kPA (4 atm.) in different anaesthetic machines (Thompson, 1968).

Anaesthetic Circuit

A typical dental anaesthetic circuit is illustrated in fig. 1. During inspiration the patient's tidal volume is supplied partly by the flow of fresh gas and partly from the reservoir

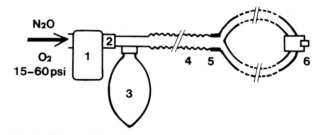

Fig. 1. Schema of dental anaesthetic circuit.
1. Vaporizer.
2. Non-return valve.
3. Reservoir bag.
4. Connecting tube.
5. Junction for attachment of nasal mask, face mask or endotracheal tube.
6. Nasal mask with expiratory valve.
N.B. 15–60 p.s.i. = 1–4 atm. = 101·3–405·2 kPa.

bag (filled during expiration). At the beginning of expiration the pressure in the circuit is below the pressure required to open the expiratory valve. The gas from the mask and the patient's airway *i.e.* the dead space which contains gas not exposed to the pulmonary circulation and having the same composition as fresh gas, re-enters the connecting tube, and assists the filling of the reservoir bag. If the flow of nitrous oxide and oxygen from the anaesthetic machine is adequate, by the time alveolar gas (containing carbon dioxide and from which oxygen has been taken up by the pulmonary circulation) reaches the nose-piece, the reservoir bag is full and the pressure in the circuit exceeds the opening pressure of the expiratory valve (*e.g.* 2–3 cm. H_2O) so that the alveolar gas is expelled through the valve. The most efficient use of the circuit is to provide a fresh gas flow low enough to allow the dead space gas to return to the delivery tubing. Since the dead space is approximately one-third of the tidal volume, the flow of fresh gas should be equal to two-thirds of the patient's minute volume:

Respiratory rate × tidal volume = minute volume; for example,

20/min. × 350 ml. = 7,000 ml./min.

2/3 × 7 l. = 4·7 l./min.

If the flow of fresh gas is too low, then alveolar gas containing carbon dioxide and deficient in oxygen may enter the connecting tubing and will be the first gas to be inspired by the patient during the next respiratory cycle (*i.e.* re-breathing occurs, the arterial P_{CO_2} will rise and the P_{O_2} may fall). For most adults a fresh gas flow of 4–6 l./min. will prevent re-breathing.

If the non-return valve is moved to the other side of the reservoir bag, between the bag and the patient, *e.g.* to the junction 5 (fig. 1), then expired gas cannot return to the connecting tubing or the reservoir bag, which will be filled entirely by the fresh gas flow and rebreathing cannot occur. However the dead space gas is also lost through the expiratory valve and the flow of anaesthetic gases must be increased by approximately one-third. Such a modification of the circuit makes it less efficient, but by preventing any possibility of rebreathing it is safer.

Vaporization of Anaesthetic Agents

The maximum concentration of a vapour which can be delivered at a particular temperature depends on the saturated vapour pressure of the substance at that temperature.

$$\text{Maximum concentration} = \frac{\text{Saturated vapour pressure}}{\text{Barometric pressure}} \times 100$$

The variation of saturated vapour pressure with temperature for several anaesthetic agents is illustrated in fig. 2. Thus at 20°C, by saturating the delivery gas, it is possible to administer approximately 1 per cent methoxyflurane, 6·6 per cent trichlorethylene, and 32 per cent halothane. However in the case of halothane this is 10 times the concentration required to induce surgical anaesthesia.

In vaporizers designed for the administration of halothane only part of the fresh gas flow is diverted to the chamber containing halothane. Figure 3A illustrates the principle of the Goldman vaporizer. Part of the gas flow blows over the surface of liquid halothane. The output of such a vaporizer depends on the relative flows of gas, the amount of halothane in the chamber, its surface area and its temperature. As the halothane evaporates its temperature falls and hence the vapour pressure and concentration administered decrease. In practice the maximum concentration which is delivered is of the order of 2 per cent.

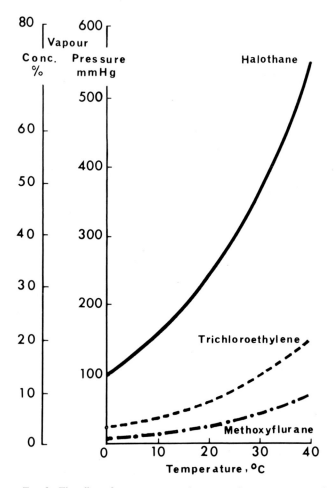

FIG. 2. The effect of temperature on the saturated vapour pressure of halothane, trichloroethylene and methoxyflurane. Percentage concentration refers to the maximum concentration which can be vaporized in dry gas at a barometric pressure of 760 mm. Hg.

i.e. $\dfrac{\text{Saturated Vapour Pressure} \times 100}{760}$ = percentage concentration.

N.B. 100 mm. Hg. = 13·3 kPa.

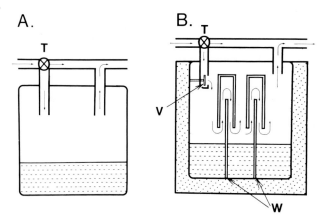

FIG. 3. Schematic representation of the Goldman (A) and Cyprane (B) vaporizers. Arrows indicate gas flow; T = tap for dividing gas flow (by allowing more gas to pass through the chamber containing the anaesthetic the concentration in the gas leaving the vaporizer is increased); V = temperature compensating valve (bimetallic strip); W = wick to ensure saturation of gas with halothane irrespective of the amount of liquid halothane in the vaporizer.

Figure 3B shows the principle of a temperature compensated vaporizer (Cyprane).

Approximately 1 per cent halothane is delivered for each 2 per cent of fresh gas flow diverted to the vaporizer. The apparatus contains a temperature compensating valve which diverts proportionately more gas to the vaporizing chamber at low temperatures and less at high temperatures, and the concentration administered remains stable over a wide range of ambient temperatures.

Factors Affecting the Uptake of Inhalational Agents

Ventilation

An increase in ventilation will increase the alveolar concentration of the anaesthetic and deepen anaesthesia. When increasing ventilation by inflating the lungs, unless the inspired anaesthetic concentration is reduced the depth of anaesthesia will be increased.

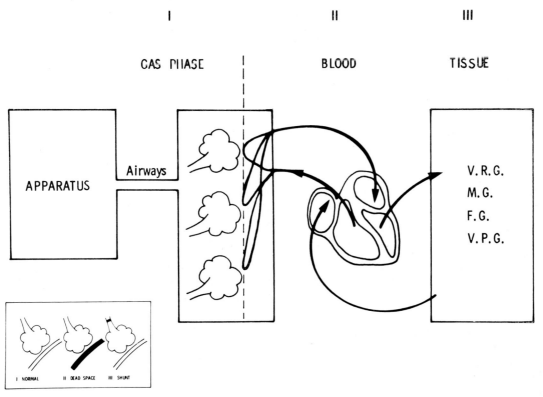

FIG. 4. Schematic representation of the 3 phases in the uptake of an inhalational anaesthetic agent, *i.e.* I. Gas; II. Blood; III. Tissues; V.R.G. very rich in blood vessels; M.G. muscle group; F.G. fat group; V.P.G. low blood flow—very poor group.
Inset I. normal, i.e. normal alveolar ventilation matched to a normal blood supply; II. ventilation without perfusion, *i.e.* increase in alveolar dead space; III. airway occlusion; blood flow without ventilation, *i.e.* a shunt.

Absorption and Distribution of Inhalational Agents

During induction of inhalational anaesthesia, anaesthetic gas is ventilated into the alveoli, enters the blood, and is transported to the tissues (fig. 4). Uptake into blood starts with the first breath. The rate of transfer into blood depends on the alveolar concentration of the agent, its solubility in blood, and the rate of blood flow through the pulmonary capillaries. The gas taken up by the blood is transported to the tissues where a second partition occurs between blood and tissues. The rate of uptake of the agent from the blood by an organ or tissue depends on its arterial tension, the vascularity of the tissue (*i.e.* blood flow per unit mass of tissue), and the solubility of the agent in the tissue.

When the tissues become saturated with the anaesthetic drug, arterial and venous concentrations are the same and approximate to alveolar concentration, and uptake ceases.

Blood Solubility

Nitrous oxide is rapidly taken up by the blood from the alveoli. However, compared to other anaesthetic agents it has a relatively low solubility coefficient in blood (*i.e.* at the same tension or partial pressure a relatively smaller mass of gas dissolves in the blood) and hence the alveolar concentration rapidly approaches the inspired concentration (fig. 5i). Methoxyflurane has a high solubility coefficient in blood and during the induction of anaesthesia the alveolar concentration rises slowly because the agent is rapidly removed by the blood (fig. 5iii). Halothane lies between these two extremes (fig. 5ii).

Concentration and Second Gas Effects

An anaesthetic gas which is highly soluble in blood is quickly taken up by the blood causing a rapid loss of gas from the alveoli, and a gradient is created between the

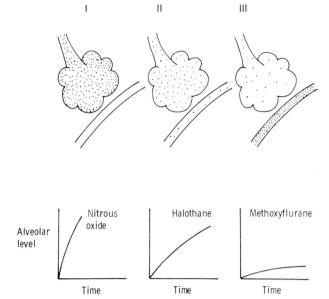

FIG. 5. Effect of the solubility in blood of an anaesthetic agent on the rate of rise of alveolar concentration:

    I. For a gas with a low solubility coefficient in blood, *e.g.* nitrous oxide, the alveolar tension rapidly equilibrates with the inspired tension.

    II. Halothane has a greater solubility coefficient in blood than nitrous oxide, hence the rate of rise of the alveolar concentration is slower.

    III. Methoxyflurane has a high solubility coefficient in blood, so that as fast as molecules of the gas arrive in perfused alveoli they are taken up by the blood and the alveolar concentration increases only slowly.

partial pressure of the anaesthetic in the inspired gas and that in the alveoli. Some of the gas taken up by blood is replaced by the additional inflow of gas down the pressure gradient without ventilation being required. At high inspired concentrations a relatively larger volume of gas is absorbed by the blood and a greater pressure gradient is created. This means that at high inspired concentrations, more anaesthetic gas enters the alveoli and is available for uptake by the blood so that the rate at which the blood becomes saturated with the anaesthetic is faster and the alveolar concentration more rapidly approaches the inspired concentration. This is called the **concentration effect.** The mechanism depends on the amount of gas absorbed, *i.e.* its solubility coefficient in blood and its inspired concentration. It is difficult to observe the phenomenon during the uptake of gases which are administered in low concentrations, *e.g.* halothane or methoxyflurane.

Because of the concentration effect the time taken for the alveolar concentration of nitrous oxide to approach the inspired concentration is several minutes slower when 50 per cent nitrous oxide (entonox) is administered as compared with an inspired concentration of 70–80 per cent.

Halothane is often administered with a high concentration of nitrous oxide. The rapid uptake of nitrous oxide has the effect of augmenting the total inflow of gas (described above). Since this gas has passed through the vaporiser the delivery of halothane to the alveoli is increased. In addition, because of the uptake of nitrous oxide (not completely compensated for by the additional inflow of gas), it has been suggested that there is a reduction in the volume of gas in the alveoli which increases the concentration of halothane. These two factors combine to create the **second gas effect** and cause an increase in alveolar concentration and uptake of any agent administered together with nitrous oxide.

Cardiac Output

When there is an increase in cardiac output (*e.g.* fever, excitement, anxiety) pulmonary blood flow is increased and a larger amount of anaesthetic is taken from the alveoli. The alveolar concentration approaches the inspired concentration more slowly, the gradient driving anaesthetic into the blood (*i.e.* alveolar tension—venous tension) is reduced, and induction of anaesthesia is slower. Conversely when the cardiac output is low as in heart disease, there is less blood flow to take up anaesthetic from the alveoli, the alveolar and blood concentrations rise more rapidly, and deeper anaesthesia is induced more quickly.

Tissue Uptake

Highly vascular tissues, (vessel rich group—VRG, fig. 4) which include the brain, heart, liver and kidney attain the same anaesthetic tension as exists in arterial blood within 5–15 min.

The muscle group of tissues (MG) has a relatively lower blood flow per unit mass and continues to absorb anaesthetic agent longer than the vessel rich group. After saturation of the muscle group further uptake depends on fatty tissues (Fat Group FG). Uptake by tissues which have a poor blood supply (Vessel Poor Group VPG), which include cartilage, tendons and ligaments, exerts a very small effect on the uptake and distribution of anaesthetic agents. For nitrous oxide, with the exception of fat, equilibrium is almost complete within 10–15 min. For halothane, uptake by the vessel rich group dominates for the first 10 min., after which the muscle group continues to take up this agent for about $2\frac{1}{2}$ hr. Halothane is highly soluble in fat, and uptake by fat and brain lipids can continue for over 36 hr.

The increase in alveolar concentration of any inhalational agent has four phases (fig. 6).

Overpressure

For a gas with a high solubility coefficient in blood the induction of anaesthesia is slow. In order to reduce induction time it is customary to start with a high inspired concentration which is subsequently reduced to the maintenance level and Harris (1951) applied the term overpressure to this technique. The principle is illustrated for halothane in fig. 7.

Age

Young children not only approach equilibrium faster but also require a higher concentration of anaesthetic than older children and adults for a comparable level of anesthesia to be attained.

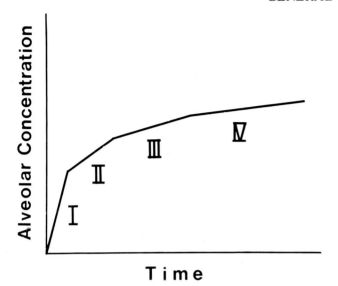

FIG. 6. The four phases in the uptake of an inhalational agent, *i.e.* equilibration with:
  I. Blood.
  II. Highly vascular tissues (*e.g.* brain).
  III. Muscle Group.
  IV. Fat.

Variations in Ventilation Perfusion Ratios in the Lungs

In patients with lung disease, and in older people, some alveoli are not ventilated, but are perfused—*i.e.* there is an intrapulmonary shunt of venous blood to the arterial circulation which is not exposed to the anaesthetic agent and hence its uptake is slower. The effect of interrupting the blood supply to parts of the lung which are ventilated is to increase the alveolar dead space and reduce the effectiveness of ventilation, thereby slowing the uptake of an anaesthetic agent.

Excretion, Metabolism and Toxicity of Inhalational Agents

Diffusion Hypoxia. During recovery, for the first few minutes a large volume of nitrous oxide enters the alveoli from the blood, dilution of alveolar gases occurs, and to prevent hypoxaemia oxygen must be administered for 5–10 min.

Duration of Elimination. Although the bulk of nitrous oxide is excreted rapidly it is possible, after anaesthesia lasting only 30 min., to detect its excretion for over 40 hr. Halothane excretion can be detected for up to 3 weeks after a single administration.

Metabolism. Until relatively recently it had been assumed that inhalational anaesthetics, with the exception of trichlorethylene, were excreted unchanged. However it is estimated that up to 20 per cent of administered halothane is metabolized, largely in the liver and to a lesser extent in the kidney. The major metabolites of halothane are chloride, bromide, and trifluoroacetic acid, none of which is toxic in the quantities produced. The metabolism of methoxyflurane may cause the release of several hundred milligrams of inorganic fluoride ion for several days, but the levels are below those normally associated with toxicity. Other metabolites of methoxyflurane include oxalic acid, and oxalate crystals have been identified in renal tubules following methoxyflurane anaesthesia.

Toxicity. It has been suggested that halothane may cause liver damage, although at present there is no evidence for this (*e.g.* Simpson *et al.*, 1971). Methoxyflurane has been implicated as a nephrotoxic drug (*e.g.* Crandell *et al.*, 1966). Prolonged exposure to anaesthetics can cause bone marrow depression.

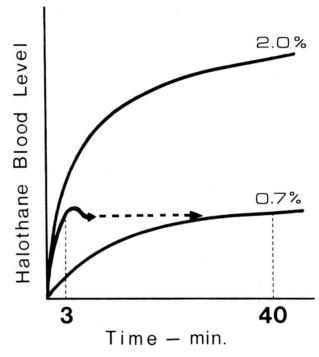

FIG. 7. "Over pressure." By commencing the administration of halothane at an inspired concentration of 2 per cent (*i.e.* after brief introductory period at a low concentration—0·5 per cent, see text) which is reduced to 1 per cent after 1½ min., it is possible to reach a blood level in 3 min. which could take over 30 min. using a concentration of 0·7 per cent from the start. The blood levels achieved during induction of anaesthesia would be represented by the arrowed line. The slight "overshoot" is caused by the time taken for the gas containing the new inspired concentration (*i.e.* 0·7 per cent started at 3 min.) to clear the previous gas mixture from the circuit.

Not only are patients exposed to anaesthetics but so too are the staff working in the patient's environment. Inhalational agents can be detected in small amounts in the breath of anaesthetists several days after prolonged exposure in the working environment. Anaesthetic agents have been shown to be teratogenic and embryotoxic in animals and there are reports of an increased incidence of abortion in female anaesthetists and operating theatre staff. Anaesthetists have a higher than normal incidence of malignancy of the reticulo-endothelial system.

Potency and Mode of Action of Anaesthetics

Anaesthetic drugs cause a decrease in the amount of neurotransmitters released within the nervous system (described above), but how this is brought about is not clear. Anaesthetic agents are soluble in the hydrophobic regions of biological membranes giving rise to membrane expansion and a critical increase in membrane surface area can be correlated with the production of anaesthesia. Exposure of anaesthetized animals (e.g. tadpoles, fish and small mammals) to high atmospheric pressures, e.g. 100–150 atm., causes a return of consciousness and this phenomenon is termed "pressure reversal". Pressure reversal is not due to the squeezing out of anaesthetic molecules from membranes but is caused by a re-ordering of the structure of the membranes to produce a configuration similar to that of the conscious state. It may be that membrane expansion prevents the normal release of vesicles of transmitter substance by the process of exocytosis and that this is the mechanism of anaesthesia.

The accurate determination of the relative potencies of various anaesthetic drugs is a relatively recent development. The minimum alveolar concentration (MAC 1) has been defined as that concentration (at equilibrium) required to prevent reflex skeletal movement in response to painful stimuli.

The best correlation of potency with a potential biological interaction is the solubility of the substance in olive oil (Table 1). This is the basis of the Overton-Meyer fat solubility hypothesis originally suggested at the turn of the century. It is proposed that "narcosis commences when any chemically indifferent substance has attained a certain molar concentration in the lipids of the cell. This concentration depends on the nature of the animal or cell but is independent of the narcotic" (Halsey and Kent, 1972).

The **three principal factors** which affect the application of a particular anaesthetic agent are its **vapour pressure** (the amount which can be administered), **the solubility coefficient** in blood and tissues (the rate of equilibration with inspired concentration) and its **potency** (the amount required).

Three other factors are of considerable importance:

(a) *Flammability and explosions.* This is a problem with ether and cyclopropane.

(b) *Irritant effects.* It is difficult to administer substances such as ether because of irritation of the tracheo-bronchial tree leading to coughing, breath-holding and laryngospasm. Halothane in concentrations above 2 per cent will cause coughing and its smell can be unpleasant to the patient. Although these effects soon disappear during induction of anaesthesia it is wise to present a patient initially with a concentration of not more than 0·5 per cent. After a few breaths, the inspired concentration may be increased.

(c) *Recovery characteristics.* Recovery after trichlorethylene and methoxyflurane anaesthesia tends to be prolonged and is associated with a high incidence of nausea and vomiting. Recovery from halothane anaesthesia is rapid and is associated with the lowest incidence of nausea and vomiting of any inhalational agent (less than 3 per cent). Sometimes shivering occurs after halothane anaesthesia.

INTRAVENOUS DRUGS

Five drugs have to be considered, *viz.* thiopentone, methohexitone, propanidid, althesin and ketamine.

Barbiturates—Thiopentone and Methohexitone

Uptake and Distribution

In 1960 Price described the kinetics of the distribution of thiopentone in the body, and other barbiturates have a qualitatively similar pattern of distribution.

In the first phase a single dose of thiopentone added to the blood forms a "central pool", and the amount of drug in the blood is lost rapidly, primarily as a result of uptake by the highly perfused viscera (heart, kidney, splanchnic area and central nervous system) so that at 1 min., 55 per cent of the drug is present in these tissues even though they represent only 6 per cent of body weight. Thus following the administration of a single intravenous dose of a barbiturate, the peak concentration in the brain will occur after 1 min. During the second phase, the drug is redistributed from rapidly perfused viscera, including the brain, to the lean body mass such as muscle and skin so that after 5 min. the maximal concentration in the brain will have been reduced by half. Fat uptake is insignificant at this stage. Recovery of consciousness is due to redistribution from the brain into lean body mass. After 30 min. the

TABLE 1

APPROXIMATE DATA OF SOME ANAESTHETIC AGENTS

Agent	Boiling Point	Vapour Pressure kPa 20°C	Solubility 37°C		Concentration for 1st Phase Surgical Anaesthesia M.A.C. 1
			Blood/Gas	Oil/Gas	
Nitrous oxide	−89°C	90	0·47	1·4	120
Halothane	50·2°C	32	2·3	224	0·74
Trichlorethylene	87°C	7	9·15	960	0·17
Methoxyflurane	104·6°C	1	13·0	825	0·20

brain will contain only 5 per cent of the injected dose, fat 18 per cent, lean body mass 75 per cent and the poorly perfused tissues, *e.g.* ligaments, tendons and cartilage play only a small part in the redistribution of the drug. During the third phase considerable uptake of the drug by the fatty tissues occurs so that 2–3 hr. after injection, the concentration there exceeds that of other tissues. Full redistribution takes 8–10 hr. at which time metabolic degradation has reduced the total amount of drug in the body to less than 20 per cent of the administered dose.

Factors Affecting Drug Requirements

Physical Characteristics of the Patient

Recovery of consciousness after a single intravenous dose of either thiopentone or methohexitone is caused largely by redistribution of the drug into lean body mass, which explains why the small muscular individual often requires a larger dose of drug, on a weight basis, than a heavier obese person. This is also one factor in the larger dose requirement of men, compared with women who have a lower ratio of muscle to fat.

Cardiac Output

When the cardiac output is increased, *e.g.* in anxious or febrile patients, the drug is diluted into a larger volume of blood during its passage through the veins and lungs, and a relatively greater proportion is distributed to tissues other than the brain. The concentration and total amount of the drug entering the brain is reduced and hence a larger amount of induction agent is required. When there is a low cardiac output, *e.g.* in heart disease or after haemorrhage, a drug which is administered intravenously is diluted into a smaller volume of blood, it achieves a higher concentration in arterial blood (a greater proportion of which is directed to the brain), and a much smaller dose of the drug is required to induce anaesthesia.

Transport in Blood

Many drugs are transported in the blood in ionized and non-ionized forms. It is only the free non-ionized form of the drug which can cross cell membranes and which is therefore the active component. Both the plasma proteins and red cells may take up the drug and reduce the amount available to the tissues. For example 73 per cent of methohexitone in human plasma may be bound to plasma proteins and a further 20 per cent of the drug may be taken up by the red cells in whole blood with a normal haematocrit. Thus only 7 per cent of the drug is free in plasma (most of which will be non-ionized, *i.e.* active). A reduction in either plasma proteins or red cell mass (*e.g.* in anaemia) will leave more drug free in an active form and reduce the amount required.

Age. Young children require a larger amount of drug administered on a weight basis to achieve the same level of anaesthesia. Elderly patients are sensitive to intravenous barbiturates, and recovery may be prolonged. It is advisable to reduce the induction dose of methohexitone to half or even a third of the normal dose in patients over the age of 65 years.

Metabolism and Excretion. Barbiturates are metabolized in the liver and the metabolites are excreted in the urine and bile. In man it is probable that over 50 per cent of a dose of barbiturate is excreted as metabolites in the faeces.

Potency. Methohexitone is approximately three times as potent as thiopentone and doses suitable for induction of anaesthesia are approximately 1 mg./kg. and 3 mg./kg. respectively.

Complications Occurring During Induction of Anaesthesia with Barbiturates

These may be classified as follows:

(a) Excitatory phenomena, *e.g.* tremors and involuntary muscle movements;
(b) respiratory upset, *e.g.* cough, hiccough, laryngospasm;
(c) respiratory depression; and
(d) cardiovascular depression.

The administration of methohexitone is more often associated with the complications in groups (a) and (b) than thiopentone. The transient "crowing" indicating narrowing of the laryngeal aperture, sometimes observed during induction of anaesthesia with methohexitone, is probably related to an increase in muscle activity and is not a serious reflexly produced laryngospasm. These complications are transient and can be minimized by avoiding large doses of the drug. Thiopentone and methohexitone have comparable effects on respiration, but methohexitone causes less cardiovascular depression than thiopentone.

Recovery from anaesthesia is more rapid after methohexitone than thiopentone and this is the principle reason why methohexitone is the drug of choice for outpatient anaesthesia. Methohexitone also causes less tissue damage if accidentally injected extravenously or intra-arterially, and it can be used intramuscularly (*e.g.* in children).

Barbiturates should never be administered to patients suffering from **porphyria,** a rare disease of porphyrin metabolism, since an acute crisis will be precipitated which can be fatal.

Propanidid is a derivative of oil of cloves (eugenol). It is quickly metabolized by cholinesterases and recovery of consciousness is rapid. After a single dose respiration is stimulated and then depressed. Occasionally it causes acute cardiovascular collapse due to a sensitivity reaction. During recovery there is a relatively high incidence of nausea and vomiting.

Althesin is a mixture of two steroids (alphaxalone and alphadolone). Induction of anaesthesia is relatively uncomplicated, but although it is rapidly metabolized more rapid recovery of consciousness can be obtained with methohexitone. Occasionally adverse cardiovascular reactions similar to those seen with propanidid occur.

Ketamine is a phencyclidine derivative. It does not cause cardiovascular depression and is associated with only minimal respiratory depression. In adults, nightmares and disorientation occur during recovery, which may be prolonged, so that it is unsuitable for routine use. It may have an indication in facio-maxillary surgery where a tracheotomy would otherwise be required.

CIRCULATORY CHANGES DURING DENTAL SURGERY UNDER ANAESTHESIA

Physiology of the Cardiovascular System

Normally cardiac output is determined by the metabolic rate of the subject.

Because of its viscosity there is a resistance to the passage of blood through the small vessels entering the tissues. The systemic blood pressure (BP) is due to the heart forcing its output (CO) through the peripheral resistance (PR); that is, $BP = CO \times PR$. Normal cardiac output in an adult at rest is approximately 5 l./min. Normal BP is 16 kPa systolic and 10·6 kPa diastolic.

Factors Affecting Cardiac Output

(a) *Blood Volume.* If there is not enough blood in the cardiovascular system, cardiac output cannot be maintained.

(b) *Venous Return.* The heart can eject only the blood presented to it. Thus cardiac output depends on venous return, and this is related to the oxygen consumption of the tissues.

(c) *Force of contraction.* The heart must provide enough energy to eject the returning blood. In response to an increase in venous return there is an increase in heart rate and stroke volume. The presystolic length of the cardiac muscle fibres is increased, which increases the amount of work which can be performed (Starling's Law) and enables the heart to eject the increased stroke volume. Increased activity in cardiac sympathetic nerves increases the amount of work which can be performed by the heart.

(d) *Heart rate.* Cardiac output = stroke volume × heart rate. If the heart rate decreases, cardiac output can be maintained by increasing the stroke volume. However there is a limit to this compensation and at low heart rates (*e.g.* below 40–50 beats/min.) cardiac output falls. At high heart rates (*e.g.* over 200 beats/min.) there is not enough time for recovery and filling and cardiac output is reduced.

Neurological Control of the Circulation

The cerebral blood flow is determined by the blood pressure in the aorta. In the upright position (*e.g.* when sitting in the dental chair), before blood can reach the brain it has to overcome the hydrostatic pressure of the column of blood in the carotid arteries (*i.e.* 1 mm. Hg. for approximately each 1·36 cm. of the column of blood in the cerebral vessels; density of blood assumed to be 1·0 and mercury 13·6 grams per cubic centimetre). The pressure in the aorta must exceed approximately 1·3–2·0 kPa before cerebral flow can occur. The structures of the cardiovascular system (*i.e.* the heart, arteries and veins) are under the control of the autonomic nervous system as illustrated schematically in fig. 8. The circulation responds rapidly to physiological changes (*e.g.* posture, blood loss, vasodilation) to maintain aortic pressure and hence cerebral blood flow.

The Baroreceptors

Stretch receptors are located in the walls of the aortic arch, the carotid sinuses, and other vessels in the neck (stippled areas fig. 8) which provide a fast feed back mechanism acting through the autonomic nervous system to stabilize the blood pressure and heart rate.

A rise in arterial pressure causes an increase in nerve impulses from the baroreceptors causing a reduction in sympathetic activity and hence peripheral vasodilation and a decrease in the rate as well as the force of contraction of the heart. Also, activity in cardio-inhibitory fibres in the vagus nerves is increased, which also causes a reduction in heart rate. A fall in arterial pressure reduces baroreceptor activity. Sympathetic activity increases and vagal activity decreases, causing peripheral vasoconstriction and an increase in the force of contraction of the heart and the heart rate which tends to restore the blood pressure to previous levels.

There are three primary events for which compensation may be required:

(1) *Loss of blood* → fall in venous return → fall in cardiac output → fall in blood pressure → reduction in baroreceptor activity → increased sympathetic activity → an increase in peripheral resistance and the force of contraction and rate of the heart.

(2) *Peripheral vasodilation* → fall in blood pressure → reduction in baroreceptor activity → increased sympathetic activity → reduction in peripheral vasodilation and in increase in force of contraction and rate of the heart.

(3) *Reduction in the force of contraction of the heart* → decreased cardiac output → fall in blood pressure → reduction in baroreceptor activity → increased sympathetic activity → peripheral vasoconstriction and an increase in the force of contraction and the rate of the heart.

Factors affecting the Circulation during Surgery under General Anaesthesia

Changes in Carbon Dioxide and Oxygen Tensions— Respiratory Obstruction

A rise in arterial carbon dioxide tension ($Pa\text{CO}_2$) or a fall in oxygen tension ($Pa\text{O}_2$) causes an increase in sympathetic activity by a direct action on the central nervous system.

During respiratory obstruction sympathetic activity is increased causing an increase in blood pressure and heart rate.

Anxiety and Nervousness

Acute anxiety causes increased sympathetic activity associated with a rise in blood pressure and tachycardia.

Control of Circulation

Baroreceptor Input   **C.N.S.**   **Autonomic Outflow**

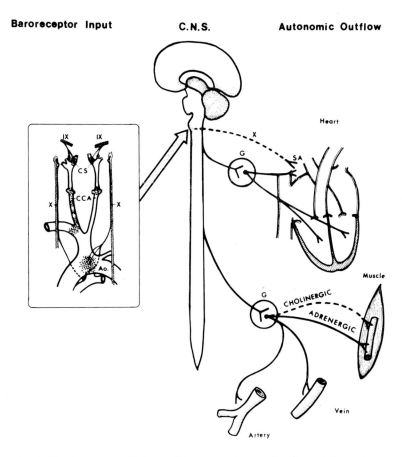

FIG. 8. Circulatory control. Inset—Baroreceptor input—stippled areas show sites of stretch receptors in the aorta and the vessels of the neck. Ao = aorta; CCA = common carotid artery; CS = carotid sinuses; IX = glossopharyngeal nerve; X = vagus nerve; G = sympathetic ganglia; SA = sino-atrial node.

The baroreceptors are a negative feed-back mechanism. They normally exert a tonic influence on the central cardiovascular neurones which inhibits sympathetic outflow and causes an increase in the activity of cardio-inhibitory fibres in the vagus nerves to slow the heart rate. A rise in arterial pressure increases these effects whilst a fall in blood pressure allows an increase in activity in sympathetic nerves and inhibits the activity in the cardio-inhibitory vagal fibres to increase heart rate.

The Effect of Anaesthetic Drugs

In general, drugs which produce anaesthesia cause cardiovascular depression and a fall in blood pressure, which may compromise cerebral blood flow, particularly in the upright position.

Anaesthetic drugs have four major effects on the circulation;

(a) reduction in metabolic rate and hence a fall in cardiac output;

(b) depression of activity of the sympathetic nervous system, causing peripheral vasodilation and a reduction in the force of contraction and rate of the heart;

(c) direct effects on the heart (causing depression of cardiac function) and on smooth muscle of the peripheral vessels (causing vasodilation); and

(d) loss of responsiveness of the heart and peripheral vessels to an increase in sympathetic activity, thereby reducing the effectiveness of the baroreceptor reflexes.

Following a small dose of a barbiturate, there is a transient fall in blood pressure which is caused largely by a reduction in sympathetic activity.

Nitrous oxide causes only a slight reduction in sympathetic activity and has minimal effect on the circulation.

Halothane and methoxyflurane both decrease the responsiveness of the myocardium to sympathetic stimulation and also cause peripheral vasodilation affecting arteries, capillaries, and veins. In addition to decreasing central sympathetic activity, halothane has ganglion-blocking properties which also reduce activity in post-ganglionic sympathetic nerves. Halothane causes a reduction in heart rate, cardiac function, peripheral resistance, cardiac output and blood pressure by a combination of its effects on the nervous system, the heart and the peripheral blood vessels.

Stimulation of Peripheral Nerves

Painful stimuli cause an increase in sympathetic activity which overcomes the depressant effects of light general anaesthesia so that during dental extractions the blood pressure rises (Whitwam and Young, 1964).

Vasovagal Attacks

A small number of patients (approximately 1 in 500, Young and Whitwam, 1964) develop this syndrome in which there is an alteration in autonomic activity. The patient becomes pale and sweaty, and feels nauseous. There is an increase in vagal activity, causing severe bradycardia, and it is also thought that the cholinergic vasodilator pathway is activated causing pooling of blood in the muscles (fig. 8). Blood pressure falls and the patient loses consciousness. Normally the cerebral circulation is protected by the subject falling to the floor, and when fainting occurs it is customary to put the patient horizontal until consciousness returns. The danger during induction of intravenous anaesthesia in the sitting position is that if the patient "faints" just as the injection commences, it may be thought that the patient has responded to the drug; the patient will then be kept in the upright position during a period of severe hypotension and cerebral damage can occur.

The Oxygen Paradox (Latham 1951)

During a period of hypoxia (*e.g.* during prolonged laryngospasm) pulmonary vasoconstriction occurs. When the subject is re-oxygenated suddenly, pulmonary vasodilation ensues and blood collects in the lungs so that there is a transient fall in cardiac output and blood pressure.

Haemorrhage

After a dental clearance the blood loss can exceed 1·5 l. (although usually much smaller than this). Cardiac output and blood pressure fall. At first this may be prevented by the baroreceptor—sympathetic reflexes so that the only evidence of severe haemorrhage may be a tachycardia. When blood is swallowed it is difficult to estimate blood loss.

Continuing haemorrhage should be considered as the cause of an otherwise unexplained tachycardia in a patient at risk (*e.g.* haemophilia, or extensive surgery).

Cardiac Dysrhythmias

These fall into two large groups, *viz.*, conduction system dysrhythmias and dysrhythmias due to "ectopic" foci.

All varieties of dysrhythmias have been described during anaesthesia. During dental surgery under general anaesthesia, dysrhythmias are common; they are often undetected and of no serious significance. Disorders of the conducting system are not uncommon during halothane anaesthesia (*e.g.* sinus bradycardia and nodal rhythm). Ventricular extrasystoles commonly occur. Persisting repeated extrasystoles may progress to ventricular tachycardia and ventricular fibrillation. Some of the factors which predispose to the development of dysrhythmias are:

(a) Pre-existing disorders in the patient: Cardiac disease. Electrolyte disturbances, *e.g.* serum potassium elevation in patients with renal failure. Acidosis (*e.g.* in renal failure). Thyrotoxicosis.

(b) The administration of an inhalational agent such as halothane, methoxyflurane, or trichlorethylene.

(c) Increased activity of the sympathetic nervous system. Anxious patients are more prone to develop serious dysrhythmias during induction of anaesthesia.

(d) A rise in Pa_{CO_2} or a fall in Pa_{O_2} (*e.g.* in respiratory obstruction). It is possible that increased sympathetic activity caused by changes in blood gas tensions is the cause of these dysrhythmias and they can be reversed with β-blocking drugs (see below).

Drugs Used in the Treatment of Dysrhythmias. If a patient develops an irregular pulse, or a persisting change in heart rate (tachycardia or severe bradycardia) administration of the anaesthetic and surgery should stop, the airway should be cleared and oxygen administered. If the dysrhythmia does not disappear its type should be determined with an ECG. While this is being arranged a short period of massage of the carotid sinuses in the neck will sometimes stop a paroxysmal tachycardia, presumably by reducing activity in cardiac sympathetic nerves.

Atropine blocks the effect of the vagus at the SA node and will correct a severe sinus bradycardia (recommended dose 0·3–0·6 mg. intravenously).

β blocking drugs (*e.g.* propanolol and practolol). These block sympathetic activity to the heart. They are used in the management of dysrhythmias but since they also reduce the force of cardiac contraction and hence the work that the heart can perform they are used in the treatment of "angina". Opinion is divided as to whether these drugs should be discontinued before surgery under anaesthesia. Because cardiac reserve is reduced, patients receiving β blocking drugs should not be anaesthetized in the sitting position. The recommended dose of practolol given intravenously to correct a dysrhythmia is 5–10 mg., given slowly in repeated doses of 1–2 mg.

Lignocaine (without adrenaline). Local anaesthetics have membrane stabilizing properties and in a dose of 1 mg./kg. given intravenously (which may be repeated), lignocaine will sometimes correct both atrial and ventricular dysrhythmias.

Cardiac glycosides. Ouabain (0·12–0·25 mg.) or digoxin (0·5–0·75 mg.) injected intravenously may sometimes be required to correct a supraventricular tachycardia. These drugs can produce ventricular fibrillation in ventricular dysrhythmias.

Clinical measurements performed on the cardiovascular system include blood pressure and heart rate. During routine dental anaesthesia a "finger on the pulse" is the simplest observation which can be made repeatedly or continuously. A fast heart rate commonly occurs during dental extraction under light anaesthesia, but it may also indicate respiratory obstruction or a serious dysrhythmia (*e.g.* ventricular tachycardia).

EFFECT OF ANAESTHETICS ON THE RESPIRATORY SYSTEM

The Control System

Normal respiration depends on the integrity of the central nervous system, the intercostal and phrenic nerves, the respiratory muscles and chest wall, the vagus nerves (feed back from pulmonary stretch receptors), and the peripheral chemoreceptors and their afferent nerves

The setting of the level of ventilation is normally determined by arterial carbon dioxide tension (Pa_{CO_2} normal range 4·8–5·7 kPa) cerebrospinal fluid pH and, to a lesser extent, by arterial oxygen tension (Pa_{O_2}). A rise in Pa_{CO_2} stimulates central respiratory neurones, the central chemoreceptors, and, to a lesser extent, the peripheral chemoreceptors, causing an increase in ventilation. A fall in Pa_{O_2} (*e.g.* to levels below 9·3 kPa) causes the peripheral chemoreceptors to stimulate respiration.

In normal sleep there is a reduction in ventilation and a rise in Pa_{CO_2} of the order of 0·5–1·2 kPa; the Pa_{O_2} falls into the range 6·7–10·6 kPa.

Inhalational Agents

These depress the responsiveness of the central respiratory neurones to a rise in P_{CO_2} and it has also been shown that halothane depresses the responsiveness of the peripheral chemoreceptors to a fall in Pa_{O_2} (Whitwam, Duffin and Triscott, 1971). Inhalational anaesthetics also sensitize pulmonary stretch receptors so that inspiration tends to be cut off at a lower lung volume. The end result is a reduction in ventilation, a tendency towards a rapid shallow pattern of respiration, and, in spite of a reduction in oxygen consumption and carbon dioxide production, there is a rise in Pa_{CO_2} (usually into the range 6·0–8·0 kPa).

Intravenous Agents

A single injection of thiopentone or methohexitone causes acute respiratory depression, often associated with a short period of apnoea which on occasions may be prolonged (up to 3 min. has been described). Usually spontaneous respiration restarts within 30–60 sec. but while the patient remains asleep respiratory depression persists.

Stimulation of afferent nerves, particularly from the periosteum causes a powerful respiratory drive. Thus the application of forceps to extract a tooth will often restart respiration during a period of drug-induced apnoea and, in the absence of respiratory obstruction, ventilation may be maintained at near normal levels during dental extraction under light anaesthesia.

Gas Exchange and the Lungs

CO$_2$ Elimination

The factors which cause carbon dioxide retention are:

(1) inadequate fresh gas flow allowing rebreathing in the anaesthetic circuit (described above);

(2) hypoventilation due to respiratory obstruction or deep anaesthesia; and

(3) increase in dead space reducing the effectiveness of ventilation.

(a) Apparatus—a full face mask may increase dead space by 150 ml.

(b) Anatomical—this is normally approximately 2·2 ml./kg. Protrusion of the jaw, *e.g.* when maintaining the airway in an anaesthetized patient, may increase the dead space by 100 ml.; tracheal intubation can reduce it by 75 ml.

(c) Alveolar dead space—this is increased during anaesthesia.

Oxygen Transfer

The principle causes of inadequate arterial oxygenation are:

(1) Failure to administer an adequate concentration of oxygen.

(2) Hypoventilation due to respiratory obstruction or deep anaesthesia.

(3) Increased venous to arterial shunting of blood. Normally up to 3 per cent of the blood returning to the heart is diverted into the arterial circulation without contact with ventilated alveoli (*e.g.* via Thebesian veins draining directly into the left heart and connections with the pulmonary veins from the bronchial and pleural blood supply). In addition, with increasing age it is believed that an increasing number of alveoli undergo closure creating an increasing pulmonary shunt and a rise in the alveolar to arterial oxygen P_{O_2} difference (*A*-a gradient).

During anaesthesia the shunt may increase to 10 per cent of cardiac output and it is believed that there is an increase in alveolar closure. Some remain closed throughout the respiratory cycle (a true shunt unaffected by variation in inspired oxygen concentration). In others, complete closure does not occur but there is a reduction of the ventilation of these alveoli, so that the blood perfusing them is not fully oxygenated when the subject is breathing air. Oxygen administration will correct this form of ventilation perfusion inequality and the inspired concentration should be increased to 30–40 per cent during anaesthesia.

Respiratory Muscles

During deep anaesthesia there is a progressive reduction of activity in the respiratory muscles with eventual respiratory arrest. The upper intercostal muscles are the first to cease functioning while diaphragmatic movement persists into deep anaesthesia.

Laryngeal Reflexes

During anaesthesia these are depressed, and inhalation of secretions, blood, and debris from the oropharynx can occur.

Assessment of the Adequacy of Ventilation

Cyanosis. The appearance of cyanosis in a patient who as normal haemoglobin and no serious cardiac or respiratory disease, implies that insufficient oxygen is reaching the tissues.

Respiratory Movement. This can be deceptive. Anaesthetic drugs depress the response of the respiratory centres to changes in blood gases, so that there may be no evidence of a respiratory problem, even in a patient who would otherwise show signs of respiratory distress.

The diaphragm descends in inspiration causing expansion of the abdomen, and this may continue in the presence of complete obstruction of the airway. However under these conditions the upper thorax will be drawn inwards during descent of the diaphragm, which also pulls the mediastinal structures downwards, causing tracheal tug which can be observed in the neck. Hence the indication that gas exchange is occurring depends on observation of the upper thorax, which should expand in phase with abdominal expansion, and of the reservoir bag on the machine. Even if the bag is being emptied and the upper thorax expands during inspiration, partial respiratory obstruction may still be present since minor degrees of respiratory obstruction are difficult to detect.

Measurement of Volume. A Wright respirometer or Drager ventimeter can be used to measure tidal and minute volumes. However such measurements require a leak free system which is not practical during routine dental anaesthesia with the mouth open.

Infra red analysis can be used to measure the end expired (*i.e.* alveolar) CO_2 concentration which under normal conditions provides an estimate of the $Paco_2$.

Blood Gas Analysis. By taking samples of arterial blood (*e.g.* from the femoral, radial or brachial arteries) under anaerobic conditions, $Paco_2$ Pao_2 and arterial pH can be determined using blood gas and pH electrodes. Such measurements would be of value where facio-maxillary injuries required treatment in a patient with multiple injuries and circulatory and respiratory complications (*e.g.* head and chest injuries).

The most important respiratory complications during dental anaesthesia are:

(a) respiratory obstruction;
(b) failure to administer sufficient oxygen;
(c) inhalation of pharyngeal contents; and
(d) hypoventilation during deep anaesthesia.

Assessment of Depth of Anaesthesia

The electroencephalogram is a poor guide to the depth of anaesthesia which at present can be assessed more effectively by observation of respiration, the eyes and responses to surgical stimulation. The system outlined in Table 2 is based on the description of the stages of anaesthesia originally introduced by Guedel.

During dental surgery, it will only rarely be necessary to deepen anaesthesia beyond plane I, stage III. During induction of anaesthesia the patient often becomes apnoeic transiently, but the question may arise as to whether the patient is too light or too deep. If the patient is in stage II

and is merely "breath-holding" the eyelash reflex may still be present, and raising the eyelids will reveal eyes which are either central or diverted with pupils which may be dilated, but which contract briskly on exposure to light as the eyelids are opened. However, if apnoea occurs, and the eyes are central with dilated pupils which are unresponsive to light, it must be assumed that cardiac arrest has occurred and this is confirmed by the absence of peripheral pulses.

If the upper thorax is not expanding during inspiration (indicated by abdominal movement) it should be assumed that obstruction of the airway has occurred. Once the airway is clear, if intercostal weakness persists the level of anaesthesia is too deep. When muscle relaxants are used, the management of anaesthesia is based on previous clinical experience.

Muscle Relaxants

Suxamethonium

This drug can be used to facilitate intubation of the trachea. It is a depolarizing muscle relaxant, and on administration causes contraction of the muscle fibres throughout the body, observed as twitching and fasciculations, followed by total paralysis. A dose of 0·5–1·0 mg./kg. will cause paralysis for several minutes during which time ventilation has to be maintained by intermittent inflation of the patient's lungs. Once intubation has been performed and spontaneous respiration returns, anaesthesia is maintained in the normal way. Over half the patients who receive suxamethonium complain of severe muscle pains for a day or so afterwards.

The drug is rapidly destroyed in the body by the enzyme pseudocholine esterase, except in rare instances of genetic origin where, because of abnormal choline esterase, paralysis may last several hours *i.e.* "scoline apnoea." Screening tests are available to detect patients with an abnormality of this type.

Pancuronium and *d*-tubocurarine

These are competitive muscle relaxants and a single dose produces paralysis for a relatively prolonged period (*e.g.* 30–60 min.). Their action is terminated by the use of the anticholine-esterase neostigmine (atropine being given first). They are used to prevent reflex skeletal movement while maintaining a light plane of anaesthesia, which has advantages in severely ill patients (*e.g.* cardiac patients or those with extensive injuries).

Malignant Hyperpyrexia

This is a rare familial condition which is often fatal. There is a primary defect of muscle metabolism which is not fully understood but in which there appears to be an alteration of calcium transport and equilibrium in muscle cells. For example after muscle contraction the sarcoplasmic reticulum fails to take up calcium ions and relaxation cannot occur. People with this condition are apparently normal until exposed to a "trigger" substance in response to which there is an increase in oxidative metabolism, which exceeds the oxygen supply, so that anaerobic

TABLE 2

ASSESSMENT OF DEPTH OF ANAESTHESIA

	Respiration		Pupils			Reflexes
	Rhythm	Volume	Size	Position	Light Reflex	
Stage I (analgesia)	Irregular	Reduced	Small	Voluntary control remains	Brisk	Response to verbal command. Eyelash reflex present*. Pharyngeal†, respiratory‡ and cardiovascular responses§. Reflex skeletal movement in response to surgical stimulation.
Stage II (excitement)	Irregular periods of apnoea	Variable shallow or deep	Large or medium	Divergent or moving	Brisk	Loss of response to verbal command. Eyelash reflex depressed. Pharyngeal, respiratory and cardiovascular responses. Reflex skeletal movement in response to surgical stimulation.
Stage III (surgical anaesthesia) Plane 1 (M.A.C. 1 Table 1)	Regular	Less than conscious state	Small	Divergent	Present	Eyelash reflex absent. Pharyngeal response absent. No reflex skeletal movement in response to surgical stimulation. Respiratory and cardiovascular responses still present.
Plane 2	Regular	Further reduced	Partially dilated	Central	Sluggish	
Plane 3	Regular	Onset of intercostal paralysis	Nearly fully dilated	Central	Absent	Loss of respiratory and cardiovascular responses to surgical stimulation. Laryngeal and tracheal reflexes abolished.
Plane 4	Jerky irregular	Onset of diaphragmatic paralysis	Fully dilated	Central	Absent	Total reflex depression.
Stage IV	Apnoea					

* Eyelash reflex—contraction of the eyelid in response to stroking the eyelashes.
† Pharyngeal response—Contraction of pharyngeal muscles in response to stimulation of the pharynx.
‡ Respiratory response—alteration of respiratory pattern or ventilation in response to surgical stimulation.
§ Cardiovascular response—changes in heart rate and blood pressure in response to surgical stimulation.

metabolism occurs (cf. the oxygen debt during severe muscular exercise). Substances which precipitate an attack include inhalational anaesthetic agents and muscle relaxants. The body temperature rises rapidly (e.g. above 42°C) and the muscles become rigid. Severe acidosis occurs and potassium is liberated from the muscle cells causing a rise in serum potassium. Cardiovascular collapse and renal failure occur. Management consists of cooling the patient, the administration of intravenous fluids and large amounts of sodium bicarbonate to correct the acidosis, artificial ventilation and haemodialysis. Recently it has been suggested that α-adrenergic blocking drugs will prevent an attack.

Sedative Techniques for Conservative Dentistry

Recent years have seen developments in the use of heavy sedation for conservative dental procedures.

Methods which have been used include:

(1) inhalation of general anaesthetics in low concentrations (*e.g.* nitrous oxide, trichlorethylene, methoxyflurane);

(2) small incremental injections of intravenous induction agents, *e.g.* methohexitone;

(3) small incremental injections of barbiturates, *e.g.* pento-barbitone (nembutal);

(4) other sedative drugs—benzodiazopines, *e.g.* diazepam (valium)—phenothazines, *e.g.* chlorpromazine, trimeprazine;

(5) analgesic drugs, *e.g.* pethidine, pentazocine (fortral), papavaretum (omnopon);

(6) belladonna alkaloids, *e.g.* scopolamine (hyoscine); and

(7) combinations of the above drugs (*e.g.* "nembutal and pethidine", "valium and fortral").

Analgesia and Antanalgesia

Inhalational anaesthetics and analgesic drugs not only alter the mood of the patient, but also elevate the threshold at which a variety of stimuli will induce unpleasant and painful sensations. The effect of other drugs is more complex. For example, after the administration of pethidine, the amount of pressure applied to the tibia which is required to induce pain is elevated; if a small dose of a barbiturate is now administered, sufficient to make the patient drowsy but not unconscious, the amount of pressure required to cause pain is reduced, *i.e.* the barbiturate reduces the analgesic effect of pethidine and the term **antanalgesia** is used to refer to this phenomenon. Barbiturates have variable effects on pain thresholds depending on the type of painful stimulus and the dose of the drug. They can reduce the sensitivity to thermal stimulation of the skin, but consistently enhance the appreciation of painful pressure on the tibia.

Diazepam has minimal effects on pain thresholds (Hall *et al.*, 1974), but is useful for the sedation of patients in pain. It is presented as an oily solution and can cause venous thrombosis, which usually occurs 5–8 days after injection.

Cardiorespiratory Effects

In general when small doses of drugs are used, there will be minimal cardiorespiratory depression. However with repeated doses or prolonged administration of any anaesthetic, complications related to unobserved respiratory obstruction, inadequate oxygenation and cardiovascular depression may occur (Mann *et al.*, 1971; Wise *et al.*, 1969). Diazepam in sedative doses appears to have a minimal effect on the respiratory and cardiovascular systems. However the response to a single dose is extremely variable, repeated doses are cumulative, and profound cardiorespiratory depression can occur when it is combined with barbiturates or narcotics.

Laryngeal Reflexes

Diazepam depresses laryngeal reflexes allowing material placed in the oropharynx to enter the lungs in a high proportion of patients in the period (5–10 min.) immediately following its administration (Healy and Vickers, 1971). The horizontal position does not prevent the inhalation of foreign material from the oropharynx. Thus the patient who is merely "sedated" requires the same standard of care as the patient who is anaesthetized.

In patients undergoing facio-maxillary surgery and in children it may be difficult to work without general anaesthesia. However dental surgery is usually of an elective, conservative nature and can be performed without the use of anaesthetic and sedative drugs which carry a considerable potential for morbidity and mortality.

REFERENCES

Hall, G. M., Whitwam, J. G. and Morgan, M. (1974), "Effect of Diazepam on Experimentally Induced Pain Thresholds," *Brit. J. Anaesth.*, **46**, 50.

Halsey, M. J. and Kent, D. W. (1972), "Molecular Mechanisms of Anaesthesia," *Anaesthesiology*, **36**, 313.

Harris, T. A. B. (1951), *Mode of Action of Anaesthetics*, p. 159. Baltimore: Williams and Wilkins.

Healy, T. E. J. and Vickers, M. D. (1971), "Laryngeal Competence Under Diazepam Sedation," *Proc. roy. Soc. Med.*, **64**, 85.

Latham, F. (1951), "The Oxygen Paradox," *Lancet*, **i**, 77.

Mann, P. E., Hatt, S. D., Dixon, R. A., Griffin, K. D., Perks, E. R. and Thornton, J. A. (1971), "A Minimal Increment Methohexitone Technique in Conservative Dentistry," *Anaesthesia*, **26**, 3.

Price, H. L. (1960), "A Dynamic Concept of Distribution of Thiopental in the Human Body," *Anaesthesiology*, **21**, 40.

Richards, C. D. (1973), "On the Mechanism of Halothane Anaesthesia," *J. Physiol.*, **223**, 439.

Thompson, P. W. (1968), "Apparatus for Dental Anaesthesia," *Brit. J. Anaesth.*, **40**, 166.

Whitwam, J. G. and Young, D. S. (1964), "Observations on Dental Anaesthesia Introduced with Methohexitone. III Blood Pressure Changes," *Brit. J. Anaesth.*, **36**, 237.

Wise, C. C., Robinson, J. S., Heath, M. J. and Tomlin, P. J. (1969), "Physiological Responses to Intermittent Methohexitone for Conservative Dentistry," *Brit. Med. J.*, **2**, 540.

Young, D. S. and Whitwam, J. G. (1964), "Observations on Dental Anaesthesia Introduced with Methohexitone," *Brit. J. Anaesth.*, **36**, 31.

FURTHER READING

Allen, G. D. (1972), *Dental Anaesthesia and Analgesia*. Edinburgh and London: Churchill Livingstone.

Feldman, F. A. and Scurr, C. F. (1974), *Scientific Foundations of Anaesthesia*, 2nd edition. London: Heinemann.

Fink, B. R. (1972), *Cellular Biology and Toxicity of Anaesthetics*. Baltimore: Williams and Wilkins Co.

Hill, D. W. (1967), *Physics Applied to Anaesthesia*. London: Butterworth.

Macintosh, R., Mushin, W. W. and Epstein, H. G. (1963), *Physics for the Anaesthetist*, 3rd edition. Oxford: Blackwell Scientific Publications.

Wylie, W. D. and Churchill-Davidson, H. C. (1972), *A Practice of Anaesthesia*, 3rd edition. London: Lloyd-Luke.

26. MORPHOGENESIS AND DEVELOPMENT OF TEETH

C. H. TONGE

EPITHELIO-MESENCHYMAL INTERACTIONS

The developmental processes, whereby specialized structures, such as teeth, differentiate, form part of a closely integrated pattern of events which progress from the initial genetic potential of the fertilized ovum and the influence of the pre-natal and post-natal environment upon it. The complex mechanisms, concerned with facial, oral and dental development, involve a series of interactions not only between specific cell components, but also between the different varieties of cells which arise during the structural and functional organization of the various tissues.

The formation of the primitive oral cavity or stomatodaeum and the perforation of the bucco-pharyngeal membrane at the end of the fourth week depend upon the contact between the oral ectoderm and the pharyngeal endoderm (fig. 1). The mucosal epithelium of the lips, cheeks, hard palate and anterior two-thirds of the tongue including its taste buds, Rathke's pituitary outgrowth, the parotid outgrowth and the odontogenic epithelium are derived from the oral ectoderm. The pharyngeal mucosa, the lining of the soft palate and the submandibular and sublingual salivary gland outgrowths, together with the epithelium covering the posterior third of the tongue, are derived from the pharyngeal endoderm.

The neural crest, which develops at the margins of the neural plates, is a constant feature of the different vertebrate classes and apart from producing pigment cells, parts of the spinal ganglia and the cranial nerve complex, it also contributes ectomesenchyme, which is distributed more extensively in the head region than in the trunk. This ectomesenchyme is concerned in the development of the cartilaginous splanchnocranium and the anterior portion of the trabeculae cranii. The neural crest can be identified histochemically by its intense RNA richness, and by means of experimental extirpation, grafts and nuclear labelling of embryonic cells with tritiated thymidine in amphibians, a

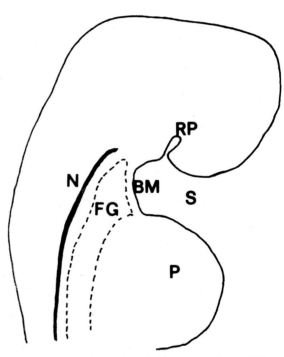

FIG. 1. Diagram illustrating primitive stomatodaeum: BM = Buccopharyngeal membrane; RP = Rathke's pouch; S = Stomatodaeum; P = Pericardium; N = Notochord; FG = Foregut.

specific region of the neural crest can be shown to be concerned with tooth development, thus identifying a sequence in which the cells of the dental papilla and the odontoblasts derived from the neural crest later influence the formation of the enamel organ. In mammalia, the evidence suggests a lesser relative quantity of ectomesenchymal tracts in the pharyngeal region.

The neural crest is not, however, the only source of mesoderm for the head, the prechordal plate and the notochordal derivatives forming a different system associated with intraembryonic mesoderm and providing the extensive mesoderm for the head.

Whatever view is taken of the contribution of the neural crest to the mesenchyme of the head, in man, primates and other mammals it occupies a restricted field limited to tracts of ectomesenchyme while the greater part of the mesoderm is derived from the primitive streak through the notochord and adjacent tissue.

It appears likely, therefore, that ectoderm, ectomesenchyme and mesoderm are involved in tooth formation and that the inductive differentiation of the cell layers of a tooth germ results from both ectodermal-ectomesenchymal and ectomesenchymal-mesodermal interactions (fig. 2).

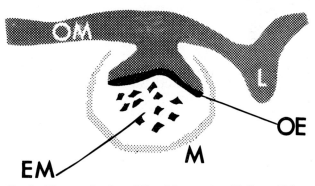

Fig. 2. Diagram showing: OE = Odontogenic epithelium; EM = Ectomesenchyme; M = Mesoderm of dental follicle; L = Lip furrow sulcus; OM = Oral mucosa.

Once the inductive mechanism has advanced to a stage where an ectodermally-derived epithelium is in contact with the "ectomesenchyme" in a potentially odontogenic area, the conditions have been established for tooth formation to occur by means of a series of epithelio-mesenchymal cellular interactions. Indeed, the ectomesenchyme may be the primary stimulus to the epithelial differentiation and a short time scale is involved in the differentiation of the odontogenic epithelium as compared with that operating in the case of the neural plate or lens. Apart from this brief initial interaction, there are more prolonged epithelio-mesenchymal interactions which promote the normal growth and differentiation of tissues throughout pre-natal life and regulate normal maintenance and repair post-natally. There is sufficient evidence obtained by *in vitro* cell and organ culture experiments to show that once a stage is reached when the initial cellular interaction has the capacity for permanence and progressive development, a tooth will form provided that the epithelium derived from ectoderm, and the mesenchyme arising from ectomesenchyme, remain in contact with one another.

The paramount importance of the ectomesenchyme in the induction of the epithelio-mesenchymal interactions involved in tooth formation has been illustrated by several experiments in which mainly embryonic mice have been used:

(i) ectomesenchyme separated from its overlying epithelium in a known odontogenic region and then recombined *in vitro* with the epithelium results in tooth formation;

(ii) ectomesenchyme from a molar area combined with epithelium from an incisor area forms a molar tooth. Similarly, ectomesenchyme from an incisor area

combined with epithelium from a molar area forms an incisor tooth;

(iii) Ectomesenchyme from a non-odontogenic area such as the developing submandibular gland combined with epithelium from a known tooth bearing area, does not form a tooth, but does form glandular tissue;

(iv) ectomesenchyme from an 11–12 day mouse embryo, when combined with odontogenic epithelium from a younger embryo (10 days) differentiates to form a tooth. Ectomesenchyme from a 10 day mouse embryo combined with epithelium from an 11–12 day embryo fails to differentiate. It is essential, therefore, for the ectomesenchyme and epithelium to be in contact, and the interaction between the cell layers only achieves its potential over a very limited period of time. An embryological factor upsetting the critical time-scale would make differentiation either impossible or incomplete.

(v) lip separation and the formation of a vestibular sulcus occurs after a specific odontogenic region has been established. The separation occurs at the periphery of the odontogenic region and the epithelio-mesenchymal interaction is limited, almost inert as compared with the extensive response observed at the developing tooth site. If, however, the dental papilla derived from the ectomesenchyme of the odontogenic area is combined with the epithelium of the vestibular lamina, then teeth will develop in the explants; and

(vi) the similarity of the reaction produced by growth suppressors such as beta-2-thienylalanine (β2T) in studies of tooth germs and the vibrissae of snout epithelium is what might be expected since skin and tooth germs are both epithelially lined areas with an underlying ectomesenchyme.

Epithelio-mesenchymal interactions in the odontogenic region give rise to the ectodermally derived enamel organ, whilst the ectomesenchyme, apart from being a primary inducer, differentiates into perhaps the greater part of the dental papilla particularly the odontoblast layer. The inducer potential continues, since dentinogenesis precedes amelogenesis. What of the relationship between the ectomesenchyme and the ordinary mesenchyme, itself a part of the mesoderm which forms the connective tissues throughout the body? This mesenchyme (fig. 2) forms a capsule, the inner layer of the dental follicle around the tooth germ (enamel organ and dental papilla) and probably provides that part of the dental papilla which forms the pulpal tissue. The mesenchyme also provides a central core of the dental follicle in which ultimately cementum and periodontal ligament will form, whilst the outer layer of the dental follicle is equivalent to the limiting layer of the periosteum which lines the bony alveolus. The significance of what is termed the inner layer of the dental follicle is its function as a capsule enabling the self-determination of tooth formation to proceed without, at this stage, the encroachment of adjacent osseous and other connective tissue elements. Salivary gland formation, hair follicle formation and even individual muscle formation also take place in similarly isolated regions.

INDIVIDUAL TOOTH PRIMORDIA

In man, potentially odontogenic epithelium, the anlage of the dentitions, can be identified in 28–30 day (ovulation age) embryos. The epithelium proliferates, giving the appearance of epithelial thickening located on the inferior borders of the maxillary processes and the superior borders

In the majority of species the odontogenic epithelium becomes invaginated relative to the underlying mesenchyme and a dental lamina is formed from which individual tooth buds arise. In man and also in *Elephantulus myurus Jamesoni* and *Tupaia javanica* the germs of the future enamel organs develop directly within the odontogenic epithelium prior to its invagination (fig. 5). The dental

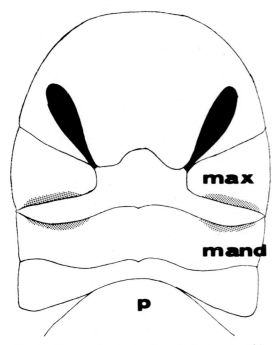

FIG. 3. Diagram showing location of odontogenic epithelium (shaded): max = maxillary process; mand = mandibular arch; P = Pericardium.

of the mandibular arches in the area forming the lateral margins of the stomatodeum (fig. 3). Beneath the odontogenic epithelium, there is an ill-defined cellular condensation. At 30–32 days, the odontogenic epithelium is 3–4 cells thick, the cells being ovoid to cuboid with little cytoplasm. The underlying mesenchyme forms an ill-defined condensation. By 32–34 days, the mesenchyme immediately beneath the odontogenic epithelium can be distinguished from adjacent mesenchyme (fig. 4).

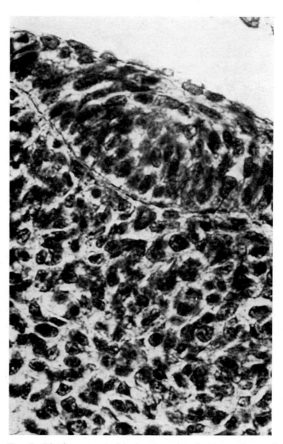

FIG. 5. The lower central incisor area in a human embryo of 36–38 days. An individual growth centre is forming within the odontogenic epithelium. × 600.

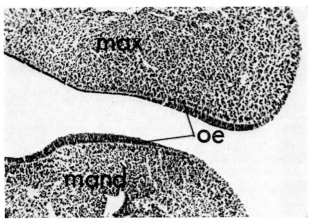

FIG. 4. The odontogenic epithelium (oe) in relation to the maxillary process (max) and the mandibular arch (mand) in a human embryo of 32–34 days ovulation age. × 100.

lamina in man is therefore a secondary formation similar to oral epithelium and derived from the epithelium adjacent to the individual growth centres for the dentitions. These growth centres are essentially regions of rapidly dividing cells with the potentiality of forming the deciduous teeth and their successors. They are associated with specific ectomesenchymal condensations which become isolated from the surrounding tissues once the inner layer of the dental follicle forms around the dental papilla. In man, by 36–38 days ovulation age, there are specific odontogenic growth centres for the central incisor teeth. Those for the lateral incisors, canines and first molars (deciduous with potentiality for first premolar) are present by 38–40 days, whilst the second deciduous molar germs and their successor potential are present by 40–44 days (fig. 6). There is some inconclusive evidence to suggest that early odontogenesis occurs in the mandibular anterior region before the maxillary differentiation and that males are possibly in advance of female embryos. The dental lamina becomes

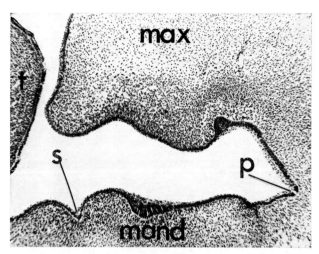

FIG. 6. Coronal section of the right side of the oral cavity in a human embryo of 40–42 days: max = maxillary process; mand = mandibular process; P = Site of parotid outgrowth; S = Groove limiting the future lingual gingival area; T = Tongue. The section passes through the first deciduous mandibular molar and the maxillary deciduous canine areas. × 114.

apparent as the odontogenic areas invaginate and constitute the internal dental epithelium. Histologically and histochemically the cells of the superficial part of the dental lamina are similar to non-odontogenic oral epithelium whilst the deeper part resembles the external dental epithelium. Once the dental lamina forms, the lip begins to separate; both processes occur at about the same time in the incisor and canine areas (fig. 7). The main vestibular sulcus forms later in the cheek region. As a result of segmentation and different depths of separation of the lips and cheeks from the future gingival alveolar processes, some individuals have septal processes within their vestibular sulci.

The rapid mitoses occurring in the individual odontogenic areas outline the internal dental epithelium, and the

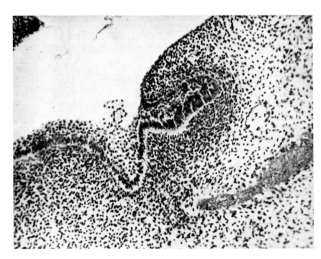

FIG. 7. Sagittal section through the lower right lateral deciduous incisor area of a human embryo of 46–48 days. The differentiation of the mesenchyme into that of the dental papilla and that forming the inner layer of the dental follicle can be seen. The vestibular sulcus is to the left of the section. × 114.

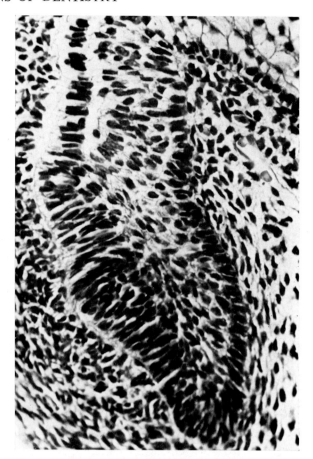

FIG. 8. Distal part of lower right central deciduous incisor in a human embryo of 46–48 days. × 300

other layers of the enamel organ become apparent (fig. 8). In epithelial regions between the individual odontogenic areas (fig. 9), although invagination occurs with the formation of a dental lamina, there is a limited and abortive differentiation of its epithelium. Supernumerary teeth forming between normal teeth could, however, arise from such sites.

Whereas the teeth of the deciduous dentition arise directly from the odontogenic epithelium of the oral cavity, acquiring a dental lamina as the odontogenic area becomes invaginated, the arrangement is different in the case of the permanent dentition. Morpho-differentiation and histo-differentiation of a deciduous tooth result in its being a separate individual structure distally, mesially and buccally. The gradual separation from the odontogenic epithelium on its lingual side leaves behind the primordium of the successor tooth which is either associated with the dental lamina or the external dental epithelium of the deciduous tooth (figs. 10 and 11).

Between 47–56 days ovulation age, the second deciduous molar and the bud for the second premolar become separately identifiable structures. More posteriorly the odontogenic epithelial extension of proliferating columnar cells with a mesenchymal condensation around it constitutes the earliest evidence of the permanent molar dentition and is connected to the surface by a long extension of the dental lamina. This development of a permanent molar tooth area takes place at the same time as the mandibular ramus begins to grow in height and the masseter, internal pterygoid, and temporalis muscles separate out from a common mesenchymal sheet. Although the primordia of the successor dentition form earlier, the first permanent molar

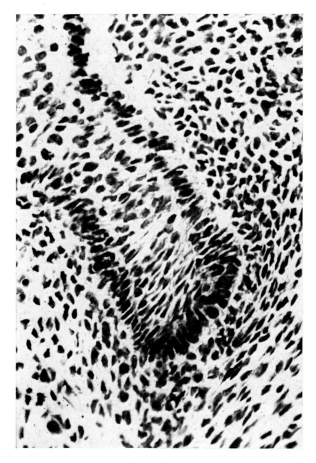

FIG. 9. Area between the lower right deciduous central and lateral incisor teeth in a human embryo of 46–48 days. × 300.

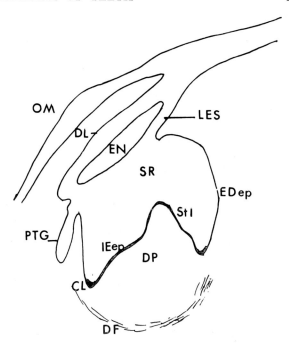

FIG. 10. Diagram illustrating the "bell stage" of tooth development: OM = Oral mucosa; DL = Dental lamina; LES = Lateral enamel strand; EN = Enamel niche; EDep = External dental epithelium; SR = Stellate reticulum; St.I = Stratum intermedium; IEep = Internal dental epithelium; CL = Cervical loop; DP = Dental papilla; DF = Dental follicle inner layer; PTG = Permanent tooth germ.

teeth show a more rapid differentiation. At 100 days, tooth buds are present and at 120 days the cell layers of the enamel organ have become differentiated, whereas at the same time the first premolar is just commencing to show an invaginated area for the dental papilla (fig. 12). There is a posterior extension of odontogenic epithelium beyond the first permanent molar tooth germ but its further differentiation to form the second and third permanent molars occurs after birth. The second permanent molars are initiated in the first year and the third permanent molars in the fourth to fifth year.

THE TOOTH GERM

The tooth germ comprises an enamel organ and a dental papilla surrounded by the inner condensed part of the dental follicle.

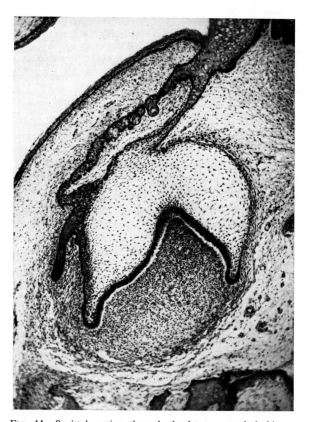

FIG. 11. Sagittal section through the lower central deciduous incisor of a 100-day-old human fetus. Figure 10 is a diagram based on this section. × 70.

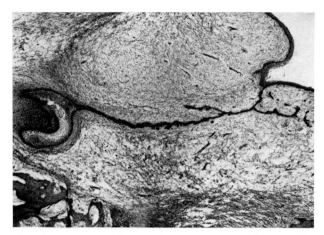

Fig. 12. First permanent human mandibular molar tooth at 120 days. × 29.

Enamel Organ

As proliferation of the cells of each odontogenic area takes place, the resultant growth is uneven, a feature which, combined with the invagination by the dental papilla on its deep aspect, leads to the formation of a cuboidal cell layer peripherally (the external dental epithelium), and a low columnar cell layer (the internal dental epithelium) adjacent to the dental papilla. Between the external and internal dental epithelia there are closely packed polyhedral cells with a small amount of intercellular fluid between them. As growth proceeds, these intervening cells become progressively separated by the accumulation between them of a mucoid ground substance rich in albumin. The cells become star shaped and are joined together by intercommunicating cytoplasmic processes, forming the stellate reticulum layer. The separation of the stellate reticulum layer appears to proceed outwards towards the margins of the enamel organ from the centre leaving for a time accumulations of cells which form both the enamel knot close to the centre of the internal dental epithelium, and the enamel cord leading from the enamel knot towards the external dental epithelium. The initial intense activity of the odontogenic epithelium, with higher ribonucleic acid level and hydrolytic and oxidative enzyme activity than that found in the glycogen richer oral epithelium, continues in the internal dental epithelium. The growth of this layer outlines the pattern of the crown of the tooth, the zone in which active mitosis first ceases becoming the first fixed part of the crown. This corresponds to the highest point of its first differentiating cusp. It is in relation to such areas that the transient structures, the enamel knot and the enamel cord, are demonstrable. They last for about a week and for the deciduous dentition are seen around 60–78 days in human embryos. As the stellate reticulum becomes expanded, 1–3 layers of squamous cells remain, as small polygonal cells with short intercommunicating processes, between the stellate reticulum and the internal dental epithelium. This layer is called the stratum intermedium and it appears to be essential to enamel formation as it fails to differentiate in relation to those parts of the internal and external dental epithelia associated with root morphogenesis.

The four layers, external dental epithelium, stellate reticulum, stratum intermedium, and internal dental epithelium form the enamel organ and are identifiable in all deciduous and permanent tooth germs.

Dental Papilla

The original ectomesenchymal condensation adjacent to the odontogenic epithelium shows active cellular proliferation and differentiation as its invagination of the early enamel organ proceeds. Acid mucopolysaccharides are demonstrable in the ground substance. Concurrently with the differentiation of the internal dental epithelial layer, the peripheral cells of the dental papilla enlarge and differentiate into odontoblasts. Between the early odontoblasts and the internal dental epithelium there is a basement membrane of reticular fibres with an acid mucopolysaccharide ground substance. At first stellate, the odontoblast becomes low columnar, whilst its nucleus migrates towards the cell base. Beneath the odontoblasts and throughout the dental papilla the undifferentiated mesenchymal cells form a network of fusiform primitive fibroblasts with linking protoplasmic processes. In the interstices between these cells there are argyrophilic fibres and intercellular ground substance. Macrophage cells also differentiate from the mesenchymal cells and there always remains a large residue of undifferentiated cells.

Dental Follicle

If the name dental follicle is given to all the tissue which lies between the tooth germ and the developing bony alveolus which surrounds it, confusion can arise unless its different parts with their different functions are identified. The inner part of the dental follicle forms a capsule of interlacing circularly arranged collagen fibres and fibroblasts around the tooth germ, being particularly marked around the margins of the dental papilla. The outer part of the dental follicle forms the collagenous limiting layer of the periosteum which lines the alveolar bone, and beneath it is the osteogenic layer. Between the outer and inner layers of the dental follicle there is a mass of loose reticular fibres, undifferentiated mesenchymal cells, a few fibroblasts and some macrophages, with a number of blood vessels and nerves traversing the area. This intermediate area of the dental follicle provides a suitable packing medium during the progressive growth of the crown of the tooth associated with continual remodelling of the alveolus. Much later, during eruption, this intermediate area is concerned with periodontal ligament formation.

Vascular Supply and Innervation

During the period of the establishment of the tooth germ, the vascular supply becomes increasingly important and its arrangement is closely related to the requirements associated with the formation of the calcified tissues, enamel and dentine. In the earliest stages the individual odontogenic areas can be located by the density of the vascular capillaries forming within the mesenchymal condensations. As the growth associated with the extension of the dental papilla into the invaginated enamel organ proceeds, the future pulpal vessels enter the dental papilla and subodontoblastic capillary networks appear as the odontoblasts differentiate. The inner layer of the dental follicle has some vessels anastomosing upon its surface and the leash of vessels runs over the entire extent of the tooth germ becoming, still within the dental follicle, applied to the outer surface of the external dental epithelium. This is really a deeply placed capillary network having some anastomosis with the vessels around the dental lamina and through them with the more superficially placed capillary network of the oral epithelium. The capillary network around the external dental epithelium never penetrates the enamel organ, which is entirely avascular. As the stellate reticulum is reduced in extent prior to amelogenesis the external dental epithelium becomes ridged with vascular capillaries pushing towards the ameloblast cells but separated from them by the other cellular layers of the enamel organ and a thin layer of connective tissue. The intermediate area of the dental follicle is traversed by blood vessels of the future supporting tissues of the tooth and the alveolus has a rich vasculature.

Once the enamel organ and dental papilla form, independent nerve bundles can be seen entering the dental papilla and forming fine nerve endings close to the developing odontoblasts. Other nerves lie across the intermediate zone of the dental follicle and there are submucosal nerve plexuses beneath the oral mucous membrane. The distribution in man of blood vessels and nerves is similar in both the deciduous and permanent dentitions.

The Enamel Niche

As the odontogenic epithelium invaginates into the underlying mesenchyme, the dental lamina is formed. It becomes arranged relative to each tooth germ so that distally it is a single stem with a proximal separation of the lamina into two limbs, the main lamina and a lateral enamel strand. This produces a space filled with mesenchyme and termed the enamel niche to appear in relation to tooth germs. The enamel niche is a cleft closed distally, bounded by the main part of the dental lamina and the lateral enamel strand and the external dental epithelium and open proximally where its contained mesenchyme is continuous with that around the tooth germ (figs. 10 and 11). As the dental lamina disintegrates so the enamel niche disappears as an identifiable feature.

The Dental Lamina

As the dental lamina elongates it acquires a superficial part which is non-odontogenic and similar to the surface epithelial lining. Its deeper part nearest to the external dental epithelium is similar to this layer and is potentially odontogenic. From the extremity of the dental lamina the permanent tooth bud arises and is lingual to its deciduous predecessor. Distally to the deciduous teeth and their successors, the odontogenic epithelium giving origin to the permanent molar teeth is connected to the surface by an extension of the dental lamina.

Crown Pattern

Once tooth development has been initiated and a tooth germ formed, the internal dental epithelium becomes actively involved in producing the detailed pattern of the crown of the tooth. The folding of the internal dental epithelium is closely associated with the arrangement of mitotic activity in its cells. This folding occurs first at its most occlusal part and gradually proceeds in a cervical direction, unequal growth of the internal dental epithelium being of significance in moulding the crown pattern. Cusps, occlusal ridges, marginal ridges and fissures arise from the activity of the internal dental epithelium. Mitosis free areas could result in enamel free areas, infrequent in man but normal in mouse molar tooth germs. The crown pattern is taking shape prior to amelogenesis and mineralization, so that a balanced arrangement is required to support the delicate cellular layers. The fluid contained within the stellate reticulum and the general protection of the tooth germ within the layers of the dental follicle may be the main sources of support.

The First Permanent Upper Molar Crown

At any stage from cusp formation until calcification on all four main cusps, the mesiobuccal (paracone) part of the tooth is the most advanced in development and the distolingual (hypocone) the most retarded. This applies not only to the cusps and ridges of the crown but also to the base of the tooth. The mesio-lingual (protocone) and disto-buccal (metacone) develop at similar times but usually the former commences to calcify before the latter. Each cusp commences its development as a rounded eminence raised only slightly above the adjacent parts of the tooth. It then develops a pointed tip which, becoming higher, begins to calcify at the cuspal tip which then becomes somewhat flatter as enamel apposition occurs on its surface. The ridges between the cusps, which start as rounded folds, soon show a prominence of the mesial marginal ridge. The buccal cingulum retains its first-defined rounded form until it calcifies. Similarly, the lingual and mesial cingula remain rudimentary, except where Carabelli's cusp differentiates.

Comparison Between First Permanent and Second Deciduous Molar Teeth

Apart from differences in size and proportion, the mandibular and maxillary first permanent molars are identical in crown morphology to the second deciduous molars. The timing is different, the maxillary second deciduous molar having three cusps calcified at 28 weeks *in utero* whereas at the same time the maxillary first permanent molar shows an enamel organ and a dental papilla with some mesio-buccal eminence, but no calcification. Similarly at 28·5 weeks *in utero* the mandibular second deciduous molar has four cusps whilst the first mandibular permanent molar has just reached a stage prior to calcification. Detailed analysis shows that second deciduous and first permanent molar teeth have similar growth patterns but that the pattern develops more slowly in the case of the first permanent molar teeth. The lag applies not only to the stages of calcification but also to the changes in the shape of the uncalcified cusps.

Pre-amelogenesis

Prior to amelogenesis the pattern of the incisal or occlusal part of the crown has been determined. The border between the internal dental epithelium and the dental papilla defines the amelodentinal junction. As the cervical portion of the crown is being outlined, and this occurs at the same time as dentinogenesis and amelogenesis of the occlusal region are taking place, the internal and external dental epithelia form the cervical loop which is an active growth area.

The external dental epithelium, with the capillary network already described, transports the materials for matrix formation and mineralization. The cells become villiform, and have increased mitochondria. The ribonucleic acid activity then becomes less marked. Once some dentinogenesis has occurred prior to amelogenesis, the stellate reticulum becomes much reduced but may show some alkaline phosphatase activity.

The stratum intermedium cell layers remain closely linked and mitotic division continues after it has ceased in the internal dental epithelium. Alkaline phosphatase and glycogen activity are marked. Amino-peptidase, cytochrome oxidase, and succinic dehydrogenase activity is also associated with the stellate reticulum and stratum intermedium cells.

The internal dental epithelium cells, at first low columnar, become taller and their nuclei are centrally situated. This pre-ameloblast stage is followed by some dentinogenesis and a resultant progressively diminishing route for nutrients reaching the enamel organ from the dental papilla. Next the ameloblast forms, with its nucleus moving basally closer to the vascular network on the surface of the external dental epithelium. As amelogenesis is due to commence the cells are tall, columnar, and have increased mitochondria and secretory granules (fig. 13).

Root Development

After the completion of the crown of a tooth the cervical loop extends apically without a stratum intermedium intervening between the internal and external dental epithelial layers of which it is formed. This rootward extension is called the epithelial root sheath of Hertwig and its function is to determine the number, size and shape of the roots to be formed and to induce the underlying cells of the dental papilla to differentiate into odontoblasts and provide the dentine of the root. As the epithelial root sheath outlines the root it constricts the dental papilla or pulp so that the resultant root canal or canals are of much smaller dimension than the pulp chamber associated with the tooth crown. The apical foramen is therefore shaped

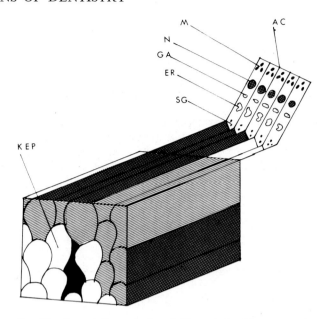

FIG. 13. General diagram of ameloblast relationship to enamel prism formation: AC = Ameloblast cells; M = Mitochondria; N = Nuclei; GA = Golgi apparatus; ER = Endoplasmic reticulum; SG = Secretory granules; KEP = Keyhole enamel prism.

by the epithelial diaphragm, the name given to that part of the epithelial root sheath which passes part of the way across the base of the dental papilla. In single rooted teeth the epithelial root sheath is a single tubular structure which determines both the size and shape of the root. In double rooted teeth there are two ingrowths from the epithelial diaphragm which fuse together; in three rooted teeth, there are three ingrowths (fig. 14). The area of fusion of the processes of the epithelial diaphragm determines the shape of the floor of the pulp chamber and the

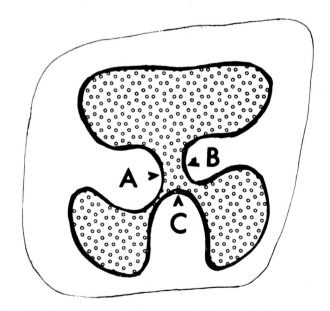

FIG. 14. Diagram to indicate how the epithelial diaphragmatic processes A.B.C. come together to form the inter-radicular region between three roots.

inter-radicular areas. The individual single roots now defined continue to grow in length by the extension of their respective root sheaths. In single-rooted teeth, root dentine formation begins at the site of the future amelo-cemental junction; in multi-rooted teeth it concurrently begins in the area of the radicular bifurcations.

As dentinogenesis follows the lengthening of the epithelial root sheath, the sheath disintegrates leaving a network of remnants, the epithelial rests of Malassez. The break-up of the sheath is associated with an insinuation of cementoblasts and fibroblasts derived from the intermediate part of the dental follicle coming to lie next to the root dentine and laying down the cemental component of the cemento-dentinal junction. Hertwig's epithelial root sheath is proliferating and functioning apically, at the same time as it is disintegrating coronally (figs. 15 and 16).

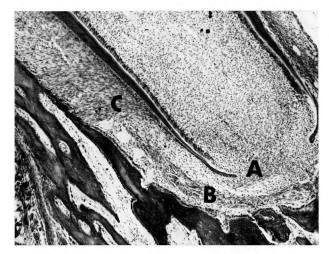

FIG. 15. The inner layer of the dental follicle A is seen in relation to the outer layer B which is the limiting layer of the periosteum. The periodontal ligament C is forming on either side of B. × 114.

Finally, the epithelial diaphragm ceases to proliferate and the apical foramen closes to the dimensions of the diaphragm, being ultimately further restricted by the continued apposition of root dentine and cementum. In some cases the epithelial diaphragmatic processes fail to fuse in the area of the pulpal floor with a resultant dentine defect. Similar defects occurring around blood vessels are associated with accessory root canals. Occasional isolated clusters of epithelial root sheath cells give origin to enamel pearls which develop on the surface of root dentine.

The Formation of Dental Arches

Teeth have a relative priority in comparison with bone when competing for space during rapid growth. The changes observed in the relative position of tooth germs indicate that normally a crowding of the dental arch takes place at a time when tooth development is more advanced than the space available to accommodate it. The upper dental arches are wide and flattened antero-posteriorly failing to conform to the usual catenary curve at 6·5–8 weeks *in utero*. Between 7·5 – 9 weeks progressive elongation and increasing depth of the dental arch occurs; but

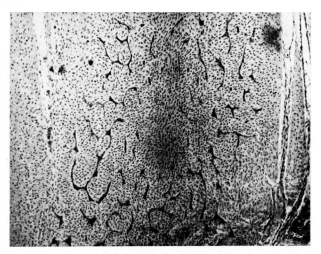

FIG. 16. Section through the epithelial rests of Malassez parallel to the tooth surface. Fibroblasts and periodontal ligament fibres are visible in between the cell networks. × 114.

the catenary curvature usual in the postnatal upper dental arch does not seem to arise earlier than 9·5 weeks *in utero*. The mandibular arch conforms to a catenary curvature around 8·5 weeks.

Developmental Remnants

Epithelial remnants (figs. 16, 17, 18, 19) may arise from:
(a) the superficial non-odontogenic part of the dental lamina as cylindrical masses continuous with the surface;

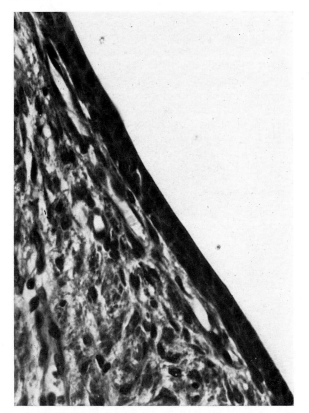

FIG. 17. Epithelial attachment of an erupting tooth near to the surface with flattened cellular layers. × 210.

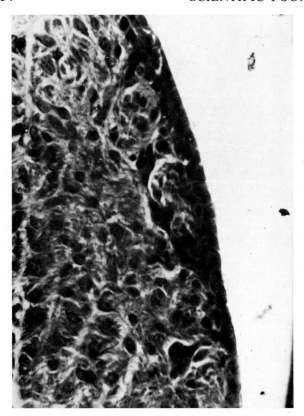

FIG. 18. Epithelial attachment of an erupting tooth near to the amelocemental junction. There is some cellular proliferation from the deeper part of the epithelial attachment into the underlying mesenchyme. × 210.

around the root of a tooth with the fibres of the periodontal ligament passing through the interstices of the network. The peristance of these epithelial remains may prevent tooth ankylosis by bony fusion with cementum. If this is the case, then the presence of the epithelial rests of Malassez could favour the orderly eruption of the tooth and prevent excessive mesenchymal activity.

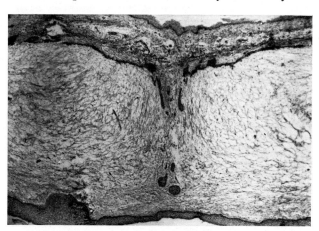

FIG. 19. Horizontal section of the superficial part of the dental lamina in the mid-line between the mandibular deciduous central incisors. There are several epithelial whorl-like structures adjacent to the mid-line. Human fetus at 120 days. × 29.

(b) independent ingrowths from the surface oral mucosa. These are coiled and tubular;

(c) the deeper part of the dental lamina as networks or clusters of cells;

(d) the breaking up of the external dental epithelium in the form of cell clusters;

(e) the epithelial attachment in the area of the amelo-cemental junction; and

(f) the breaking up of the epithelial root sheath of Hertwig. This forms the epithelial rests of Malassez

REFERENCES

Butler, P. M. (1971), "Growth of Human Tooth Germs," in *Dental Morphology and Evolution*, p. 3 (A. A. Dahlberg, Ed.). University of Chicago Press.

Mathiessen, M. E. (1968), "Comparative Enzyme Histochemical Studies on the Development of Teeth in Man and in the Mouse," *Acta anat.*, **70**, 14.

Nery, E. B., Kraus, B. S. and Croup, M. (1970), "Timing and Topography of Early Human Tooth Development," *Arch. Oral Biol.*, **15**, 1315.

Provenza, D. V. and Sisca, R. F. (1971), "Electron Microscopic Study of Human Dental Primordia," *Arch. Oral Biol.*, **16**, 121.

Tonge, C. H. (1966), "Advances in Dental Embryology," *Int. dent. J.*, **16**, 328.

Tonge, C. H. (1971), "The Role of Mesenchyme in Tooth Development," in *Dental Morphology and Evolution*, p. 45 (A. A. Dahlberg, Ed.). University of Chicago Press.

27. AMELOGENESIS AND THE STRUCTURE OF ENAMEL

A. BOYDE

The enamel referred to in this chapter is the shiny, off-white, semi-opaque layer which covers most or much of the working surfaces of the teeth of mammals. Not all mammals have teeth, and not all the teeth have an enamel layer. The enamel covering is incomplete, or is breached at an early stage in the functional life of teeth that are subject to heavy wear, such as the grinding molars of herbivores. Nevertheless, dental enamel reduces the rate of attrition of tooth substance, the other dental tissues, dentine and cement, always wearing at a greater rate. This resistance to abrasion is also important in the function of teeth that are comparatively much less subject to wear. The latter are the sharp, blade-like or pointed, piercing and cutting teeth of carnivorous and insectivorous mammals. The sharp curvatures of the biting points or blades would not survive as such if they were made of material as soft as dentine.

Mammalian teeth have, in general, to survive greater functional lifetimes than those of the reptilia, teleost and elasmobranchs, which are usually replaced many times over during one lifespan; the structure of the enamel is considerably more complex. The main components of enamel are calcium phosphate (hydroxyapatite), water and some special proteins which apparently have no equivalent elsewhere. The singular feature of enamel constructed from these materials is that the composite has important properties possessed by neither of the two main components. Above all, it is remarkably resistant to brittle fracture: enamel is hard, yet tough. Apatite is hard and comparatively brittle: a thin layer of apatite on a basis of elastic dentine would soon crack and crumble. The aim in this chapter will be to approach the understanding of the completed structure by examining some features of the development of enamel, and to relate the structure of the adult tissue to its known properties.

ORIGIN OF ENAMEL

Enamel is the secretory product of cells which differentiate from the aboral poles of the oral epithelial ingrowths which form the basis of tooth germs. The whole epithelial ingrowth which moves into the adjacent embryonic connective tissue or mesenchyme is involved to some degree in enamel formation—and the whole is known as the enamel organ. It is, however, evident that only the innermost (or inner enamel epithelium) cells are in contact with the developing tissue and that they secrete or pump the necessary building blocks for the developing enamel, but this is not their sole function.

Experimental and observational studies of tooth development show that the inner enamel epithelium cells interact with the adjacent mesenchymal cells—which are comparatively greater in number per unit volume near the future enamel organ—and induce them to differentiate into the cells which form the main substance of the teeth, namely the dentine. The nature of the exchange of information between epithelial and mesenchymal cells is under intensive investigation (Slavkin, 1972), but that it is an exchange of messages may be deduced from the observation that inner enamel epithelial cells do not go on to produce enamel unless dentine has formed first. In some mammals enamel does not form at all, but dentine may not be formed by the differentiated mesenchymal cells, or odontoblasts, unless dental epithelium is present. Examination of the enamel-free regions of the crowns of certain mammalian teeth, and the enamel-free (cement covered) roots of most mammalian teeth, shows that absence of enamel formation follows from a relative lack of growth and differentiation of the odontogenic epithelium. Thus the epithelium (enamel organ) capable of making enamel shows, before enamel formation, four distinctive layers—the inner enamel epithelium, the stratum intermedium, the stellate reticulum and the outer enamel epithelium whereas the dental epithelium capable only of inducing dentine formation has just two layers—the inner and outer epithelia.

THE AMELODENTINAL JUNCTION (EDJ)

Chapter 26 provides details of the growth and development of the tooth germ and the formation of dentine. It needs to be mentioned here that the "mould" or "form" against which the first dentine is deposited is the line of junction with the inner enamel epithelial cells. This, it may be speculated, is a rather flexible mould, but the consistency of the procollagen released by the odontoblasts is more or less that of a liquid, and is unlikely to deform the junction. Once the dentine collagen has formed into fibrils, and mineralization has begun, the future ameloblasts have a rigid mould against which to lay their own secretion. This form is again that of the original line of junction between pre-ameloblasts and odontoblasts, now the surface of the dentine, but the enamel matrix gel has the advantage of setting, by crystal growth within it, on a stable base.

The serrated or scalloped junctional plane of enamel and dentine serves to minimize the chances of cracks developing along the junction, potential cleavages being stopped by the numerous changes of direction of the EDJ. The penetration of the enamel by thin spurs of dentine—the so-called enamel spindles (fig. 1)—would serve to improve the anchoring of enamel to dentine in particularly critical locations.

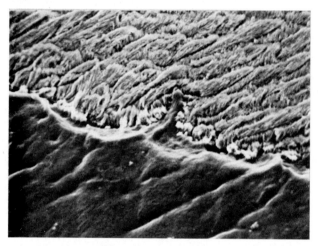

FIG. 1. Etched section through enamel (top)—dentine junction, showing base of a "spindle" of dentine penetrating the enamel. Picture width 69 μm.

The EDJ is also penetrated by cell process spaces which, owing to their similarity to the equivalent spaces in dentine with which they are usually in continuity, are called enamel tubules (Lester, 1970). Enamel tubules are tunnel-like vacancies in the enamel structure, in man about 0·5 μm. in diameter and varying in length from a few microns up to about 50 μm. It is a peculiarity of marsupial mammals that, with the exception of wombats, they all have large numbers of enamel tubules which penetrate a long distance into the enamel, but never reach its surface.

AMELOBLASTS

The cells of the oldest part of the inner enamel epithelium are the first to complete their differentiation into secretory cells. They are the first to induce the differentiation of odontoblasts from adjacent mesenchymal cells, and are the first to be induced, in turn, to become ameloblasts.

Fully differentiated ameloblasts are typical columnar epithelial exocrine secretory cells in most respects (fig. 2).

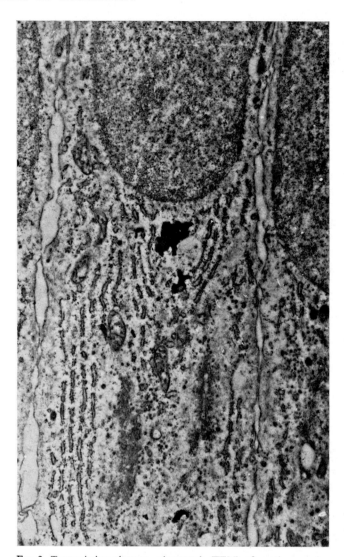

FIG. 2. Transmission electron micrograph (TEM) of monkey ameloblast, showing Golgi region and rER. Picture width 7 μm.

They obviously differ in being backed up by a multilayered epithelium (the other layers of the enamel organ) rather than lying in close contact with a basal lamina with the adjacent connective tissue, and in the fact that they secrete towards the original basal lamina, i.e. towards the connective tissue to which they lie closest. In earlier stages of tooth germ development, pre-ameloblasts have centrally placed nuclei with their centrioles and Golgi regions on the side of the nucleus towards the remainder of the enamel organ. This is the polarity seen in most exocrine secretory cells. It is also associated with the development of continuous belts of junctional attachments between all pre-ameloblasts at the same level in each cell, namely near their junction with the stratum intermedium. Again, these terminal bars are placed at the would-be secretory pole of other exocrine cells, away from the basement membrane. This set of outer* terminal bars is retained by the amelo-

* The terms inner and outer will be used in the same sense as inner and outer enamel epithelia to avoid the confusion which often follows the use of the terms basal, distal, proximal and apical for cell polarity.

blasts, but in the process of completing their differentiation into enamel secreting cells they reverse their polarity and develop inner terminal bars at the real secretory pole. Ameloblasts are apparently unique in possessing two sets of terminal bars. Functionally, the presence of the terminal bars would seem to indicate that nothing (except perhaps small ions) can penetrate the potential intercellular gaps between ameloblasts and, conversely, that everything in the enamel must pass through these cells.

The reversal of polarity of ameloblasts occurs synchronously with their change to a tall columnar form. Their nuclei move towards their outer ends and the Golgi and centrioles move to the inner side of the nucleus. At the same time, and continuing afterwards, there is a great development of rough-surfaced endoplasmic reticulum (rER) that packs the main part of the cell body from the inner terminal bars and associated web of cytoplasmic filaments to the nucleus, and enwraps the growing Golgi zone. A thin peripheral layer of cytoplasm remains virtually free of rER.

Microtubules are a prominent component of the inner pole cytoplasm during the movements of organelles at the reversal of polarity (Katchburian and Holt, 1972). Prior to the development of the rER, i.e. in the undifferentiated IEE cells, the cytoplasm is occupied by many free ribosomes and polyribosomes, indicating that the cells are engaged in manufacturing protein for internal use. The main protein which becomes evident internally is that of the microtubules (Katchburian and Holt, 1972).

Material which is identical in appearance with the extracellular granular or stippled material eventually secreted by the ameloblasts (fig. 3) accumulates in the cisternae of the granular ER even before the migration of the Golgi apparatus is complete, and at early stages of differentiation it is not found in the smooth-surfaced sacs or vesicles of the Golgi zones. This enamel matrix precursor material may sometimes be found in extracellular locations before the development of the usual association of Golgi apparatus and rough ER, which appears to represent an early, abortive attempt of the differentiating ameloblasts to secrete the matrix by a route which bypasses the Golgi complex (Katchburian and Holt, 1972). However, in the fully differentiated cell, the mechanism of release of the matrix appears to be via packaging in the Golgi zones; secretory granules of characteristic morphological forms migrate to the secretory poles of the ameloblasts, where they fuse with the cell membrane and liberate their contents into the extracellular space. The lysosomes and multivesicular bodies which have been reported to be present in and near the secretory ends (the Tomes' processes) of rat molar and incisor ameloblasts could be associated with destruction of the surplus membrane which arrives in this pole of the cell as the membranes of the secretory granules.

NATURE OF THE ENAMEL MATRIX PROTEIN

The contents of the secretory granules are thus liberated between the inner ends of the ameloblasts and the surface of the dentine. Biochemical and biophysical analyses show that the new enamel consists of a complex mixture of proteins with a characteristic amino acid composition in which the cardinal features are a high proline content, unusually high glycine, and a ratio of the basic amino acids histidine: lysine: arginine of 1:7:9 (Eastoe, 1965). The developing enamel matrix proteins are soluble in cold water at physiological conditions of pH and ionic strength at 37°C. They appear to be globular proteins which may form aggregates of 20–30 million molecular weight (Simmons, 1972). These aggregates dissociate, releasing small subunits of ca. 10,000 mol. wt. if the pH of the solution, originally pH 7·4, is raised or lowered by as little as 0·5. The ease with which large aggregates dissociate probably accounts for both the observed thixotropic (degelling upon mechanical disturbance) properties of the enamel protein matrix gel and the apparently complicated nature of the mixture, with so many fractions running separately upon biochemical analysis. It seems improbable, however, that the matrix protein is in fact a complicated series of distinct proteins, since this would require matching complexity in the necessary messenger RNA.

From a morphological viewpoint, the important features of existing analyses of the organic matrix of the enamel seem to be the ease with which it may be degraded by physical disturbances or by a relatively minor change in the local pH—such as might occur at the surface of a growing hydroxyapatite crystal within the matrix. Enamel contains a lot of protein when it is first secreted, but this labile gel material is literally a "mother medium"—it has little place in the adult tissue. The greater part of the protein secreted as new enamel by ameloblasts is eventually lost from the enamel, perhaps under the control of the ameloblasts or perhaps mediated by forces generated within the enamel itself. It is highly probable that the loss of enamel matrix protein from within a given unit of new enamel is a continuous process, since the converse increase in mineral content is demonstrably so. This means that it is not possible to know exactly how much and what sort of protein is present in the newly secreted matrix gel, because it is not possible to obtain measurable quantities of this exceedingly thin layer: but studies of bulked young enamel have led to measurements of 15·9 per cent by weight, compared with bulked mature enamel at 0·6 per cent by weight. It is probably safe to extrapolate backwards and guess that the concentration might be much higher—perhaps even as high as 30 per cent, but guesswork does not help towards the understanding of underlying principles.

It should be understood that the organic matrix provides a temporary home for growing enamel crystals that is just sufficiently rigid to allow them to grow in length and width and, apparently, sufficiently undisturbed. Some important physical properties of enamel depend upon the great length of the apatite crystals, and mechanical disturbance would lead to interruption of this seemingly perfect crystal growth. However, stability of the young enamel matrix is largely due to the apatite crystals themselves, which grow into and invade newly secreted matrix within a short morphological and temporal interval.

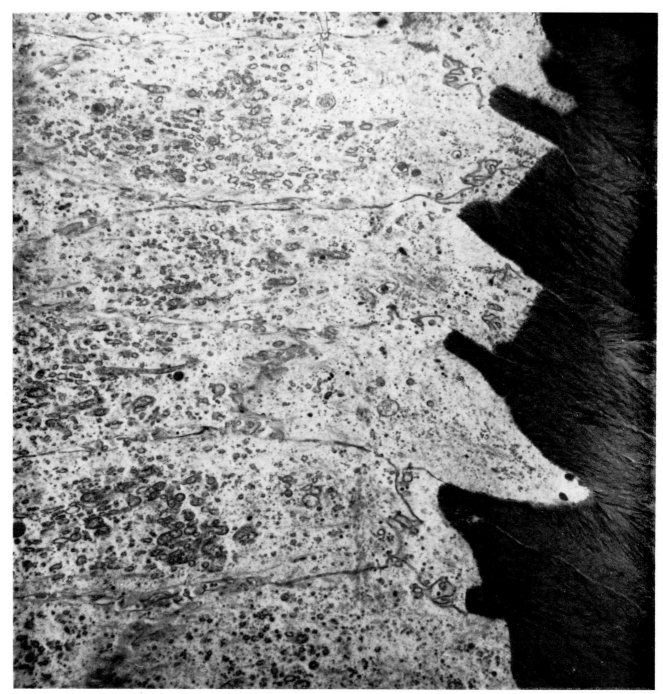

Fig. 3. TEM of monkey ameloblasts and developing enamel surface with Tomes' process pits. ×7,000.

NATURE OF THE ENAMEL MINERAL

The mineral component of mammalian dental enamel bears the closest resemblance to a particular calcium phosphate species called hydroxyapatite. It may be considered, crudely, to be an impure form in which various ions, but notably Mg and Sr, may substitute for the Ca; CO_3 may substitute for PO_4; and F for OH. Furthermore, the ratio of Ca:P is never that of the theoretical pure solid. Evidence for the apatitic nature of enamel mineral comes from the near but not exact similarity in the value for the discrepancy between the refractive index measured parallel with the crystal C-axis (the long axis) and perpendicular to it, and the same discrepancy—which is known as the birefringence—for mineral apatite. Enamel mineral gives the same X-ray diffraction pattern as apatite and, in suitable preparations, the same electron diffraction pattern. Thus the main reasons for its description as "apatite" came from physical rather than chemical analytical methods. Spectroscopic methods, particularly infra-red spectroscopy, are able to provide some insight into the details of the ionic substitutions which may occur in the solid solution of enamel apatite.

The form of the crystals in enamel is easily described. They are long and thin and, on average, oriented perpendicularly to the surface of the developing tissue (figs. 4, 5 and 6). In cross-section, they appear as flattened hexagons in early development, but a regular hexagonal form may be lost in many fully grown crystals in the matrix enamel. They thus resemble ribbons or laths, rather than needles during early development.

Each crystal has a long developmental history, lasting in human enamel for months, with important changes occurring during weeks, because no new crystals grow in the enamel that were not present in a particular unit volume within a few hours of its elaboration The increase in the quantity of mineral in enamel, then, is due to the growth in diameter of the crystals already in it (figs. 4, 5 and 6): and is not, as is the case with bone, dentine and cement, due to the nucleation and growth of new crystals.

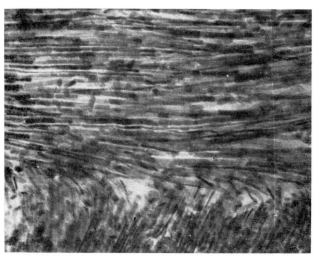

FIG. 5. Same, deeper in enamel, *i.e.* further away from the formative front, showing the increase in the diameter of the crystallites. Enamel that is significantly harder than this cannot be cut with glass knives—and, in any case, suffers too much distortion as a result. ×48,500.

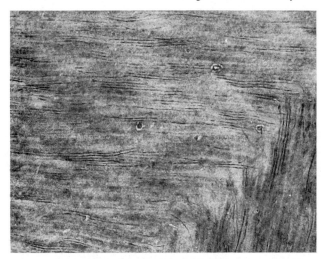

FIG. 4. Developing enamel, close to formative front. Prism boundary change of orientation can be seen towards lower left. Coypu rat. TEM of methacrylate embedded glass-knife-cut section. ×48,500.

to put the case in reverse, *viz.,* that growth of the apatite crystals in enamel is limited by the absence of new protein matrix gel to grow into.

Enamel crystallites close to the developing surface may have diameters of less than 10 nm. This increases to 20 nm. within a few microns of the surface and continuously and gradually until the mature diameter of 40–60 nm. is reached (figs. 4–6). Thus, the spacing between the centres of crystals at the developing front is the same as that in the completed tissue—what changes is their width. Each crystal may therefore be regarded as a long tapered wedge whose incremental growth maintains its previous shape.

Enamel crystals are found in the first thin layer of matrix laid down on the surface of the dentine. It is possible that the first crystals are dentine crystals that grew on or in the dentine collagen, and outwards into the enamel. However, it is improbable that the enamel matrix is entirely incapable of allowing or inducing the formation or nucleation of new crystals, since we can deduce that some new crystals develop throughout amelogenesis to replace those which end (see later) at prism boundaries. The first enamel crystals appear as elongated dark lines in electron micrographs of ultra-thin sections of the developing enamel. They are not all perfectly parallel but they are close to perpendicular to the relatively smooth and flat surface of the first formed layer of enamel (figs. 4, 12 and 14). They may be seen at less than 0·05 μm. from the surface of the enamel matrix at its junction with the secretory process of the ameloblast. In man, enamel is secreted at a rate of slightly more than 4 μm. per day. Thus crystals may grow into newly secreted enamel matrix in less than one-quarter of an hour. For most practical purposes, it may be said that the deposition of mineral begins with the formation of matrix but it would be neater, conceptually,

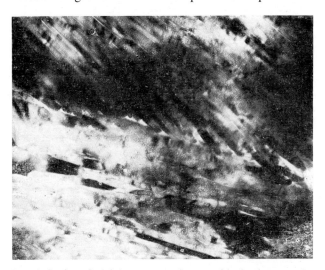

FIG. 6. Section of adult human enamel prepared by ion beam machining. The "frothy" appearance of the crystals is due to ion beam damage, but the crystals are intact and undeformed. Note that they can be traced over long distances. The dark bands crossing some of the crystals are Bragg extinction contours, which result when certain lattice planes are oriented so as to diffract the electron beam outside the limiting aperture. They move along the crystals when the specimen is moved or tilted with respect to the electron beam, thus proving that the crystals are elongated single crystals. A prism boundary discontinuity runs along the centre of the field. TEM ×48,500.

A number of such crystals may be regarded as imposing pressure upon the intervening matrix protein and water, which will lead to their expulsion back towards the developing surface. It is not known whether a certain economy in the use of enamel matrix results from such a mechanism, but it has been put forward as an explanation for the loss of protein during enamel mineralization.

This description also implies that the final size of adult enamel crystals is determined by whatever determines the inter-crystalline spacing at the developing front, and by the limiting thinness to which the enamel matrix protein may be squeezed between and by the growing crystals.

SHAPE OF THE DEVELOPING ENAMEL SURFACE AND CRYSTAL ORIENTATION WITHIN IT

After layers of enamel a few microns thick have been produced, the interface between the young enamel and the secretory ameloblasts takes on a characteristic inter-digitating form (figs. 3, 7, 8 and 9). Detailed features of the interface are different in several of the different taxonomic groups of the mammals (fig. 10), and are related to important differences in the resultant enamel structure at an intermediate structural level. The shape of the pits also differs in different regions of one tooth type, for example, in different regions in a single human tooth; but in the following, emphasis will be placed on the form of the ameloblast : enamel interface found during the development of the bulk of the lateral enamel of human teeth.

Each ameloblast develops a projection, roughly conical in form, at the secretory pole of the cell. The projection is known as Tomes' process; it is limited by the band-like terminal bar attachment of each cell to its six neighbours. Internally, Tomes' process is partially de-limited by the web of filaments running into the cytoplasm from the terminal bar, a thickening of the cell membrane. ER and mitochondria are rarely found in Tomes' processes, which are usually filled with large numbers of different sorts of secretory granules, amongst which numbers of criss-crossing microtubules may be found (Katchburian and Holt, 1972).

Each Tomes' process is surrounded by the enamel which it has produced and thus occupies a pit in the surface of the new enamel which conforms to its averaged external shape—that is, excluding minor and temporary undulations in the surface of Tomes' process. In the following, the term **pit** will be used to mean the depression in the developing enamel surface caused and occupied by one Tomes' process (Boyde, 1964).

CRYSTAL ORIENTATION DISCONTINUITIES— THE ORIGIN OF PRISM BOUNDARIES

The crystals which grow immediately beneath the surface of the developing enamel can no longer all be perpendicular to all of the surface, but they still tend to be perpendicular to that part of the surface below which they are growing. This tendency is responsible for the subdivision of enamel into units whose size is an obvious reflection of the size of the formative cells.

The two adjacent faces of a single pit meet at a sharp angle—roughly at right angles. Thus crystals growing normal to these two faces will, where the faces merge, collide with each other (fig. 12). There is a sharp change in the orientation of the (subsurface) crystals corresponding to the sharp change in orientation of the surface of the developing enamel. Crystals growing beneath parts of the surface which are flat or curve gently are parallel to one another or undergo only a slight change in orientation over a considerable distance. The important discontinuities in enamel organization are, therefore, the planes at which the crystallite orientation changes suddenly between adjacent domains, at whose peripheries the orientation was different. These discontinuities are the prism boundaries or junctions and are the sites where the prism sheath will develop during enamel maturation. For the moment, however, we shall continue to refer to them as discontinuities in order to emphasize the point that the definition of prisms (to follow) belongs as much to human language and custom as it does to reality.

In the bulk of human enamel, the crystal orientation discontinuities are not continuous with one another. The enamel structure is therefore not perfectly divided into prisms whose limits are neatly defined. The reason why discontinuities are not usually continuous is that the surface concavities which generate the discontinuities are usually found only within the pits. The pit wall margins are convex, and convexities generate a fan-like spread of crystal orientations in the underlying enamel rather than discontinuities. However, the pit walls are thin, ca. 1 μm. across, and even thinner in the relevant critical zone referred to below. This means that the prism boundary discontinuities approach close to each other at some places and it has become customary to join them up in the mind's eye —thus creating either separate prisms with all the enamel belonging to prisms if adjacent, separate discontinuities formed in different pits are joined: or circumscribed prisms, separate from each other, and a continuous inter-prismatic phase if the two ends of each discontinuity are joined in a circle. The latter arrangement can and does exist, for example in the enamel immediately overlying the amelodentinal junction at the cusps of human teeth, where there are completely circumscribed prism boundary discontinuities. The former sometimes exists, yet even where it does not, the shape of the prism boundary that it suggests is the most common in human enamel. This means that human enamel can be regarded as a single continuous phase, an idea having the practical usefulness that it dispels the conceptual errors which result from conceiving of separate prismatic and interprismatic phases in the enamel. All of the enamel is, to begin with, equal; and the main differentiation which occurs within it during its further mineralization is the concentration of protein at the prism boundary discontinuities leading to the development of prism "sheaths". If prism boundary discontinuities were continuous with each other it would then be possible to regard the prism sheath protein concentration regions as something interprismatic. Historically, this usage has been made by certain authorities and may need to be borne in mind when interpreting earlier findings.

Pattern 1 Prisms

In human early cuspal enamel (and most of the enamel of the Insectivora Sirenia and some of Cheiroptera and lemurs) the pits are nearly straight cylinders with flat floors. The prism boundary discontinuities represent the paths traced out by the sharp corners of the roughly cylindrical Tomes' processes. Each prism sheath of the adult tissue, then, shows the course which an individual ameloblast traced throughout the formative part of its life cycle. Prisms are separated from one another by a continuous interprismatic region which formed the mutual walls of the pits at the formative surface and which was secreted between and by the sides of adjacent Tomes' processes (figs. 7 and 10A). The prismatic regions were secreted at the (inner) ends of the Tomes' processes.

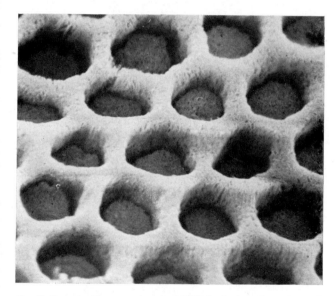

FIG. 7. Scanning electron micrograph (SEM) of mineralizing front of dog molar enamel showing Pattern 1 type pits. Anorganic, freeze dried. Picture width 18 μm.

The prismatic crystals growing in the flat pit floors and in the tops of the interpit walls are nearly perpendicular to these surfaces and parallel to the direction of movements of the ameloblasts. The crystals which grow in the new matrix close to the cell-matrix interface at the side walls of the pits are apparently influenced by the shearing, sliding translation that occurs there. These crystals are not parallel to the interface, but are slewed round in a direction more nearly parallel with the direction of progress of the ameloblasts.

Pattern 1 enamel is thus simple in its organization. It occurs where the plane of the developing surface is parallel to the EDJ and there is no component of movement of the ameloblasts across the surface they are producing. However, such circumstances are not usual, so that Pattern 1 enamel is uncommon.

Pattern 2 Prisms

Pattern 2 prisms may occur locally in human enamel. They are even less common than Pattern 1. Most, if not all, ungulates and marsupials have Pattern 2 enamel, and the basic structure of the enamel of rodents is also of this kind. In Pattern 2 and 3 enamel, the ameloblasts are not perpendicular to the surface. The pits enter the surface obliquely so that the floor of a pit becomes tilted and forms the missing part of the wall.

In both Patterns 2 and 3, the floor is the cervical side of the pit if there is no lateral inclination of the prism direction (lateral ameloblastic movement) such as occurs in the development of prism decussation, and the cuspally inclined, continuously curved, wall encloses the lateral and cuspal sides of the pits.

The pits in developing Pattern 2 ameloblast matrix interfaces are aligned in rows parallel with the longitudinal axis of the tooth. The thick, longitudinal inter-row walls often form ridges more prominent than the intra-row partitions. Concavities of the surface may therefore form at the border of the partitions and the inter-row sheets, in which case longitudinal rows of prisms are clearly separated from longitudinal inter-row sheets of an interprismatic phase. If, however, the intra-row partitions are confluent with the inter-row walls, then the prism discontinuities are not joined to each other and the enamel may be regarded as one continuous phase. Crystals in the floors of Pattern 2 pits grow parallel with the direction of movement of the ameloblasts. The majority of the crystals in the inter-row sheets grow perpendicularly to the tops of the inter-pit walls which are in the general plane of the developing surface. Since the axis of net ameloblastic movement (prism direction) is inclined to the general plane of the surface, the crystals in the prisms and inter-row sheet interprismatic regions are similarly inclined to each other, but they are remarkably parallel within each region.

Each ameloblast contributes one prism boundary discontinuity to Pattern 2 enamel, but each prism is formed between two ameloblasts—even though one of them forms the overwhelming part. The interprismatic sheets are contributed equally by the adjacent cells (fig. 10B).

Pattern 3 Prisms

Pattern 3 pits are also inclined to the general plane of the ameloblast:matrix interface because the cells have a marked component of movement across the formative surface in addition to the backwards movement due to their elaborating the matrix. Pattern 3 pits are arranged in transverse rows, though the row axis is rotated in areas where the net cell movement has a lateral as well as cuspal component. The floor—again the cervical side of the pit—merges inconspicuously with the interpit wall next to it (instead of adjoining the next cervical wall as in Pattern 2) (figs. 9 and 10). The prism boundary discontinuity again forms at the margins of the inclined floor, but it is deficient on the cervical side facing the next inter-pit region, which would be a truly interprismatic region in Pattern 1. It is now current practice, therefore, to attribute an inter-pit wall region to the prism cuspal to it. Since such a region has three prism boundaries—counting the two lateral to it and the one cervical—and since it is joined to a prism core, body, or head which is (partly) defined by another, fourth

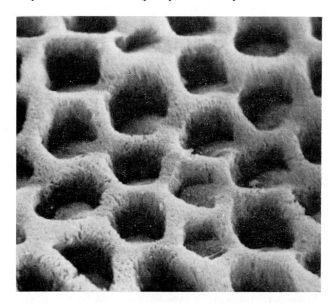

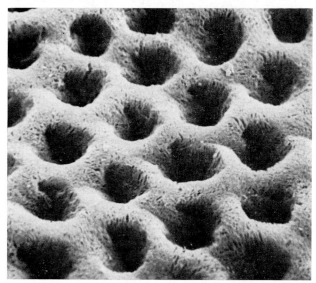

Fig. 8 (*above*). SEM of mineralizing front of dog molar enamel with some Pattern 1 and some Pattern 3 type pits, illustrating the transition between these forms. Picture width 18 μm.

Fig. 9 (*below*). Same, showing Pattern 3 pits. Picture width 18 μm.

prism boundary, it follows that each prism is contributed to by four ameloblasts and that, conversely, each ameloblast contributes to four prisms (fig. 10C). It should be emphasized that this is according to the definition of prism, and it may not be justifiable to assume that this is a natural definition.

Summary of Prism Patterns

In all the prism patterns the bulk-average orientation of the crystals in the centre of the region circumscribed by the

prism boundary (the core, head, or body) is parallel with the prism direction, *i.e.* parallel with the resultant direction of movement of the ameloblasts; the crystal orientation in the centre of the inter-pit walls is normal to the general plane of the surface (defined by the tops of these walls); and the ameloblasts are responsible for only one prism boundary.

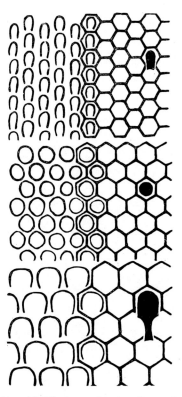

Fig. 10. Diagrams showing form of Patterns 1, 2 and 3 prisms (*left*) and their relationship to the formative cells, the ameloblasts (*right*). The horseshoe-shaped, curved lines are the prism boundaries or sheaths: the hexagonal areas are the secretory territories of the ameloblasts. The black shapes are prisms.

Only in Pattern 1, where the ameloblast movement is nearly perpendicular to the developing surface, is the crystal orientation the same in the centres of the inter-prismatic and prismatic regions. In Pattern 2, where two ameloblasts make each prism, there are also two predominant crystal orientations, *viz.*, that of those in the prisms and that of those in the interprismatic sheets. Since prisms are inclined at angles of 45–60° to the developing surface, the two major groups of crystals are in sheets normal to the surface and in bundles at 45–60° to the surface.

In Pattern 3 the same extreme range of crystal orientations exists as in Pattern 2 but the orientation in the interprismatic (winged process or tail) regions of the prisms merges gradually into that in the prism body proper. The tail regions are what was the inter-pit wall and contain the crystals which grew mostly in relation to the tops of the inter-pit walls and thus normal to the general plane of the developing surface—the orientation of which is retained in the completed adult tissue as the incremental growth lines, or brown striae of Retzius. The crystals in the prism body centres are parallel with the prism direction, so that there must be a span of orientations between the body and the tail at least as great as the angle of inclination of the prisms with respect to the developing surface. However, the crystals in the most cuspal side of the prism may diverge cuspally towards the next prism by some 5 or 10°; and those few which grow in the limited amount of new matrix added along the long cuspal wall of the pits (*i.e.* in the far cervical, fan-shaped part of the tails of the prisms) diverge cervically towards that surface, so that the total fan angle of orientations from top-of-head to bottom-of-tail of Pattern 3 prisms may exceed 60°. The same span of orientations from side to side of the prism is only a few degrees.

Nature of the Varicosities of Enamel Prisms— The Cross Striations

Enamel prisms may be studied by light microscopy of ground sections of the completed, adult tissue (fig. 11) or by scanning electron microscopy (SEM) of the surfaces of fractured preparations. In both cases it is possible to see

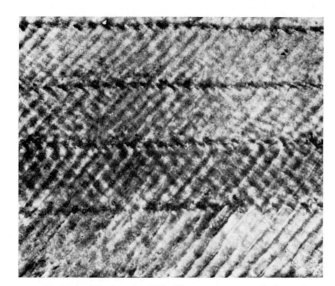

FIG. 11. Light micrograph of LS of human permanent incisor, showing prisms, their cross striations, and the incremental lines of Retzius. Prisms are *ca.* 6 μm wide.

that the prism boundary discontinuities, known as prism sheaths in the completed tissue, show slight sinusoidal undulations with a wavelength of usually from 4–8 μm. These varicosities of the prisms correspond to the cross striations of alternate lighter and darker bands which can be seen with ordinary light microscopy, are prominent when examined by polarized light microscopy and become even more prominent with both methods during the early stages of destruction in the carious lesion (see Chapter 32). Although a complete developmental study of these features has yet to be published, it seems reasonable to infer

the following from what is known of the adult structure and from the developmental information that is available. The distance between them corresponds to the rate of deposition of enamel matrix in human teeth. They are caused by circadian variation in the rate of enamel matrix

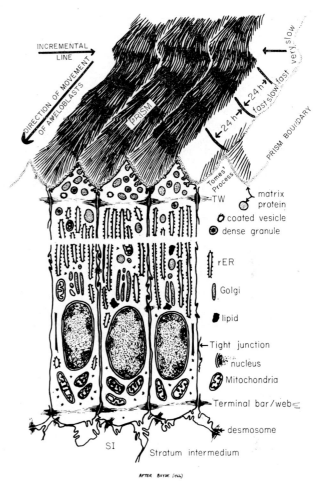

FIG. 12. Diagram showing some essential features of amelogenesis as seen in near LS TEMs of Pattern 3 developing enamels. The tall, columnar, secretory ameloblasts are interrupted—they would be much longer than is shown here. Prisms are bundles of *ca.* 10^4 apatite crystals which grow into the protein matrix gel secreted by the ameloblasts (shown here as stippled areas). The cross-striations of the prisms are seen as sinusoidal undulations of the crystal orientation discontinuities or prism sheaths. Incremental lines of Retzius may be severe cross striations. (After Boyde, 1964).

release by the ameloblasts. The explanation for the influence of a rate perturbation on the external form of the prisms and on the orientation or changes in the relative proportion of regions of the prisms containing differently oriented crystals follows from a consideration of events in the lateral and cuspal wall portions of the Tomes' process pits (figs. 12 and 14).

It has already been indicated that little new enamel is added to the walls of the pits below a region close to their tops. This can be inferred from the relatively constant shape of the pits. Furthermore, such crystals as do grow in those sites are oriented by the shear movement of the cell membrane of Tomes' process past the surface of the matrix. Thus these sites which are the most nearly aligned with the axes of cell movement appear to be unusually influenced by cell movement, show the greatest influence of that movement on crystal orientation, and are also the least favourable sites for the release of new matrix from the ameloblasts.

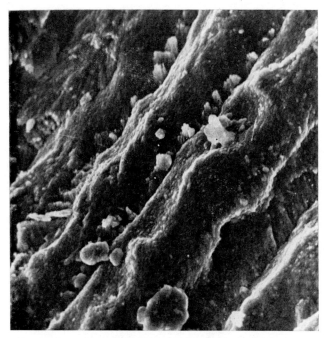

FIG. 13. SEM of fractured human enamel, showing undulations (varicosities or cross striations) of prism boundaries. Picture width 25 μm.

Consider now a reduction in the total rate of matrix release: this is synonymous with a reduction in the rate of (backward) cell movement. The lateral and cuspal wall sites must now be slightly less unfavourable sites for matrix release, and may grow slightly at the expense of the floors. Further, the crystals which grow in this new matrix may have orientations which deviate to a slightly greater extent from the direction of cell movement (figs. 12 and 14).

The situation is reversed during the succeeding more rapid phase of amelogenesis. The lateral and cuspal wall sites again become unfavourable sites for matrix release, and the floors grow at the expense of the walls.

The walls in this analysis are the tails of Pattern 3 prisms: the floors are their heads. Thus the cross-striations of the prisms are expansions of the prism heads at the expense of the tails (fig. 14). Depending on whether the prisms are sectioned longitudinally in the head-to-tail or side-to-side direction, so the external prism form will appear as snake-like (figs. 12 and 13) or repetitively bulbous (varicose) (fig. 14).

Tortuous Course of the Prisms (Decussation)

At the commencement of amelogenesis in lateral regions of human teeth, the pits are oriented as intimated by the nomenclature for the pits used so far, viz., the continuous lateral and cuspal walls are the cuspal sides of the pits, and the floors are cervical. This soon changes, so that after a

few more microns of enamel have been added, the pits can be seen to enter the surface obliquely from one side or the other as well as from the cuspal aspect. Belts or zones of pits behave in unison and there is a gradual change in the entry direction of the pits—which is, of course, the exit direction of the ameloblasts—from zone to zone. The zones are disposed roughly in the circumferential direction

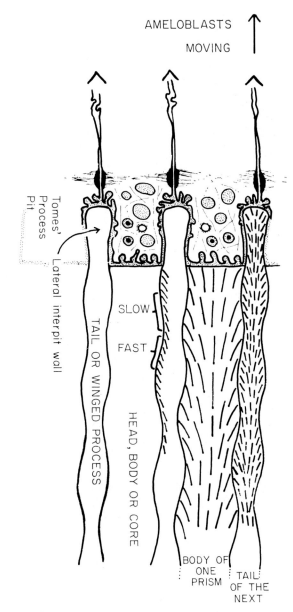

FIG. 14. Diagram showing enamel formation as seen in oblique transverse sections of developing Pattern 3 enamels and/or any plane of section normal to the surface of developing Pattern 1 enamels. The section is parallel with the prism direction, i.e. the direction of movement of the ameloblasts, but cuts from wall to wall of the pits. The inter-pit wall regions are the interprismatic regions of Pattern 1 (and 2) enamels and the tail or winged process of the prisms regions in Pattern 3 enamels. The material forming in relation to the floors of the pits corresponds to prism bodies or heads. According to the hypothesis of Boyde (1964), expansion of the wall regions at the expense of the floors occurs during the relatively slower matrix release phase of the 24 hr. cycle. This effect is somewhat exaggerated in the diagram.

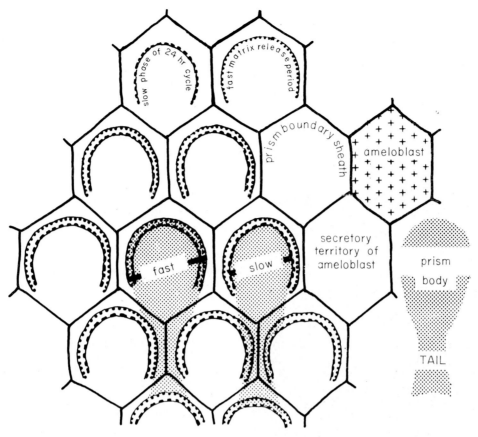

FIG. 15. Diagram showing the variation in the cross-sectional form of human (Pattern 3) enamel prisms. During slow phase of the matrix release cycle the prism tails expand at the expense of the heads. Stippled areas are prisms. Curved lines are prism boundaries or sheaths—double, because viewed at two different levels. Hexagonal areas are the secretory territories of individual ameloblasts.

of the tooth and are of the order of 10 or more pits wide. They show that belts of ameloblasts, corresponding to the zones of pits, are moving in opposite lateral directions with respect to the surface. This component of ameloblast movement is responsible for the complex and tortuous course of the enamel prisms from a level near the EDJ to another well below the final surface of the enamel in human teeth.

It is unusual to encounter adjacent pits entering the surface in opposite directions in human enamel, but this is common in the developing tissue of many other mammals. If this situation is found, it implies that the corresponding prisms defined by the discontinuities forming within these pits will cross one another at an angle, like the Roman numeral X. This is the origin of the term, decussation of enamel prisms. Although strict decussation is not found in human enamel, the term is still used because the phenomenon of relative change of prism boundary direction due to relative difference in the direction of ameloblastic movement is homologous with that leading to real decussation in other mammals.

Light microscopic and SEM studies of the adult tissue must again be used to fill in the gaps in the developmental story with respect to decussation. Transverse ground

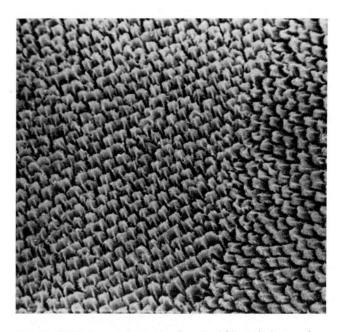

FIG. 16. SEM showing Pattern 3 prisms in African elephant molar. Two decussating zones of prisms are seen. Picture width 175 μm.

sections of mid-lateral enamel show that an equal number of prisms diverge to the right and to the left shortly after leaving the EDJ. Longitudinal sections show belts in which the prisms are more longitudinally sectioned (**parazones**), and belts in which the prisms are more transversely sectioned (**diazones**). Two parazones and two diazones then encompass one wavelength of the cyclical change in lateral movement direction of the ameloblasts that can be seen at the developing surface.

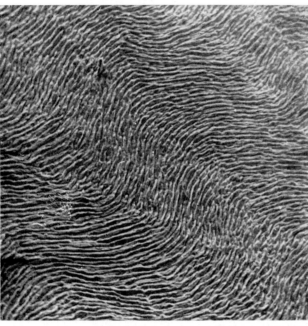

FIG. 17. SEM of oblique transverse section of human enamel (HCl etched), showing gradual change of orientation between prisms in adjacent zones. Picture width 235 μm.

They also show that the prism axes are not parallel with the diazones and parazones and/or the related phenomenon of the Hunter Schreger bands (HSB). Thus prisms cross from one zone or HSB to the next, and since zones are distinguished by different common degrees or properties of lateral movement, we can infer that prisms deviate from side to side a few times in the passage from the EDJ to the surface of the tooth. This inference may be confirmed directly by the examination of a suitable oblique-transverse section for light microscopy or a polished and etched preparation examined in the SEM, when the sinusoidal lateral movements of the prisms can be seen (fig. 17).

Hunter Schreger Bands

Hunter Schreger bands are seen in the inner four-fifths of the enamel in longitudinal sections of human teeth. Differently oriented groups of enamel prisms reflect light in different directions and to different degrees. Some bands appear dark and the alternating ones light, but these may be reversed by altering the direction of illumination; as, for example, by viewing by reflected light instead of transmitted light, or by rotating the section through 180° when it is obliquely illuminated.

Prism Sheaths

The increase in the amount of apatite present within a volume of enamel continues steadily from the time of its secretion. The process of continuing mineralization is called **maturation.** It goes on long after the shape of a given part of a tooth has been determined in the form of the partly mineralized matrix, but it begins long before that shape is completed. To emphasize this point, some of its features will be considered before examining the form of the completed enamel surface.

The surplus water and protein present in newly secreted enamel matrix must move back towards the tooth surface, parallel with, and in the spaces between, the crystals. The crystals are long and do not apparently end within the centre of the prism except perhaps in the more severe growth disturbance lines (see later). A certain proportion do, however, end at the prism boundary discontinuities, since that is the essential nature of the latter. Protein migrating back towards the forming surface may thus accumulate at the prism boundaries, to which a proportion of it is squeezed. The packing of the ending crystals at the prism peripheries is certainly far less perfect than that of the parallel crystals within, and the potential spaces appear to become partly filled with more protein, rather than with more mineral. Thus, decalcified sections of mature enamel show matrix concentrations in the prism sheaths, with little recoverable matrix from the prism cores, whereas decalcified sections of newly secreted enamel show no greater concentration of matrix at the prism boundary discontinuities than in the prism centres (figs. 4 and 5).

Tufts and Lamellae

The so-called tufts and lamellae bear such strong resemblances to geological fault lines that, in the absence of any developmental information, "faulting" may be regarded as one causative factor. They are features seen to good advantage in transverse and tangential sections of the enamel, but rarely in midline longitudinal sections—indicating that they are radial-longitudinal structures.

Tufts are groups of dark prisms and prominent prism sheaths seen in ground sections, apparently emanating from the enamel dentine junction. The tuft plane usually extends through one-quarter to one-third of the thickness of the enamel, and waves from side to side at its outer end.

Lamellae extend through the entire thickness of the enamel. They are usually thinner than the tufts and often appear to consist of accentuated widened prism sheath regions.

Tufts and lamellae are retained if a ground section (or a whole tooth) is carefully decalcified on the microscope stage. There is thus no doubt that they contain more than the particular critical concentration of matrix protein necessary to survive this ordeal, and their resemblance to the prism sheaths is immediately suggested. It is further indicated in the negative observation that this protein concentration has never yet been found in the newly formed enamel in which the tufts and lamellae may develop. It therefore seems that the high protein concentration in tufts and lamellae—relative to the rest of the surrounding normal enamel—is acquired due to either the remobilization of enamel matrix proteins from underlying and surrounding regions, and/or to the defective mobilization or removal of the original protein level contained in these regions. Why extra protein should move into these regions or the usual protein removal should be hindered is not known; it has been suggested that readjustments of the relative positions of longitudinal blocks of young, immature enamel may occur to relieve internal strain built up probably as a result of dimensional changes due to the intermediate stages of influx of minerals into the enamel matrix. Faulting occurs, and either the normal exit routes for the matrix protein are interrupted and/or spaces are created which may become filled with surplus matrix protein (Boyde, 1964). Lamellae evidently represent late readjustment occurring after the full thickness of the enamel matrix has been produced, but the stage at which the tufts form is not apparent.

CESSATION OF AMELOGENESIS: FORMATION OF THE SURFACE ZONE

The end of the secretory phase of the life cycle of an ameloblast is as carefully programmed as any other stage. The secretory phase may last (say) 300 days with an average of 4·5 μm. of matrix deposited per day during that period.

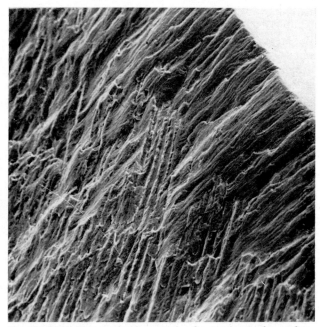

FIG. 18. SEM of human deciduous molar, fractured normal to surface (top right) in longitudinal direction: cervical is to bottom right. Note thick true surface zone or prism-free layer. Picture width 200 μm.

A few days before complete cessation, the rate slows down considerably with an associated reduction in the prominence of Tomes' process. The loss of the associated pits in the matrix surface with the loss of the sharp changes in orientation of the surface leads to the disappearance of the prism boundary discontinuities. The developing crystals

all take on an orientation perpendicular to the matrix surface and the prismatic structure of the enamel disappears. The orientation of the crystals in this surface zone enamel is thus parallel with the tail (inter-prismatic, inter-pit wall) crystals of the immediately subjacent layer and the two appear to merge. The prism boundary discontinuities contain more water-filled, permeable space than the remainder of the tissue and may function as one sort of selective diffusion pathway in the enamel; their absence in the true surface zone implies that this may function as a peripheral seal to the underlying prismatic enamel.

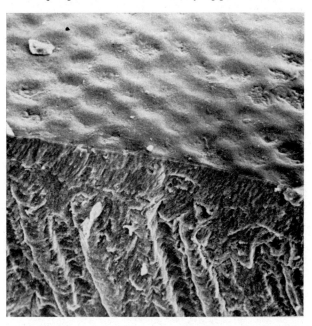

FIG. 19. SEM of human permanent premolar enamel fractured normal to mid-lateral surface. Note thinner true surface layer (prism-free) and shallow surface pits. Picture width 83 μm.

The true surface zone in human deciduous teeth (at *ca.* 30 μm.) is much thicker than it is in the permanent enamel (*ca.* 5 μm.), but it is also much more constant in its appearance (figs. 18 and 19). It is not known why the former should be so, but the latter is evidently a consequence of the much longer developmental history of the permanent teeth, with the increased chance of minor pathological changes (see section on incremental lines).

Ultrastructure of Ameloblasts at End of Amelogenesis: Maturation

All published reports on the ameloblasts during the phase of maturation have been based on studies of the rapidly growing teeth of non-humans. The details of the process in such teeth are likely to be rather different from those in human teeth because on-going mineralization during matrix formation is not so evident, and the whole thickness of the enamel may exist at one stage as a soft material. Studies of non-human material, then, have given rise to the concept that maturation begins only at the end of matrix synthesis. The following descriptions of maturation changes in ameloblasts may therefore need to be modified in the case of human teeth, and particularly permanent human enamel, but certain underlying principles will hold good for the human case.

Fully differentiated secretory ameloblasts have a great concentration of mitochondria in the outer pole of the cell, that is, between the nucleus and the stratum intermedium end of the cell, whereas few mitochondria are found amongst the ER and Golgi zones at the secretory end of

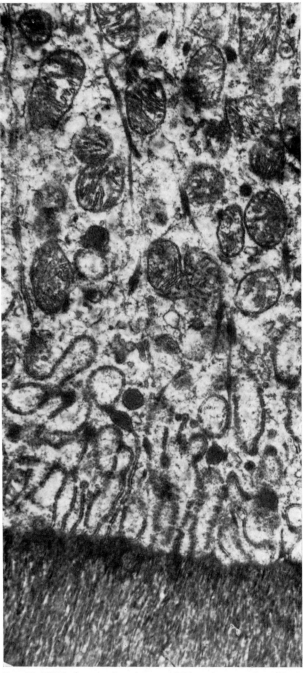

FIG. 20. TEM of maturation phase ameloblasts (post matrix synthesis phase) of rat incisor, showing complex invagination of plasma membrane and absorptive granules containing material similar in appearance to that on the surface of the enamel: this is presumed to be the protein matrix component that is re-absorbed by the ameloblasts. Note numbers of mitochondria and filament bundles. ×18,000.

the cell. At the end of amelogenesis numbers of mitochondria appear throughout the cell and at the same time the ER and Golgi become progressively less evident as the length of the cells is severely reduced (fig. 20).

In rodents about 10 per cent of the late secretory stage or early maturation stage ameloblasts appear to undergo a process of self destruction, via the formation of autophagosomes and cytosegresomes. (Boyde, 1964; Reith, 1970 and Moe and Jessen, 1972). Resulting cell debris may be phagocytosed by SI cells and by macrophages (Moe and Jessen, 1972). It is probable that these cells fail to limit processes which are normal for ameloblasts at the end of amelogenesis, whereby a large part of the protein-manufacturing (rER) and secreting apparatus (Golgi and granules) which were required during matrix secretion is dismantled.

Intercellular spaces, which were common in undifferentiated IEE cells but rare between fully differentiated secretory ameloblasts, again become conspicuous during the change to the maturation phase. The inner terminal bar apparatus may disappear temporarily, so that the intercellular space between the ameloblasts is continuous with the enamel matrix space. Large numbers of microvilli appear on the lateral cell surfaces, so that they resemble the stratum intermedium in this respect. The ameloblasts become joined to each other by a larger number of desmosomes and tight junctions than was the case during active matrix formation, when the parallel lateral cell membranes were closely positioned but only showed occasional definitive attachments.

Whereas occasional hemidesmosomes or attachment plaques have been reported to attach secretory ameloblasts to the surface of the formative matrix, these are rarities. Large numbers of such plaques form to attach the ameloblasts to the completed enamel surface, prior to the development of a deep invagination of their inner poles. At the same time, the inner terminal bar apparatus reforms, thus probably separating the enamel matrix extracellular space compartment from the lateral intercellular space compartment once more. The striated border formed by invagination of the enamel pole of the cells can be seen to contain clumps of granular material apparently identical to material which forms a layer on the surface of the enamel, and the current assumption is that this is the enamel matrix protein being absorbed by the ameloblasts—the granules may therefore be called "absorptive" (Reith, 1970). Mitochondria are common near the striated border (fig. 20). The outer terminal bar apparatus disappears before or during the phase of maturation, so that the lateral intercellular space compartment is in communication with that of the stratum intermedium. Ameloblasts are joined to each other by tight junctions as well as desmosomes and to the SI cells by tight junctions.

Late Maturation Phase

The enamel matrix protein absorption phase of maturation eventually gives way to a stage when mineral ions continue to be transported by the ameloblasts into the enamel, but there is no evidence of macromolecular or polymeric material coming out. The ameloblasts at this stage contain numerous large mitochondria with many internal cristae and some granules. Their lateral surfaces show numerous microvilli, and still face on to a common extracellular space shared with the SI cells, to which they are now attached mainly by desmosomes. It seems likely that their main function at this stage lies in pumping mineral ions into the enamel, and water out.

Reduced Enamel Epithelium

During the late maturation phase, and afterwards, the ameloblasts are separated from the surface of the mineralized enamel by a 40–80 mm. gap containing basal lamina material, which they presumably synthesized, and are attached to this by hemidesmosomes or attachment plaques. Further changes in cell organization occur through the development of numerous bundles of tonofilaments in the cytoplasm, which may find attachment to

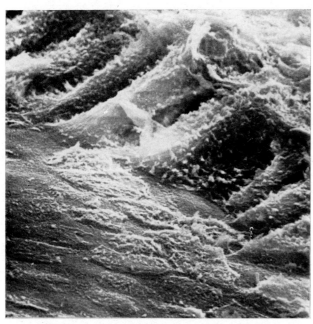

FIG. 21. Reduced ameloblasts, partially removed from surface of unerupted developing human third permanent molar. Note numbers of microvilli and/or intercellular bridges and adherent end plates of some cells. SEM. Picture width 45 μm.

the numbers of desmosomes developing to form intercellular bridges between these cells and those of the reduced stratum intermedium. Filament bundles are also found in the cytoplasm of the secretory ameloblasts, but it is not yet clear whether these are of the same material. The tonofilaments in reduced enamel epithelium cells seem to be equivalent to those formed in stratified squamous epithelial cells in general.

The reduced enamel organ (REE) remains attached to the enamel surface of human teeth, at least until late stages in the eruption of the tooth. The functions of the REE during this period appear to include that of separating the enamel from cells of the surrounding connective tissue,

and of allowing, if not being actively engaged in, a continuation of the maturation process. The space left in enamel for the continued influx of mineral ions is at this stage small, but not negligible, and this process may even continue passively after the tooth has erupted.

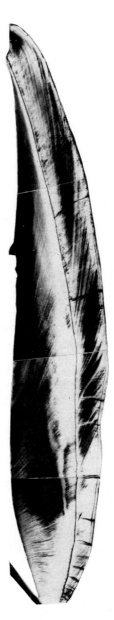

FIG. 22. L/M LS of labial half of forming human upper central permanent incisor. Note pattern of the incremental lines of Retzius.

The REE may be isolated from an unerupted tooth by acid decalcification, and the resulting membrane is named after Nasmyth. If the REE is dissected from an unerupted tooth, the inner ends (end-plates) of the reduced ameloblasts tear away from the remainder of the cell and remain attached to the enamel surface; together with the basal lamina material they constitute a thin cuticle (fig. 21).

Incremental Lines

Incremental, or disturbed growth lines are a prominent feature of the enamel of most human permanent teeth. They are less prominent in post-natal deciduous enamel and unusual in pre-natal enamel. There can be no doubt that the underlying cause of incremental lines is systemic rather than local, since the same pattern can be found in all parts of all the enamel forming at the same time in different teeth of an individual. So reliable is this matching that it has been used to provide forensic evidence that two or more teeth have come from the same individual; this also implies that the pattern of the growth lines is characteristic for the individual. The causes of the brown striae of Retzius and the perikymata—as the internal and external surface features of the growth lines are generally called—are not known. The growth lines are frequent in the low lateral and cervical enamel of human permanent teeth, suggesting that these ameloblasts are unusually sensitive to whatever might be the causative factor.

The incremental lines may be seen in longitudinal and transverse ground sections, as orange to black layers using transmitted light and as blue to white when viewed with reflected light. The orange hue is due to the Rayleigh scattering effect which has a strong dependence on the wavelength of the scattered light and the size of the scattering elements. Growth lines that appear black totally reflect transmitted light and appear white by reflected light. These optical effects suggest that enamel structure is less uniform in the plane of the growth lines, but do not prove that the overall composition of the enamel is changed. However, other evidence does indicate a higher protein and higher space (water) content for many brown striae. For example, growth lines may be seen in decalcified sections of immature enamel and they are more permeable to stains in ground sections; carious lesions tend to track sideways along the plane of some growth lines, and enamel tends to fracture along the plane of the growth lines when subjected to clinical instrumentation in certain ways. If the organic matrix of the enamel is first dissolved in a strong alkali, the tendency to break along the incremental layers is increased.

EM studies have not indicated that crystals are absent from the growth lines, or even reduced in number, but it is possible that they are constricted or thinned. The brown striae may be merely accentuated cross striations with all the prisms margins taking an extra large kink owing to the greater or longer change in the rate of matrix production.

Perikymata (circumferential wrinkles) and imbrication (overlapping) lines are the surface equivalent of the internal growth lines. Terminal phase ameloblasts do not recover after a disturbance of matrix production, and fail to secrete the true surface zone matrix. The result is a slight deficiency (*ca.* 2 to 10 μm) in the total enamel thickness. The usual developmental surface type of pit is thus found in the troughs of the circumferential wrinkle pattern, since these ameloblasts still had Tomes' processes.

Morphological evidence suggests that the recovery of near-terminal ameloblasts is an all or none process: either the cell makes no new matrix, or—in the adjacent cell

cervically—it makes the full amount of surface zone matrix. Thus overlapping layer (imbrication) lines are a feature of this pattern. They are, however, much more common in the low-lateral and cervical regions of human permanent teeth, where growth lines are marked even in the true surface zone enamel (fig. 23). Thus imbrication

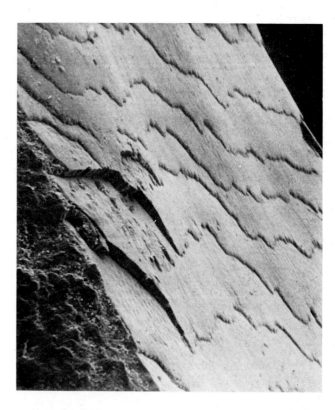

FIG. 23. SEM of low lateral enamel surface of human permanent molar showing shallow overlapping perikymata or imbrication lines. Instrumentation of Class II box cavity margin (lower left) has caused fracture parallel with the incremental lines. Picture width 250 μm. Cervical to top left.

lines in the cervical enamel are not usually associated with troughs showing developmental type pits: all the enamel is of the Tomes' process pit-free type. There are merely shallow (0·1 to 0·2 μm.) pits indicating the previous location of the ameloblasts on the surface.

Perikymata are not found on the tips of cusps, since growth lines here are parallel with the surface. They increase in frequency towards the cervix. Because relatively more enamel is being formed at one time in deciduous teeth since more ameloblasts have differentiated, the growth lines in the lateral enamel are more nearly parallel with the EDJ and the tooth surface, so that the frequency of perikymata is low. All deciduous enamel has a thick true surface zone (fig. 18) and the most severe type of superficial incremental growth manifestations are overlapping layer lines in the surface enamel. Deep, developmental pits are thus not seen on deciduous tooth surfaces.

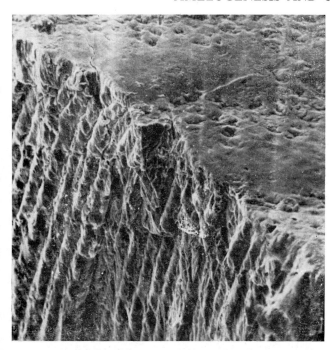

FIG. 24. SEM of longitudinal fracture normal to surface (seen at top right) of human premolar. Note smooth wave crests of surface and pitted trough. Incremental lines meet surface at imbrication lines. Cervical to top left. Picture width 120 μm.

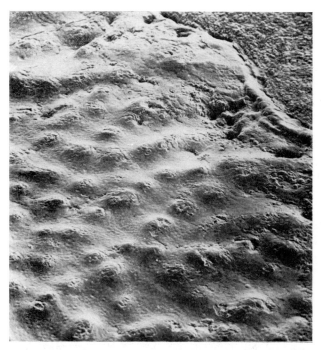

FIG. 25. Cervical enamel surface of unerupted human premolar showing brochs (see text). The root cementum surface is seen in the top right corner. Picture width 590 μm.

Some Common Abnormalities of the Enamel Surface

Linear, circumferential enamel hypoplasias, which are especially deep perikyma-troughs, are common in certain human populations. Severe infectious diseases (*e.g.* scarlet fever) lead to complete, non-recoverable, cessation of enamel matrix synthesis at a much earlier stage in the ameloblast's life history. The enamel surface in the exceptionally deep troughs remains in the typical developmental morphology.

Brochs. This term has been coined to describe low, volcano-shaped projections of the cervical enamel of some human permanent teeth, with an incidence perhaps as high as 30 per cent in premolars. They project about 10 to 15 μm. above the level of the surrounding surface and may be crowded together at intervals of 30 to 50 μm. in a band 500 to 1000 μm. wide at the cervix. The enamel in this band is slightly deficient in thickness. Brochs are characterized by absence of the most superficial strata of the surface enamel, so that the surface enamel fails to extend to the peak of the projection (fig. 25).

Surface overlapping projections (SOPs) and isolated deep pits (IDPs).

Surface overlapping projections (SOPs) may be found anywhere on the tooth surface, but they are particularly common on lateral enamel surfaces. They are nearly always found in close association with irregular clefts or pits in the surface, whose form does not resemble the Tomes' process pits, and which are much deeper: hence the term isolated deep pits (IDPs) (fig. 26).

SOPs and IDPs will be found all around a tooth at a particular series of developmental levels and thus represent a generalized local disturbance of enamel production—it is not yet known whether they have a systemic origin. In mid-lateral enamel, where perikymata are clearly defined,

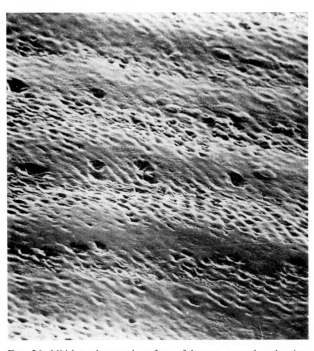

FIG. 26. Mid-lateral enamel surface of human premolar showing Tomes' process pits in wave troughs of perikymata and smooth crests: isolated deep pits and surface overlapping projections are seen on the smooth, true surface zone wave crests. Picture width 166 μm.

it can be seen that they occur only on the smooth wave crests of true surface zone enamel and not in the defective-thickness zones or troughs.

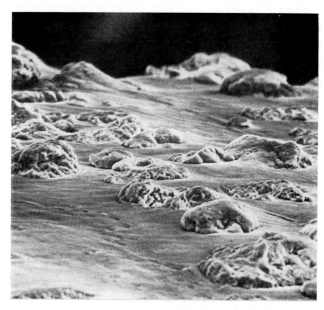

FIG. 27. Large surface overlapping projections on the lateral enamel surface of a human permanent canine tooth. Picture width 185 μm.

SOPs vary in form from flattened features overlapping the surrounding enamel to rounded protuberances; and in size from what appears to be the product of one ameloblast to what must have been the result of a concerted action by several tens of cells (fig. 27). The SOPs can often be found half broken away, revealing an IDP underneath, and the succession of intermediate forms that can be traced strongly suggests that IDPs have just this origin. The fact that so many SOPs break away with so little known cause suggests that the IDP is a vacancy in the enamel structure—perhaps a gas bubble or an enclosure of too watery or non-mineralizable matrix.

REFERENCES

Slavkin, H. C. (1972), *Developmental Aspects of Oral Biology*. New York: Academic Press.

Lester, K. S. (1970), "On the Nature of 'Fibrils' and Tubules in Developing Enamel of the Opossum, *Didelphis marsupialis*," *J. Ultrastructure Res.* **30**, 64.

Katchburian, E. and Holt, S. J. (1972), "Studies on the Development of Ameloblasts," *J. cell Sci.*, **11**, 415.

Eastoe, J. E. (1965), *Tooth Enamel* (M. V. Stack and R. W. Fearnhead, Eds.). Bristol: Wright.

Simmons, N. (1972), *The Comparative Molecular Biology of Extracellular Matrices*, pp. 284–289 (H. C. Slavkin, Ed.). New York: Academic Press.

Boyde, A. (1964), "The Structure and Development of Mammalian Enamel," Ph.D. Thesis, University of London (For extensive enamel bibliography).

Reith, E. J. (1970), "The Stages of Amelogenesis as Observed in Molar Teeth of Young Rats," *J. Ultrastructure Res.*, **30**, 111.

Moe, H. and Jessen, H. (1972), "Phagocytosis and Elimination of Amelocyte Debris by Stratum Intermedium Cells in the Transitional Zone of the Enamel Organ of the Rat Incisor," *Z. Zellforsch.*, **131**, 63.

Weinstock, A. and LeBlond, C. P. (1971), "Elaboration of the Matrix Glycoprotein by the Secretory Ameloblasts of the Rat Incisor as Revealed by Radio-autography After Galactose-3H Injection," *J. cell Biol.*, **51**, 26.

28. DENTINE AND PULP

N. B. B. SYMONS

DENTINE

Dentine is a highly calcified tissue which constitutes the greater bulk of the human tooth. Normally, dentine is covered by enamel in the crown of the tooth and by cement (cementum) in the root area. In the centre of the tooth, dentine forms the walls of the pulp cavity which is occupied by the pulp tissue. The pulp is derived developmentally from the dental papilla and acts as the formative organ for the dentine and also serves as the pathway by which nutrition reaches the dentine.

Composition

Dentine has an organic content amounting to 19–21 per cent by weight, which is considerably more than that of enamel but rather less than that of bone or cement. This organic matrix is similar in its composition to that of bone and cement. It contains a considerable proportion of collagen fibres, which constitutes 18 per cent of the total dentine weight, with about 0·9 per cent of citric acid, and approximately 0·2 per cent each of insoluble protein, mucopolysaccharide, and lipid.

In the outer part of the dentine the collagen fibres are arranged at right-angles to the surface and are coarser than the fibres in the main, inner, part of the dentine where they are finer and have a course at right-angles to the dentinal tubules. It is usual to refer to the outer narrow zone of dentine with the coarser fibres as the mantle dentine and the rest of the dentine as the circumpulpal dentine.

The inorganic content of dentine amounts to 75 per cent and the rest of the total weight is accounted for by water. It is generally accepted that the inorganic content of dentine, in common with the other mineralized tissues, is in the form of hydroxyapatite crystallites, for which the empirical formula is $Ca_{10}(PO_4)_6(OH)_2$. The apatite crystallites in dentine are of similar size to those in bone and cement, having a length of 20–100 nm. and a width of about 3 nm.

Formation

Although dentine is largely formed during the phase in which the tooth lies in a developmental position in the jaws or during the period of active eruption of the tooth it is possible for dentine formation to continue throughout the life of a tooth at a greatly reduced rate. As long as dentine formation takes place there is a narrow unmineralized zone at the inner, pulpal, surface of the dentine. This zone is known as the predentine and it is constituted by the organic matrix of the dentine. At the predentine–dentine junction a rapid mineralization takes place so that in histological sections the junction is sharply defined.

During the active formation of dentine a distinction can be made between a layer of young (early) predentine and one of old (late) predentine on account of the differing staining reactions shown by the predentine next to the odontoblasts from that adjacent to the mineralized dentine. The differences in staining occur both with ordinary histological staining methods and with certain histochemical techniques. The significance of this observation is at present unknown.

Odontoblasts

The cells which are related to the deposition of dentine are the odontoblasts, a layer of specialized cells which lie on the surface of the pulp against the internal surface of the dentine. The odontoblasts have long been considered to be of mesodermal origin but some authorities believe them to be of ectomesenchymal nature since it has been shown, in amphibians, that the odontoblasts are derived from neural crest tissue. In a fully formed tooth the odontoblasts are arranged as a single layer of closely packed cells which are somewhat pyriform in shape (fig. 1). As the cells are of different lengths and the nuclei therefore appear at different levels in the layer an erroneous impression of stratification results.

Each odontoblast possessed a long process which passes from the distal end of the cell into the substance of the dentine where it is housed in a fine canal, the dentinal tubule. The dentinal tubules run, roughly parallel to each other, from the pulpal surface almost as far as the outer surface of the dentine and show numerous lateral branchings along their course. It is generally accepted that the whole length of the dentinal tubules is occupied by an odontoblast process. However, this concept has more recently been questioned, for although the presence of an undoubted cytoplasmic process has been demonstrated with the electron microscope in the predentine and the inner part of the mineralized dentine there is no certainty that the odontoblast process extends peripherally beyond this. So far, the problems of fixation and sectioning of such a dense calcified tissue have precluded any demonstration of an undoubted process in the outer part of the dentine.

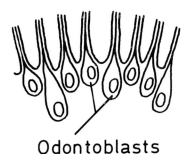

Odontoblasts

FIG. 1a. Diagrammatic representation of
the odontoblasts and their relationship
to the dentine.

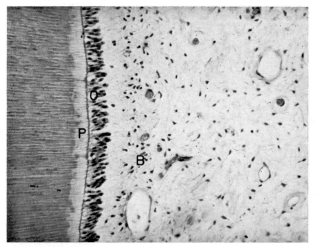

FIG. 1b. Section of human tooth showing dentine and pulp tissue.
O, odontoblasts; P, predentine; B, cell-rich layer deep to relatively
acellular basal layer of Weil. Original magnification × 200.

The odontoblast shows the features typical of a protein-forming and secreting cell, namely the presence of a well-defined rough-surfaced endoplasmic reticulum and Golgi complex together with numerous free ribosomes (fig. 2). These features are, of course, to be seen best during the phase of active formation of dentine, that is of the primary dentine, compared with the subsequent period when secondary dentine formation takes place at a slower rate. Experimental evidence for the secretory activity of the odontoblasts has been provided by radio-active isotope studies in which tritiated proline has been traced from the endoplasmic reticulum to the Golgi complex of the odontoblast and then to the odontoblast process and into the predentine matrix.

The large rounded or ovoid nucleus is situated near the basal (proximal) end of the cell and close to it there is a concentration of rough-surfaced endoplasmic reticulum which is connected to a similar concentration at the distal end by strands of reticulum which run parallel and close to the cell membrane. The centrally situated Golgi complex is surrounded by the endoplasmic reticulum. Mitochondria and free ribosomes are to be found scattered throughout the cytoplasm. Some globules are present amongst the basal, subnuclear concentration of endoplasmic reticulum and similar globules appear in the distal concentration when the cell is active (fig. 2). The nature of these globules is unknown.

Where the odontoblast process lies in the predentine a few mitochondria, some endoplasmic reticulum and ribosomes may be present, but otherwise the process is occupied by a finely stippled material and numbers of microfilaments, microtubules, some dense granules, and large vacuoles with a finely granular content. In the mineralized dentine immediately adjacent to the predentine the odontoblast process still shows a ribosomal content, vacuoles and microfilaments, though virtually all signs of endoplasmic reticulum and mitochondria have disappeared (fig. 3). Further into the dentine a marked change becomes evident in that the process becomes occupied by a large vacuole which compresses the cytoplasm into a peripherally placed ring. Progressively this narrow ring of cytoplasm takes on a hyaline appearance. In the mineralized dentine close to the predentine there is commonly a periodontoblastic space between the tubule wall and the membrane of the odontoblast process. This space is occupied by a more or less granular material and frequently unmineralized collagen fibrils are also present.

Dentinal Tubules and Peritubular Dentine

The numbers of dentinal tubules is very considerable, for at the pulpal surface of the dentine there are 30,000–70,000 tubules per sq. mm. Since the external surface of the dentine is of a considerably greater area than the pulpal surface, the tubules are more widely spaced towards the external surface where there are about 15,000 tubules per sq. mm.

It has been estimated that mid-way between pulp and enamel the total cross-sectional area of the dentinal tubules corresponds to a tube of a diameter of 0·3 mm. for each square millimetre of dentine. This degree of porosity could allow of a considerable movement of fluid within the dentine and experimental work on teeth both *in vivo* and *in vitro* has supported this concept. The application of various stimuli to the surface of exposed dentine results in the outward or inward movement of fluid in the dentinal tubules. Removal of fluid at the exposed surface through evaporation by air blast, dehydration of the surface by hypertonic solutions or by absorbent material, or the application of cold, all produce an outward movement of fluid. Heat, applied via a heated fluid, on the other hand produces an inward flow towards the pulp.

The dentinal tubules constitute a system in which capillary forces can act. The loss of fluid at the dentinal surface is made good by fluid transported by capillary action along the tubules. This can occur at considerable rates, for it has been found that the maximum rate of flow can reach 2–4 mm. per sec. The displacement of fluid in the dentinal tubules is probably related to the production of pain by the distorting effect produced on the nerve endings situated either in the dentinal tubules or close to them in the pulp. This matter is considered in detail in Chapter 22.

The fluid in the dentinal tubules contains large quantities of sodium and chloride but very little potassium. This large Na/K ratio indicates that the dentinal fluid is extracellular; and this lends support to the possibility that only a limited part of the dentinal tubule is occupied by an odontoblast process in the completed tooth.

When first formed the dentinal tubules have a diameter of several micrometres but this is quickly reduced to a diameter

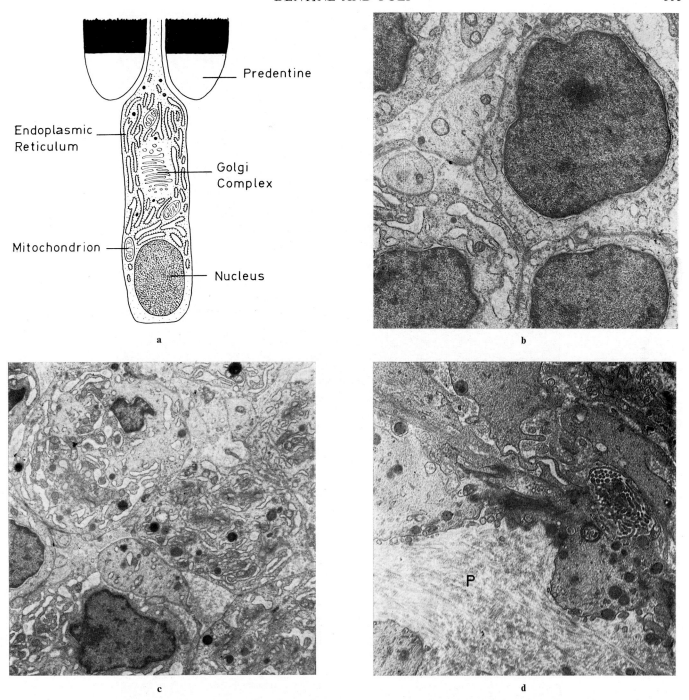

FIG. 2a. Diagrammatic representation of an odontoblast as seen with the electron microscope. b-d: Three electron micrographs of transverse sections through the odontoblast layer of a human tooth. b. At the level of the nuclei of the odontoblasts. c. At the level of the endoplasmic reticulum close to the distal pole of the nuclei. Numbers of mitochondria and dense globules are also visible in the cells. Original magnification × 2500. d. Where the odontoblast and their processes are approaching and entering the predentine (P). Numerous dense globules are present in the odontoblasts. Original magnification × 4000.

of about 1·5 μm. by the deposition of a zone of very highly calcified dentine within the original or primary tubule. This tissue is called the peritubular dentine from its relationship to the tubule in the completed tooth (fig. 4). However, from a developmental point of view it would be better described as intratubular dentine. The peritubular dentine shows a number of differences compared with the rest of the mineralized dentine, or intertubular dentine. The peritubular den-

tine is much more highly mineralized than the intertubular dentine; the level of mineralization is such that the peritubular dentine is completely broken down and disappears on being subjected to routine decalcification methods. As a result of the high mineral content, it shows as a strongly radiopaque ring surrounding the tubules in microradiographs of ground sections of dentine cut perpendicular to the course of the tubules, and in ground sections seen by

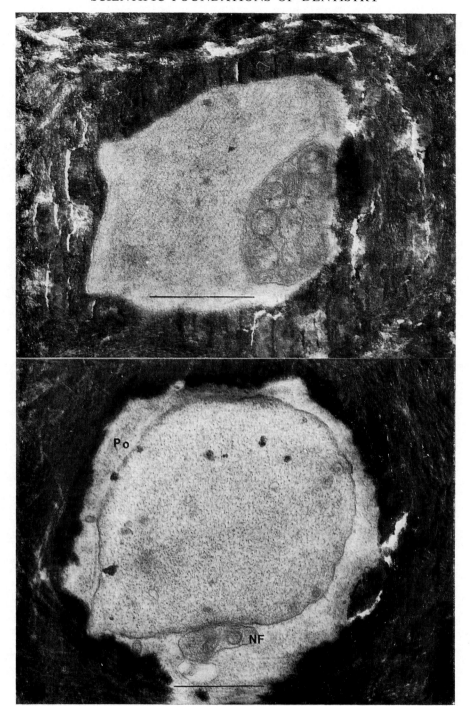

FIG. 3. Electron micrographs of odontoblast processes in dentinal tubules. In both cases a nerve
fibre is closely related to the odontoblast process. In the upper figure (×29,000) the nerve fibre contains numerous mitochondria. In the lower figure (×25,000) the nerve fibre contains two mitochondria. NF, nerve fibre; Po, periodontoblastic space. (From Symons, 1968, by courtesy of
Professor R. M. Frank and the University of Dundee.)

transmitted light the peritubular dentine shows up as a
strongly translucent zone (figs. 5 and 6). Unlike the intertubular dentine, no collagen fibrils have been demonstrated
in peritubular dentine. The small amount of organic matrix
in peritubular dentine contains acid mucopolysaccharide in
contrast to the intertubular dentine.

In the intertubular dentine, the collagen fibrils are grouped
together in dense bundles or fibres. The fibres have a lattice-

like arrangement, coursing in gentle curves between the
tubules and their peritubular zones (fig. 4). Since the figures
for the content of inorganic material in dentine are derived
from the whole tissue it is obvious that these are raised by
the high mineral content of the peritubular dentine. It may
well be that the intertubular dentine has a mineral content
equal to that of bone or cement.

During the active formation of dentine the peritubular

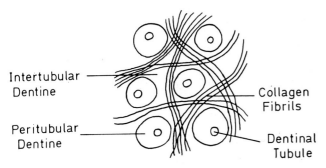

FIG. 4. Diagrammatic representation of a section of dentine cut transversely to the dentinal tubules, showing the peritubular dentine and the collagen fibrils of the intertubular dentine.

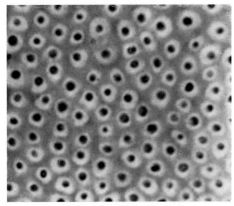

FIG. 5. Ground section of dentine cut transversely to the dentinal tubules and showing the peritubular translucent zones. Original magnification ×1200. (From Scott, J. H. and Symons, N. B. B., *Introduction to Dental Anatomy*, 6th Ed., 1971, by courtesy of Churchill Livingstone.)

dentine reaches to the predentine-dentine junction, but in the crown of the newly erupted tooth the peritubular dentine stops a distance of some 60–100 μm. short of this junction (fig. 7). Since newly erupted teeth extracted for orthodontic reasons rather than unerupted teeth are the common source of human material certain difficulties in interpretation have arisen. It was thought originally that the deposition of peritubular dentine always lagged behind the mineralization of the intertubular dentine, but clearly this is not so during the earlier stages of tooth formation (fig. 7).

Moreover, in such newly erupted teeth there is a deeply reactive layer of intertubular dentine of a width of about 20–25 μm. immediately adjacent to the predentine (fig. 8). As this zone stains intensely with both alcian blue and the PAS method, a high content of both acid mucopolysaccharide and other carbohydrate-containing material is indicated. In view of its reactivity and position, this zone was thought to represent the region where the intertubular dentine mineralized, the intermediate dentine of some authorities, but it is clear that this view is incorrect for two reasons. Firstly, it is not found in the unerupted tooth where dentine formation is actively progressing and secondly it persists unaltered in the fully formed tooth which has been present for many years in the mouth.

Between this zone and the region where the peritubular dentine stops is a further narrow zone of intertubular dentine which shows no content of acid mucopolysaccharide

(fig. 8). These two zones show optical differences compared with the main mass of the dentine when unstained ground sections are examined by transmitted light (fig. 8). It seems likely that they represent the layer of dentine which has been called physiological secondary dentine (see p. 358).

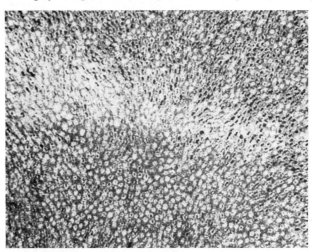

FIG. 6. Microradiograph of a transverse ground section through an incisor from an elderly subject. A belt of occluded tubules runs across the field. Elsewhere the peritubular dentine shows as radiopaque rings surrounding the radiolucent dentinal tubules. Original magnification ×80. (From Scott, J. H. and Symons, N. B. B., *Introduction to Dental Anatomy*, 6th Ed., 1971, by courtesy of Churchill Livingstone.)

In their course from the pulp cavity towards the external surface of the dentine the dentinal tubules generally show two shallow curvatures, the primary curvatures. The curvature in the pulpal half of the dentine is directed convexly rootward, whereas the curvature in the outer half of the dentine is directed with its convexity crownwards (fig. 9). The primary curvatures are particularly marked in the coronal and cervical dentine apart from those tubules which arise from the roof of the pulp cavity and take a relatively straight course towards the occlusal surface or incisive edge. Progressively, the tubules in the root also become arranged in a straight course as the apical region is approached. In the crown and cervical region the double-curved course of the tubules is so arranged that the tubules finish considerably farther pulpward compared with their commencement at the outer dentine surface. This feature has an important bearing on cavity preparation in clinical practice. Most of the tubules involved in cavity preparation are those which have been cut off from the pulp cavity and pulp tissue by sclerosis and occlusion or by a deposit of irregular secondary dentine at their pulpal ends. However, in shaping a cavity on an approximal surface for purposes of retention it is almost unavoidable that fresh tubules, not isolated from the pulp cavity in these ways, will be involved. These tubules will be those situated more incisally or occlusally to the carious lesion (fig. 10). Particularly when silicate cements are to be used in the restoration, care will be necessary to cover these exposed tubules with a protective lining.

In addition to the primary curvatures, each tubule shows numerous small secondary curvatures along its course. These are produced by the spiral course taken by the odontoblast or its process in the laying down of the dentine.

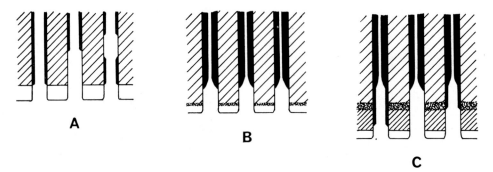

A

B

C

■ = Peritubular Dentine

▨ = Intertubular Dentine

▨ = Physiological Secondary Dentine

▨ = Later-formed Physiological Secondary Dentine

☐ = Predentine

FIG. 7. Diagrammatic representation of three stages in the deposition of the coronal dentine. A, during the formation of the primary dentine; B, shortly after the tooth has appeared in the mouth; C, after the tooth has been present in the mouth for a considerable number of years. (From Symons, 1968, by courtesy of the University of Dundee.)

At the outer dentine surface, the dentinal tubules usually show a division into two main branches. These or further fine branchings unite with the branchings of adjacent processes to form a plexus close to the outer surface of the dentine. In the crown, especially in the cuspal regions, a few tubules show prolongations, known as enamel spindles, which pass a short distance into the enamel. In the root,

many of the dentinal tubules end in the granular layer of Tomes; some may pass into the cement and link up with the canaliculi there.

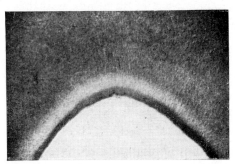

FIG. 8a. Ground section cut horizontally through the crown of a recently erupted premolar and stained with Alcian Blue–P A S method. The narrow dark zone adjacent to the pulp cavity is Alcian Blue and P A S positive; the narrow lightly stained zone shows only a P A S positive reaction. Original magnification ×20. (From Symons, 1968, by courtesy of the University of Dundee.)

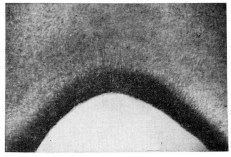

FIG. 8b. The same section as in Fig. 8a but unstained. Original magnification ×20. (From Symons, 1968, by courtesy of the University of Dundee.)

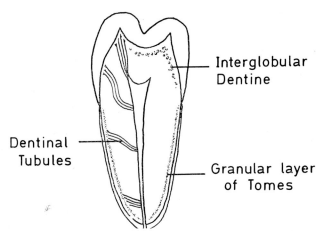

FIG. 9. Diagrammatic representation of a vertical section through a tooth to show the arrangement of the dentinal tubules and the granular layer of Tomes.

Incremental Lines

Certain features which are seen in histological examination of ground (undemineralized) sections of dentine are produced by variations in the pattern of mineral deposition in the organic matrix. These include incremental lines, interglobular dentine and the granular layer of Tomes. Variations in mineralization may be produced by a disturbance in calcium metabolism which is associated with dietary deficiencies, birth or certain diseases. A number of experimental procedures, such as the injection of fluoride, vitamin D or strontium produce a severe disturbance of dentine formation which is known as the calciotraumatic response.

The incremental lines run at right-angles to the dentinal

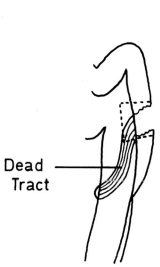

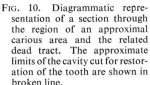

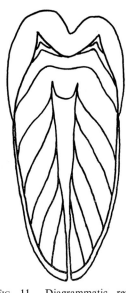

FIG. 10. Diagrammatic representation of a section through the region of an approximal carious area and the related dead tract. The approximate limits of the cavity cut for restoration of the tooth are shown in broken line.

FIG. 11. Diagrammatic representation of a vertical section through a premolar to show the arrangement of the incremental lines (the contour lines of Owen) in dentine.

tubules but are not parallel to the outer surface of the dentine (fig. 11). They correspond to the position of the inner or pulpal surface of the dentine at successive stages in its formation and are about 16 μm. apart. Strictly speaking, the incremental pattern should represent phases in the laying down of the organic matrix of the dentine but histologically the incremental lines are observable because of variations in the degree of mineralization at their sites. Since the advancing front of mineralization is always parallel to that of the forming matrix, the two correspond spatially. The incremental lines in dentine are often known as contour lines of Owen.

In certain teeth, namely the deciduous teeth and the first permanent molar, mineralization has begun before birth and a particularly accentuated incremental line is to be found between the dentine formed before and that formed after birth. The line is known as the neonatal line and it is believed that it is produced by the disturbance in nutrition and external environment of the infant at birth. In the great majority of teeth the incremental lines in dentine, including the neonatal lines, are much less well defined than the corresponding lines in enamel.

Interglobular Dentine

The mineral material is laid down in dentine in the form of globular concentrations, known as calcospherites, which normally fuse together rapidly so that a relatively homogeneous area of mineralized dentine is produced. In certain teeth, however, the fusion may not take place completely in all situations and so areas of interglobular dentine are found. These areas represent small patches of non-mineralized organic matrix of dentine which are bounded by the rounded outlines of unfused calcospherites. Interglobular dentine is found, to some degree, in the crowns of

most teeth not far from the amelodentinal junction (fig. 11). Sometimes the incremental lines are accentuated by areas of interglobular dentine. Those dentinal tubules which traverse areas of interglobular dentine show no peritubular dentine in that part of their course (fig. 12).

An additional situation from which evidence of the calcospherite pattern of dentine mineralization may be obtained is at the predentine–dentine junction. In some teeth, unfused or partially fused calcospherites can be observed in stained sections instead of the usual sharp line of junction between predentine and mineralized dentine.

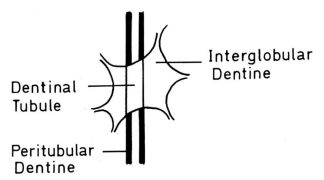

FIG. 12. Diagrammatic representation of an area of interglobular dentine and a dentinal tubule passing through it. The curved lines bounding the interglobular dentine represent the outlines of calcospherites.

Granular Layer of Tomes

Beneath the cement, a narrow layer of dentine of a granular appearance is constantly found in ground sections (fig. 9). This is known as the granular layer of Tomes and is seen in such sections because of variations in the level of mineralization in the layer which give the appearance of a concentration of numerous minute areas of interglobular dentine. Over the years, a number of different hypotheses have been put forward in explanation of the origin of this layer but none of them appear to be completely satisfactory.

External to the granular layer of Tomes there is a narrow zone of an amorphous and hyaline appearance which appears to be a part of the dentine and to separate the granular layer of Tomes from the cement. It has recently been shown that there is a delayed mineralization at the outer, root surface of the dentine before cement deposition occurs and that the mineralization of this region takes place parallel to the root surface. This area showing mineralization different in direction from that of the bulk of the dentine would seem to correspond to the narrow zone of dentine external to the granular layer of Tomes.

Secondary Dentine

The formation of dentine may continue throughout life though the rate can vary considerably. It is customary to classify the formation of dentine into several types though opinions on this differ. It is generally accepted that the dentine which produces the bulk of the tissue and the typical basic form of the tooth should be described as primary dentine. This dentine is laid down rapidly during the development of the tooth and is characterized by having a very orderly or regular arrangement of the dentinal tubules. In man the rate of deposition is of the order of 4μm. per day. The dentine which is laid down later is known as secondary dentine (figs. 13 and 14). It is generally agreed that secondary dentine can show various degrees of regularity depending on the arrangement of the dentinal tubules. In some secondary dentine the tubules may be as numerous and as regularly arranged as in primary dentine, whereas there may be few tubules present or sometimes none at all. It is also generally accepted that secondary dentine may be physiological, that is, it is not produced as a response to any

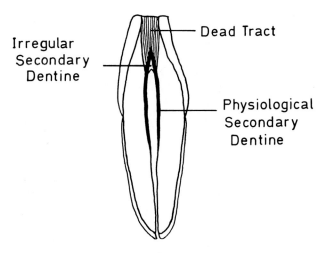

FIG. 13. Diagrammatic representation of a vertical section through an incisor with attrition which has exposed some coronal dentine, and the related dead tract and secondary dentine.

external stimulus, whereas the deposition of some secondary dentine is the result of the opening up of dentinal tubules at the external surface of the dentine by some agent such as attrition, abrasion or caries. Difficulties arise, however, when attempts are made to correlate the morphology of the secondary dentine with its origin. It is frequently stated, for example, that physiological secondary dentine can be recognized as a narrow zone of dentine with usually regularly arranged tubules internal to the primary dentine over the whole pulpal aspect of the dentine. However, it is possible to find limited areas of secondary dentine of physiological origin in some teeth. Moreover, although the secondary dentine found in relation to attrition, abrasion or caries is usually of an irregular variety, yet in relation to the early stages of occlusal caries a regular form is generally deposited.

The deposition of secondary dentine is an advantage in helping to prevent exposure of the pulp, whether it be by wear, caries, or by cavity preparation, especially as it quickly occludes the pointed cornua of the pulp cavity. Presumably, the deposition of regular secondary dentine is a better protection to the pulp than the more irregular forms as the regular variety naturally contains the normal number of odontoblast processes through which some warning is transmitted to the pulp should this layer be approached by a destructive agent. There is no doubt that successive layers of secondary dentine can frequently be observed in relationship to occlusal caries.

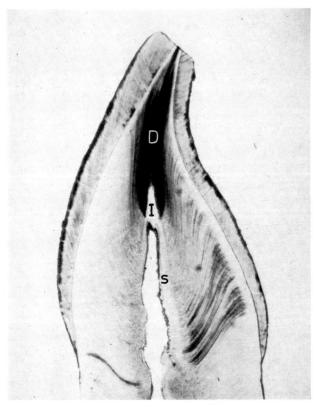

FIG. 14. Ground section cut vertically through an incisor with a limited amount of attrition. D, dead tract; I, irregular secondary dentine. S, physiological secondary dentine. Original magnification ×10.

Translucent Dentine

Changes can also take place within dentine as a result of external stimuli (fig. 6). In some instances, notably in relationship to occlusal caries, the dentine reacts by the production of a sclerosed area beneath the carious cavity. In such an area the dentinal tubules are occluded by mineral deposits with the result that the sclerosed dentine has a more uniform refractive index than normal dentine (see Chapter 32).

When viewed by transmitted light the sclerosed dentine appears more translucent than normal dentine and so the term translucent dentine is commonly used to describe it. There is some evidence to suggest that the mineral material in tubules occluded as a response to caries is not in the form of hydroxyapatite but is present as crystallites of octacalcium phosphate. The ability to produce translucent dentine varies but where it is well developed it presumably must act as a barrier to the rapid spread of caries towards the pulp. The production of areas of translucent dentine occurs progressively in the roots of teeth, and here it must be considered as an age change.

Dead Tracts

More commonly, the response within the dentine to external stimuli is the production of the so-called "dead tract" (see also Chapter 29). Such areas reach from the affected surface of the dentine to the pulp surface; they appear dark when seen by transmitted light and are bounded at the pulpal surface by a deposit of irregular secondary dentine (fig. 13, 14 and 15). It is believed that the dentinal

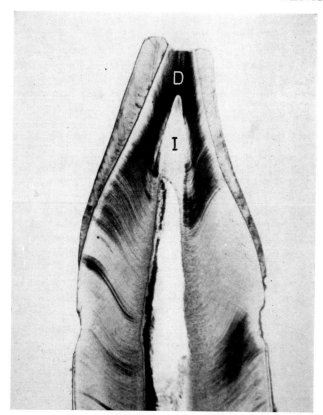

FIG. 15. Ground section cut vertically through an incisor with considerable attrition. D, dead tract; I, irregular secondary dentine.

stimuli from the tooth to the central nervous system where, irrespective of the nature of the stimulus, the sensation of pain is experienced.

Cells and Fibres

There are three kinds of cells, apart from those connected with the vascular channels and nerve fibres, to be found in the pulp. These are the odontoblasts which have already been described (see p. 353), the fibroblasts, and the defence cells. Beneath the covering layer of odontoblasts there is often a cell-free zone, the basal layer of Weil, and deep to this a relatively cell-rich zone which is best seen during

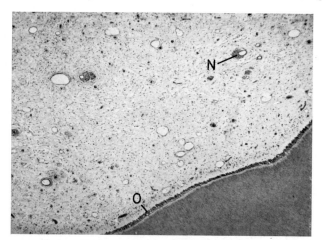

FIG. 16. Section of pulp tissue and adjacent dentine. O, odontoblast layer, N, nerve fibre bundle. Original magnification × 32.

tubules are empty in the area of the dead tract. Each dead tract is surrounded by a narrow zone of sclerosed dentine. Dead tracts are commonly found in relationship to attrition which has involved the dentine. Yet there is some doubt as to a causal relationship between the two, for dead tracts have been demonstrated beneath the incisive edge of teeth which have never erupted. Moreover, it is a common observation that in incisor teeth with attrition the dead tracts involve an area of dentine which is more extensive than that containing the tubules which have been opened up by attrition (fig. 14). It may be that the presence of dead tracts in certain areas must be thought of as an age change which possibly is accelerated by attrition. It is believed that in some teeth dead tracts may be caused by the death of odontoblasts crowded in narrow pulpal cornua.

In relation to cervical caries, the initial response is often the production of a narrow zone of sclerosed dentine followed at a later stage by a dead tract at a deeper level in the dentine. Whereas the usual response to occlusal caries, especially in the initial stages, takes the form of sclerosed dentine, a dead tract is produced in approximal caries.

PULP

The pulp tissue is composed of loosely arranged connective tissue on the surface of which there is a layer of specialized cells, the odontoblasts, which are the formative cells of the dentine. Throughout the life of the tooth the pulp tissue subserves the nutrition of the dentine by virtue of its rich vascular supply. The nerve fibres of the pulp transmit

primary dentine formation (figs. 1b, 16). The basal layer of Weil would not appear to be an artefact for it can be demonstrated in both fixed and unfixed undecalcified sections. Apart from these layers, the rest of the pulp tissue shows a uniform arrangement of its cellular constituents. The fibroblasts are by far the most numerous pulpal cells and have an irregular distribution. They are large flat cells with an oval nucleus, but seen from the side they have a narrow spindle-shaped appearance. They have narrow elongated processes which, though widely separated, come into relationship with the processes of adjacent fibroblasts, and give the cells a somewhat stellate appearance. The electron microscope has shown that there are desmosomal attachments at the junction of the processes. With the light microscope and routine staining with haematoxylin and eosin, the exact limits of the fibroblasts are difficult to distinguish.

Between the fibroblasts there is an amorphous ground substance which contributes the gelatinous nature to the pulp tissue. In the ground substance there are numbers of collagen fibrils which are distributed singly or in delicate fibre bundles. With the light microscope these fibres are not readily seen except when they are impregnated with silver for which they have considerable affinity. The von Korff fibres which pass from the sub-odontoblastic layer of the pulp between the odontoblasts to reach the predentine, especially in the initial stages of dentine formation, show this argyrophilic feature particularly well.

The defence cells, which are represented by histiocytes,

undifferentiated mesenchymal cells and wandering lymphoid cells, are scattered irregularly throughout the pulp tissue, some of them in a perivascular situation. In inflammatory conditions of the pulp tissue the histiocytes act as macrophages. These cells are not easily distinguishable in sections prepared by routine histological methods.

Blood Vessels

The largest blood vessels on the arterial side in the pulp tissue are arterioles and these are characteristically thin-walled showing a minimum of muscle fibres in the tunica media. The small arterioles are very difficult to distinguish from capillaries. The arterioles enter the pulp tissue at the apical foramina, in groups of three or more. These vessels tend to run in the long axis of the pulp and give off branches which anastomose with those of adjacent arterioles and others entering the pulp cavity by separate roots. The major branching takes place in the pulp chamber. Although the great bulk of the blood vessels enter the pulp via the apical foramina, it is not uncommon for small arterioles or occasionally larger ones to enter the pulp from the periodontal membrane at other levels in the roots. There is usually a close relationship between the larger arterioles and the pulpal nerve bundles; especially in the apical region the arterioles are often embedded in the nerve bundles (fig. 16).

The arterioles give rise to a rich sub-odontoblastic capillary plexus, from which looping branches pass between the odontoblasts towards the predentine. The capillary plexus drains into fairly large thin-walled venules, which come together to form several large veins which leave the pulp through each apical foramen.

The thin-walled nature of the pulpal blood vessels make them particularly liable to dilatation. In inflammation of the pulp the accompanying hyperaemia and exudative changes lead to a great increase in pressure due to the unyielding walls of dentine which form the pulp cavity. This compresses the blood vessels and tends to occlude them particularly at the apical foramina. The pain produced by pulpitis is largely due to the effect of this pressure on the nerve fibres of the pulp.

Nerve Fibres

The nerve fibres found in the pulp are of two kinds:

(a) unmedullated fibres which are part of the autonomic nervous system and run along the blood vessels for the control of the contraction of the smooth muscle in their walls; and

(b) medullated fibres which are sensory somatic nerves and carry sensation to the sensory cortex of the brain.

The sensory somatic supply of the pulp is rich. Two or three large trunks as well as several small bundles enter each root. Most of the nerve bundles travel direct to the pulp chamber where considerable branching takes place. In the pulpal cornua of incisors and canines the nerve fibres arrive by a fairly direct course from the main nerve trunks. In other regions of the pulp, most of the nerve fibres change their course abruptly on approaching the cell-rich zone deep to the odontoblasts. The fibres turn in random directions and many of them divide, some frequently. This produces an interlacing network of fibres, the plexus of Raschkow, situated beneath the roof and walls of the pulp chamber. From this plexus fibres arise which cross the cell-free zone of Weil obliquely to reach the odontoblast layer, where they either turn sharply between the odontoblasts towards the predentine or turn back towards the pulp. At the surface of the predentine most of the fibres bend again and divide into numerous branches to form a plexus, the marginal plexus, on the predentine surface. The fibres of the marginal plexus are unmyelinated, and most of the fibres of the plexus of Raschkow have also lost their myelin sheaths. From the marginal plexus fibres have been traced into the predentine. Some are embedded in the substance of the predentine, others lie in tubules in which they may reach some distance into the mineralized dentine. The presence of unmyelinated nerve fibres in the inner part of the mineralized dentine has been confirmed in studies with the electron microscope. The nerve fibres are in close relationship to the odontoblast process and in some instances show complex invaginations of the odontoblast processes at the external limit of the inner third of the dentine. At these places cellular attachments between the plasma membranes of the nerve fibres and odontoblast processes are present which have a similarity to junctional complexes. There is considerable doubt as to the exact role played by these nerve endings in the sensitivity of dentine; the matter is considered in detail in Chapter 22. Not all tubules in the inner part of the dentine contain nerve fibres; it would seem likely that random growth towards the dentine of the nerve endings could account for this arrangement.

REFERENCES

Bradford, E. W. (1967), "Microanatomy and Histochemistry of Dentine," in *Structural and Chemical Organization of Teeth*, p. 3. New York: Academic Press.

Brännstrom, M. and Aström, A. (1972), "The Hydrodynamics of the Dentine; its Possible Relationship to Dentinal Pain," *Int. dent. J.*, **22**, 219.

Eastoe, J. E. (1967), "Chemical Organization of the Organic Matrix of Dentine," in *Structural and Chemical Organization of Teeth*, p. 279. New York: Academic Press.

Frank, R. M. (1966), "Etude au microscope electronique de l'odontoblaste et du canalicule dentinaire humain," *Arch. Oral Biology*, **11**, 179.

Gaunt, W. A., Osborn, J. W. and Ten Cate, A. R. (1971), *Advanced Dental Histology*, p. 75. Bristol: John Wright and Sons Ltd.

Johansen, E. (1967), "Ultrastructure of Dentine," in *Structural and Chemical Organization of Teeth*, p. 35. New York: Academic Press.

Symons, N. B. B. (1968), *Dentine and Pulp: Their Structure and Reactions*, p. 67. University of Dundee.

29. AGE CHANGES IN DENTAL TISSUES

A. E. W. MILES

General principles

Attrition
   Other age changes in enamel

The pulp-dentine complex
   Vascular supply
   Odontoblasts
   Reticular atrophy
   Calcific degeneration
   Age changes in dentine
   Generalized change
   Translucent dentine
   Dead tracts
   Translucent root tip dentine

Cementum

Ageing or senescence may be defined as the progressive loss of homeostatic efficiency that occurs at the latter end of the life span. There is now a good deal of evidence to suggest that this state of ultimate decline is characteristic of most, if not all, forms of metazoan life. It is certainly seen in domesticated and laboratory-maintained species, as well as in man.

Living organisms are unlike engines, the moving parts of which are bound to wear out in the course of time. Living tissues have powers of repair and, at a cellular or sub-cellular level, most if not all parts are gradually being replaced all the time. Injury and disease, by interference with essential metabolic processes, could be expected to impair these processes and undoubtedly this plays a part in what are described as age changes. Nevertheless the sum of evidence suggests that senescence is not simply due to the cumulative effect of partial recovery from environmental injuries. The term, intrinsic age change, is employed for the concept of change attributable to the passage of time *per se* however well the organism may be protected from its environment.

It is conceivable, for example, that in the same way that the fertilized ovum carries a "programme" for its development into a complex organism, it might carry a programme that ensures the ultimate decline and death of the organism. There appears to be a limit to the number of times fibroblasts will undergo population doubling (roughly equivalent to mitoses) in cell culture, and this appears to be related to the life span of the species. It has been observed that, whereas cell cultures of fibroblasts from human embryos died out after about 50 population doublings, those from young adults seemed to be limited to about 30 doublings. Embryonic fibroblasts from short-lived species, such as chicks and rats, survived only for about 15 doublings.

Whether or not a species-specific finite life span is characteristic of cells in culture, this does not appear to be true of organized tissue because both skin and prostate have by serial transplantation from old to young mice been kept alive for 6–7 years, that is for longer than twice the normal life span of the mouse. It must be assumed that something in the nature of programmed cell death is involved in a number of other phenomena. For instance, precisely timed cell death is a feature of many processes of embryonic development. Examples are the degeneration of the tadpole tail at metamorphosis and the degenerative changes that occur in the embryo at the surfaces of the palatal shelves during their fusion in the midline, and perhaps even in the final stages of the life cycle of ameloblasts which, having become reduced enamel epithelium and involved in the epithelial attachment, finally disappear.

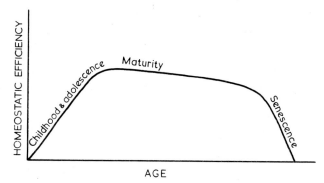

Fig. 1. A diagrammatic representation of the human life span.

Figure 1 depicts the human life span in a simple way. There is a gradual development of increasing body efficiency in childhood and adolescence until maturity is reached. After a long period of little change, there is a gradual decline in powers. The time at which age changes become evident is variable but many tissue changes associated with, or the cause of, the decline occur early. Almost as soon as adolescence has ended, deterioration begins in some tissues. What must be regarded as deteriorative changes can be detected in joints as early as 25–30 years. Similarly, minor vascular changes similar to those of old age can be detected almost as soon. Other changes, such as loss of muscle strength, begin much later.

Changes in articular cartilage tend to occur earlier and more severely in weight-bearing joints and provide an example of the difficulty of distinguishing the cumulative effect of wear and tear from intrinsic age change. The vascular changes that are one of the most constant features of advancing age illustrate the need to distinguish secondary changes from first causes. Because efficient function of every organ depends upon its blood supply, these widespread changes undoubtedly lead to widespread impairment of function. Nevertheless changes in vessel walls must be secondary to some underlying cause.

Current ideas about the ultimate cause or mechanisms concerned in senescence broadly involve the concept of somatic mutation. In its simplest form, this proposes that the accumulation of minor imperfections in the replication of the gene material of cells leads to an irreversible deterioration in the efficiency with which cells operate. In the case of cells that are constantly dividing throughout life, this is easy to understand. Every fault in mitosis would be transmitted to the descendants of cells and the accumulation of occasional errors would, in the course of many generations, become serious. Errors in replication of the genetic DNA code can be compared with errors made by a typist copying an original script. The cumulative errors made in repeated typings, or replications, would eventually change the meaning of words or of sentences. The prevalence of abnormal chromosomes among liver cells, which undergo mitosis only occasionally when cells are damaged, appears to increase with age.

Epidermis is typical of tissue which is continuously undergoing mitosis and therefore at first sight might be expected to show more rapidly the effect of cumulative errors of chromosome replication. Although there is some evidence that mitotic activity in epidermis does lessen in advanced age, the reduction is not particularly marked. This could be because in such a tissue a process akin to natural selection would seem likely to apply; that is, the cells most affected by chromosomal aberration would tend to die or not to reproduce themselves and the least affected would have correspondingly more descendants. In other words, as in a population of competing organisms, the less fit to survive and reproduce would tend to be eliminated.

Apart from cell division, the replication of DNA, RNA and analogous molecules is a continuous feature of cell metabolism. The cumulative effect of random errors in such replications can obviously in the course of time be very large and lead to change in the nature or quality of the products of the cell. This effect could be particularly great in populations of non-dividing cells because of the absence of the mechanism, referred to in the previous paragraph, whereby unfit cells can be eliminated during mitosis.

Neurones are the outstanding example of cells that do not divide; it has been said that we are as old as our nerve cells. By the same token, we are also as old as our odontoblasts because, although there is some evidence to suggest that odontoblasts may occasionally reproduce themselves in repair of traumatic injuries to the pulp, the vast majority do not.

Auto-aggressive immune reactions may play a part in the ageing process. Mutations or errors of replication in somatic cells may give rise to clones of lymphoid cells or of target tissue cells which interact with one another.

ATTRITION

The most conspicuous change in the teeth with advancing age is, of course, attrition (fig. 2). The dentition is the notable exception to the statement that living tissues have the capacity to repair or renew themselves. Given enough use for long enough, the crowns of teeth must wear away as inevitably as the moving parts of a machine. In general, however, food consumed in most European-type communities contains so little roughage that wear of the tooth is minimal, although notable exceptions are encountered. The amount of wear present by the time advanced age is reached differs a great deal, due no doubt to variations in the type of occlusion present in the first instance, variations in habit, muscular power and type of food. Wear is also much influenced by loss of teeth, and opportunities to study complete dentitions in the later years of life are relatively few, so that most of our knowledge of patterns of tooth wear derive from studies of ancient peoples and primitive contemporary ones.

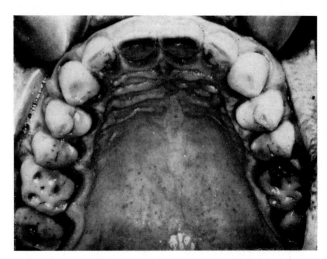

FIG. 2. Unusually marked attrition in a male of 55 years.

The first part of the permanent dentition to show wear is the mesiobuccal cusp of the mandibular first molar where it occludes with the second deciduous molar. As molar wear increases, there is a gradual flattening of the helicoidal curve which is characteristic of the occlusal plane of the unworn human dentition and a gradual loss of the incisor overlap. Closure of the inter-jaw relationship by wear, associated with loss of the incisor overlap, tends to advance the mandible so that the incisors gradually assume an edge to edge relationship. In the relatively unworn dentition, the occlusal surfaces of the upper first permanent molars face outwards a little. The second molar occlusal surfaces incline outward a little more and those of the third molars more still, producing the curve of Spee. In the course of wear, this inclination is gradually diminished by a greater amount of wear on the lingual than buccal cusps of the upper molars and, in the lower molars, greater wear of the lingual cusps, so that a stage is reached when, in the coronal plane, the occlusal surfaces first of the first molars, and later of the other molars, are horizontal. The differential rates of wear between lingual and buccal cusps continue so that, in due course, in the coronal plane the originally outward inclination of the occlusal surfaces of the first molars becomes inclined inward; thus there is a gradual reversal of the original helicoidal curve of the occlusal plane.

Wear is not confined to occlusal surfaces. Because teeth are capable of some degree of independent movement, during mastication there is slight rubbing together of the approximal contact surfaces, which produces facets of wear. The amount of approximal wear is always proportional to that of the occlusal surfaces and in due course can lead to a considerable reduction in the mesiodistal dimensions of the teeth. A reduction in this dimension also occurs because the teeth taper from the approximal contact points to the cervix so that, once occlusal wear passes beyond the level of the contact points, the crown becomes narrower and there is a reduction in the size of the occlusal surface. This is particularly marked in the case of the incisors.

Under normal circumstances, mesial movement of the teeth in their sockets maintains the teeth in approximal contact. Approximal attrition can reduce the length of each dental arcade by as much as 8–10 mm.

Other surfaces of the teeth, besides the occlusal and approximal, also suffer some loss of substance as a result of wear which is contributed to by the use of the toothbrush, so that the tooth surface becomes more smooth and polished with advancing age. Furthermore, in people who consume large quantities of fruit or fruit juices or other acid drinks, loss of tooth substance may be considerable through chemical erosion.

Needless to say, wear of the occlusal surfaces of the extent described tends to produce occlusal surfaces which fit together more closely than is the case in the unworn dentition. The occlusal surfaces are not truly flat because, as dentine is softer than enamel and therefore wears away at a greater rate, the occlusal surfaces tend to be cupped out with a raised, often sharp rim of more or less unsupported enamel.

Although severe degrees of attrition can be harmful, it can be argued that moderate wear of tooth cusps is beneficial, allowing freedom of mandibular excursion during function and reducing lateral stresses on the teeth; such stress may be particularly damaging where there is lengthening of the clinical crowns as a result of gingival recession. On this basis, there are those who advocate the artificial simulation of tooth wear by cusp grinding. In order to apply this prophylactic measure with proper discrimination, it is necessary to be familiar with the normal pattern of natural wear.

A question that arises in connection with tooth wear is whether, as occlusal tooth substance is lost, the inter-jaw relationship is substantially altered. The rest position of the mandible in general tends to remain constant so that, when the occlusal surfaces become much worn, the freeway space would be expected to increase. There is, however, a good deal of evidence that, as a compensation for occlusal wear there is axial movement of the teeth by appositional growth of bone on the alveolar surfaces, active eruption in fact, though it is probable that in some cases this compensatory mechanism is imperfect. The evidence rests upon cross-sectional studies involving measurements of facial height in skulls showing degrees of tooth attrition. Longitudinal studies of living subjects would be more convincing but obviously difficult to carry out, especially over the periods of 30 years or so that would be needed.

Age Changes in Enamel

Apart from loss of substance due to wear, enamel undergoes intrinsic change after eruption. The colour of the teeth becomes darker with age. It is said that this is due mainly to a deepening of the colour of the dentine which shows through the slightly translucent enamel but it is possible that enamel itself either becomes darker with age or more translucent.

Even in freshly erupted teeth, a layer about 0·1 mm. thick at the outer surface has characteristics slightly different from the rest of the enamel. The surface enamel is slightly harder and often lacks prism structure. As age advances, however, the differences in composition between the surface and the rest of the enamel increases and the width of a surface zone with special characteristics gradually increases. This is well demonstrated by the etch characteristics of the surface zone in ground sections of various ages (fig. 3).

Studies of the permeability of enamel to water, dyes, inorganic salts and organic substances, sometimes isotope-labelled, show that the enamel in a young tooth behaves as a semi-permeable membrane; that is, it permits the slow passage of water and dissolved substances of relatively small molecular size but does not permit the passage of large molecules. From this it may be deduced that enamel contains a system of minute spaces or pores smaller than large molecules (see Chapter 32). The most striking demonstration of enamel permeability is contained in the work of Bergman who noted that, if enamel of a freshly extracted tooth is dried and then covered by a thin film of oil, within 2 or 3 hr. 2–4 μm. droplets of fluid exude from the enamel surface and accumulate under the oil (fig. 4). These experiments would appear to be repeatable *in vivo*.

The permeability of enamel decreases with advancing age in association with changes in the composition of the enamel. There is now a good deal of evidence of a qualitative difference in composition of the outer layer of enamel which is acquired or increased after eruption of the tooth. There is, for example, a progressive increase with age in the fluoride content of enamel, reaching a peak at about 30 years. However, this peak does not represent the saturation point of enamel for fluoride because, in areas of high fluoride in the water supply, the fluoride content of enamel continues to increase after 30 years. Many other ions, tin, copper, iron and lead appear or increase in amount after eruption, tin, unlike the others, being related to the presence of amalgam fillings.

The use in recent years of micro-analysis of minute samples from selected areas of the enamel surface *in vivo* has greatly added to knowledge of the changes that occur in the surface of enamel, and it is certain that many substances are taken up from the fluids of the oral environment, including saliva.

Some analyses suggest a steady increase in nitrogen in enamel, particularly in the enamel of white and brown

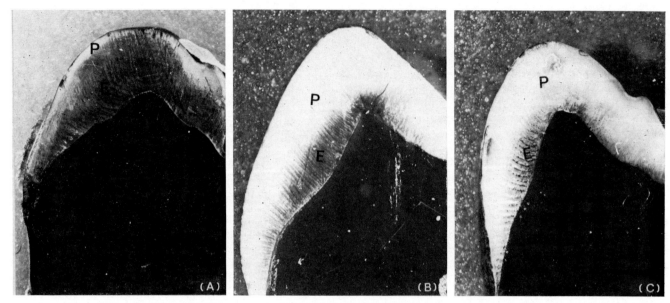

FIG. 3. Ground surfaces of human teeth of various ages after exposure of the surfaces to acid for a standard time and then stained with Alizarin red: A. 11-year-old subject. The whole thickness of the enamel, *e*, has been etched apart from a narrow acid-resistant zone, *p*, at the enamel surface which has remained smooth and unstained, and therefore white in the photograph. B. 35-year-old subject. The acid-resistant zone, *p*, is wider. C. 58-year-old subject. The acid-resistant zone is wider still. (Reproduced from Yonan and Fosdick, 1963.)

spots found approximally. These areas of altered enamel are common in elderly people and are indicative of arrested enamel caries. As the proportion of pores in early enamel caries may increase by as much as 40 times, it is easy to envisage a process by which these pores could be entered by organic matter from the oral environment. Until such organic matter can be characterized, it is impossible to be sure whether it is derived from salivary protein, food, or products of bacterial plaque on the enamel surface, or from a combination of these.

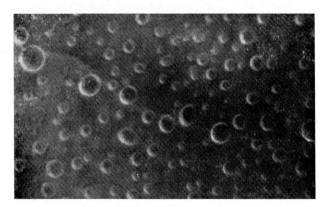

FIG. 4. Drops of enamel fluid, 4–8 μm. in diameter, which have emerged from the surface of the enamel of a human tooth 12 hr. after extraction. The cleaned and dried tooth surface was covered with oil to prevent evaporation of the fluid. (Reproduced from Bergman, 1963.)

There is an interesting hypothesis that the special characteristics of the enamel surfaces of erupted teeth are brought about by the cumulative effect of intermittent compression stresses during chewing, a change similar to the work-hardening of metals and other inanimate substances. Alterations in the properties of matter resulting from

increases in pressure, and the observation that the uptake by the enamel of rhesus monkeys of intraperitoneally injected ^{32}P is greater in functional teeth than in those rendered non-functional, form a basis for the theory that temporary compression of enamel during mastication could produce changes in the nature and velocity of biochemical processes occurring within its substance or on its surface.

In ultra-violet light, the crowns of human teeth fluoresce with a bluish-white light. The character of this fluorescence is said to change in advanced age. This needs to be explored further but it seems likely that absorption of organic matter by white and brown spot enamel would be associated with changes in fluorescence.

THE PULP-DENTINE COMPLEX IN MATURITY AND SENESCENCE

The dental pulp bears the same relation to dentine as bone marrow to the calcified matrix of bone. In terms of function, pulp and dentine should be regarded as a single tissue, the pulp-dentine complex. Nevertheless in what follows it is inevitable that pulp and dentine are to some extent treated separately.

The pulp continues to lay down dentine slowly throughout life so that as age advances the volume it occupies diminishes and, in advanced age, it may be reduced to a slender thread of tissue in the root extending only a short distance into the crown beyond the cervix. On completion of the apex, the opening at the base of the tooth remains as a narrow canal or system of canals which in time become more narrow and attenuated, partly by the continued deposition of dentine and partly by the growth of cementum. These changes in the size and morphology of the pulp are associated with changes in its structure and composition.

Deposition of dentine proceeds more or less evenly over the whole of the pulp surface but in molars and premolars rather more dentine is deposited on the floor and roof of the pulp chamber then elsewhere. Sometimes the dentine formed during the early years, approximately up to the time of eruption of the tooth, is demarcated from the latter formed dentine by a darkly staining line in which the dentinal tubules may abruptly change direction (figs. 5 and 6). More often the junction is much less distinct but the dentine formed after the tooth has become functional roughly corresponds with the change in direction of the tubules to form the final portion of the open S-shaped curves. The dentine on the outer side of such a line of demarcation is known as primary dentine and that on the pulpal side as secondary dentine, or, in order to distinguish this type of dentine from that which is formed as a reaction to injury, as physiological secondary dentine.

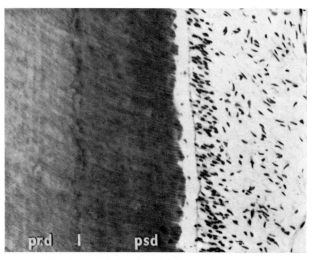

FIG. 6. Pulp–dentine border in the crown of tooth of a 20-year-old subject. Stained haematoxylin and eosin. ×96. pr.d = primary dentine; l = line of arrest; psd = physiological secondary dentine.

cell inclusions and is often poorly calcified (fig. 7). Not uncommonly the dentine formed as a reaction to injury is entirely without tubules and no recognizable odontoblasts are then found on the pulp surface.

Enclosed as it is within an unyielding chamber and having only slender communication with the rest of the body via narrow apical foramina, the pulp is in a situation unmatched by that of any other tissue of the body. The

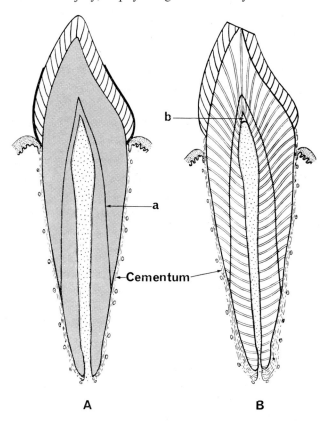

FIG. 5. A. Young tooth. a indicates a line of junction sometimes seen between dentine formed before the completion of eruption (primary dentine) and that formed after eruption (physiological secondary dentine). B. Tooth in advanced age. Reactionary dentine at b has formed in response to wear, the gingival margin has receded, the cementum is thickened and the pulp cavity is reduced in size. (Reproduced from Miles, 1962.)

As a result of irritation to the peripheral dentine by attrition, caries, or other gradual loss of surface substance, the rate of formation of dentine by the pulp cells in relationship to the irritated tubules is accelerated. Dentine formed under these conditions is known as reactionary dentine or reactionary secondary dentine and usually contains fewer tubules than primary dentine owing to death of odontoblasts from the injury. Reactionary dentine may contain

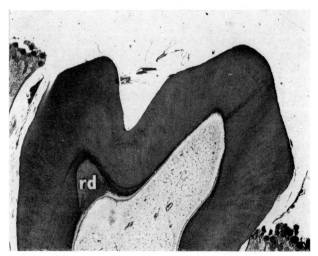

FIG. 7. "Reactionary dentine" (rd) in tooth from ovarian cyst, unassociated of course with any peripheral lesion of dentine. Stained haematoxylin and eosin. ×9.

influence of these unique circumstances on the hydrodynamic and hæmodynamic aspects of the physiology of the pulp has not been fully explored but, because the volume of the whole pulp cannot be increased, a critical balance must exist between the entry and exit of fluids and the intercellular pressures in the pulp. There must be a reciprocal relationship between the volume of circulating blood and that of the other fluid constituents, inter- and intra-cellular, of the pulp. It is well-known that a pulp which becomes acutely inflamed is liable to become necrotic. This is probably because of obstruction to the blood flow by increased pressure of intercellular fluid or inflammatory exudate rather than by dilatation of the arterioles and capillaries of the pulp.

tissue pressure directly, and for deducing the capillary blood pressure, in both laboratory animals and human subjects. However, these have yet to be applied to teeth in disease and advanced age.

Sectioned material shows that, in the young pulp, even the main arterioles have thin walls, the endothelium abutting directly on a thin membrane of elastin; the media consists of a few smooth muscle cells and a few elastic fibres and the adventitia is composed of a slight condensation of the mainly precollagen network of the

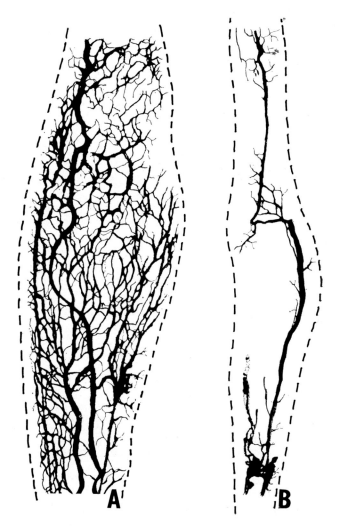

FIG. 8. Vascular architecture of the pulp injected with Indian ink. The dotted lines indicate the approximate position of the dentine surface. A. Mandibular incisor of a 30-year-old subject. The primary vessels are centrally located and there is a system of peripheral arcades related to the odontoblasts. This system is not as rich as in a younger tooth. B. Mandibular incisor of a 61-year-old subject. The vascular architecture is greatly reduced and peripheral arcades are almost totally absent. (From Bennett, Kelln and Biddington, 1965.)

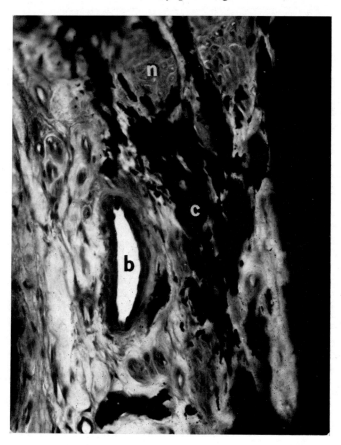

FIG. 9. Transverse section through the pulp in the apical region of a canine tooth of a 40-year-old subject. b is a blood vessel; c indicates areas of calcification. Calcification has encircled a small nerve fasciculus at n. Verhoeff's iron haematoxylin stain. × 150. (Reproduced from Bernick, 1967.)

Vascular Supply

The young pulp has a complex vascular architecture with terminal capillary loops beneath, and to some extent among, the odontoblasts (see Chapter 28). As age advances there is a considerable reduction in the size and complexity of this vascular pattern which appears to be greater than is commensurate with the reduction in its size. There is in particular a considerable loss of the peripheral odontoblastic capillary plexus which must be indicative of a reduction in odontoblast activity, real and potential (fig. 8).

Methods are available for measuring *in vivo* the pulp

body of the pulp with, in addition, a few collagen fibres. In the young coronal pulp, the walls even of the largest vessels, arterioles and venules, resemble those of capillaries, consisting of an endothelial lining with some supporting fibrous tissue and no very evident media or adventitia.

In older pulps, the arterioles in the radicular pulp show various changes; these include thickening of the endothelial intima with an increase of PAS-positive material and hyperplasia of the elastic layers. Calcification in the walls of the radicular arterioles and less commonly in the coronal pulp becomes common, apparently commencing in the adventitia and gradually extending to the media and intima (fig. 9). These changes, with the possible exception of calcification, are those of arterio-sclerosis or, to use a term many regard as more precise, degenerative hyperplastic sclerosis. Although these changes appear to be related to advancing age, they, or vascular changes indistinguishable from them, have a close relationship with hypertensive cardio-vascular disorders, the prevalence of which is certainly greater in the aged than in the young though its cause is multifactorial. Hence, it cannot be taken for granted that degenerative changes of this sort found in the vessels of the pulp are age or senile changes.

The vascular changes described in the pulp lead to reduction in the bore of vessels supplying the pulp and hence, if not producing actual ischaemia, render the pulp less able to become active, for instance, to produce reparative dentine in response to some stimulus.

Before considering some of the finer detail of the structure of the pulp, reference must be made to the difficulty of securing adequate fixation of the tissue. Unless fixative solution reaches a tissue quickly, for fine detail even within minutes, various artefacts appear, due mainly to the release of lytic enzymes by the cells following their death (autolysis). The enclavement of the pulp within virtually impermeable dentine walls with access solely via the apical canals means that adequate fixation cannot be achieved by simply dropping the tooth into fixative solution. It is necessary to divide the root transversely with wire cutters or an abrasive rotating disc so that the fixative can penetrate the pulp from three directions, apical canals and two cut surfaces. The nearer the cervix the level of division the better. Alternatively, or in addition, the tooth can be ground under plenty of cooling water until the greater part of the pulp can be seen through a thin layer of dentine. Naturally, precautions of this sort are taken in most instances of pulp research.

Odontoblasts

Odontoblasts in the mature pulp are very different from the columnar cells with plenty of basophilic cytoplasm characteristic of recently differentiated odontoblasts. As the surface area of the pulp diminishes, the odontoblasts become crowded together as a layer two to four or even more cells thick (fig. 6). The cell outlines of mature odontoblasts are very difficult to discern and they have relatively little cytoplasm which is neither granular nor basophilic.

In adult pulps, the nuclei of the odontoblasts are in a state of relative inactivity, and are typically homogeneously staining so that no chromatin network and only an occasional nucleolus can be distinguished. There is some evidence that odontoblasts revert to a condition resembling that of more youthful odontoblasts if they resume activity, as in the formation of reactionary dentine.

Odontoblasts are highly specialized, long-lived cells and do not under normal circumstances reproduce themselves; that is they are, like nerve cells, long-lived fixed post-mitotic cells. Mitotic figures among odontoblasts and adjacent pulp cells have, however, been described in scorbutic guinea pigs. There is furthermore other evidence suggesting that odontoblasts may differentiate from some

other cell type in the pulp. Following the surgical removal of a part of the pulp, the dentine laid down on the raw surface may sometimes contain tubules associated with cells on the pulp surface having the morphology of odontoblasts. These could be odontoblasts that survived the operative procedure, they could be derived from adjacent odontoblasts by mitosis or migration, and it has been suggested that they might be odontoblasts that have re-emerged after being displaced into the substance of the pulp by the original trauma. Alternatively the possibility has to be considered that they have differentiated from some primitive cell-type in the pulp. The last possibility would seem unlikely in view of evidence that the organizing influence of ectoderm is required for the differentiation of odontoblasts.

The sensitivity of the pulp and dentine appears to diminish in advanced age and there is a great deal of evidence to explain this. Nevertheless it has been claimed that the response of tooth crowns of elderly persons to electrical stimulation is about the same as that in younger adults. However, this can be explained by the fact that the electrical conductivity of dentine is unaffected by whether it is living or dead-tract dentine or has undergone sclerosis. This probably applies to thermal conduction also so that, providing the tooth contains some pulp capable of responding to gross thermal change, response of an aged tooth to the crude clinical stimulus of hot and cold may be similar to that of a young tooth although presumably where the tooth contained an aged retreated pulp there would be some delay in the response.

As far as dentine is concerned, reduction of its sensitivity could be explained on the basis of conversion of the greater part of the coronal dentine to sclerosed or to dead-tract dentine (p. 372). However, it has been shown that, as age advances, there is a reduction in the nerve supply distributed to the coronal pulp and this is associated with the involvement of the main nerve bundles by calcific changes in the apical part of the radicular pulp (fig. 9).

In the young pulp, the connective tissue that supports the blood vessels is insubstantial and consists of relatively few stellate fibroblasts in a matrix containing delicate reticulin fibres. The young pulp contains little mature collagen. In adult pulps, and even more so in those from old people, it is common to find appreciable amounts of mature collagen with a proportionate reduction in the number of cells and amount of ground substance. There is little doubt that the tendency for the pulp to undergo fibrosis as age advances is independent of the cumulative effects on the pulp of injuries to the dentine; for example, fibrosed pulps are common in teeth that have remained buried and uninfected in the jaws for many years. It is of interest that the collagen and ground substance in the aged pulp show increased resistance to proteolytic digestion and in general their chemical reactivity is reduced. These changes are characteristic of collagen in old age and are attributable to an increase in cross-linking between its long-chained molecules. It has been suggested that changes of this sort affecting many protein and other complex molecules throughout the body are, if not the ultimate cause of senescence, one of the main mechanisms involved.

It is possible that progressive fibrosis of the pulp is secondary to disturbance of its blood supply by the gradual narrowing of the apical canals resulting from continuous additions to the thickness of cementum on the root surface. It has been suggested also that, in the case of erupted teeth, the intermittent pressure exerted on the tooth apex during mastication could produce interruptions of the vascular supply and lymphatic drainage of the pulp and thereby induce fibrous and other changes in the pulp.

The progressive decrease in volume of the pulp with advancing age, which is greater than the reduction of its surface area, is not associated with an increase in its cellularity, but rather the reverse, so there must be a progressive loss of cells from the central part of the pulp. Similarly the apparent increase in fibrous elements that occurs as age advances need not necessarily be the result of the formation of additional fibres, but could simply reflect the persistence of the fibrous elements of an originally larger pulp. However, the frequent localization of fibrosis in the aged pulp in relation to blood vessels, and the fact that the fibres are collagen and not reticulin as in the young pulp, suggest that the changes are more complex than this.

The difficulty of interpreting fibrosis in the pulp, and elsewhere, is enhanced by the findings that if the pulps of dogs were treated *in vivo* with saline before fixation, there was an increase in the amount of perivascular collagen in the stained sections; it has been suggested that saline aggregates tropocollagen, the precursor of collagen, into collagen. If saline does this, it would seem likely that fixative solutions can similarly produce collagen *in vitro*.

It is extremely common to find intra- and inter-cellular vacuolation in the odontoblast layer and less frequently elsewhere in sections of pulp, even when a special effort has been made to secure good fixation. In young teeth with open or incomplete roots, vacuolation among the odontoblasts and a disorderly arrangement of the cells is relatively uncommon, whereas, in teeth with closed apices, some vacuolation of the cytoplasm, nuclear vacuoles, and intercellular spaces distorting the cells, are almost invariably present. There appear to be three chief possible explanations of the difference. Firstly, in the case of teeth with closed apices, in spite of cutting off the apex or making an opening into the pulp, fixing reagents may be unable to reach the more inaccessible parts of the pulp quickly enough to prevent post-mortem changes. This would apply particularly to older pulps. Other technical considerations such as shrinkage of pulp tissue fixed to walls of more rigid dentine may play a part. Secondly, in a critical evaluation of pulp changes, the possibility has to be taken into account of movements of the tooth during extraction, or even grasping it in forceps, so interfering with the circulatory systems in the pulp as to produce accumulations of intercellular fluid; for example, the nuclei of odontoblasts are sometimes found in the dentinal tubules of extracted teeth, having been driven or sucked up by pressure changes in the pulp set up by rocking the tooth in its socket during extraction.

The pulp in a tooth with a narrow apical foramen would seem to be more liable to suffer from pressure changes set up by the rocking motion involved in tooth extraction than one with a wide apical opening. Local anaesthesia employed in tooth extraction can produce oedematous changes in the pulp. Thirdly, the completion of the root apex may perhaps lead to some change, not necessarily abrupt, in the structure of the pulp by reducing a relatively free blood supply to one in which the pulp is more confined and is supplied by vessels which reach it via one or more narrow canals. The term end-organ can be more appropriately applied to the adult pulp than to any other organ or tissue in the body.

Reticular Atrophy

A degenerative condition of the pulp known as reticular atrophy is common in the pulps of teeth with complete apices. It is most common in the coronal portion of the pulp where it may be met with not uncommonly in the

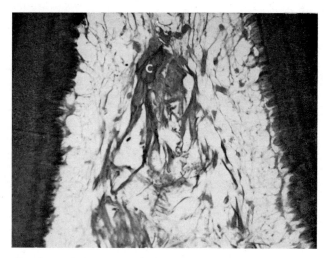

Fig. 10. Reticular atrophy of pulp of incisor of a 45-year-old subject. *c* indicates collagen bundles. Stained van Gieson. ×54. (Reproduced from Miles, 1962.)

intact teeth of young persons. As a more widespread apparent degeneration of the pulp, its incidence increases with age. The earliest sign of reticular atrophy is the presence of fine droplets of fat in the odontoblasts, in the nuclei of the fibroblasts of the pulp, and in the walls of capillaries. Accumulations of intercellular fluid forming large vacuoles appear at intervals between the odontoblasts pushing them aside so that they come to be arranged in bundles—the so-called wheatsheaf appearance of odontoblasts. Spherical spaces or vacuoles appear between the pulp cells and the total number of cells in the pulp is reduced (fig. 10). Blood vessels and nerve bundles become reduced in size and number. In the fully developed condition of reticular atrophy, the whole pulp consists of a system of large vacuoles in a reticulum of collagen fibres with few pulp cells. Typical columnar odontoblasts are entirely absent but there may be a few flattened cells, which are presumably altered odontoblasts, on the surface of the pulp. The pulpal surface of the dentine is irregular and a zone of predentine may be absent. Occasionally the pulp may contain cystic spaces which appear to be formed by the confluence of vacuoles.

The changes of reticular atrophy are closely simulated by post-mortem change due to delay in fixation. While it is not intended to suggest that reticular atrophy is not a real entity, it must be pointed out that the most widely quoted works on this subject were done before it was fully realized how difficult it is to secure adequate fixation of the pulp. At least in the advanced forms of true reticular

Calcific Degeneration

Calcification in the pulp, either of diffuse character or consisting of discrete nodules, is common in pulps of all ages (fig. 11A). Whereas traces only may be found in the young, 90 per cent of pulps from subjects over 50 years may be affected and to a more severe degree than in young subjects. Although caries and other dentine injuries undoubtedly increase the incidence, calcification can certainly be induced by other factors.

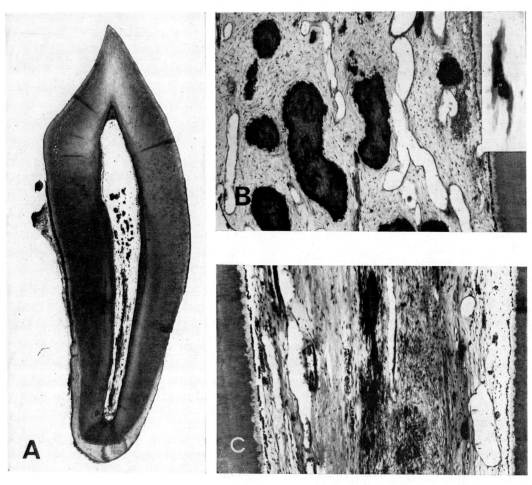

FIG. 11. A. Longitudinal section of pulp of male aged 41 years. Stained haematoxylin and eosin. ×4. B. Strongly periodic-acid-Schiff-positive borders to the pulp nodules. ×48. C. Diffuse calcification in root portion. The dust-like particles are stained deeply with Weigert's iron haematoxylin. ×60. Inset: Calcified particle in diffuse calcification. The tissue has not been demineralized and there is a positive von Kossa reaction for calcium at the centre of the particle. ×1,020. (From Miles, 1962.)

atrophy where there has been a progressive disturbance of pulp function over a long period of time, it is reasonable to expect to find some disturbance of the predentine zone, either complete absence of predentine or a zone of irregular width. Apparent reticular atrophy with vacuolation in the substance of the pulp and "wheatsheafing" of odontoblasts associated with a normal predentine zone, such as is commonly found in a random selection of sections of pulps where there have been no special precautions to secure good fixation, is probably the result of poor fixation.

Pulp nodules or stones are relatively large discrete masses of calcified tissue commonly found in the coronal part of the pulp and more rarely in the root portion. Typically they are of rounded outline with a concentrically laminated structure and large examples which may almost entirely replace the coronal pulp usually consist of a conglomeration of smaller laminated nodules. Pulp stones, especially at the periphery and the lines between the laminations give a more intense periodic acid-Schiff reaction than primary dentine (fig. 11B). Sometimes small central deeply staining bodies, perhaps the remains of dead cells, can be identified at the centres of the laminations.

In diffuse calcification, which is usually found only in the root portion of the pulp, the pulp is "dusty" with small calcified particles among which are larger masses, usually elongated in the long axis of the pulp and evidently formed by aggregation of the smaller particles (fig. 11C). The tissue in which diffuse calcification occurs often appears to have undergone previous fibrous change and as a rule the changes are confined to the central areas of the pulp, the peripheral zone related to the odontoblasts being free of the dustlike calcified particles. Diffuse calcification sometimes appears to be related to blood vessels, sometimes taking the form of calcification in the vessel wall with almost complete obliteration of the lumen. As has already been mentioned, calcification may affect the sheaths of nerve bundles.

Both types of calcification, which are possibly no more than morphological variants resulting from essentially similar processes, consist of calcified organic or fibrous matrix. Usually the matrix of pulp nodules is collagen although the peripheral layers may consist of reticulin fibres. The staining properties of the material formed in the pulp in diffuse calcification suggest that it consists of a concentration of cement substance, possibly in relation to a matrix of reticulin fibres, in which mineral salts are deposited; for instance, it gives a strong periodic acid-Schiff reaction, is metachromatic with thionin, and in undecalcified sections gives a strong von Kossa reaction. Particles of strongly periodic acid-Schiff positive material may be found with von Kossa positive material at the centre (fig. 11 inset). It seems probable that, as in the case of bone, dentine and cementum formation, there is an organic phase consisting of reticulin fibres in a matrix of metachromatic ground substance which precedes the phase of calcification.

Age Changes in Dentine

Quantitative X-ray absorption studies of sections, specific gravity measurements and chemical analysis suggest that the density or mineralization of dentine of both crown and root increases with age. Furthermore, there is some evidence that hardness of dentine increases and its crushing strength or brittleness decreases with age. The staining character of dentine changes with age in a way that suggests changes in its mucopolysaccharide ground substance.

In young teeth, the dentinal tubules in predentine have no peritubular zone but, especially in sections through the tubules at some distance from the pulp, the tubules have a lining of peritubular dentine and the diameter of the odontoblast process is proportionally decreased. These changes within the tubules accord well with, and account for, the changes in chemical composition and physical properties already referred to.

In teeth in advanced age it is a common observation that much of the dentine of the crown and of the apical region of the root has undergone change in its optical properties. In the root dentine, these changes are relatively uncomplicated and are dealt with under the heading translucent root tip dentine. In the crown the changes are more complex and, although translucency may be the predominant change, zones of apparent increased opacity or of dead-tract dentine also occur. Questions of semantics also arise because such terms as metamorphosed dentine have been used without precise definition.

In addition to the formation of reactionary dentine, various forms of peripheral irritation to the pulp-dentine complex give rise to two kinds of change in dentine already formed. These two types of change or reaction are translucency or sclerosis of dentine and dead-tract reaction.

Translucency or Sclerosis of Dentine

Beneath slowly destructive lesions of dentine, such as attrition or the more chronic type of caries where the peripheral stimulus is mild, there is frequently a zone of dentine which in ground sections is particularly translucent when viewed in transmitted light but which may be darker than normal in reflected light. The impermeability of this dentine to dyes, the constancy of its optical properties when immersed in fluids of various refractive indices, its X-ray opacity and increased hardness, all indicate hyper-mineralization and justify the term sclerosis.

In considering the significance of translucency of dentine, it is necessary to bear in mind that when a ground section of dentine is thoroughly dehydrated and mounted in Canada balsam the whole section becomes translucent and it is difficult to discern any structures at all. This is because the balsam, which has a refractive index similar to that of the calcified matrix of the dentine, has penetrated and filled the tubular system. The older dental literature abounds with reference to "translucency" and "opacity" of dentine with no record of the thickness of sections or of the medium in which they were mounted.

In translucent sclerotic dentine, the odontoblast processes have been replaced by peritubular dentine. As the peritubular dentine occluding the tubule has about the same refractive index as the intertubular dentine, transmitted light is not refracted or reflected at the interface and thus the translucency of the dentine is increased and the occluded tubules are difficult to discern in ground sections.

Dead-tract or Metamorphosed Dentine

This type of reaction appears to result from irritation of greater severity. The odontoblast process in the whole length of the injured tubule degenerates and at the same time is sealed off at the pulpal end by a deposit of reactionary dentine.

The dentine of dead tracts is more opaque than normal to transmitted light because the "empty" tubules often contain bubbles of gas or air. The tracts of changed dentine are bordered by narrow bands of translucent or sclerosed dentine so that the dead tract is walled off by an impermeable layer. Once such tracts are opened into, however, the tubular system is freely permeable to dyes.

Fat has been demonstrated in the tubules of dead-tract dentine but it is uncertain whether this is derived from the degeneration of the original odontoblast process or is a fatty substance that has entered the tubules from the mouth.

It is probable that dead-tract dentine as originally described by Fish corresponds to the "opaque sclerosed dentine" and "metamorphosed dentine" of other writers. Chemical analyses of opaque dead-tract dentine have shown less organic matter and a lower percentage of calcium and phosphorus than normal dentine from the same teeth. The lowered percentage of organic matter would be consistent with loss of the protoplasmic odontoblast processes from the tubules. It could be that the difference in mineral content is due to a change in the adjacent living dentine rather than in the dead-tract dentine; while the latter remains unchanged, living dentine undergoes a slight natural increase in mineralization with age as a result of increase in the width of the peritubular zones.

Dead-tract dentine, in accord with the view that it results simply from relatively abrupt death of the odontoblast processes within the tubules, would not be expected to show any change in X-ray absorption. It has, however, been recorded that light-opaque "attrition cones", which appear to correspond with dead tracts beneath attrition, show slightly increased radiopacity. A narrow dead tract is in fact a solid inverted conical structure composed of diverging tubules with its apex towards the pulp. The radiopacity could perhaps be explained by the fact that, as has been mentioned, such cones of dead-tract dentine have a peripheral layer of sclerotic dentine.

As age advances, there is a tendency for more and more of the coronal dentine to be translucent, often in patches but sometimes diffusely. Areas of dead-tract dentine occur also. Much of this change is due to the accumulation of episodes of response to peripheral irritation. For instance, many of the patches of translucent dentine can be ascribed to identifiable peripheral lesions, such as tooth wear or dental caries. In other instances, there may be no evidence of peripheral lesions. Nevertheless, even in such cases the translucency could be due to some environmental cause; for instance, the crowns of the teeth during mastication are exposed to mechanical stresses and to considerable changes of temperature.

Authentic instances have been described of dead tracts and "reactionary" dentine (fig. 7) in unerupted teeth and in teeth which though erupted have never been in occlusion or subjected to wear.

The fluoride content of dentine, from districts with either high or low fluoride in the water supply, increases progressively with age, reaching peaks by about 55 years at a level is much higher in the high fluoride districts. It appears that at about 55 years of age a state of equilibrium is reached in the dentine, perhaps because by that age permeability is reduced by peritubular dentine formation and therefore the F ions are less likely to reach the substance of the dentine from the vascular system in the pulp.

Translucent Root Tip Dentine

If a tooth from a subject of middle or advanced age is held to the light, the apical portion is usually seen to be translucent. The root tip translucency is also evident in ground sections (fig. 12). Occasionally root tip translucency may affect more than half of the root. This change (fig. 13) is more closely correlated with age than any of the other features that are used in the Gustafson (1966)

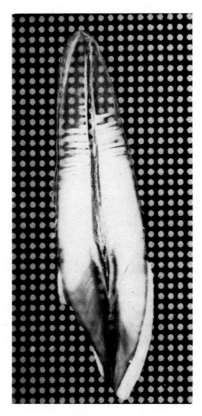

Fig. 12. Longitudinal ground section of upper incisor of man aged 52 years. (From Miles, 1963.)

method of age assessment for forensic purposes, namely attrition, size of pulp, thickness of cementum, areas of resorption on the root surface and distance of the gingival attachment from the cervix.

Root apices affected by translucency are usually brittle and liable to break off during tooth extraction. The affected dentine is impermeable to dyes and in fact exhibits the features of sclerotic coronal dentine mentioned earlier. Chemical analysis has not produced clearcut evidence of hypermineralization but this may be due to the fact that the dentine of the root in a young tooth is slightly less mineralized than that of the crown so that chemical analyses of root dentine are not likely to be helpful unless compared with unaffected dentine from the same tooth.

Where the apical dentine is completely translucent, no predentine layer is found; in its place there is usually an irregular zone of haematoxyphilia at the pulp surface of the dentine. Furthermore odontoblasts are absent. Hence, it seems that the changes of translucency in apical dentine are associated with the ultimate disappearance of the odontoblasts (fig. 14).

The only explanation of the cause of this condition, apart from the suggestion that it is an age change independent of environmental influences, is that it is related to periodontal disease and is due to the reaction of odontoblasts to bacterial toxins derived from the gingival

peripheral ends of the tubules were obliterated, toxins could not penetrate further.

AGE CHANGES IN CEMENTUM

Cementum is deposited intermittently throughout life and its deposition in later life is probably to a large extent in response to stresses to which the tooth is subjected; for instance, the continuous deposition of cemen-

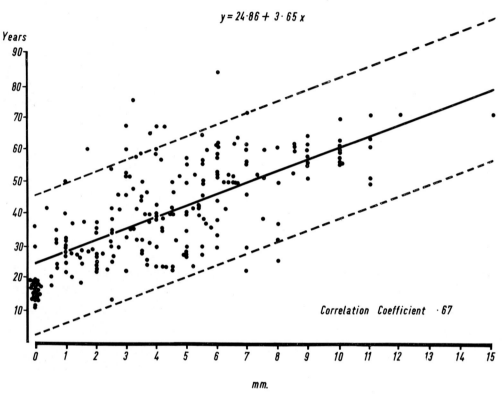

FIG. 13. The relation of age to length of translucent root in longitudinal sections of 454 incisor teeth: ———(solid line) calculated regression line. – – – –(broken line) 95 per cent confidence limits.

margin. As slowly progressive periodontal disease in some degree is almost universal, starting in young adult life, this would explain the correlation of apical translucency with age. It might be supposed that toxins reach the apical pulp as a result of the pumping action of tooth movement during mastication. Occasional pumping action of greater force could carry toxins further into the pulp and these would tend to produce a gradually extending effect because, like all random events, they would tend to accumulate with time.

It is necessary to postulate some fairly direct action on the bodies of the odontoblasts rather than something acting at the peripheral ends of the tubules, for two reasons; firstly, because dyestuffs and bacterial toxins cannot penetrate the root surface except in the apical region itself; secondly, because if anything did act at the periphery to produce obliteration of the tubular system in the dentine, it would be self-limiting, *i.e.* once the extreme

tum provides a means for the attachment to the root surface of new suspensory fibres of the periodontal ligament. Formation of cementum is also much influenced by disease; for instance in periodontal disease the cementum over the whole of the root surface tends to be unusually thick. Similarly, following infection and death of the pulp, thickening of the apical cementum commonly occurs. The intermittent character of cementum formation is manifested by a pattern of irregularly spaced incremental lines and, as a record of changes in the direction of the stresses to which teeth have been subjected during successive periods of formation, Sharpey's fibres often change direction in successive layers.

The deposition of cementum is by no means completely dependent upon the stimulus of functional stress and relatively thick layers of cementum are found on the roots of unerupted teeth in aged persons. There is certainly a loose correlation between the thickness of cementum and age; cementum thickness therefore forms one of the criteria on which Gustafson (1966) bases his method of age assessment.

When deposition is active, a zone of uncalcified matrix, comparable to an osteoid seam, is found on the surface and cells resembling osteoblasts may be identified between the fibres of the periodontal ligament around which the

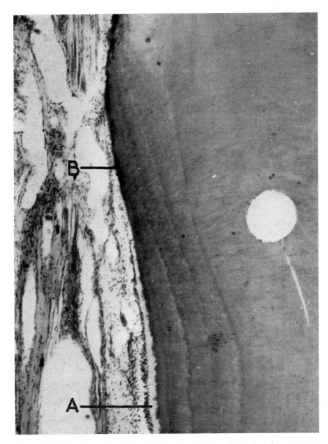

FIG. 14. Demineralized longitudinal section of tooth of a woman aged 42, of which the apical 4·2 mm. were translucent. A marker hole is situated at the junction of translucent (above) and non-translucent dentine (below). There is a predentine zone associated with odontoblasts at A but, at the level of the marker hole, the odontoblasts have disappeared and the predentine zone narrows. At B there is a zone of haematoxyphilia which becomes more pronounced apically. Haematoxylin and eosin. ×10, 6.

cementum is formed. Over the greater part of the root, cementum contains no cells or lacunae (acellular cementum) but, where the cementum is normally thicker than elsewhere, namely at the root apex and in the root bifurcations of multirooted teeth, it contains cells in lacunae similar to those of bone, though distributed in a less orderly pattern.

When cellular cementum is thick, living cells may be found only in the lacunae of the surface layers, those of the deeper layers being empty or containing pyknotic nuclei. It is evident that the pathway whereby nutritive substances reach the cells is a tenuous one and when cementum becomes thick the cells furthest away from the source of nourishment die.

Experiments on monkeys and dogs have shown that, although in young animals dyes may pass slowly *in vivo* from the dentine into the cementum, in adult animals the cementum-dentine junction is resistant to the passage of dyes. There might nevertheless be free passage of small molecules like those of water and inorganic salts. The site of the impermeable barrier appears to be between the granular zone of Tomes and the cementum.

In human teeth it has been shown that, at least in adult teeth *in vitro*, penicillin inserted in pulp cavities does not penetrate to the root surface. The commonplace clinical observation that, when pulp cavities become the site of profuse growth of pathogenic bacteria, inflammatory changes in the periodontal membrane are as a rule confined to the region of the apical canals, serves to strengthen the evidence that a relatively impermeable barrier between dentine and cementum exists in human teeth.

The number of areas of active and past resorption of the roots of teeth is correlated with advancing age. Local injuries or mechanical stresses are the most likely cause of the resorption which, in most cases, is repaired by the deposition of new cementum. Since root resorption leaves, in the outline of Howship's lacunae, a record of even greater permanency than similar records in bone, it is to be expected that records of resorption from past injuries would accumulate with age and there seems to be no reason to believe that the susceptibility of roots to undergo resorption increases with age.

The fluoride content of cementum, like that of other mineralized tissues, increases with age, there being a particularly large increase in the acellular cementum of the cervical region, probably because this tends to be exposed to the oral environment and so directly acquires ingested F and F by topical absorption.

A comprehensive review of the literature on age changes in oral tissues, with references, is available in Miles (1962).

REFERENCES

Gustafson, G. (1966), *Forensic Odontology*. London: Staples Press.
Miles, A. E. W. (1962), "Ageing in the Teeth and Oral Tissues," in *Structural Aspects of Ageing*, pp. 355–397 (G. H. Bourne, Ed.) London: Pitman.
Quigley, M. B. (1971), "Functional and Geriatric Changes of the Human Pulp," *Oral Surg.*, **32**, 795.

30. THE EFFECTS OF TRACE ELEMENTS ON THE CALCIFIED TISSUES

G. N. JENKINS

Clinical effects of fluoride

Effects of fluoride overdosage

Mode of action of fluoride in reducing caries

Effects of fluoride on tooth morphology

Effects of fluoride on plaque and bacteria

The significance of the multiplicity of effects of fluoride

The fluoridation controversy

Alternatives to fluoridation

Trace elements other than fluoride

Trace elements and bone

INTRODUCTION

The importance of trace elements in the physiology of the dental tissues became clear about 1930 when the water-borne substance responsible for mottling of enamel, whose existence had been established some 20 years before, was identified as fluoride. When, during the following decade, the relation between fluoride and caries became established, it was realized that trace elements might be a major factor in dental health.

CLINICAL EFFECTS OF FLUORIDE

The main clinical effects of 1 p.p.m. of fluoride in water are so well-known and so widely documented that they do not require detailed discussion here. The following is a brief summary of the main findings and includes a few points which have received inadequate attention. For its full effect, of about 50 per cent reduction in DMF, fluoride must be taken during the formation of the teeth (*i.e.* up to eight years) and continued after this period and presumably for life. Experimental studies show that the placenta acts as a partial barrier to fluoride so that fetal concentrations are always low and most of the clinical data show that fluoride taken during pregnancy has a negligible effect on caries in the offspring. If children first receive fluoridated water one or two years after their deciduous teeth are already erupted they derive about one-third of the full benefit (Ministry of Health, 1962); if received within a few months of eruption the benefit is greater. Post-eruptive benefits of fluoride in drinking-water have also been reported in mature adults (U.S. servicemen). If fluoride is received before and after tooth formation the effects last into adulthood and, although no really thorough survey has been carried out in areas with 1 p.p.m., the benefits are detectable, at least with 2 p.p.m., throughout the whole life span. The occlusal surfaces are less protected than the approximal surfaces. It is not known whether this reflects the easier access of fluoride to the approximal areas than to occlusal fissures or whether this element, although the most powerful single anti-caries substance yet proven, is not powerful enough to protect areas as susceptible as the fissures of molars.

The total intake from all sources, of fluoride and other trace elements, rather than the concentration in water, probably determines the degree of systemic protection, although for some effects, *e.g.* possible interactions between water-borne fluoride and plaque or the enamel surface (whether these occur is discussed later) may be governed by the concentration. Food usually contains so little fluoride (not more than 0·5 mg. a day) that the total intake is dominated by the level in the drinking water (although in some communities the issue is complicated by the presence of on average 1 p.p.m. of fluoride in tea, even when brewed with fluoride-free water). The fluoride intake cannot be estimated from the concentration in the water unless the total fluid intake is known (usually estimated as 1·5 l., but widely variable) and the proportion taken as tea. In the absence of data on these points there seems no alternative but to refer loosely to the effects of "1 p.p.m." or of living in a "high fluoride area" when what is meant is the average total intake when the water contains 1 p.p.m. of fluoride. In experiments on rats, 5 p.p.m. of fluoride added to the food exerted a larger post-eruptive protection against caries than did 20 p.p.m. in water, but the feasibility and safety of adding fluoride to human foods has not yet been fully considered.

The effects of doses higher than that provided by about 2 p.p.m. in the water, when assimilated during enamel formation, are liable to produce dental fluorosis (a preferable term to mottled enamel) in a proportion of the teeth of some children, characterized by areas of chalky whiteness (usually bilateral) visible as the teeth erupt. In severe cases, these patches acquire a yellow or brown pigment some years after eruption owing to the increased permeability of the enamel to oral fluids arising from slight hypomineralization, believed to result, in turn, from defects of the matrix. It is not known why only some people residing in a fluoride area (2–4 p.p.m.) should be affected nor why the severity varies within a population; differences in water (and therefore fluoride) intake or in sensitivity of the ameloblasts to the fluoride ion are possible, unexplored explanations.

The measurement of very mild dental fluorosis has been confused by the discovery of a very similar condition present in the absence of fluoride in the water (idiopathic enamel opacities) and its prevalence is, curiously enough, reduced by intake of water containing 1 p.p.m. fluoride. This condition was not detected by earlier observers and the classifications of fluorosis they suggested (very mild, mild, moderate) presumably erroneously included the idiopathic opacities.

It is often assumed that 1 p.p.m. in the water provides the optimum intake for caries reduction. This is certainly not true in Britain where approximately 2 p.p.m. (the original level in Hartlepool, now reduced to 1·5 p.p.m.) was significantly more effective than 1 p.p.m. American data are somewhat ambiguous on this point. However, 1 p.p.m. is the best compromise, producing a very substantial, if suboptimal reduction in caries, virtually no dental fluorosis and a reduction of idiopathic opacities. The maximal effects of fluoridated water can be supplemented by other methods of applying fluoride in high concentrations as dentrifrices, rinses and gels (discussed by Geddes, Jenkins and Stephen, 1973).

Small reductions in the extent of malocclusion have been reported in fluoride areas probably arising from the fewer premature extractions of deciduous teeth as a result of the lower caries incidence.

EFFECTS OF FLUORIDE OVERDOSAGE

As already mentioned, the cells which seem to be most sensitive to fluoride are the ameloblasts or, at any rate, their toxic response can be observed in the form of enamel opacities—it is conceivable that other cells respond but that the result is invisible. There is no agreed explanation of their sensitivity; possibly their proximity to the high fluoride concentrations in partly mineralized enamel, or in stores of mineral, may lead to higher levels within the cell (although these circumstances would be expected to apply also to odontoblasts and osteoblasts, but no changes in dentine or bone have been found with intakes associated with enamel fluorosis).

Somewhat higher intakes lead to changes in the bone consisting of large areas of resorption accompanied, at first sight rather paradoxically, by the extensive deposition of new bone, sometimes as exostoses. The radiological appearance is of a thickening of the bone and this has given rise to the false impression that the bone is more dense than normal. The additional bone is now known to be undermineralized. A suggested explanation of these changes is that fluoride enters the bone mineral and makes it less soluble (see later) leading to a tendency for plasma calcium (partly maintained by the dissolution of bone mineral) to fall slightly. This, in turn, leads to the release of increased parathyroid hormone (PTH) which then increases bone resorption, presumably occurring mostly in areas with low fluoride concentration, and is compensated for by the formation of new bone—imperfect because the bone cells are affected by the fluoride. Some workers have reported evidence for increased PTH release, others have failed to detect it, and until this question is settled the validity of this otherwise plausible hypothesis remains in doubt. Mild fluorosis in bone does not cause any symptoms and may even be beneficial as it is believed to protect against osteoporosis.

Two populations with fluoride intakes estimated as about 12–15 mg. a day have been studied and skeletal changes were detected radiologically in some of them. In Bartlett, Texas, with a water supply containing 8 p.p.m., 10–15 per cent were affected and in an aluminium factory whose workers were excreting an average of 9 mg.F a day (probably equivalent to an intake of at least 15 mg. allowing for skeletal storage and loss in sweat) 25 per cent were affected, but no members of either population suffered any disability.

With even higher fluoride intakes, mineralization of joints may occur, causing serious interference with mobility. "Poker-back" (ankylosis of the vertebrae) is an incapacitating result of prolonged daily intake of about 20 mg. or more and is common in areas of India with water supplies very high in fluoride.

MODE OF ACTION OF FLUORIDE IN REDUCING CARIES

The fluoride ion possesses numerous properties all of which, if they act *in vivo*, could contribute to its effect in reducing caries. One group of properties is concerned with the solubility of enamel which, several studies have shown, is reduced slightly by an intake equivalent to 1 p.p.m. (for references, see World Health Organization, 1970).

Fluoride has a great affinity for hydroxyapatite crystals which it enters at the expense of the hydroxyl ion, the resulting fluorapatite being usually regarded (but not by all workers) as a less soluble crystal than hydroxyapatite. All calcified tissues, including pathological structures such as kidney stones or calcified arteries, contain fluoride throughout their depth. Bone and the dental tissues acquire fluoride during their development and the concentration on the outer surface of enamel continues to rise by uptake from tissue fluid during the interval (of several years duration in some teeth) between the completion of development and eruption, eventually reaching values of five to ten times that of the enamel as a whole. In some areas of the enamel, the acquisition of fluoride continues after eruption by ionic exchange with the fluoride of the oral fluids (see later).

The bones of animals which have received high doses of fluoride contain larger apatite crystals than do those of control animals and their carbonate concentration is lower. It is believed that carbonate tends to "poison" the growth of apatite crystals, thus limiting their size and favouring imperfections in their form while fluoride, by competing with carbonate, tends to exclude it so allowing the crystals to become larger and more perfect. The same process may occur in enamel, although it has not been convincingly shown in the one attempt to demonstrate it and if so, the larger crystals would be less soluble because their surface area would be smaller.

If fluoride, even at concentrations below 1 p.p.m., is added to a saturated solution of calcium and phosphate which is on the verge of precipitation, then the precipitation is favoured; there is also a greater tendency for the precipitate to be in the form of apatite (as opposed to other crystalline forms of calcium phosphate such as octacalcium phosphate, brushite or whitlockite), including a proportion of fluorapatite. The caries process is thought to comprise alternate dissolution and precipitation of apatite crystals. The phase of dissolution occurs when the pH of plaque reaches a level sufficiently low (about 5·5) to disturb the equilibrium between calcium and phosphorus in plaque and apatite in enamel. The phase of remineralization results from the precipitation of apatite as pH rises between periods of carbohydrate ingestion. The higher the fluoride concentration of the plaque, whether acquired from oral fluids or from dissolved enamel, the greater would be the expectation of precipitation and thus the slower would be the progress of the carious lesion. Electron micrographs of early cavities show two types of crystal strongly suggestive of the original enamel crystal and of those formed by remineralization.

Thus, the formation of the less soluble fluorapatite, perhaps as larger crystals during enamel development, and an increased tendency for remineralization once caries begins may have additive effects in the caries-reducing action of fluoride.

Although in sound enamel the fluoride concentration on the surface exceeds that within, once the surface is breached by caries or injury fluoride begins to accumulate within the damaged enamel as do other trace elements. In other words, the fluoride accumulates where it can be most effective—at the site of incipient caries. It has been known for many years that "altered enamel" (i.e. early carious enamel containing inclusions of plaque matrix and bacteria) is less soluble in acid than intact enamel and, for example, leaves a visible residue when decalcified before histological sectioning. More recent work shows that the inorganic parts of "altered" enamel are also less soluble than whole enamel, the difference being even more marked in fluoride areas, suggesting that at least one factor reducing its solubility is the rise in fluoride concentration. Two other possible factors are preferential dissolution of the more soluble enamel leaving behind the less soluble, and the protection of apatite crystals surrounded by invading organic matter. Changes during age in the concentration of fluoride on the surface of enamel are mentioned later.

EFECTS OF FLUORIDE ON TOOTH MORPHOLOGY

Fluoride shares with some other trace elements (molybdenum and boron) the property of influencing the formative cells of dental tissues in such a way that the teeth are smaller and more rounded in contour. This effect was observed in experiments in which large doses of salts of these elements were injected into rats at the time their molar teeth were forming; the teeth were sectioned after eruption and certain measurements were made from the sections. Similar measurements, made either in vivo or from plaster models, of human molars from carefully matched high- and low-fluoride areas have confirmed the existence of this morphological trend—although two surveys have shown the reverse tendency (larger teeth with fluoride) but factors other than fluoride may have operated. At 1 p.p.m., the effect is probably too small to be of much practical importance in making the tooth more self-cleansing.

It has been shown that the injection of 0·1mg. F/kg. of body weight into four-day-old rats causes slight distension of the endoplasmic recticulum of the ameloblasts, probably indicating interference with the synthesis of the amelogenins of the matrix; the effect is very marked with higher doses

(3 and 7 mg/kg.). If this occurs in man with daily doses of about 3 mg. it might account for the changed morphology in fluoride areas and, with higher doses, for enamel opacities. Changes in cusp shape would, however, only be expected if there were differential effects on neighbouring cells so that some produced more, and others produced less, matrix. A detailed study of the response to fluoride of different parts of the forming tooth has yet to be made.

EFFECTS OF FLUORIDE ON PLAQUE AND BACTERIA

One of the most surprising discoveries about fluoride is that dental plaque, the source of the carious attack, contains higher concentrations of fluoride than any structure in the body other than the mineralized tissue. Values of 10–20 p.p.m. are normal, of which less than 1 p.p.m. is present as fluoride ions. In areas with fluoride in the water, plaque concentrations are higher. It must be borne in mind that the absolute amount of fluoride in 10 mg. of plaque, a typical yield from one month after 24 hr. without toothbrushing, is so low (0·2 μg. would be typical) as to be near the limits of accurate detection. Different methods of analysis give different figures, suggesting that the fluoride is combined in two or more ways, one fraction being more tightly bound than the other. Figures for plaque fluoride must therefore still be regarded as very approximate. The high fluoride concentration in plaque (and incidentally its considerable ability to accumulate calcium and phosphate) might suggest that plaque protected, rather than damaged, the teeth and that its removal should not be encouraged. The overall effect of plaque in most members of modern communities is, however, to form acid and therefore produce caries. It seems likely that the fluoride apparently present in all plaques, even from people without fluoride in their drinking water, exerts some restraining influence on bacterial activity. This means that the usual measurements of the effect of fluoride—comparisons of caries scores in high- and low-fluoride areas—are underestimates, since residents in the low-fluoride area probably enjoy some benefit both from the fluoride in plaque and in enamel.

Although the question is still controversial, it is believed that most of the plaque fluoride is bound to bacteria where it exerts a small inhibitory effect on the pH drop which occurs with sugar. Plaque collected from high- and low-fluoride areas and incubated with sugar in vitro showed a slightly slower pH drop in the high-fluoride plaque, a result which was repeated when plaque from residents of Durham was compared with that from Newcastle before and some weeks after Newcastle water supply was fluoridated in 1968. Previous experiments in vitro had shown that fluoride at concentrations within the range of those in plaque had several effects on bacteria which might contribute to its anti-caries action; it reduces acid production, it accelerates the removal of lactate by its conversion into other acids less highly ionized, it increases base production (probably the formation of amines by the decarboxylation of amino acids) and reduces the synthesis of intracellular polysaccharides. Except for the last-mentioned, these effects are all very small individually but, collectively, they might influence plaque pH sufficiently to contribute to the reduction in caries.

The question arises as to the source of plaque fluoride. Arithmetical considerations show that it is unlikely to be derived from the fluoride of the enamel surface. If it were, the constant removal of plaque by tooth-brushing would denude enamel of its fluoride and its concentration would reach zero quite quickly. The greater part of the enamel surface does lose fluoride with ageing but it has recently been shown that the cervical areas, which are covered by the thickest plaque, gain fluoride with advancing age. This is strong evidence that fluoride is gradually removed, probably mechanically (since the affinity of fluoride for apatite is so great that it is unlikely to diffuse out) from those surfaces of enamel which are vigorously brushed, but that enamel is replenished with fluoride from the plaque. It must be assumed that plaque gains its fluoride from the saliva or from assimilated fluids, of which tea is an important source if fluoride is not present in the water. Food is an unlikely source as the daily intake usually contains only about 0·5 mg. (diluted in two or more kilos of food!), most of which is bound and not readily soluble in saliva. The concentration in saliva is extremely low (0·01–0·02 p.p.m. are typical figures for whole saliva; if collected from the duct, free of cells and debris, it is even lower, less than 0·01 p.p.m.), but it has been shown to rise following the experimental ingestion of 1 mg. doses of fluoride. The effect of water at 1 p.p.m. consumed in a normal way, raises the concentration in whole saliva (*e.g.* from 0·011– 0·033 p.p.m.) but has a much smaller effect, of doubtful significance, on duct saliva raising it, in one series of experiments, from 0·007–0·009 p.p.m. In spite of its low concentration, saliva seems the only available source of plaque fluoride in areas without fluoride in the water or where tea is not usually taken; perhaps the additional plaque fluoride in fluoridated areas comes directly from the water.

THE SIGNIFICANCE OF THE MULTIPLICITY OF EFFECTS OF FLUORIDE

There is at present no means of deciding the relative contributions of all the numerous properties of fluoride to the anti-caries action of 1 p.p.m. in water. It seems reasonable to suggest that those involving plaque cannot account for more than one-third of the total effect because this is the approximate proportion observed when fluoridated water is received by teeth already erupted. The remaining two-thirds are presumably effected by the various actions of fluoride built into the enamel. This distinction must be approximate, of course, because some post-eruptive fluoride may be incorporated into the enamel and exert "enamel-type" effects even if plaque fluoride may be necessary for this as an intermediary.

One point that does emerge tentatively is that fluoride may be effective because, unlike most other suggested anti-caries substances, it does act in this multiplicity of ways. In looking for alternative or additional preventive measures, it may be essential either to find other measures with a similar wide range of effects or to apply simultaneously several measures each with a limited effect. This history of

attempts at caries prevention, as well as these more theoretical considerations, give little hope that any one measure with a single property will be wholly successful.

THE FLUORIDATION CONTROVERSY

In view of its practical importance, some comments on the main issues of the fluoridation controversy are appropriate.

The grounds for objection to this measure can be classified into three groups: (a) that fluoride is ineffective or has too small an effect to warrant the expense and alleged risk; (b) that its safety cannot be guaranteed; (c) that it interferes with the freedom of the individual.

The first objection arises from a biased selection of part of the evidence. The DMF figures for the 8- and 11-year-old children in the report after 11 years of fluoridation in the U.K. (Department of Health and Social Security, 1969), for example, have been interpreted to indicate that fluoride merely postpones the caries in one tooth by one year (Table 1). This interpretation ignores the facts: (a) that

TABLE 1

AVERAGE NUMBER PER CHILD OF DECAYED, MISSING AND FILLED TEETH IN FLUORIDATED AND CONTROL AREAS FOR DIFFERENT AGE GROUPS 11 YEARS AFTER THE INTRODUCTION OF FLUORIDATION IN THE U.K.

Age	Before F	After F	% Reduction or Increase	Comments
3–7 years	Fluoride 5·3 Control 4·9	2·7 4·0	55 19	Full temporary dentition for 3- and 4-year-olds, temporary canine and molars only for 5-, 6- and 7-year-olds
8–10 years	Fluoride 2·8 Control 2·8	1·8 2·7	36 5	The basis of the criticism that only one tooth is saved
11–14 years	Fluoride 5·9 Control 5·4	4·7 5·9	21 +9	Only the 11-year-old children had fluoride throughout their lives

at eight years, only the molars, the teeth which receive least protection, are at risk and (b) that DMF does not indicate the extent of the caries, and cavities may be smaller and more amenable to conservation in fluoride than in control areas. The figures for the 11–14-year-old group refer, of course, to children who did not receive fluoride throughout the whole of their lives and would not have enjoyed the full benefit. There can be no reasonable doubt about the effectiveness of natural and artificial fluoridation if the worldwide evidence is taken into account.

The question of the safety of fluoridation (or of any other measure) can never be proved conclusively because it is logically impossible to prove a negative, including the proposition that fluoride has no harmful effects. Unfortunately, much of the debate on the safety of fluoridation has not been at a scientific level and completely false, grossly misleading, and biased statements or interpretations abound. Nevertheless, there has been insufficient investigation into the type of minor effects which fluoride might, from its known properties, conceivably produce. Too much emphasis has been given to demonstrating that the vital statistics, or the prevalence of killing diseases like coronary thrombosis, are similar in high- and low-fluoride areas; this information would not be expected to be relevant quite apart from the doubtful reliability of data based on routine death certificates. There has also been considerable reliance on the argument that "no harmful effects have ever been reported" when, without a carefully controlled study, they would be most unlikely to be detected.

The really important question is whether residents in fluoride areas with the highest fluoride intake, either because they are heavy tea-drinkers or ingest large volumes of water, suffer any deleterious effects, the most likely being an increased stiffness and pain in their joints, bearing in mind that daily intakes in the region of 12–15 mg. are the maximum tolerable. Attention has been drawn to the frequency of tea drinking among children, although conclusions that this could be excessive are not unchallenged. The influence of tea on fluoride intake of adults has not been extensively studied but the results of a survey of tea consumption among residents of fluoridated Newcastle was reassuring. All except one of a group of people describing themselves as heavy tea-drinkers were consuming fewer than 12 cups of tea a day and their urine contained 4–5 mg. of fluoride over 24 hr., indicating (assuming the storage of one-third of the intake) a probable ingestion of 7 mg.—well within the safety margin. One man, apparently highly exceptional, drank 22 cups of tea a day and four pints of beer; his urinary excretion of 6·5 mg. (in 4·5 l.) represented the ingestion of perhaps as much as 10 mg. This is clearly approaching the undesirable level and if there are individual variations in sensitivity to fluoride, as there are to most substances, a resident of a fluoridated area who ingested this amount of tea during an adult lifetime, and who happened to be more sensitive than usual, might be at risk of some early fluorotic changes. This combination of circumstances is, however, likely to be rare.

The possibility of hypersensitivity to fluoride (sometimes loosely referred to as an allergy), so that normally harmless intakes may affect certain individuals adversely, has received more attention and has been reported, but never authenticated. Unfortunately, some who claim that symptoms develop from small doses have refused to submit to double-blind tests.

The position on the safety of fluoridation may be summarized as follows: no major deleterious effect has ever been observed in spite of considerable epidemiological study, no minor symptoms have been discovered although the search has perhaps not yet been sufficiently thorough, nor have any claims of hypersensitivity been established. The beneficial effects on dental health far outweigh the hypothetical possibility of undesirable effects which, if they exist at all, must be either rare or mild or both.

The third group of objections based on value judgements

about the freedom of the individual is outside the scope of this chapter.

ALTERNATIVES TO FLUORIDATION

In view of the limited adoption of fluoridation, arising from the opposition to this measure, much attention has recently been given to various alternative methods of applying fluoride. Preparations available in the U.K. have been described by Geddes et al. (1973). The mode of action of these methods is not known exactly but presumably the mechanisms mentioned for natural fluoride are also operative; in view of the gross difference in concentration between fluoridated water and the solutions used topically (some reaching as much as 10,000 p.p.m.), the relative importance of the various actions may be different.

TRACE ELEMENTS OTHER THAN FLUORIDE

The presence of many trace elements in dental tissues was detected spectroscopically in the 1930s but doubts existed about their significance. Some elements were probably derived fortuitously from filling materials in neighbouring teeth and by contamination from instruments used in extraction or in grinding the samples before analysis. Some trace elements (Fe, Pb, Sb and Zn) share with fluoride a higher concentration on the outer enamel surface than in the deeper layers which tends to increase with age, probably because they can enter the apatite lattice or form tight bonds with it. Some elements (Na and Mg, not strictly trace elements) tend to be dissolved out slowly by the oral fluids and their concentration in outer enamel is lower than within; other trace elements (Sr, Cu, Al, K) are uniformly distributed. The concentrations vary from as little as 0·01 to tens of parts per million except for Sr, Si, Pb and Zn which (in that ascending order) may vary from 100–1,000 p.p.m.

The most important issue relating trace elements to the teeth refers to effects on caries. Epidemiological evidence showing that caries is less prevalent in some areas than others has produced some correlations with trace elements in the environment but the evidence is incomplete and cannot be related to known physiological functions of these elements. The importance of water as a source of fluoride has misled dental research workers into the belief that trace elements in general are derived from water. With a few exceptions, trace elements are obtained from food rather than water.

The most striking results emerge from three independent surveys in very different parts of the world. In the U.S.A., the childhood residences of 360 caries-free naval recruits were investigated and the majority came from three areas (two in Ohio and one in South Carolina) with water supplies subsequently shown to contain high concentrations of boron, lithium, molybdenum and strontium. A survey of caries in children in some of these areas confirmed a correlation between low caries scores and high levels of boron and strontium in the drinking water. The second survey in New Zealand related areas with high and low caries prevalence to the trace element composition of sweet vernal, a plant whose composition was known to be related to the type of soil on which it was grown. Once again, low caries was associated with high levels of boron, molybdenum and strontium. A classification of villages in New Guinea into those whose population had high and low caries scores followed by an analysis of the surrounding soils revealed high levels of lithium, strontium and a high pH (which favours molybdenum uptake by plants). These results are summarized in Table 2 and illustrate the similarities of the trace elements associated with a low caries incidence in these very different environments.

TABLE 2

SUMMARY OF TRACE ELEMENTS WITH HIGH CONCENTRATIONS IN THE ENVIRONMENT ASSOCIATED WITH LOW CARIES PREVALENCE

New Zealand (*plants*)[1]	U.S.A. (*water*)[2]			New Guinea[3] (*soils*)
	Ohio (1)	Ohio (2)	S. Carolina	
B	B	B	B	—
—	Li	Li	—	Li
Mo	Mo	Mo	—	—
Sr	Sr	Sr	Sr	Sr
High pH in soils	—	—	—	High pH

[1] Cadell (1964).
[2] Losee and Adkins (1969).
[3] Barmes (1969).

Three surveys, from Hungary, New Zealand and England, have specifically related a high molybdenum intake to low caries prevalence. Experiments in animals confirmed an anti-caries effect of molybdenum at the same concentration as in the water in the Hungarian survey (0·1 p.p.m.—much higher than in other waters containing molybdenum) and in the ash of the plants in the New Zealand study.

A tendency for low caries associated with unusually high intakes of vanadium (0·1–0·22 p.p.m. in the water) has been reported on a small scale survey and several surveys as well as an experiment on monkeys have suggested that selenium may increase caries. Apart from the distribution of individual constituents, a tendency has emerged for caries to be high in areas with leached or acid soils whereas arid areas, or those near river mouths, with rich alluvial deposits are associated with a low incidence.

The circumstantial nature of all this evidence must be emphasized. The link between the presence of these trace elements in water, soil or plants and intake is often tenuous and the link with the teeth frequently non-existent. Even if the association of these elements with low caries activity is eventually established it would not necessarily mean that all these elements had anti-caries properties. It is quite possible that only some (or even one) are active and the others happen to be associated with it in soils or water.

Over 100 animal experiments on various trace elements and caries have been recorded but the results are mostly inconclusive or contradictory. Unfortunately, many of these animal experiments have been badly designed. Among the factors which have led to confusion are the following:

(a) lack of information about the trace elements already present in the basal cariogenic diet;

(b) failure to realize the complex interactions between certain trace elements, *e.g.* copper and sulphate antagonize the effect of molybdenum: the effect of added molybdenum depends therefore on the concentration of all three in the diet;

(c) trace elements often exist in several combinations and it is rarely known which occurs naturally (*e.g.* molybdenum occurs as molybdates and as paramolybdates and in foods is probably bound to protein as a co-enzyme);

(d) the trace elements have usually been fed after the teeth are erupted but caries may be reduced only if they are assimilated before eruption, or even pre-natally;

(e) very high doses have sometimes been fed which may have non-specific effects, *e.g.* imparting an unpleasant taste to the cariogenic food so that less is eaten.

In view of the confused state of knowledge concerning the influence on dental tissues of trace elements, it is not possible to present any clear ideas of their mode of action except in regard to fluoride. At physiological concentrations few have been found *in vitro* to possess any properties comparable with those of fluoride and none exhibits the multiplicity of its properties.

Although workers with experience in this field are convinced that trace elements are of great importance in the epidemiology of caries an immense amount of work is necessary before any practical applications can be expected to match the undoubted benefits of fluoride.

TRACE ELEMENTS AND BONE

Although animal experiments have shown that deficiency of certain trace elements (Cu, Mn and Zn) may have deleterious effects on bone these are not specific but simply a manifestation of effects produced throughout the body. The explanation of these effects is still obscure but it probably related to the function of these elements as co-factors for enzymes.

Certain trace elements (Ba, F, Ni, Pb and Sr, including, of course, ^{90}Sr) are bone-seekers and tend to become bound or incorporated in bone mineral and to increase in concentration with age (Sr), or after increased ingestion (Pb). Becker, Spadaro and Berg (1968) have published one of the few complete analyses of trace elements in bone and reported the consistent presence (in ascending order of concentration) of Cu, Fe, Al, V, Si, Zn and Sr, the presence in some specimens of Mn, Ag, Sb and failure to detect other elements (F is invariably present but would not be detected by the method used). The concentration of Pb was some ten times greater in modern bone than in archaeological samples from ancient Peru.

REFERENCES

Barmes, D. E. (1969), "Caries Etiology in Sepik Villages—Trace Element, Micronutrient and Macronutrient Content of Soil and Food," *Car. Res.*, **3**, 44.
Becker, R. O., Spadàro, J. A. and Berg, E. W. (1968), "The Trace Elements of Human Bone," *J. Bone J. Surg.*, **50A**, 326.
Cadell, P. B. (1964), "Geographic Distribution of Dental Caries in Relation to New Zealand Soils," *Aust. Dent. J.*, **9**, 32.

Department of Health and Social Security (1969), "The Fluoridation Studies in the United Kingdom and the Results Achieved after Eleven Years," *Reports on Public Health and Medical Subjects No. 122*. London: H.M.S.O.

Geddes, D. A. M., Jenkins, G. N. and Stephen, K. W. (1973), "The Use of Fluoride in Caries Prevention," *Brit. dent. J.*, **134**, 426.

Kruger, B. J. (1970), "The Effect of Different Levels of Fluoride on the Ultrastructure of Ameloblasts in the Rat," *Arch. Oral Biol.*, **15**, 109.

Losee, F. L. and Adkins, B. L. (1969), "A Study of the Mineral Environment of Caries-resistant Navy Recruits," *Car. Res.*, **3**, 23.

Ministry of Health (1962), "The Conduct of the Fluoridation Studies in the United Kingdom and the Results Achieved After Five Years," *Reports on Public Health and Medical Subjects No. 105*, London: H.M.S.O.

World Health Organization (1970), *Fluorides and Human Health*. Geneva: W.H.O.

31. DENTAL PLAQUE AND THE BACTERIOLOGY OF CARIES

W. H. BOWEN

Infectious and transmissible nature of dental caries

Development of oral flora

Plaque
  Definition
  Formation of plaque
  Plaque matrix
  Chemistry of plaque
  Metabolism within plaque
    Acid production
    Formation of alkali
    Polysaccharide synthesis

Influence of diet on plaque formation and caries

Bacteriology of caries

Caries activity tests

INFECTIOUS AND TRANSMISSIBLE NATURE OF DENTAL CARIES

Despite the overwhelming weight of evidence to the contrary, there are many who still believe that dental caries develops solely as a result of dietary indiscretions in the form of frequent consumption of readily fermentable carbohydrate. Since the time of W. D. Miller it has been known that micro-organisms are essential in the pathogenesis of dental caries. As early as 1924 J. K. Clarke suggested that dental caries was caused by a single type of streptococcus which he termed *Strep. mutans*. This hypothesis did not receive wide support and the belief prevailed that dental caries was caused by a group of micro-organisms termed *Lactobacillus acidophilus*. For more than two decades this view persisted and almost certainly hampered advances in studying the microbial aetiology of dental caries.

The introduction of antibiotics and gnotobiotic techniques contributed greatly to the understanding of the importance of micro-organisms in the pathogenesis of dental caries. It was observed that when low concentrations of antibiotics active against Gram-positive micro-organisms were incorporated in the diet of rodents they remained caries-free. These observations provided indirect proof that micro-organisms are essential in the pathogenesis of dental caries. In addition they implicated those that are Gram-positive.

Unequivocal proof of the necessity of micro-organisms in the pathogenesis of dental caries came with the observation that rodents housed under germ-free conditions failed to develop caries even when fed a normally cariogenic diet. When rats of the same strain, on the same diet, were infected with a streptococcus and an unidentified pleomorphic rod dental caries developed rapidly. These observations have been confirmed and extended by many investigators. However, two investigations warrant particular mention because their results may have great relevance to humans.

It was Keyes (1960) who demonstrated that caries in hamsters is an infectious and transmissible disease. A litter of hamsters taken from a strain which had been caries-active for four generations was divided into two groups. One half was given antibiotics in its feed to suppress the cariogenic flora; the other half constituted the control. The antibiotic-fed group remained caries-free, while the other animals developed rampant decay. A litter was obtained from a female in each group. That from the caries-inactive animals was divided into two; half the litter was housed alone and the other half with the litter from the caries-active animals. The half-litter housed alone remained caries-free whereas the remaining animals developed rampant caries.

The significance of this experiment for humans became clearer when Zinner *et al.* (1965) observed that rodents infected with specific streptococci isolated from carious lesions in humans developed rampant dental caries. The streptococci used by Zinner's group appear to be identical with those described by Clarke and have by almost universal agreement been named *Strep. mutans*.

These observations may be of more significance for humans than would first appear. A clear correlation has been demonstrated between the caries score of siblings and that of their parents. It has also been observed that parents and siblings of caries-free adults had significantly less caries than those of the caries-active control adults. The prevalence of caries in sons and daughters was compared with that in mothers and fathers, in a population living on a remote Pacific island. It was found that a significant similarity existed between the caries scores of mothers and sons and between those of mothers and daughters, but not between those of fathers and their children. These observations support the belief that dental caries in humans is an infectious and transmissible disease. It is often forgotten that the mouth of the new-born infant, be it Caesarean-derived or born naturally, is devoid of micro-organisms. Yet in a short time after birth an "oral flora" develops. The alternative to a doctrine of spontaneous generation is that these micro-organisms are derived from a person in most intimate contact with the infant. It seems probable that if the mother of the neonate has active carious lesions she is more likely to transmit a cariogenic flora to her child than a mother who is caries-free. However, the essential components of a caries-promoting flora are obligatory periphytes (i.e. they require a surface on which to multiply).

DEVELOPMENT OF ORAL FLORA

The mouth is probably the first mucous membrane area of the body to develop a flora after birth. Occasionally, contaminants from the vagina are isolated within a few minutes of birth but they usually disappear rapidly. Substantial numbers of micro-organisms are not found in the mouth until 8–9 hr. post-partum. A great variety of micro-organisms can be isolated after this period and include many species of streptococci, pneumococci, micrococci, enterococci, staphylococci, veillonella, sarcina, anaerobic streptococci, coliforms, lactobacilli, bacillus subtilis and neisseria. Many of these are probably transients and do not become part of the established flora. An exception to this, however, is *Streptococcus salivarius* which normally finds its ecological niche on the dorsum of the tongue and thus does not require the presence of such surfaces as teeth before becoming established in the mouth. It has been observed that *Strep. salivarius* becomes established in many infants within 24 hr. after birth regardless of the diet they receive. *Strep. salivarius*, however, makes up less than one per cent of the total cultivable flora. An extensive study carried out on infant monkeys being fed a human-type milk formula showed that aerobic and anaerobic micro-organisms were present even before teeth erupted. Micrococci, alpha and gamma haemolytic streptococci, and lactobacilli were isolated. However, neither *Strep. sanguis* nor *Strep. mutans* were isolated in large numbers from mouths before the teeth erupted. Following eruption the enamel surface was quickly colonized; the flora changed rapidly during the period following eruption.

Although the term "oral flora" is frequently used, it is important to realize that there are many oral floras. Organisms found in saliva in profusion may be sparse in plaque; the lactobacilli and *Strep. salivarius* are good examples of this phenomenon. In contrast, *Strep. mutans* and *Strep. sanguis* are regularly isolated from plaque and are infrequently found in saliva in large numbers. Further instances of micro-organisms inhabiting different parts of the mouth

are seen in the localization of actinomyces and candida. For example, *A. israelii* was isolated from 12·5 per cent of mucosal scrapings, 56·1 per cent of plaque, 52·2 per cent of

TABLE 1

PERCENTAGE DISTRIBUTION OF ORGANISMS ON DIFFERENT SITES IN THE HUMAN MOUTH (SOCRANSKY AND MANGANIELLO, 1971)

Organism	Supra-gingival Plaque	Tongue	Gingival Crevice	Cheek	Saliva
Strep. mutans	3·9	0·3	ND	0·5	0·2
*Strep. sanguis**	75·0	9·0	ND	29·0	47·0
*Strep. salivarius**	0·7	55·3	0·5	10·7	47·4
B. melaninogenicus†	0·3	0·4	4·5	0·3	0·42
Spirochaetes‡	0·1	ND	1·5	ND	ND
Lactobacillus	0·0001	ND	ND	ND	0·01

* % of facultative streptococci
† % of total cultivable flora
‡ % microscopic count
ND Not Determined

samples from gingival crevices but from only 28·9 per cent of saliva samples. *Candida albicans*, in contrast, was isolated most frequently from saliva. Thus it can be seen that a single sample of saliva will be as representative of the various microbial aggregations in the mouth as a bucket of water taken at Tower Bridge would be of the River Thames.

PLAQUE

Definition

It is difficult to contrive a definition of plaque which is universally acceptable. For the present discussion it will be defined as soft tenacious material found on tooth surfaces and not readily removed by rinsing with water. This definition however could be inadequate for investigational purposes; it would then be necessary to stipulate at least the period for which the plaque was allowed to accumulate, and the time elapsed since the last intake of food.

Formation of Plaque

Following thorough cleansing with abrasive paste, a pellicle quickly re-forms on the cleaned tooth surface. This is usually virtually free of bacteria and is found on electron histochemical examination to be structureless. Available evidence suggests that the material is derived from saliva, although which gland makes the major contribution is not agreed. Immunoelectrophoretic techniques and electrophoresis indicate that the material is composed of at least four proteins. It is of interest that the material adsorbed on to dentures or plastic differs in chemical composition from that adsorbed on to tooth enamel. The pellicle has been shown to be rich in the acidic amino acids and especially glutamic acid and to be low in sulphur-containing amino acids, although recent studies suggest that the material adsorbed on teeth near the orifice of the sublingual gland is rich in sulphated glycoproteins. It seems unlikely that bacteria are directly involved in this initial formation of pellicle because it develops with such rapidity and because a similar process can be demonstrated *in vitro* using pure secretions in the absence of bacteria. Nevertheless, it is probable that bacteria play a part in the later formation of pellicle and of the protein matrix of plaque.

Saliva is rich in glycoproteins which confer on saliva its viscous nature. These substances consist essentially of a protein backbone to which are attached short side chains of carbohydrate. The side chains are negatively charged. There are many bacteria present in the mouth capable of removing these side chains by means of the enzyme neuraminidase. When this happens the negative charges on the glycoprotein are removed, the isoelectric point of the molecule alters, and the material comes out of solution readily. Sialic acid and fucose are always found to occur in terminal positions in the short side chains. The absence of these substances from plaque is frequently taken as evidence to support the concept that the action of bacterial neuraminidase on salivary glycoproteins is of major consequence in the formation of the protein component of plaque. There is, however, little direct evidence that this is so.

The cell-free layer is quickly covered by colonies of micro-organisms and indeed individual colonies can be identified on the pellicle up to 24 hr. after its initial formation. The microbial population of the plaque after 24 hr. ranges from 72–103 million per mg. wet weight, and increases after three days to 80–132 million. The predominant organisms are Gram-positive cocci usually *Strep. mitis*, *Strep. sanguis* and *Strep. mutans*. They comprise approximately 84 per cent of the cultivable flora after 24 hr. and 70 per cent of the plaque flora after 72 hr. As the plaque gets older filamentous forms of micro-organisms appear and these form the largest group as a rule after the streptococci. The veillonella which are Gram-negative anaerobic cocci also contribute significantly to the population of plaque. They also have the ability to metabolize lactate to CO_2 and H_2.

This outline account of the chronological appearance of particular micro-organisms on the tooth surface leaves unanswered the question of why such selection and adherence occurs. The oral environment has been compared to a fast-flowing stream, an analogy which is particularly apt when it is considered that up to 1·2 l. of saliva can be secreted per day. It is clear that unless mechanisms exist which enable micro-organisms to adhere to surfaces such as teeth and mucous membranes there would be few bacteria in the mouth. The evidence suggests that the ability of micro-organisms to adhere to tooth surfaces is intimately related to the surface structure of bacteria, its interaction with some salivary components and, of course, with the tooth surface itself.

The addition of micro-organisms to pure, sterile parotid or submandibular saliva results in their aggregation and this phenomenon is enhanced by the presence of calcium ions. Some micro-organisms such as lactobacilli which are found in plaque in small numbers do not aggregate *in vitro* readily; in addition it has been observed that the aggregating factor(s) are species specific. The addition of

one species of micro-organism to saliva does not necessarily remove the ability of the saliva to aggregate other types of micro-organisms. It has also been observed that some species of micro-organisms will adhere to enamel powder which has been treated with saliva. This ability has been associated with the possession of a fibrillar fuzzy coat in *Strep. mitis* (*mitior*) which can be removed by treatment with trypsin. If the aggregation factors were identical with the salivary protein adsorbed on to the enamel surface, a ready explanation would be available for the early colonization of the tooth surface and pellicle. However, it is possible that the streptococci which first appear on the tooth surface do so because of some nutritional advantage which they gain from a presumed ability to utilize the adsorbed protein. A similar situation has been reported to occur when micro-organisms are placed in a nutritionally inadequate medium. Following the provision of a surface to which nutrients in the medium can be adsorbed, the micro-organisms grow upon it readily.

Other mechanisms also exist which may encourage the colonization of tooth surfaces. It has been observed that dextran (a polymer of glucose formed by bacteria such as *Strep. mutans* and *Strep. sanguis* from sucrose) will adhere readily to hydroxyapatite treated with saliva. It has further been reported that the addition of small amounts of dextran to a suspension of glucose-grown *Strep. mutans* results in their rapid aggregation. It seems unlikely however that this phenomenon is the primary ecological determinant in the development of the plaque flora although there seems little doubt that it could play an important secondary role. The processes which lead to the appearance of other micro-organisms in plaque have not been well studied. A major factor could be the ability of different species of micro-organisms to adhere to each other. In addition, it is easy to explain how the metabolism of glucose to lactate could confer a nutritional advantage in veillonella. Likewise, the negative Eh (as low as −200 mV.) found in plaque resulting from the dense clumping of micro-organisms would favour the appearance of anaerobic types such as fusiforms.

Plaque Matrix

Plaque thickens on tooth surfaces through the adherence of additional organisms and also as a result of micro-organisms dividing in the plaque. Cell divisions have been observed in the depths of plaque even as old as 14 days. A major factor in the growth of plaque is the formation of extracellular matrix. This can be particularly abundant when sucrose is being consumed frequently and in large quantities although other sugars too can enhance its formation.

Based on electron histochemical examination, a large proportion of the volume of the extracellular matrix of plaque seems to be composed primarily of polysaccharides. The structure of these polysaccharides varies, depending on the type of bacterial colony with which they are associated. Dense and heavily staining polysaccharides are found primarily around Gram-positive and Gram-negative cocci.

The polysaccharides found in plaque are usually of the levan and dextran types. (Their formation and structure are discussed in Chapter 34.) The ratio of micro-organisms to matrix is usually of the order 2:1.

Chemistry of Plaque

The chemical composition of plaque depends, like its bacterial composition, on its age and the circumstances of its formation; it differs, too, in different areas of the mouth. Plaque contains approximately 80 per cent water which can be readily removed; when removed from the mouth, it rapidly loses moisture making wet-weight determinations difficult. The protein content of dried plaque is approximately 40 per cent. The available evidence suggests that a substantial amount of it is of salivary origin; bacteria also contribute significantly. Although the amount of protein in plaque is dependent on the composition of the diet there is little evidence to suggest that diet contributes directly to the protein content. Plaque formed under several different dietary regimens has essentially the same amino acid content. The carbohydrate moiety of plaque varies between 10–20 per cent approximately and is dependent on the age of the plaque, the type of diet consumed and the time elapsed since the last intake of food. Water-soluble polyglucan usually makes up the bulk of the polysaccharide in plaque. Lesser amounts of water-insoluble polyglucan are also found. However, if the diet lacks sucrose, polysaccharides of different types may be found. When plaque has recently been exposed to sucrose, polyfructan, both water-soluble and insoluble, will be found. (The importance of these polysaccharides in the pathogenesis of caries will be discussed later.) The levels of these polysaccharides in plaque are highly variable because those which are water-soluble are readily metabolized by plaque bacteria. The levan is utilized easily by a wide variety of micro-organisms. Indeed there are micro-organisms in plaque which under some circumstances can synthesize levan from sucrose, and later break down the material which they had earlier formed. Approximately 50 per cent of water-soluble hexose can be metabolized over 24 hr.

Significant levels of calcium and phosphorus are present in plaque. The levels are dependent on the age of the plaque, its site of collection, and the composition of the diet. The level of calcium varies from approximately 2–30 μg./ mg. dry weight of plaque and that of phosphorus from 10–40 μg./mg. of plaque. Higher levels of calcium are found in young plaque. This is probably because adsorbed saliva has a high affinity for calcium; indeed, it appears that calcium may be tightly bound to some salivary proteins. Plaque collected from teeth near the orifices of the salivary ducts has a higher level of calcium and phosphorus than that from other areas of the mouth. It also appears that the level of calcium and phosphorus in plaque is inversely related to the amount of sugar in the diet; this observation could be of particular significance in relation to the pathogenesis of caries.

Significant levels of fluoride may be found in plaque. Concentrations reported range from 16 p.p.m. to as high as 80 p.p.m. There is little doubt that the level of fluoride in plaque is dependent on the amount consumed either in the diet or drinking water. It appears to be independent of the level in the tooth surface. There is evidence to indicate that at normal pH values little of the fluoride in plaque is available in the ionic form and that some of it may be tightly bound to organic material in plaque.

Small amounts of magnesium too are present in plaque, concentrations varying from 1–10 μg. per mg. dry weight of plaque. Research into the significance of this ion will increase with the recent observation that magnesium-rich mineral is one of the first materials to be removed from enamel during the initial carious attack.

Metabolism Within Plaque

Acid Production

Because of the acknowledged importance of plaque in the pathogenesis of dental caries, a cult has developed which implies that plaque itself is a disease. The mere physical presence of plaque will not *per se* give rise to disease. However, under the circumstances in which plaque normally forms, *i.e.* associated with the consumption of high levels of carbohydrate, it does have pathogenic potential. Following the application of simple sugar solutions to such a plaque its pH value will fall rapidly and substantial amounts of acid will be formed. In many instances the pH will fall to as low as 4·0. It is generally agreed that pH values lower than 5·5 at the tooth surface initiate demineralization. After approximately 15–20 min. the pH in plaque starts to rise. It is not certain whether this rise is attributable to dissolution of the tooth surface leading to the neutralization of the acid, to alkali production by components of the plaque, to the inherent buffering capacity of the plaque, to diffusion of acids out of plaque or to a combination of all four. Protein and calcium phosphate are the most important buffers in plaque, but from the levels of calcium and phosphorus in plaque it can be seen that the buffering capacity is not substantial. The age of plaque also influences its acid-producing ability. One-day-old plaque has little capacity to lower the pH of a sugar solution; however the capacity increases with age, the maximum being reached after approximately three days.

The types of acid formed in plaque have received scant attention considering their potential importance. *In vitro* studies have shown that the concentrations of lactic acid formed are the same as or less than those of acetic or propionic acids. However, it must be remembered that a large population of veillonella in plaque would lead to the rapid disappearance of lactic acid. The fall in pH values of the plaque cannot be correlated with the concentration of lactic acid. Further investigation of plaque formed *in vivo* has shown that the concentration of lactate in plaque following the chewing of sugar was 4·6 m. $\times$ 10^{-5} mmoles/mg. wet weight and that most of the acid was in the D form.

Formation of Alkali

Although most attention has been focused on acid production by plaque, it would be an error to neglect the ability of plaque components to form alkali from a number of substrates. The pH of plaque not exposed to carbohydrate substrate for 24 hr. is frequently found to be as much as 1 pH unit higher than that of surrounding saliva. This raised pH is almost certainly due to the deamination of amino acids giving rise to the production of ammonia. Decarboxylation of amino acids can occur at low pH values which will also give rise to alkali and help to overcome the untoward effects of acid.

A substance termed "pH rise factor" has been identified in saliva. This substance, the exact chemical composition of which has not been defined, stimulates the uptake of oxygen by plaque thus accelerating the removal of lactic acid by promoting the formation of acetic acid and carbon dioxide. The presence of small amounts of urea in saliva also helps to overcome the ill-effects of acid, for it is broken down to ammonia and carbon dioxide. Indeed, the incorporation of small amounts of urea in glucose solution prevents the decline in pH values when the solution is applied to plaque.

Polysaccharide Synthesis

If dental caries arose simply as a result of acid production on the tooth surface it should not, in theory at least, be difficult to prevent. The buffering capacity of saliva under normal circumstances is more than adequate to overcome the deleterious effects of acid production. However, not only is acid formed following each ingestion of sugar but substantial amounts of polysaccharide are also formed; this is formed both intracellularly and extracellularly, and its presence does much to exclude the beneficial action of saliva.

The intracellular polysaccharide formed is of the amylopectin type and stains with iodine. It can be readily metabolized to acid by plaque micro-organisms when extraneous sources of carbohydrates are lacking. Available evidence suggests that the synthetic pathways involved are particularly sensitive to fluoride although it is probable that the effect of this ion is to inhibit glucose from entering the bacterial cell, thereby blocking the availability of the substrate.

The extracellular polysaccharides found in plaque are primarily dextrans and levans. Their precise role in the pathogenesis of caries is not clear. Some of the extracellular polysaccharide is easily metabolized, but it seems probable that the most deleterious effect of extracellular polysaccharide in plaque results from its ability to prevent the ready diffusion of neutralizing substances through plaque. This raises the question of why, if a molecule such as sucrose can readily diffuse into plaque, it is not possible for a comparatively small molecule such as bicarbonate to diffuse and neutralize acid. Recent evidence has shown clearly that polysaccharides formed in vitro by Strep. mutans move readily in disc electrophoresis indicating that they have a charge. Furthermore, chemical analysis has shown that phosphate is tightly bound to the polysaccharides. If a similar situation exists in plaque, it seems likely that the net effect would be that charged molecules such as bicarbonate would diffuse through with difficulty whereas uncharged substances such as sugars could diffuse through readily.

In all probability therefore the polysaccharides in plaque (fig. 1) contribute to the adhesiveness of plaque, also protect the micro-organisms from influences inimical to them, and serve to exclude acid-neutralizing substances from the tooth surface.

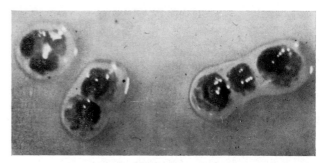

Fig. 1. Colonies of *Strep. mutans* growing on mitis-salivarius sucrose agar, showing viscous emanations of extracellular polysaccharide.

INFLUENCE OF DIET ON PLAQUE FORMATION AND CARIES

The formation of plaque is greatly influenced by the type of diet consumed and it is important to realize that not all plaques have equal capacity to produce disease, nor is diet essential for their formation. For example, plaque forms rapidly in patients and also in animals that receive their entire diet by stomach tube. When plaque thus formed is exposed to glucose solution (fig. 2) it fails to lower the pH of the solution; it has less polysaccharide (fig. 3), and more

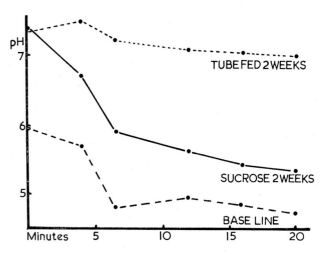

Fig. 2. The effect of a glucose rinse (administered at 0 minutes) on the pH of plaque from (a) an animal fed by stomach tube; (b) one which received sucrose by mouth; and, (c) a control fed on a high carbohydrate diet.

calcium and phosphorus than plaque formed under more conventional circumstances. Animals so fed do not develop dental caries.

In other investigations plaque that formed when glucose or fructose was the only substance in contact with the tooth surfaces (the remainder of the diet being given by stomach tube) formed acid rapidly when exposed to sugar solutions. In addition, substantial amounts of polysaccharide were

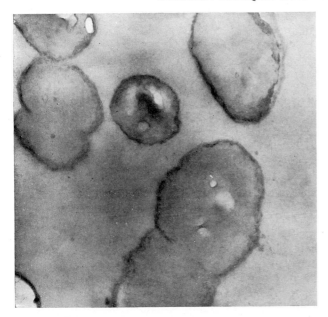

FIG. 3. Electronhistochemistry of plaque from a tube-fed animal. Note absence of extracellular and intracellular polysaccharide. Despite absence of extraneous substrate, there is evidence of cell division. Original × 3,000.

The influence of particular vitamins and minerals on plaque formation has not been studied in detail. There is, however, clear evidence that substances such as calcium glycerophosphate and sodium phytate, both of which occur naturally, can reduce the amount of plaque both present and potential possibly by desorbing protein pellicle from the tooth surface. In addition calcium glycerphosphate has a substantial buffering action. Such plaque as is formed when calcium glycerophosphate is included in the diet has significantly increased levels of calcium and phosphate.

BACTERIOLOGY OF DENTAL CARIES

There is now overwhelming evidence that *Strep. mutans* can induce caries in susceptible animals fed a high carbohydrate diet. Nevertheless, there are still many who question the importance of this micro-organism in the pathogenesis of dental caries in humans.

In experiments carried out in primates it has been observed that minimal caries develops in animals not infected with *Strep. mutans* but fed a high sugar diet. This is in marked contrast to the situation which prevails when animals of the same species fed on the same diet are infected with *Strep. mutans*; extensive carious lesions then develop

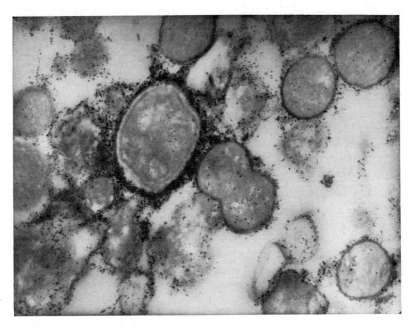

FIG. 4. Electronhistochemistry of plaque formed in presence of glucose and fructose only; note much extracellular polysaccharide and some intracellular polysaccharide. Original × 3,000.

found in this plaque (fig. 4) although its composition differed from that of plaque formed under conventional circumstances. These observations provide no support for speculation that caries can be prevented by substituting glucose or fructose for sucrose.

Proteins too can have a profound effect on plaque formation. Plaque formed in the presence of casein, a phosphoprotein present in milk, exhibits little capacity to form acid but rapidly undergoes transformation to calculus.

rapidly. In addition, the results of numerous studies have demonstrated the importance of *Strep. mutans* in the pathogenesis of dental caries in rodents. It is true that other micro-organisms too have been shown to have the ability to produce caries in rodents; these organisms include *Lactobacillis acidophilus*, *Lactobacillus casei*, *Actinomyces* species, and certain types of *Strep. sanguis*. It is of particular interest that all the micro-organisms produce extracellular polysaccharide from either glucose or sucrose. However, in no instance has the level of caries activity reached that associated with *Strep. mutans* infection. Furthermore, in many instances the experiments continued for 90 days. Considering that the thickness of rodent enamel is approximately 0·1 mm. and that of human enamel is 2·7 mm. it would on this basis take approximately 6·5 years for a lesion to penetrate the enamel of a human tooth. However, this observation should not be interpreted to mean that these micro-organisms do not contribute to the overall cariogenic activity of plaque. Plaque is never composed of a pure culture of micro-organisms except under specific experimental circumstances. Clearly, any organism in plaque that is capable of forming acid from sugar can contribute to the carious attack.

There are many studies which show a positive correlation between the development of caries and the numbers of *Strep. mutans* in plaque. However, many of these have been of a cross-sectional type and their validity can rightly be questioned. As a carious lesion takes months to develop, the bacteriological analysis of plaque taken after a lesion has formed may not be a reflection of conditions when the cavity was forming. Some short-term longitudinal studies have been carried out and the results of these investigations support the importance of *Strep. mutans* in the pathogenesis of caries. Five serotypes of *Strep. mutans* have been identified (a–e) but all have at least one common antigen, which has not been identified. Studies have also shown that the numbers of lactobacilli increase in plaque only after carious lesions have developed; *L. casei* is the lactobacillus most frequently found in plaque. In addition substantial numbers of actinomyces have been isolated from plaque in patients with rampant caries; *A. naeslundi* and *A. israelii* were those most frequently found.

When caries has penetrated into dentine the flora associated with the advancing lesion differs markedly from that which occurs in plaque. A much simpler type of flora is found. *Actinomyces odontolyticus* is usually seen at the advancing front of the dental lesion. Large numbers of lactobacilli too are found in carious dentine. They frequently comprise 25 per cent of the cultivable flora in contrast to the situation in plaque and saliva when they usually comprise substantially less than 1 per cent of the total flora. Streptococci are usually isolated, both *Strep. mutans* and *Strep. sanguis* being present. Micro-organisms capable of destroying dentine must not only possess the ability to produce acid, and to survive in aciduric conditions, but must also be able to break down the protein structure of dentine.

Root surface caries has been receiving an increasing amount of attention because of the problems it causes in elderly patients. In animals, this type of lesion is associated with the presence of *Actinomyces viscosus*. This microorganism forms substantial amounts of levan from sucrose, and in addition elaborates levanase, which breaks down pre-formed levan.

CARIES ACTIVITY TESTS

Of many caries-activity tests in use, none involves the use of plaque; all are carried out on samples of saliva. The salivary flora is not, however, representative of the microbial population of all parts of the mouth and largely comprises washings from the mucosal surfaces. Many of the tests are simple to carry out; but although they are useful when applied to groups, they are generally valueless when used to investigate individual patients. The two which are the most popular are the lactobacillus test and the Snyder test.

The lactobacillus test was introduced almost 40 years ago. It was based, at that time, on the belief that lactobacilli are the prime bacteriological initiators of dental caries. The test is carried out by collecting a known volume of paraffin-stimulated saliva from a fasting patient and diluting it 1:100 in nutrient broth at pH 5. 0·1 and 1 ml. samples of this dilution are used to prepare pour plates using Rogosa's medium, which is selective for lactobacilli. The plates are incubated in an atmosphere of increased carbon-dioxide tension at a temperature of 37°C for four days. The number of lactobacilli per millilitre of saliva is then estimated.

Some difference of opinion exists concerning the population of lactobacilli in saliva that constitutes a positive result. A count of 10,000 per ml. of saliva from children and 40,000 in adults is usually regarded as positive. Subjects with counts higher than these have significantly more caries than those with fewer lactobacilli in their saliva.

The lactobacillus count can be correlated with caries incidence (number of new lesions in a given period of time) in 67–90 per cent of instances. It cannot be used to predict caries development beyond one year and, in addition, it does not enable a prediction to be made about the number of new lesions likely to develop. It has also been shown that 71–79 per cent of children with negative lactobacillus counts developed less than three newly-decayed tooth surfaces in 12 months. Sixty-two per cent of those with positive counts develop three or more carious surfaces over a similar period.

Because of technical difficulties in carrying out the lactobacillus test Snyder developed a simpler method for determining caries activity. The interpretation of the test is based on the degree and rate of colour change in a bacteriological culture medium containing bromocresol green as a pH indicator. The test is not difficult to carry out. In addition it has the advantage that micro-organisms other than lactobacilli are included. A sample of paraffin-stimulated saliva is collected from a fasting patient. 0·1–0·2 ml. of saliva is added to 5 ml. of Snyder test agar at 45°C. The saliva and the agar are mixed thoroughly, then cooled rapidly to 37°C, incubated, and examined at 24, 48 and 72 hr. The test is positive when green is no longer the predominant colour in the medium; this change indicates that acid has been produced in the medium. A subject with a positive test after 24 hr. is regarded as being highly caries-active. A negative test after 72 hr. suggests that the subject is not caries-active. The available evidence suggests that there is no difference in the number of new carious surfaces developed by patients with strongly positive Snyder tests and those with weakly positive tests. However, those with negative tests, *i.e.* in which the medium remains green after 72 hr., developed fewer lesions than those patients with either strongly or weakly positive tests. The Snyder test may be used to predict whether or not a group of individuals is likely to develop more or less new lesions than average. Like the lactobacillus test, this test cannot be used to predict beyond a 12-month period; nor can it be applied with confidence to individual patients.

One of the major problems facing research workers and clinicians is the difficulty of determining whether plaque taken from a patient at a particular time is caries-promoting. Longitudinal studies on plaque samples from defined areas of the tooth go some way towards overcoming the difficulty. Even so, however, an element of assumption is inseparable from a procedure which correlates plaque taken at a precise moment in time with lesions which become manifest only long afterwards; moreover there is an implied assumption that caries is a continuous process whereas, in fact, there is abundant evidence to indicate that it is not.

There is clearly a need for the development of a simple

and reliable caries-activity test which can be applied with confidence to individual patients. The availability of such a test could result in the testing *in vivo* of many more substances possessing anti-caries potential. Such an advance would hasten the day when caries could to a large measure be brought under control.

REFERENCES

Clarke, J. K. (1924), "On the Bacterial Factor in the Aetiology of Dental Caries," *Brit. J. exp. Path.*, **5**, 141.
Keyes, P. H. (1960), "The Infectious and Transmissible Nature of Experimental Dental Caries," *Arch. Oral Biol.*, **1**, 304.
Socransky, S. S. and Manganiello, S. D. (1971), "The Oral Microbiota of Man from Birth to Senility," *J. Periodontol.*, **42**, 485.
Zinner, D. D., Jablon, J. M., Aran, A. P. and Saslaw, M. S. (1965), "Experimental Caries Induced in Animals by Streptococci of Human Origin," *Proc. Soc. exp. Biol.* (*N.Y.*), **118**, 766.

32. THE STRUCTURE OF CARIOUS LESIONS

L. M. SILVERSTONE

Caries in enamel
  Translucent zone
  Dark zone
  The body of the lesion
  The surface zone
  Organic matrix
  Ultrastructural studies

Caries of dentine
  Lesions deep to intact enamel
    Translucent zone
    The body of the lesion
    Reactionary dentine
  Lesions after cavitation of enamel
    Translucent zone
    The body of the lesion
    Zone of demineralization
    Zone of penetration
    Zone of destruction
  Arrested caries

CARIES IN ENAMEL

The earliest macroscopic evidence of smooth surface caries may be seen on an extracted tooth where it appears as a small opaque white region on the approximal surface, usually situated at the cervical margin of the interdental facet. This "white spot" lesion contrasts with the translucency of adjacent sound enamel (fig. 1). The enamel surface overlying the white spot lesion is hard and shiny, and cannot be distinguished from the surface of adjacent sound enamel when examined with a sharp dental probe. Intact surface lesions may also appear brownish and are then

described as "brown spot" lesions. The extent of discolouration or staining is dependent upon the degree of exogenous material adsorbed by the porous region. It has often been stated that the degree of discolouration is related to the length of time the lesion has been present in the mouth. Thus, stained white spots have been assumed to be lesions of slow progress. However, factors such as smoking, and other habits, must also play a part in the degree of staining of the original white-spot lesion.

The smooth surface enamel lesion is conical in section, having its apex pointing towards the dentine. On reaching the amelodentinal junction, spread of the carious process is usually rapid along this plane. In the case of smooth-surface lesions, lateral spread along the amelodentinal junction results in a broad base to the dentine lesion. In this manner the carious process undermines sound enamel, a process termed secondary caries of enamel.

With fissure caries, the enamel lesion broadens as it approaches the underlying dentine since it is guided by prism direction. With lateral spread at the amelodentinal junction, the area of involved dentine is larger than with smooth-surface lesions. The lesion of fissure caries is not initiated at the base of the fissure, but occurs bilaterally on the walls of the fissure, giving the appearance of two small smooth-surface lesions (fig. 2). Eventually the lesions increase in size, coalescing at the base of the fissure.

The histological features of the small carious lesion in human dental enamel have been described by a number of workers. The small lesion has been divided into zones based upon its histological appearance when longitudinal ground sections are examined with the light microscope. The number of zones described has varied from three to seven, the larger subdivision probably being due to varying degrees of overlap. It is most convenient to subdivide the small enamel lesion into four zones, each clearly distinguishable from the others (figs. 3 and 4). There is a translucent zone at the inner advancing front of the lesion whilst just superficial to this is found a dark zone. The body of the lesion is the third zone and lies between the dark zone and the apparently undamaged enamel surface. This third zone shows marked demineralization and provides the greater mass of the small lesion. The relatively unaffected surface zone superficial to the lesion is the fourth zone. Since the small

tissue. However, this zone is seen in only about half of the lesions examined by conventional histological methods. It is best demonstrated when a ground section is examined in a clearing agent, such as Canada balsam or quinoline, having a refractive index similar to that of the enamel (1.62). Canada balsam was the medium used by earlier histologists but quinoline is more suitable since its refractive index is identical to that of the enamel. When a ground section

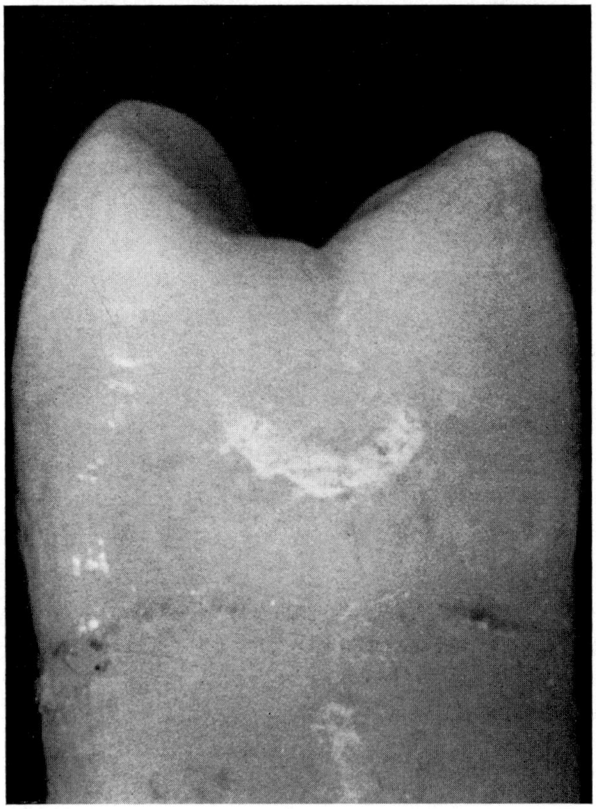

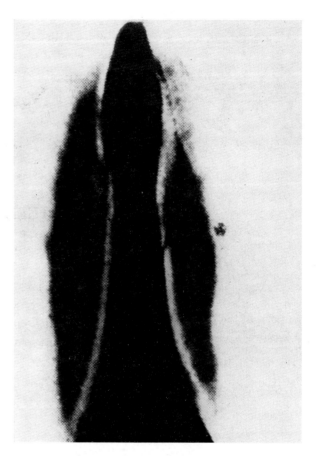

FIG. 1. A premolar tooth showing a white spot lesion on the approximal surface. The lesion is situated just cervical to the point of contact with the adjacent tooth.

FIG. 2. Microradiograph of a longitudinal ground section through the occlusal fissure in a molar showing a small carious lesion. The radiolucent areas of the lesion are seen to be situated bilaterally on the walls of the fissure, and not at its base ($\times$ 100). (By courtesy of Dr. K. V. Mortimer.)

lesion in enamel consists essentially of these four easily recognizable zones, it is convenient to describe the structure of carious enamel, at the light microscope level, on this basis.

The histological features of caries in deciduous enamel are essentially similar to those in the enamel of permanent teeth. However, enamel in deciduous teeth is approximately half the thickness of that in permanent teeth and the pulp chambers are relatively much larger. Thus, caries progresses a shorter distance to reach the pulp in a deciduous molar than in a molar of the permanent series.

Zone 1: The Translucent Zone

The translucent zone of enamel caries lies at the advancing front of the lesion and there is full agreement that, when present, it represents the first observable alteration in the

is examined in transmitted light after imbibition with quinoline, the translucent zone appears structureless, its translucency being well demarcated from normal enamel with its structural markings, on its deep aspect, and the dark zone (Zone 2) on its superficial aspect (fig. 3).

The zone appears translucent because the spaces, or pores, created in the tissue in this first stage of enamel caries are located at prism boundaries, and other junctional sites. Therefore, when the pores are filled with a medium, such as quinoline, having the same refractive index as enamel, normal structural markings are no longer visible (figs. 3 and 4).

Several workers have shown that the translucent zone is situated deep to the region of visible radiolucency seen on microradiographs (fig. 4). From this it was assumed that there was no demineralization in the translucent zone. Other workers claimed that the translucent zone was produced by a loss of soluble protein from enamel, but this has not been substantiated. By means of polarized light it was shown that the translucent zone is more porous than sound enamel, having a pore volume of 1 per cent compared with about 0·1 per cent found for sound enamel. More detailed examination of microradiographs of carious enamel revealed changes in density corresponding in posi-

the advancing front of the lesion than is the translucent zone, occurring in 85–90 per cent of lesions in permanent enamel, and about 85 per cent of lesions in deciduous enamel. Polarized light studies showed that the dark zone has a pore volume of 2–4 per cent. When examined with the polarizing microscope after imbibition with quinoline, the dark zone shows positive birefringence in contrast to the negative birefringence of sound enamel, and a reduced

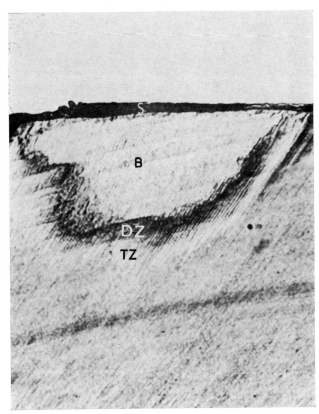

FIG. 3. Longitudinal ground section through a small lesion of enamel caries examined in quinoline by transmitted light (× 50). TZ = translucent zone, DZ = dark zone, B = body of the lesion, S = enamel surface.

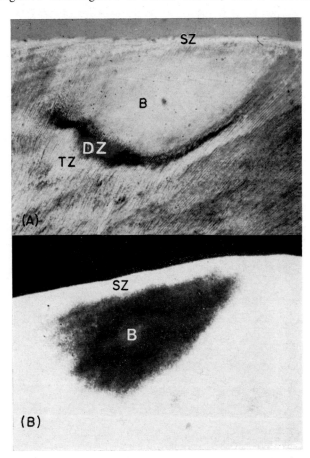

FIG. 4. A. Ground section showing a small enamel lesion in quinoline (polarized light × 50). TZ = translucent zone, DZ = dark zone, B = body of the lesion, SZ = surface zone. The dark zone shows positive birefringence in contrast to the negative birefringence of both sound enamel and the rest of the lesion. B. Microradiograph of the above section showing the subsurface nature of the lesion. SZ = surface zone, B = body of the lesion.

tion to the translucent zone indicating, for the first time, that mineral loss had occurred in this region. In recent studies the histological zones from ground sections of enamel lesions have been separated by micro-dissection and subjected to chemical analysis. It was found that carious attack had preferentially removed magnesium- and carbonate-rich mineral from the translucent zone but there was no evidence of protein loss, thus providing direct evidence that the spaces created in the translucent zone are caused by the removal of mineral and not organic material.

Zone 2: The Dark Zone

The dark zone lies just superficial to the translucent zone. The zone appears dark brown when examined by transmitted light after imbibition with quinoline or Canada balsam (fig. 3). The dark zone is a more constant feature of

negative birefringence of the rest of the lesion (fig. 5). Hence, it is often referred to as the "positive" zone.

This effect was shown to be due to the presence of very small pores in the zone in addition to the relatively large pores which are present in the first stage, the translucent zone. Therefore, when a ground section is examined in a mounting medium such as quinoline or Canada balsam, the relatively large molecules of the medium are unable to penetrate the micropore system of the dark zone. This effect has been described as a "molecular sieve".

Since the micropores remain "filled" with air or vapour, light is scattered on passing through the zone, causing the brown discolouration of the dark zone (fig. 3). In a similar manner, the presence of a medium of low refractive index within the micropores is responsible for the reversal of birefringence from negative to positive in the dark zone when examined in polarized light (figs. 4 and 5). If a ground section is examined in an aqueous medium having small molecules which penetrate the micropores, the dark zone is no longer seen.

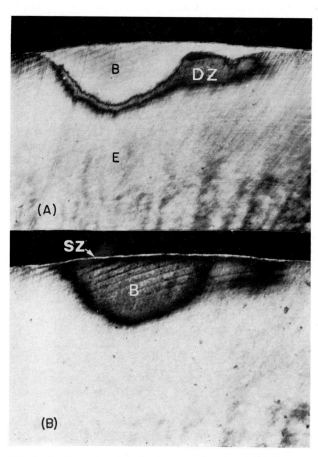

FIG. 5. A. Ground section showing a small carious lesion in outer enamel (polarized light ×40). The dark zone (DZ) shows positive birefringence when viewed in quinoline in contrast to the rest of the lesion (B) and sound enamel (E) which appears negatively birefringent. B. Same section as above now examined in water with polarized light. The body of the lesion (B) shows positive birefringence in contrast to the relatively unaffected surface zone (SZ) which is negative in sign.

The above work led to the conclusion that the formation of a micropore system must be regarded as a result of demineralization. This was consistent with evidence from microradiography where the region of visible radiolucency extended into the region of the dark zone.

In experimental studies on the remineralization of enamel caries, lesions were exposed to either saliva or a synthetic calcifying fluid *in vitro*. After exposure, there was a significant reduction in porosity, giving the histological appearance of a much earlier stage in lesion formation than that existing previously. The most obvious change was a broadening of the dark zone as a result of its extension back towards the enamel surface, into the region identified previously as the body of the lesion (Zone 3). In addition, lesions with no dark zones showed, after experiment, dark zones

positioned at the appropriate site between the translucent zone and the body of the lesion. Therefore, part of the body of the lesion (Zone 3) had reverted to the histological characteristics of the dark zone (Zone 2).

Prior to this finding the dark zone had been regarded as a breakdown stage successional to the translucent zone and preceding the body of the lesion. If some of the relatively large pores of the body of the lesion could, in effect, become the minute ones of the dark zone, then this could indicate that the micropores may not be formed by a simple process of demineralization. The zone may not be a stage in the sequential breakdown of the tissue, but may be formed by "remineralization" whereby the size of the large pores is reduced by the deposition of material. If this were so, it would lend support to the concept that the carious process in enamel is a dynamic one, comprising alternate phases of demineralization and remineralization, rather than a more simple process of continuing dissolution. The role of remineralization in the mechanism of carious dissolution of enamel has been dealt with in greater detail elsewhere (Silverstone, 1973).

Zone 3: The Body of the Lesion

The body of the lesion is the largest proportion of carious enamel in the small lesion, consisting of the whole area superficial to the dark zone and deep to the relatively unaffected surface of the enamel. When a longitudinal ground section is examined in quinoline with transmitted light, the body of the lesion appears relatively translucent compared with sound enamel (figs. 3 and 4). However, the striae of Retzius within this region are well marked and therefore appear enhanced in contrast to the translucency of the area. When the section is examined with polarized light after imbibition with water, the body of the lesion shows as a region of positive birefringence in contrast to the negative birefringence of the rest of the lesion and sound enamel (fig. 5). This region shows a minimum pore volume of 5 per cent of spaces, at its periphery, increasing to 25 per cent or greater in the centre of the small intact surface lesion.

When the section is examined by microradiography, the region of visible radiolucency corresponds closely with the size and distribution of the body of the lesion. However, when examined in more detail, the advancing front of the radiolucent region is seen to extend deep to the body of the lesion, into the dark zone. Superficially, the radiolucent region is limited by the presence of a well mineralized, radiopaque layer at the surface of the lesion (fig. 4). Alternate radiolucent and radiopaque lines can be seen passing obliquely through the subsurface region. The radiolucent lines, showing an apparent preferential demineralization, are spaced about 30 μm. apart. Many workers consider them to be the striae of Retzius. Within the radiolucent region a pattern of alternating radiolucent and radiopaque lines can also be seen running approximately at right-angles to the enamel surface (fig 6). These structures are spaced 6–8 μm. apart and are parallel to prism structure. In addition, many regions show a pattern of radiolucent lines at right-angles to prism direction. Since these are spaced at approximately 4 μm., they are thought to represent the cross striations of the prisms. Microradiographs of sections of carious enamel prepared in a direction transverse to prism structure show a pattern of circles having radiolucent centres with narrow radiopaque borders (fig. 7). The radiolucent circles have a diameter of about $5\,\mu$m. and have been interpreted as demonstrating a preferential demineralization of the prism cores.

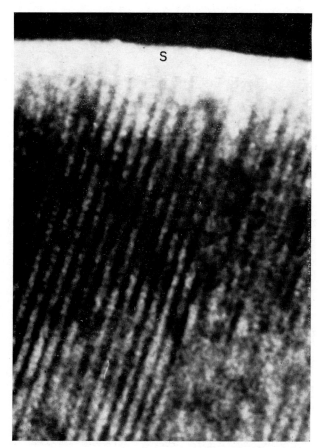

FIG. 6. Microradiograph showing the surface (S) and body of the lesion in a section of enamel caries ($\times 150$). Radiolucent and radiopaque lines are seen almost at right angles to the enamel surface, indicating a pattern of demineralization in relation to the long axes of the prisms.

Not all workers agree that the striae of Retzius are necessarily the channels along which there is a preferential demineralization. The appearance has also been explained on the basis that alternate bands are demineralized in relatively fixed proportions. The alternate incremental banding may therefore be only a reflection of an existing structural relationship "unmasked" by the process of demineralization.

Zone 4: The Surface Zone

One of the important characteristics of caries of human dental enamel is that the greatest degree of demineralization occurs at a subsurface level, so that the small lesion remains covered by a surface layer which appears relatively unaffected by the attack. When a small lesion is examined with the polarizing microscope after imbibition with a medium having a refractive index remote from that of the enamel (*e.g.* water), although the porous subsurface enamel is seen to be positively birefringent (fig. 5), the surface zone retains a negative birefringence. This relatively unaffected surface zone is also identifiable on microradiographs as a radiopaque surface layer, approximately $30\,\mu$m. in depth, sharply demarcated from the underlying radiolucent subsurface region of the lesion (fig. 4). The greater resistance of the surface enamel to carious dissolution has been explained as being due, in part at least, to its higher degree of mineralization compared with subsurface enamel. This, together with a higher fluoride content, and perhaps a greater amount of insoluble protein in the surface enamel, may explain why it is less soluble than subsurface tissue.

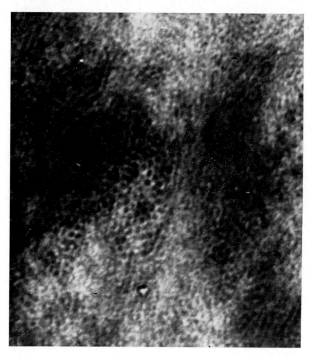

FIG. 7. Microradiograph of a section of carious enamel prepared transverse to prism structure ($\times 100$). Where prisms have been cut transversely, a pattern of circles having radiolucent centres with narrow radiopaque borders can be seen.

However, several workers have removed part of the natural enamel surface prior to *in vitro* experiments with acid buffer solutions in order to see if a surface zone would form superficial to the lesion on the new enamel surface. Artificial lesions created on such abraded enamel surfaces, which had up to $500\,\mu$m. of surface enamel cut away prior to experiment, showed well-mineralized surface layers (fig. 8) overlying subsurface regions demonstrating high degrees of dissolution.

These observations suggest that the special physical and chemical properties of surface enamel, relative to subsurface enamel, are not entirely responsible for the presence of a well-mineralized surface zone above the small carious lesion. The suggestion is that the surface zone remains intact and well mineralized because it is a site where calcium and phosphate ions, released by subsurface dissolution, become reprecipitated. This process is referred to as remineralization. The high fluoride concentration of surface enamel, presumably released at the initiation of solution of outer enamel, would favour remineralization. The surface zone is thus maintained at a relatively low level of demineralization throughout lesion formation and progression. Eventually, the surface zone is demineralized, usually at the stage when the lesion has penetrated some way into the dentine. This attack upon the surface itself has been reported as being a late stage in the carious process in enamel, and commences from the outer contour of the surface zone inwards.

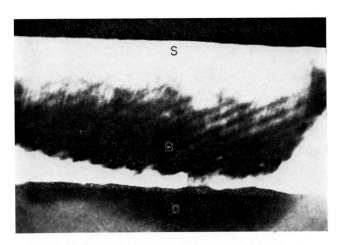

Fig. 8. Microradiograph of an artificial lesion created on abraded enamel (× 50). About 500 μm of the original enamel surface was ground off the tooth prior to lesion formation. There is marked demineralization in the subsurface enamel (B) and in the underlying dentine (D). However, the surface overlying the lesion shows a well mineralized surface zone (S).

The Organic Matrix

The outer layer of enamel, whether intact or carious, has a higher organic content than deeper layers but there is widespread agreement that the organic content of carious enamel overall is greater than that of the sound tissue. The organic material is amorphous and may be of bacterial, or mixed salivary and bacterial origin. Many workers have reported the penetration of exogenous organic material into defects in the surface enamel overlying the small carious lesion. These plaque-filled defects vary in size but are about 3 μm. in width, penetrating the tooth surface to depths of 5–10 μm. (fig. 9). Decalcified ultra-thin sections of carious enamel from the body of the lesion reveal a network of organic material. The spaces within this network are comparable in size and shape to the mineral crystals in the section before decalcification. This gives the impression that the organic network forms envelopes which ensheath the crystals. There is clearly a lack of detailed information on the specific composition of the organic material in carious enamel. The organic matrix could play a more important role in the initiation and progress of the lesion than is generally thought.

Ultrastructural Studies on Carious Enamel

It was hoped that the introduction of ultrastructural techniques would help to resolve some of the problems of interpretation which have existed at the light microscope level. However, progress has been slow, mainly because of technical difficulties involved in the preparation of ultra-thin sections from such a hard tissue.

It has, however, been shown that carious enamel exhibits a diffuse demineralization, with an increase in intercrystallite distance affecting all areas within the prisms and

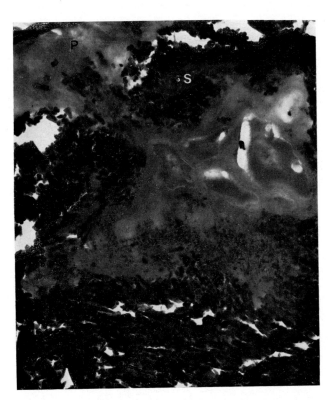

Fig. 9. Electron micrograph showing the enamel surface (S) from a small carious lesion demonstrating a typical surface defect about 3 μm in diameter containing a few bacteria, and filled with a hyaline material continuous with the surface pellicle (P) (× 31,500). (By courtesy of Dr. N. W. Johnson.)

interprismatic enamel (fig. 10). Several workers have observed narrow channels, 50–100 nm. wide, partially surrounding the prisms in the carious tissue when examined in transverse section (fig. 10). The effects of caries on individual crystals in enamel appear to be of two types. Firstly, mineral is removed from the external surface of the crystals, seen as an irregularity of their margins. In the second type, central defects are found, the preferential loss of crystal centres resulting in the appearance of "hairpin" shapes due to longitudinal splitting of the crystals (fig. 11). In transverse section, the damaged crystals are seen as hollow hexagons or rectangles.

In addition to damage to crystals, several workers have also recorded the frequent finding of large crystals at prism borders when examining carious enamel in transverse section. These thicker and more electron-dense crystals are larger than those found in sound enamel and are thought to be formed as a result of remineralization.

Studies reported by a number of electron microscopists indicate that carious destruction of human dental enamel may not be as dependent on the structural detail of the

as identified with the polarizing microscope, cannot be distinguished from sound enamel by ultrastructural means. Therefore, the first area of change from sound enamel seen with the electron microscope appears to coincide with the body of the lesion.

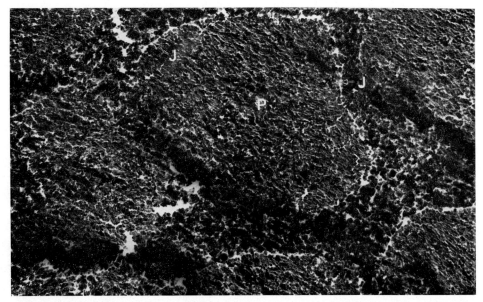

FIG. 10. Electron micrograph through the body of a lesion of enamel caries cut transversely to prism direction ($\times 17,700$). P = prisms, J = narrow channels present at prism junctions. The channels are not artefact since they contain embedding material. A diffuse demineralization is present throughout the tissue.

tissue as has previously been believed. However, such an interpretation must be viewed with caution since many structural features readily visible with the light microscope, cannot be identified by transmission electron microscopy. Tissue changes within the first two stages of enamel caries,

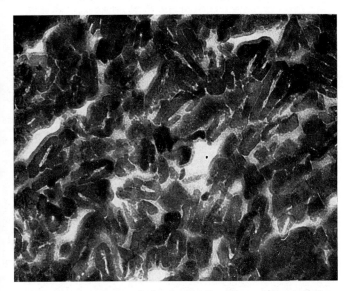

FIG. 11. Electron micrograph showing details of the apatite crystals from the body of the enamel lesion ($\times 106,250$). The external outlines of the crystals are irregular due to surface etching. Many crystals have central defects which appear as longitudinal splitting, giving the crystals a "hairpin" shape. (By courtesy of Dr. N. W. Johnson.)

CARIES OF DENTINE

Whilst caries in enamel is clearly a dynamic process, the tissue is devoid of cells and is therefore incapable of reacting in a vital manner. However, this is not the case with dentine which must be considered as integral with the pulp and therefore capable of defence reactions.

The Small Dentine Lesion Deep to An Intact Enamel Surface

When the advancing front of the enamel lesion reaches the ameloduntal junction, the enamel surface is still intact. In the case of smooth-surface lesions, lateral spread of the lesion along the ameloduntal junction results in a broad base to the dentine lesion. The dentine lesion follows the primary curvature of the dentinal tubules so that its narrow apex approaches the pulpal surface at a level cervical to the point at which the lesion enters the dentine (fig. 12). Thus, the established dentinal lesion is conical with its base on the ameloduntal junction and its truncated apex pointing towards the pulp (fig. 12).

In the case of fissure caries, lateral spread of the enamel lesion at the ameloduntal junction results in the area of involved dentine being larger than that seen in smooth surface lesions. However, because the tubules are relatively straight over the occlusal aspect of the pulp chamber, the lesion does not taper so much towards the pulp. Thus a relatively large area of dentine is affected, in spite of an apparently small lesion in the occlusal surface. Although the enamel surface is intact when the lesion reaches the amelodentinal junction, acids are able to diffuse to the dentine via carious enamel, which is extremely porous compared with sound enamel. This, together with other chemical stimuli, causes the pulpo-dentinal unit to respond. At this early stage, the initial dentine lesion consists of two main zones.

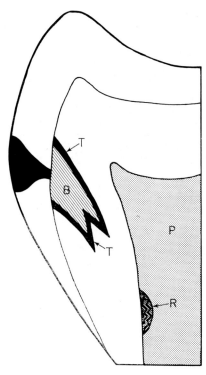

FIG. 12. Diagram of a small lesion of dentine caries below an intact enamel surface. T = translucent zone, B = body of the lesion, R = reactionary dentine, P = pulp.

Firstly, there is a zone of sclerosis walling off the lesion from the surrounding normal dentine. This zone of sclerosis is often referred to as the translucent zone, which is a defence reaction on the part of the pulpo-dentinal unit. A further defence reaction can be seen some distance from the lesion. A region of reactionary, or reparative, dentine is laid down on the pulpal aspect of the lesion as shown in fig. 12. This latter defence reaction effectively increases the depth of tissue between the invading lesion and the pulp.

Contained within the sclerotic, or translucent, zone and limited by the amelodentinal junction is the second zone, the body of the lesion.

The Translucent Zone

The translucent zone, or zone of sclerosis, is formed as a result of mild stimulation. In this zone, mineral is laid down within the dentinal tubules to form a barrier of sufficient density to inhibit the diffusion of acids (figs. 13 and 14). Later, this barrier also limits the diffusion of proteolytic enzymes and the progress of bacteria along the tubules towards the pulp. This has been confirmed by isotope and

dye diffusion studies. The zone of sclerosis shows as a clear translucent zone when ground sections are examined by transmitted light (fig. 13). This is because light passes through the more homogeneous region relative to adjacent areas in which the light is scattered. The sclerotic zone is therefore referred to as the translucent zone, but should not be confused with the translucent zone in the enamel lesion. The translucent zone tends to occur at the periphery of the dentine lesion where the stimulus is reduced. In microradiographs of ground sections, the translucent zone is seen to be radiopaque relative to normal dentine, showing it to be hypermineralized.

It is believed that the calcified matrix within the tubule may be formed by an acceleration of the normal physiological process of peritubular dentine formation. This

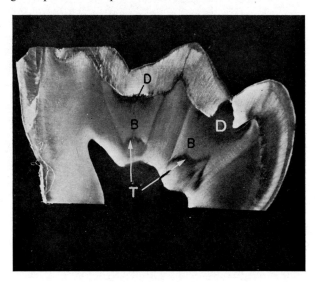

FIG. 13. Ground section from a deciduous molar examined in water by reflected light showing two carious lesions (×10). T = translucent zone, B = body of the lesion, D = zone of destruction. (By courtesy of Drs. N. W. Johnson, B. R. Taylor and Prof. D. S. Berman.)

would occur in response to relatively mild stimulation such as might be expected at the periphery of a lesion. Electron diffraction studies have suggested that the mineral is apatite. The crystals appear identical to those found in normal peritubular dentine when examined by electron microscopy (fig. 14). However, in demineralized ultra-thin sections, the organic matrix within the occluded tubules is not always the same as that seen in the peritubular dentine since it appears much denser and more homogeneous. For this reason, the process of sclerosis in the translucent zone cannot be regarded as identical to the normal process of peritubular dentine formation. Both the peritubular matrix and the intertubular matrix appear normal at this stage.

The Body of the Lesion

This region is not, as yet, infected since bacteria cannot gain access until a cavity forms in the overlying enamel. In the superficial part of the body of the lesion, both the peritubular dentine and intertubular dentine are partially demineralized. Tubules towards the centre and base of the cone-shaped lesion, in which irritation of their processes caused death of many odontoblasts, form the so-called "dead tract". This is associated with the deposition of an acellular calcific obstruction, termed "eburnoid", within the tubule at the pulpal end of the affected area. Tubules within the dead tract probably contain remnants of odontoblast processes together with air. Since air has a low refractive index, the dead tract in a ground section will appear dark in transmitted light.

It is at this stage that the lesion can first be detected on clinical "bite-wing" radiographs. Although the dentine has already been demineralized, the lesion would only appear as a wedge-shaped region of radiolucency confined to the outer enamel. It is essential that the clinician appreciates the true extent of the lesion at this stage, but it is not implied that such lesions must necessarily be restored immediately. If preventive measures are instituted, the lesion can remain static or even regress. However, such lesions must be examined radiographically at regular intervals. If evidence

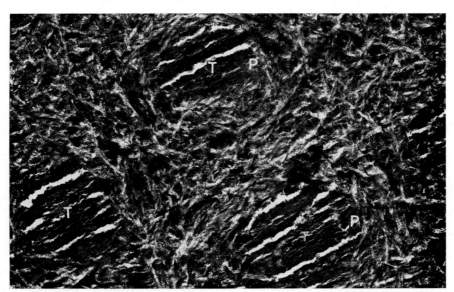

FIG. 14. Undemineralized ultra-thin section from the translucent zone of a lesion of dentine caries (×18,000). The tubules (T) are filled with crystals indistinguishable from those in the surrounding peritubular dentine (B). Gaps within the tubules are sectioning artefacts. (By courtesy of Drs. N. W. Johnson, B. R. Taylor and Prof. D. S. Berman.)

Reactionary Dentine

Reactionary dentine is a layer of tubular dentine formed at the surface of the pulp chamber deep to the dentine lesion. Sometimes referred to as secondary dentine, it varies in structure from well-formed tissue, indistinguishable from adjacent primary dentine, to severely dysplastic tissue in which there may be few tubules and many interglobular areas. Regular reactionary dentine is formed in response to a mild stimulus. With increasing degrees of stimulus, there is a greater chance of damage to odontoblasts. This in turn leads to increased dysplasia of the tissue formed. No reactionary dentine will be formed when the stimulus is sufficiently severe to cause the death of large numbers of odontoblasts, although occasionally other cells in the pulp differentiate to produce a layer of atubular calcified tissue.

Thus the changes, or regions, which occur in the tissue at this stage and are shown diagrammatically in fig. 12 can be listed, from the pulp outwards, as:

(a) A mild degree of irritation in the pulp;
(b) production of a zone of reactionary dentine;
(c) a region of normal dentine;
(d) a translucent zone;
(e) the body of the lesion.

of their progression is found, the decision to restore should be made.

The Lesion of Dentine Caries After Cavitation of the Enamel

Once the enamel lesion becomes a cavity, bacteria are able to penetrate into the tissue and the rate of progression of the dentine lesion increases. The pathway for invasion of the dentine by the pioneer organisms is along the dentinal tubules. The first wave of bacteria infecting the dentine are primarily acidogenic. The acid they produce diffuses deep to, and in advance of, the organisms causing demineralization as far as the translucent zone. It has been suggested that the bacterial invasion of dentine occurs in two waves. The first wave consists of lactobacilli which occupy tubules towards the periphery of the lesion, but without enlargement of the tubules. The second invasion is a mixed one which produces widening of the occupied tubules and considerable damage to the surrounding dentine. Towards the amelodentinal junction, there is a more mixed bacterial population in which proteolytic and hydrolytic enzymes are added to the effect of acid production, resulting in destruction of the organic collagenous matrix of the tissue.

At this stage too, the dentine lesion can again be described as consisting of a translucent zone and the body of the lesion.

The pulp will show a mild degree of inflammation, and a further layer of reactionary dentine is deposited on the pulpal aspect of the lesion. However, tissue changes at this stage are more complex than in the previous stage where the surface of the enamel was still intact. Thus the body of the lesion may be conveniently divided into three regions, giving a total of four discrete zones in the dentine lesion (fig. 15).

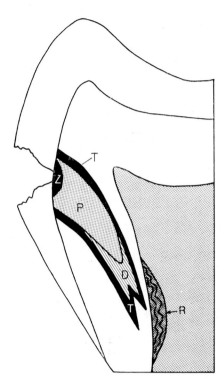

Fig. 15. Diagram of a dentine lesion deep to a small carious cavity in the enamel. Z = zone of destruction, P = zone of penetration, D = zone of demineralization, T = translucent zone, R = reactionary dentine.

1. The Translucent Zone

The translucent zone is the most deeply placed zone and still walls off the rest of the lesion from sound dentine.

The body of the lesion is once again contained within the translucent zone and the amelodentinal junction, but may now be divided into three areas, representing zones, 2, 3 and 4 in the lesion.

2. The Zone of Demineralization

The deep edge of the body of the lesion is usually bacteria-free. This region superficial to, but contiguous with, the translucent zone has been demineralized and may therefore be referred to as the zone of demineralization (fig. 15). Large plate-like crystals have been found within the tubules in this region of the lesion. It was concluded that they were produced as a response to mild stimulation and the consensus of opinion is that they are octacalcium phosphate.

3. The Zone of Penetration

The zone of penetration refers to the region of the body of the lesion which contains bacteria. Many of the tubules within this area are enlarged. The advancing front of the bacterial infection is usually superficial to the translucent zone. Over large areas of the zone of penetration, bacteria are confined to the tubules. In many tubules, the organisms have multiplied to such an extent that they show varying degrees of degeneration (fig. 16). It is thought that as the bacteria multiply, so they out-run their nutritional

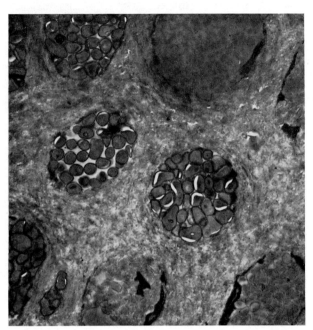

Fig. 16. Electron micrograph from the zone of penetration, demineralized and stained with phosphotungstic acid (×7,500). Both the intertubular and peritubular dentine are heavily demineralized. Whilst some tubules contain viable bacteria, others show bacteria in varying degrees of degeneration. (By courtesy of Drs. N. W. Johnson, B. R. Taylor and Prof. D. S. Berman.)

requirements. Remnants of densely mineralized tissue are usually present in bacteria-filled tubules, usually positioned at the periphery of the tubule (fig. 17). The crystal structure of these regions is indistinguishable from that of the peritubular dentine, and the sclerosed tubular matrix of the translucent zone. These areas have been interpreted as residues of either one component or the other. In the zone of penetration, the intertubular dentine is extensively demineralized. Typical banding is still present on collagen fibres but this does not preclude the possibility that substantial changes may have taken place in the matrix, particularly in its mucopolysaccharide component. There is also histochemical evidence to show that the lipid component of the matrix has been released from its binding to protein.

4. The Zone of Destruction

Finally, a zone of destruction is seen at the amelodentinal junction forming the base of the body of the lesion (figs. 13 and 15). It is heavily discoloured and little of the normal

THE STRUCTURE OF CARIOUS LESIONS 399

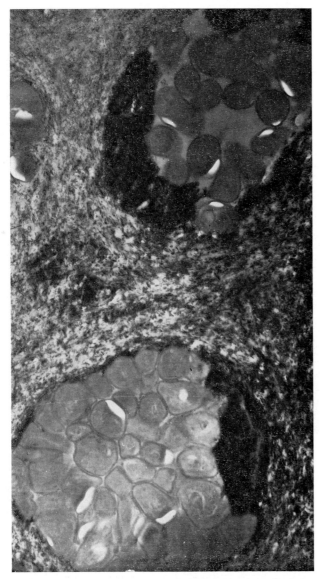

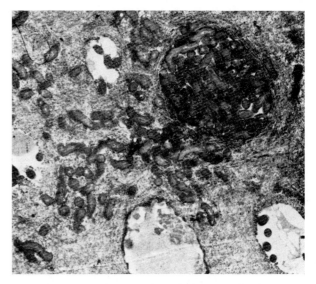

FIG. 18. Electron micrograph from the border region between the zone of penetration and the zone of destruction (×3,500). Adjacent to a bacteria-filled tubule the intertubular dentine is invaded by numerous bacteria. (By courtesy of Prof. N. B. B. Symons.)

FIG. 17. Electron micrograph of an ultra-thin section from the zone of penetration in dentine caries (×14,500). Remnants of densely mineralized tissue are present in the bacteria-filled tubules. The crystals are similar to those of peritubular dentine, and the sclerosed tubular matrix of the translucent zone. (By courtesy of Drs. N. W. Johnson, B. R. Taylor and Prof. D. S. Berman.)

arrested. Organisms will invade the reactionary dentine, finally to reach the pulp.

Arrested Caries

In the advanced dentine lesion, lateral spread of the carious process along the amelodentinal junction undermines much of the sound enamel. Eventually the unsupported enamel fractures, giving rise to a large cavity. If the exposed softened dentine is removed by attrition, the affected surface eventually appears smooth and polished and the carious process becomes arrested. Whereas actively progressing dentine caries is light brown and soft, arrested dentine caries

architecture of dentine remains. In this zone, microbial action has completely destroyed the substance of the dentine. Little or no mineral remains and micro-organisms, initially confined to tubules and their lateral branches, now invade the peritubular and intertubular dentine (fig. 18). Aggregations of bacteria and necrotic tissue coalesce in the softened matrix to form areas known as liquefaction foci (figs. 19 and 20). Destruction of the tissue is often more advanced along the incremental lines of growth, producing transverse clefts (fig. 21). This is the reason why carious dentine can be excavated with hand instruments in large sheets in a plane parallel to the amelodentinal junction.

The degree of inflammation in the pulp increases progressively. Any reactionary dentine formed will be extremely dysplastic and eventually dentinogenesis will be

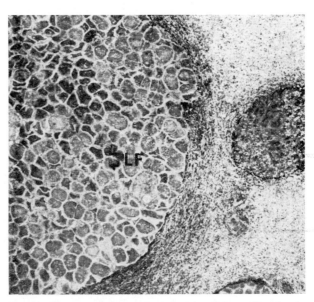

FIG. 19. Electron micrograph from the zone of destruction showing a large bacteria-filled cavity, a liquefaction focus (LF). The size can be compared with the enlarged tubule to the right-hand side of the field (×3,500). (By courtesy of Prof. N. B. B. Symons.)

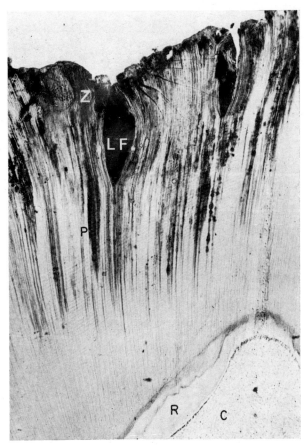

FIG. 20. Demineralized section of carious dentine examined in transmitted light (H & E, ×30). Z = zone of destruction, P = zone of penetration, LF = liquefaction focus, R = reactionary dentine, C = inflammatory cells in pulp.

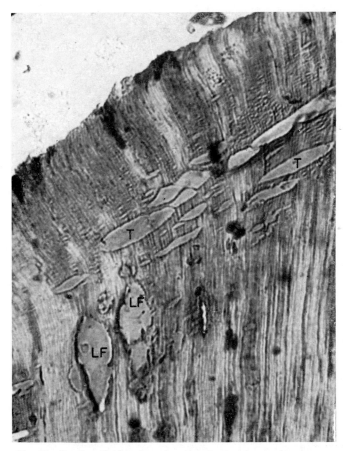

FIG. 21. Demineralized section of carious dentine showing transverse clefts (T) and liquefaction foci (LF) (×50).

appears dark brown, and has a tough leathery texture. This is due to the accumulation of organic and mineral deposits from oral fluid.

REFERENCES

Silverstone, L. M. (1973), "Structure of Carious Enamel, Including the Early Lesion," in *Oral Sciences Reviews* (A. H. Melcher and G. A. Zarb, Eds.). Copenhagen: Munksgaard.

33. THE EPIDEMIOLOGY OF DENTAL CARIES

D. J. BECK

Epidemiology may be defined as a science that deals with the incidence, distribution, and control of disease in a population. This chapter will deal with the first two of these topics—the incidence (or, more correctly in this context, the prevalence) and distribution of dental caries in the world's population, today and in historical times, with some discussion of the control of the disease.

Dental caries affects different population groups to differing extents. In some instances it occurs as a rampant destructive disease while in some fortunate people the disease is totally absent. Between these two extremes lies a variable pattern of severity.

Scientific knowledge has only limited explanations for the varying patterns of distribution of this disease. Some gross oversimplifications can be made—the more fermentable carbohydrate a population group consumes, and the more frequently it is consumed, the more dental caries appears. But this **is** an oversimplification. There are those who eat frequent meals and snacks containing sucrose, the 'arch criminal in dental caries', and yet remain caries free. Like so many biological phenomena, a frequency distribution of the prevalence of dental caries takes the shape of a normal curve; at one tail of the bell-shaped curve are the caries immune individuals; at the other end of the curve are individuals with rampant dental caries. The known attacking forces of dental caries (notably carbohydrate consumption) and the established preventive agents, (notably fluorides), can shift this normal curve along the base line, left or right, but a spectrum of the disease persists. Rampant dental caries still occurs in areas of long term optimum water fluoridation (rarely, however, as the fluoride ion has shifted the normal curve to the left) and the habitual sugar eater without the benefits of fluoride intake may occasionally be shown to be caries immune. This complexity of the normal curve contributes to making the epidemiology of dental caries an interesting subject. Invariably a spectrum of intensity is found in any one population group. This is probably one of the reasons that many people—dentists included—hardly think of dental caries as a disease at all. Erroneously, it is thought of as a petty annoyance that mankind must simply put up with. This erroneous belief, in turn, leads to a widespread disinterest in, and suspicion of, the available, workable means of preventing dental caries. A process such as water fluoridation obviously does not eradicate the disease in the way a successful programme of immunisation against poliomyelitis can. With a sample size of one the effect of water fluoridation may be obscure. Only in population groups may the useful shift of the normal curve of caries prevalence in the direction of prevention and control be detected.

THE MEASUREMENT OF DENTAL CARIES: THE TOOLS OF EPIDEMIOLOGY

The dental epidemiologist, unlike his colleague the clinician, turns his back on the problems and needs of individual dental patients. Instead he directs attention to groups of people, grouped in any logical fashion that he chooses, and so grouped that some specific research enquiry about the distribution of disease will be answered by the study undertaken. The grouping may be geographic, by age and sex or other such stratifying factors, or chronological—the examination of prehistoric or historic skulls for dental caries being an example of the latter. It is this interest in groups of people rather than individuals that distinguishes the epidemiologist from the clinician. From it follow two important characteristics of how the epidemiologist goes about his work. The first of these is that he must have some sort of measure or index by which to gauge the extent and severity of dental caries in the group under investigation. For the clinician who at any one time is dealing with a sample size of one—an individual patient—the conventional dental record card is an adequate measure of dental caries. For the epidemiologist, a pile of a hundred or a thousand such clinical record cards would be an unwieldy research tool indeed. From such a series of tooth charts it is difficult to gain an impression of the

SCIENTIFIC FOUNDATIONS OF DENTISTRY

characteristics of dental caries in the group. The epidemiologist needs to know two things in summary about this group of people. He wants to know the mean level of intensity of dental caries—central tendency—and he wants to know how much variability in this intensity occurs within the group—scatter. So he substitutes for the clinician's record card an index for dental caries, the aim being to express for each individual a single numerical figure (for ease in data processing) that measures the intensity of past and present dental caries attack in that individual. Central tendency can then be measured by a simple mean, and scatter by any suitable measure, commonly the standard deviation.

The second characteristic of the epidemiologist's work that results from his dealing with groups of people rather than individuals is that the result of the dental examination he undertakes may be dissimilar from the dental examination undertaken at the same time by the patient's own dentist. This must be so as the examinations are done for different reasons. When the clinician charts a tooth surface as carious he is saying that in his professional judgement the tooth surface requires restoration or some other treatment. The epidemiologist, on the other hand, is not committing himself or anyone else to therapeutic procedures for any surface he charts as carious—nor for that matter to standing idle about any surface he charts as sound. The epidemiologist has entirely different goals, the most important of which are reproducibility and reliability of examination.

This fundamental difference between the two types of dental examination was clearly illustrated in a recent epidemiological study undertaken by the World Health Organization. The protocol for this study allowed for the recording of a sound tooth (caries-free) with, at the same time, the tooth being recorded as having a requirement for restoration. This rather strange event occurred when the epidemiologist, using the epidemiological criteria established for the study, decided that the tooth did not meet the criteria for dental caries and was accordingly sound. Then, to get the most realistic estimate of treatment needs in the community, the epidemiologist started thinking like a clinician when deciding treatment needs. He looked at the tooth again and asked himself the question, "If this were my own patient in dental practice, and not a survey subject, would I fill that tooth now?" If the answer to that question were "yes" then he dictated to his recorder the appropriate treatment need. Such a filling would normally be a prophylactic or very early therapeutic one.

Percentage Prevalence

The epidemiology of dental caries is more complex than that of many diseases in that normally multiple lesions are, or have been present in the dentition; in the epidemiology of poliomyelitis, lung cancer, or traffic accidents the condition is often simply recorded as present or absent in each member of the community. Such point prevalences (the prevalence at one point in time) is not normally helpful in regard to dental caries for in most samples studied the figure arrived at is close to 100 per cent. Prevalence of dental caries expressed as a percentage of persons affected finds its main usefulness in three situations where the percentage figures can be expected to be considerably less than 100 per cent and so more meaningful; it has been used to report caries prevalence in skulls of people who lived in earlier centuries when caries was a far less prevalent disease; it has also been used in studying primitive people not exposed to a modern diet; and it has been used in surveys of young children (up to the age of three or four years) who have not experienced the full attack of dental caries. For most other groups a more sensitive measure than this simple head-count is required.

The Tooth as a Counting Unit

The tooth provides an obvious and useful counting unit for dental caries and it is a unit of considerably more sensitivity than merely counting the numbers of people suffering from caries. This disease is, of course, an irreversible one; a cut finger or a boil on the neck heal completely and the affected tissue is usually restored to complete functional normality. This is not so with dental caries. Once a tooth has been attacked by dental caries the "scars" of that attack persist. Such a "scar" may take one of three main forms: firstly, it may be in the form of a carious lesion—active or arrested—still present and untreated on the tooth; secondly, it may be a filling where the diseased tooth tissue has been removed and a restoration made; and thirdly, the ultimate fate may have overtaken the tooth—there is a gap in the arch and the tooth is missing. This, of course, is the basis of the classical index for dental caries using the tooth as the unit of measurement—the DMF (decayed, missing, and filled) index. This index is sometimes called DMFT to indicate that the unit of measurement is the tooth and to distinguish it from the equivalent surface index, DMFS. The index for an individual is simply calculated as the sum of the numbers of decayed teeth, missing teeth, and filled teeth.

The DMFT Index

The DMFT index has come to be almost universally accepted as the most effective and reliable measuring system in the epidemiology of dental caries. Challenges from other systems, notably the DMFS index, have never been strong. Just as changing from point prevalence, where the unit of measurement is the person, to DMFT increases sensitivity of the measuring device, so changing from DMFT to DMFS in turn also increases sensitivity. But the price for this increased sensitivity is reduced reliability and reproducibility. Sensitivity may be even further increased compared with that of DMFS by again reducing the size of the unit and counting individual carious lesions rather than tooth surfaces but again reliability is reduced. The inverse relationship between reliability and sensitivity as the unit of measurement is increased or decreased in size is illustrated in fig. 1.

Most agree that for epidemiological work the tooth, that is DMFT, has optimum sensitivity and reliability. On the other hand, in the clinical testing of caries-preventing agents where greater sensitivity is required to detect sometimes small differences in caries increments between control and experimental groups of subjects, the DMFS index is often the index of choice; but such work demands great scientific discipline on the part of the investigator because of the innate relatively low reliability and reproducibility of the DMFS index.

make the best clinical judgement he can regarding the reason for tooth loss. If, in his judgement, he concludes that caries was the major reason for the loss, the tooth is classified M; if on the other hand, he concludes that periodontal disease was the major reason, the tooth is classified A (absent for reasons other than caries). This latter solution, currently recommended by the World Health Organization, at least avoids the spurious data of the type shown in fig. 2, even if it does confront the examiner with a few difficult decisions in the field.

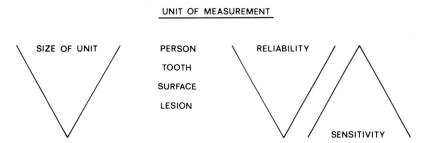

UNIT OF MEASUREMENT

SIZE OF UNIT   PERSON   RELIABILITY
                    TOOTH
                    SURFACE
                    LESION
                                               SENSITIVITY

FIG. 1. Relationship between sensitivity and reliability of dental caries measuring systems as the unit of measurement increases or decreases in size.

Rules for the DMFT Index

Many ground rules governing the DMFT index have been developed. For instance, each tooth is only counted once so that a tooth that has a filling and also is carious is counted as a decayed tooth and the presence of the filling is ignored. Unerupted teeth, teeth lost by trauma, congenitally absent teeth, and teeth extracted for orthodontic reasons are excluded from the survey, commonly being coded "A" (for absent) in the field. Teeth that have been lost for periodontal reasons pose a particular problem in the DMFT index. Often in adult subjects, particularly of middle-age or older, tooth spaces are encountered where it is difficult to decide whether the tooth was lost for periodontal reasons, because of dental caries, or, as is commonly the case, because of a combination of both diseases. Two solutions to this problem have been used. The first ignores the problem altogether—all such teeth are classed as M. This poses few difficulties in children but can be dangerous in adults. This danger is clearly seen in fig. 2 showing the DMFT, by age groups, for a group of subjects from the Tokelau Islands in the South Pacific. These people were relatively untouched by western civilisation and showed the low level of caries attack to be expected under such conditions. Although fig. 2 is concerned with DMF and, therefore, assumedly caries, the most significant feature of the curves, the steeply rising slope from middle-age onwards, is at least influenced by periodontal disease. Certainly in this population there does indeed appear to be an increase in caries activity in later life (a rather unusual finding) but some of the steepness of the slope can be attributed to tooth loss as a result of periodontal disease with consequently an artificially expanded M component of the DMF.

The second solution to the problem of the tooth lost for periodontal reasons requires the examiner in every case to

Teeth that are difficult or impossible to examine are excluded from the investigation (coded X in the field). This group includes teeth that have been restored for reasons other than caries (trauma or aesthetics), teeth used as bridge abutments, banded for orthodontic reasons, and impacted teeth.

Many of the ground rules of the types discussed here for DMFT are given in the World Health Organization (1971) publication *Oral Health Surveys. Basic Methods*, a volume that should be regarded as the authoritative sourcebook in all such matters.

Refinements of the DMFT Index

Further refinements of the DMFT have been suggested and used. A common one today, recommended by WHO, is to subdivide the category D into a new D, which becomes decayed teeth that can be saved by restoration or other means, and I, which is a category of teeth indicated for extraction because of caries. Even further elaboration of DMFT is possible and a recent survey conducted by WHO probably took this process to its most advanced stage so far—teeth being categorised into no fewer than 12 groups: sound (S), traumatised (T), decayed (D), filled and primary decay (K), filled and secondary decay (Y), filled (F), crowned (C), crowned and decayed (Q), missing due to caries (M), missing due to periodontal disease (P), other absent (A), and excluded (X). The DMFT index has evolved into the STDKYFCQMPAXT index! Interestingly, in this advanced elaboration of DMFT, the category I (indicated for extraction) has been deleted. The reason for this is that the protocol for this study called for the recording, by rather elaborate codes, of the treatment needs of each tooth as well as its DMFT status. Computer processing of the data would therefore allow the computation of the category I if it were required.

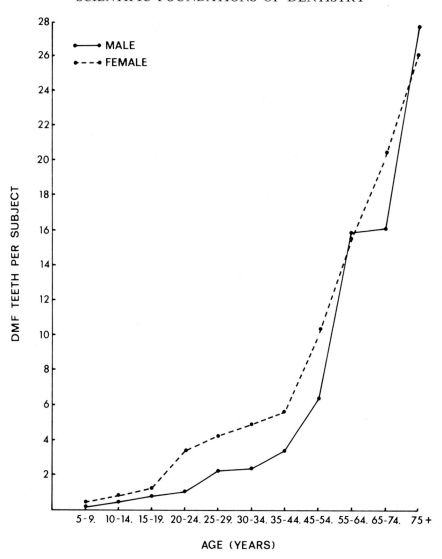

Fig. 2. The numbers of decayed, missing and filled (DMF) teeth per subject in a group of Tokelau Islanders, by age and sex. (Data from Beck and Ludwig, 1966.)

Problems with the DMFT Index

In designing the protocol of any epidemiological study involving DMFT much attention must be given to detail, the aim being consistency. As many problems as possible should be anticipated; inevitably however, some will be overlooked and will only appear once field work starts. When these problems arise it usually does not matter much what decision is taken, so long as the decision is made known to all participating epidemiologists—no matter how trivial the point appears to be—and they all abide by the decision throughout the study. An example of such little problems—and they are legion—is the exfoliated deciduous tooth; should it be scored as that or as an unerupted permanent tooth? Similarly, how are erupted supernumerary teeth to be handled? If a tooth is both traumatised and carious, in which of those two categories should it be placed? It certainly cannot be placed in both. Is a three-quarter crown a crown or a filling (if the DMFT technique being used makes a distinction between the

two)? In many of these cases flipping a coin is often as useful a way of making a decision as any but, once having been made it should be communicated—in writing—to all participating, abided by, and preferably made mention of in the report originating from the study, unless this course would lead to impossible verbosity.

Data on DMFT may be expressed in three main ways: as the total number of DMF teeth among the sample studied, the mean number of DMF teeth per person (by far the most usual method), or as the mean number of DMF teeth per hundred erupted teeth. The latter technique reduces fluctuation in the DMFT in children due to varying numbers of teeth at risk for dental caries, as more teeth erupt into the mouth. In calculating the value for DMFT per hundred erupted teeth care is required in deciding what the denominator should be; the numerator is no problem, being merely the sum of DMFT for the whole sample examined. The denominator is the sum of sound teeth and DMF teeth for the whole sample; in other words, the denominator, "erupted teeth", includes some teeth that are not present at all, M teeth. However, excluded from the denominator and the whole calculation are teeth coded A (unerupted teeth, teeth lost as a result of trauma, periodontal disease, or as a part of orthodontic treatment, and congenitally absent teeth) or X (teeth restored because of trauma or aesthetics, bridge abutments, or teeth banded for orthodontic reasons).

Versatility of the DMFT Index

The DMFT index is a remarkably versatile one for it may be manipulated in many ways to accentuate various facets of the pattern of dental caries in a community. The relative magnitude of the three independent components of the index, D, M, and F, is often of interest and this applies also to the category I when this has been included in the study design. A large value in this latter category indicates a need for better treatment service as the community under study is not even receiving an adequate extraction service, to say nothing of a restorative or preventive service. The percentage of subjects in various DMF categories is also often interesting. Examples of these are percentages of subjects with no D teeth (no restorative dentistry is required), percentage of subjects with no M teeth (intact dentitions), and percentage of subjects with 10 or more D teeth (taking this as an arbitrary but quantitative measure of rampant dental caries or at least those subjects with a need for extensive restorative dentistry). The ratio of F to DMF, expressed as a percentage, which has been called the "Care Index", is a useful measure of the adequacy of dental caries treatment service as F is a unit of success for a community's treatment services whereas D and M represent units of failure by the service. The closer the ratio F to DMF approaches 100 per cent the more efficient is the treatment service.

The Two Dentitions

Data on dental caries prevalence for the two dentitions, deciduous and permanent, should nearly always be expressed specifically. Probably the only justifiable exception to this rule is in young children for whom a percentage is expressed of those who, at the time of examination, were completely free of dental caries in both dentitions.

Separate indices, characterized by the use of lower case letters, have been established for the deciduous dentition. Because of the difficulty in distinguishing an exfoliated tooth, among the excluded teeth (x), from a tooth that has been extracted because of dental caries (m), it is often now recommended simply to exclude both groups of teeth and report results in the df index rather than the dmf index. As in its permanent counterpart, d teeth may be subdivided into two groups, a new d group composed of carious deciduous teeth which can be saved and i teeth, carious teeth indicated for extraction; this subdivision produces a dif index which has also been called a def index. The latter is a confusing term best avoided as in various authors' hands e has stood both for teeth indicated for extraction and teeth that had been extracted (i.e., m teeth).

THE ANTIQUITY OF DENTAL CARIES

Dental caries has affected mankind for a very long time. The disease is largely one of modern, westernized civilization—probably associated with diet—but it is by no means uniquely modern or westernized. The disease occurred many thousands of years ago in people living on a diet we would today regard as "non-cariogenic". The resistance of teeth to post-mortem destruction allows a study of the prevalence of dental caries through history as we can study no other disease. The prevalence and distribution of lung cancer, influenza, or syphilis 2,000 years ago is largely unknown; the prevalence of dental caries 2,000 years ago is fairly well established. Certainly the disease occurred then, and for many thousands of years before that, but it was relatively mild and infrequent. It did however, at times, progress to gross destruction of the tooth crown. Toothache must be a long-standing burden man has borne.

Probably the earliest established dating of the occurrence of dental caries is that reported in hominoid skulls of some half a million years ago. One particular skull from 10,000 to 50,000 years ago—Rhodesian Man—must once have belonged to an unfortunate individual very prone, for his population group, to dental caries; he would have fallen well out to the right of the normal curve of dental caries intensity for his group. Of Rhodesian Man's 15 teeth, 12 were carious and in five of these caries had advanced to complete destruction of the crowns. It is interesting, if idle, to speculate just what this man did about his toothache.

RACE, HEREDITY AND CARIES

The extent and severity of dental caries—or the location of the normal curve of dental caries distribution on the base-line—varies widely on a geographic basis. Dental caries is a much more serious problem in some racial groups than in others. The multifactorial aetiology of the disease makes it difficult to assess the extent to which this variability is associated with the many factors possibly involved. It is again possible to make simplistic generalizations, such as that dental caries tends to be a much more prevalent disease in westernized societies than it is in more primitive societies. But the question as to whether one racial group has an intrinsically greater resistance to this disease than another is difficult to answer. The most likely answer is that external variables such as food habits and dietary patterns, trace element (especially fluoride) intake, and even such diverse influences as climate and soil type are far more important in establishing the intensity of dental caries in a racial group than any innate, hereditarily determined susceptibility.

The Food-caries Relationship

In recent years simple sugars, notably sucrose, have received most attention as caries-producing agents. There is more than enough evidence based on laboratory and clinical investigation and epidemiological observation to establish as fact that sucrose intake is involved in the carious process. The recent focusing of attention on sucrose by dental research workers is largely attributable to the discovery that sucrose may be involved in two ways: its traditional role as a substrate for bacterial degradation to organic acids resulting in the decalcification of hard tooth tissue, and its more recently discovered involvement in plaque formation through the polymerization of sucrose to dextrans and levans which may well be important components of plaque contributing to its 'stickiness'. Sucrose may have a further role yet in dental caries: it may be polymerized by cariogenic bacteria to polysaccharides of the glycogen-amylopectin group for the intracellular storage of carbohydrate. Later bacterial catabolism of this stored carbohydrate may produce further acid and so possibly prolong the low pH conditions of plaque and encourage further decalcification.

Such interesting speculation has certainly furthered our knowledge of the relationship between food and dental caries but, at the same time, the enthusiasm to label sucrose as the arch-criminal in dental caries may have obscured the importance of other food components, especially starches, in the aetiology of dental caries. The epidemiological evidence of dental caries in different racial groups certainly suggests that we should be considering the total carbohydrate character of the diet rather than just the sucrose content. Among these characteristics are the frequency of carbohydrate consumption, the ratio of solid to liquid carbohydrate foods and, perhaps of central importance, the staple cereal of the diet, usually predominantly one of the three: wheat, rice, or corn. An interesting recent speculation is that some of the variation in caries between different racial groups may be attributable to the traditional method of cooking cereals; the high temperatures of baking, through dextrinisation of starch, may render it a more suitable substrate for bacterial degradation to acid than the lower temperatures of boiling which breaks the starch granules (gelation) for easier digestion but leaves the starch molecules intact. The fact that in any one cultural group dental caries tends to be more prevalent in more temperate climates than in warmer climates may be associated with the greater consumption of baked cereal-based foods in the cooler areas. Of course confectionery consumption may also be involved in this climatic variation in dental caries.

It would be rash to discredit entirely the suggestion that social differences in dental caries are at least related to the fact that different racial groups have different staple cereals in their diet. The Chinese boil their rice, the Italians boil or sometimes bake their wheat-based pasta, the Americans bake their wheat-based bread and cookies, the Tokelau Islander, with virtually no cereal in his diet, obtains most of his carbohydrate from coconut and breadfruit. Such fundamental racial differences in the carbohydrate component of diets would be most unlikely not to be associated with differences in the patterns of dental caries prevalence.

In this complex relationship between dietary carbohydrates and dental caries it is probably still appropriate to comment that the primary dietary factor in determining racial levels of dental caries is in all likelihood sucrose, but it would be wrong to regard it as the only factor involved.

The Westernization of Primitive Peoples

A great many instances have been reported of the deterioration of dental health of primitive peoples as they are introduced to western civilization. This process in many cases has not involved a change in location of the population concerned, and therefore no climatic or other environmental differences are involved; often their general way of life (such matters as clothing and housing) changes little during the "westernization" process. What does change rapidly and significantly is the diet, with the introduction of pleasant tasting carbohydrate foods of the western type. The observation that this dietary change is followed by a rapid increase in the prevalence and severity of dental caries has been made so frequently as to suggest strongly that it is a cause and effect relationship. This subject, admirably reviewed by Bibby (1970), represents one of the clearest pieces of evidence available indicting refined, westernized carbohydrate foods as the major factor in the onslaught of dental caries in contemporary civilized man. Similar dental disasters have overtaken African tribes, Eskimos, and the Polynesians of the Pacific Basin, including New Zealand's Maoris. One of the sadder cases reported is that of the Tahitians, a happy race of people living in one of the most pleasing spots on this earth. Two hundred years ago Captain Cook was greatly taken by the flashing, white teeth in the mouths of smiling Tahitian maidens. Today Baume (1965) describes the dental health of Tahitians as "catastrophic" with many teenagers edentulous or still dentate merely for the want of an extraction service. This type of dramatic deterioration in dental health by no means requires the passage of two hundred years; just a generation or two is often sufficient. And it is a change that is already in progress in many parts of the developing world.

One facet of this "westernization" process is a fairly frequently reported difference in the levels of dental caries between urban and rural areas of developing countries. The trend is a clear one in the direction of less dental caries in rural areas than urban areas. The explanation of this phenomenon, that the impact of "westernization" on the diet would appear first and more markedly in the cities and towns than in the villages and countryside, seems an entirely reasonable and acceptable one.

Findings such as those related to the dental effects of "westernization" of primitive societies strongly suggest that the different levels of dental caries in different races are to a large extent a reflection of different dietary patterns from race to race rather than any innate, genetically determined racial immunity or susceptibility to caries. Bibby (1970) has re-discovered in the literature Pickerill's (1924) delightful aphorism which, although fifty years old, still gives an excellent summary of this aspect of the epidemiology of dental caries. Pickerill said that the main hereditary factor in dental caries is the inheritance of the family cookbook!

AGE AND CARIES

Dental caries is a markedly age-dependent disease. One result of this is that data presented on dental caries prevalences, such as DMF data, must always be age-specific. (WHO [1971] recommends that age should be recorded as age last birthday, and results should be reported separately for each age group, year by year, from birth to age 14, for half decade groupings from age 15 to 34, for decade groupings from age 35 to 64, and a final group of those 65 years of age and over.)

In contemporary man it is fair to comment that dental caries is largely a disease of childhood. Certainly it is in childhood that the disease poses the greatest public health

By age 15 years in this set of data the DMFT is 15·5. It is apparent that there is no way in which this intense caries attack could continue, with an increment of 15·5 DMF teeth every decade. Such a farcical extrapolation would give a value for the DMFT of 31 at age 25 and 46·5 at age 35! So it is a simple biological and arithmetical fact that a caries attack rate that has produced 15·5 DMF teeth by age 15 must regress as patients grow older. This regression in caries attack rate in the passage from childhood to adulthood may simply be due to the fact that all the most susceptible sites have already been attacked by age 15 years or broader issues may also be involved, such as changes in dietary preferences with increasing age; the possibility of immunological or even of some hormonal

TABLE 1

CARIES PREVALENCE IN THE PERMANENT TEETH OF NEW ZEALAND CHILDREN EXPRESSED BY THE D, M, F, AND DMF INDICES
(Data of Beck, 1967)

Age	Number of Subjects*	Decayed (D) Permanent Teeth		Missing (M) Permanent Teeth		Filled (F) Permanent Teeth		Decayed, Missing, Filled (DMF) Permanent Teeth	
		Mean D per Subject	S.E.†	Mean M per Subject	S.E.†	Mean F per Subject	S.E.†	Mean DMF per Subject	S.E.†
6	71	0·15	0·05	0·00	—	0·96	0·17	1·11	0·18
7	92	0·42	0·08	0·00	—	1·91	0·17	2·34	0·19
8	93	0·62	0·12	0·00	—	2·84	0·18	3·46	0·20
9	93	0·97	0·14	0·02	0·02	3·91	0·23	4·90	0·27
10	96	0·71	0·09	0·03	0·02	4·82	0·23	5·56	0·25
11	92	2·04	0·26	0·03	0·02	4·84	0·24	6·91	0·35
12	101	2·74	0·27	0·14	0·06	6·50	0·35	9·39	0·47
13	92	3·85	0·33	0·07	0·04	7·57	0·39	11·48	0·53
14	90	4·44	0·31	0·13	0·06	8·62	0·46	13·20	0·57
15	85	4·53	0·34	0·18	0·07	10·75	0·58	15·46	0·57

* The number of subjects does not include those younger children who have no permanent teeth erupted.
† Standard error of the mean.

problems. This is in contrast to the situation in earlier centuries where the pits and fissures and proximal surfaces in children showed remarkable immunity and caries mainly appeared in adulthood, commonly in the cervical area (probably following gingival recession) or following fracture of the enamel associated with marked attrition.

The changing intensity of caries attack between childhood and adulthood in contemporary "westernized" man has been frequently observed but little explanation for this change has been offered—a pity, as study of this fundamental characteristic of the disease could well provide new information on the aetiology of this complex disease.

One set of data (Table 1) on dental caries, more or less typical for civilized groups in areas where the water supply is fluoride-deficient (in this case drawn from New Zealand) indicates the progression of caries through childhood. The value of the DMFT at age five years must obviously be zero as there are no permanent teeth "at risk" at that age.

factors altering the balance of caries resistance needs to be considered. These promising areas of research have received little attention.

PREVALENCE IN MALES AND FEMALES

In any one population group, it is nearly always found that there is a higher DMF level in girls than boys. Traditionally this has been partly or wholly attributed to earlier eruption times for teeth in females than in males. However other factors, notably dietary differences between the sexes, are possibly involved. In adults, sex differences in dental caries prevalence are much more obscure. Again, if such differences exist, they can in all likelihood be largely attributable to variations in dietary habits between the sexes. One concrete example of this is again derived from the Tokelau Islands. Beck and Ludwig (1966) found that Tokelauan males had considerably fewer DMF teeth than females (fig. 2), at least up to 54 years of age, beyond which age the loss of teeth for periodontal reasons obscured the situation with regard to dental caries. The differences in DMF between the sexes ranged as high as 70 per cent (in the age group 20–24 years). Similar differences have been reported by other investigators in the Pacific region. These differences are so great that factors other than differences in post-eruptive tooth age must be involved. The explanation may lie in the fact that in the Tokelauan community males have greater freedom and can indulge in pursuits such as fishing which are often forbidden to the female. This probably results in higher consumption of fish and other sea-foods by males as some of the catch is consumed raw in the canoes by the exclusively male crews.

No such sex differences in the Tokelauans could be demonstrated for the deciduous dentition possibly due to the fact that the susceptibility of the deciduous teeth may be largely influenced by maternal nutrition which could be expected to be equal between offspring of both sexes.

TRACE ELEMENTS AND CARIES

The centrally important role of the fluoride ion in establishing optimum caries resistance is an established scientific fact and fluoridation of public water supplies clearly represents the most effective method of altering the epidemiological pattern of dental caries in the direction of benefit. Other trace elements may well be involved in caries resistance but the evidence is by no means as clear-cut or overwhelmingly convincing as that supporting the action of fluoride. The interesting observation of Ludwig, Cadell and Malthus (1964) in the Napier–Hastings area of the North Island of New Zealand, clearly suggests that an association exists between the trace element pattern of soil and the caries resistance of the people on the soil. The drainage of an extensive saltwater lagoon in Napier during a calamitous earthquake in 1931 provided the city with a large area for suburban growth on an unusual soil type, a saline gley of recent marine origin. Lower caries levels in children have been found in these areas compared with those in the areas of recent alluvial soil in neighbouring Hastings. Different patterns of trace elements in the two soils have been implicated in the differences in caries; in vegetables grown on the two soils no pronounced differences in major element levels were found but considerable variation occurred in trace elements with Napier vegetables being higher in molybdenum, aluminium, and titanium and Hastings vegetables being higher in manganese, copper, barium, and strontium. Associations of this type, between trace elements other than fluoride and dental caries have been supported by studies undertaken in the United States of America, the United Kingdom and South Africa. One of the more interesting pieces of supporting evidence is that reported by Anderson (1965); low caries rates in children were associated with high (200 p.p.m.) molybdenum soil known as "Teart pasture" in central Somerset. The demonstrated association of varying trace elements in soils and varying caries prevalence cannot yet be regarded as a cause and effect relationship. It is however fair to conclude that some of the epidemiological patterns of the disease observed globally may well be associated with varying caries resistance resulting as an effect of trace element intake.

INTRAORAL DISTRIBUTION OF CARIES

It is well known that the distribution of caries on the surfaces of teeth is far from random. Specific sites tend to be attacked (Jackson, 1972). The fact that some teeth and some tooth surfaces are more caries susceptible than others is a matter of routine day to day observation by all dentists. In general terms, the lower first molar is the most frequently attacked tooth in the permanent dentition and the lower canine and lower incisor teeth are the least frequently attacked. The caries attack rate for the whole dentition, tooth by tooth, follows a regular pattern partly explainable by the aetiology of the disease so far as it is known. Those sites in the dentition that from their morphological characteristics encourage stagnation and plaque accumulation are the most susceptible to dental caries. However this simplistic statement by no means explains all the fascinating patterns of intra-oral distribution of the disease. The fact that the most frequently attacked tooth and one of the least frequently attacked teeth are both located in the same jaw, separated merely by a couple of premolars, is an interesting observation for which there is no convincing explanation.

Bilateral Symmetry of Caries

In any one mouth dental caries often attacks the dentition unilaterally but in groups of people the attack tends to be reasonably bilateral and any minor divergence from bilateral symmetry appears to be merely a chance fluctuation. Of the many studies reported on intra-oral patterns of dental caries attack, one study of some 4,000 Minnesota university students serves to illustrate the point of bilateral symmetry: in males, 38·9 per cent of teeth of the right side of the mouth were affected by dental caries and 38·8 per cent of teeth on the left side were affected; in females 40·8 per cent of teeth on the right and 41·1 per cent of teeth on the left were affected. Such symmetry is not only of interest epidemiologically but is also of relevance to the evaluation of toothbrushing in the prevention of dental caries. If the toothbrush is of value, data should demonstrate lower caries rates on the side of the mouth most people clean more effectively, that is, the left. However, no such difference has been reported.

Caries Attack in Upper and Lower Teeth

Dental literature is replete with reports on the relative susceptibility to dental caries of teeth in the upper and lower jaws. The conclusion is virtually unanimous that upper teeth are more susceptible than lower teeth. Again, the study of Minnesotan students is adequately representational of the whole literature. In males and females respectively, 44·4 per cent and 47·5 per cent of upper teeth were attacked and 33·1 per cent and 34·4 per cent of lower teeth were attacked. An examination of the reasons for this noticeable variation between maxilla and mandible brings no revealing conclusion. The points of entry of saliva into the mouth have been often suggested as being implicated but no convincing theory has emerged.

Susceptibility of Individual Teeth

As the attack of dental caries in an individual mouth progresses with the passage of time, so individual teeth tend to be attacked in a roughly predictable order. In nine of ten studies reviewed by Finn (1952), the lower first permanent molar was the most frequently attacked tooth and in eight of the ten studies the upper first molar was the second most frequently attacked. The lower second molar was commonly third in the ranking of frequency of carious attack. Other teeth commonly near the top of the ranking were the upper premolar teeth and the lower second premolars with the lower first premolar often considerably lower down the list. The lower canine tooth and the two lower incisor teeth commonly, in the ten studies reviewed, vied for the last three places in the ranking of susceptibility. The lower canine was the tooth most frequently reported to be least susceptible of all.

Susceptibility of Tooth Surfaces

The widely varying susceptibility to dental caries of various types of tooth surface is another area well documented in the literature reviewed by Finn (1952). One large study in children reported that 43 per cent of all involved tooth surfaces were occlusal, 17 per cent mesial, 14 per cent distal, 13 per cent buccal, and 13 per cent lingual. The occlusal type of surface with its obvious sites for caries initiation, the pits and fissures, is clearly the most commonly attacked surface. However the proportion of each type of surface attacked changes with age. The susceptibility of the occlusal surface to attack in childhood declines in adulthood if for no other reason than that most of the occlusal surfaces have already been attacked by the end of childhood. In some American data, the attack of dental caries on the proximal surfaces of premolar teeth reached a peak at age 30 to 34 years and then declined while buccal cavities tended to rise in numbers fairly smoothly throughout life.

Caries on adjacent proximal surfaces has also been the subject of considerable study. In broad terms, in some 75 per cent of cases both abutting proximal surfaces are carious and in 25 per cent of cases only one surface is attacked.

The subject of the relative susceptibility of the different tooth surfaces in the mouth poses far more questions than it answers. Research in this area could lead to further light being cast on the aetiology of this complex but fascinating disease of dental caries.

REFERENCES

Anderson, R. J. (1965), "Dental Caries Prevalence in Teart Pasture Areas of Great Britain," in *Advances in Fluorine Research and Dental Caries Prevention*, Vol. 3, p. 165 (J. L. Hardwick, H. R. Held and K. G. König, Eds.). Oxford: Pergamon Press.

Baume, L. J. (1965), "Assessment of Dental Health Problems Around the World," *Ned. Tandbld*, **20,** 197.

Beck, D. J. (1967), "Evaluation of Dental Care for Children in New Zealand and the United States," *N. Z. dent. J.*, **63,** 201.

Beck, D. J. and Ludwig, T. G. (1966), "Sex Differences in Dental Disease in Polynesian Peoples," *N.Z. dent. J.*, **62,** 279.

Bibby, B. G. (1970), "Inferences from Natural Occurring Variations in Caries Prevalence," *J. dent. Res.*, **49,** 1194.

Finn, S. B. (1952), "Prevalence of Dental Caries," in *A Survey of the Literature of Dental Caries*, p. 161 (G. Toverud, S. B. Finn, G. J. Cox, C. F. Bodecker and J. H. Shaw. Washington, D.C.: National Academy of Sciences—National Research Council.

Jackson, D. and Burch, P. R. J. (1972), "Non-random Distributions of Caries Attacks Among Mesial and Distal Surfaces of Human Permanent Maxillary Incisors," *Arch. oral Biol.*, **17,** 119.

Ludwig, T. G., Cadell, P. B. and Malthus, R. S. (1964), "Soils and the Prevalence of Dental Caries," *Int. dent. J.*, **14,** 433.

Pickerill, H. P. (1924), *The Prevention of Dental Caries*. New York: Hoeber.

World Health Organization (1971), *Oral Health Surveys. Basic Methods.* Geneva: World Health Organization.

34. THE CHEMISTRY OF CARBOHYDRATES

P. CRITCHLEY

Chemical structure

Distribution, structure and function
    Food storage polysaccharides
    Skeletal polysaccharides
    Protective polysaccharides

Biosynthetic pathways

Significance in dental disease

The term carbohydrates refers to the family of organic molecules composed mainly of carbon, hydrogen and oxygen which, together with lipids, proteins and nucleic acid, are major components of all living matter. In this chapter the distribution of carbohydrates in nature will be related to the structure, physical properties and functions of the molecules. Mention will be made of the pathways of biosynthesis of carbohydrates, and the significance of specific types of these molecules to dental workers will be emphasized.

The carbohydrate family can be sub-divided, on the basis of molecular size, into monosaccharides (often called sugars), oligosaccharides (which contain less than ten monosaccharide units linked together), and polysaccharides. Typical examples are listed in Table 1. Polysac-

TABLE 1

COMMON MONO-, OLIGO- AND POLYSACCHARIDES

Monosaccharides	Oligosaccharides	Polysaccharides
Glucose	Maltose	Starch
	Cellobiose	Cellulose
Fructose	Sucrose	Dextran
		Levan
Galactose	Lactose	Galactan
Glucosamine	Chitobiose	Chitin
N-Acetyl		
galactosamine		Mucopolysaccharides
Glucuronic acid		

charides formed from glucose alone are called glucans *e.g.* dextran, starch and cellulose. Polymers of fructose, *e.g.* levans and inulin, are called fructans. These are all examples of homoglycans, polysaccharides made up of only one type of sugar. In contrast, many polysaccharides are composed of a number of different monosaccharides linked together in a repeating pattern. These polymers are called heteroglycans. Many of the seaweed mucilages, plant gums, bacterial cell-walls, extracellular slimes and the mammalian mucopolysaccharides are heteroglycans.

CHEMICAL STRUCTURES AND LINKAGES

The structure of glucose (and other monosaccharides) has been known for many years and is shown in fig. 1. The D signifies that the sugar is stereochemically related to D-glyceraldehyde (dextro-glycerose). The different monosaccharides normally occur in the ring form, which is a hemiacetal for glucose and galactose, and a hemiketal for fructose. Acetals and ketals are formed from aldehydes and ketones respectively, and it is this chemical group that makes the C1 group of the sugar so reactive compared with

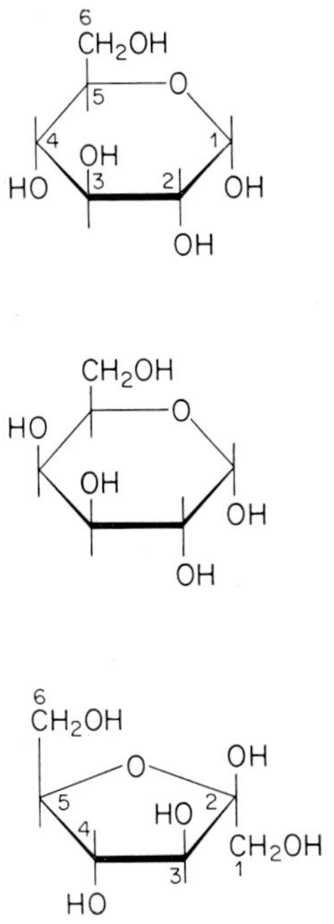

FIG. 1. The structure of common monosaccharides.

the other hydroxyl groups around the ring. The ring can open to produce the aldehyde or ketone form of the sugars; since both are reducing agents this provides the basis of most quantitative and qualitative tests for sugars.

The structures of some polysaccharides, such as starch and hyaluronic acid, have been deduced but for many polysaccharides only the ratios of the component sugars are known and the exact sequence of sugars and the linkages present have yet to be determined.

When sugars are linked together to form polysaccharides it is the reactive C1 hydroxyl group that forms the linkage to another carbon atom in the ring of another sugar unit. The position of this linkage is characteristic for a particular polysaccharide. Thus, cellulose is a linear chain of units of the disaccharide cellobiose, which is O-*β*-D-glucopyranosyl- (1 → 4)-D-glucopyranose (fig. 2).

The pyranoside indicates that a six-membered ring is present in contrast to a five-membered furanoside like that of the fructose molecule shown in fig. 1. Rings are conventionally drawn as seen from above, so that the back of the ring, which contains the oxygen bridge is at the top of the diagram.

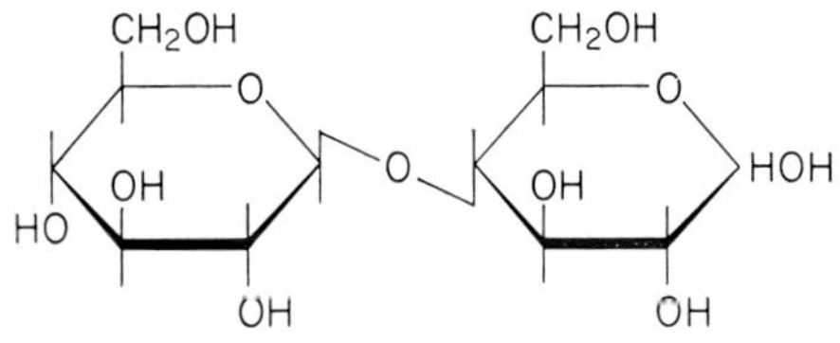

O-β-D-Glucopyranosyl-(1 → 4)-D-glucopyranose

FIG. 2. The structure of the disaccharide cellobiose.

Each hydroxyl group around the ring is written above or below and the particular orientations of these hydroxyl groups are characteristic for each particular sugar. The hydroxyl group on the first carbon atom can be in either of the two possible positions in a monosaccharide, representing the α-form when the hydroxyl is downwards, and the β-form when it points upwards. The optical rotation of each form is different.

When a disaccharide linkage is formed between two sugars water is lost and the orientation of the oxygen on the first carbon atom of one of the sugars is fixed in either the α or β position depending on the disaccharide. The formation of this linkage involves the reducing group of one of the sugars producing a reducing and a non-reducing end to the molecule. These terms are often referred to in polysaccharide chemistry. Sucrose is an exception to this rule because it has no reducing properties. The reducing end of glucose is linked to the reducing group of fructose.

Many polysaccharides are branched rather than linear polymers thus providing several non-reducing ends and only one reducing group per molecule. Because these molecules are so large it is difficult to detect any reducing activity. On analysis the branch points give rise to a smaller number of linkages different from those found in the chain. Thus, in dextran, which has an O-α-D-glucopyranosyl-(1 → 6)-O-α-D-glucopyranose repeating unit, a few of the glucopyranoside rings have short chains attached to the hydroxyl on carbon 3 or carbon 4 (fig. 3).

THE DISTRIBUTION, STRUCTURE AND FUNCTION OF POLYSACCHARIDES IN NATURE

Polysaccharides occur in almost all forms of life, the type of molecule present depending on its function and the cell which produces it.

Food Storage Polysaccharides

Granules of starch are found in many plant cells, whereas in animal and bacterial cells glycogen is the normal food reserve. In some plant cells, for example dahlia tubers, a fructan called inulin provides the food reserve. A related fructan, levan, is synthesized outside the cells of a number of bacteria and some species break down this polysaccharide as the organisms start to grow.

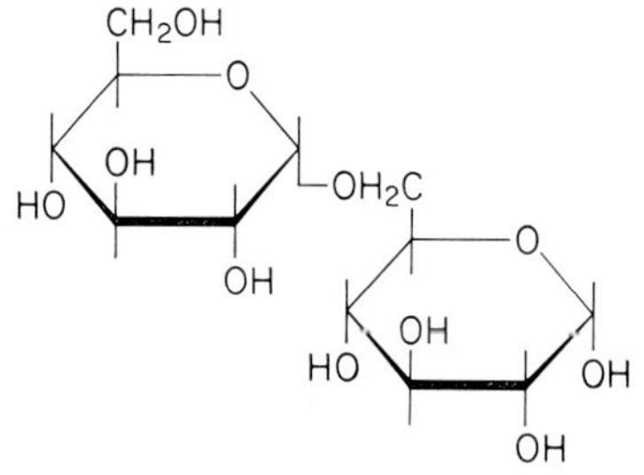

O-α-D-Glucopyranosyl-(1 → 6)-O-α-D-glucopyranose

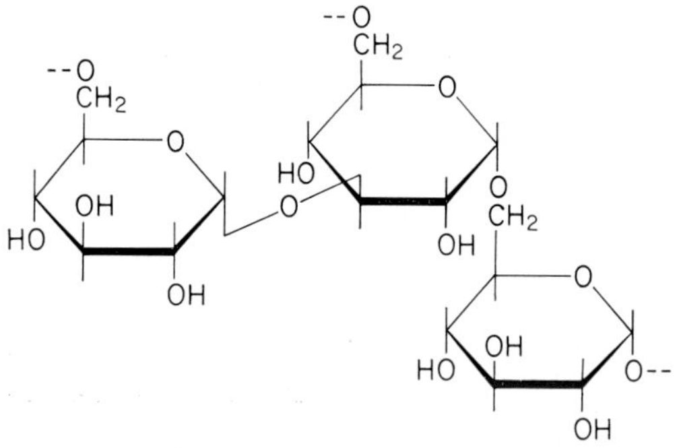

α-Glucosyl branch on position 3

FIG. 3. Typical saccharide units of dextran.

The structure of the food storage polysaccharides varies but they are normally homoglycans composed of either glucose or fructose with a low degree of branching. Many of the polymers have a high affinity for water and consequently they dissolve or form gels fairly readily. These molecules are broken down rapidly by the appropriate enzyme or enzymes (usually only one or two are required) to liberate glucose or fructose which is subsequently metabolized to produce energy, as well as carboxylic acids and other components required by cells. In particular, lactic acid is formed by the glycolytic pathway (see Chapter 7). In some cells the acid may be metabolized further to produce more energy.

Skeletal Polysaccharides

Various polysaccharides are present in different living organisms as major constituents of the skeletal tissues. In plants, the cell walls, which give the cell much of its rigidity and shape, are composed of layers of cellulose laid-down on a middle lamella of pectic substances. These pectic substances are present in all plant cell walls and are a complex mixture of at least three different polysaccharides cross-linked to each other. One is a linear polymer of α1 → 4 linked D-galacturonic acid units, present in nature as the methyl ester and therefore insoluble in water. The other two polysaccharides are a linear galactan of β 1 → 4 D-galactopyranose units and a branched araban composed of α1 → 5 L-arabinofuranose units with 1 → 3 branches on about half of the main chain units.

The cell walls of yeasts contain chitin (β 1 → 4 *N*-acetyl glucosamine units) with cellulose, mannan or galactan hydrogen bonded to the basal layer. In contrast, bacterial

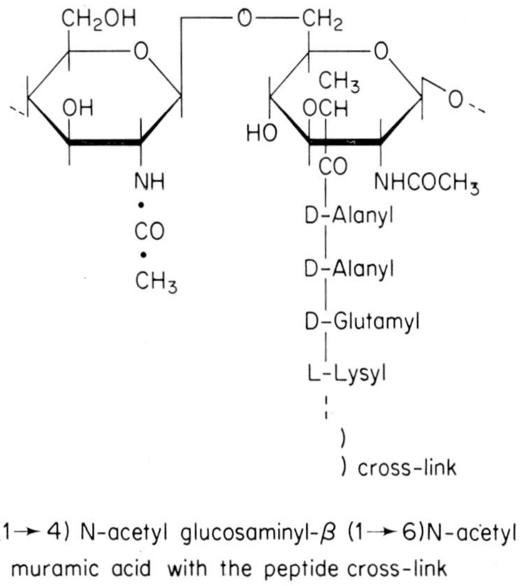

β (1→ 4) N-acetyl glucosaminyl-β (1→ 6)N-acetyl muramic acid with the peptide cross-link

FIG. 4. The repeating unit of a mucopeptide from bacterial cell walls.

cell walls are based on mucopeptide (murein) linked to various polysaccharides. If the wall of the cell is broken by enzymes or prevented from forming by antibiotics, the resulting bacterial cell (enclosed in its cytoplasmic membrane) takes up a spherical shape, provided that the osmotic pressure is compatible with that of the cell. Under these conditions even a bacillus changes into a coccoidal shape. The bacterial mucopeptide structure is a polysaccharide chain of βN-acetyl glucosaminyl 1 → 6 N-acetylmuramic acid units with short chains of 5–10 amino acids attached to the lactate ether of C3 of the muramic acid residue (fig. 4). These amino acids are unusual in that many of the residues are in the D not the L form normally found in proteins. The amino acids form the bridges between the polysaccharide chains making a three-dimensional structure.

The skeletal polysaccharides are insoluble and highly cross-linked either to other polysaccharide chains, as in plant cell walls, or through side chains of amino acids as in the mucopeptides of bacterial cell walls. This tight cross-linking of the polysaccharides satisfies most of the hydrogen bonding regions and tends to exclude water. Many of these regions of highly organized cross-links are therefore crystalline. Inorganic material, such as calcium carbonate, may be incorporated into the polysaccharide network to harden it, *e.g.* the calcified chitin of crab shells. The resulting complex of mineral matter coupled with the cross-linked, insoluble polysaccharide is highly resistant to enzymic or chemical attack.

Protective Polysaccharides

Many polysaccharides, particularly extracellular polymers, protect the plant or animal that synthesized them from attack by other life forms or from dehydration. For example, many trees produce an exudate when they are injured. This fluid is rich in polysaccharide and on exposure to air it becomes sticky or is converted to a hard glassy material which seals the wound. The formation of a "scab" may protect the tree against loss of sap as well as infection by bacteria and virus.

Many species of bacteria produce slimy capsules or extracellular polysaccharide around the cell wall. There is no major difference between a capsule and an extracellular polysaccharide. Both types of material are located outside the cell wall but the capsule usually follows the shape of the cell and is tightly bound to the wall whereas the extracellular polysaccharide spreads away from the cell and can be removed more easily. Bacterial slimes protect organisms against phagocytosis, attack by bacteriophage and dehydration.

Lubrication is another protective function of polysaccharides. In mammals a protein-carbohydrate complex often fulfils this role. Thus, salivary glycoproteins coat food particles and protect the soft tissues of the mouth, oesophagus and stomach from damage.

The physical characteristics of protective polysaccharides are more difficult to define. They are normally extracellular heteroglycans which have charged groups such as glucuronic or galacturonic acid residues at regular intervals along the chain. Moreover, these groups frequently occur in the terminal positions of the branching side chains. Structures of this type have an extended shape resulting from both steric hindrance and electrical repulsions of side chains. Even in dilute solutions most of the polysaccharide chains interact with other chains producing a viscous solution. At higher concentrations a gel is produced and on dehydration many of the molecules produce a glassy solid which is sticky when moistened.

BIOSYNTHETIC PATHWAYS

Simple sugars are primary products of the fixation of carbon dioxide and water, using the energy of sunlight and the catalyst chlorophyll, present in green plants.

The biosynthesis of polysaccharides can be effected by either of two major routes:

(a) the intracellular pathway involving the breakdown of nucleoside pyrophosphate sugar intermediates to provide the energy to drive the reaction; and
(b) the transglycosylase pathway which often occurs outside the cell and involves an enzymic transfer of a sugar from one glycoside to another (fig. 5).

Reactions proceeding by the first pathway, involving the nucleoside pyrophosphate sugar intermediates, are almost exclusively intracellular reactions because nucleoside triphosphates such as adenosine triphosphate (ATP) are

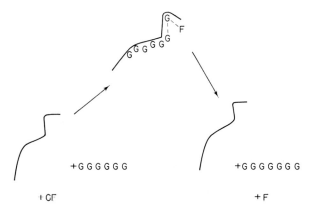

FIG. 5. Transfer of glucose units from sucrose to dextran by dextransucrase. ($\int$ is the dextransucrase.)

involved in forming the intermediates and a large number of different enzymes are necessary to effect the transformation. Most polysaccharides, including the complex heteroglycans found in bacterial cell walls and capsules, are synthesized by the nucleoside pyrophosphate pathway. Cells have the ability to transform glucose, or other simple monosaccharides, into different sugars, using the nucleoside phosphate intermediates. Therefore, glucose entering the cell may be metabolized by the glycolytic pathway and generate ATP and acid, or it may be converted to intracellular glycogen food storage. A further alternative is that some glucose is converted to the nucleoside pyrophosphate glucose intermediate, which may then undergo one of a number of fates (fig. 6):

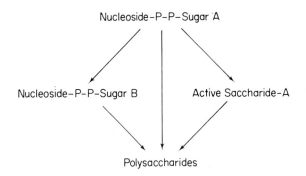

FIG. 6. Synthesis of polysaccharides from nucleoside pyrophosphate intermediates.

(a) the glucose part of the intermediate may be transformed into a different sugar by a series of steps while still attached to a nucleoside diphosphate carrier;

(b) the sugar may be transferred to a growing polysaccharide chain as the next residue to be added; and

(c) one nucleoside pyrophosphate sugar intermediate may transfer its sugar residue to another intermediate to produce an "activated" di- or oligosaccharide which in turn will transfer the repeating unit synthesized to a growing polymer on a membrane.

In the transglycolase pathway it is the "free-energy" liberated when one glycoside bond is broken, e.g. that between glucose and fructose in the sucrose molecule, that drives the reaction forwards. A mathematical expression for the change of "free-energy" during a reaction can be derived from the second law of thermodynamics. Any system that possesses "free-energy" is capable of doing work to change spontaneously into a system of greater stability. As mentioned earlier, sucrose is exceptional in that the reactive reducing function of both the component sugars is linked together. This bond is easily broken to liberate the more stable sugars glucose and fructose together with "free-energy". It is this energy that is harnessed by the extracellular enzymes dextransucrase, amylosucrase or levansucrase to transfer glucose or fructose units from the sucrose to a growing polymer chain of dextran (fig. 5), amylopectin, or levan respectively. In this type of reaction, provided that sucrose or another suitable substrate is present, no cellular energy is required once the enzyme has been synthesized and secreted. The products are homoglycans.

THE SIGNIFICANCE OF SPECIFIC TYPES OF CARBOHYDRATES IN DENTISTRY

Each tooth in the mouth exists in an environment containing carbohydrate. For example, the dermis of the gingiva is composed mainly of the protein collagen with some mucopolysaccharide. Carbohydrates also make up a significant proportion of salivary glycoproteins, acquired pellicle, and dental plaque.

The polysaccharides involved in mesodermal tissues such as the corium of skin and gingiva, and mineralized tissues such as bone and dentine, are heteroglycans having negative charges at frequent intervals along the chain (e.g. hyaluronic acid and sulphated mucopolysaccharides such as chondroitin sulphate). Cartilage contains a high proportion of chondroitin sulphate, which gives it elasticity, whereas synovial fluid owes its lubricating property mainly to hyaluronic acid.

Dental plaque has been discussed in Chapter 31. This chapter will deal with the metabolism of carbohydrates by bacteria present in plaque, and the relationship between the physical properties of the polysaccharides (synthesized by these bacteria) and tooth diseases.

When carbohydrates are eaten the bacteria present in plaque are provided with food. The availability of dietary carbohydrate to plaque bacteria depends on a number of factors. The most important of these are:

(a) the oral retention of the carbohydrate, which depends on the physical properties of the food consumed;

(b) penetration of the carbohydrate into plaque—e.g. sucrose and glucose are small, neutral molecules that diffuse rapidly, whereas larger or charged molecules may be excluded; and

(c) as a corollary to (a) and (b) carbohydrates with long oral retention, which can be broken down easily by oral bacteria, or by salivary amylase in the specific case of starch or glycogen, will penetrate into plaque.

The carbohydrates eaten most frequently are sucrose and starch. Clearly, sucrose is the most dangerous sugar because bacteria are fed by between-meal snacks of foods rich in sucrose and large amounts of this sugar penetrate plaque rapidly. As soon as sucrose enters the plaque, bacteria break part of it down to glucose and fructose which enter the cell and are converted to acid and energy. In addition, a large quantity of intracellular polysaccharide is formed thus ensuring the survival of the organisms over the fasting period of the human host (particularly overnight). The amount of intracellular polysaccharide formed is increased when the growth of some bacteria is limited because insufficient nitrogenous food is available. Under these conditions some bacteria synthesize more of the cell wall polysaccharides and can be recognized in the electron microscope because they have thicker cell walls than similar organisms growing rapidly.

Some of the sucrose is transformed to glucans and fructans outside the cells by the transglycosylase pathway discussed earlier. Little is known about the structures of the polysaccharides formed in plaque. The work published so far suggests that a number of different homoglycans are formed from sucrose by the various species of organisms in the plaque. The size, branching and solubility of the molecules synthesized can vary depending on the local conditions of pH (acidity), ionic strength, the particular ions present and the different strains of bacteria in the sample. In cultures, plaque organisms synthesize both soluble and insoluble dextrans and levans. A particularly insoluble glucan, called mutan, is produced by strains of *Streptococcus mutans* and in this polysaccharide $\alpha 1 \rightarrow 3$ linkages predominate; it cannot therefore, be classed as a dextran which has $\alpha 1 \rightarrow 6$ linkages.

When glucose is eaten instead of sucrose for a day or two the plaque bacteria produce acid and intracellular polysaccharide; cell wall, but little extracellular polysaccharide, can be detected. However, if glucose or invert sugar is substituted for sucrose in the diet for several weeks, large amounts of extracellular polysaccharides can be found in the plaque. Extraction and analysis of these polysaccharides show that they are heteroglycans composed of fucose, glucose, galactose, mannose, N-acetyl hexosamine and hexuronic acid. These polysaccharides are synthesized by the nucleoside phosphate pathway. The presence of these polysaccharides has been demonstrated in plaque from monkeys and humans fed on glucose instead of sucrose. Also, cultures of plaque streptococci, grown on a simple medium to avoid polysaccharide contaminants, produce similar heteroglycans.

Plaque is composed of a network of protein chains in which many different kinds of bacteria are trapped. Some of these organisms reproduce and grow through the network whereas others survive and metabolize but they multiply only slowly, if at all. Within this structure polysaccharide is synthesized whenever suitable substrates for the bacteria are eaten by the host. Only certain bacteria are capable of producing polysaccharides and the

nature of these polymers will vary according to the local conditions. Moreover, some bacteria can degrade dextrans and levans so that a rapid synthesis will occur when sugar is present, followed by a slow loss of some polysaccharide.

The role of polysaccharides in the pathogenesis of caries, and therefore the significance of these findings, is not completely understood. However, if one considers the properties of polysaccharides of known structure it is possible to predict to some extent what may happen in the plaque.

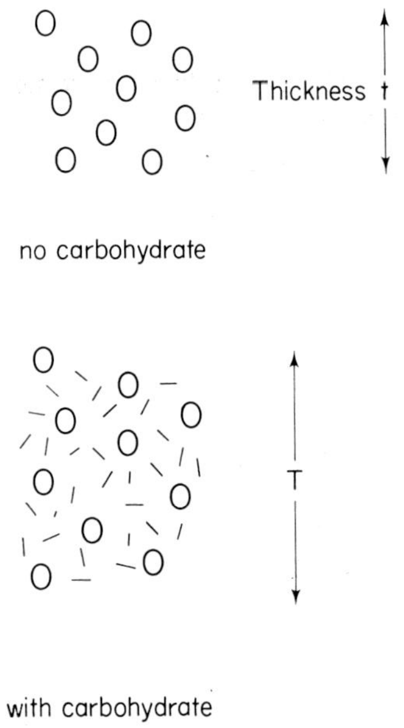

FIG. 7. The expansion of plaque volume by polysaccharide. (– the short bars in the lower picture represent polysaccharide formed *in situ*; acid is also found under these conditions.)

Many polysaccharides dissolve or swell considerably in water. This results in gel formation. In high concentrations even soluble polysaccharides form a network of chains that interact with each other at "junction-zones". Gels of this type are formed by dextrans and many negatively charged heteroglycans, like the extracellular polysaccharides formed in plaque from glucose. These gels exclude large molecules such as proteins and polysaccharides. They can also concentrate ions. The negatively charged polymers, like hyaluronic acid, are more effective than dextran in their ability to exclude molecules. This ability to concentrate ions and prevent loss or entry of large molecules into plaque may be of fundamental importance in the mechanism of caries where acid is generated in large quantities within the plaque and only slowly neutralized by saliva (fig. 7).

Another important property of polysaccharides that may be relevant to the caries mechanism is the volume-expanding property. The use of dextrans in blood transfusions and soluble cellulose derivatives in slimming foods that swell and make the stomach feel full is well known.

Voluminous plaque has been described by a number of workers and in at least one instance it has been shown that less bacteria are present per unit volume in plaque formed during frequent intake of sugar. This suggests that the formation of polysaccharide *in situ* may expand the volume of plaque from within, producing a thicker deposit and thereby increasing the distance that acid must travel through the plaque to be neutralized; or, conversely, that salivary buffers must penetrate into the thicker deposit to neutralize the acid completely (fig. 7).

It may well be that thicker layers of plaque retain more molecules potentially toxic to the gingiva and so facilitate the progression of gingival disease as well as caries.

An attempt has been made in this chapter to introduce non-chemists to the essentials of carbohydrate chemistry in order to explain current views on the relationship of carbohydrates in dental plaque to caries. This particular area of dental research has become a centre of attention over the past few years and it can be expected that some of the current hypotheses will come to be validated or dismissed.

FURTHER READING

Critchley, P., Saxton, C. A. and Kolendo, A. B. (1968), "The Histology and Histochemistry of Dental Plaque," *Caries Res.*, **2**, 115.

Critchley, P. (1970), "The Local Effects of Foods, Effects on Bacterial Metabolic Processes," *J. dent. Res.*, **49**, suppl. 6, 1283.

Critchley, P. and Saxton, C. A. (1970), "The Metabolism of Gingival Plaque," *Int. dent. J.*, **20**, 408.

Critchley, P. (1971), "The Microbiology of Dental Plaque with Special Reference to Polysaccharide Formation," *Dtsch. zahnärztl. Z.*, **26**, 1155.

Hassel, Th. M. (1971), "pH-Telemetrie der Interdentalen Plaque nach Genuss von Zucker und Zuckeraustauschstoffen," *Dtsch. zahnärztl. Z.*, **26**, 1145.

Laurent, T. C. (1964), "The Interaction Between Polysaccharides and Other Macromolecules. 9. The Exclusion of Molecules from Hyaluronic Acid Gels and Solutions," *Biochem. J.*, **93**, 106.

Rees, D. A. (1969), "Structure, Conformation and Mechanism in the Formation of Polysaccharide Gels and Networks," *Advanc. Carbohyd. Chem. Biochem.*, **24**, 267.

Stacey, M. and Barker, S. A. (1960), *Polysaccharides of Microorganisms*. London: Oxford University Press.

Whistler, R. L. and Smart, C. L. (1953), *Polysaccharide Chemistry*. New York: Academic Press.

Wilkinson, J. F. (1958), "The Extracellular Polysaccharides of Bacteria," *Bact. Rev.*, **22**, 46.

35. BIOLOGICAL PROCESSES IN TOOTH ERUPTION AND TOOTH MOVEMENT

A. H. MELCHER

Cellular activity in the functioning periodontium
  Turnover
  Functional cells

Eruption of teeth
  Intrinsic force
  Changes in the ligament
  Penetration of gingival connective tissue

Tooth movement
  Osteoblasts and osteoclasts
  Fibroblasts and "fibroclasts"
  Control of osteogenesis
  Remodelling of connective tissue
  Effect on dental pulp

INTRODUCTION

Both eruption and movement of teeth involve trans-location of a tooth from one situation in the jaw to another. The forces that move the tooth during eruption, and which as yet have not been identified clearly, are produced within the periodontium and are therefore intrinsic. Tooth movement on the other hand, results from forces being applied to the crown of the tooth during physiological, pathological or therapeutic processes, and these forces are extrinsic. Notwithstanding the nature of the forces, it is impossible for a tooth to be relocated as a result of either eruption or applied force without intervention of the cells of the periodontium. This is because an enduring alteration of the position of the tooth in the jaw, as distinct from a reversible displacement of the tooth, cannot occur unless the periodontium is remodelled, and remodelling can be effected only by cells. This axiom is most graphically illustrated by a simple example. Suppose that identical orthodontic appliances are applied to the teeth of two similar animals, one of which is alive and the other freshly killed, to relocate a given tooth in each animal. Immediately after application of the appliances both teeth will be displaced similarly, but thereafter only the tooth in the live animal will be moved to, and retained in, the desired situation. This conclusion may appear self-evident, or even elementary, but it is often forgotten that it is not sophisticated orthodontic appliances that actually relocate teeth; teeth can be moved to and retained in new positions in the jaw only through the intervention of cells. Consequently, to escape from explanations of tooth movement that are purely mechanistic, the role of cells in these processes must be explored, and it is with this question that the present chapter will largely be concerned.

CELLULAR ACTIVITY IN THE FUNCTIONING PERIODONTIUM

Comprehension of cellular behaviour and homeostasis in the functioning periodontium is a pre-requisite to understanding the activity of cells during movement of teeth.

Turnover in the Periodontium

The periodontium is an organ comprising four connective tissues, two of which are mineralized and two of which are soft. The former tissues comprise cementum and alveolar bone, and the latter the periodontal ligament and the lamina propria of the gingiva. The cementum attaches the periodontium to the dentine of the root of the tooth. The alveolar bone, which is a thin shell of bone surrounding the socket of the tooth, attaches the periodontium to the bone of the jaws and forms part of the alveolar process. The alveolar process comprises alveolar bone and external cortical plate, and varying amounts of spongiosa. The alveolar bone and external cortical plate may be fused and largely indistinguishable from one another, or they may be separated by cancellous bone, the spongiosa. In the latter case, they are continuous with one another at the alveolar crest. The differing architecture of alveolar process reflects a relationship between the degree of development of the supporting bone and the forces being exerted on the tooth. For example, a fused alveolar bone and external cortical plate is seen on the labial surfaces of lower incisors, while discrete alveolar bones and cortical plates, with relatively large amounts of spongiosa between, are found supporting molars. In the latter situation the trabeculae of the spongiosa act as a buttress between the alveolar bone and the external cortical plate, increasing the strength of the bony structure. Separation of the two plates of bone may be complete or partial, and the trabeculae of the spongiosa vary in number and size. It is important that these differences in architectural form be recognized if the identity of the bone cells that respond to movement of a tooth are clearly to be understood. Where the alveolar bone is separated from the external cortical plate, two surfaces of the alveolar bone can be distinguished. These are the periodontal surface that forms the wall of the periodontal space, and the spongiosa surface that forms the central wall of the spongiosa and which is covered by endosteum (fig. 1). No spongiosa surface can be distinguished where the alveolar bone and external cortical plate are fused. The external surface of the alveolar bone and the external surface of the alveolar process are, in this case, the same and this surface is covered by periosteum.

The periodontal ligament occupies the periodontal space and provides continuity between the cementum and alveolar bone and, as will be discussed below, it is the major source of the cells that are responsible for homeostasis in the periodontium. The periodontal ligament and lamina propria of the gingiva are continuous at the level of the crest of the alveolar process.

The constituents of many tissues in the body undergo turnover. Turnover is a physiological process in which a given constituent is continually being removed and replaced without apparent change in the architecture of the tissue or loss or gain of the constituents. The periodontal ligament

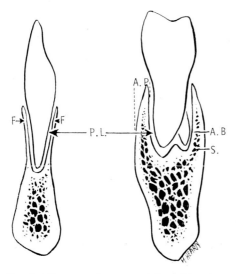

FIG. 1. Diagrammatic representation of two types of alveolar process. Note that the alveolar process (F) on the left contains no spongiosa and that the alveolar bone and external cortical plate are fused. The alveolar bone on the right (AB) is separated from the cortical bone of the alveolar process (AP) by the spongiosa (S) and exhibits a periodontal ligament (PL) surface and a spongiosa surface.

of teeth of limited eruption in small rodents and monkeys has a comparatively high rate of turnover of extracellular protein, but the rate at which this occurs is not uniform throughout the ligament. In particular, turnover appears to be higher in the peripheral part of the ligament than centrally. This means that cells of periodontal ligament are continually resorbing and synthesizing extracellular protein and carbohydrate in the ligament, and therefore have the capacity to produce collagenase and other enzymes that can depolymerize the constituents of the extracellular substance. It also means that the cells in some part of the ligament are more active than are those in others. This knowledge is central to the discussion that is to follow, and it also raises two questions: firstly, why the periodontal ligament has such a high turnover of protein; and secondly, why the rate of turnover is not the same throughout the ligament. There do not appear to be any data to shed light on either of these questions. It has been suggested that sites of elevated turnover in the periodontal ligament coincide with the areas where stress is greatest, but there is no direct evidence to support this contention.

Turnover in tissue involves cells as well as extracellular substance. It has been shown using radioautography and ^{3}H-thymidine (which is incorporated into forming DNA) that synthesis of DNA occurs in cells of the functioning periodontal ligament, and that the number of cells synthesizing DNA also varies in different sites. Synthesis of DNA usually presages cell division, but it must be emphasized that synthesis of DNA does not always guarantee that the cell will divide. This observation may therefore not provide direct information on turnover of cells in the ligament, but it does suggest some degree of cellular proliferation.

If division is a slow continual process among cells of functioning periodontal ligament, it is important to know the identity of the dividing cells. There appear to be no data on this question, but it is conceivable that a population of progenitor cells, as in other connective tissues, constitutes the source of new cells. The precise location of the progenitor cells in the ligament is unknown, but unless this tissue is different from other connective tissues, they may be confined to perivascular sites. It is believed that when a progenitor cell divides to produce two daughter cells, one differentiates into a functional form while the other remains as an undifferentiated progenitor.

The cells of the periodontal ligament are also involved in turnover of alveolar bone and deposition and resorption of cementum. Turnover of alveolar bone is believed to be relatively high, occurring at a greater rate than elsewhere in the jaws. Cementum behaves differently, however, and while apposition apparently continues throughout life, this process is not normally accompanied by resorption. Resorption of cementum can occur, but this is generally associated with abnormal function or pathological change.

Turnover of extracellular substance of gingiva appears to be independent of that of periodontal ligament, but the evidence on its rate of turnover appears to be conflicting. However, it is important to realize that the constituents of gingival connective tissue do turn over, and that the cells possibly have an origin different from that of periodontal ligament and may therefore exhibit differences in functional characteristics.

Functional Cells in the Periodontium

Data on turnover of extracellular material in the periodontium show that a number of different types of cells are present and function in the organ, and that these are present mainly in the periodontal ligament. It is also evident that progenitor cells in the ligament must have the capacity to differentiate into functional forms when and where required. Turnover is effected by active synthetic and resorptive cells, so that cells of the periodontal ligament must have the capacity to synthesize and resorb the extracellular substance of periodontal ligament and alveolar bone, and also to synthesize and, on occasions, to resorb cementum. It is well known that fibroblasts are present in the ligament. There is also some evidence for the presence of mononuclear cells that bear some cytological resemblance to fibroblasts, but that apparently are engaged in resorption of collagen fibrils. Osteoblasts and osteoclasts may be seen on the periodontal surface of the alveolar bone and cementoblasts, and on occasions cementoclasts, are found on the surface of the cementum. The questions that now arise concern the origin of these cells and the mechanisms whereby their differentiation and activity are controlled.

While it is clear that these functional cell-types must differentiate from progenitor cells in the ligament, the identity of the precursor of each differentiated cell is not known and it is impossible to say whether the periodontal ligament contains more than one population of progenitor cells. Thus, it is not known whether one form of progenitor cell can differentiate into all of the different functional types or whether the progenitor cells are each of specific type capable of giving rise only to particular functional types. Elucidation of the nature of the progenitor populations in the periodontal ligament is fundamental to the understanding of the mechanisms that control differentiation and distribution of the specialized cells in the periodontal ligament. This need is also closely related to understanding control of turnover in the ligament and to understanding control of cellular activity responsible for eruption and movement of teeth.

Information available on the derivation of different functional forms of bone cells may be applicable to cells in the ligament. It has long been held that all types of bone cells are interchangeable; that is, that osteoblasts, osteoclasts and osteocytes are all derived from a single type of progenitor, and that each of these functional forms can revert to a progenitor or change to a different functional type. Recent evidence questions the accuracy of this concept. For example, it has been claimed that osteoblasts and osteoclasts each have a morphologically distinctive progenitor cell, both located perivascularly. More recently, it has been suggested that osteocytes are end cells, and that they die when released from their lacunae. These observations are of course also applicable to the bone cells of the periodontium, and suggest that more than one type of progenitor cell may be present in the ligament.

The origin and interchangeability of the fibroblasts and "fibroclasts" seen in the periodontal ligament is obscure. Similarly, there is a paucity of information about cells associated with cementun, but it is probable that their origin is similar to that of cells found in bone.

The cells that cover the periodontal surface of alveolar bone have received little attention. All bone surfaces are covered by cells. These are in different states of differentiation depending upon whether osteogenesis or osteoclasis is occurring at that particular site. The internal surfaces of bone are covered by a cellular layer termed the endosteum. The external surfaces of bones are covered by a three-layered structure, the periosteum, and this comprises an internal cellular layer in contact with the extracellular substance of the bone, a tenuous intermediate layer consisting of elastic fibres, and an external fibrous layer. The internal cellular layer, termed the cambium or osteogenic layer of the periosteum, is continuous with the endosteum at the external orifices of bone canals. The cambium layer of periosteum and the endosteum comprise a unitary system of cells covering all bone surfaces, with the outer two layers of the periosteum forming a stocking that encloses the external surface of bones. Electron microscopic observ-

ations on the periodontal surface of alveolar bone show clearly that this surface is not covered by a periosteum. It must then be assumed that, like all internal surfaces of bone, this surface is covered by an endosteum, but one that is penetrated by Sharpey's fibres from the periodontal ligament.

If one examines the bony wall of the periodontal space in the light microscope, it is evident that it is not a flat continuous surface. The wall is often rough, and is penetrated in many areas by canals which transmit blood vessels that course between the spongiosa of the alveolar process and the periodontal ligament. The endosteum that lines these canals is continuous with the endosteum covering both the periodontal surface and the spongiosa surface of the alveolar bone. It is therefore probable that both the cells of the endosteum lining the periodontal space, and those of the endosteum lining the vascular canals, act as progenitors for specialized cells that remodel the alveolar bone. If this is true, the cells of the vascular canals can be expected to play an important role in tooth movement.

The potential of the cells of the lamina propria of the gingiva is another question that requires exploration, but about which at present little appears to be known. The developmental origin of the gingival connective tissue is different from that of the cells of the periodontal ligament (which arise from the dental follicle), and functionally the gingival cells appear to have the capacity only of producing, and probably removing, fibrous connective tissue, unlike the cells of the periodontal ligament. It is not known what differences there are between the cells at the junction of the periodontal ligament and the lamina propria of the gingiva, nor whether there are biological interactions between the two groups of cells that influence homeostasis in the periodontium. These questions are important in relation to the events that occur in eruption and tooth movement, as well as changes attributable to periodontal disease and periodontal therapy.

Having discussed the different specialized cells of the periodontium and their origins, there remains the most tantalizing question of all: what are the factors that control the differentiation and function of these cells? This problem, about which so little is known, is pursued below in the section on tooth movement.

ERUPTION OF TEETH

The topic of eruption has recently been reviewed well and it is intended here to deal in detail only with aspects of the subject that appear to be relevant now.

The Intrinsic Force That Effects Eruption

The motive force for tooth eruption has been attributed to a variety of developmental and physiological phenomena. These include:

(a) Events during tooth development such as proliferation of dental epithelium, root formation (including dentinogenesis), pulp constriction, and deposition of alveolar bone;

(b) blood pressure; and
(c) the hammock ligament.

However, none of these suggestions has withstood experimental investigation. Indeed, there is evidence that excludes the role of most of them. Experiments in which resection of the growing end of the continuously erupting incisor of the rat failed to prevent eruption of the tooth, point strongly to the probability that the force of eruption resides in the periodontal ligament. Although these experiments were performed on teeth of continuous eruption, it seems unlikely that the mechanisms responsible for eruption of such teeth are different from those responsible for teeth of limited eruption. If it is true that the force of eruption resides in the periodontal ligament, then the possible sources of the force are narrowed to three:

(a) The blood supply to the ligament;
(b) the extracellular substance of the ligament; and
(c) the cells of the ligament.

As mentioned above, there does not appear to be any solid evidence to support the hypothesis that blood-pressure provides the force for eruption, although it may play a part in supporting the teeth and in returning a depressed tooth to its occlusal position. It has been claimed that a contractile force in maturing collagen fibres pulls the tooth out of its bony socket. However, there is no evidence to support the belief that collagen fibres do contract during the chemical cross-linking associated with their maturation. Finally, it has been suggested that the force may reside in the cells of the ligament. Unfortunately there is no direct evidence to support this belief either, although sufficient circumstantial evidence is available to make this a fruitful field for future investigation. Some of the reasons why fibroblasts of the ligament may provide the force will therefore be outlined.

It is well known that a wound in skin contracts after a few weeks of healing, and there is evidence to support the belief that the motive force for this contraction resides in the capacity of the fibroblasts of the young connective tissue occupying the wound to contract. There is also evidence for the presence of a contractile apparatus in the cytoplasm of fibroblasts. The protein that is responsible for contraction of muscle is actomyosin. The actin component occurs in muscle as fine filaments, and under appropriate conditions these contract in the presence of myosin. However, it is not only in muscle cells that cytoplasmic constituents have the capacity to react with myosin; it has been shown that when the active fraction of myosin is introduced under experimental conditions into a number of cell types, including fibroblasts, microfilaments which are present in the cytoplasm of these cells will bind the myosin fraction. The microfibrils having this binding capacity have a diameter of $\sim$4–6 nm., and are usually found adjacent to the plasma membrane. It has been shown in some cells *in vitro* that the microfibrils which bind the myosin fraction can be depolymerized by cytochalasin B and that this change in the microfibrils halts these cells when they are migrating. These findings suggest that the microfibrils have contractile properties.

The capacity of fibroblasts to emulate muscle cells by contracting is reflected in the ultrastructural appearance of contracting connective tissue. It has been shown that the cells of young connective tissue in an actively contracting wound exhibit some ultrastructural characteristics of smooth muscle cells. Unfortunately, since none of the descriptions of the ultrastructure of cells of periodontal ligament associated with erupting teeth mentions more than an occasional characteristic of those catalogued for cells in a contracting wound, there is still no direct evidence to support the view that cells of periodontal ligament contract and, by traction on collagen fibrils attached to bone and to tooth, pull the tooth out of its socket. However, it is difficult to ignore the possibility that a mechanism so active elsewhere performs a similar function in the periodontium, but it must be stressed that until direct proof to support the idea is obtained, the concept must be regarded as no more than an attractive hypothesis. It is likely that the most promising approach to the solution of this problem will come from *in vitro* studies of the periodontium.

Changes in the Ligament During Eruption

Eruption of teeth of limited eruption occurs in two different circumstances; firstly, as young developing teeth move from their crypts in the jaw to the occlusal plane, and secondly, when functioning teeth lose their occlusal contact and eruption is reactivated.

Phenomena that must be explored are firstly, the orientation of the fibres of the developing periodontal ligament, secondly, the changes that occur in the supporting tissues of the teeth during eruption and finally, the need for an erupting tooth to be supported while it moves in an occlusal direction.

There is still argument over the relationship between the time of orientation of the fibres of the developing periodontal ligament and the stage of eruption of the developing tooth. It has been claimed that the fibres of the ligament are orientated in response to the tooth becoming loaded axially or to the tooth meeting resistance from overlying tissues as it erupts. However, there is also evidence that orientation of fibres occurs as the tooth starts to erupt, and this seems more likely. It is generally agreed that orientation is first seen in the cervical region and that this then proceeds apically.

As to the changes in the supporting tissues of the teeth during eruption, it is evident that the fibres, ground substance, blood vessels and nerves of the formed periodontal ligament must undergo rearrangement, and perhaps disruption, as a tooth erupts. Alterations in the extracellular substance, particularly the collagen fibres, involve resorption and synthesis, and are accompanied by a noticeable change in architecture; these changes are termed remodelling, as distinct from turnover. For many years there was a strong belief that, in the formed ligament, the fibres embedded in cementum and in bone are spliced together in an "intermediate plexus". The "intermediate plexus" was regarded as the site where fibres could be depolymerized to make the two halves of the ligament discontinuous, and synthesized to re-establish its continuity. Consequently, it was thought that the adjustments that must occur in the ligament if a tooth is to be allowed to erupt (or to be moved in any other direction), take place in the "intermediate plexus". This view also suggests, by implication, that the "intermediate plexus" is the seat of highest metabolic activity in the ligament. As has been discussed above, it is evident that the highest metabolic activity is located in the peripheral part of the ligament and not in an "intermediate plexus". This finding makes it likely that the remodelling of the ligament takes place on the bone side, and there is light microscope morphological evidence that this is the case in reactivated eruption. Consequently, belief that an "intermediate plexus" provides the site for remodelling of the periodontal ligament is no longer tenable. All that can be said of the "intermediate plexus" in the formed ligament is that it is an appearance resulting from plane of section. Evidence that there is no physiologically significant "intermediate plexus" in the developing ligament is also beginning to accumulate.

The extent of resorption of collagen fibres at any given time during eruption is of importance. If a large proportion of the peripheral fibre matrix were resorbed, and not simultaneously replaced, the tooth would loosen, as occurs in scurvy. Although nothing is known about the topic, it is clear that the resorption and synthesis occurring during eruption must take place very rapidly in continually changing sites in the ligament. This would permit the tooth to retain its attachment to bone throughout eruption, while allowing the fibres of the ligament first to be distorted as a result of the movement of the tooth, and subsequently to be remodelled and reconstituted in a new orientation to accommodate to the new position of the tooth.

The extent to which the ground substance, the blood vessels and nerves are remodelled during eruption is not known. There is evidence that during reactivated eruption of teeth of limited growth the fibres of the central part of the ligament are carried occlusally on the tooth, while those in the peripheral part of the ligament are remodelled. This means that the contents of the peripheral part of the periodontal space remain spatially static, whereas those more central move. Vessels and nerves in the central part of the space are presumably able to stretch sufficiently to accommodate their dislocation. Alternatively, the vessels in particular may proliferate, as occurs, for example, in wound healing. Once more, this is a question that requires solution.

It is reasonable to suppose that the processes that are responsible for the remodelling of the periodontal ligament during eruption are the same as those that effect its turnover during normal function. The difference between the two processes is probably quantitative and not qualitative, but the nature of the stimuli that increase the rate of resorption and deposition to the level of that which occurs during eruption is unknown.

An erupting tooth whose crown lies in the mouth is subject to extrinsic forces which may originate from mastication or from the oral musculature, so that the tooth must be supported during eruption. It is obvious that the intrinsic force of eruption acting on the tooth is sufficient to overcome the extrinsic occlusal forces, or the tooth would stop erupting. This is not so say that the force of eruption is greater than occlusal forces, but rather that the occlusal forces are intermittent, whilst the eruptive force is continuous.

For the tooth to be supported during eruption it clearly must be attached to the alveolar bone, and the periodontium must be able to resist the pressures that are exerted upon the tooth. Maintenance of the attachment between tooth and bone during eruption has been discussed above. It seems likely that despite the remodelling that is taking place in the periodontal ligament of the erupting tooth, support for the tooth (as distinct from attachment of the tooth to bone) will still be provided by blood pressure, interstitial fluid, cells, ground substance, and collagen fibres, the last-named acting as a "cushion" rather than as guy-ropes.

Penetration of Gingival Connective Tissues by the Erupting Tooth

A tooth erupting from its crypt has to penetrate the fibrous connective tissue of the overlying gingiva, and this is permitted by destruction of the gingival connective tissue and epithelium. The manner in which this occurs is not clear, but it may be expected that the process of removal is in part the same as that which occurs in the resorptive phase in turnover of the periodontal ligament and, presumably in gingival lamina propria. Once again, the question to be posed concerns the nature of the stimulus that presumably depresses synthesis and enhances resorption by the connective tissue cells. This stimulus could be provided by pressure on the overlying connective tissue exerted by the erupting tooth, acting directly or indirectly by interfering with the blood supply. Alternatively, some interaction between the dental epithelium and the overlying connective tissue, arising from increased pressure in the area, could be responsible. A further possibility is that the epithelium plays a part in resorption of the extracellular substance, as epithelial cells are known to have the capacity for phagocytosis. The cells in the connective tissue overlying the erupting crown eventually die, and it seems likely that their disruption results in shedding of enzymes, including collagenase, that are able to digest the extracellular substance of the gingival connective tissue, an occurrence which would provide another mechanism for its removal.

TOOTH MOVEMENT

In this section the descriptive knowledge of tooth movement will be discussed briefly, and this will be followed by an attempt to look at the cellular activity that occurs in response to extrinsic pressure being applied to a tooth.

If a tooth is moved, say from lingual to labial by an extrinsic force, it will eventually be located in a new position in the jaw and, if stabilized there, will be supported in its new situation by a remodelled periodontium with a periodontal space of normal width. The events that occur from the time movement is initiated to the end of the process are illustrated in fig. 2. For simplicity of description it will be assumed that the tooth is moved bodily, that it is not tipped, and that the distance moved is short. Application of the force will move the tooth towards the labial aspect of the socket. As a result, the periodontal space on the lingual aspect of the root will be widened and that on the labial aspect narrowed, and the crest of the alveolar bone will be bent, that on the lingual aspect being pulled

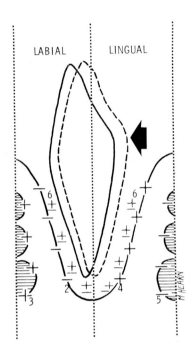

FIG. 2. Diagrammatic representation of a tooth that has been moved bodily from lingual to labial illustrating on its labial aspect resorption of the periodontal surface of the alveolar bone (2) and deposition on the spongiosa surface of the alveolar bone (3), and on its lingual aspect deposition on the periodontal surface of the alveolar bone (4) and resorption from the spongiosa surface (5). Remodelling of the periodontal ligament (6) probably occurs peripherally. (+ indicates deposition of extracellular substance, — indicates resorption of extracellular substance.)

labially and that on its labial aspect pushed labially. If the tooth is now stabilized in its new position, a number of cellular processes will be activated. On the lingual aspect of the periodontal space, that is on the side away from which the tooth has been moved, cells will differentiate into osteoblasts and deposit new bone on the periodontal surface of the alveolar bone. New bone will continue to be deposited, and will perhaps be remodelled, until the width of the space has returned to normal limits. It is important to note that the osteogenesis is controlled, and that it does not continue unabated until the periodontal space is obliterated, a phenomenon that will be taken up again below. Apposition of bone on the periodontal surface of the alveolar bone may be accompanied by resorption from its spongiosa surface or, where alveolar bone and external cortical plate are fused,

from the periosteal surface, so that the preoperative dimension of the alveolar bone is largely maintained. It is to be expected that coincidental with osteogenesis, remodelling of the ligament, particularly the collagen fibres, will occur. Movement of the tooth must be expected to change the orientation of fibres of the ligament and the arrangement of ground substance on all aspects of the tooth. This remodelling would involve resorption of collagen and ground substance in appropriate sites and their replacement by material deposited in the desired orientation and arrangement.

Movement of the tooth will narrow the periodontal space on its labial aspect. This will be followed in a few days, in areas of the periodontal ligament that have not been devitalized by compression, by differentiation of osteoclasts and resorption of bone from the periodontal surface of the alveolar bone. Coincidentally, new bone will be deposited on the spongiosa aspect of the alveolar bone or, where the alveolar bone and external cortical plate are fused, subperiosteally. These processes, accompanied by remodelling of the periodontal ligament bring about restoration of the dimensions of the periodontal space, maintenance of the thickness of the alveolar bone and restoration of the architecture of the periodontal space on the labial aspect of the tooth. Similar changes may be expected to occur on the mesial and distal aspects of the tooth.

If compression of the periodontal ligament is of a degree sufficient to cause its necrosis, and this appears to be a common occurrence in orthodontic movement of teeth, then resorption of the alveolar bone is effected by osteoclasts that differentiate on its spongiosa surface or, where this does not exist, on the periosteal surface, and not on its periodontal surface. This resorption, so-called "undermining resorption", results in formation of a wide periodontal space that is later restored to normal dimensions by deposition of new bone. The necrotic periodontal ligament must be invaded by cells which then resorb its remains and synthesize new extracellular substance for its reconstitution. The osteoblasts that lay down the new bony wall probably originate from the adjacent spongiosa and periosteum, and possibly from cells of the newly-formed periodontal ligament.

The basic processes described above occur universally, irrespective of whether the distance through which the tooth is moved is short or long, or whether the force is applied briefly or for a protracted period. The cellular activities that effect these processes will now be discussed.

Differentiation of Osteoblasts and Osteoclasts

The stimuli directly responsible for the differentiation of osteoblasts and osteoclasts from cells of the periodontal ligament in response to pressure on a tooth are not known. A number of possible stimuli need to be discussed, but the first question that should be raised is the behaviour of progenitor cells prior to the differentiation of specialized cells.

It is self-evident that there must be a continual supply of new osteoblasts and osteoclasts to remodel the periodontium as a tooth is moved, and that these must be provided by division of progenitor cells. Experiments have shown that cells of the ligament incorporate ^{3}H-thymidine, and that the rate of incorporation is increased when teeth are moved. There is also an accompanying increase in mitotic rate, but this is lower than the rate of incorporation of ^{3}H-thymidine, which raises the question as to whether rate of ^{3}H-thymidine incorporation can be equated with rate of mitosis. What are the stimuli that increase synthesis of DNA and mitotic activity?

Control of mitosis in tissues other than the periodontium has received considerable attention. One of the mechanisms that appears to be concerned with controlling mitotic activity involves an inhibitor, termed a chalone, which is secreted by cells of the same type as its target cells. It is therefore tissue-specific, and it requires adrenaline as a cofactor. There is evidence that removal of cells from a tissue by wounding decreases the amount of inhibitor that is being secreted by the tissue as a whole. As a result, inhibition of mitosis is decreased and, as a consequence, there is a burst of mitotic activity in the cells in the vicinity of the wound. It is easy to understand how such a mechanism could account for increased mitotic activity following wounding, but not so easy to understand how it could promote increased mitotic activity in response to movement of a tooth except when death of ligament cells occurs following application of excess force. The availability to the cells of adrenaline and the presence of receptor sites for adrenaline on the cell surface play a part in the activity of the chalone. Perhaps alterations in the availability of circulating hormone or alterations in the surface of the cells of the ligament could occur in response to tooth movement. In this connection, it is of interest that alterations in circulating hormone are thought to play a role in the diurnal rhythm of mitosis.

In addition to chalones, there are other substances believed to play a role in the control of mitosis, and these include calcium ions, hormones and cyclic AMP. As will be discussed briefly below, in relation to differentiation of osteoblasts and osteoclasts, it is possible that other mitotic inhibitor or stimulator substances could be produced or activated by local cellular activity or changes in cell surface in response to alterations in the conditions of the periodontal space.

A number of stimuli have been shown to influence the differentiation of osteoblasts and osteoclasts in general. *In vitro*, under given experimental conditions, oxygen tension has been shown to influence resorption and deposition of bone, and heparin has been shown to enhance resorption. As is well known, parathormone stimulates resorption of bone and calcitonin stimulates osteogenesis. One of the prostaglandins (E_1) is believed to stimulate local resorption of bone and it has recently been suggested that lymphocytes stimulated by endotoxin produce an "osteoclast activation factor" which promotes resorption of bone. These last observations raise the important possibility that, in response to appropriate stimuli, cells of the periodontal tissues could secrete substances capable of stimulating differentiation of osteoclasts and perhaps osteoblasts.

It is not possible to discuss factors that stimulate resorption and deposition of bone without mentioning the effect of biophysical stimuli such as streaming potentials, and

particularly piezo-electricity, both of which have been demonstrated in bone. Piezo-electricity is charge produced by deformation of an asymmetrical crystal. Such crystals include hydroxyapatite, and collagen and other fibrous proteins. Much has been written in this field, and the changes that occur in alveolar bone in response to movement of a tooth have been interpreted against this background. It has been shown that if a long bone is bent, the convex surface will become positively charged and the concave surface negative. A positive charge is believed to stimulate osteoclasis and a negative charge osteogenesis, and this results in restoration of the contours of the bone to those existing before deformation (fig. 3). The crystalline

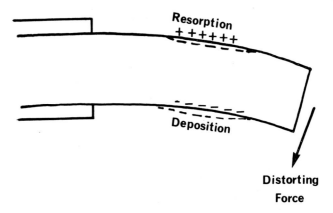

FIG. 3. Electrical effects and bone remodelling. When bone is subject to a distorting force it becomes bent in a curve. The convex face acquires a positive charge and is resorbed while the concave face develops a negative charge resulting in bone deposition.

constituent which produces this changed charge structure in bone is the collagen, and not the hydroxyapatite crystals. Attempts have been made to correlate patterns of osteogenesis and osteoclasis with the bending of bone that is known to occur as a result of movement of teeth and with the relative changes in distribution of charge on bone surfaces that result (fig. 4). However, while such a mechanism may be important, there is no direct evidence that changes in relative charge on surfaces of alveolar bone can be correlated precisely with differentiation of osteoblasts and osteoclasts following tooth movement *in vivo*. Furthermore, piezo-electric phenomena do not explain the fact that, in the absence of damage to the ligament, bone is normally deposited on the spongiosa surface of the alveolar bone on the "pressure side" whereas, when the ligament becomes necrotic, there is resorption from this surface.

Some of the other mechanisms that may be responsible for the behaviour of cells in response to application of a force to a tooth should now be considered. For many years it has been believed that pressure in the periodontal space results in interference with blood supply, and that this leads to formation of osteoclasts and resorption of alveolar bone. Conversely, it is held that increasing the width of the space leads to increased tension in the fibres of the periodontal ligament and to dilatation of blood vessels, and that this results in differentiation of functioning osteoblasts and osteogenesis. Although basically acceptable, such a concept is, in the light of current knowledge, too facile an explanation. Shortly after application of a force to a tooth, there is compression of periodontal blood vessels in the parts of the periodontal space where pressure is increased, and the vessels are dilated in the sites where the space is widened. However, after a few days, capillary loops are seen to have developed in the vicinity of the bony wall on the compression side, and this change is accompanied by the differentiation of osteoclasts. No sprouts are given off from the dilated vessels and osteoblasts differentiate on the bony wall associated with these. A number of interpretations may be placed on these observations:

(a) The changes in oxygen tension resulting from alterations in circulation in the ligament are responsible for differentiation of these cells. This possibility must be considered, but there are many other physiological changes occurring in response to movement of a tooth that cannot be ignored;

(b) changes in circulation could be expected to be followed by changes in pH in the micro-environment, and the effect of these changes in pH on the progenitor cells must be considered;

(c) mast cells are present in normal functioning periodontal ligament. These mast cells may degranulate under pressure or changes in blood supply, and release heparin which could stimulate osteoclasis;

(d) pressure and tension may conceivably have a direct effect on the connective tissue cells of the ligament. It is now known how susceptible these cells are to changes of this sort. For example, it has been found that *in vitro*, where blood supply is not a factor to be considered, a single short sharp application of force to a tooth will result in necrosis of the affected area of the ligament in 2–3 days. On the other hand, a limited increase in pressure or tension could result in secretion by the cells of local active factors such as prostaglandins or "osteoclast or osteoblast activation factors" that act on progenitor cells; and

(e) the changes in the charge structure that follows deformation of bone, and possibly deformation of collagen fibres of the periodontal ligament, could affect progenitor cells indirectly through changes in intercellular communication, cellular secretion of locally active factors, or by some other means.

If too great a pressure is applied to a tooth, the ligament will be compressed between bone and tooth in some sites, and necrosis will occur. How much pressure is needed to produce necrosis is not known, but it is evident that this depends in part on the manner in which the tooth is being moved. It is conceivable that the phenomenon occurs following deprivation of blood supply resulting from occlusion of vessels, but the degree to which cells are able to withstand increases in pressure *in vivo* is not known. The most obvious sequel to necrosis of areas of the ligament is the failure of osteoclasts to differentiate on the surface of the associated alveolar bone. The reason for this is obvious: if the cells of the part have been killed, there can be no source of osteoclasts. The outcome of this state of affairs is the differenti-

ation of osteoclasts on the spongiosa aspect of the affected area of alveolar bone. When forces of lesser magnitude are applied to the tooth, it is osteoblasts that develop at this surface. This raises the question of the nature of the stimuli that result in osteoclasts differentiating in a site where, when similar events are less traumatic, osteoblasts differentiate. The enigma of the possible role of piezo-electric stimuli in this situation has already been mentioned. Another

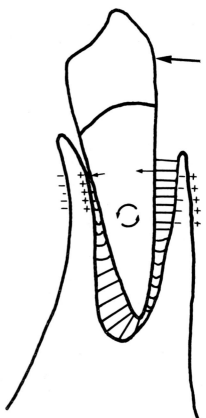

FIG. 4. Electrical effects on bone remodelling in orthodontic treatment. When the tooth is subjected to a sideways thrust (large arrow) it is resisted by the tissues of the socket so that the effect is that of a couple. The bone on the inner edge of the socket on the left hand side is distorted becoming more convex. Hence it becomes positively charged and is resorbed. The bone on the inner edge of the socket to the right is under tension from the periodontal fibres. Hence it becomes more concave, acquires a negative charge and new bone is deposited there. As a consequence the tooth moves towards the left.

mechanism that could be considered involves possible communication between cells in bone and those covering its surfaces. Signals may be transmitted between the osteocytes of viable alveolar bone and the cells covering its surfaces, and there is morphological and physiological evidence obtained from bone elsewhere to encourage this view. These signals could stimulate progenitor cells to differentiate into osteoblasts or osteoclasts in response to changes in cellular environment or cellular physiology. Such a situation is thought to occur elsewhere in the skeleton. It therefore seems reasonable to suppose that necrosis of cells arising out of movement of a tooth could lead to communication of a specific message directing progenitor cells on the spongiosa surface to differentiate into osteoclasts, whereas resorptive activity on the periodontal surface would result in communication by the osteocytes of a different message that would stimulate differentiation of osteoblasts on the spongiosa surface. This communication might be effected by substances being passed from one cell to another via specialized intercellular contacts, gap junctions, that have been identified between communicating cells elsewhere, or through released substances being taken up by adjacent cells, or through changes in surfaces of adjacent cells.

Differentiation of Fibroblasts and "Fibroclasts"

Remodelling of the periodontal ligament involves differentiation of fibroblasts and "fibroclasts", the stimulus for whose differentiation is not understood. Much of what can be said about the topic has been set down above and in the section on eruption. One point that should be raised, however, is this: if piezo-electric stimuli arising out of deformation of bone originate in the collagen fibres, does deformation of the ligament by moving the tooth have an effect on the charge-structure in the ligament? This question has not received much attention.

Control of Osteogenesis in the Periodontal Ligament

Despite considerable remodelling of bone and periodontal ligament during tooth movement, the width of the periodontal space is eventually restored to normal limits. Unfortunately, it is not known how this control is exercised, nor by what tissue or cells. There is some evidence to support the belief that control of osteogenesis is vested in the periodontal ligament. If a sufficient amount of the periodontal ligament is removed or killed experimentally or by accidental trauma, cells will invade the affected part of the periodontal space, and new bone will obliterate the space and ankylose the root of the tooth to the bone of the jaw. It is not known what constituent of the ligament is responsible for this control, the cells, the fibres, or the ground substance. It is known that the presence or absence of hyaluronic acid plays an important role in controlling cellular movement and differentiation in some developmental processes, and that collagen is thought by some investigators to play a similar role in others. This means

that extracellular substance as well as cells could contribute to the homeostatic processes of the periodontal ligament. It seems probable that the cells of the ligament are responsible for this control. Even if the extracellular substance does play an important role in this control mechanism, it is the cells that are responsible for the quantitative and qualitative make-up of the extracellular substance and which respond to changes in environment by changes in their secretion.

It may eventually be found that the resorption of cementum that sometimes accompanies tooth movement, and for which there does not appear to be an explanation, occurs as a result of loss or alteration of the homeostatic mechanisms discussed above. However, pressure on the tooth has been observed to change the distribution of charge on the surface of the root so that piezo-electricity may be implicated in the process.

(d) Remodelling of Gingival Connective Tissue

It is well known that teeth that have been rotated tend to return to their former position. Surgical incision of the gingiva apparently prevents, or at least modifies, the extent of this relapse. This suggests the possibility that, for reasons unknown, the collagen fibres of the gingival lamina propria are not remodelled as rapidly or as readily as those of the periodontal ligament. If the turnover of the extracellular substance of gingival connective tissue is slower than that of the periodontal ligament, the tardy remodelling of gingival fibres following rotation of teeth would easily be explained, but the evidence on this point is currently confused. Furthermore, it is well known that repair of wounds in gingiva is rapid, and consequently one could expect to see active remodelling, but this does not appear to be the case. It seems that this is a phenomenon requiring careful examination, and its solution could provide useful information for the clinician.

Effect of Tooth Movement on Dental Pulp

In conclusion, it should be mentioned that movement of teeth can cause damage to the dental pulp. This may become apparent in dentinogenesis, formation of pulp stones, or even death of the pulp. Interference with the apical vessels, and consequently with the blood supply to the pulp, is the likely cause of these changes.

36. GINGIVAL TISSUE

H. E. SCHROEDER

DEFINITIONS AND SUBDIVISIONS OF GINGIVAL TISSUE

Gingival tissue is defined as that portion of oral mucous membrane which, in the complete post-eruptive dentition of a healthy young individual, surrounds the neck of the tooth and covers the alveolar bone crest coronally and externally. Its existence is a function of the presence of erupted teeth. Its development begins at the moment when the most coronally situated portion of a tooth, during its eruption, has created the initial break in the continuity of the oral epithelium, *i.e.* when the tip of the crown makes its appearance in the oral cavity. It serves deciduous as well as permanent teeth. It is the most peripheral portion of the periodontal tissues at large.

Clinically as well as histologically the gingival tissue is subdivided into three portions. These are classically termed the **free**, the **attached** and the **interdental gingiva.** These terms, in the course of recent history, were neither always unequivocally clear nor of generally accepted meaning. For example, depending on the views prevailing about the existence and nature of the epithelial attachment and the definition of the gingival sulcus, the free gingiva was either regarded as almost non-existent under normal conditions or defined as that tissue located coronal to the contour of the cemento-enamel junction.

Free (marginal) gingiva (fig. 1) is the most peripheral comprising a narrow, smooth rim, which follows the cervical contours of the tooth orally and facially. Its width ranges between 0·5–2·0 mm. Coronally, the free gingiva terminates at the gingival margin, a line passing through the most coronal points of the tissue surrounding the neck of the tooth. Apically, its borderline is at the gingival groove which demarcates free and attached gingivae externally. The gingival groove is most pronounced and more frequently found on the vestibular side. Under normal conditions, it never really comprises a solid continuous furrow but rather is a result of a series of irregularly aligned surface stipples. An imaginary line connecting the gingival groove

with the cemento-enamel junction (fig. 1) represents the internal level of demarcation between free and attached portions. It is the tissue located coronally to this line which deserves the clinical impression of being free, *i.e.* mechanically movable against and/or from the tooth surface. In other words, the term "free" is a clinical designation and relates to a clinical "property" of the gingival rim. From a biological point of view, the free gingival tissue portion, through the mechanism of epithelial attachment, is united to the tooth surface rather than free, *i.e.* disconnected. Although biologically attached, the peripheral portion of the gingiva is clinically still subject to mechanically displacing movements. Therefore, it appears unreasonable to deny the clinical existence of a freely movable gingival rim, even if there is no sulcus gingivae present.

Attached (stippled) gingiva (fig. 1) is located apical to the free gingival tissue portion. This portion is confined mainly to the labial aspects of the upper and lower jaws. On the palatal aspect, the attached gingiva is part of the overall attached mucosa of the hard palate. On the lingual aspect, the attached portion extends to the floor of the mouth. The attached gingiva ranges in width from a few up to about 10 mm. Its amount and compactness vary within one and between different individuals. In general, the attached portion is most obvious labially in relation to anterior teeth of the upper and lower jaw and diminishes in width distally. Its coronal border is the gingival groove. Apically it merges into the alveolar mucosa at the mucogingival junction (fig. 1). The latter does not exist on the palatal aspect. The surface pattern of the attached gingival portion is characterized by numerous stipples. These pitlike surface indentations appear randomly scattered and reflect a peculiar cross-over of inserting collagen fibres. Stipples are encountered over sites where the epithelial ridges of the epithelium-connective tissue interface interconnect. The term "attached", therefore, refers to the fact that this tissue is comprised mainly of collagen fibre bundles which arise from the cervical root surface as well as from the periosteal surface of alveolar bone, and insert into subepithelial connective-tissue papillae. This fibre arrangement results in the firmness and immobility of the attached tissue portion.

Interdental (papillary) gingiva (fig. 6) is that tissue located at and within the interproximal space of adjacent teeth. Its shape and contour depend upon the position of adjoining teeth, whether the teeth are in contact, and how wide diastemata extend. Between contacting posterior teeth, the interdental gingiva comprises two elevated tissue portions, the vestibular and lingual papillae, and an apically curved col between them. While the vestibular papilla, in general, extends more coronally than the lingual one, the shape of the col which lies apical to the contact point depends on the linguo-buccal extension of the contacting teeth. By definition, and for topographical and clinical reasons, the coronal part of the interdental gingiva is regarded as free gingival tissue, although it differs in shape and contour, while the apical part, lying below the cemento-enamel junction, should be categorized as attached tissue. That is, the interdental tissue is a combination of free and attached gingiva especially adapted to the topographical situation prevailing within the interproximal space.

partly through the same collagen fibre bundles, is also connected and attached to the cervical root surface.

The attached gingiva varies considerably in width and extent. There are no data to indicate that its pattern reflects certain or general anatomic situations such as the coronal level of alveolar bone. Formerly, it was sometimes alluded

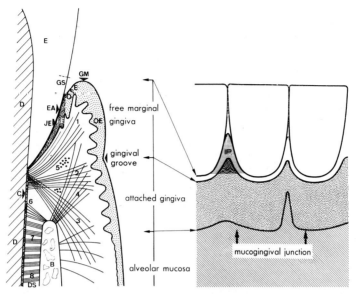

FIG. 1. Clinical features and schematic section of labial/buccal gingival tissue. B = bone; C = cementum; D = dentine; DS = periodontal ligament; E = enamel; EA = epithelial attachment; GM = gingival margin; GS = gingival sulcus; IP = interdental papilla; JE = junctional epithelium; OE = oral epithelium; OSE = oral sulcular epithelium. 1 = cemento-gingival fibres; 2 = cemento-gingival fibres, horizontal portion; 3 = cemento-gingival fibres, alveolar portion; 4 = alveolo-gingival fibres; 5 = circular fibres; 6 = cemento-alveolar fibres; 7/8 = differently oriented periodontal fibres.

Clinical *vis-à-vis* Structural Aspects

From a biological point of view, the differentiation into free, attached, and interdental gingiva appears unnecessary and somewhat misleading. Differences in shape, contour and clinical properties appear to be minimal in tissues which are normal, and are the result of tissue adaptation to the particular topographical relations between the teeth and the alveolar bone crest rather than a reflection of structural originality. Stippling, under normal conditions, extends very close to the gingival margin. The smoothness of the peripheral gingival rim can conceivably be attributed to epithelial curvature and a particular fibre arrangement rather than to a different type of epithelium. The clinical impression of handling a freely movable tissue is an apparent one because, as discussed later, the peripheral tissue is subject to epithelial rather than to fibrous attachment. The demarcating effect of the gingival groove rests on an irregular distribution of isolated stipples. The connective tissue fibres arising from the alveolar bone crest and the cervical root surface radiate into free as well as attached gingiva. In fact, in a normal freely movable gingival rim, the connective tissue is composed of the same dense meshwork of collagen fibres as is that of the attached gingival portion. Ultimately, the free tissue portion, in a similar sense and

to under the general, unfortunate term "masticatory mucosa". The attached gingiva is, however, a product of genetically determined factors rather than of environmental influences.

For all these reasons—and similar arguments apply to a separation of the interdental portion—the gingival tissue should be regarded as a unit, and, if subdivision is necessary, it should be on a topographical basis. The gingival unit could thus be defined as that tissue which is located around the neck of the tooth and is demarcated coronally by the gingival margin, interdental col and papillae, and by the muco-gingival junction apically. A line connecting the muco-gingival junction with the bone crest and the tooth surface apical to the cemento-enamel junction would separate the gingival tissue from the periodontal ligament and the alveolar mucosa. This definition is not valid for the palatal gingiva which does not offer a landmark such as the muco-gingival junction. At this site, the freely movable gingival portion is nothing more than the peripheral rim of the overall attached palatal mucosa.

Normality

Under everyday conditions strictly normal gingival tissue is rarely found in humans. While antigens and the microbial flora occur, but do not concentrate, clinically and histo-pathologically normal gingival tissue can be maintained under strict, chemical or mechanical, oral hygiene procedures. A vibrating massage and mechanical stimulation of the gingival tissue is unnecessary to maintain normality, provided that microbial and antigenic injury does not surpass a rather low, unspecified threshold level. In germ-free animals, normal gingival tissue is usual.

The following features characterize normal gingival tissue histologically (figs. 2a, b and 7a): Keratinizing oral epithelium covers the tissue up to the gingival margin. The latter is located at the enamel surface and terminates edgewise. There is no gingival sulcus. A smooth strip of junctional epithelium, practically free of transmigrating leucocytes, extends coronally to the gingival margin. The classical sulcus bottom, *i.e.* the free surface of junctional epithelium, coincides with the gingival margin. The collagen fibre meshwork directly supports the junctional epithelium. There is no sign of either acute inflammation or of chronic cellular infiltration.

Clinically the following criteria have all to be met: The tissue is basically pale pink (unless pigmented). It slopes coronally into a thin edge, forming a scalloped pattern marginally, the papillae declining into and filling the interproximal space to the contact point. Its surface reveals a consistent stippling extending close to the gingival margin. The tissue is firm and flat. A periodontal probe would pass 0·5–2·0 mm. below the gingival margin until it meets resistance. No sulcus fluid can be harvested. Leucocytes are rare when examined by intraepithelial (junctional epithelium) strip or loop sampling.

A clinically healthy gingiva cannot, however, be equated with tissue normality. Gingival tissue which fulfils all the above-mentioned requirements for health might still deviate histologically from a strictly normal pattern. A typical feature to be encountered in clinically healthy and even histologically non-inflamed gingiva is focal infiltration by lymphocytes and macrophages of some portions of the junctional and oral epithelium (fig. 2c, d). This infiltration involves mainly basal and immediately suprabasal layers of the junctional epithelium as well as a narrow zone of the underlying connective tissue. It is far removed from the gingival margin and the sulcus bottom, and resembles a partly infiltrated portion of tonsillar crypt epithelium. In addition, or as a separate feature, a small population of probably transmigrating neutrophilic granulocytes may be found within the intercellular spaces of the junctional epithelium without accompanying signs of acute inflammatory reactions in the connective tissue, *i.e.* without changes from clinical normality. In man, particularly in children and adolescents, a moderately infiltrated junctional epithelium in combination with a narrow zone of infiltrated sub-epithelial connective tissue can be concealed in gingival tissue which is clinically close to normal (fig. 2e, f). In such cases, the non-epithelial cell population residing within the junctional epithelium consists, by average volume, of 45 per cent neutrophilic granulocytes and 60 per cent mononuclear cells, mostly lymphocytes and macrophages (Schroeder, 1973). The connective tissue infiltrate would be comprised of up to 75 per cent lymphocytes (Schroeder, Münzel-Pedrazzoli and Page, 1973). Clinical leucocyte sampling would, however, reveal the presence of an elevated number of inflammatory cells within the junctional epithelium. It appears that initial changes in colour, contour, texture and consistency mainly reflect the state and extent of acute inflammatory reactions. The latter being minimal, partly infiltrated gingival tissue might still appear clinically close to normal. The threshold level up to which a deviation from strict histological normality would remain undetectable clinically is difficult to determine and unknown at present.

Structural Components

Gingival tissue which meets most of the requirements of clinical health, *i.e.* gingiva of a clinical status which can be achieved by everyday oral hygiene procedures and then reflects "normality" in man, deviates in its structural composition slightly but in part significantly from strict normality as outlined above. Clinically normal gingiva in man is generally characterized by a shallow gingival sulcus, and no more than a narrow zone of cells infiltrating the connective tissue (figs. 1 and 3a). In gross histological terms, gingival tissue is composed of stratified epithelium and densely collagenous and highly vascularized connective tissue. Gingival epithelium includes two types of stratified epithelia (non-keratinizing and keratinizing) which, for topographical reasons, are termed junctional epithelium, oral sulcular epithelium and oral epithelium (figs. 1 and 3). The junctional epithelium provides the epithelial attachment which unites the gingival tissue to the tooth surface. The oral sulcular epithelium is the coronal portion of the epithelium which lines the gingival sulcus laterally and is continuous with and structurally similar to the oral epithelium. The latter covers the gingival tissue at vestibular, lingual and palatal sites. The gingival connective tissue, including a number of preferentially oriented collagen fibre bundles, provides tone and tensile strength to the tissue and unites it to the cervical cementum surface as well as to the alveolar bone crest. It often harbours a small cellular infiltrate immediately beneath the junctional epithelium and in close topographical relationship to the sulcus bottom (fig. 3a). By volume, the gingival tissue, on the average, is comprised of 4 per cent junctional epithelium, 27 per cent oral sulcular and oral epithelium, and 69 per cent connective tissue. The latter may include an infiltrated portion of approximately 3–6 per cent of gingival tissue volume (Schroeder *et al.*, 1973).

The coronal portion of the gingiva–tooth interface, which in young individuals covers part of the cervical enamel surface, is maintained by epithelial cell-attachment, while that portion located between the cemento-enamel junction and the alveolar bone crest comprises a collagenous fibre attachment. In ideal situations, the epithelial cell and fibre-attachment meet at the cemento-enamel junction (figs 1, 2a, c, e and 3a). However, both the structure and the topography of the junction vary along the circumference of a particular tooth as well as between different teeth. Not only may the junctional epithelium terminate at various points up to 1 mm. coronal to the cemento-enamel junction or slightly overlap the root cementum (Schroeder and

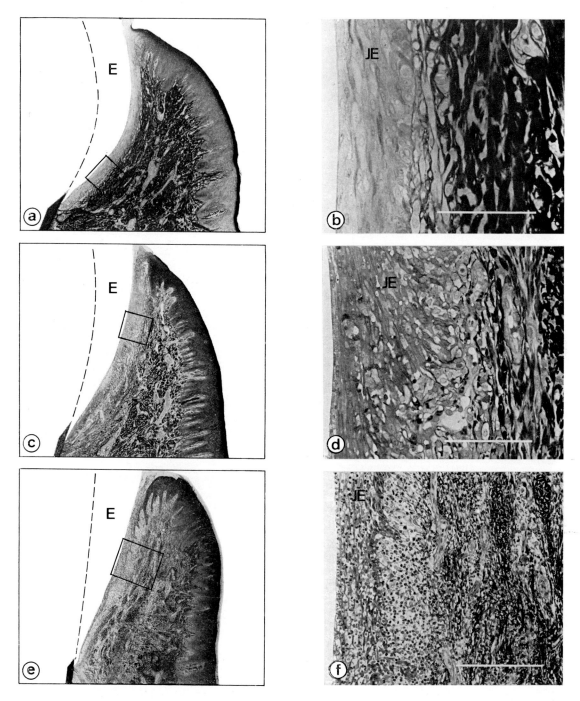

Fig. 2. Histological features of clinically healthy, buccal gingival tissue. (a) Dog gingiva after several weeks of toothbrushing. Junctional epithelium and underlying connective tissue completely free of transmigrating or infiltrating inflammatory cells. No gingival sulcus present. Outlined area is shown in (b). E = enamel. ×30. (b) Higher magnification of area outlined in (a). Adjacent to junctional epithelium (JE) is infiltrate-free connective tissue. Narrow zone of subepithelial vascular plexus is enmeshed and supported by fibre bundles. ×270 (white bar = 100 μm.). (c) Dog gingiva after several weeks of tooth-brushing. Junctional epithelium is heavily infiltrated with lymphocytes. No gingival sulcus present. Outlined area is shown in (d). E = enamel. ×30. (d) Higher magnification of area outlined in (c). Junctional epithelium (JE), exhibiting indistinct border with connective tissue, is heavily infiltrated by lymphocytes; these also appear extravascularly within subepithelial vascular zone which is supported by collagen fibres. ×240 (white bar = 100 μm.). (e) Clinically healthy human gingiva. Narrow sulcus bordered by infolding oral epithelium. Predominantly lymphoid round cell infiltrate within zone of vascular plexus. Outlined area is shown in (f). E = enamel. ×23. (f) Higher magnification of area outlined in (e). Junctional epithelium (JE) infiltrated with migrating neutrophil granulocytes as well as lymphocytes. Epithelium-connective tissue interface is indistinct. Subepithelial zone harbours lymphoid infiltrate, and fibres have almost disappeared. Fibre bundles underlying infiltrated zone less dense than in (d). ×240 (white bar = 100 μm.).

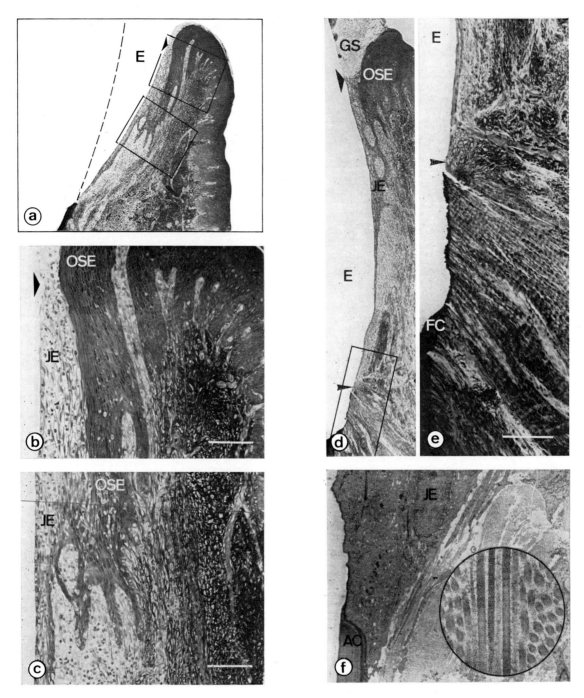

FIG. 3. (a) Section of clinically healthy human buccal gingiva revealing deeply infolding oral sulcular epithelium and shallow sulcus (arrow marks sulcus bottom). Lymphocyte infiltrate at apical termination of junctional epithelium bordered by infolding oral epithelium. Fibre bundles reach into gingival margin. Areas outlined are shown in (b) and (c). E = enamel. ×30. (b) Higher magnification of upper area outlined in (a). Apical to sulcus bottom (arrow) junctional epithelium (JE) is fused to infolding oral sulcular epithelium (OSE) which is supported by collagen network. ×120. (white bar = 100μm.). (c) Higher magnification of the lower area outlined in (a). Lymphocyte infiltrate at apical termination of interface between JE and OSE. ×120 (white bar = 100 μm.). (d) Section of clinically healthy human buccal gingiva. Enamel (E) is covered by a thin layer of fibrillar cementum to which collagen fibres attach. Junctional epithelium (JE) does not reach cemento-enamel junction; apical half is narrow; coronal portion displays epithelial proliferation, fuses with oral sulcular epithelium (OSE) and forms base (arrow) of the gingival sulcus (GS). Outlined area is shown in (e). ×30. (e) Marginal enamel (E) covered by fibrillar cementum (FC) and a two-cell layer of junctional epithelium. Arrow demarcates termination of epithelial and beginning of collagenous attachment. ×135 (white bar = 100μm.). (f) Junctional epithelium (JE) terminating at the cemento-enamel junction formed by spur of afibrillar cementum (AC). Collagen fibre bundles seen in longitudinal and cross-section (inset) under the epithelium. ×2,900. Inset: ×27,400.

Listgarten, 1971), but the latter, not infrequently, overlaps the enamel surface. The cementum which covers part of the enamel surface may be composed of either a coronally advancing spur of afibrillar cementum (fig. 3f) which does not, at least primarily, serve as a stratum for fibre attachment, or a narrow sheet of fibrillar cementum which does carry attachment fibres (fig. 3d, e). Both, the afibrillar cementum spur and the fibrillar cementum sheet, arise from and are continuous with the cementum investing the root surface. In addition, large cervical areas of enamel may be encountered which are covered neither by epithelium nor cementum, but simply faced by connective tissue (Schroeder and Listgarten, 1971). These structural variations along the gingiva–tooth interface, although of minor importance *per se*, probably result from deviations in the ideal course of developmental and eruptional events, and may have clinical implications. The latter indicate that the distance between the gingival margin and the cemento-enamel junction is not generally reflected by the depth to which a periodontal probe can easily be advanced into the gingival sulcus.

Junctional epithelium on the one hand and connective tissue on the other are considered the key components of gingival tissue. Knowledge of their structure and physiological behaviour is essential for any attempt to understand gingival tissue in health and disease.

GINGIVAL EPITHELIUM

The integument of the gingival tissue essentially is a stratified, squamous epithelium derived from the ectodermal layer investing the anterior two-thirds of the mouth. For structural, functional and topographical reasons, it must be differentiated into two different types, the non-keratinizing junctional epithelium and the keratinizing oral sulcular and oral epithelium.

Junctional Epithelium

The term junctional epithelium (formerly called epithelial attachment, attached epithelial cuff, attachment epithelium) designates the epithelial collar which surrounds the neck of the tooth and, in most parts of the tooth circumference, extends from the region of the cemento-enamel junction to the bottom of the gingival sulcus. It provides the epithelial attachment to the tooth surface and is continuous with but structurally distinct from the oral sulcular epithelium (fig. 3). The junctional epithelium must not be confused with what was formerly called crevicular epithelium. The latter, most often, was a term applied to a combination of oral sulcular epithelium and an artificially (during gingivectomy) torn portion of the junctional epithelium lacking its interface to the tooth surface.

Around fully erupted teeth, the bandlike junctional epithelium is 2–3 mm. wide (*i.e.* in the apico-coronal direction); it faces the enamel and/or, in cases of recession, the root surface. At its apical termination it may comprise 1–3 cell layers, while beneath the gingival sulcus it may be 15–30 cells thick.

The junctional epithelium is derived from the reduced enamel epithelium (Schroeder and Listgarten, 1971). Under artificial conditions, *i.e.* after a complete removal by gingivectomy, it can be reconstituted *de novo* by cells derived from the oral epithelium (Listgarten, 1972). During the transforming process, which prior to, during, and after tooth eruption progresses sequentially from the coronal to the cervical sites of the crown and involves reduced ameloblasts as well as the external cells of the reduced enamel epithelium, the cytoplasm of all cells becomes reorganized. The structural features typical of reduced enamel epithelium cells are turned into those characterizing junctional epithelial cells. During this course of development and while the tooth erupts, the former reduced ameloblasts, because of re-established proliferative activity in the former external cells of the reduced enamel epithelium and as a result of regained epithelial turnover, eventually become displaced by daughter cells of the new basal cells of the junctional epithelium. It has to be appreciated that, while both epithelial transformation and tooth eruption take place, there is never an interruption of the epithelial attachment which is established prior to the onset of eruption.

The junctional epithelium is composed of two strata, the stratum basale and the stratum suprabasale. Except for the rather cuboid basal cells, all suprabasal cells are flattened and oriented in a plane parallel to the tooth surface (fig. 4a, b). In contrast to the oral epithelium, cells of the junctional epithelium are interconnected by only a small number of desmosomes. The intercellular space comprises up to 18 per cent of the epithelial volume and may contain a variable number of inflammatory cells. The epithelium–connective tissue junction is generally straight (fig. 3a, c, d), and the epithelium–tooth interface replicates the tooth surface pattern, *i.e.* the enamel perikymata and lines of Pickerill (fig. 4a). The coronal extremity of the junctional epithelium comes to constitute the base of the gingival sulcus as is shown in fig. 3d.

In the interdental gingival portion between contacting teeth the junctional epithelia, which belong to the mesially and distally positioned teeth, fuse coronally to form the surface of the col (figs. 6 and 7a). It is for this reason that the col epithelium lacks keratinization and, as is typical for junctional epithelium, is more easily penetrated by foreign substances. As a result, the subepithelial connective tissue of the col region, which generally lacks cellular infiltrates in germ-free animals (fig. 7b), reflects earlier and most often more advanced symptoms of established chronic gingivitis than that of other gingival regions in man (fig. 7c, d).

All cells constituting the junctional epithelium display a similar cytoplasmic composition. The cytoplasm of junctional epithelial cells is characterized by a prominent Golgi apparatus, extended cisternae of endoplasmic reticulum and scarceness of cytoplasmic filaments. The parameters for volumetric and surface densities reveal that in these cells the Golgi apparatus and rough endoplasmic reticulum are two- to threefold more voluminous and richer in membrane-bound surfaces than in basal cells of the oral epithelium. In contrast to cells of the oral epithelium, which accumulate an increasing volume of cytoplasmic filaments as they approach more distal positions, cells of the junctional epithelium appear to maintain a stable density of cytoplasmic filaments and synthesizing organelles regardless of their

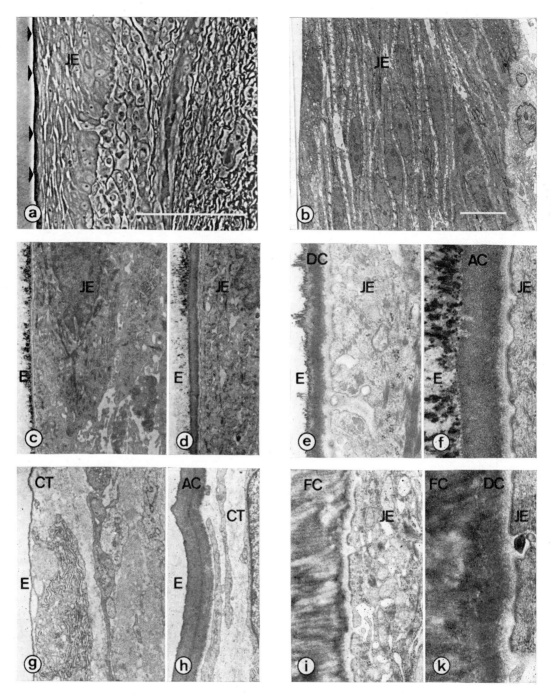

Fig. 4. (a) Section through junctional epithelium (JE). Surface facing enamel replicates perikymata and lines of Pickerill (arrows). Vascular plexus and collagen fibres subjacent to JE. ×300 (white bar = 100 μm.). (b) Higher magnification of junctional epithelium (JE). Basal cells ovoid and columnar; suprabasal cells elongated and parallel to tooth surface. A basal lamina connects JE to enamel surface (left) and to connective tissue (right). ×1,200 (white bar = 10μm.). (c) Internal basal lamina and hemi-desmosomes attach elongated epithelial cells (JE) to crystalline enamel surface (E). ×6,700. (d) Internal basal lamina and hemi-desmosomes attach JE cells to layer of afibrillar cementum which covers crystalline enamel surface (E). ×6,700. (e) Internal basal lamina and hemi-desmosomes attach JE cells to layer of dental cuticle (DC) which covers crystalline enamel surface (E). ×18,500. (f) Internal basal lamina and hemi-desmosomes attach JE cell to cuticle accumulated on afibrillar cementum (AC) which covers crystalline enamel surface (E). ×31,900. (g) Connective tissue (CT) rich in fibroblasts directly opposed to the crystalline enamel surface (E). ×6,700. (h) The connective tissue (CT) apposed to layer of afibrillar cementum (AC) which covers the enamel surface (E). ×25,500. (i) Internal basal lamina and hemi-desmosomes attach JE cells to fibrillar cementum (FC). ×31,900. (k) Internal basal lamina and hemi-desmosomes attach JE cell to dental cuticle (DC) which covers fibrillar root cementum (FC). ×18,500.

actual position. In addition, junctional epithelial cells, especially when positioned beneath the sulcus bottom, contain a remarkably high number of lysosomal bodies and display an appropriate acid phosphatase activity. Not infrequently, they can be observed to have engulfed intercellular débris such as membrane-bound bodies probably derived from transmigrating granulocytes and microorganisms.

Basal cells of the junctional epithelium are attached to the underlying connective tissue by means of a basal lamina and half-desmosomal junctions. As demonstrated for other ectodermal epithelia, anchoring fibrils are regularly associated with the lamina densa at the interface between the junctional epithelium and connective tissue. Part of the basal lamina material, as demonstrated by ruthenium-red and lanthanum labelling, is continuous with the intercellular substance as provided by extraneous cell surface coats. This material, which also fills intermittent gap junctions, is, furthermore, continuous with the basal lamina substance formed at the epithelium-tooth interface. The external (connective tissue side) and the internal (tooth surface side) basal laminae are structurally alike and merge at the apical termination of the junctional epithelium.

At its coronal extremity the junctional epithelium fuses with the oral sulcular epithelium (figs. 1, 2a, c, e and 3a to d). The zone of convergence varies in length depending on the presence, depth and configuration of the sulcus. In clinically healthy gingiva, the coronal epithelial portion frequently narrows between the tooth surface and the oral sulcular epithelium. Because of distinctly different densities of cytoplasmic filaments, the two merging epithelia can easily be distinguished tinctorially (fig. 3a to d).

Junctional epithelium, as measured by autoradiographic techniques in non-human primates, has a remarkably high rate of cellular turnover which is actually double that of the oral epithelium. In this context, it has to be realized that the junctional epithelium serves as the preferential pathway for the emigration of inflammatory cells, especially neutrophilic granulocytes, acting non-specifically in host defence.

The Gingival Sulcus

Under strictly normal conditions there is no gingival sulcus present in man or other mammalian species. In clinically healthy gingiva, the gingival sulcus is defined as the shallow groove between the tooth surface and the gingival tissue, which extends from the sulcus bottom to the level of the gingival margin (fig. 1). On the average, this groove, as measured histologically in clinically close-to-normal tissue of man and dogs, is 0.4 ± 0.1 mm. deep. This shallow groove is lined in part by the free surface of the junctional epithelium forming the sulcus bottom, and in part by the oral sulcular epithelium which provides the lateral wall (fig. 3a, d). Depth, configuration, and the surface proportions provided by either of the epithelia vary around one particular tooth and from one tooth to the next.

The bottom of the sulcus is located at the level up to which the epithelial attachment extends, and the junctional epithelium maintains its integrity and coherence. All junctional epithelial cells bound to exfoliate at this level

approach the sulcus bottom in a vertical position with their edged "end" rather than their flattened surface, which is in contrast to the more usual horizontal orientation of cells at surfaces of stratified squamous epithelia. Not infrequently, the most apical site of the gingival sulcus is located somewhere within the epithelial surface rather than at the site of the tooth surface. Along the latter attached cells can still be encountered coronal to the sulcus bottom prior to being detached from the tooth surface.

All daughter cells of the junctional and the oral sulcular epithelium desquamate at the surface of the sulcus. In addition, the sulcus bottom is the point of entry into the mouth for most of the granulocytes found in saliva. In view of the high rate of desquamation of junctional epithelial cells and the exclusiveness of this epithelium as a pathway for leucocyte transmigration, large numbers of cells can be expected to proliferate, desquamate and transmigrate into the gingival sulcus.

The structural pattern prevailing in the sulcular area escapes routine clinical observations. A probe designed to reinforce clinical diagnostic measures is, in fact, trapped by a tissue which, because of its structural and functional peculiarities, does not resist mechanical challenge. Due to its structural characteristics, the junctional epithelium and its free surface represent the weakest site of the sulcular lining. Not only does it not offer noticeable mechanical resistance but it also is most readily disrupted. The level of the sulcus bottom, therefore, is impossible to determine by routine clinical probing (fig. 5). The latter will result in a pseudo-reversible but reparable disruption within the junctional epithelium rather than a disconnection of cells from the tooth surface. "The distance such a probe will travel through the tissue will vary a great deal, depending on such factors as thickness of the probe, pressure applied, degree of inflammatory cell infiltrate in the junctional epithelium and adjacent connective tissues, degree of connective-tissue fibre destruction, thickness of junctional epithelium and curvature of the tooth surface" (Listgarten, 1972). The clinical measurement of sulcular depth cannot be expected to reflect structural reality.

Epithelial Attachment

The term epithelial attachment refers to a biological phenomenon which operates at but is not unique to the gingiva–tooth interface. It is the means by which epithelial cells adhere to an epithelial or non-epithelial substratum, and the morphologically recognizable components are hemidesmosomes and a basement lamina (fig. 4). It is a product elaborated and constantly maintained by cellular activity, but is non-specific because a variety of different tissues such as connective tissue, enamel, dentine, cementum, can serve as a substratum (fig. 4c to f, i, k). It is needed in order to seal the surface of the oral integument around teeth, and it thus serves to maintain the continuity of the epithelial covering.

Regardless of the substratum against which it is built up, the attachment consists of hemidesmosomes and a basement lamina divided into lamina lucida and lamina densa, both of which, on the average, are 119 ± 19 nm. wide, ranging between 90 and 150 nm. It is structurally similar to the external basement lamina being produced at the interface of junctional epithelium or other epithelia and the connective tissue. Cells facing the tooth surface assume a rather smooth membrane along the basement lamina, which is apposed by elongated hemidesmosomes. The latter are rarely equipped with internally inserting cytoplasmic filaments.

The epithelial attachment extends from the apical termination of the junctional epithelium to and often somewhat beyond the level of the sulcus bottom. In the absence of a gingival sulcus, it extends to the edgelike gingival margin.

junctional epithelium contacts fibrillar cementum of the root surface, the epithelial attachment apparatus is again the same as described above (fig. 4i). When the junctional epithelium terminates at enamel surface sites located coronally to the cemento-enamel junction, connective-tissue contacts the enamel directly or indirectly through the interposition of afibrillar cementum. An epithelial attachment in then lacking (fig. 4g, h).

It has to be appreciated that, being a product of epithelial cells, the epithelial attachment (i.e. the internal basement lamina) is a constantly rebuilt arrangement rather than a static structure. The coronal movement and gliding of

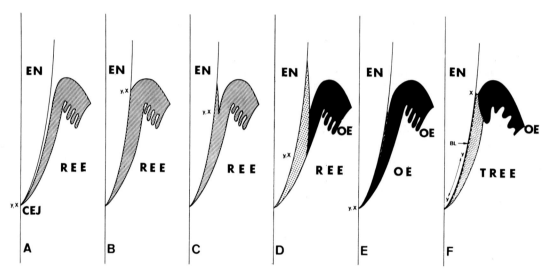

FIG. 5. Schematic drawing illustrating historical and current concepts of the gingival sulcus. EN = enamel; CEJ = enamel-cement junction; REE = reduced enamel epithelium; OE = oral epithelium; TREE = transformed reduced enamel epithelium; BL:basal lamina; x = sulcus (crevice) bottom defined histologically; y = sulcus (crevice) bottom defined clinically. A = G.V. Black, 1915; B = B. Gottlieb, 1921; C = O. Weski, 1922; D = H. Becks, 1941; E = J. Waerhaug, 1952; F = H. E. Schroeder and M. A. Listgarten, 1971. (Adapted from D. Lange, 1972.)

Because of structural irregularities, the epithelial attachment prevailing around a particular tooth does not always unite epithelial cells to the enamel surface proper (fig. 4c). These irregularities consist of the diversified occurrence of two different cellular products covering parts of the enamel surface, i.e. afibrillar cementum and the dental cuticle. The presence of both is highly unpredictable. Afibrillar cementum, in the form of spurs, isolated islands or continuous thin sheets, is a frequently found, mineralized deposit of lamellated structure. It probably develops prior to or during tooth eruption at sites where the enamel surface becomes denuded of its epithelial covering and contacted by connective tissue. It is assumed to be the product of cementoblasts. In the course of further development and eruption, it may become re-covered by junctional epithelium. The epithelial attachment at the afibrillar cementum surface is structurally identical to that found on enamel (fig. 4d, f). The same is true for an epithelial attachment contacting a dental cuticle (fig. 4e, k). The latter, conceivably a product of epithelial cells, is a non-mineralizing, homogeneous, non-lamellated, brittle sheet of varying thickness, which is found covering enamel, dentine, or afibrillar and fibrillar cementum surfaces (fig. 4c, k). When

epithelial cells along the tooth surface necessitates a continuous dissolution and reformation of hemidesmosomal junctions as well as a rearrangement of basement lamina material maintaining a rather constant width.

In contrast to former belief, the importance of the epithelial attachment is not reflected by its physical strength. The latter is large enough to withstand attempts to disconnect junctional epithelial cells from their substratum mechanically, for example, by pulling on gingival tissue. It is also of secondary importance with regard to pathogenic mechanisms operating in this region. The junctional epithelium by providing and maintaining the epithelial attachment, and so sealing the surface around teeth, plays the key role at the gingiva-tooth interface. Because of the structural pattern explained above, its functional abilities and properties are visualized as follows: The junctional epithelium is a loosely knit tissue formed by cells which lack rigidity due to a meagre cytoplasmic filament content. Its cells are equipped with a relatively large set of synthesizing organelles, so that it can maintain two basement laminae located along its internal and external interfaces. It proliferates rapidly, has a rapid turnover and its cells are desquamated at a proportionally narrow free surface. The latter is approached by cells in a vertical position and constitutes the weakest point mechanically for intrusion of foreign bodies. The junctional epithelium serves as the preferential pathway for leucocyte emigration. It adheres rather strongly to both tooth surface and connective tissue, but is readily disrupted internally. For all these reasons the junctional epithelium has to be considered as a weak, readily permeated and easily penetrated, but rapidly repairable membrane through which molecular and cellular movements occur, some of which serve to defend and others to harm the gingival tissue.

Oral Epithelium

The oral epithelium **of the gingival tissue** extends from the gingival margin to the muco-gingival junction buccally or to the floor of the mouth lingually. It is a typically stratified squamous, keratinizing epithelium which closely resembles that of the hard palate where the oral epithelium continues as palatal epithelium. It consists of four strata: stratum basale, stratum spinosum, stratum granulosum and stratum corneum.

The oral epithelium which is firmly attached to the underlying connective tissue has a characteristically undulating subsurface. The connective tissue extends with ridges and/or fingerlike papillae, often running more or less parallel to the gingival margin, into respective depressions of the oral epithelium. When the epithelial lamellae embracing the connective tissue ridges intersect or furcate, small circular depressions, termed stipples, develop at respective sites of the free epithelial surface. Along the undulated epithelium–connective tissue interface, a basement lamina, product of the basal cell layer, separates the two tissues. The basement lamina is typically comprised of a lamina densa and a lamina lucida. These vary in thickness between 34 and 57 nm., or 24 and 43 nm., respectively. This basement lamina is only part of what is known in light microscopy by the term basement membrane. The latter refers to a subepithelial zone, 0.5–1.0 μm. in width, which includes the basement lamina, anchoring fibrils inserting into the lamina densa, and a variety of loosely arranged small fibrils of random orientation. The basement membrane, histochemically, characteristically reacts with PAS and silver stains indicating a condensation of polysaccharides.

The four strata of the oral epithelium reflect its keratinizing properties. Basal cells attached to the basement lamina by means of hemidesmosomes and acting as the germinative layer maintain the epithelial turnover which, as measured in non-human primates, completes one renewing cycle in about 8–15 days. Because the oral epithelium as well as the junctional epithelium comprises a constantly renewing cell population, the number of daughter cells leaving the stratum basale equals the number of desquamating cells. On its way from stratum basale to the stratum corneum, each epithelial cell undergoes a co-ordinated, precisely timed differentiation process, known as keratinization. The most undifferentiated basal cell already reveals, in part, indications of the future fate of its daughter cells. Cytoplasmic filaments, a major constituent needed for keratinization, occupy approximately 20 per cent of the cytoplasmic volume. Compared to the junctional epithelium, basal cells of the oral epithelium appear, therefore, already in part differentiated and classified as future keratinocytes. The cytoplasm of basal cells, by volume, is characterized by 20 per cent cytoplasmic filaments which often gather into fibrils and bundles traversing the cytoplasm and inserting into desmosomal attachment plaques, 9 per cent mitochondria, 2·9 per cent rough endoplasmic reticulum, and 0·8 per cent smooth membrane-bound vesicles including the Golgi apparatus.

With increasing distance from the basal layer, the keratinocytes change in shape and cytoplasmic composition. These changes as reflected, for example, by an increasing volume of cytoplasmic filaments, and a decreasing volumetric and surface density of synthesizing and energy-providing organelles indicate the preparatory, quantitative and productive steps taken by each single cell prior to its qualitative and sudden shift toward the horny squama. This process of keratinization involves the production and intracellular accumulation of a number of constituents such as cytoplasmic filaments, hydrolytic enzyme-containing, so-called membrane coating granules (Odland bodies), proteins rich in sulphur, keratohyaline granules, and a variety of enzymes. While this happens, cells and nuclei flatten considerably in a plane parallel to the epithelial surface and all cells traverse through the stratum spinosum and stratum granulosum, approaching the interface between stratum granulosum and stratum corneum. These strata are arbitrarily defined and their structural characteristics are provided by cells which have reached a certain stage on their differentiating pathway towards keratinization. During this series of events contiguous cells maintain contact by desmosomes and gap junctions. Desmosomes are closely associated with bundles of cytoplasmic filaments which insert into their attachment plaques. All cell surfaces are covered by a fuzzy, ruthenium-red-positive material, the extraneous cell surface coat, which contains proteins such as surface antigens and polysaccharides and provides most if not all of the intercellular substance.

As a result of these strictly co-ordinated, intracellular, single-cell phenomena, the oral epithelium produces a stratum corneum of varying density and homogeneity. The keratinized cells are very flat, closely apposed to each other and still united by demosomal junctions. In a fully orthokeratinized stratum corneum, nuclei and synthesizing, energy-producing cytoplasmic organelles are absent, probably lost because of enzymatic breakdown.

The entire cell is then composed of a dense rather homogeneous mat of filaments enmeshed in amorphous ground substance. A parakeratinized stratum corneum still contains flat and structurally altered nuclei as well as remnants of cytoplasmic organelles. As keratinization proceeds independently in individual cells, a single almost non-keratinized and considerably less dense cell may enter and/or pass through the stratum corneum unchanged.

In oral gingival epithelium of man parakeratinization appears to prevail. Apparently, superficial mechanical stimulation has little influence on the degree of keratinization. In fact, the best possible result of the keratinization process appears to be attained when the gingival tissue functions in the absence of clinical and subclinical inflammation and immunological reactions.

In contrast to junctional epithelium, the oral gingival epithelium regularly contains two cell populations different from keratinocytes, namely melanocytes and Langerhans cells. These are described in Chapter 38.

GINGIVAL CONNECTIVE TISSUE

The connective tissue comprises the bulk of gingival tissue. By volume, it occupies approximately 70 per cent (Schroeder *et al.*, 1973). Its most important and most voluminous constituents are collagen fibrils, which occupy 56 per cent of the total connective tissue fraction. The connective tissue provides and maintains important functional properties of gingival tissue such as tone, tensile strength, rigidity and protection; in time of injury, it harbours and reacts with the cell population that responds to injury.

Cell Population

Gingival connective tissue contains a variety of freely mobile cells, some of which are present in the healthy state while others act in host defence. The most important and most numerous cell type present is the fibroblast. Per unit volume of $1\,cm.^3$ connective tissue there are, on the average, 202×10^6 fibroblasts. They range in size between 100 and $800\,\mu m.^3$ The population of fibroblasts is irregularly scattered between bundles of collagen fibrils and around vessels. Fibroblasts produce the connective tissue substances including collagen, proteoglycans and elastin, and essentially maintain the integrity of the tissue.

Large numbers of mast cells are also regularly encountered in normal gingival connective tissue, especially in close topographical relationship to blood vessels. In addition, small numbers of leucocytes are found in normal connective tissue, predominantly located around and along blood vessels. The most numerous of these cells are the medium-sized lymphocytes, followed by small lymphocytes and plasma cells. Neutrophilic granulocytes, monocytes, macrophages and immunoblasts are rarely encountered. Leucocytes do not normally occur in clusters (forming inflammatory infiltrates) but appear to act in isolation and to fulfil scavenging functions.

Blood Supply, Lymphatics and Innervation

Besides freely mobile, single cells the gingival connective tissue includes those cellular elements which form the blood and lymphatic vessels and protect nerve axons and fibres.

The gingival connective tissue is highly vascularized. The primary blood supply arises from the posterior superior alveolar arteries and the anterior superior alveolar branches of the infraorbital arteries in the upper, and from the inferior alveolar arteries in the lower jaw. These vessels give off branches which traverse the interseptal bone and reach the gingiva through numerous foramina in the cortical plate.

Other branches enter the gingival tissue via the periodontal ligament. An additional supply is through terminal branches of the greater palatine arteries in the upper, and through those of the lingual and mental arteries in the lower jaw. These branches reach the gingival tissue from the vestibular fornix, the floor of the mouth and the hard palate. This additional blood supply is of particular importance with regard to gingival flap surgery. Within the gingival connective tissue, the terminal blood vessels assume particular structural arrangements along the connective tissue–epithelium interface. Beneath the oral epithelium and the oral sulcular epithelium, capillary loops arise from larger vessels and extend into the periphery of connective tissue papillae. Lateral to the circular collar of the junctional epithelium a capillary network termed the gingival plexus forms a vessel basket rich in anastomoses. The gingival plexus which also comprises a great portion of post capillary venules is subject to early structural alterations in case of inflammatory reactions to injury.

Venous return runs more or less parallel to the course taken by arteries. The pterygoid plexus serves to collect the blood returning from the gingival tissue of the upper and lower jaws. Lymphatics from the gingival tissue eventually drain into the deep cervical lymph nodes. Densely arranged lymphatic vessels generally accompany the blood vessels. Lymphatic capillaries arising in the gingival tissue of the lateral vestibulum drain into the submandibular nodes while those from the anterior lower vestibulum drain through the submental nodes. Lymphatic vessels of the palatal gingival tissue carry the lymph directly into the deep cervical nodes while all the former reach the cervical nodes only by passing through either submental or submandibular nodes.

Sensory innervation is provided through branches of the superior alveolar and anterior palatal nerves in the upper and of the lingual, inferior alveolar and mental nerves in the lower jaw. While entering the gingival connective tissue in a myelinated form, peripheral supply is embedded in a Schwann cell sheath through numerous non-myelinated axons. Within the connective tissue papillae extending into epithelial depressions a variety of nerve endings can be encountered. Among these the corpuscles of Meissner and Krause are the most outstanding structures serving touch and pain perception.

Collagen Fibres

The extracellular matrix of the gingival connective tissue comprises various fibrous proteins such as collagen, reticulin, very little elastin, and the ground substance. The latter is composed mainly of proteoglycans, hyaluronic acid, glycoproteins and water. Collagen is the predominant structural constituent which is of particular importance in health and disease. It is a product of fibroblasts, the most numerous cell population in gingival connective tissue. Although there is a histochemical difference between collagen and reticulin fibres, they are identical when viewed with the electron microscope.

Structurally, collagen fibrils are normally organized into bundles of fibres with preferential orientation. On the basis of orientation and sites of insertion these bundles are described as dento-gingival, dento-periosteal, alveolo-gingival, circular and transseptal fibre groups (figs. 1 and 6).

The **dento-gingival fibres** (fig. 1) inserting in the cementum of the root apical to the cemento-enamel junction (fig. 7g, h) spread out into the gingival tissue, taking three major routes (fig. 1). One group radiates coronally to the gingival margin, passing in part directly beneath the junctional epithelial collar (fig. 2a, b). Another group follows a rather horizontal course, extending into the connective tissue ridges and papillae penetrating into the oral epithelium. A third group, the alveolar portion of **dento-periosteal fibres**, bends apically over the alveolar crest, inserting in the periosteum (fig. 7g, i). The **alveolo-gingival fibres** (figs. 1 and 6) arise from the alveolar bone crest and radiate coronally into all sites of the free and attached gingival portions. The **circular fibres** (figs. 1 and 6) circulate around the neck of the tooth

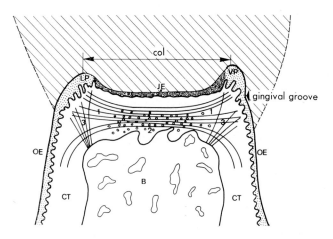

FIG. 6. Schematic linguo-buccal cross-section of interdental gingival tissue. B = bone; JE = col epithelium, comprised of junctional epithelium; CT = connective tissue; LP = lingual papilla; OE = oral epithelium; VP = vestibular papilla. 1 = circular fibres; 2 = transseptal fibres; 3 = alveolo-gingival fibres.

and, within the interdental gingival portion, cross over to connect bundles of one to those of the contacting tooth. Dento-gingival as well as circular fibres have been observed to traverse the interdental gingival portion to spread into the buccal or lingual tissue of adjacent teeth (Page and Schroeder, 1975). **Transseptal fibres** (fig. 7a) originate from the cervical cementum on one tooth, traverse the interdental tissue in a mesio-distal direction, and insert into the cervical cementum of the adjacent tooth. Collectively, the transseptal fibres are termed the interdental ligament which interconnects all adjacent teeth of one arch. Most of the fibre groups can rarely be encountered as separate bundles. In general, they are enmeshed with each other to form a rather densely spliced collagenous mat.

In strictly normal gingival connective tissue, this meshwork of collagen fibre bundles is homogeneously distributed throughout the entire free and attached gingival portions (fig. 2a, b). However, with the onset and spread of acute

inflammatory and chronic infiltrative reactions the structural pattern and the density of collagen fibres become altered. Within a narrow zone beneath and along the junctional epithelium the formerly dense fibre bundles appear to thin out or to disappear completely (fig. 2c to f). When a small and narrow area of infiltration has established itself beneath the junctional epithelium, the collagen pattern definitely deviates from the normal (fig. 3a). Within the infiltrated area only a few, very fine residual collagen fibres can be found. At the periphery of the infiltrate collagen fibres appear thinned out and indistinct. Beneath the oral epithelium the collagenous meshwork is still unchanged. The structural differences between the macerated, fuzzy collagen fibres at the infiltrate periphery and those of normal appearance are demonstrated in fig. 7e and f. These structural alterations are difficult to explain at present.

"In both human and marmosets the size of the salt-soluble collagen component" (representing the newly synthesized, non-crosslinked collagen) "in clinically normal gingiva is several times larger than that of skin, indicating that the gingiva may contain an unusually large pool of recently synthesized unstable collagen" (Page and Schroeder, 1975). Furthermore, rate of collagen production, maturation and breakdown have been measured by following the course of the radioactively labelled precursor C^{14}-proline into and out of the gingival connective tissue of mature marmosets with time (Page and Ammons, 1974). In comparison to palate, skin, tendon and granulation tissue proliferating into implanted foam rubber sponges, the newly synthesized salt-soluble collagen fraction in gingival tissue is many times greater than that in all other tissues except granulation tissue. This fraction does not become degraded as seen in tendon, skin and palate, but persists with time. In addition, the insoluble collagen fraction of gingival connective tissue is remarkably different from that of other tissues in expressing symptoms of unusual instability. In fact, connective tissue in the gingiva behaves much more like that of the involuting uterus and healing wounds *i.e.* sponge granulation tissue, than it does in an immediately neighbouring tissue such as that of the palate.

These new data on gingival connective tissue metabolism imply that the collagenous constituent of gingival tissue is unusually unstable and may turn over, even under normal conditions, at an inordinately high rate. Gingival fibroblasts obviously produce a pool of newly synthesized molecules with rapid turnover rates from which molecules can be withdrawn for purposes of maintenance and repair. And, "the gingival connective tissue differs from other tissues in that a far greater portion of the newly synthesized molecules is subsequently required for incorporation into insoluble collagen" (Page and Ammons, 1974) which in itself represents an unstable and rapidly changing fraction.

These observations "might help to explain the high potential for regeneration and repair in gingiva as well as the mechanisms by which the general structure and architectural features of the gingival connective tissue and the periodontium are maintained during tooth eruption, mesial drift, and inflammatory disease" (Page and Schroeder, 1975). They might even serve to better understanding of the collagen loss observed in early and advanced stages of

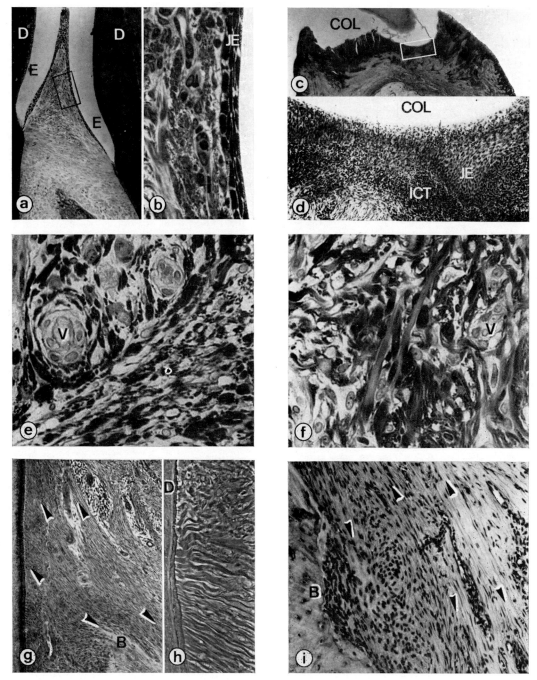

FIG. 7. (a) Mesio-distal section through interdental gingiva of germfree rat. Smooth and narrow junctional epithelia fuse
to form surface of interdental col. Transseptal fibres interconnect teeth coronal to interdental bone crest.
E = enamel, D = dentine. The outlined area is shown in (b). ×60. (b) Higher magnification of area outlined
in (a). The three-cell layer junctional epithelium (JE) smoothly apposes connective tissue including the vascular
plexus. ×420. (c) Bucco-lingual section through interdental gingiva of posterior human teeth. The col lies
between the vestibular (right) and lingual (left) papillae. Col epithelium (fused junctional epithelium) is
pathologically altered and subepithelial connective tissue is infiltrated by plasma cells. Outlined area is shown
in (d). ×7·5. (d) Higher magnification of area outlined in (c). Junctional epithelium (JE) heavily infiltrated with
leucocytes. Connective tissue (ICT) loaded with plasma cells. ×60. (e) Connective tissue at periphery of slightly
infiltrated area of buccal human gingiva. Collagen fibre bundles appear cross-sectioned and reveal fuzziness.
V = vessel. ×450. (f) Connective tissue beneath oral epithelium of human buccal gingiva. Strong collagen fibre
bundles predominate. V = vessel. ×450. (g) Collagen fibre bundles connecting attached buccal gingiva to
cementum surface. Arrows indicate course of collagen fibre bundles. B = alveolar bone crest. ×75. (h) Insertion
of gingival connective tissue fibre bundles in root cementum. D = dentine. ×300. (i) Insertion of gingival connective tissue fibres into bone periosteum (B = alveolar bone crest). Arrows indicate the course of fibre bundles
radiating from the root surface into the attached gingiva. ×75.

chronic gingivitis. Any event which is likely chronically to disturb the peculiar conditions of collagen production and degradation, even when leading to relatively minor alterations, can eventually result in dramatic changes of collagen content, clinical symptoms, and the functional properties of the tissue.

Gingival tissue, a small peripheral portion of the oral mucous membrane which, in the complete post-eruptive dentition of a healthy young individual, surrounds the neck of the tooth and covers the alveolar bone crest, not only has several remarkable features of its own but also appears to be well adapted for the lifelong battle between local microbial challenge and host defence. An even better and more complete understanding of its functional properties than is possible today might eventually result in a scientific foundation for more simple, more precise and more specific clinical measures to support natural ways of protecting the periodontal tissues, maintaining the stability of teeth, and providing efficient masticatory function in young and aged individuals.

REFERENCES

Listgarten, M. A. (1972), "Normal Development, Structure, Physiology and Repair of Gingival Epithelium," *Oral Sciences Reviews*, **1**, 3.

Page, R. C. (1972), "Macromolecular Interactions in the Connective Tissues of the Periodontium," in *Developmental Aspects of Oral Biology*, pp. 291–308 (H. C. Slavkin and L. Bavetta, Eds.). New York: Academic Press.

Page, R. C. and Ammons, W. F. (1974), "Collagen Turnover in the Gingiva and Other Mature Connective Tissues of the Normal Marmoset *Saguinus oedipus*," *Arch. Oral Biology*, **19**, 651.

Page, R. C. and Schroeder, H. E. (1975), "The Normal Periodontium," in *Management of Periodontal Disease* (S. Shluger R. C. Page and R. Youdalis, Eds.). Philadelphia: Lea & Febiger. In press.

Schroeder, H. E. and Listgarten, M. A. (1971), "Fine Structure of the Developing Epithelial Attachment of Human Teeth," in *Monographs in Developmental Biology*, **2** (A. Wolsky, Ed.). Basel: S. Karger.

Schroeder, H. E. (1973), "Transmigration and Infiltration of Leucocytes in Human Junctional Epithelium," *Helvetica odontologica Acta*, **17**, 6.

Schroeder, H. E., Münzel-Pedrazzoli, S. and Page, R. C. (1973), "Correlated Morphometric and Biochemical Analysis of Gingival Tissue in Early Chronic Gingivitis in Man," *Arch. Oral Biology*, **18**, 899.

37. THE ESSENTIAL NATURE OF PERIODONTAL DISEASE

B. COHEN

The course of the disease

Changes associated with ageing

Relationship to dental caries

Plaque, calculus and gingivitis

The role of bacteria

Destructive potential of the immune response

Morphological factors

Vulnerability of the interdental area

THE COURSE OF THE DISEASE

Periodontal disease is the term commonly used to describe a slowly progressive disruption and irreversible disintegration of the tissues supporting the teeth eventually resulting, if not arrested, in the affected teeth becoming so loose (and their surrounding tissues so septic) that they may be spontaneously exfoliated.

Because the tissues attaching teeth to their sockets are, for the most part, robust, and because the healing capacity of oral soft tissue is redoubtable, periodontal destruction is not rapidly accomplished. Next, because the course of the disease extends over many years—sometimes to be measured in decades—its progress will be governed in some measure by vicissitudes within the body as a whole. Intercurrent disease, unrelated to the oral lesion, may indirectly promote an exacerbation of periodontal disease—for example, by general lowering of resistance as occurs in anaemias or in diabetes—and this may give an erroneous impression of a cause and effect relationship. Changes in the local environment too, may modify the course of the disease, and thus it comes about that a wide variety of clinical appearances can be encountered over a period of many years and a wide variety of terms has been coined to describe stages of what is essentially a continuing process.

The term pyorrhoea alveolaris, old-fashioned to dentists but still accepted usage to their patients, is an apt description of the terminal phase of the disease, for by the time the teeth have become loose the crevice has become abnormally wide and deep, and suppuration is almost inevitable, so that pus flows, as the term implies, from the region of the alveolus.

Much more is known about the terminal stage of this disease than about its earlier phases. The histological appearance of advanced periodontal disease displays the features of local bone resorption, disintegration of the fibrous ligament, and foci of suppuration superimposed upon a chronic inflammatory process. Microscopic appearances are however, no more than a static portrayal of a formalin-fixed moment in time. To this disadvantage must be added the fact that periodontal disease is notoriously unsuitable for microscopic study in its earlier stages because a satisfactory section of the periodontal tissues necessitates the removal, *en bloc*, of at least two teeth and the intervening tissue that supports them; small wonder, then, that the availability of human tissue for studies is extremely limited and that recourse must be made to examining the tissues of experimental animals in order to determine early changes in the evolution of this disease.

The evidence accruing from such studies as well as clinical and radiological observations has clearly established that the disease process originates coronally and spreads in an apical direction. Destruction of the bony socket supporting the tooth can occur in a variety of conditions of which hyperparathyroidism is a notable example (see Chapter 48), and this will usually be accompanied by loosening of the teeth. The significant feature characterizing such destruction of the supporting tissues (commencing apically rather than coronally) is that the effect is reversible; if the cause is removed (for example, the parathyroid adenoma) new bone will be deposited and the teeth will become firmly reattached. In the contrary situation, as is seen in periodontal disease, the best that can be achieved is to arrest the destructive process; a new attachment apparatus, with regeneration of bone, is not normally achieved. It may seem paradoxical that bone loss of extreme severity due to hormonal disturbance, or tooth mobility of rapid onset and marked degree (as seen when orthodontic forces are injudiciously applied), are both reversible; whereas the much more gradual expression of these two features in periodontal disease is, in the untreated case, inexorably progressive.

The reasons for failure of repair—which are equally those that account for the irreversible nature of periodontal disease—call for careful consideration. In advanced periodontal disease three components of the periodontium exhibit damage: the epithelial surface is ulcerated, and in an attempt at repair downgrowths of epithelium extend apically; fibrolysis occurs within the periodontal ligament, thus weakening the attachment of tooth to bone and tooth to adjacent tooth; and alveolar bone undergoes resorption. In order for fibrous–osseous repair to be successful it is necessary not only for new fibres and new bone to be formed, but for a new fibrous attachment to the surface of the tooth to be effected. That these formidable requirements can be met is demonstrated by the fact that teeth which have been loosened by trauma, by mechanical forces, or by metabolic disease can become firm again if the underlying cause is eliminated.

There are two fundamental reasons why this does not occur in periodontal disease, and both are related to the epithelial component of the periodontium. The first is that as long as the epithelial integument is incomplete, the factors responsible for fibrolysis and bone resorption persist; as long as fibres and bone are exposed to contamination from the oral environment, the integrity of both fibres and bone remains at risk. The second and perhaps

more subtle reason is that epithelial downgrowths intervene between the ligament and the cementum, and thus prevent the reattachment of periodontal fibres to the tooth. The process of apical migration of epithelium is depicted in fig. 1. This proliferation could be interpreted as a reflection of an inherent capacity of epithelium to cover a denuded surface; it seems probable that such a protective reaction is primarily directed towards covering the damaged soft tissues (from which, indeed, the epithelial

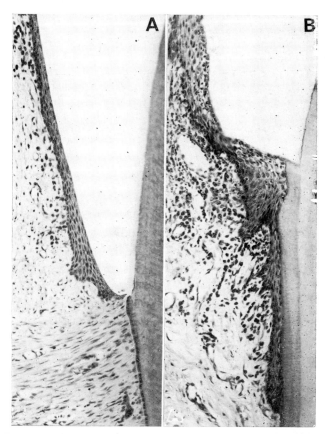

Fig. 1. Periodontal tissues of monkey. A. The appearance of the epithelial attachment in the healthy periodontium. The apical extremity is located at the junction of cementum and enamel (dissolved out in the course of preparation). Fibres of the periodontal ligament are inserted into the coronal extremity of cementum. B. Coronal fibres have disintegrated and an infiltration of inflammatory cells is present. Junctional epithelium has extended apically to cover the denuded area and has thus come to segregate a portion of cementum that previously afforded attachment to fibres. Haematoxylin and eosin × 115.

cells derive their nutrition) rather than the cementum, as is sometimes inferred from histological appearances. In fact, far from being protected by epithelialization, the tooth is being excluded from the internal environment—so that the epithelial downgrowth can be likened to the first footsteps on the pathway to ultimate exfoliation.

CHANGES ASSOCIATED WITH AGEING

The exposure of cementum is not a phenomenon peculiar to periodontal disease for the attachment of periodontal tissues at the level of the cemento–enamel junction is rarely

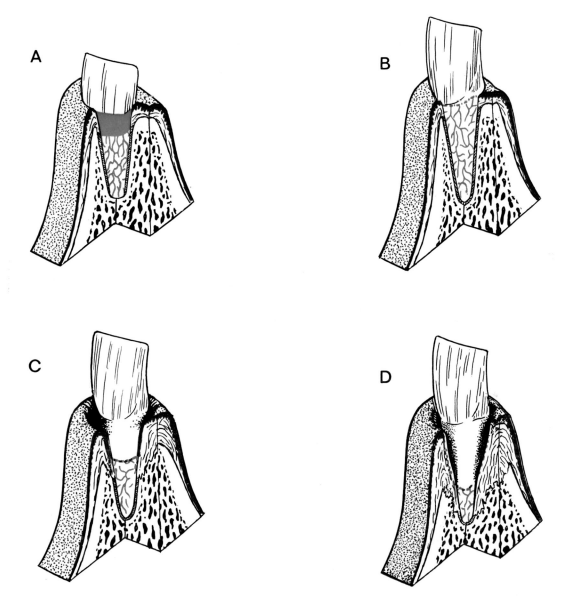

PLATE I. Red denotes oral stratified squamous epithelium. Green denotes epithelium of odontogenic origin. A. Erupting tooth. B. Eruption completed. C. Recession and early pocket formation as seen in ageing. D. Advanced pocket formation with loss of fibre attachment, bone resorption, and epithelial downgrowth.

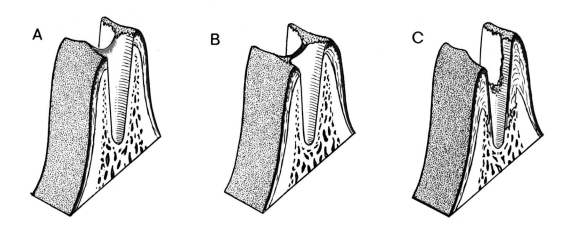

PLATE II. Diagrams depicting the structure of the interdental col. Red denotes oral epithelium. Green denotes epithelium of odontogenic origin. A. Immediately following the eruption of contiguous teeth. B. In normal health, after physiological recession has permitted the reunion of lingual and facial papillae, separated in the course of eruption. C. In pathological circumstances where an interdental ulcer has developed.

maintained beyond middle age. Before assuming that periodontal disease is a universally prevalent disease, allowance should be made for the wear and tear inevitably associated with the process of ageing. A progressive deterioration and loss of structural integrity is an inexorable accompaniment of senescence in most, if not all mammalian species. Important though they are to survival (except, perhaps, in the case of modern man) the tissues which attach the teeth are not uniquely privileged in respect of the ravages of time. This being so it is inevitable that estimations of the prevalence of periodontal disease, no matter how they are scored, will be inflated by the intrusion of data reflecting changes attributable to ageing; what may be regarded as normal in the middle-aged periodontium would be pathological in the young, and beyond reasonable expectation in the elderly. Until the more gross signs of periodontal disease are reached, such as overt tooth mobility, the assessment of periodontal health demands allowance for age changes. The accurate standardization of such changes is not easily achieved. To define the boundary between truly pathological change and alteration that can reasonably be attributed to wear and tear, is one of the besetting problems confronting research into periodontal disease; it calls for an assessment not only of the dentition at the time of examination, but of its past history and sometimes, indeed, for an evaluation of prognosis since true periodontal disease, unlike senile recession, cannot be expected to progress in step with the advance of time. Plate IA, B, C and D depict the changes occurring in normal and pathological recession.

It is probably true to say that the prevalence of periodontal disease in a population is progressively less amenable to accurate estimation as average age increases. However, although tooth morbidity may be difficult to measure, there is much less difficulty about determining the effect of periodontal disease on tooth loss, and this is more than sufficient to establish the serious effect of the disease on the human dentition.

RELATIONSHIP TO DENTAL CARIES

Since the commonest causes of tooth mortality are periodontal disease and dental caries, it is inevitable that a comparison should be made between these two diseases, and that aetiological factors common to both should be sought.

At one time it was widely held that an inverse relationship existed between the incidence of periodontal disease and that of caries, but no great weight of statistical evidence has been adduced to support this proposition. The fact that tooth mortality as a consequence of caries is likely to eventuate at a much earlier age than that attributable to periodontal disease, can introduce a spurious impression of antagonism between the two diseases. However, whereas caries arising in enamel is a specific and recognizable lesion, the loss of periodontal attachment is a much less distinct deviation from the normal. It follows, therefore, that coexistence of the two diseases may not easily be identified.

In populations that are not susceptible to caries there will certainly be more teeth at risk to periodontal disease

in later life. It is beyond question that the successful implementation of caries-preventive measures would enhance the demand for therapy to combat periodontal disease.

Although theories of an inverse relationship between caries and periodontal disease have not progressed beyond the status of unsubstantiated conjecture, it may seem equally speculative to postulate that these two diseases share anything in common other than the oral environment and their capacity to destroy dentitions. A major advance in the understanding of the carious process followed a series of discoveries concerning the formation and physico-chemical properties of dental plaque. This has led to a great volume of research effort being concentrated on plaque in relation to periodontal disease. Since plaque is part of the oral environment in which the disease is presumably initiated, it seems logical that such research should be done. Less acceptable, however, is any tendency to regard plaque as the totipotent forerunner of all diseases affecting the teeth. To do so is to encourage the notion that all plaque is a pathological entity, which is manifestly untrue. Since dental plaque begins to form on a tooth surface within hours of thorough cleaning and independently of the presence of bacteria or food, it must be regarded as within the range of the normal so far as the oral environment is concerned. It may well be that a particular type of plaque is pathogenic in relation either to the development of caries or of periodontal disease, but most probably not both. Certain dietary constituents, notably and notoriously sucrose, are acted upon by mouth bacteria in such a way that a substantial carbohydrate component is added to the glycoprotein matrix derived from saliva. There is good reason to believe that this phenomenon is of prime importance in the pathogenesis of caries, but similar evidence implicating the carbohydrate component of plaque in the development of periodontal disease has not been forthcoming.

PLAQUE, CALCULUS AND GINGIVITIS

The notion that plaque, or calculus, is in some way responsible for periodontal destruction is not difficult to accept by anyone who has had the common clinical experience of witnessing an overnight transformation in the appearance of the gingivae following the careful removal of subgingival and circumgingival deposits. However, this immediate change, dramatic though it may appear, reflects no more than the resolution of marginal gingivitis—and illustrates, incidentally, the remarkable reparative capacity of gingival tissues.

To assume, because marginal gingivitis responds to debridement, that plaque removal is a means of preventing or treating periodontal disease, is to equate marginal gingivitis with periodontal disease. There is strong evidence to support the view that marginal gingivitis can progress to chronic gingivitis and thence to periodontal disease proper; there is nothing like the same evidence to justify the assumption that the course of periodontal disease follows this pattern invariably. An equally fallacious extrapolation is embodied in such beliefs as "plaque is a necessary prerequisite to periodontal inflammation"—a misconception derived from the oft-confirmed observation that preventing the accumulation of plaque helps to prevent marginal gingivitis.

The implication of plaque in the pathogenesis of periodontal disease is in many ways analogous to the belief that calculus plays a causative role; this view, once widely expounded, has to some extent been supplanted by the increased attention paid to plaque in recent years. However, the distinction between calculus causing the disease or merely constituting a concomitant phenomenon, has not been established, and the same is true in some degree of the coexistence of plaque and periodontal disease. Experiments have shown that gingival fluid provides a more satisfactory substrate for the proliferation of bacterial plaque than does saliva, and as inflammatory exudate is the chief component of such fluid there are grounds for suggesting that gingivitis or periodontitis of long duration may indeed be a cause as well as a consequence of the accumulation of plaque. Also, as will be mentioned later, the presence of immunoglobulins in oral fluids could indirectly contribute to the aggregation of bacterial deposits.

Clinical experience, supported by numerous epidemiological studies, has established an association between poor oral hygiene and periodontal disease to an extent that is incontrovertible. There are two inferences that can be drawn from this association: the first is that poor oral hygiene plays a causative or contributory role in the pathogenesis of periodontal disease; an alternative is that the existence of periodontal disease interferes with the normal maintenance of oral hygiene. Various studies have shown that impaired hygiene has an important part to play in the development of marginal gingivitis. Several schools of thought have postulated that untreated marginal gingivitis is the first stage in the development of periodontal disease proper and it is claimed that some evidence in support of this has been adduced from animal studies.

However, the pattern of distribution of periodontal disease in the mouth does not support the hypothesis that poor oral hygiene necessarily or inevitably leads to periodontal disease. For example, the accumulation of calculus on mandibular incisors is considerably greater than on maxillary incisors—yet, paradoxically, tooth loss as a consequence of periodontal disease is somewhat more common in the upper anterior region of the mouth than it is in the lower. The areas of the mouth most susceptible to periodontal destruction do not always correspond to the sites of maximum incidence of calculus accumulation.

Whether or not plaque can be held responsible for periodontal breakdown depends largely on whether marginal gingivitis can be regarded as the forerunner of periodontal disease. There are many important differences between the two conditions, none of greater significance than the fact that gingivitis is capable of resolution, with the affected tissue reverting to normal structure and function, whereas periodontal disease is irreversible. It is likely, to say the least, that in some instances the progression from gingivitis to periodontal destruction does take place; it might, however, be important to concentrate research endeavour on those cases where recurring or long-standing marginal

gingivitis is not followed by periodontal destruction and, conversely, those instances in which periodontal destruction has occurred without overt evidence of antecedent gingivitis. The essential difference distinguishing the two conditions is that in periodontal disease there is denudation of cementum, loss of collagen fibres, and resorption of alveolar bone whereas marginal gingivitis is no more than superficial.

THE ROLE OF BACTERIA

There is strong circumstantial evidence to support the belief that bacteria are implicated in the development of marginal gingivitis, and the nature of the oral *milieu* is such that micro-organisms are inevitably involved in the progress of periodontal disease. Most mouth organisms are not pathogenic (as discussed in Chapter 15), and many investigators have sought in vain for evidence to incriminate a bacterial invader capable not only of breaching the epithelial defences of the periodontium but also of destroying the collagenous framework of the periodontal ligament, and even resorbing the bone of the alveolar crest. The likelihood of a single pathogen with so broad a spectrum of potency being associated with so commonplace a disease is remote, to say the least.

From time to time attention has been directed to one particular species or another which appears to meet the exacting criteria of a causative organism for periodontal disease. In recent years, for example, first *Bacteroides melaninogenicus* and then *Actinomyces viscosus* have been chosen to audition for this role but neither has been found to fill the part. More recently, refinements in technique have led to the isolation of unusual Gram-negative anaerobic rods from the depths of pockets in cases of the type customarily referred to as periodontosis. Interest in these findings has been enhanced by experiments in which extensive destruction of periodontal tissue was observed following mono-infection with these organisms in gnotobiotic rats.

It is conceivable that the periodontium could be especially vulnerable to the effects of particular organisms, and should this possibility be substantiated in regard to Gram-negative anaerobic rods, the way will be opened for the introduction of new therapeutic measures directed towards checking the acceleration of periodontal destruction. This would not mean, however, that periodontal disease could be prevented by the elimination of this or any other particular organism. Indeed, it is important to recall that some of the earliest germ-free studies showed unequivocally that the absence of micro-organisms did not prevent the development of periodontal disease in rats. Since that time many gnotobiotic studies have shown that the introduction of different organisms has increased the rapidity and the severity of periodontal destruction, which illustrates their importance in the progress of the disease but cannot be interpreted as an indication of total responsibility.

It may well be that the initiation of periodontal disease is associated with injury and that the end-result is the same, regardless of the nature of the injury; in rodents, for example, there is strong evidence to suggest that sharp particles of food or impacted hair may breach the outer integument of the periodontium (fig. 2), and, whether or not micro-organisms are capable of similar penetration, they are certainly likely to be incidentally introduced. What can be inferred from germ-free experiments, however, is that periodontal disease is not a specific infection. It is a common misconception to equate inflammation with infection—and because inflammation is an invariable accompaniment of periodontal disease that does not necessarily mean that the disease is infective in origin. Even when infection has been superimposed, as inevitably it must be, the possibility that a specific pathogen can be held responsible for changes occurring over the lengthy duration of this slow and chronic disease, is less than likely. Once the oral surface of the periodontium is breached, or even damaged to a minor degree, organisms which are harmless commensals in normal circumstances may assume the significance of pathogens. The proliferation of organisms on an ulcerated surface or even within the sub-epithelial tissues, must be expected to give rise to tissue damage; many of the metabolic products of bacteria are likely to be cytotoxic in tissues not normally exposed to them. Nor should it be assumed that collagenolytic enzymes must necessarily be present to bring about dissolution of the periodontal ligament. Various studies have shown that collagen in this site is rather more labile than was previously recognized, and the toxic influence required to inhibit replacement may well be less potent than that which would be postulated for lysis. This subject is dealt with in greater detail in Chapters 35 and 36, and toxic activities are discussed in Chapter 15.

DESTRUCTIVE POTENTIAL OF THE IMMUNE RESPONSE

Much attention has been devoted in recent years to immunological factors in relation to different diseases, and periodontal disease has come under close scrutiny. It is a well-recognized fact that in the course of confining and neutralizing harmful foreign material, the inflammatory process may exert deleterious effects upon the tissues of the host. Any circumstance which serves to initiate or to sustain inflammation within the periodontium even indirectly, could therefore contribute to periodontal breakdown. The antigenic load existing at the periodontal surface is enormous, both in variety and in volume, and especially, perhaps, when plaque is abundant. This has led to the belief that products of the plaque may serve to provoke periodontal damage.

There are several ways in which this could occur. Bacterial endotoxins could collect within the plaque and (always providing that they could gain ingress to the periodontium) would exert a potent inflammatory effect. Another possibility is that repeated exposure to plaque antigens could provoke an Arthus-like reaction; in other words, antigen in plaque could react with precipitating antibody already present as a result of recurrent previous exposures to the same antigen, resulting in the formation

(in the presence of complement) of antigen–antibody complexes, and giving rise to persistent inflammation. Secretory immunoglobulin could contribute to any ill-effects of plaque accumulation by virtue of its capacity for causing bacteria to aggregate and could thus add to the bulk of marginal deposits—a further instance of the possibility mentioned previously, that excessive plaque could as likely be a consequence as a cause of periodontal inflammation. Perhaps most important of all, periodontal destruction could conceivably constitute a manifestation of delayed hypersensitivity, in which macrophages might be predominantly responsible for the dissolution of connective tissue elements.

Extensive research has been carried out with the purpose of examining the above possibilities. Immunological technique has flourished in recent years, and a battery of *in vitro* tests has become available for investigations of this sort. Many of these are described in detail in the Chapters of Section III, and they can be referred to only briefly here. It must suffice to say that many experiments have been carried out to examine the effects of plaque and plaque extracts on tissue culture systems, that lympho-proliferative factors have been isolated from several mouth bacteria, and that lymphoproliferative responses in patients with severe periodontal disease have been found to differ from those detectable in normal subjects; so far as macrophages are concerned they have been shown to synthesize and release enzymes in response to exceedingly dilute homogenates of dental plaque, and electronmicrographic evidence has been adduced to support the belief that they are capable of phagocytosing collagen within the periodontal ligament. As mentioned previously, however, the loss of collagen occurring in periodontal disease may not necessarily be a result of collagenolysis. Such is the rate of replacement within the periodontal ligament normally, that cessation, or even a slowing down of fibrogenesis, would be sufficient to result in disruption of the normal periodontal architecture. Thus cytopathic effects upon fibroblasts could conceivably evoke a condition superficially resembling collagen destruction.

In addition to loss of collagen fibres, resorption of bone is an essential part of the dissolution of tooth-supporting structure. It has been conjectured that this too can be attributed to effects of the immune response. *In vitro* studies have disclosed the release from sensitized lymphocytes of a substance that stimulates osteoclastic activity. There is, however, nothing novel in the observation that inflammation predisposes to bone resorption, and the part played by osteoclasts in this process is of course in no sense peculiar to alveolar bone. *In vitro* studies have also been used to illustrate the effect of prostaglandins in promoting bone loss, and the likelihood that such agents would be synthesized and released in the vicinity of periodontal lesions is inescapable. Either of these mechanisms could account for the bone resorption seen in periodontal destruction, but neither can be regarded as anything more than a non-specific accompaniment of a local inflammatory state.

Investigations seeking to establish host–antigen reactions as a basis for periodontal disease, are an offshoot of the prodigious volume of new research in immunopathology. It has to be realized, however, that there is nothing remarkable in the demonstration that immune responses operate in respect of periodontal disease. The same is true of most pathological processes in the body and, what is more, not merely those of infective origin. The fact that immunoglobulins are present in crevicular exudate is by no means an indication that periodontal inflammation is immunologically induced. Likewise, the fact that serum contains antibodies to plaque bacteria, and that peripheral lymphocytes from patients with periodontal disease have been found to be sensitized to plaque antigens, provides no information of how (or even whether) the bacteria or the antigen penetrated the periodontal integument; they could conceivably have been absorbed from the gut following fortuitous ingestion.

The characteristically conspicuous concentration of plasma cells and lymphocytes in periodontal tissue, even at a stage of early damage, suggests a pronounced B cell response, but considering the formidable concentration of antigen in the immediate proximity of the periodontal surface it would be remarkable if immunological stimulation were not in evidence. The crucial question to be answered concerns the circumstances in which the defence system of the internal environment comes to make acquaintance with the foreign material of the external *milieu*, and there is immunological as well as clinical evidence to suggest that periodontal disease is by no means the only portal of ingress.

MORPHOLOGICAL FACTORS

It is in respect of this latter question that the topography and anatomy of the periodontium assumes especial importance. Whether bacteria are directly involved or not, and whether or not the inflammatory response is self-injurious, the pathological changes seen in periodontal disease are not intrinsically different from those seen in many other diseases; in periodontal disease it is the anatomy of the affected part that is unique, not the nature of the pathological change. Nowhere else in the body does so complex a relationship exist between soft and mineralized tissue; nowhere else is connective tissue separated from a hostile outer environment by so tenuous an epithelial integument; and in no other part of the skeleton is cancellous bone so ineffectively shielded from extraneous contamination. Upon a clear understanding of the micro-anatomy of the area, progress in the understanding as well as the treatment of the disease depends.

The advent of electronmicroscopy has done much to clarify problems of periodontal structure that were previously unsolved. There now appears to be a reasonably general measure of acceptance in regard to the nature of the epithelial components of the periodontium and the reader is referred to the detailed description provided in Chapter 36. Judged by the direction of destruction from the cemento–enamel junction towards the root apex, it is in this epithelial surface that the initial lesion of periodontal disease should be sought. There are at least two possibilities in this respect, and they are not mutually exclusive.

The first is that periodontal disease begins with frank ulceration and the second is that the epithelial surface is permeable to the seepage of toxic material from surrounding plaque. In regard to the first possibility ulceration can arise from direct injury, as is commonly seen in periodontal disease affecting laboratory animals whose diet includes

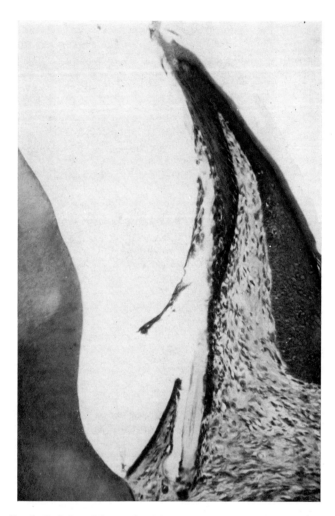

FIG. 2. Periodontal damage in a laboratory rat caused by a sharp particle. Oral epithelium is amply protected against such injury but the vulnerable junctional epithelium has been lacerated. Haematoxylin and eosin × 130.

sharp particles (fig. 2), or in horses living in drought-stricken areas where dry pastures include sharp penetrating fragments; ulceration can also persist in the inter-dental area, possibly as a consequence of impaired epithelialization of the col, after the eruption of contiguous teeth.

The second alternative could well be the dominant mechanism in the more slowly progressive type of periodontal disease that is particularly associated with poor oral hygiene. If seepage of toxic material from plaque is to occur through apparently intact epithelium it seems likely that the deficiency resides in the junctional epithelium. This epithelium (*see* Chapter 36), originally derived from vestiges of enamel organ but capable of regeneration (possibly by having recruited cells from oral epithelium), constitutes that part of the periodontal integument least suited to resist penetration either by trauma or by seepage. Normally, however, it is well protected from assault by an umbrella of robust stratified squamous epithelium extending into the depth of the gingival sulcus, by the bulbous configuration of teeth deflecting particulate matter away from the sulcus and, interdentally, by the overlying area of contact of adjacent teeth. Various authors have made different claims concerning the ability of this epithelial surface to act as a barrier against the ingress of bacteria or even small molecules of their products. Whatever the truth of the matter, junctional epithelium is likely to be more vulnerable at its apical or coronal extremities. The apical extremity abuts the most coronal of the periodontal fibres, while the coronal end becomes confluent with the stratified squamous epithelium lining the gingival sulcus (see fig. 3d, Chapter 36).

The likelihood that the apical extremity is especially vulnerable is suggested by the existence of epithelial downgrowths, possibly as a consequence of a sudden or severe movement rupturing or detaching the most coronal of the transseptal fibres; whatever the cause, the apical extension of epithelium is interpreted as akin to a healing reaction and therefore as an indication of prior injury. A further indication of vulnerability at the coronal extremity is provided by the remarkably constant feature of cells characterizing the immune response being preferentially concentrated beneath the confluence of the junctional and sulcular epithelia; so much so, in fact, that in earlier writing this was referred to by the apt term "zone of injury".

The structures, the properties, and the function of junctional epithelium are dealt with in the preceding Chapter; in considering the pathology of periodontal disease, it must be thought of (see p. 435) as "weak, readily permeated, and easily penetrated". This being so, an explanation is afforded for the particular susceptibility of the interdental area to the onset of periodontal disease, for it is between the teeth that the periodontium is covered to the greatest extent by junctional epithelium.

THE VULNERABILITY OF THE INTERDENTAL AREA

The structure of the interdental area is difficult to study histologically because, as explained previously, a block of at least two teeth is required. Moreover, interpretation of the histological appearances necessitates a three-dimensional conception, for the appearance of a section cut in the mesiodistal plane differs considerably from that of a buccal-lingual section. Bucco-lingual sections disclose the appearance of a col (Chapter 36, fig. 7c) whereas the mesiodistal plane (fig. 3) provides no indication of the saddle-shaped configuration of the interdental septum. In addition, the appearance of a mesio-distal section is largely determined by its position in relation to the vestibular and lingual embrasures. When a mesio-distal section is cut at a point approximately equidistant from the two embrasures, the appearance between recently erupted teeth is that

shown in fig. 4. This shows that the interdental periodontium has, as its surface protection, no more than the junctional epithelia of the two adjacent teeth, perhaps fused together at their coronal extremities, but certainly a frail integument at best. The situation illustrated in fig. 3 shows that in normal circumstances the surface of the interdental

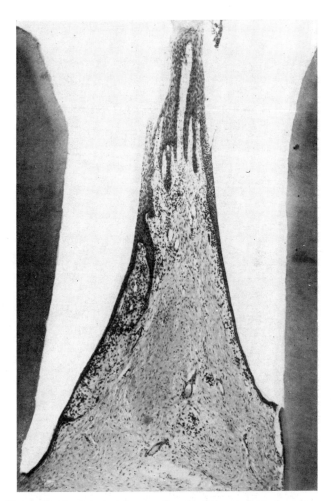

Fig. 3. Monkey interdental area sectioned in the mesiodistal plane. Junctional epithelium separates the periodontal tissues from the enamel on each approximal surface, but immediately below the contact point the surface of the septum is composed of parakeratinized stratified squamous epithelium. Haematoxylin and eosin × 49.

septum comes to be covered by stratified squamous epithelium; junctional epithelium persists, of course, but only in the region where soft tissues attach to the teeth—as described in the previous chapter.

It should be understood that the replacement of junctional by squamous epithelium illustrated in fig. 3 although apparently covering only the tip of the interdental periodontium does, in fact, extend along the entire length of the col from the vestibular papilla to the lingual papilla. Until oral epithelium has joined the two papillae in this fashion the integrity of the interdental periodontium must inevitably be at considerable risk. A selection of circumstances occurring interdentally is depicted in Plate IIA, B and C. The appearance shown in IIA is that of a col between two contacting teeth, one of which has recently erupted. A section cut through the middle of this col in the mesiodistal plane will provide the appearance shown in fig. 4. Once this vulnerable surface has been replaced by stratified sqamous epithelium (as shown in fig. 3) the appearance of the col is that depicted in Plate IIB. The third diagram of this series (Plate IIC) illustrates the circumstances obtaining when the col area is injured, or becomes ulcerated

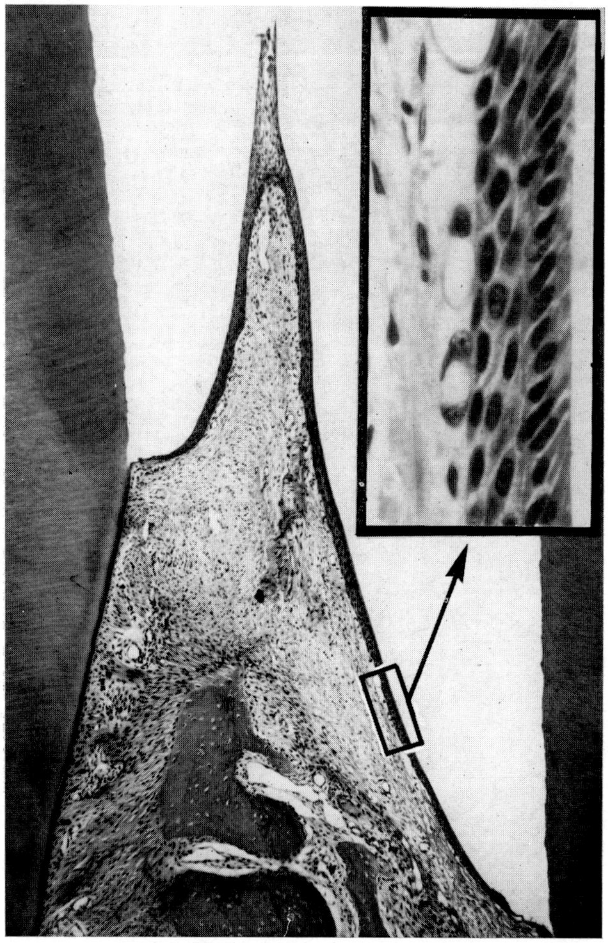

FIG. 4. Mesiodistal section of the interdental area in a young monkey. The tooth on the right side is in the course of eruption. The periodontium is covered by the fused interproximal junctional epithelia of the two teeth. Haematoxylin and eosin × 49. Inset × 540 shows the reduced enamel epithelium in which the ameloblast layer is still recognizable.

before the epithelia of the opposite embrasures have become rejoined. It should be noted that ulceration in this area not only permits the ingress of foreign material—whether products of plaque, food debris or any other contaminant—but also constitutes a barrier to the through-growth of oral epithelium from embrasure to embrasure.

It is clearly not possible to determine, by histology, the length of time during which junctional epithelium forms the interdental surface. It seems likely, however, that a failure of oral epithelium to effect the replacement is an important factor in the development of severe periodontal

disease in young subjects. Among the factors that should be considered in order to account for epithelial failure in the interdental area, none is more obvious than topography.

The topographical relationship of teeth to one another in the dental arch determines the size and the shape of the interdental area, and the degree of cervical constriction of the teeth themselves determines the shape and volume of the embrasure. Thus, where teeth show marked cervical constriction (fig. 5) the embrasure will be large, but the

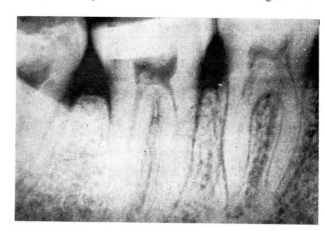

FIG. 5. Radiograph of the lower molars of an adult Australian aborigine showing wide embrasures associated with marked cervical constriction.

embrasure will be much less voluminous when the area of contact between adjacent teeth is more extensive. Broad contacts and meagre embrasures are characteristically seen in the dentitions of animals in which periodontal disease is common—such as horses and short-muzzled dogs. This feature could perhaps account for an apparent predisposition to periodontal disease in certain human races, and should be remembered as a possible cause of iatrogenic periodontal disease (fig. 6).

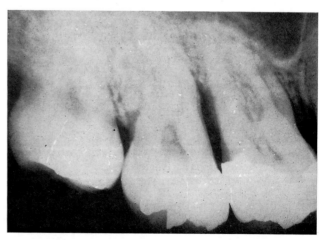

FIG. 6. Radiographs of an intrabony pocket between first and second molars of a young adult. Failure to restore the approximal contours of the first two molars has obliterated the embrasure.

Several investigations have provided data to support the commonplace clinical observation that crowded arches and malposed teeth are often associated with poor periodontal health. The extent to which crowding may be a contributory factor is not accurately reflected in cases of advanced periodontal disease for, once the process has affected transseptal fibres, teeth become displaced by masticatory and occlusal forces. Thus it comes about that teeth which may have been in abnormally close contact at the time of inception of the disease, appear to be widely separated by the time that gross signs of periodontal disease are in evidence.

CONCLUSION

The search for initiating factors of periodontal disease, as distinct from those which exacerbate the disease or accelerate its progress, appears to emphasize the importance of local rather than systemic factors, and of morphological rather than physiological considerations. From the viewpoint of the pathologist the interest and the complexity of periodontal disease resides in the unusual inter-relationship of several different but inter-dependent tissues—two separate epithelia, an intricate pattern of fibres, cortical and trabecular bone, and, of course, the teeth: all this in an environment where both functional demand and extraneous constituents pose a constant challenge to the integrity of the tooth-supporting tissues. In essence, however, pathological interpretation is irresistibly directed towards the identification of an initial failure in the periodontal integument. There is nothing in the clinical or microscopical features of periodontal disease that is incompatible with the presence of a leak in the epithelial surface permitting contamination of the underlying fibres, cementum and bone. Whether this leak takes the form of an obvious epithelial discontinuity or merely slow seepage through a surface incompetence, the ultimate result, if the defect persists, will be the same, although the duration of the disease will differ according to the circumstances.

There should be a clear clinical distinction between these two types of epithelial inadequacy, for gingival bleeding is the all-important diagnostic sign. Bleeding is not a characteristic of either acute or chronic inflammation, but it is inevitably associated with ulceration. If, therefore, bleeding either occurs spontaneously during mastication or tooth-brushing, or can be elicited by gentle exploration of the sulcus with a blunt probe, the existence of ulceration is unquestionable. If, alternatively, tooth mobility and the presence of pathologically deepened gingival sulci exist in the absence of bleeding, the associated inflammatory process could be attributed to seepage of toxic matter through the periodontal integument.

The course of the disease depends, to some extent, on the nature of the epithelial deficiency, but may be profoundly influenced by a wide variety of extraneous factors. The degree to which this disease can be prevented, arrested, or treated must eventually depend, however, on recognition of the fundamental nature of the lesion and the complex anatomical situation in which it occurs.

SECTION IX

THE ORAL MUCOSA

38. THE STRUCTURE AND FUNCTION OF THE ORAL MUCOSA

JULIA MEYER, O. F. ALVARES AND S. J. GERSON

Structure and function of oral mucosa
  Protective
  Sensory

Histology of oral epithelium
  Traits common to all regions
  Regional variation
  Differences within major classes of epithelium
  Non-keratinocytes

Histology of connective tissue
  Junction of epithelium and connective tissue
  Fibroblasts and connective tissue fibres
  Use of fibres in the construction of the lamina propria
  Innervation

Maintenance of oral mucosa
  Characteristic features of the metabolism of oral mucosa
  Blood supply
  Nutritional requirements and the influence of hormones
  Control of cell renewal
  Estimates of epithelial turnover time
  Regional differences in mitotic activity
  Renewal of melanocytes and Langerhans cells
  Connective tissue turnover

INTRODUCTION

The oral mucosa is the lining organ which separates the interior of the oral cavity from the complex of underlying organs. Like skin and the mucosa lining other body cavities, oral mucosa serves to protect the underlying organs and to receive and transmit stimuli from the environment. These functions are shared by two anatomically separated components, a multilayered epithelium and a species of loose connective tissue. Protection against exchange of substances between environment and organism is provided by the epithelium, mechanical protection by both, and sensory innervation largely by the connective tissue.

The epithelial cells must be able to form a protective surface and to provide for cohesion between themselves. In a tissue exposed to an aggressive environment, injury and death of cells is an everyday occurrence, and the cells must be able to provide for replacements. Cells having the properties which enable them to form protective surfaces are, however, not capable of division. These two

requirements determine the major features in the biology of the cells. A steady population of new cells, arising by division of relatively undifferentiated cells at the base, migrates towards the surface while differentiating into surface-adapted cells. Control of cell division at the base and of cell desquamation at the surface must be so interrelated as to result in a constant number of component cells.

Reflecting these features, this chapter is divided into two major sections, the first dealing with the two component tissues and the second with the maintenance of these tissues. These two sections are preceded by a brief discussion of the functions of oral mucosa.

FUNCTIONS OF ORAL MUCOSA

Man and the animals considered in this chapter are organisms in whom functions are distributed among organs or organ systems, and the functions of each organ or system are the contributions it makes to the economy of the whole. This definition, though oversimplified, is nevertheless helpful in distinguishing the functions and functionally adaptive structures of an organ from what might be called its accidental qualities. This latter term designates those attributes which are derived from the organism's past history and which, while they do not interfere with the function of the organ, do not make a contribution to it. The functions common to oral mucosa and skin are to protect underlying parts from noxious effects of the environment while admitting and relaying needed information about external events. In addition to these local functions, skin has a systemic function in the regulation of the body temperature. Oral mucosa has a temperature-regulating function in panting animals but not in the human. Another systemic function of skin is the synthesis and secretion of vitamin D and cholesterol. Oral mucosa does not participate in the former and is an unknown in respect to the latter. Insofar as receptors in oral mucosa participate in the thirst mechanism, oral mucosa has a systemic function not shared by skin.

Melanocytes in skin have a light protective function and sebaceous glands a lubricating function. Both these structures are present in oral mucosa; should a function therefore be ascribed to them?

If, as seems likely, both skin and oral mucosa have neither excretory nor ingestive functions, their permeability to various substances should be regarded as existing in spite of their barrier function and, frequently enough, endangering the latter even though the pharmacologist may be pleased at having a quick route for drug adminstration.

Their impermeability characteristics, on the other hand, are essential to their barrier functions.

Protective Functions of Oral Mucosa

During mastication, the hard palate is chiefly exposed to forces of compression, the gingiva to shear, and all mobile regions to distension. Adaptations to resist compression, to resist friction, and to allow distension determine the great regional variability of oral epithelium. Connective tissue shares in the function of mechanical protection, hence structural arrangements implementing the required regional adaptations are reflected in the great range of regional differences of this tissue as well.

In contrast to the great regional variation needed for mechanical protection, the barrier function of oral mucosa could be provided by rather uniform structures since in this respect the oral cavity represents a rather uniform environment. The barrier to exit is entirely and the barrier to entry largely the task of the epithelium. The defence system in the lamina propria is available in case the epithelium does not succeed in barring unwanted entrants. It is, therefore, not surprising to find that protein molecules applied to the epithelial surface do not penetrate beyond a superficial level in both non-keratinized and keratinized regions of mucosa, and that the barrier in both regions may be provided by cell organelles of similar life history and ultrastructure. As regards smaller molecules, the rapid entry of sublingually administered drugs is well known, while little is known about their entry in other regions. There is, however, nothing to suggest that oral mucosa anywhere serves a physiological absorptive function.

Although excretory functions, if any, seem confined to salivary glands, little is known about the effectiveness of oral epithelium in barring the exit of substances from the lamina propria. The exit like the entry of protein molecules seems to be barred at the same level and by the same mechanisms in both keratinized and non-keratinized regions. Retention of water, which in epidermis is a major function in protecting terrestial animals from dehydration, is of no importance in the oral cavity. If water were to seep through oral epithelium, it would, like saliva, be swallowed and reabsorbed in the intestinal tract. At any rate, oral epithelium seems to be effective in preventing the exit of water, if one may judge by the xerostomia associated with salivary gland disease.

Sensory Functions of Oral Mucosa

Sensory functions of oral mucosa are the same as those of skin in the sense that both receive and convey pain, cold, heat, touch and pressure, and elicit responses of the organism to these stimuli. Responses unique to the oral apparatus are swallowing and gagging, and perhaps mobilization of the thirst mechanism. Unique to oral mucosa is the sense of taste.

HISTOLOGY OF ORAL EPITHELIUM

Traits Common to All Regions

The epithelium of oral mucosa belongs to the class of stratified squamous epithelia. Both keratinized and non-keratinized types occur in human oral mucosa. The epithelium of both types contains cells which produce keratin (keratinocytes) and cells which do not (non-keratinocytes). In each stratum, keratinocytes are by far the most numerous cells. Differences between the keratinocytes in different strata, rather than the uneven distribution of the non-keratinocytes, give rise to the stratified appearance of the epithelium. To acquire surface-adequate properties young cells undergo a process of maturation. During this process their morphology changes and they move towards the epithelial surface. Since this movement occurs as a fairly orderly progression, cells in successive layers represent a succession of ages and of stages in the maturation process.

In all regions of stratified squamous epithelium the cells still capable of division exhibit the main features by which keratinocytes differ from the cells of other tissues. These are the features of cells specialized for the synthesis of proteins which are retained in the cell and, in addition, the features of cells specialized for mutual cohesion. Thus basal and parabasal cells show a predominance of free ribosomes over rough endoplasmic reticulum and Golgi apparatus. The chief of the retained products of synthesis, the tonofilaments, are already present, as are the specialized intercellular attachments, the desmosomes.

The maturational changes common to all regions are an increase in cell size and a sequence of changes in shape. The increase in size is associated with the continued synthesis of synthetic machinery and of the previously synthesized product: further, it is associated with the appearance of some new synthetic products, i.e. Odland bodies (membrane coating granules, microgranules) and keratohyalin granules, and also with the continued formation of desmosomes. Also common to all regions and levels is the synthesis of cell-coating substances and of lytic enzymes. The latter are, at least in deeper cell rows, probably contained in lysosomes. Common to all regions is the eventual extrusion of the contents of the Odland bodies into the intercellular space, the thickening of the internal aspect of the cell membrane at some superficial level, and the loosening of desmosomal attachments at or near the epithelial surface.

Regional Variation in Oral Epithelium

The list of regional differences in the epithelium of oral mucosa is longer than the list of common traits. Moreover, these differences cover a wider spectrum than in epidermis, unless specializations like nail or hair are included. Conventionally, the mucosa is divided into masticatory, lining, and specialized types. Masticatory mucosa covers the hard palate and most regions of gingiva (see Chapter 36). The lining type constitutes the oral surface of the cheeks and lips, the buccal and labial sulci, the floor of the mouth, the ventral surface of the tongue, and the soft palate. Specialized mucosa lines the dorsal surface of the tongue. The term masticatory mucosa thus refers to the lining of immobile regions, while both lining and specialized mucosa cover mobile regions.

Differences between the epithelia associated with these three classes ought to reflect regional differences in the required performance. The epithelium of masticatory mucosa should show adaptations to the forces of pressure and friction to which it is subjected during mastication, and that of lining mucosa to its distension during the use of the oro-facial musculature. Specializations on the surface of the tongue should accommodate the sense of taste, the interaction between tongue and palate during mastication, and also distension of the organ.

Mobile and immobile regions include a wide sub-range of regional differences in the degree of functional stress. Thus in lining mucosa, the cheek, especially in the occlusal plane, is subject to friction and to frequent injury during chewing, and also to far greater distension than the lining of the floor of the mouth. The latter region is in a protected location and comparatively immobile.

In the human oral cavity, the greatest part of the masticatory mucosa is orthokeratinized, a smaller portion (of the gingiva; see Chapter 36) is ortho- or para-keratinized, lining mucosa is essentially non-keratinized, and specialized mucosa is a mosaic of both.

The keratinocytes of non-keratinized epithelium, beginning as smaller basal cells, soon attain far greater size than those of keratinized epithelium. Synthesis of mitochondria, ribosomes, and tonofilaments does not keep pace with the increase in cell size. As the concentration of these constituents decreases, glycogen accumulates and in part persists to the surface. Water also accumulates and the density of cell dry matter decreases towards the surface. In keratinized epithelium a high concentration of synthetic equipment persists for more cell rows, the concentration of tonofilaments increases towards the surface, dry matter density shows a progressive increase, and glycogen is not demonstrable.

Early cessation of protein-synthesizing activity in non-keratinized epithelium is reflected in the condensation of chromatin and a decrease in size of the nucleolus due to decreased amounts of ribosomal precursors. In keratinized epithelium chromatin dispersal and RNA precursors in the nucleolus persist in more cell rows.

The tonofilaments of non-keratinized epithelium remain dispersed in all, including surface cells, and only short tufts are associated with the attachment plaques of desmosomes. In keratinized epithelium, tonofilaments are organized into bundles and prominent bundles are associated with the desmosomes.

Keratohyalin granules (KHG) of the non-keratinized epithelium begin as infrequent electron-dense small rounded particles surrounded by ribosomes and eventually reach large size, still surrounded by ribosomes. It has been suggested that eventually they contribute to the thickening of the internal aspect of the cell membranes. From similar beginnings, KHG of the keratinized epithelium increase in number and size so that the cells containing them form a distinct granular layer. At this level they associate with bundles of tonofilaments. They are thought to contribute an embedding matrix for the fibrillar component in the keratin layer.

Odland bodies of the non-keratinized epithelium show a lighter zone between an electron-dense core and a bounding membrane; upon extrusion, non-lamellated material appears in the intercellular space. Odland bodies of keratinized epithelium appear striated and give rise to lamellated material in the intercellular space. Despite these differences, the extruded material is thought to constitute the barrier to the passage of protein in both types of epithelium.

In non-keratinized epithelium the Golgi zone is found in many cell rows. PAS-positive intercellular material is progressively more prominent. In keratinized epithelium, such material is less prominent between all, especially the more superficial cells, in which a Golgi zone is rarely seen.

In the superficial rows of non-keratinized epithelium, cytoplasmic organelles may show signs of degeneration, dry matter density is low, and long stretches of highly convoluted cell membrane are seen between short desmosomes. All maturational changes are gradual, hence they appear as inconspicuous differences between successive cell rows. In keratinized epithelium, the junction between granular and keratin layers appears as a sharp break in pattern, mediated at most by infrequent transitional cells. At this junction, cell size decreases abruptly, dry matter density undergoes a sudden marked increase, nucleus and cytoplasmic organelles disappear, and tightly packed, matrix-embedded bundles of tonofilaments are the sole content of the flattened squames of the keratin layer. Few further changes occur, except for the gradual disintegration of the desmosomes.

Keratins, as a class of proteins, are distinguished by their high content of the sulphur-containing amino acids, cysteine and cystine. Oxidation of two cysteine residues within or between the polypeptide chains supplies a cross-linking cystine residue, and hard keratins such as wool owe their resistance to chemical attack to the large number of such links. The concentration of these amino acids is lower in oral than in epidermal keratins. Oxidation of cysteine is probably more complete in keratinized than in non-keratinized regions, but the site of the resulting cross-links within or between tonofilaments is not established.

Some of the differences just presented are readily interpreted as functional adaptations. Of obvious value in permitting the distension of non-keratinized epithelium are the dispersed tonofilaments, the high water content, the reserve of cell surface area created by folding of the plasma membrane, and finally, the large amount of mucinous intercellular material, which facilitates gliding movements between the stretched cell membranes. Similarly, in keratinized epithelium exposed to compression or shear, a surface layer of multiple rows of squames composed of tightly packed tonofilaments and capable of resisting swelling in a fluid environment is of evident adaptive value.

Comparative histology of oral epithelium is helpful in deciphering the significance of some of the other differences noted above. In the rat, mouse, and hamster, the entire oral cavity is lined by orthokeratinized epithelium. In epithelium lining mobile regions, disintegration of nucleus and organelles at the junction of granular and keratin layers is abrupt and complete and eosinophilia of the keratin layer is as sharply demarcated as in palatal epithelium. Dispersal of tonofilaments, however, persists in all cell layers and in the keratin layer as well. Although cell size and cell dry weight decrease at the granular-keratin junction, cell density does not increase and cells near the surface swell through uptake of fluid from the oral cavity. A sharply demarcated, thick keratin layer and complete, sudden hydrolytic processes may thus be found in distensible as well as in rigid epithelia. Conversely, there are parakeratotic regions of human attached gingiva in which the keratin layer differs from that of ortho-keratinized regions by nothing more than the retention of nuclei. Resistance to swelling of the superficial keratin squames is not dependent on an embedding matrix furnished by KHG, for it is found in the epithelium of the hard palate in the rabbit, which has neither KHG nor matrix. It has, however, a well demarcated keratin layer consisting of multiple rows of flat squames which contain tightly packed tonofilaments.

In contrast to these examples of species differences, persistent dispersal of tonofilaments is seen in the epithelium of mobile regions of all species and early bundle formation in all rigid regions. It seems that persistent dispersal precludes the eventual formation of a stable keratin layer, perhaps because enough water cannot be eliminated to allow for tight packing of tonofilaments. Early organization of the tonofilament bundles thus seems to be a critical precondition of a resistant surface layer.

Differences Within the Major Classes of Epithelium

Functional requirements differ in degree within the distensible and rigid classes of mucosa. Adaptations to different magnitudes of compression or friction are brought about mainly by differences in the number of cell rows, in particular of the keratin layer, and also in the tightness of packing of the tonofilaments. A good example of the latter is seen in the dorsum of tongue, when posterior and anterior surfaces of the filiform papillae are compared. Adaptations to different degrees of distension are also brought about mainly by variation in the number of cell rows and by variations in cell size. Within both classes, however, a wide range exists in the rates of cell proliferation. Thus functional stress is only in part taken care of by the construction of the epithelium, and faster exfoliation and replacement are needed to meet the remaining needs.

The differences which exist between and within the major classes of oral mucosa reflect numerous variables in the epithelium of separate regions. Each region, however, maintains its own features constant, so that the same maturation process is repeated each time a new cell arises. This means that the same unique pattern of genome activation is repeated in each new cell, ensuring that the characteristic cell size, rate of tonofilament synthesis, and organelle disintegration are attained. Attempts to unravel this pattern by inducing changes in genome activation have

shown that simultaneous changes may occur in a few of these variables, which suggests that more than one variable may depend on a single event in the sequence of genome activation. However, the large variety of naturally occurring combinations of these variables argues that the normal sequence of genome activation must include a number of independent events.

Non-keratinocytes

Non-keratinocytes include melanocytes, Langerhans cells, Merkel cells and migrating inflammatory cells. They are estimated at about 10 per cent of the epithelial cell number, but the frequencies of all four types show great mutually independent regional variation. Their common trait is their failure to produce tonofilaments; their cytoplasm therefore is far more electron-lucent than that of the keratinocytes and they appear as "clear cells", i.e. cells with clear cytoplasm, in light-microscopic preparations.

Melanocytes and Langerhans cells are dendritic cells with widely branching dendrites. Both the cell bodies and the processes fail to form desmosomes with keratinocytes. This is true for migrating inflammatory cells also, whereas Merkel cells form infrequent desmosomal attachments to neighbouring keratinocytes. Melanocytes and Langerhans cells differ in the specific ultra-structural organelle each produces: the melanosome and the Langerhans granule. These organelles, when present, permit cell identification in electron microscopic preparations. In the absence of identifying planes of sectioning or of cell-specific organelles, dendritic cells can only be classified as indeterminate, and some authors believe that this class is indeed a third cell type.

Melanocytes are early immigrants from the neural crest. They are confined to the basal layer and closely apposed to the lamina densa but do not form hemidesmosomes (see below).

The melanosome is the membrane-bound end organelle of melanin synthesis and collection. Melanosomes, singly or grouped, are transferred to adjacent keratinocytes, the keratinocyte perhaps being the more active partner. Oral like epidermal melanocytes are thought to be no more numerous in dark- than in light-skinned persons but to be more active. In the epidermis of light-skinned persons ultraviolet radiation activates melanin synthesis and melanosome transfer; control and function of oral melanocytes are unclear.

Langerhans cells seem to be more frequent in middle than in deeper cell rows and have not been observed apposed to the basal lamina. The ultrastructural organelle identifying the Langerhans cell is similar in size to the melanosome; it also is membrane-bound and more electron opaque in its centre than at the periphery. The structure of the central density and the shape of the granule in melanocytes and Langerhans cells are distinctly different, and no transitional forms between the two organelles have been observed. Fusion of the organelle membrane with the cytoplasmic membrane has been observed in the case of the Langerhans granule, not the melanosome.

The content of Langerhans granules has not been identified and the origin and function of the cell have remained a matter of debate. Most authorities think that the cell is not of neuroectodermal origin and is not a later stage in the life of melanocytes. Regarding function, it is suggested that the cells might participate in the organization of groups of keratinocytes into units differentiating within coordinated epithelial columns, that they might participate in the process of cell determination eventuating in keratinized or non-keratinized epithelium, that they are the cells synthesizing mitosis-regulating substances, and finally that they participate in allergenic processes. Earlier suggestions of a sensory or a specialized phagocytic role are no longer accepted. The current suggestions of the role of Langerhans cells might all apply to oral epithelium as well as to epidermis, although the precise stacking of keratin squames seen in epidermis does not occur in oral epithelium.

Merkel cells, now accepted as sensory receptor cells, will be discussed in the section on innervation.

Intra-epithelial inflammatory cells (most commonly lymphocytes) are short-lived immigrants from the subjacent connective tissue. It is, however, exceptional to see a histological section of epithelium of any oral region without at least a few of these migrants, even when their number in the lamina propria is low. Hence their presence must be considered as "normal", at least in the statistical meaning of the word.

HISTOLOGY OF CONNECTIVE TISSUE

The structural elements of connective tissue are fibre-producing cells and an assortment of fibres, cells of the defence and repair systems, blood and lymph vessels, sensory receptors, and nerve endings and nerve fibres. The characteristics of cells of the defence and repair systems are the same in oral mucosa as in their counterparts in other organs, and will not be described in this chapter.

Since temperature regulation is not one of the functions of oral mucosa in man the supply of blood should correspond to local nutritional needs and will therefore be treated in the section on tissue maintenance.

Junction of Epithelium and Connective Tissue

The zone of tissue in which connective tissue papillae interdigitate with epithelial ridges is termed the papillary layer. The upward projections of connective tissue between the downward projections of epithelium can be likened to connective tissue septa, since they carry vessels and nerves and also act to attach the epithelium to the lamina propria. Height and/or frequency of ridges and papillae are far greater in masticatory regions, where external forces tend to separate epithelium and connective tissue, than they are in lining regions, where mucosa and underlying muscles undergo simultaneous elongation.

The attachment of the two tissues is greatly strengthened by a sub-microscopic structure, the "basal complex". The basal complex includes the lamina densa, a continuous sheet of protein and glycoprotein of ultra-microscopic thickness, which is now thought to be a product of the epithelial basal cells. The lamina densa is separated from the basal cell plasma membrane by the lamina lucida, a zone of density akin to that of intercellular spaces in the deeper epithelial layers. The lamina lucida is interrupted by "peripheral densities" or "hemidesmosomes". The peripheral densities face attachment plaques on the internal aspect of the basal cell membrane which are associated with tufts of tonofilaments. A system of finest filaments, perhaps originating within the basal cell, traverses the lamina lucida and lamina densa and emerges as a fine fibril. This is the so-called anchoring fibril, which is thought to form a loop beneath the lamina densa and then to re-enter it. Fine collagen fibrils arising in the lamina propria can be seen to enter such loops and to return to the lamina propria.

Because of the greater height and closer spacing of interdigitations in masticatory than in lining mucosa, a far greater area for attachment of anchoring fibrils is provided in the former. The filaments at each anchoring site are said to be more numerous in lining mucosa, which might in part compensate for the smaller total area of the junction.

Fibroblasts and Connective Tissue Fibres

The fibres of the lamina propria carry a large share of the protective functions of the mucosa. Reticular, collagenous and elastic fibres vary in amount in different parts of the mucosa as fits regional needs. Fibroblasts produce the required quantities of these fibres, as well as the glycoproteins of the ground substance of the lamina propria but the mechanisms controlling fibrogenesis are not known. These same fibroblasts, moreover, are the source of regionally differing determinants for the overlying epithelium and perhaps of chalones regulating not only their own mitotic rates but influencing that of the epithelium as well.

Fibroblasts have the ultrastructural characteristics of cells synthesizing proteins for export at a rapid rate; that is, large quantities of rough endoplasmic reticulum, prominent Golgi zones, numerous mitochondria and prominent nucleoli. They have an extremely high ratio of surface area to volume due to multiple long cytoplasmic processes, hence are in a favourable position for uptake of nutrients. Although highly differentiated, they are capable of division and thought to be capable of turning into phagocytosing cells.

Reticular and collagenous fibres are both thought to be secreted as tropocollagen molecules undergoing, when outside the cells, lateral and longitudinal aggregation to reticular and collagen fibres respectively, as well as association with glycoproteins. Reticular fibres show the ultrastructural periodicity typical for aggregated tropocollagen molecules; they are thought to owe their affinity to silver to a high proportion of glycoproteins. Primary collagen fibres form interlacing bundles with one another.

Elastic fibres consist of an electronlucent amorphous core of light microscopic dimensions and numerous fine tubular filaments forming acute angles with the core. Elastic fibres branching in close contact with the ends of collagen fibres have been demonstrated in oral mucosa. While the modes of secretion of collagen are well known, that of elastic fibres seems to be unknown. Embryological studies have shown that the filaments are secreted first and form a solid cylinder, and are subsequently separated by the progressive secretion of the amorphous core. Oxytalan fibres may be immature elastic fibres rather than a distinct fibre type.

Use of Fibres in the Construction of the Lamina Propria

Masticatory mucosa is protected from deformation by the resistance provided by collagen fibres. These fibres do not stretch, and potential elongation in all directions is counteracted by interlacing of fibre bundles. Collagen fibres take a straight course in these bundles. Deeper fibres eventually enter the hard tissues. The amount of collagen varies regionally in relation to the imposed load. Elastic fibres are absent or sparse in such areas.

In lining mucosa overlying muscles and glands the lamina propria may be thin. The primary collagen fibres are of smaller diameter than in masticatory mucosa and form delicate wavy bundles. Elastic fibres are numerous and may lie close to collagen fibre bundles. Collagen and elastic fibres of the lamina propria interweave with the connective tissue fibres of the muscle bundles. Thus, lamina propria and muscle layer remain closely approximated whether the muscles are elongated or contracted. When the mucosa is distended, the collagen fibres straighten first, then elastic fibres are stretched. During return to their resting position, the muscles act to restore the mucosa to its resting dimensions and recoil of elastic fibres restores the slack of the collagen bundles.

The mucosa of the buccal and labial sulci is only loosely attached to underlying structures and here distension occurs through the action of distant muscles. Hence restoration to the resting state depends on elastic recoil and elastic fibres are plentiful, especially in the region of the muco-gingival junction, where they form a dense network.

Innervation of Oral Mucosa

The structural components of the nervous system located in oral mucosa are the peripheral extremities of afferent fibres. In the case of taste, and perhaps in part in the case of touch, cells in the epithelium specialized for reception of stimuli precede the first afferent neurone. With these exceptions, stimuli are received by terminal specializations (organized endings) or simply by the first nonmyelinated stretch of the afferent fibre (free endings).

Organized endings are more or less complex structures which may be enclosed by a connective tissue capsule. They are named after the authors who first described them and are located in the papillae or the subpapillary layer of the lamina propria. According to current opinion, each of these structures and also free endings are differentially sensitive to a particular sensory modality, e.g. Meissner's corpuscles to touch and Krause's end bulbs to cold, but are not the sole receptor for the given modality.

Free endings are numerous in the lamina propria and are frequently seen in the epithelium. They may be branched or unbranched in both locations. Fibres in the epithelium usually converge to fibres in the connective tissue papillae which may also be joined by organized and free endings from the lamina propria. Electron microscopy shows that free endings contain numerous mitochondria and that intraepithelial free endings usually lie between epithelial cells.

The two sensory cells of oral mucosa are cells of taste buds and the Merkel cell. Taste buds are located in the epithelium of fungiform, foliate, and circumvallate papillae of the dorsum of the tongue and, in some mammals, in the epithelium of the soft palate. They consist of 30–60 dark- or light-staining spindle-shaped cells, the longer axes of which lie perpendicular to the epithelial surface, and of numerous nerve fibres. The superficial plasma membranes of dark and light cells form numerous microvilli facing a shallow depression in the epithelial surface, the taste pore.

The functional significance of dark and light cells is debated. Electron-microscopically, light cells differ from dark in having rounder nuclei with more dispersed chromatin and larger amounts of smooth endoplasmic reticulum; while dark cells contain many bundles of fine filaments and numerous electron-opaque, membrane-enclosed granules resembling small secretion granules. Numerous unmyelinated nerve fibres are seen adjacent to dark and light cells, and synapse-like structures between cell membrane and nerve have frequently been observed. The nerve fibres converge in the lamina propria to fewer fibres, which eventually join the cranial nerves. There is no complete agreement that taste bud cells rather than nerve endings are receptive to the chemicals mediating taste. As of old, taste modalities are thought to be sweet, sour, salty and bitter. The distribution of these modalities over the taste buds is as yet not clear. Taste bud cells seem singularly dependent on trophic stimuli from their afferent nerves, but do regenerate following nerve regeneration.

The status of the Merkel cell as a tactile sensory cell is open to more doubt than that of the taste bud cells as taste receptors. Like the dark cells of taste buds, the Merkel cell contains numerous electron-opaque membrane-bound granules, which are usually clustered in regions of cytoplasm near nerve endings. A synapse-like structure, and fusion of the membranes of granules with the plasma membrane opposite this structure, has been reported in a Merkel cell from rabbit palatal epithelium. Considering the respective sizes of synapses and plasma membranes, multiple electron-microscopic observations of this sort are not likely.

Somatic sensory endings in oral mucosa are more numerous in anterior than in posterior regions, and sensitivity parallels this distribution. The anterior portions of tongue and hard palate were found to be more sensitive to touch than the fingertips, and two-point discrimination was closer at the tip of the tongue than in the fingertips.

Temperature perception, as in skin, is mediated by separate cold- and warmth-sensitive spots. It is acute in the vermilion zone of the lip and the tip of the tongue, but rather poor in posterior regions.

No comparative data seem to be available for pain sensitivity. Pain is mediated by free endings of specific thin myelinated and slower unmyelinated fibres, which perhaps are stimulated by liberation of substances from damaged cells or the activation by such substances of pre-existing pain mediators in the lamina propria.

Excepting smooth muscle in blood vessels, oral mucosa itself has no effector organs, but stimuli from its receptors participate in the initiation of swallowing, gagging and retching reflexes and give rise to withdrawal and salivary gland reflexes, and in addition, of course, to responses involving higher centres in the central nervous system. One of the latter may be mobilization of the thirst mechanism.

Touch receptors in the soft palate, though chiefly receptors in the oropharynx, initiate the swallowing reflex. Gagging and retching reflexes seem to be initiated by differing constellations of stimuli from the same sites. Taste stimuli reaching higher centres may aid in determining which of these responses occurs and may facilitate the reflex sequence. Withdrawal reflexes and perhaps salivation occur in response to painful stimuli. Taste stimuli seem to be the chief initiators of salivary reflexes.

MAINTENANCE OF ORAL MUCOSA

Characteristic Features of the Metabolism of Oral Mucosa

The metabolic requirements of oral epithelium reflect features discussed in the preceding sections: rapid cell division, rapid protein synthesis, and rapid catabolic activity, and in addition the separation of the epithelium from direct blood supply. Associated with high rates of cell division and marked increase in cell size are high rates of synthesis of nucleic acids and of membrane lipids.

Basal cells reaching the granular layer in 3 or 4 days may during this time have increased their dry weight as much as 29 times, indicating rates of protein synthesis comparable to the rate in pancreas. There is electron-microscopic and histochemical evidence for a moderate concentration of RNA in all cellular layers of keratinized oral epithelium and in the deeper layers of non-keratinized epithelium. Ribosomes from gingival, palatal and buccal mucosa of rabbits and cattle are as active in directing the incorporation of amino acids as those from the liver.

Compared to epithelium, the connective tissue of the lamina propria is metabolically inert. Autoradiographic sections show almost no labelling with tritiated thymidine and much less labelling with tritiated proline than is seen in the epithelium, suggesting slow cell turnover and less protein synthesis.

The synthesis of proteins, lipids and nucleic acids requires energy, and oral epithelium has a relatively high capacity for energy conversion. Lactate dehydrogenase, which is a rough indicator of the level of anaerobic glycolysis, is about 20 per cent more active in isolated oral epithelium of the rat than in rat kidney glomeruli. Malate dehydrogenase, an indicator of aerobic oxidation, is 60 per cent more active in the epithelium than in the glomeruli and nearly the same in oral epithelium as in liver.

Glycolysis. In the absence of a blood supply, anaerobic glycolysis must be significantly increased. This is seen when oral epithelium is compared with other tissues. Thus, the ratio of lactate to malate dehydrogenase should be high in tissues depending on anaerobic energy conversion, and indeed in rabbits is about twice as high in oral epithelium as in striated or smooth muscle. The isoenzymes of lactate dehydrogenase in human oral epithelium show the pattern that characterizes anaerobically metabolizing tissues. The oxygen quotient of oral epithelium is considerably lower than that of liver, muscle, and kidney cortex. Different species were, however, used in this comparison.

A progressive decrease in oxygen tension with distance from the lamina propria is reflected in the decreasing concentration of mitochondria and in the distribution pattern of enzymes obtained from ultramicroassays at successive epithelial levels. The indicator enzymes for anaerobic and aerobic energy conversion both show decreasing activity towards the surface, but the decrease is less steep for enzymes of anaerobic glycolysis than for those involved in aerobic oxidation.

Pentose Phosphogluconate Pathway. The pentose phosphogluconate pathway (hexose monophosphate shunt) is rather active in oral epithelium. Generally, the main function of this pathway is the production of NADPH, which serves as a source of hydrogen in biological reductions and is a necessary co-enzyme in lipid synthesis. The pathway also produces ribose which can be used in ribonucleic acid synthesis and metabolites that can enter the glycolytic pathway.

In isolated oral epithelium of the rat the activity of glucose-6-phosphate dehydrogenase (G_6PDH), which catalyzes the first step in the shunt pathway, is 3 to 9 times as high as in kidney glomeruli and 4 to 13 times as high as in liver. In all regions of oral epithelium of laboratory animals and humans in which micro-assays at successive levels were made, the distribution of this enzyme was strikingly different from that of the enzymes in the energy conversion pathways. While these enzymes invariably decrease in activity between basal and spinous cells, G_6PDH showed markedly elevated levels in the spinous and even in the granular layer, the latter especially in keratinized epithelium. This distribution parallels the high levels of lipid and RNA synthesis in the upper cellular layers. A specific role of lipids in the final keratinization process has often been suggested. The high level of G_6PDH activity in the granular layer of keratinized epithelium is compatible with this suggestion.

Catabolic Activity. In keratinized epithelium, disintegration of cell organelles and nuclei is complete, while in non-keratinized epithelium progressive though partial disintegration of organelles occurs. In view of the high cell turnover rate this organelle distintegration reflects a high level of lytic activity. Using acid phosphatase as an indicator enzyme, levels of activity in rabbit oral epithelium were found 4 to 14 times as high as in striated muscle. Keratinized regions showed 2 to 9 times greater activity than non-keratinized regions. Numerous histochemical and some quantitative studies have shown that acid phosphatase activity is higher in the granular than in deeper cell layers of keratinized epithelium.

It is true that part of the epithelial acid phosphatase activity is located in the Odland bodies and appears in the intercellular spaces upon their extrusion. This fraction, and possibly other lytic enzymes, are thus lost to the cytoplasm before major organelle disintegration occurs. There is, on the other hand, no reason to postulate that all disintegration occurs through the release of pre-existing lytic enzymes from lysosomes. Indeed, there is evidence to show that oral epithelium of the rabbit contains acid phosphatase with the properties usually found in the lysosomal enzyme as well as the form usually unassociated with lysosomes.

Regional Differences in Metabolic Requirements. Regional comparisons are complicated by differences in cell size, cell dry weight, and tonofilament concentration. These factors complicate comparisons between deeper and upper cell layers, and between different regions as well. Since tonofilaments constitute an inert contribution to the dry weight of cells, comparisons of enzyme activities per unit dry weight are distorted when tonofilaments are present in greatly differing concentrations. Enzyme activities per unit DNA, on the other hand, may not at all reflect the true levels of metabolic activity in different tissues.

Taking these factors into account, keratinized epithelium has higher levels of glycolytic activity, higher levels of lytic activity, and higher levels of glucose-6-phosphate dehydrogenase activity than non-keratinized epithelium, especially in the upper cellular layers. It is also clear that the activity of the pentose shunt is much higher in upper than deeper cell rows.

Blood Supply

The vascular components of the microcirculation are smallest artery; arteriole; terminal arteriole; metarteriole; capillary; venule; small vein. For nutrient and oxygen supply, capillaries are the only directly significant vessels. This is true also for return of carbon dioxide and metabolites, the latter supplemented by lymph capillaries.

Differences in blood supply other than those determined by the size of the vascular bed, relative to the size of the organ, are brought about by differences in the distribution of sympathetic constrictor and dilator fibres to arterioles and precapillary sphincters, by the presence or absence of parasympathetic dilator fibres, and by the local responsiveness of muscle fibres to changes in oxygen, carbon dioxide and pH and other metabolic changes of their environment. Due to events upstream, flow through a capillary may fluctuate between zero and the maximum corresponding to its full dilatation. In intermittently active organs, *e.g.* skeletal muscles, a small proportion of capillaries is open at rest and all are open at maximal activity.

Different organs vary greatly in their degree of arteriolar constriction and thereby in their contribution to the total peripheral resistance, that of brain being perhaps the smallest, that of skin the greatest. Blood flow through human skin is chiefly under central nervous control in accordance with the regulation of body temperature. The vascular capacity of the skin, and usually also blood flow, far exceeds local tissue needs, as is seen from the small arterio-venous oxygen difference. When cooling is needed, blood flow is maximal through the numerous arterio-venous shunts in the skin of hands and feet and through capillaries in other areas. The reverse is true when heat is to be conserved.

This brief sketch may serve to recall the complex interrelation of variables entering into the blood supply of a given organ. Present knowledge of the blood supply of oral mucosa is too fragmentary for a description in these terms, even though the anatomy of the microcirculation is fairly well known. Most regions of oral mucosa are inaccessible to *in vivo* observation, and there are hardly any regions in which circulatory parameters can be measured in mucosa in isolation from the underlying muscles or other organs.

The most frequently studied region in man and animals is the gingiva. Also studied by *in vivo* methods in man are labial alveolar mucosa and filiform papillae of tongue. An extensively studied region, because it is free of muscles, glands, and adnexa, is the blind end of the hamster cheek pouch.

All vessels comprising the microcirculation are present in the lamina propria, with the probable exceptions of arterio-venous shunts in all oral regions in man, and in the cheek pouch and gingiva of hamsters. A plexus of smallest arterial vessels lies close to the epithelium. True capillaries arise at right angles from metarterioles and from preferential channels and form a hairpin-shaped loop into the connective tissue papilla. The venous limb of the loop connects with venules forming a dense network in the subreticular layer. The frequency and length of the capillary loops thus parallels spacing and height of the papillae. Blind beginnings of the lymphatic capillaries also reach the height of the papillae. Vasomotor innervation of mucosal vessels seems similar to that of other organs. Arterioles of the gingiva and capillaries of the tongue respond in the same way as those of other regions to stimulation of sympathetic nerves and vaso-active drugs. Precapillary sphincters, though present, seem to be less responsive than those in skin. Vasodilator fibres, believed absent in skin, may be present in buccal mucosa.

Generalizing from the following fragmentary observations, the blood supply of oral mucosa seems to exceed local tissue needs. High oxygen tension persists in gingiva of the dog even when systemic and gingival metabolic activity are made to increase several fold. All capillaries in hamster gingiva and cheek pouch are simultaneously open, gingival capillaries remaining open even when gingival arterioles participate in induced vasoconstriction. Healing of mucosal wounds generally seems faster than in skin, and better blood flow is thought to be a major contributing factor. In oral mucosa, a fragmentary quantitative study has suggested a relation between the distribution of capillaries per surface area and thickness of the overlying epithelium. Since thickness of epithelium is correlated with mitotic activity, blood supply in oral mucosa may also be related to mitotic activity.

Nutritional Requirements and the Influence of Hormones

Effects of nutritional deficiencies, as well as those associated with hormonal dysfunction, are mentioned in Chapter 40, and will not be dealt with here.

Control of Cell Renewal

The thickness of oral epithelium in the adult varies widely from region to region, but is remarkably constant in each. Thus in each region the rate of cell division must be matched by an equal rate of cell desquamation. Little is known about the control of desquamation, but the rate of cell proliferation and its control have been studied in great detail. The life cycle of cells undergoing repeated mitosis has come to be divided into the following four phases: M, the mitotic phase; G_1, the post-mitotic phase; S, the DNA synthesis phase; G_2, the post-DNA synthesis phase. The duration of DNA synthesis, the time interval between synthesis and entrance into mitosis, and that of mitosis itself are fairly constant in cells of different tissues and species. They are approximately estimated as $S = 8$ hr.; $G_2 = 3$–4 hr.; $M = 1$ hr. The duration of G_1, the post-mitotic interval, varies from a few hours, *e.g.* in regions of intestinal epithelium, to a few weeks, *e.g.* in some regions of skin. In a histological section, which represents but a single point in time, the number of cells in each phase is proportional to the duration of the phases, hence cells in mitosis will always be smallest in number. The duration of G_1 is the main variable in the length of the cell cycle, and its duration is most often affected under altered conditions. It appears that DNA synthesis, once begun, proceeds to completion and similarly, cells that have entered mitosis will proceed to the formation of two daughter cells. There seem to be three points in the cell cycle at which "decisions" are made: before the beginning of DNA synthesis, after completion of synthesis, and after completion of mitosis. Following mitosis, the two daughter cells may remain in the population of dividing cells and re-enter the cell cycle at G_1 or proceed to differentiation, migration, and eventual exfoliation. It has recently been proposed that there is a time interval before the choice between these two alternatives is made, a phase termed G_0, which follows mitosis. Daughter cells entering this phase are said to be in a "resting state".

The principle by which cell proliferation is controlled is through inhibition by negative feedback. Cells are thought to retain their embryonic capacity to divide and to be restrained by inhibitory substances, termed chalones, which they or their fellows elaborate. Attempts are being made in several laboratories to isolate and purify chalones, and to elucidate their mode of action. Unlike hormones, chalones are thought to be produced in the tissues on which they act, but like hormones they are thought to be fairly tissue-specific although not species-specific. Thus, appropriate extracts of pig epidermis will decrease the mitotic rate of rat epidermis and of the epithelium of rat tongue as well. Inhibiting substances may be elaborated at different cellular levels and act at different points in the cell cycle. Differentiating cells at higher levels in rat epidermis have been shown to contain substances inhibiting entrance into the DNA synthesis phase and basal cells have been shown to contain substances inhibiting entrance into mitosis.

The rate of cell division follows a diurnal rhythm corresponding to the sleep-wake cycle of the animal. This dependence was thought to be mediated by the fluctuating level of circulating adrenaline. Adrenaline *in vitro* indeed enhances the mitosis-inhibiting effect of chalones but perhaps not *in vivo*. Adrenaline has, however, been shown to stimulate the formation of cyclic-3′, 5′-adenosine monophosphate (cyclic AMP), and the increased intracellular concentration of the nucleotide was followed by decrease in mitotic rate. Glucocorticoids also enhance the effect of chalones *in vitro*, but their role *in vivo* is not clear. The mitosis-stimulating effect of oestrogen in the vaginal and uterine lining epithelia of mice is brought about by decreasing the duration of the G_1 and S phases.

Estimates of Epithelial Turnover Time

If the number of cells in a given volume of epithelium be K, its turnover time may be defined as the time required to produce K new cells by division. This time equals the average lifespan of the cells in this region. Turnover times can be determined by a number of techniques including the use of colchicine or related compounds, and of tritiated thymidine. Colchicine arrests mitosis in metaphase, and the percentage of epithelial cells entering metaphase during a known time period can be used to compute the time for total renewal. The uptake of tritiated thymidine by DNA-synthesizing cells can be used to count the number of the tagged cells by means of autoradiography. Changes with time in their numbers and location in the epithelium enable the average lifespan of cells and other parameters to be computed. Turnover times of oral epithelium in a variety of experimental animals have been reported. In comparing such data, attention must be given to the dimensions used by different authors. Computations sometimes refer to the turnover time of the entire epithelium, but sometimes to the so-called progenitor compartment only. This compartment includes only those deepest rows of cells all of which are assumed to undergo division. In human buccal mucosa, turnover times of eight days for the progenitor compartment and of 25 days for the whole epithelium have been reported. Generally speaking, the lifespan of cells of oral epithelium is longer than that of the cells of the intestinal lining and shorter than that of epidermal cells.

Regional Differences in Mitotic Activity

As has been pointed out above, the structural adaptations of oral epithelium do not suffice to compensate for the regional differences in functional stress. Different rates of cell renewal are required to maintain a constant cell population in every region. This is best seen when numbers of mitoses per unit area are compared. In the rabbit, the rate so computed is lowest in epithelium of the ventral surface of the tongue, 1·53 times as high in epithelium of the hard palate, and 4·33 times as high in buccal epithelium. In the mouse, daily epithelial growth increments have been computed as 1·05 μm. for floor of the mouth, 2·7 μm. for hard palate and 7·24 μm. for cheek. In both of these species the thickness of the epithelium varies in the same direction as the mitotic rate, though not in proportion to it.

Renewal of Melanocytes and Langerhans Cells

There is evidence for DNA synthesis in epidermal melanocytes, and melanocytes undergoing mitosis have been observed, as also their proliferation at the edges of epidermal wounds. Quantitative data on their lifespan are not available. Extraction of a melanocyte-specific chalone from a transplantable mouse melanoma has been reported.

Proliferation of Langerhans cells after wounding has been reported, but cell division in physiological circumstances does not seem to have been observed.

Connective Tissue Turnover

Information on turnover of connective tissue is scanty. Fibroblasts are known to be capable of division, but because of the small number per microscopic field, fibroblasts in mitosis will rarely be seen in physiological circumstances. The rate of collagen turnover is usually inferred from the specific radioactivity of hydroxyproline measured in isolated collagen after administration of labelled proline. Collagen from guinea pig oral mucosa showed much higher activity than collagen from the skin of the animal. Guinea pig oral mucosa also showed far greater collagen depletion than skin following the inhibition of synthesis by vitamin C deprivation. Comparison of the rate of collagen synthesis in gingiva and palate of marmosets showed the rate of incorporation of amino acids into the insoluble and soluble fractions to be greater in gingiva than in palate.

39. NON-INFECTIOUS LOCAL DISEASES OF THE ORAL MUCOSA

R. DUCKWORTH

Benign migratory glossitis

Black hairy tongue

Median rhomboid glossitis

Papillary hyperplasia

Focal epithelial hyperplasia

Developmental white lesions
  Leukoedema
  White sponge naevus

Melanotic pigmentation

Recurrent aphthous ulceration

Herpetiform ulceration

Allergic contact stomatitis

Submucous fibrosis

There are numerous non-infectious local diseases of the oral mucosa and they have widely different characteristics. Some of these disorders, notably many of those with inflammatory or neoplastic origins, may arise not only in the mouth but at any of several sites in the body. In this group a particular type of lesion tends to have similar features whatever its site. Thus, because these lesions tend not to have unique features which make them of special nterest when occurring in the mouth they will not be described here. On the other hand, some local disorders are peculiar to the mouth and have features which are not met with in lesions occurring elsewhere in the body. This chapter will deal with some of these changes.

BENIGN MIGRATORY GLOSSITIS

(Erythema migrans, Geographical tongue)

This is an ill-understood condition virtually limited to the mucosa covering the dorsal surface of the tongue, although there have been one or two reports of similar changes affecting the mucosa of the cheeks and lips. In the United States about 1 per cent of adolescents and young adults have been found to be affected.

Benign migratory glossitis is an intractable inflammatory process, which gives rise in some patients to a persistent but low-grade burning sensation or soreness. One or more tongue lesions appear, often at the lateral margins, and spread over the dorsal surface (fig. 1). The white or yellowish inflamed zone at the advancing edge of a lesion may be followed by a second or third concentric zone spreading across the tongue. These may intersect with the edges of other zones of inflammatory change giving rise to the irregular pattern suggested by one of the synonyms.

At the edge of the lesion there is a zone of acute or subacute inflammation characterized by spongiosis of the

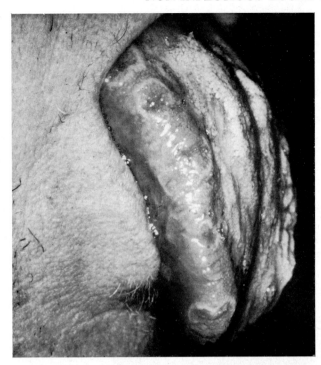

FIG. 1. Benign migratory glossitis. Zones of inflammatory change arranged in an annular pattern arising at the lateral border of the tongue.

epithelium and the accumulation within it of many polymorphonuclear leucocytes. Within this peripheral zone the mucosa is thinned and it loses many of its filiform papillae. Gradually, as the front of the lesion spreads over the tongue surface and eventually fades away, these papillae regenerate. For variable periods the tongue may resume a more or less normal appearance until new

inflammatory zones arise once more and spread over its surface. These cycles of activity may vary in length from a few days to, more usually, a slower change extending over a period of weeks.

The aetiology of benign migratory glossitis is obscure. Searches for specific infective agents, nutritional factors and allergens have been unrewarding although there is some evidence in young adults that emotional factors may play a part. A familial tendency has been demonstrated, for in one study 42 per cent of the families of patients were affected, whereas only 9 per cent of the families of control subjects showed evidence of the disorder. There is no consistently effective therapy to relieve tongue soreness.

BLACK HAIRY TONGUE

This is another simple condition of the tongue which disturbs patients mainly because of its appearance (fig.2). The essential change is probably a failure of epithelial cells to desquamate which results in a great elongation of the filiform papillae over the central part of the dorsum of the tongue. These elongated papillae become discoloured yellow, brown or black, possibly because of the proliferation of chromogenic bacteria and the staining effect of foods and smoking. This condition, which is more common in men than women, is long lasting and resistant to treatment although the application of friction via a toothbrush or spoon may shorten the papillae and thereby make the tongue look cleaner. Treatment with acids or enzymes is not to be recommended although the keratolytic effect of urea in solution may aid the cleansing action of a toothbrush.

A less florid and transient form of hairy tongue may follow antibiotic therapy, especially when a tetracycline is

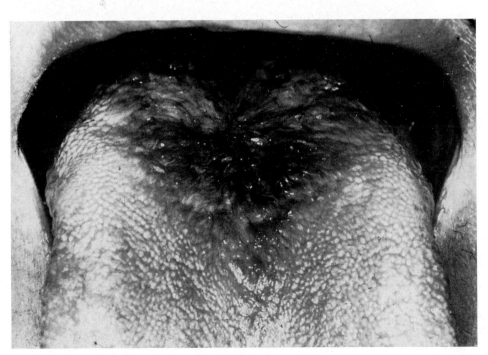

FIG. 2. Black hairy tongue. Elongated and stained filiform papillae lying on the dorsum of the tongue.

used locally for periods in excess of 7 days. There is soreness of the tongue but no real elongation of the papillae. The dorsum is covered by soft yellowish material in which *Candida albicans* is readily identified. Thus, this is a form of acute candidiasis created by the supression of tetracycline sensitive organisms and the consequent overgrowth of *Candida*. It responds simply to the withdrawal of the antibiotic; antifungal agents are rarely required.

MEDIAN RHOMBOID GLOSSITIS

This is believed to be a developmental condition upon which inflammatory changes are superimposed. In the embryo the anterior part of the tongue forms from the centrally placed tuberculum impar and the adjacent ventro-medial portions of the first pharyngeal arches.

of filiform papillae and the epithelium has much elongated and narrowed ridges penetrating deeply into the corium. Chronic inflammatory changes are always found histologically but more acute exacerbations of inflammation may occur and give rise to symptoms in this otherwise symptomless defect. If warranted, excision of the affected area with closure of the defect will prevent these recurrent and painful inflammatory episodes.

PAPILLARY HYPERPLASIA

(Papillomatosis)

This change is relatively common in only one site—the mucosa of the hard palate—but it is occasionally found arising from the alveolar mucosa of either jaw. Although it usually occurs in denture wearers (a prevalence of 3–4 per cent has been noted in such patients) it is seen

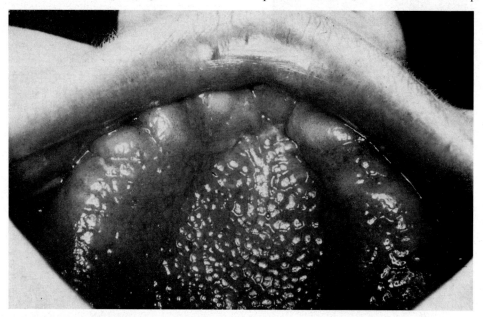

FIG. 3. Papillary hyperplasia. Multiple papillae arising from the mucosa covering the central part of the hard palate.

Normally the tuberculum impar contributes little to the substance of the tongue as the lingual swellings overgrow it. It is generally believed that should this not occur, or be incomplete, an altered area of mucosa persists on the dorsal surface, immediately in front of the site of the foramen caecum.

The prevalence of this defect amongst adults has been reported to be of the order of 1–2 per 1,000. However, because no cases were found in a study of over 10,000 subjects, most of whom were aged 16 or less, there is doubt about the role of maldevelopment in its causation.

Often this area of indurated, altered mucosa is rhomboidal in shape but it may be irregular in outline. Commonly, the dark red surface of the lesion is slightly depressed below the level of the surrounding normal mucosa although there may be fissuring and nodularity in grosser defects. The latter lesions have sometimes been mistaken for carcinomata. The affected mucosa is devoid

occasionally in those who have never worn dentures and in some such instances involvement of members of the same family has suggested a genetic basis. However, a causal role of the dentures worn by most affected patients tends to be substantiated by the fact that hyperplasia of this type is much more prevalent in those who wear their dentures while sleeping than in those who do not; also, removal of ill-fitting dentures, or their replacement, favours regression of lesions, especially when these are small.

Papillary hyperplasia affects mainly the more horizontal parts of the hard palate, tending not to spread to the mucosa covering the sloping surface of the alveolus (fig. 3). The individual papillae are less than 1 mm. in diameter and are made up of a core of inflamed connective tissue covered by hyperplastic epithelium often showing pseudo-epitheliomatous changes. Intra-epithelial keratinization is commonly found.

Because of these last two features some authors have

stressed the malignant potential of papillary hyperplasia of the palate but this seems not to be a real hazard. The prevalence of papillomatosis would suggest that palatal carcinoma arising from it should be a clearly recognized entity but there are few, if any, well-documented reports of this association.

As mentioned above papillary hyperplasia of minor degree is often controlled or reversed by the insertion of a well-fitting denture but in more severe hyperplasia denture construction should be preceded by the removal of excess tissue. Of the many methods used for this cryosurgery appears to give the best results.

formation of elongated bulbous ridges and some spongiosis and ballooning of cells in the superficial epithelial layers. Inflammatory changes in the corium are slight.

The recent interest in this lesion stems mainly from the demonstration in electronmicrographs of tissue from some lesions of virus-like particles within the nuclei of cells in the upper prickle-cell layer. The morphology of these particles and of the apparently associated changes in cytoplasmic organelles suggests that they are members of the Papova virus group—a group containing the viruses found in verruca vulgaris, canine oral papilloma, and the Shope rabbit papilloma. However, until more direct

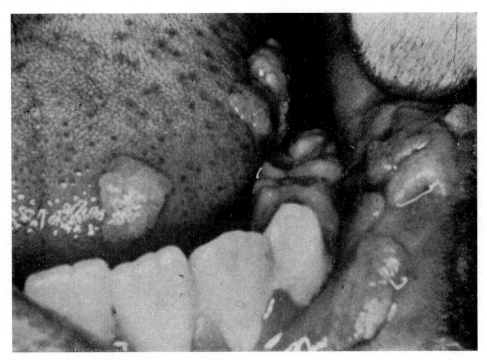

FIG. 4. Focal epithelial hyperplasia. Asymptomatic lesions in an eight-year-old Guatemalan Indian. Courtesy of Dr. C. Lopez, University of Guatemala.

FOCAL EPITHELIAL HYPERPLASIA

Focal epithelial hyperplasia of the oral mucosa is a condition which has come into prominence only recently, although sporadic reports have been published over the last 15–20 years. A geographical distribution, and involvement of particular ethnic groups, have been suggested but better recognition of the disorder has now led to its being reported in populations distributed around the world.

Clinically, numerous fine granulations and larger sessile swellings are seen arising from any part of the oral mucosa (fig. 4). There may be an associated gingival hyperplasia. The hyperplastic tissue is normal in colour and it retains the softness and elasticity of the healthy mucosa. Unless traumatized, inflammatory changes are not found. Usually, the lesions are first noticed in childhood and they tend to have a familial distribution but this is not genetically based.

The histological appearances are unremarkable at the light microscope level, there being acanthosis with the

evidence of pathogenicity is forthcoming, the mere presence of the virus in some of these hyperplastic epithelial lesions does not prove that it has a causal role.

DEVELOPMENTAL WHITE LESIONS OF THE ORAL MUCOSA

These are distinguished from white lesions which have an infective or other local cause largely by their clinical features, their histological appearances and sometimes by the demonstration of genetic factors. However, there is some confusion between the members of the group because of overlap of certain characteristics. This confusion tends to be heightened by the large number of different terms which have been applied to the relatively few types of lesion reported. Simplification can be achieved by excluding those intra-oral white lesions which form part of more widespread syndromes and concentrating attention upon two disorders with predominantly oral changes—leukoedema and the white sponge naevus.

The principal significance of these two developmental disorders of the oral mucosa is their differentiation from the more sinister leukoplakic changes. Although clinical findings may go some way towards diagnosis, biopsy is necessary to exclude histological characteristics which would suggest the potential for more aggressive behaviour.

Leukoedema, in its common form, appears bilaterally in the cheek mucosa as a diffuse whitish-grey film. The whole mucosa tends to be covered by this film which obliterates the outline of the underlying vessels. Stretching of the mucosa makes the film less apparent. In addition, thicker, coarsely wrinkled changes have been described but their clear differentiation from other white lesions is not certain.

There is an increased thickness of the prickle-cell layer with many cells showing intra-cellular oedema. The surface layer is parakeratotic and there is no evidence of a prominent orthokeratotic layer. The corium is virtually free of inflammatory changes.

The frequency with which this condition is encountered —in two surveys of selected adult subjects it was found in 90 per cent or more of the individuals surveyed—does suggest that it is an anatomical variant rather than a pathological entity. The dependence of its recognition upon lighting conditions during examination and the relatively minimal deviation of the histological appearances from the normal also throw doubt upon the pathological significance of leukoedema.

The White Sponge Naevus, although far less common than leukoedema, has better defined characteristics. It appears as a whitish thickening, often widely distributed over much of the oral mucosa. The surface layers are usually folded and spongy and it is sometimes possible to scrape off sheets of sodden epithelium. In nearly every case there is involvement of the cheek mucosa. In patients with oral lesions similar changes may be found in the mucous membranes of the nose, larynx, labia, vagina and rectum.

Nearly all lesions are discovered accidentally because they do not produce symptoms. They are found shortly after birth or in the first few years of life. They may enlarge up to puberty but new lesions do not form in adult life. Familial involvement is widespread in many of the reported case histories. An autosomal dominant gene with irregular penetrance appears to be responsible.

The histological appearances are unremarkable except for extensive vacuolation of cells in the thickened prickle-cell layer. The surface cells are parakeratotic and the corium relatively free of inflammatory change.

MELANOTIC PIGMENTATION OF THE ORAL MUCOSA

During development the primitive melanoblast from the neural crest migrates to the embryonic skin and oral mucosa to become by the 12th–14th week of intrauterine life the dermo-epidermal melanocyte. Melanin synthesized in this cell from tyrosine is transferred to adjacent basal epithelial cells by cytocrine activity or by epithelial phagocytosis. Melanotic pigmentation of the oral mucosa may be due to excessive deposition of melanin by these

mechanisms in otherwise normal cells (melanosis), to hyperplasia of melanocytes or to their neoplastic proliferation with an increase in their attendant pigment.

Racial pigmentation, usually symmetrically distributed over the gingiva and palatal mucosa, is the commonest form of melanosis. Simple developmental pigmentation of this type is however not limited to the darker skinned ethnic groups, for one or more discrete patches of brown or black pigmented mucosa may occasionally be found in those of Caucasian stock. Uncommonly, melanosis may be related to underlying Addison's disease, to the Peutz-Jeghers syndrome, to incontinentia pigmenti or to haemochromatosis in which deposits of both iron and melanin contribute to bronzing of the mucosa. However, melanotic patches or more proliferative lesions may be encountered without any underlying factor being discovered. It is then essential to distinguish between harmless developmental pigmentation and pigmentation arising in naevi or malignant melanomata. This differentiation is the principal reason for concern with any pigmented lesion in the mouth.

Clinically, the distinction is based upon the macular nature of the developmental lesion and the constancy, over a long number of years, of its size, shape, and surface in contrast to the more proliferative form of the pigmented naevus and the often rapidly changing character of the malignant melanoma. However, the latter is not always overtly aggressive for in one recently reported series a quarter of the malignant lesions had appearances initially which suggested benign behaviour.

There are four types of pigmented or cellular naevi. They may be dermal in type, where clumps or cords of naevus cells lie entirely within the corium or junctional, where the naevus cells, many of which show clear-cell activity, lie at the corio-epithelial junction. In compound naevi the naevus cells are present at both levels. In the blue naevus the melanocytes assume a spindle form and lie deeply in the lamina propria.

There are few reports of benign intraoral melanotic lesions and this has led some authors to conclude that they are less common than malignant ones. It is more likely that because many benign lesions are symptomless they are not removed for biopsy; therefore any survey of pathological material will give an erroneous impression of the relative proportions of cellular naevi and malignant melanomata. Most of the naevi which have been reported have arisen from the keratinized mucosa of the vermilion border of the lip, the palate (the principal site for the truly intraoral ones), and the gingiva, but the significance of this distribution is unclear.

A malignant melanoma may arise on a previously unblemished mucosal surface, although the presence of a microscopic precursor lesion cannot be ruled out, or it may be superimposed upon a pre-existing pigmented lesion, most likely a junctional naevus or the junctional component of a compound naevus. In either case, rapid proliferation of the lesion, often with early intensification of the colour change due to deeper spread of pigment, and the formation of satellite pigmented spots at its periphery (fig. 5) plus some of those features of malignancy commonly associated with intraoral carcinoma are signs virtually diagnostic of malignant melanoma. Most often this will be a primary lesion although a secondary deposit metastatic to bone and overlying oral mucosa can occur. Rare cases of amelanotic malignant melanoma have been reported.

More certain diagnosis of the melanotic pigmented lesions of the mucosa can only be made by histological examination of tissue. The presence of melanin may be confirmed by the "dopa" test on fresh tissue, or by the reduction of silver nitrate by melanin in fixed tissue. Excisional biopsy of relatively small lesions with clinical characteristics suggesting a benign neoplastic process

RECURRENT APHTHOUS ULCERATION

This is one form of recurrent ulceration affecting the oral and pharyngeal mucous membranes. Because of its prevalence it is the most important one. It is known by a variety of synonyms coined by different authors but there is little to be gained from debating which of these is the most appropriate.

Aphthous ulceration is characterized by the appearance of crops of painful ulcers which heal after a few days or weeks only to be followed by further attacks after variable periods of remission. A useful clinical distinction has been

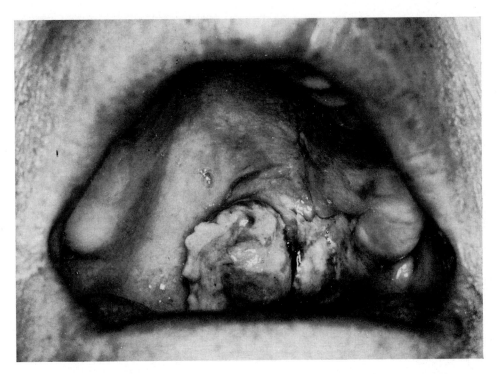

FIG. 5. Malignant melanoma. A proliferative and partly pigmented lesion of the palatal mucosa.

should be carried out. However, there is debate about the wisdom of taking a biopsy of a lesion thought to be a malignant melanoma. Many would argue that pre-operative biopsy disseminates more widely the cells of this most malignant neoplasm and therefore that histological examination should be confined to the examination of frozen sections at the time of definitive surgery.

Most developmental pigmented lesions require no treatment although removal of lesions in the anterior part of the mouth, especially those in the lips, is sometimes requested by patients for cosmetic reasons. Cellular naevi should be excised not least because of the potential of some to undergo malignant change. In patients with primary malignant melanoma of the oral cavity the prognosis is poor, 5 year survival being uncommon, but wide excision of the affected area with removal of a major portion of the maxilla (about 80 per cent of reported intra-oral malignant melanomata have arisen in the maxillary alveolar and palatal mucosa) seems to offer the best prognosis.

drawn between major and minor aphthae. The common minor form is characterized by the presence of up to 4 or 5 ulcers at a time, each one being only a few millimeters in diameter although larger lesions may arise by confluence. Individual ulcers last for 10–14 days but may be painful for only half this period. They tend not to involve the keratinized mucosa of the hard palate, dorsum of the tongue, and gingiva and they heal without scarring.

In major aphthous ulceration the lesions are less numerous, larger, more likely to involve both the pharyngeal mucosa and any part of the oral mucosa; they last for several weeks and may be painful for much of this time. These major aphthae tend to heal with some scarring, especially at the lateral borders of the tongue (fig. 6).

Periods of remission are extremely variable. Crops of ulcers may appear after variable periods of freedom from ulceration lasting months or even years, or crops of new ulcers may appear before previous lesions have healed. Major aphthae are more likely to behave in this latter way.

In extreme cases nutrition may suffer because of pain during mastication and deglutition.

In clinical practice, occasional patients with aphthous ulceration also exhibit one of a variety of ulcerative conditions affecting other parts of the gastro-intestinal tract or the body more generally. However, with the exception of the aphthous-type of recurrent oral ulceration which is a part of Behcet's syndrome, almost all affected patients are adolescents or young adults free of other disorders. In women, there is evidence that ulceration reaches its maximum incidence in the post-ovulation phase of the menstrual cycle. This has been related to oestrogen

and the results of laboratory studies have complemented earlier clinical and histological findings. Epidemiological studies have enlarged our understanding of the disease in individuals who do, and do not, seek treatment, whereas laboratory investigations have demonstrated the immunological phenomena within the oral mucosa and the possible relationship of these to the aetiology of aphthous ulceration.

Epidemiological investigations of aphthous ulceration in individuals randomly selected from total populations have not yet been undertaken but studies of selected populations have given information beyond that obtained

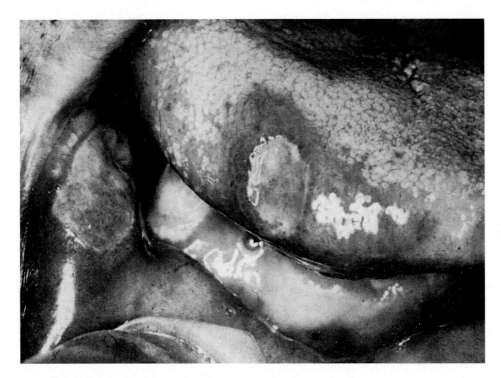

FIG. 6. Recurrent aphthous ulceration. Major aphthae affecitng the lip mucosa and tongue.

withdrawal affecting the degree of cornification of the oral epithelium, to progesterone secretion, or to a relative neutropaenia occurring pre-menstrually. It is claimed that pregnancy leads to a remission.

Individual ulcers begin at a site which can often be detected by the patient up to 24 hr. before ulceration occurs. At this early stage a red macule develops on the mucosa and is quickly replaced by an ulcer without any intervening vesicular phase. Yellowish ulcers with red margins persist until the base becomes pink and cleaner prior to healing. Histological appearances, particularly the nature of the cellular infiltrate, depend upon the time of the biopsy in relation to the life history of the ulcer. A mononuclear infiltration is the first to appear but polymorphonuclear leucocytes become numerous once ulceration occurs. Plasma cells are found in the later stages.

For a century or more the aetiology of aphthous ulceration has puzzled clinical observers of the condition. However, in the last decade epidemiological investigations

from afflicted patients. Because aphthous ulceration is, in most cases, only a minor threat to the health of the individual, it is probable that of those afflicted few seek formal advice and may not be representative of all patients with the condition. Consequently, it may be unwise to draw conclusions solely from clinical data relating to patients. Thus, for certain purposes, data from epidemiological studies are more satisfactory although the long remissions which may occur in aphthous ulceration limit the value of oral examinations of large numbers of subjects. Therefore reliance has had to be placed upon standardized interview/questionnaire techniques. For small groups the data obtained in this way have been verified by demonstrating their close correlation with findings obtained in later longitudinal studies of the same groups in which prevalence and incidence of ulceration have been determined by oral examinations.

Among the information which has emerged from these studies, most of which have been carried out in North

America, is the relationship of aphthous ulceration to socio-economic group, to other ulcerative processes, to familial factors and to recurrent herpes simplex infections. Middle and upper social class professional students appear to be much more often affected than individuals in lower social classes—the prevalence range for males was 5–56 per cent and for females 13–60 per cent. A possible influence of a class factor has been noted in another way. Low social class dental students, without previous history of aphthous ulceration, have been shown to develop the condition before graduation and it has been postulated that this is related to changes in their status associated with the acceptance of professional standards and responsibilities.

In clinical practice, occasional patients have established diagnoses of ulcerative conditions of the gut or report symptoms which are suggestive of gastro-intestinal disorders. However, most seem to be free of these other processes and there is a tendency to attribute the presence of co-existent lesions to chance. Epidemiological data do however suggest positive associations between aphthous ulceration, ulcerative states of the gut, and vulvo-vaginal ulceration.

There is an increased risk of the offspring of affected parents having aphthous ulceration. When there was a history of both parents being afflicted, 90 per cent of the offspring gave a history of aphthae; if one parent gave a positive history, 60 per cent of the offspring also reported recurrent ulceration; but when neither parent reported ulceration, only 20 per cent of the offspring had experienced attacks.

Although earlier workers have sometimes confused ulcers of the aphthous type with those occurring in herpetic infections there is no evidence that minor or major oral aphthae have a viral aetiology. The incidence of recurrent aphthae has been shown to be similar in those with antibody to the herpes simplex virus and those without, but those with antibody may be further sub-divided into those who experience recurrent attacks of herpes labialis and those who do not. Those with recurrent herpes have been shown to have an incidence of aphthae which is twice that occurring in the group with antibody but who are free from recurrent herpetic lesions. However, this finding must be interpreted with caution because the increased incidence of oral ulceration noted in this study may have been due to intra-oral recurrent herpes and not to recurrent aphthous ulceration.

There has been recent speculation over the possible role of the Merkel cell in aphthous ulceration. This dendritic epidermal cell has cytoplasmic granules of a type which suggest that it is a member of the chromaffin system, producing catechole amines. It has been postulated that under appropriate, perhaps psychogenic, stimuli substances released by this cell could cause necrosis of the oral mucosa, although evidence for this is lacking.

Over the past decade immunological responses to oral mucosal antigens have been extensively investigated. Most of this work has been directed towards obtaining a better understanding of the role of autoimmune processes in the pathogenesis of recurrent aphthous ulceration. Auto-immune disorders are usually characterized by the presence of mononuclear cell infiltrations in the lesions, circulating auto-antibodies, raised immunoglobulins, therapeutic responses to corticosteroid drugs, and association with other immunological diseases. In aphthous ulceration there is some evidence for the presence of all but the last of these characteristics although the response to corticosteroids, if any, is weak. Thus, humoral antibodies to fetal oral mucosa and raised titres of some immunoglobulin fractions have been found. In the pre-ulcerative phase of the lesion there is a predominance of mononuclear cells in the corium. This histological finding is consistent with the process being a delayed hypersensitivity reaction, a concept supported by some experimental data demonstrating that oral mucosal fractions may stimulate this cell-mediated response.

Humoral antibodies to oral mucosal antigens have been demonstrated by haemagglutination and other techniques although these antibodies are not specific for oral mucosa. The prevalence of these antibodies and the titres reached are significantly greater in the sera of patients with recurrent aphthous ulceration than in the sera of control subjects. However, the close association of these antibodies with the disease process is weakened by the fact that in patients with antibody the titres are inconsistently related to exacerbations and remissions of ulceration.

In view of this lack of correlation between titres of circulating antibody to oral mucosa and the incidence of ulceration, recent work has been directed towards an examination of the possible role of delayed hypersensitivity in the pathogenesis of aphthous ulceration. The ability of oral mucosal homogenates to stimulate peripheral blood lymphocytes, taken from aphthous ulcer patients and from control subjects, to transform in culture into "blast" cells has been determined. In one investigation, stimulation of lymphocyte transformation, indicated by the up-take of C-14 labelled thymidine, was found in 10 out of 19 cultures from different patients afflicted by ulceration, a frequency of stimulation which was much greater than that found in lymphocyte cultures from control subjects. In addition, transformation was stimulated in 9 out of 10 patients during the active phase of ulceration, there being no demonstrable stimulation during healing or in remissions. Thus, there seems to be a closer association between the clinical phases of aphthous ulceration and cell-mediated immune responses to oral mucosal antigens than there is between the disorder and humoral responses.

In autoimmune disorders a variety of auto-antibodies may be found. One of these is the antinuclear factor. This is more prevalent in the non-organ specific autoimmune disorders than in those in which there is a specific target organ. Therefore, it is perhaps not surprising that the incidence of antinuclear factor in the sera of aphthous ulcer patients and control subjects is not different. This suggests that aphthous ulceration does not result from a central immunological mechanism. However, it does not eliminate the possibility that local immune responses may play a part.

Further evidence for this has been obtained by determining the percentages of adult gingival epithelial cells surviving in tissue-culture systems exposed to sera or peripheral blood lymphocytes. The addition of sera from subjects with aphthous ulceration, or from those without ulceration, failed to influence the survival rates of the cultured epithelial cells. However, viable epithelial cells disappeared from the culture at an increased rate when lymphocytes from patients with ulceration were added. This cytotoxic action of the probably sensitized lymphocytes upon the epithelial cells was reduced by their pretreatment with antilymphocyte serum. Lymphocytes from control subjects did not accelerate the destruction of the cultured epithelial cells. Again these findings suggest the importance of cell-mediated immunity in aphthous ulceration.

In another approach to the same problem the histological characteristics of experimentally induced lesions of the Arthus type (a localized vascular reaction to antigen-antibody complexes) and the delayed hypersensitivity type (a reaction dependent upon the presence of sensitized lymphocytes) have been compared with those of naturally occurring oral aphthae. The closest resemblance was between the appearances of the aphthae and DNCB induced delayed hypersensitivity lesions. There is further support for the importance of this latter mechanism from the observation in human lesions that slow degranulation and loss of mast cells occurs during the first 48 hr. of the existence of a lesion whereas these changes would be expected to occur much more rapidly in an acute vascular reaction.

Thus far, the evidence for the role of autoimmune phenomena in the pathogenesis of recurrent aphthous ulceration is largely circumstantial. The mode of release of oral mucosal antigens, if this is the initial stimulus, has still not been satisfactorily explained, nor have attempts been made to identify more exactly one or more specific antigenic components in mucosal homogenates.

Claims have been made that a streptococcus (*Strep. sanguis* type 2A) initiates aphthous ulceration. These claims have been based on the frequent isolation of the streptococcus from oral aphthae, the production by its inoculation into animals of aphthous-like lesions, and the ability of killed organisms to stimulate delayed hypersensitivity responses in sensitized guinea pigs and the skin of patients with aphthous ulceration. Hypersensitivity to 2A has been demonstrated *in vitro* by means of the leucocyte migration test. On the other hand the presence of this organism in substantial numbers in many normal mouths and in those with disorders other than aphthosis, the limitations of some of the clinical data because of insufficient numbers of controls, and evidence which shows the streptococcus not to stimulate lymphocyte transformation make it unlikely that this organism is anything more than one factor in a condition which requires many for its initiation. A suggestion that mycoplasmas are associated with aphthous ulceration is not supported by their low rate of recovery from the mouths of affected patients.

However, the possibility remains that microbial antigens could cross-react with oral mucosa and stimulate humoral or cell-mediated immune responses capable of inducing pathological change. The major factor appears to be a cell-mediated response in which the lymphocyte may damage the oral epithelial cell.

The management of patients with aphthous ulceration continues to present difficulty. During the last 15 years a range of drug treatments has been evaluated, mostly in double blind controlled clinical trials, but few advances have been made.

Although a useful therapeutic effect of locally applied hydrocortisone hemisuccinate has been reported, later work with more potent corticosteroid drugs has not provided clinically significant evidence of their value. Among those tested for their topical effects have been triamcinolone acetonide in the adhesive vehicle carboxymethyl cellulose, betamethasone disodium phosphate, and betamethasone-17-valerate, both in pellet form for local use. Carbenoxalone sodium, another anti-inflammatory agent, proved to be no better than a placebo at controlling aphthous ulceration. In the face of these unrewarding results it is of interest to note that hydrocortisone succinate sodium, an analogue of the hemisuccinate which has been used therapeutically, stabilizes oral epithelial cells in tissue culture when they are exposed to the cytotoxic action of lymphocytes from patients with aphthous ulceration.

Care has to be exercised when using corticosteroids for the treatment of this condition. Suppression of plasma cortisol levels by treatment with topically applied betamethasone disodium phosphate, in daily doses of 0·3–0·4 mg., has been described but in normal therapeutic daily doses of hydrocortisone hemisuccinate (10 mg.), betamethasone-17-valerate (0·4 mg.), or triamcinolone acetonide (1 mg.) evidence of adrenal suppression has not been found.

Although the full significance of autoimmunity in aphthous ulceration is still uncertain the therapeutic effect of azothioprine, an immunosuppressive agent, has been tested. Because of its possibly dangerous effects this was given topically in low dosage, but in a double blind trial no benefits were observed.

On the basis that the post-ovulation prevalence of aphthae is related to oestrogen withdrawal, oestrogens have been used in the treatment of aphthous ulceration. In an uncontrolled clinical trial a good improvement was claimed in 30 out of 33 women treated with various oestrogens for periods up to 3 years. However, it is doubtful whether this regimen, in which oestrogens were administered systemically in doses sufficient to inhibit ovulation, would find favour with many clinicians.

Antihistamines, given systemically to prevent the effects of a possible allergen, have not proved successful in controlling aphthous ulceration. Antibiotics of the tetracycline group have frequently been reported to assist healing in severe attacks and objective evidence of this has been provided for chlortetracycline mouth rinses. However, this agent did not reduce the incidence of new lesions and in consequence patients experienced little or no subjective improvement from its use.

HERPETIFORM ULCERATION

This is a variety of recurrent oral ulceration with certain characteristics which distinguish it from the minor and major forms of aphthous ulceration. "Herpetiform" is an unfortunate adjective for in its clinical features it bears only a superficial resemblance to herpetic stomatitis and the herpes simplex virus has not been identified in the lesions.

In comparison with aphthous ulceration, herpetiform ulceration has its onset in patients who are approximately 10 years older (in the third and fourth decades) and about three-quarters of these are female. Individual lesions are tiny (1–2 mm. in diameter) but they may coalesce to form larger ulcers. They are widely distributed over the oral mucosa, including the well-keratinized surfaces of the palate and gingiva and the mucosa of the oro-pharynx (fig. 7). The number of lesions is much in excess of the

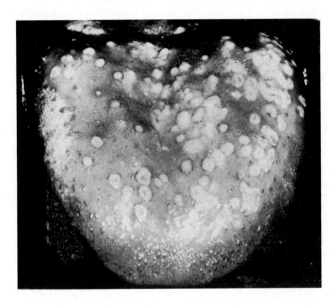

FIG. 7. Herpetiform ulceration. Numerous tiny vesicles and ulcers covering the dorsum of the tongue.

number found in minor aphthous ulceration. Herpetiform ulcers have been found to scar more frequently than minor aphthae but are not as likely to do so as in the major form of ulceration. The recurrence rate in herpetiform ulceration is higher than in major aphthous ulceration.

In electronmicroscope studies intra-nuclear inclusion bodies and vesicles have been found in epithelial cells adjacent to the ulcers. There is little evidence for the role of autoimmunity in the pathogenesis of herpetiform ulceration. Circulating autoantibodies to oral mucosa are not significantly raised in herpetiform ulceration and lymphocytes from patients are less frequently stimulated to transform by oral mucosal homogenates. On the basis of these clinical, histological and immunological findings a viral aetiology for herpetiform ulceration has been suggested.

The response to tetracycline mouth washes is said to be more dramatic than the response of aphthous ulcers but evidence of this in a controlled clinical trial appears to be lacking.

ALLERGIC CONTACT STOMATITIS

Allergic contact stomatitis or contact cheilitis arises in the mouth or lips when, after more than one local application of an agent, an inflammatory reaction is initiated at the site of contact by a hypersensitivity mechanism. The contacting agent is usually of low molecular weight and is not itself allergenic. However, by interaction with epithelial cell protein an allergenic complex is formed and induces sensitization over a period of 1–4 weeks. Further exposure to the sensitizing agent in sufficient concentration leads, within 24–48 hr., to a clinical reaction or flare.

Numerous substances have been incriminated in the causation of contact stomatitis and cheilitis. Most of these appear to gain access to the oral tissues because of their use in toothpastes, mouthwashes, lozenges or cosmetics. Some may be contained in foods as preservatives or may be materials used in dental treatment. Although many case reports have been published not all provide convincing evidence that the oral changes described were due to allergic contact stomatitis. For this diagnosis the following criteria should be fulfilled:

(1) the stomatitis or cheilitis should have clinical features consistent with contact allergy;
(2) the changes should resolve rapidly on removal of the allergen;
(3) on renewing contact with the allergen signs of inflammation should reappear within a few hours; and
(4) there should be evidence on intraoral patch testing that the agent will cause a reaction.

Although the number of possible allergens is large the type of reaction initiated in the oral mucosa to the different allergens is relatively limited. It is the severity of response which differs. This may depend upon the nature of the allergen, its concentration at the site of contact, and variability in immunological reactions between different individuals. The oral changes may vary from an initial burning sensation in the mucosa which is followed by moderate and localized inflammatory change, to gross oedema of the mucosa with vesiculation and ulceration and with considerable swelling of the peri-oral tissues.

In management every attempt should be made to identify the allergen, to prove its allergenic role and to isolate the patient from further contact with it. The prevention of further contact is not always easy because a given agent may appear in several different vehicles, the constituents of which are not always disclosed. The acute symptoms can be controlled by antihistamine drugs.

SUBMUCOUS FIBROSIS

This is a disorder almost entirely limited to Indians but Europeans who have adopted Indian cultural habits may also be affected. Within India the prevalence of the disorder varies according to the community studied but has been reported to be as high as 1 per cent. The changes are usually seen in adult life but they have been observed in childhood. Both sexes are affected.

Submucous fibrosis is a clinical entity associated with

characteristic histological changes. Atrophic changes in the mucosa of the mouth and sometimes the pharynx and oesophagus predominate. A burning sensation and disordered taste are frequently the first symptoms. The mucosa loses its elasticity and eventually palpable fibrous bands, which may limit mobility, form within the substance of the cheeks, soft palate and lips. Vesiculation, ulceration and blanching of the mucosa with depigmentation are common. Tongue papillae may atrophy and leukoplakia may co-exist.

The principal change appears to be in the juxta-epithelial connective tissue where collagen fibres swell and become hyalinized. At first there are associated chronic inflammatory changes although later the lesions lose much of their cellularity. Vessels are narrowed or obliterated. Atrophic changes in the epithelium appear to be secondary to the changes in the lamina propria. Vesiculation occurs with the formation of subepithelial collections of fluid. The connective tissue changes have some resemblance to those in scleroderma but the skin and visceral changes of that condition are not found in patients with submucous fibrosis. At the electron microscope level collagen fibrils of narrower diameter than usual have been found—a finding which is also present in scleroderma.

The striking racial distribution of submucous fibrosis has prompted a search for its cause in the dietary or other habits of Indians. Chilli, betel and tobacco have all been considered to play a part. Although some clinical evidence and data from animal studies suggest that chilli has a role no comparable condition is seen in Central America where chilli is also consumed in quantity. It is possible that local irritants or allergens from food are insufficient in themselves to cause mucosal lesions unless there are associated changes in nutrional state or an underlying predisposition.

Submucous fibrosis of the oral mucosa may be a precancerous condition. The evidence for this is that leukoplakia is much more prevalent in Indian patients with submucous fibrosis than in those free of this change; epithelial atypia has been found in substantial numbers of biopsies from patients with submucous fibrosis and the latter change has been found in 40 out of 100 consecutive patients with oral carcinoma. In addition, histological evidence of carcinoma has sometimes been found in biopsies from patients with submucous fibrosis who are free of clinical evidence of carcinoma. It has been suggested that the association between submucous fibrosis and carcinoma may depend upon the greater vulnerability to carcinogens of the thinned atrophic epithelium. These may at first stimulate epithelial atypia, later hyperplasia, and eventually frank neoplasia.

40. NON-INFECTIOUS SYSTEMIC DISEASES

F. F. NALLY

Immunological disorders

Pemphigus
Benign familial chronic pemphigus
Bullous pemphigoid
Mucous membrane pemphigoid
Pemphigoid-like conditions
    Dermatitis herpetiformis
    Other non-infectious bullous conditions
Lupus erythematosus
Scleroderma
Behcet's syndrome
Crohn's disease

Metabolic diseases

Endocrine dysfunction
Nutritional disorders
    Vitamin A deficiency
    Hypervitaminosis A
    Vitamin C
    Thiamine
    Nicotinic acid
    Riboflavin
    Pyridoxine
Amyloidosis

Blood dyscrasias

Iron deficiency
B_{12} deficiency
Folic acid deficiency
Other disorders

Developmental anomalies

Peutz-Jegher syndrome
Albright's syndrome
Melkersson-Rosenthal syndrome
Epidermolysis bullosa

Idiopathic anomalies

Stevens-Johnson syndrome
Erythema multiforme
Sarcoidosis

Many systemic diseases can give rise to lesions of the oral mucosa. Immunological disorders such as pemphigus and lupus erythematosus may become manifest initially in the mouth; metabolic diseases and blood dyscrasias can first become apparent as mucosal breakdown and there are developmental and idiopathic anomalies whose oral clinical features can lead to the diagnosis. Careful examination of the mucosa can therefore yield important and sensitive clues to a wide variety of systemic diseases.

IMMUNOLOGICAL DISORDERS

Pemphigus

Pemphigus is an uncommon dermatological condition which usually starts insidiously as bullae and erosions on the oral mucosa; indeed, the oral lesions may precede those on the skin by months or years. Acantholysis is the

produced by extensive skin burns could become antigenic, before healing has occurred, and so induce a transient epithelial antibody response. Myasthenia gravis may be associated with Hashimoto's disease, systemic lupus erythematosus, antibody to the A-band in skeletal muscle and thymus gland abnormalities. These findings lend support to the probable autoimmune nature of pemphigus where an antigen-antibody reaction may account for acantholysis in squamous epithelium.

However, an autoimmune mechanism cannot completely account for acantholysis. It has been shown that if pem-

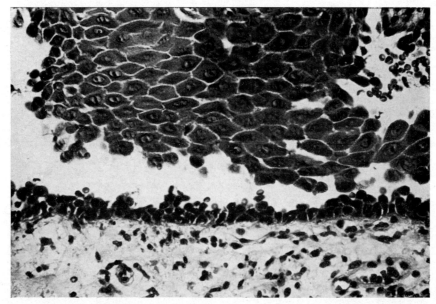

FIG. 1. Pemphigus: Characteristic histological features. ×300. (Courtesy of the Editor of Irish J. Med. Sci.)

essential cytological feature and probably results from the destruction of a substance located between the cells of squamous epithelium. This substance appears to act as a cementing agent and the site of maximum acantholysis is in the Malpighian layer (fig. 1). The basal cells are left intact so that supra-basal clefts occur and an intra-epithelial bulla is formed. Acantholytic cells can be demonstrated in scrapings from the base of a ruptured bulla (fig. 2).

Although extensive research has been undertaken and viral, metabolic and immunological factors have been reported, the cause is still obscure. Encouraging results have recently been obtained from immunological studies. An antibody to an intercellular substance of squamous epithelium has been demonstrated in serum by immunofluorescence techniques and the titre parallels the severity of the disease (fig. 3). Its essential autoimmune character has been proved by the capacity of the antibody to react with antigenic material taken from the patient (direct immunofluorescence technique) although this is not necessary for routine titre estimation; the indirect immunofluorescence technique is usually sufficient for diagnostic purposes. The antibody exhibits a remarkable specificity for pemphigus patients although it has also been identified to a limited extent in patients with severe burns and in sufferers from myasthenia gravis. It is possible that substances

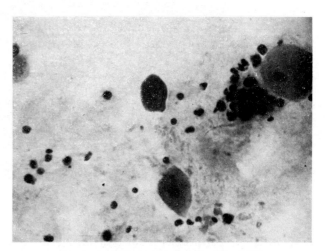

FIG. 2. Pemphigus: Acantholytic cells. ×285.

phigus serum is injected into monkey's skin, intercellular fixation of antibodies occurs but no acantholysis, and intercellular antibodies have been located in unaffected skin taken from pemphigus patients. This suggests that, in addition to the presence of specific autoantibodies in the intercellular region of squamous epithelium, some other mechanism is necessary to increase tissue permeability and

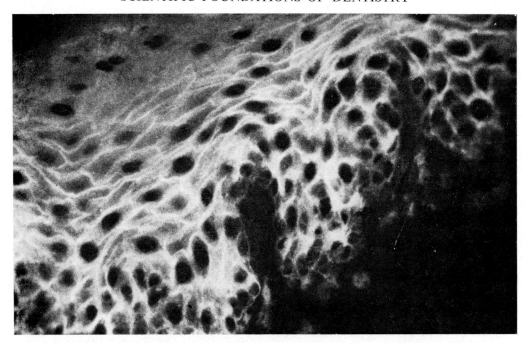

FIG. 3. Pemphigus vulgaris: Positive indirect immunofluorescent staining of epithelium by intercellular antibody. (Courtesy of Dr. S. Alexander.) × 500.

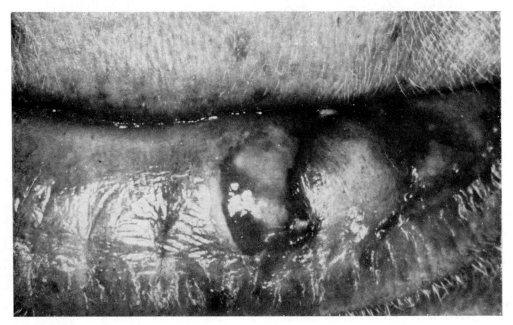

FIG. 4. Pemphigus.

allow complement and cytotoxic agents to trigger-off acantholysis. When this factor has been identified it will bring about a better understanding of this serious disease.

Clinical Considerations

The clinical features of fragile bullae (fig. 4) and erosions in an elderly patient usually suggest the diagnosis and confirmatory procedures include biopsy, cytological examination of scrapings from an intact bulla, and estimation of intercellular epithelial antibody titre. Early diagnosis is imperative because the mortality rate in untreated patients is considerable. Systemic corticosteroids are used to control the lesions. Recently immunosuppressive agents including azathioprine and methotrexate have been tried with beneficial results and this demonstrates the probable autoimmune nature of the disease.

Benign Familial Chronic Pemphigus

Although no immunological abnormalities have been demonstrated in benign familial chronic pemphigus (Hailey-Hailey disease) it has been included in this section for comparison with the previous condition. It is an uncommon hereditary disease in which bullae are mainly found on specific areas of skin and, more rarely, on the oral mucosa. Genetic transmission usually occurs as a Mendelian dominant trait. The exact nature of this inborn defect is uncertain but the tendency to acantholysis may result from faulty synthesis of desmosome complexes or intercellular cementing substance. The intercellular antibody found in pemphigus has not been demonstrated in this disease. External factors also appear to be important in precipitating the condition, for example, friction, sunlight and secondary infection, especially with staphylococci and *Candida albicans*.

Clinical aspects

A positive family history, the persistent localization of lesions in a young person, the histological changes showing supra-basal cleft formation or an intra-epithelial bulla and the absence of circulating intercellular antibody should be sufficient evidence to make the correct diagnosis. The course is usually protracted and sometimes permanent; however, long periods of remission often occur, and the condition tends to regress after the age of fifty. Antibiotics, topical corticosteroids and occasionally small doses of X-rays have given much benefit. Rarely, surgical excision and skin grafting are necessary.

Bullous Pemphigoid

The clinical features and histological findings in bullous pemphigoid are different from those of pemphigus. There is evidence that it may be an immunological disorder, as an antibody to epithelial basement membrane can be demonstrated by the indirect technique in most patients. The antibody can be found in serum IgG, it is capable of binding complement, and localization takes place at the site of tissue breakdown, *viz*. the basement membrane area. On the other hand it is not possible to transfer the disease passively and the antibody titre does not consistently reflect the severity of the clinical condition.

It is usually possible to differentiate the condition from pemphigus on clinical grounds. Perhaps the most significant feature is the absence or minimal involvement of the oral mucosa in bullous pemphigoid (one in every five patients) in contrast to the extensive and severe mucosal lesions seen in pemphigus. The diagnosis can be confirmed histologically by the absence of acantholysis and by the identification of a circulating antibody to basement membrane using the indirect immunofluorescence technique.

Bullous pemphigoid tends to be chronic and may last for many years. The mortality rate is much lower than in pemphigus and systemic corticosteroids are effective in controlling it. Methotrexate can also give considerable benefit, which suggests an immunological abnormality as a basis for the disease. Spontaneous remissions can occur in some patients while others may die from intercurrent infection or the complications of therapy.

Mucous Membrane Pemphigoid

This is mainly a disorder of mucous membranes with occasional skin involvement and is characterized by tense bullae which lead to extensive scarring of the affected area. The cause is unknown although an antigen-antibody reaction in the basement membrane area of epithelium has been demonstrated by Bean *et al*. (1972) using the direct immunofluorescence technique. It is possible that this condition may be a variant or less severe form of bullous pemphigoid.

The diagnosis is usually made on finding oral bullae (fig. 5) in an elderly patient which, on healing, leave scars; additional diagnostic features are the absence of any constitutional upset and the demonstration of a subepithelial

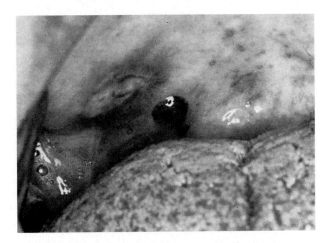

FIG. 5. Mucous membrane pemphigoid.

bullae with no acantholysis (fig. 6). If cicatrization of the conjunctiva is also present the diagnosis becomes obvious. Patients remain surprisingly healthy in spite of the locally distressing nature of this condition. Relapses and remissions occur over many years and the symptoms are usually controlled by topical corticosteroids. Systemic administration may occasionally be necessary if scarring is extensive as, for example, in adhesions of the eyes and scarring of the face and mouth.

Severe and persistent oral bullae may indicate the presence of an underlying malignant lesion; for example, carcinoma of the rectum. The reason for this is not clear but it is always a wise precaution to suspect neoplasia in all patients with pemphigoid, especially those with extensive involvement of the oral mucosa.

Pemphigoid-like Conditions

Dermatitis Herpetiformis

The oral mucosa is rarely involved in dermatitis herpetiformis. If bullae occur they usually appear after the cutaneous lesions although they can be the first feature of the disease. Oral lesions are transient and the diagnosis is usually made on the symmetrical extensor distribution of skin lesions in young adults, the benign and recurrent nature of the disease, and the demonstration that the bullae

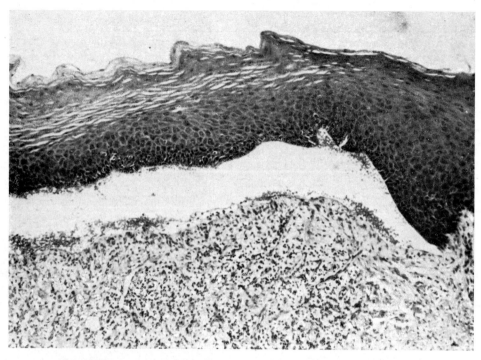

FIG. 6. Mucous membrane pemphigoid: Intact subepithelial bulla found on biopsy.

are subepithelial. Localization of antibodies in the basement membrane area of epithelium is a rare finding by indirect immunofluorescence. However, by using the direct immunofluorescence technique IgA-complement complexes can be demonstrated in uninvolved skin but not in the lesions. Their absence in the lesions may be due to phagocytosis by the extensive polymorphonuclear infiltration in the area.

Other Non-Infectious Bullous Conditions

Bulla formation can result from direct burns of the mucosa or as a reaction to the intake of certain foods and drugs in hypersensitive individuals. Gingivitis is a common finding in pregnancy but bullae can also occur, especially if the patient has concomitant skin lesions. If this happens the condition is known as "herpes gestationis" or toxic eruption of pregnancy and mucosal lesions can occur in one out of every five patients. Attacks occur in successive pregnancies or if contraceptive therapy containing progesterone is prescribed. Rarely, oral bullae can be associated with lichen planus, submucous fibrosis, Darier's disease, porphyria, and bullous papular urticaria; the association with internal malignancy has been mentioned.

Lupus Erythematosus

Lupus erythematosus has a wide range of clinical manifestations and the several patterns recognized comprise discoid and disseminated types, and the systemic chronic and acute forms. This variation has led some authorities to regard systemic and discoid lupus erythematosus as separate entities, but in view of more recent findings this is no longer tenable. The cause is uncertain, although lesions induced by drug therapy are well recognized and there is considerable evidence that genetic factors may play a part. An autoimmune mechanism has been suggested because of the development of multiple serum antibodies which apparently can destroy host tissues especially the nuclear material of cells. Some patients have a positive Wassermann cardiolipin reaction. A specific phospholipid is used in this test and is present in many diseases including multiple myelomatosis and carcinomatosis. However, if these diseases are not present and these antibodies are found in the absence of syphilis, lupus erythematosus should be considered. The VDRL test also appears to have the same basic characteristic. Acquired haemolytic anaemia, confirmed by a positive direct Coombs' test, has been noted in five per cent of patients with systemic lupus erythematosus, and leucopenia is also a common finding. It has been shown that leucocytes and platelets, as well as erythrocytes, can be agglutinated by antiglobulin serum having anticomplement specificity, and the globulin appears to be IgG.

Unlike pemphigus, the titre of autoantibodies does not necessarily parallel the severity of the condition. One reason for this is that the antigenic nuclear material is intracellular and so is not readily available to serum antibodies and there is little evidence to show how antibodies can enter a cell to produce a destructive reaction. Tuffanelli (1969) has demonstrated localization of gamma globulin and bound complement on the dermal-epidermal junction in both affected and healthy tissue taken from patients with lupus erythematosus. Perhaps the same argument put forward in pemphigus should be considered here and a more deliberate search undertaken for the mechanism whereby cell membrane damage occurs.

Clinical and Diagnostic Aspects

The oral mucosa is affected in up to half the patients and oral lesions may be present in both the discoid and systemic forms. In the early stages discrete erythematous areas of mucosa which eventually coalesce may be seen. As the condition progresses white elevated striated plaques develop in the centre, and these white areas differ in appearance from those of lichen planus (fig. 7). Telangiectasis may be present at the margins of these lesions, but this is not a constant feature. Painful mucosal ulceration can also be present which tends to be chronic and leads to scar formation. Lesions can develop anywhere in the mouth, but the buccal mucosa is most often involved. A "butterfly"

atrophy of the prickle cell layer, degeneration of the basal cells, a predominantly lymphocytic infiltration in the lamina propria which is usually perivascular, and degeneration of collagen and elastic fibres. However, similar changes can also be found in other forms of oral keratosis. The deeper and more patchy perivascular cellular infiltration in lupus erythematosus contrasts with the more uniform distribution in lichen planus. It should be emphasized that histological features alone are not usually diagnostic of lupus erythematosus and continuous assessment is necessary. One should be aware of the possible development of systemic signs of the disease. The antinuclear antibody test is a more sensitive one than the L.E. cell

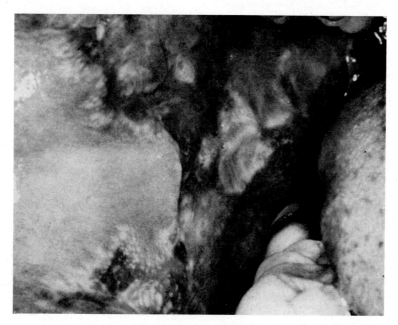

FIG. 7. Lupus erythematosus.

pattern may occasionally be present in the palate and it corresponds to the location of the glands in this area. A generalized non-specific stomatitis together with destructive lesions in the nose and pharynx can occur in systemic lupus erythematosus.

Disorders associated with lupus erythematosus include Sjögren's syndrome, rheumatoid arthritis, bullous pemphigoid, anaemia, coagulation abnormalities of blood, especially idiopathic thrombocytopenic purpura, and lymphogranulomatosis. Carcinoma can rarely occur in scar tissue but one must be careful not to interpret the pseudoepitheliomatous appearance of discoid lupus erythematosus as a true malignant change.

Although problems associated with the diagnosis of systemic lupus erythematosus have received considerable attention, the discoid form is less well delineated. Because of the variety of oral lesions the diagnosis can be difficult. The histological findings together with other specific investigations may help. Then, by a process of elimination, the underlying condition will become apparent. The histological features in the oral mucosa are more variable than those of skin. The changes include hyperkeratosis,

inclusion phenomenon, and it may be positive in discoid lupus erythematosus.

Scleroderma

Scleroderma is a condition which may affect the oral mucosa and skin only; it can occur in a number of conditions including Sjögren's syndrome, lupus erythematosus and dermatomyositis and it is present in progressive systemic sclerosis. This wide variation makes the diagnosis of "scleroderma" an unsatisfactory one. It is probably better to limit the term to local or generalized cutaneous lesions and to regard progressive systemic sclerosis as a separate entity. A more acceptable classification, therefore, is localized scleroderma, generalized scleroderma and progressive systemic sclerosis. The causes of cutaneous scleroderma and progressive systemic sclerosis are unknown. Although the clinical behaviour patterns are different examination of affected skin by histological, histochemical and autoradiographic techniques, and X-ray diffraction analysis, show the same results in both conditions. A familial tendency has been noted in some patients but the main emphasis is now placed on immunological findings. There is a group of auto-immune diseases that can be associated including Sjögren's syndrome, systemic lupus erythematosus, dermatomyositis, myasthenia gravis, acquired haemolytic anaemia and Hashimoto's thyroiditis. In addition, it may be significant that human embryo fibroblasts in tissue culture can be killed by lymphocytes obtained from patients with progressive systemic sclerosis.

Clinical Aspects

The oral mucosa can be affected in cutaneous scleroderma and progressive systemic sclerosis. The tongue and soft palate are often partially immobilized giving rise to difficulty in eating, talking and swallowing. Function is further inhibited by progressive involvement of the facial skin, muscles of mastication and the temporomandibular joints. Significant widening of the periodontal space occurs in about half the patients with systemic sclerosis. Examination of the oral mucosa will probably reveal atrophic epithelium and the affected tissue will feel indurated. In the early stages macroglossia is usual but as fibrosis occurs the tongue becomes small, hard and immobilized.

The diagnosis is essentially a clinical one. The mode of onset, the induration of affected tissues and the possible development of widespread systemic lesions are characteristic. Histological changes include atrophic epithelium, degenerative changes in collagen, perivascular lymphocytic infiltration and a reduction in fibroblasts and elastic tissue. Blood analysis is non-contributory in cutaneous scleroderma. The findings in progressive systemic sclerosis can include anaemia, a raised erythrocyte sedimentation rate, hypergammaglobulinaemia, a positive Wassermann reaction, antinuclear antibodies, and a positive rheumatoid arthritis factor.

The prognosis for both types of cutaneous scleroderma is favourable in most cases, but is invariably poor for progressive systemic sclerosis and patients may die from functional impairment of vital organs or from intercurrent infection. It should be emphasized that submucous fibrosis is a different disease, although many of the oral changes are similar to those seen in scleroderma.

Behcet's Syndrome

Behcet's syndrome consists of recurrent oral ulceration together with genital and ocular lesions. Since the original syndrome was described other disorders have been associated with it, including lesions of blood vessels, skin, the nervous system, joints and viscera. An immunological disorder should be considered in this syndrome because of the clinical behaviour pattern and laboratory findings. The widespread involvement, the intermittent nature of the condition, and the frequent association with other immunological diseases including ulcerative colitis and rheumatoid arthritis, is probably significant. Lehner (1967) has demonstrated haemagglutinating, complement-fixing and precipitating antibodies to fetal oral mucosa in blood from affected patients.

Pathology

Non-specific inflammatory changes are seen in biopsies of mucosal ulcers. Perivascular infiltration is a common finding and is probably associated in some way with the high incidence of thrombophlebitis. Scattered areas of necrosis may also be found in many parts of the nervous system including the brain stem, ganglia and optic tracts and, more rarely, a chronic non-specific meningo-encephalomyelitis; these findings probably account for the neurological abnormalities in severely affected patients.

Clinical and diagnostic aspects

The diagnosis is essentially a clinical one. If there is a history of severe recurrent oral ulceration and genital involvement Behcet's syndrome should be considered. When ocular lesions, pyoderma, and neurological signs develop the diagnosis becomes obvious. The prognosis is unpredictable, and spontaneous remissions have been reported. More often repeated attacks can lead to blindness and other complications. Involvement of the nervous system is always serious and most fatalities result from it.

Crohn's Disease

Crohn's disease is a non-specific chronic granulomatous condition which can involve any part of the gastro-intestinal tract and, rarely, the oral mucosa. Many causes have been put forward to account for this condition including tuberculosis, foreign irritants, defective blood supply, sarcoidosis and hypersensitivity; most of these have not been proven. Remissions tend to occur with the restriction of certain proteins, especially dairy produce; this suggests hypersensitivity, and the hypothesis that an antigen-antibody reaction affects the intestinal cells is an attractive one. Mowbray et al. (1973) have demonstrated circulating IgG immune complexes in 9 (28 per cent) out of 32 patients with Crohn's disease. The question remains as to whether these complexes play a causative role or are only secondary to the disease process.

Clinical aspects

The cutaneous manifestations include erythema nodosum, anal and perineal ulceration, pyoderma gangrenosum and non-specific skin lesions due to malnutrition. Non-specific oral ulceration, swollen gingivae (fig. 8) and glossitis can occur.

Crohn's disease can be difficult to diagnose. The histological features tend to be complex because of the effects of long-standing inflammation, ulceration and repair. Tortuous lymph vessels and non-caseating giant cell granulomata are the most striking findings. It is often difficult to differentiate between sarcoidosis and Crohn's disease.

Findings in sarcoidosis include a marked deficiency in cell-mediated immunity. Contact sensitivity to dinitrochlorbenzene is absent and delayed-type hypersensitivity reactions of skin are reduced. The lymphocyte transformation test is diminished together with increased activity of serum complement, and these are dependent on the severity of the disease. Added to this there appears to be an increased tolerance to homografts. The Kveim test consists of the injection of a suspension of sarcoid tissue into the upper dermis of patients. If the test is positive a papule will appear in about three weeks and this should be biopsied in six weeks. Examination should show the characteristic histological changes of sarcoidosis. The immunological mechanism causing this local sarcoid is probably cell mediated against the antigen, the active component of which has not yet been found. Perhaps the identification of the active principle of the Kveim test will ultimately lead to a better understanding of sarcoidosis.

tion, probably due to elevated plasma levels of melanin-stimulating hormone (MSH).

Diabetes mellitus is a chronic disorder of carbohydrate metabolism. Changes in protein, fat and electrolyte metabolism also occur. The lesions of the oral mucosa are similar to changes occurring elsewhere. The cause is either a deficiency or decreased effectiveness of insulin. Atrophy of the β cells of the islets of Langerhans in the pancreas can usually be demonstrated at *post mortem* examination. However, failure to produce insulin is not the whole story; in some instances insulin may be produced but its effectiveness is diminished. The reason for

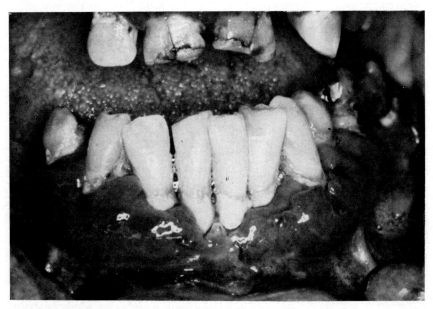

FIG. 8. Crohn's disease.

The Kveim test is negative in Crohn's disease. In the absence of oral and skin lesions radiographic and surgical exploration of the abdomen may be required to establish the diagnosis.

METABOLIC DISEASES

Endocrine Dysfunction

All tissues in the body are influenced to some extent by hormones either during development or in the maintenance of health, and the oral mucosa is no exception. The effects of pituitary dysfunction depend on the age of onset, the type of hormone concerned, and its rate of production. Malocclusion and gingivitis are frequently found in hypopituitarism and changes in the oral mucosa typical of old age may start in the third decade of life. If excess growth hormone is produced the lips and tongue are considerably enlarged and inflammatory changes may also be present in other areas of the oral mucosa; these can be attributed, in part, to mouth breathing and malocclusion. Additional mucosal changes may include Addisonian type pigmenta-

this is not clear, but the anti-insulin hormones may play a part, for example, an increased output of growth hormone, ACTH, thyroxine, the glucocorticoids, adrenaline or glucagon.

The oral lesions are non-specific. There is usually a reduced resistance to trauma and healing is poor. Candidal stomatitis and severe periodontal disease are often present. The increased susceptibility to infection is probably due to elevated sugar content in tissues, alteration in the amino-acid pool upsetting antibody production, disordered electrolyte metabolism with a tendency to acidaemia because of increased fat breakdown, vascular changes and peripheral neuropathy.

In congenital hypothyroidism (cretinism) the skin is coarse with suborbital swelling, a flat nose, enlarged lips and the tongue may protrude from the mouth. The skin is pale, dry, thickened and cold and the limbs may show a cyanotic livedo. A large cranium with small jaws is usual; this results in delayed eruption, malocclusion and gingivitis. There is also a reduced resistance of the oral mucosa to trauma and infection. In adult hypothyroidism (myxoedema) similar skin and mucosal changes are found. The disease may occur after an incomplete thyroidectomy, irradiation, or thyroid suppressive therapy. Spontaneous deficiency also occurs, and an immunological disorder is demonstrable in Hashimoto's disease.

In severely affected patients the diagnosis is made on the clinical features. It is more difficult to make in mild cases and there is no specific investigation that will confirm the diagnosis. There are many causes for a raised serum cholesterol and it can be normal in thyroid deficiency, as may the basal metabolic rate. The protein-bound iodine is low in most cases but can be normal, especially if iodine contrast media have been used in radiological examinations or when iodine or contraceptive therapy has been prescribed. Radioactive iodine uptake by the gland is also low in most patients. Skin biopsy may assist by showing degenerative changes in the dermis and sweat glands, and thyroid antibodies may be demonstrated in some cases. There is a high incidence of antibodies to colloid antigen

Hypoparathyroidism is often due to damage to the glands or their removal during thyroidectomy. More rarely, it may be familial. In such cases an association with cutaneous and oral candidiasis is usually found and there may be a coexisting adrenal and thyroid deficiency. In some instances circulating antibodies to the parathyroid, thyroid and adrenal glands have been described, suggesting an autoimmune process (Nally, 1970).

Primary hyperparathyroidism is usually caused by a functioning parathyroid adenoma. More rarely, generalized hyperplasia of all four glands, multiple adenomata, or carcinoma may be responsible. Secondary hyperparathyroidism can occur in chronic renal disease with phosphate retention. Histological examination of an epulis showing giant cells may lead to the diagnosis if confirmed by finding hypercalcaemia, hypophosphataemia, elevated alkaline phosphatase, hypercalciuria and hyperphosphaturia.

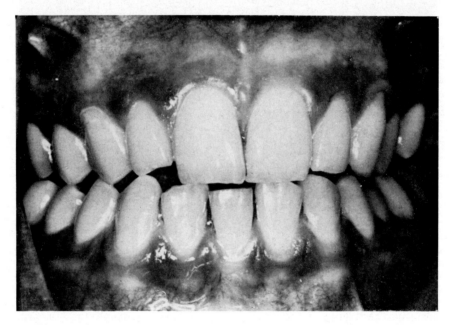

FIG. 9. Addison's disease.

and thyroid microsomes in patients with persistent oral ulceration, although the reason for this is not clear.

Cutaneous vasodilatation is usually present in hyperthyroidism and the skin feels warm, smooth, soft and moist. Pigmentation and vitiligo may develop on the skin and occasionally melanin deposition occurs in the oral mucosa. Although the cause is unknown in most cases, familial, neurological and immunological factors should be considered. Overactivity of the pituitary or a functioning adenoma of the thyroid may sometimes be present. The diagnosis is usually a clinical one. It is confirmed by a raised basal metabolic rate, low serum cholesterol, elevated protein-bound iodine and increased uptake of radioactive iodine by the gland. Occasionally, specific circulating thyroid antibodies are demonstrable, suggesting an auto-immune process; if this is so, it is most unusual to have overactivity of tissue induced by antibody production.

Deficient output of adrenocorticoids may result from primary atrophy or secondary involvement of the glands by tuberculosis, amyloidosis, haemochromatosis or neoplasia. Circulating antibodies to the cytoplasm of cells in the adrenal cortex can be demonstrated in fifty per cent of patients with primary atrophy (Addison's disease). Pigmentation of skin and mucous membranes usually occurs early and can be the most obvious clinical evidence of the disease; it is due to increased secretion of melanocyte-stimulating hormone. The oral mucosa is commonly involved and the distribution is usually an exaggeration of the normal pattern (fig. 9). If Addison's disease is suspected, the response to ACTH should be investigated. The output of urinary 17-ketosteroids and 17-hydroxycorticoids is measured after the injection of ACTH; a normal subject will increase the output but in Addison's disease there is virtually no response.

In adrenal hyperfunction (Cushing's syndrome), caused by pituitary overactivity, pigmentation of MSH pattern may also be present in the skin and oral mucosa.

Experimental evidence in animals has shown that excess oestrogens, but not androgens, will increase pigmentation. Oestrogens also influence the metabolic activity of squamous epithelium and changes in the oral mucosa are often seen at puberty, and during pregnancy and the menopause; use of the contraceptive pill may induce similar changes.

Nutritional Disorders

Insufficiency of essential nutrients can result from defective diet, malabsorption from the gut, factors inhibiting blood transport or uptake in the mucosa, inadequate storage, increased metabolic need or from excessive loss from the body. In chronic malnutrition depression of the pituitary, thyroid, adrenal glands and gonads results. Addisonian pigmentation of the oral mucosa and skin is not uncommon. Kwashiorkor occurs in severe protein deficiency and is endemic in certain parts of Africa. The skin is dry and cracked, and a patchy vitiligo may be present together with areas of hyperpigmentation. Mucosal changes are similar and a generalized stomatitis is usually present. Mucoviscidosis and acrodermatitis enteropathica are rare disorders of protein metabolism and are probably familial. Striking cutaneous manifestations can occur in both diseases together with non-specific stomatitis.

Vitamin A deficiency

If the deficiency is mild, only night blindness, xerophthalmia, and xerostomia may be noted. As it progresses hyperkeratotic changes occur in the skin and mucous membranes. Squamous metaplasia in the trachea, bronchi, renal pelvis, conjunctiva and salivary glands have been described in severe cases. The diagnosis can be confirmed by an isolated blood examination. The normal serum level of vitamin A is between 30 and 100 units per ml. A more accurate method is to estimate the fasting vitamin level; then the patient is given 200,000 i.u. by mouth and a further blood sample is taken 3 to 5 hours later. This time serum vitamin A should be twice the fasting level; if it is not, the cause is probably lack of absorption and not dietary.

Excess vitamin A may produce a transition of squamous to columnar secreting epithelium in tissue culture and deficiency can cause the reverse.

Hypervitaminosis A

Symptoms of hypervitaminosis A occur if the daily intake constantly exceeds 50,000 i.u. The usual findings are a low grade fever, nausea and weight loss. Enlargement of the liver and spleen can also occur. Bone and joint pain is common and periosteal thickening may be seen on radiographic examination. Gradual loss of hair occurs and the skin, lips and oral mucosa become dry. If progressive, pigmentation, erythema, follicular keratosis and purpura will develop. An increased level of vitamin A in the serum confirms the diagnosis.

Vitamin C

Biosynthesis of vitamin C occurs in most animals; the exceptions are guinea pigs, primates and man. It is associated with tyrosine and folic acid metabolism, with many oxidation-reduction processes, progesterone excretion, hyaluronic acid metabolism and with collagen formation. It is also concerned in the absorption of iron from the small intestine and the formation of haemoglobin. A high concentration of the vitamin is found in the pituitary, adrenals, pancreas, wall of the small intestine and in white blood cells.

Mild deficiency states are often recognized by changes in the oral mucosa especially those occurring in the gingivae. Generalized gingival swelling starts in the interdental areas and bleeding, either spontaneous or on slight provocation, is a striking feature. As the condition progresses cutaneous manifestations occur and are characteristic. Perifollicular haemorrhages, multiple petechial haemorrhages and a sudden ecchymosis into a muscle or joint may occur. The diagnosis is made on the dietary history, clinical features, the vitamin C saturation test and, if necessary, plasma level estimation. Treatment not only consists in administering vitamin C; other factors must be considered including mental stress, adrenocortical function, and infection. It is known that stimulation of the adrenal cortex rapidly reduces the vitamin stored in the gland. Adrenal hyperactivity occurs in anxiety states and following burns and severe injuries. Vitamin C is catabolized in excess in rheumatoid arthritis and in some infections. Hence vitamin C deficiency should not be regarded as an isolated entity.

Thiamine (B_1)

Thiamine is converted in the mucosa of the small intestine into thiamine pyrophosphate, an important coenzyme in carbohydrate metabolism. Deficiency will cause beri-beri and occurs in people who exist largely on polished rice. The characteristic features include muscle pain and tenderness especially during exercise, peripheral vasodilatation, cardiac symptoms, oedema and neurological changes. There are no striking changes in the mouth although mucosal hypersensitivity may occur. If lesions such as non-specific stomatitis are present it is more likely that multiple deficiency exists. A raised blood pyruvate is found in thiamine deficiency. This is the result of a hold up in carbohydrate metabolism; thiamine pyrophosphate is one of the factors that converts pyruvate to acetyl coenzyme A. Hence the increased pyruvate level is the result of the thiamine pyrophosphate deficiency and not the cause of the disease. The diagnosis can be confirmed by estimation of blood pyruvate before and after the administration of glucose. The level of thiamine pyrophosphate in blood and urine should also be determined. The measurement of thiamine excretion in the urine during the four hours after injecting one mg. is another useful diagnostic procedure; in normal subjects more than 50 μg. are excreted. These tests may be conclusive in most patients but the estimation of the level of blood transketolase is probably the most sensitive method.

Nicotinic acid

Nicotinic acid can be synthesized to some extent by micro-organisms in the small intestine and excess dietary tryptophan can also be converted into nicotinic acid in the body. It is essential for many oxidation reactions including lactic acid, pyruvic acid, β hydroxybutyric acid, the citric acid cycle and in the generation of adenosine triphosphate.

Deficiency of nicotinic acid will cause pellagra which is mainly a disease of maize eaters. It can occur in malabsorption syndromes such as sprue or coeliac disease and Hartnup disease, which is a rare familial recessive disorder of protein metabolism. Isoniazid, used in the treatment of tuberculosis, has caused pellagra in some patients probably by substrate competition. A carcinoid tumour can also induce pellagra as the neoplasm requires trytophan in the manufacture of excessive amounts of 5-hydroxytryptamine (serotonin).

The classical triad of pellagra comprises dermatitis, diarrhoea and dementia which develop gradually in that order. Erythema, scaling, and increased pigmentation occur in exposed skin. Mucous membranes are involved early and the oral mucosa can be severely affected. The tongue may be red, swollen, smooth and inflamed, with atrophy of the filiform papillae. As the condition progresses the rest of the mucosa becomes inflamed and ulcerated. Acute ulcerative gingivitis is a common secondary complication. In humans the clinical features are usually associated with other nutritional deficiencies such as vitamin A, riboflavin, iron and protein. Kwashiorkor, porphyria, drug hypersensitivity and neurodermatitis should be considered in the differential diagnosis.

The diagnosis can be confirmed by estimating the level of nicotinic acid in the blood or its methylated derivative in urine. However, the dietary and social history together with the clinical findings are usually sufficient to make the diagnosis.

Riboflavin (B$_2$)

Riboflavin can be synthesized in the gut. It is essential for the flavoprotein enzyme system which is responsible for the carriage of hydrogen ions in nucleotides by cytochromes. Deficiency can arise from defective intake, such as malabsorption due to lack of phosphorylation by the intestinal mucosa, and it can be associated with chronic infection, other metabolic disorders, cirrhosis of the liver, pellagra and neoplasia. Tissues of ectodermal origin are mainly affected; conjunctivitis and corneal vascularization, non-specific glossitis and angular cheilitis, together with a seborrhoeic dermatitis around the eyes, nose, ears, vagina and rectum have been reported in experimental deficiency in human volunteers. The diagnosis is made on the dietary history and clinical findings, and may be confirmed by estimation of the urinary vitamin excretion.

Pyridoxine (B$_6$)

Pyridoxine acts as a coenzyme for many metabolic reactions including the conversion of tryptophan to nicotinic acid to 5-hydroxytryptamine and the formation of nor-adrenaline and histamine. Deficiency may result from poor intake. Isoniazid therapy, hyperemesis gravidarum and iron deficiency anaemia have been associated with pyridoxine deficiency. The clinical manifestations are ill-defined but convulsions in infants, dermatitis, acrodynia and angular cheilitis have been reported. Mental confusion, depression, albuminuria and leukopenia have been found in human volunteers. An excessive amount of xanthurenic acid in the urine after administering tryptophan can indicate a deficiency of this vitamin.

Deficiency of vitamins D and E do not appear to have a direct effect on the oral mucosa. Prolonged hypervitaminosis D will produce some of the findings described in hyperparathyroidism. Vitamin K is essential for prothrombin synthesis in the liver and deficiency may occur in obstructive jaundice, malabsorption, liver disease and during anticoagulant therapy. Considerable amounts are also produced by the intestinal flora and prolonged antibiotic therapy can depress this source of the vitamin. The only significant finding in the mouth is a haemorrhagic tendency. The diagnosis is confirmed by an increased coagulation time that is decreased by administration of the vitamin.

Amyloidosis

Deposition of amyloid material in tissues may occur as an isolated finding or as a complication of many identifiable diseases. As a result the terms primary and secondary amyloidosis have been extensively used in the past. Amyloid consists of protein-polysaccharide complexes whose exact chemical composition is unknown. It may be formed locally in skin and oral mucosa and be relatively harmless or it can be deposited from circulating protein precursors in many organs and tissues in the more serious forms of the disease. In every case, however, there is an upset in protein metabolism which may be genetically transmitted and several types of hereditary amyloidosis are recognized. In other instances an acquired factor may disturb protein synthesis and act locally or systemically producing the characteristic signs. Available evidence from experimentally induced lesions in animals points to a derangement of reticuloendothelial function and abnormal immunoglobulin synthesis.

Clinical types

Local amyloidosis is mainly confined to the skin and is known as cutaneous amyloidosis. It may arise spontaneously or be associated with existing chronic inflammatory lesions or tumours. The diagnosis can be confirmed by histological findings. The prognosis of cutaneous amyloidosis is usually favourable, but it should also be regarded as a "cutaneous marker" of a possible underlying systemic disorder, for example, internal malignancy.

Several forms of familial systemic amyloidosis have been described; peripheral nerves, heart and kidneys may be involved together with the cutaneous lesions. It affects mainly the Jewish and Armenian races in association with familial Mediterranean fever and is transmitted as a recessive Mendelian trait. The prognosis is poor and eventually there may be renal failure caused by amyloid deposits.

Oral lesions are among the most common findings in primary systemic amyloidosis. Macroglossia caused by gross infiltration with amyloid can cause discomfort, and examination may reveal yellowish nodules distributed along the lateral border of the tongue. Plaques and papules can also be present together with haemorrhagic lesions. It is probable that trauma to the tongue occurs more readily because of its increased size. Other areas of the oral mucosa, the lips, and the pharynx can be affected but the lingual disturbance is usually the most striking. The skin of the face and body flexures may show similar changes in addition to erythema, petechial haemorrhages and occasional bulla formation. The cause is uncertain but there is a close association with myelomatosis. It may arise from somatic mutation of plasma cells which can result in dysproteinaemia, systemic amyloidosis, or myelomatosis and each may occur as an isolated entity in some patients or in combination in others. The prognosis is invariably poor and death from cardiac failure or multiple myeloma usually occurs within two to three years.

Secondary systemic amyloidosis results as a complication of a wide variety of chronic diseases, for example, tuberculosis, syphilis, osteomyelitis, Hodgkin's disease, rheumatoid arthritis, severe chronic psoriasis and carcinoma. Amyloid is deposited mainly in the reticuloendothelial system and the liver, spleen, and adrenal glands are primarily involved. The mouth and skin are rarely affected. It is important to distinguish between secondary and primary systemic amyloidosis because if the underlying disease process is successfully treated a considerable improvement can occur in the secondary type.

The diagnosis depends on the identification of amyloid deposits in affected tissues. Rectal mucosal biopsy is usually recommended as the procedure of choice in systemic amyloidosis because amyloid deposits are nearly always found in the rectal submucosa. However, amyloid infiltrates will be found in the oral mucosa of a high proportion of affected patients, the biopsy procedure is simple, and amyloid can be demonstrated around small arterioles. If this is negative, rectal biopsy is a logical alternative. The absence of demonstrable amyloid by either method does not rule out the diagnosis and renal or hepatic biopsies may be necessary. In addition, serum and urine estimation of proteins by electrophoresis and immunoelectrophoresis together with bone-marrow biopsies for plasma cell dyscrasia are also useful diagnostic procedures.

BLOOD DYSCRASIAS

Blood dyscrasias may have a profound effect on the oral mucosa.

Iron Deficiency

The skin of anaemic patients is pale, but this important sign is more obvious in the conjunctiva and oral mucosa. Oral manifestations are common and many patients complain of a burning sensation especially on the tongue, a dry mouth, angular cheilitis and, more rarely, difficulty in swallowing. Epithelial atrophy will be most evident on the tongue giving it a smooth glazed appearance. These mucosal changes probably result, in part, from a defect in the cytochrome oxidase system which normally requires a constant supply of iron. Infection with *Candida albicans* producing a glossitis or angular cheilitis is not uncommon because a defect in cell-mediated immunity occurs in this anaemia. The histological changes confirm atrophy of the lingual papillae and a chronic inflammatory cell infiltration in the corium is usual. An increase in the size of nuclei together with prominent nucleoli and an irregular chromatin pattern may be seen in the epithelial cells of the buccal mucosa. These changes are also seen in vitamin B_{12} and folic acid deficiencies and suggest some interference in cell division.

Vitamin B_{12} Deficiency

Normally vitamin B_{12} is absorbed in the terminal ileum as a bound complex with intrinsic factor secreted from the gastric parietal cells. Specific receptors are thought to exist on the ileum for absorption to occur. Within the mucosa the vitamin is released again, enters the blood, is then attached to α globulin and stored in the liver. Anything that interferes with this mechanism may produce a deficiency state.

Pernicious anaemia is the commonest of the vitamin B_{12} deficiency anaemias. It is caused by a lack of production of intrinsic factor in the stomach and often appears to be familial. A histamine-fast achlorhydria is also present. Circulating parietal cell antibody is present in ninety per cent of cases, suggesting an immunological abnormality. Alternatively, antibody production could be the result of progressive structural changes in the gastric mucosa in the same way as intercellular epithelial antibody develops in response to extensive burns of the skin.

Lesions of the oral mucosa may precede changes in the peripheral blood by months or years. Later, mild jaundice may be apparent in the conjunctiva, soft palate (fig. 10) and then in the skin. Cutaneous markers also include vitiligo, premature grey hair, and Sutton's naevus; the incidence is higher in blond people with blue eyes, and subacute combined degeneration of the spinal cord is a serious neurological complication.

Although the role of vitamin B_{12} in cellular metabolism is uncertain it is known to have many functions including purine biosynthesis, protein and fat metabolism. It is also necessary for methionine, DNA, RNA and collagen metabolism. These facts suggest that B_{12} deficiency has a marked inhibiting effect on epithelial cell activity.

Folic Acid Deficiency

Folic acid deficiency may also cause a macrocytic anaemia and the clinical features, except for spinal cord damage, are similar to those found in vitamin B_{12} deficiency. There are many causes including defective diet, malabsorption associated with lesions of the small intestine, pregnancy, haemolysis, liver disease, and therapeutic agents that antagonize folic acid (such as sodium phenytoin and cytotoxic agents used in leukaemia). Folic acid is reduced to tetrahydrofolic acid in the body and it is necessary for the synthesis of purines, methionine and thymidine for DNA production. A deficiency is confirmed on finding a macrocytic anaemia, normal gastric secretion, and the presence of a low plasma and red blood cell folate level. .

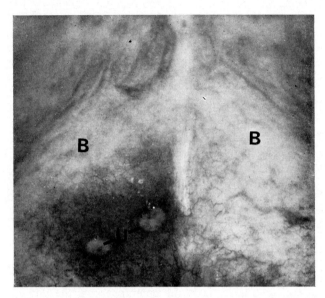

FIG. 10. Pernicious anaemia: Bilirubin staining (B) and ulceration (U).

Other Disorders

A macrocytic anaemia may occur in prolonged ascorbic acid deficiency. It is possible that many factors are responsible including defective intake of protein and minerals as well as ascorbic acid. Bone marrow biopsy does not usually show the changes described in pernicious anaemia. Anaemia can also occur in pituitary, thyroid and adrenal deficiency states and responds to endocrine therapy. It may also occur in diets low in copper and pyridoxine.

Degenerative changes in the oral mucosa have also been noted in aplastic and haemolytic anaemias.

Although the cause of polycythaemia vera is unknown there is a familial background in some patients. The oral mucosa is usually cyanotic and congested, especially the gingivae and tongue. Spontaneous bleeding and submucous petechiae may be found. Cutaneous cyanosis is also found and this is due to the presence of more than 5 gm. of reduced haemoglobin per 100 ml. of blood.

Lesions of the oral mucosa may occur in leukopenia and usually take the form of a non-specific infective process. The severity will depend on the underlying cause. Leukopenia is often associated with aplastic anaemia.

The reaction of the oral mucosa in leukaemia is usually striking; gingival bleeding and enlargement are the usual findings. Extensive ulceration and necrosis occurs as the condition progresses. The reason is that the white cells are no longer capable of carrying out their normal protective function and there is a lowered immunological resistance; herpes zoster, for example, is not infrequently associated with leukaemia. Cutaneous bullous lesions have

also been described. Although the cause remains unknown remarkable advances have been made in chemotherapy.

Haemorrhagic diseases may be caused by a deficiency of platelets, defects in the clotting mechanism, or increased capillary fragility. Thrombocytopenia may result from exposure to radiation or drug therapy. It can also occur in hypersplenism and may be associated with aplastic anaemia, leukaemia, and carcinomatosis. Defects in the clotting mechanism are dealt with in Chapter 56. Bleeding in the oral mucosa is a finding common to all the haemorrhagic diseases.

DEVELOPMENTAL ANOMALIES

Peutz-Jeghers Syndrome

This syndrome consists of distinctive mucocutaneous pigmentation associated with gastrointestinal polyposis and is inherited as a Mendelian dominant trait. However, oligosymptomatic and normal carriers are recognized. Pigmentation is most obvious on the lips and buccal mucosa, gingiva and palate. It can also occur on the hands, feet and abdomen. Cutaneous pigmentation tends to fade after puberty but mucosal lesions remain unchanged. Histological examination of maculae reveals an increase in the number of melanocytes in the basal layer and pigment-containing macrophages are found in the dermis. Polyp formation is usually present in the small intestine but benign adenomatous hamartomas can occur anywhere in the gastrointestinal tract.

Although the condition may be suspected from the abdominal symptoms the lesions in the oral mucosa are the most constant feature. They are particularly important in differentiating it from the Cronkhite-Canada syndrome which consists of gastrointestinal polyposis and diffuse pigmentation of the hands but in which the oral mucosa is not affected.

Albright's Syndrome

Cutaneous and mucosal pigmentation also occurs in this syndrome. Fibrous dysplasia and precocious puberty are also present. Extensive areas of cutaneous pigmentation develop early in life and have an irregular outline. They commonly occur on the abdomen and thighs.

Melkersson-Rosenthal Syndrome

The triad of recurrent non-inflammatory swelling of the lips, peripheral facial paralysis and fissured tongue is known as the Melkersson-Rosenthal syndrome. It is a rare condition and little is known about the aetiology although it appears to be genetically determined in most instances. Tissue swelling, similar to angioneurotic oedema, is an early and constant finding. At first it is intermittent but with repeated attacks a permanent swelling occurs. Early histological changes show oedema and perivascular infiltration, and later sarcoid-like granulomata are usually found.

Epidermolysis Bullosa

Epidermolysis bullosa includes a number of inherited conditions, in which the major characteristic is bulla formation spontaneously or following minimal trauma. It can be serious and the oral mucosa is often affected. Several distinct forms are recognized and these can be classified as epidermolysis bullosa simplex, dystrophic epidermolysis bullosa and epidermolysis bullosa letalis.

The simplex type is inherited as a Mendelian dominant trait and usually commences in the first year of life. The oral mucosa can be affected, but not severely. Healing

oral mucosa is nearly always affected and death usually occurs in early infancy.

Acquired epidermolysis bullosa is not a well recognized entity. However, there appears to be a condition in which bullae confined to the oral mucosa occur spontaneously or can easily be produced by gentle friction, and then tend to fill with blood (fig. 11). In addition a blunt probe can be inserted under the edge of a ruptured bulla and no resistance is felt as the instrument moves under the epithelium, thus indicating loss of adherence of epithelium to underlying structures (fig. 12). A subepithelial bulla is found on biopsy but no circulating epithelial antibodies

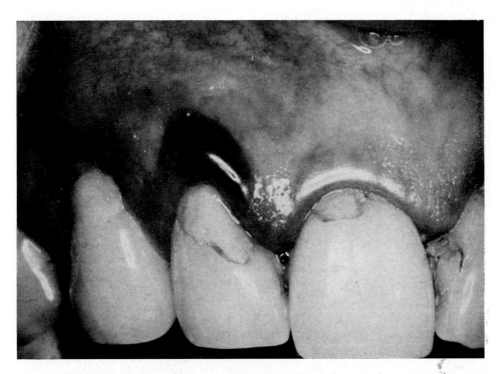

Fig. 11. Acquired epidermolysis bullosa.

takes place without scar formation and general development of the patient is otherwise normal. The condition is usually permanent although some patients improve in the second decade.

Dystrophic epidermolysis bullosa may be transmitted as a dominant or recessive trait. In the dominant type scar formation follows healing but physical and mental growth remain unaffected. Bullae on the oral mucosa can leave hyperkeratotic plaques as well as considerable scarring. Other mucous membranes including the larynx, pharynx and oesophagus may be involved. Carcinoma developing in scar tissue is not uncommon. Associated findings include dystrophic changes in the nails, hair and teeth. Severe anaemia and amyloidosis usually gives this type an unfavourable prognosis.

Epidermolysis bullosa letalis is caused by a recessive gene. There is a high incidence of abortion and stillbirths but if the infant is born alive extensive bullae usually develop rapidly and there is little tendency to heal. The

can be demonstrated. Healing occurs without scar formation. The disease occurs usually in middle-aged patients and there is no familial history. The condition gradually disappears and as it does so the probe test becomes more difficult to demonstrate. These findings are not characteristic of mucous membrane pemphigoid or bullous pemphigoid and one can only regard the condition as idiopathic. The term acquired oral epidermolysis bullosa has been suggested.

IDIOPATHIC ANOMALIES

Stevens-Johnson Syndrome

Stevens and Johnson in 1922 reported a mucocutaneous syndrome which occurred in two children and was unlike anything previously described. They labelled it as an "eruptive fever associated with stomatitis and ophthalmia". The children suddenly developed a purulent conjunctivitis complicated by blindness in one of them. Extensive bullous lesions were noted in the mouth and a circumscribed maculo-papular skin rash was found which became necrotic centrally. Resolution occurred within three weeks. From the description of the clinical features this syndrome should be regarded as a variant of erythema multiforme.

Erythema Multiforme

Erythema multiforme is an acute recurrent inflammatory condition which can affect the oral mucosa and skin.

The cause is still obscure and many factors have been suggested including drug hypersensitivity, emotional disturbances, heredity and a virus. There are isolated reports that herpes simplex virus and *Mycoplasma pneumoniae* may play a part in the aetiology.

recovery in a few weeks, the diagnosis becomes apparent. In the absence of the characteristic skin lesions diagnosis is more difficult and a biopsy may be necessary in some cases. Because this is a complex disease treatment is still empirical. However, efforts should be made to identify and eliminate specific allergens, for example, sulphonamides and barbiturates. Secondary infection is usually present if the mouth is affected and antibiotic therapy is often indicated. Occasionally systemic corticosteroid therapy may be necessary. The condition is seldom fatal and in most instances complete remission eventually occurs.

Sarcoidosis

This is a systemic granulomatous disease which may affect almost any tissue or organ in the body. Lymph nodes,

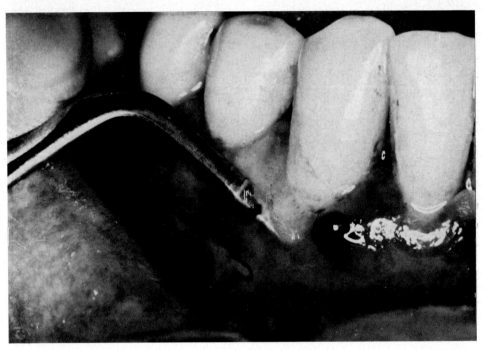

FIG. 12. Acquired epidermolysis bullosa.

Pathology

The most obvious areas of destruction are in the region of the basement membrane. Vasodilatation, oedema and chronic perivascular inflammatory cell infiltration are noted in the early stages followed by rupture of small blood vessels. Degenerative changes then occur in the lower epidermis and either subepithelial bullae or frank ulcers result. Electronmicroscopic studies have shown that the basement membrane forms the floor of the bulla. Similar changes may be found in the gastrointestinal and respiratory tracts.

Clinical aspects

The diagnosis is usually made on the clinical features and the absence of any specific laboratory findings. If there is a history of repeated and sudden attacks of skin (fig. 13) and oral bullae and ulceration associated with general malaise in a young person, followed by complete

lungs, skin, eyes, and bones are most frequently involved and, more rarely, the oral mucosa. The wide spectrum of clinical manifestations and histological findings can lead to a diagnostic dilemma as local lesions indistinguishable from sarcoidosis can be caused by many other agents including micro-organisms, parasites, chemicals, and foreign bodies. Added to this, sarcoid-like lesions may be seen in association with disorders of collagen and in neoplasia including Hodgkin's disease. It is apparent, therefore, that other granulomatous conditions should be excluded before a definitive diagnosis of sarcoidosis can be made. The essential features of the condition include the generalized nature of the disease process (an isolated granulomatous lesion is not diagnostic), all the affected tissues should show similar histological changes, the Kveim tests should be positive, and other specific serological and immunological findings may be present. Finally, in addition to their protean nature the clinical features, although protracted, are benign in most cases.

The cause is still unknown and sarcoidosis cannot be reproduced in animals. In the past it was considered to be an atypical form of tuberculosis but this has not been proved. More recently a multiple aetiological background has been suggested and attention has been drawn to the immunological aspects of the disease.

Clinical and diagnostic aspects

The wide variation in clinical manifestations in the early stages makes an accurate description difficult. However, a high proportion of patients complain of weight loss, lethargy, and general malaise. Cough, fever, and night sweats are also common. Three stages of the disease can be described. The first is usually transient and includes the

of laboratory findings, and the exclusion of other causes of granulomatous lesions is necessary before a confident diagnosis can be made. A biopsy should be carried out if the affected tissue is accessible, for example, the oral mucosa, lip, or skin. Changes similar to tuberculosis will be found, but caseation and necrosis do not occur. Masses of epithelioid cells with some multinucleated giant cells in fibrous granulomatous nodules are the main histological features. The Kveim test may be negative in the less active stages of the disease and should be repeated a number of times. Blood investigations may reveal anaemia, leucopenia, eosinophilia or monocytosis, and thrombocytopenia. A raised erythrocyte sedimentation rate is also found in the active stages and hypergammaglobulinaemia commonly

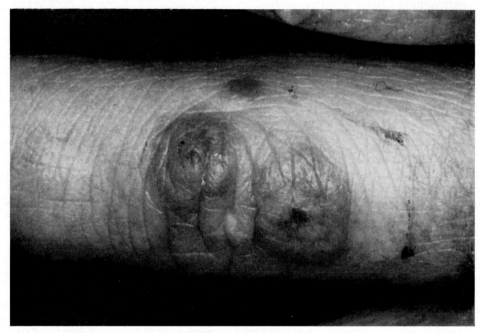

Fig. 13. Erythema multiforme.

above features. Skin and mucosal changes together with salivary gland lesions may be noted but spontaneous resolution tends to occur and the diagnosis can be missed. The next stage, which may last for years, consists of subacute inflammatory lesions in many organs. Ultimately, many patients reach the chronic stage which is characterized by fibrosis and atrophy resulting in progressive functional impairment of affected organs. A fatal outcome, however, occurs only in a relatively small number of patients.

Although sarcoidosis affecting the oral mucosa is said to be rare, lesions may be found more often when looked for. The mucous membrane of the cheeks, palate and tongue may be ulcerated, and may exhibit nodular hyperpigmented areas or pale yellow plaques. The nasal mucosa and larynx can be similarly affected.

Correlation of the clinical manifestations, the results

occurs in the chronic stage. Chest radiographs, and liver and kidney function tests should also be carried out to determine the extent of the disease.

FURTHER READING

Bean, S. F., Waisman, M., Michel, B., Thomas, C. I., Knox, J. M. and Levine, M. (1972), "Cicatricial Pemphigoid", *Arch. Derm.*, **106,** 195.

Lehner, T. (1967), "Autoimmunity and Management of Recurrent Oral Ulceration", *Brit. dent. J.*, **122,** 15.

Mowbray, J. F., Holborow, E. J., Hoffbrand, A. V., Sheah, P. P. and Fry, L. (1973), "Circulating Immune Complexes in Dermatitis Herpetiformis", *Lancet*, **i,** 400.

Nally, F. F. (1970), "Idiopathic Juvenile Hypoparathyroidism with Superficial Moniliasis", *Oral Surg.*, **30,** 356.

Tuffanelli, D. L. (1969), "Dermal-epidermal Junction in Lupus Erythematosus", *Arch. Derm.*, **99,** 652.

41. INFECTIONS OF THE ORAL MUCOUS MEMBRANE

R. A. CAWSON

A wide variety of infections affect the skin and at least in theory a variety of infections can affect the oral mucosa. In practice however, although dental caries and gingivitis are universal, mucosal infections are relatively few. Viruses (especially herpes simplex and Coxsackie strains) and fungi (especially *Candida albicans*) account for the vast majority. Virtually the only important bacterial infections are tuberculosis and syphilis which, though they should not be forgotten, are rarely seen today.

VIRAL INFECTIONS

Herpes Simplex—Primary Herpetic Stomatitis

Herpetic stomatitis is not the only manifestation of primary herpetic infection but in the case of Type I virus it is certainly the commonest. This infection may however be subclinical, or dismissed as "teething" in an infant. Formerly the primary infection was in infancy or childhood but, like tuberculosis, the pattern has changed. In Britain the primary infection is often not acquired until adult life or even middle age. By contrast in countries where there are large urban communities with a low standard of living, surveys have showed 70–90 per cent to have positive antibody titres during early childhood. By contrast in London, the incidence of positive titres among 5–10-year-olds, according to surveys at the Hospital for Sick Children, has fallen from 60 per cent in 1949 to 40 per cent in 1969 (Dudgeon, 1970).

Transmission of herpes is by close contact, from labial lesions for instance, and herpetic whitlow is also a well known occupational hazard especially among nurses and occasionally in dentists. Occasional small outbreaks affecting a group of children living closely together have been described but infectivity is far lower than in the case of hand-foot-and-mouth disease.

Pathology

The earliest recognizable lesion is the vesicle; the pre-vesicular changes are not known.

The vesicle is sharply defined and forms in the upper epidermis (fig. 1). The roof is several cells thick. The vesicle is therefore relatively strong and intact vesicles are often seen in the mouth. The cause of this collection of intra-epithelial fluid is not clear from the histology as the amount of recognizable viral damage to the epithelium at this stage appears small in relation to the size of the vesicle. Only a small number of pleomorphic nuclei with obvious ballooning degeneration and some multinucleate cell formation can be seen in the epithelium in the floor of the vesicle, while only scanty epithelial cells showing signs of viral damage may be seen floating in the vesicle fluid.

Progressive proliferation of the virus and colonization of the epithelium is followed by rupture of the vesicle and the development of a brief pre-ulcerative stage. This is easily recognizable clinically as a flat coin-like yellowish lesion of the same size as the vesicle. At this stage the epithelium is of virtually normal thickness but, within sharply defined margins, all the cells show severe viral damage and there is gross inter-cellular oedema (fig. 2). Finally the damaged and dying cells are shed, leaving an ulcer with a granulating base and edges that are still well-defined (fig. 3). Irregular ulcers are sometimes formed by the fusion of multiple closely-set lesions.

Involvement of regional lymph nodes presumably results

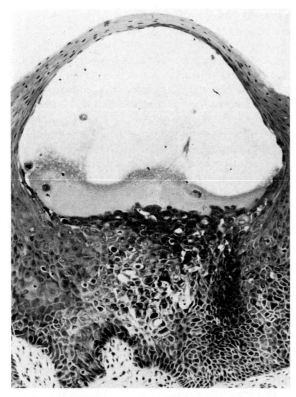

FIG. 1. Intact herpetic vesicle showing nuclear changes in infected epithelial cells in its floor. (H and E × 150.) (Reproduced from *Essentials of Dental Surgery and Pathology*, by kind permission of the publishers, Messrs. Churchill Livingstone.)

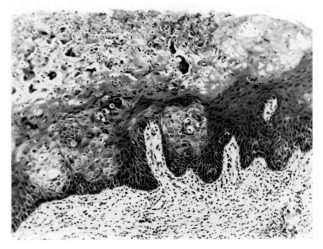

FIG. 2. Pre-ulcerative stage of the herpetic lesion at the stage before complete breakdown of the epithelium but with widespread viral damage and liberation of large numbers of infected cells. (H and E × 98.)

from local spread of the virus but the gingivitis is unexplained; it is not seen with the mucosal lesions of zoster or hand-foot-and-mouth disease. In addition, many patients are febrile and have moderate to severe systemic disturbance with malaise which may be prolonged. Viraemia, however, is said not to be a feature except in rare instances when the infection becomes disseminated. Herpetic encephalitis is a rare sequel to herpetic stomatitis but the factors precipitating this dangerous complication are not clear. Disseminated herpetic infection is an uncommon complication even among patients having immunosuppressive therapy. In these patients, herpetic infections tend to be severe but localized to the mouth and sometimes the adjacent skin.

Clinical and Diagnostic Aspects

The clinical features of typical primary herpetic stomatitis are too well known to need further description, but occasionally the disease may be atypical. Thus inflamed and engorged gingivae may dominate the picture or ulceration may affect the gingivae to an extent that mimics acute ulcerative (Vincentiform) gingivitis. Occasionally the lips may be grossly swollen with blood-stained crusting, and the appearances simulate erythema multiforme exudativum. Further to complicate the issue the latter may also follow or (it is said) be precipitated by herpetic infection.

Finally, there may be confusion between established

herpetic ulcers (after the vesicles have disappeared) and aphthous stomatitis. Examination of the distribution of lesions is usually helpful in that herpetic commonly, but aphthous very rarely, affect the vault of the palate, the gingival margins and the dorsum of the tongue. Systemic upset and enlarged regional nodes also suggest herpetic infection. If, on the other hand, there is a clear history of recurrent herpes labialis the diagnosis of herpetic stomatitis is highly unlikely.

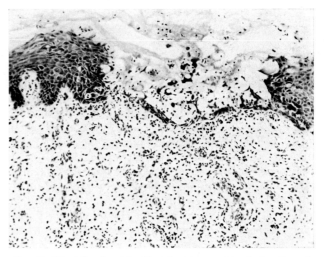

FIG. 3. Herpetic ulcer showing almost complete destruction of the full thickness of the epithelium. The sharply defined borders of the lesion and the surprisingly mild inflammatory reaction are noteworthy. (H and E × 20.) (Reproduced from *Essentials of Dental Surgery and Pathology*, by kind permission of the publishers, Churchill Livingstone.)

The diagnosis of herpetic infection can be assisted or confirmed in the following ways:

1. Direct Smears. The finding of viral damaged nuclei (swelling, ballooning, degeneration and multinuclear cells) is for most practical purposes adequate for diagnosis. It is not specific, and herpes cannot be distinguished from zoster in this way but the difference in clinical appearance is such that these will rarely be confused. The main limitation of this simple test is that it is so often negative. This may possibly be due to sampling at too early or too late a stage, since histology suggests that the largest numbers of viral damaged cells are present in the pre-ulcerative stage.

2. Electron Microscopy and Fluorescent Antibody Treatment of Smears. Both of these are elaborations of the simple direct smear technique but also depend on finding infected epithelial cells. The fluorescent antibody technique is specific though it does not seem to have established itself very widely as a diagnostic technique.

3. Isolation of the Virus. This can readily be carried out in a virology laboratory. Herpes virus can be grown on chick chorioallantoic membrane or tissue cultures and produces characteristic plaques. These experimental infections can be inhibited by specific antisera.

Growth of the herpes virus may leave doubt, however, as to whether the patient is merely a carrier.

4. Antibody Titration. The detection of a rising titre of antibodies to herpes virus is the most convincing evidence for the diagnosis of this infection. The mere presence of antibody in an adult's serum is of little value except as an indication that there had been a primary infection at some time in the past. When antibodies are minimal at the onset of the infection, but reach a significant titre during convalescence two to three weeks later, the diagnosis of herpetic infection can be made with confidence.

Recurrent Herpetic Infections

Herpes Labialis

After the primary infection (which may have passed unrecognized) it is estimated that about 30 per cent of patients are subject to recurrent infections, of which by far the commonest is herpes labialis. After what seems to be some insult to the defences, the infection becomes reactivated. The best recognized precipitating factor is another infection—classically in the past, lobar pneumonia—hence the English familiar name "cold sore" and the American "fever blister". Exposure to sunshine, sea air and many other factors can trigger attacks in a particular individual.

Once the virus is reactivated the clinical changes follow a remarkably uniform course. The site for the attack declares itself by a premonitory pricking or burning sensation. This is followed, within an hour or two, by a cluster of vesicles at some point along the junction between the skin and the vermilion border of the lip or on the skin adjacent to the nostrils. The blisters grow, coalesce and may weep exudate. After two or three days the vesicles rupture and the raw area crusts over. Healing is usually complete in about ten days after the first symptoms.

Repeated recurrences of viral infections are unusual since they usually provoke production of neutralizing antibodies with long-lasting protection. Herpetic infection shows a similar immune response but this fails to protect some patients against recurrent infections. In these

subjects, the virus appears to persist in the body in a latent form and to be reactivated by certain stimuli.

There has been for some time a suspicion that the trigeminal ganglion plays a role in the latent stage of herpes. Recurrent infections may occasionally accompany attacks of trigeminal neuralgia but more frequently follow intracranial operations for this disease when the sensory root of the trigeminal ganglion is sectioned. These recurrences are, however, dependent on the peripheral sensory fibres of the ganglion remaining intact. Moreover, recurrent herpetic infection may occasionally be distributed in a zoster-like fashion with lesions confined to the related dermatomes. This circumstantial evidence seems to have been confirmed by recent findings that the virus could be isolated from trigeminal ganglia taken at autopsy after prolonged culture *in vitro*. Only a minority of patients from whom these ganglia came had a history of recurrent herpetic infections, and this suggests that persistence of the virus need not necessarily mean that reactivation is inevitable. This in turn is in keeping with clinical experience that there appears to be a wide spectrum of response to reactivation. At one extreme there are patients who have frequent recurrences at the slightest provocation, while others have recurrences exceedingly infrequently.

Many questions about this disease remain unanswered. While it seems likely that recurrent herpetic infections result from the reactivated virus tracking to the periphery along sensory nerve fibres the nature of the process of reactivation is not known nor is the state of the latent virus. It is not known whether it is the intact virus or if it is in some incomplete (provirus) form. It is also particularly puzzling that in the vast majority of patients recurrences develop not in the mouth but within so limited and sharply defined an area, on the lips. The fact that either side can be affected in any given patient also suggests that both trigeminal ganglia harbour the latent virus.

Intra-oral Recurrent Herpes

Though herpes labialis is by far the commonest recurrent form of the disease it can occasionally be intra-oral. In the past there has been confusion between this infection and aphthous stomatitis. When recurrent herpes affects the oral cavity the hard palate is often affected, but this is a rare site for aphthae. The diagnosis should, however, only be made if there is clear evidence of vesicles preceding the ulcers and if there is positive evidence of viral damage, *e.g.* in direct smears. Intra-oral recurrences of herpetic infection seem to be self-limiting and do not seem to follow the pattern of aphthous stomatitis, or of herpes labialis, that is with intermittent ulceration going on for years. The term "herpetiform" ulceration is an unfortunate one which refers to a clinical variant of recurrent aphthae but not to true herpetic infection.

Hand-Foot-and-Mouth Disease

This is a relatively recently recognized viral infection of the oral cavity. It appears to be appreciably more readily transmitted and commoner than herpetic stomatitis; an outbreak ultimately involving no fewer than 800 children and adults in South Wales was described by Evans and Waddington (1967). The reason why relatively few cases are seen by the dental surgeon is the fact that the oral symptoms may be slight while the rash, though usually also mild, determines the patient's path to the doctor's surgery.

Hand-foot-and-mouth disease is caused by Coxsackie viruses, usually of group A and most often type 16; A5 and A10 and occasionally others have been isolated from particular outbreaks. In Britain the incidence has shown upswings at three year intervals with 1973 being the most recent peak year.

Epidemiology and Clinical Features

The incubation period appears to be between three and ten days. Outbreaks frequently affect a relatively large number of children in a school. Parents and teachers may also become infected.

The main clinical features are a painful vesicular stomatitis and a vesicular rash mainly affecting the extremities. In general the infection is mild and the symptoms are much less severe than those of primary herpes. Though the mouth alone may be affected in hand-foot-and-mouth disease (Cawson and McSwiggan, 1969), its epidemic nature, the mildness of the lesions, and the lack of gingival involvement help to distinguish it from herpes simplex. The diagnosis can however, be confirmed virologically.

Although most cases are exceedingly mild, severe or fatal complications, including meningo-encephalitis, paralytic disease and myocarditis have been reported.

Virology

The virus can be isolated from vesicle fluid (if obtainable), saliva (if suitably prepared), and faeces. The virus will grow in tissue culture and has a cytopathic effect. A neutralizing antibody is also produced in a rising titre by infected patients. Direct smears to find viral damaged cells do not appear to be useful and the histopathology of these lesions seems not to have been investigated in detail.

Management

There is no specific treatment available but in most cases the disease is mild and recovery takes only a few days.

Antiviral Chemotherapy

The last ten years have seen the development of specific antiviral agents which have at least some potential clinical usefulness.

In the case of herpes simplex and zoster topically applied idoxuridine has been used successfully for superficial lesions while intravenous idoxuridine and cytarabine have been used for herpetic encephalitis. Another agent with certain advantages is vidarabine but this has not yet been adequately evaluated.

Idoxuridine has been most beneficial in the treatment of dermal and ocular lesions where it can be readily applied in a vehicle (dimethyl sulphoxide) which ensures absorption. This agent has also been used for herpetic stomatitis, and though some studies have not confirmed the effectiveness of this agent it seems reasonably certain that, when properly applied in an appropriate vehicle, it does expedite healing. The necessity for painting idoxuridine frequently on to the intra-oral lesions is, however, a drawback.

CANDIDIASIS

Candidiasis (or less usually but more correctly, candidosis) is a fungal infection with a wide variety of clinical manifestations which can be broadly divided into superficial and systemic infection. In general these remain distinct, and the superficial infections do not progress to disseminated candidiasis (which will not be discussed further here) even in those cases where the infection has been persistent for years. Though almost any part of the body may be affected, the mouth is the most frequent site of candidiasis.

Candida albicans exists in yeast and hyphal forms; it is the latter which actively invades the tissues in mucocutaneous candidiasis. Though many regard it as the pathogenic form of the organism there is no firm evidence on this point.

Candidiasis is often described as an opportunistic infection. The organism is a common inhabitant of the normal mouth—approximately 40 per cent of healthy adults may be carriers—and mild or severe candidal infections can result from disorders which weaken the resistance of the host. While the concept of candidiasis as (in Trousseau's expression) a "disease of the diseased" is a useful reminder that some latent underlying disorder should be looked for, it must also be appreciated that persistent candidiasis can affect healthy patients in whom no systemic disease can be found or becomes evident after years of observation. In another group of patients an underlying disorder (particularly of iron metabolism) is present but latent and has little overt effect upon the patient's health.

Thrush is the best known form of candidiasis and was recognized in antiquity. Candidiasis is a disease with many clinical variations and associations, and while these cannot all be discussed in detail it may be useful to summarize their main features in the hope of providing a broader view of this infection and its possible implications. At the same time it is important not to lose a sense of proportion. The dentist is likely to see only the commoner localized forms of candidiasis, but even these should be investigated as occasionally familial mucocutaneous candidiasis for instance, may affect the mouth alone and remain unrecognized until late in life; in other patients significant but latent systemic disorders may be found.

The forms of candidiasis which are most likely to be seen among the ordinary run of out-patients are (in order of frequency), denture stomatitis, candidal leukoplakia (*i.e.* late onset "idiopathic" candidiasis) and thrush. The last may, in some cases, be a complication of corticosteroid or other drug therapy or any of the disorders known to precipitate this infection. Thrush however, is commoner among the newborn and infants, *i.e.* at one extreme of life, and debilitated patients (especially those having cytotoxic or immunosuppressive therapy) at the other. Among the latter some have generalized superficial inflammation of the oral mucosa and angular stomatitis with the complaint of severe soreness. This variant first became well known as a drug-associated disease in the early days of antibiotic therapy, when it was regarded as a hypersensitivity to penicillin or a vitamin B group deficiency secondary to interference with the gut flora by broad-spectrum antibiotics. These hypotheses have never in fact been established, and if the mouth in a case of "acute antibiotic stomatitis" is carefully examined patches of thrush will usually be found, especially in protected sites such as the upper posterior buccal sulcus. In addition to mycological evidence of candidiasis, the condition responds rapidly to adequate topical antifungal therapy.

Clinically, most forms of candidiasis are characterized by the formation of whitish plaque, either soft and friable in the case of thrush, or firm and leukoplakic in the chronic disease.

Angular stomatitis is, however, a particularly characteristic sign of candidiasis and is common to all the many variants of the disease. Though angular stomatitis is often

(a) Acute candidiasis: Thrush
(b) Chronic candidiasis: Denture stomatitis
                          Candidal leukoplakia

Candidiasis can also be classified in relation to aetiological factors, in so far as they are known (Higgs and Wells, 1973).

While such a classification (or any other) should be regarded as tentative, and useful only in relation to the present state of knowledge on the subject, it forms a useful framework into which the main clinical types of the disease can be fitted.

Chronic Mucocutaneous Candidiasis as the Predominant Disease

1. Familial Chronic Mucocutaneous Candidiasis

In this form of the disease candidiasis is present early in life; certainly in infancy, and perhaps in the neonatal

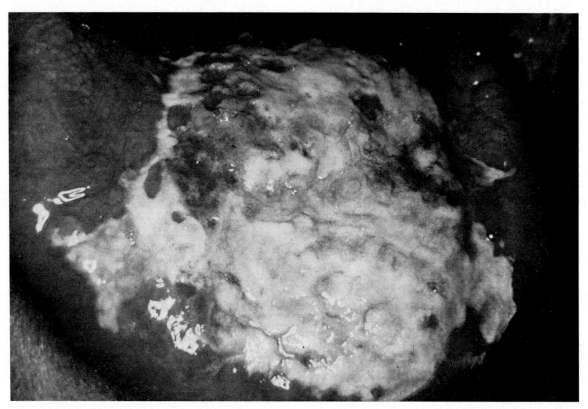

FIG. 4. Familial muco-cutaneous candidiasis (Group I). There is extensive candidal leukoplakia on this man's tongue. The candidal nature of the lesion was not recognised until the patient was middle-aged and the familial background not appreciated until considerably later. There were two affected sisters and the parents were first cousins. All three patients were sideropenic. (Reproduced from the *British Journal of Dermatology* by kind permission of the Editor.)

regarded as a typical sign of anaemia it is present in only a minority of anaemic patients, but anaemia (or latent iron deficiency) and candidiasis are not infrequently associated.

Classification of the various types of candidiasis is difficult, even when only those which affect the mouth are considered.

The main clinical types of oral candidiasis are as follows:

period. The mouth is invariably affected and may be the only site in the less severe cases. Widespread whitish mucosal plaques, especially on the tongue and buccal mucosa, are thrush-like, *i.e.* soft and friable initially but become progressively firmer in texture and acquire the clinical features of leukoplakia. Angular stomatitis is also a regular feature, but dermal lesions are usually mild or may be absent (figs. 4 and 5).

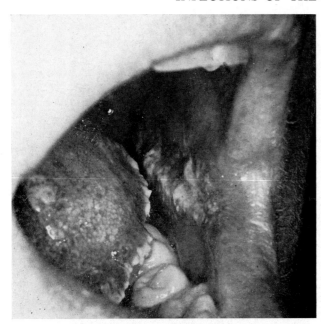

FIG. 5. Familial muco-cutaneous candidiasis (Group I). This is an example of fairly severe disease in a child with extensive candidal leukoplakia of the buccal mucosa and edges of the tongue.

2. Diffuse Chronic Mucocutaneous Candidiasis

Diffuse chronic mucocutaneous candidiasis is the most severe form. Lesions may extend from the mouth down the pharynx and larynx and into the gastro-intestinal tract. In addition, the mouth and nails, the skin of the face, scalp, and other parts may be affected, sometimes with grossly proliferative lesions (fig. 6). Though such lesions have been called "candidal granuloma" this is a misnomer, since they are the result of epithelial, not connective tissue, proliferation.

The oral lesions are clinically similar to those in familial chronic mucocutaneous candidiasis but tend to be more severe, giving rise to widespread candidal leukoplakia even in childhood.

These patients are often also abnormally susceptible to other infections, either fungal or, more often, bacterial, especially of the respiratory tract.

3. Candida Endocrinopathy Syndrome

As in the preceding groups these patients have candidal infection of early onset, affecting the mouth and nails especially, but generally of lesser severity. In addition, however, these patients develop endocrine deficiencies, most often hypoparathyroidism but also others such as hypoadrenalism. The endocrine disorder may be delayed in its appearance until years after candidiasis has become obvious, and though this has led some to postulate that the endocrine disorder is the result of the infection the nature of the relationship between the two is in fact unknown.

4. Late Onset "Idiopathic" Mucocutaneous Candidiasis

These are the commonest types of chronic candidiasis. Denture stomatitis and candidal leukoplakia can be conveniently grouped together under this heading. Most

of these patients are apparently well, but anaemia or sideropenia can also be associated as in other forms of candidiasis. As mentioned earlier, denture stomatitis and candidal leukoplakia are the commoner types of candidiasis that the dentist will see (fig. 7).

Within these groups the first and third show a strong genetic influence and are probably inherited as autosomal recessives. In addition, a significant majority of patients overall (though least often in the last group) show a defect of iron metabolism, particularly sideropenia, or less often overt anaemia, resistant to conventional forms of treatment.

In addition there are immune defects associated with this disease, but it should be made clear that chronic

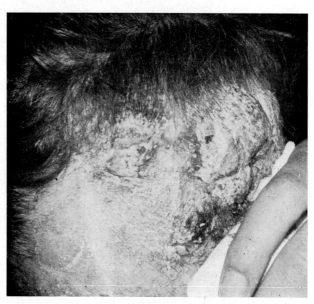

FIG. 6. Diffuse muco-cutaneous candidiasis (Group II). A grossly proliferative epithelial plaque—a so-called granuloma—characteristic of this form of the disease is seen on the forehead of an affected child.

mucocutaneous candidiasis is not simply the result of an immune deficiency state. Many patients have no detectable immune defect, and in some that do the defect appears to be secondary either to antigenic overload by the persistent infection or to iron deficiency. Among the remainder it might be expected that the strong genetic influence would mean that there was a single identifiable immunological disorder; in fact, the immune defects, when present, are variable in character (Valdimarsson et al., 1973).

These patients must therefore be clearly distinguished from those with primary immune deficiencies or defects of the polymorphonuclear leucocytes (as described below) who may develop candidiasis. In these cases, this infection is merely one complication among many others.

Mucocutaneous Candidiasis Secondary to the Primary Immune Deficiency States

This comprises a group of rare conditions where candidiasis may be a prominent or occasional feature, as follows:

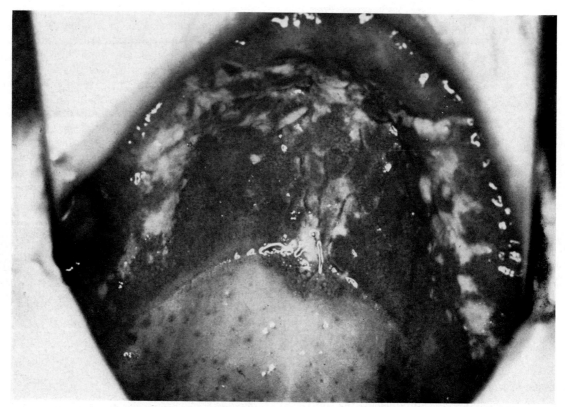

Fig. 7. Late onset candidiasis (Group IV). In a middle-aged woman with a chronic iron and folate deficiency there was, as shown here, denture stomatitis with persistent, widespread thrush and angular stomatitis.

1. Swiss-type Agammaglobulinaemia

This is a genetically determined disease where there is failure of thymic development and antibody production. As a consequence, there is severely diminished resistance to infections of all types. Recurrent oral candidiasis is a prominent and characteristic complication, and this infection may occasionally become systemic. These patients do not usually survive beyond the first year of life.

2. Hereditary Thymic Dysplasia

Cell-mediated immunity is impaired but antibody production is normal in these patients, who are particularly susceptible to viral infection but also to severe candidiasis. Patients generally do not survive beyond the first two years of life.

3. Chronic Granulomatous Disease

Unlike those just described, the underlying defect is of polymorphonuclear leucocyte function, *i.e.* it is not therefore an immunological disorder. Phagocytosis takes place but there is failure to kill some bacteria and Candida species. Recurrent infections are the chief clinical characteristic of this disease and though chronic candidiasis may be a feature, bacterial infections are commoner and more prominent.

4. Di George Syndrome

This is not genetically determined, but there is defective development of the third and fourth branchial pouches so that thymus and parathyroid glands fail to form. There is usually, therefore, (among other features) a defect of cell-mediated immunity but normal antibody production. These patients are susceptible to recurrent bacterial infections and sometimes to candidiasis; it is important to note that though candidiasis may be associated with hypoparathyroidism in the Di George syndrome this is not the same disease as the candida endocrinopathy syndrome mentioned earlier. In this latter disease the mechanism of the association between candidiasis and hypoparathyroidism is unknown, and the endocrine defect may appear relatively late in the course of the disease.

It is pertinent to comment here that this association between chronic candidiasis and hypoparathyroidism, apparently coincidentally in two otherwise different diseases, has probably given rise to statements that hypoparathyroidism is an aetiological factor in candidiasis. There is at present no evidence that this is the case.

Pathology

Candidiasis shows some remarkable features. Firstly it appears by invasion of the tissue to provoke epithelial hyperplasia. This is a characteristic feature of candidal lesions and can be reproduced experimentally. Secondly, when *Candida albicans* invades epithelia it becomes an intracellular parasite and grows within the cytoplasm of the epithelial cell.

Denture stomatitis, however, forms an exception and in

this special case the organism proliferates in the interface between denture and mucosa, provoking an apparently non-specific inflammatory response.

The histopathology (fig. 8) of the two main types of oral candidiasis which may be conveniently termed thrush and candidal leukoplakia has been described on several occasions and it is only necessary to emphasize some salient features.

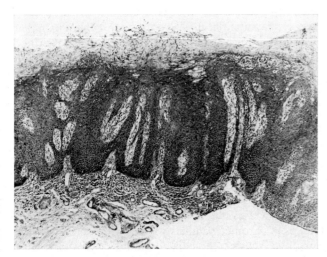

FIG. 8. Chronic muco-cutaneous candidiasis (candidal leukoplakia). This low power view shows one of the various histological patterns. The superficial infected plaque with microabscesses at its base, severe acanthosis of the epithelium and inflammatory infiltrate in the corium can be seen. (PAS × 36.)

In both acute candidiasis (thrush) and candidal leuko-plakia an essentially similar response is seen to invasion by this fungus. The differences can be partly explained in terms of the duration of the infection, and transitional stages between thrush and candidal leukoplakia can be seen.

The main pathological features of mucosal candidiasis are as follows:

1. Epithelial Plaque

This, the characteristic clinical feature of the disease, consists of a thickened layer of parakeratinized epithelium which is invaded by the candidal hyphae. The latter are not, of course, easily seen with conventional haematoxylin and eosin staining and it is not surprising, therefore, that so many cases of candidiasis went unrecognized in the past.

One obvious feature of this plaque is the presence of an inflammatory infiltrate—both fluid and cellular—at an unusually superficial level. This infiltrate is within the parakeratinized zone but tends to be particularly intense at the base of the plaque at its junction with the glycogen-rich zone.

2. Hyphal Invasion

By use of periodic acid-Schiff stain hyphae can be clearly seen invading the superficial plaque, growing downwards at right angles (figs. 9 and 10) to the surface and reaching

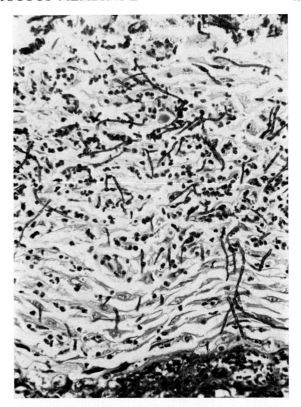

FIG. 9. Thrush. A higher power view of the plaque showing the epithelial cells separated by the widespread inflammatory exudate and the hyphae growing down through them. Many of the epithelial cells nevertheless retain good nuclear structure. (PAS × 300.)

(but rarely entering) the glycogen-rich zone. The hyphae are often surprisingly straight, allowing the plane of section to pass through the long axis for a considerable length in some instances. Due to the intracellular growth of the organism the hyphae do not, of course, insinuate themselves along the intracellular boundaries.

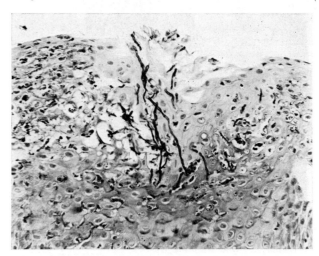

FIG. 10. Candidal leukoplakia. This higher power view shows the parakeratotic nature of the plaque and in this area the inflammatory exudate extending up to the surface. The comparatively straight, vertical course of the hyphae is also characteristic. (PAS × 200.) (Reproduced from the *British Journal of Dermatology*, by kind permission of the Editor.)

3. Spinous Layer and Corium

Acanthosis of some degree is invariable, together with cellular changes in keeping with the degree of epithelial proliferation and associated inflammation. Frank atypia or dysplasia are uncommon but have been reported. The form of the epithelial downgrowths that seems to be most common is that of rounded or bulbous processes.

The basement membrane may be broken up by inflammatory cellular infiltrate at one or two points, but in most PAS stained specimens it is unusually prominent or appears thicker than normal.

The corium is infiltrated by chronic inflammatory cells, usually both plasma cells and lymphocytes, but either may predominate.

The clinical lesion of thrush is a plaque of hyperplastic epithelium, as is that of candidal leukoplakia. The acute lesion is, however, more heavily infected with hyphae and shows a more florid inflammatory response. Gross inflammatory oedema separates the cells of the plaque which is, as a result, loose and friable in texture. The concentration of acute inflammatory cells and fluid exudate at the base of the plaque is sufficient to form a plane of cleavage, allowing the plaque to be wiped off the deeper epithelium. The latter is attenuated, and in place of the

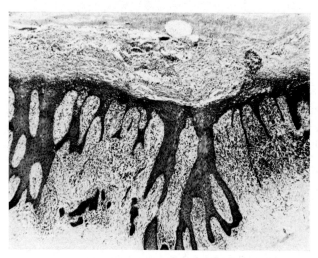

Fig. 11. Thrush. There is a superficial plaque but the epithelium immediately underneath shows alternating acanthosis and thinning along its length compatible with rapid production and shedding of its surface layers. The inflammatory infiltrate in the corium is moderately dense. (H and E × 33.)

more massive hyperplasia characteristic of the chronic lesion the epithelial downgrowths are deep but slender. The appearance is suggestive of rapidly proliferating epithelium and is in keeping with the clinical experience that plaques of thrush can appear within a matter of days or even hours (fig. 11).

Iron Deficiency and Candidiasis

It has been shown that among the four groups of mucocutaneous candidiasis, approximately 70 per cent of patients are iron deficient. This is either latent (sideropenia) or less often, overt anaemia. Sideropenia is particularly

common in familial mucocutaneous candidiasis and may affect all siblings with the disease. Overt anaemia was found in all patients examined with diffuse CMCC ("candidal granuloma") the most severe type of this disease.

The cause of this iron deficiency is unknown, but iron deficiency is known to have dystrophic effects on the oral mucosa and other epithelia affected by candidiasis, such as the nails. There seems, however, to be a defect of iron metabolism and iron is poorly absorbed or utilized. If, however, parenteral iron is given this contributes materially to clinical improvement. The response to oral iron is exceedingly slow and, in severe late onset candidiasis, clinical improvement may not be obvious until as long as two years of such treatment.

Iron deficiency is less often found in late onset candidiasis (denture stomatitis and candidal leukoplakia) when compared with other forms of mucocutaneous candidiasis. It has been shown independently, however, that there is a significant association between angular stomatitis and sideropenia, but not overt anaemia. Haematological examination of these patients should not therefore be neglected.

A further recent finding that appears relevant to the findings in chronic candidiasis is that iron deficiency itself leads to defective cell mediated immunity (Joynson et al., 1972).

Candidiasis as a Cause of Proliferative Epithelial Lesions

Experimental and Ultrastructural Aspects

There has been a curious reluctance to accept the idea that candidiasis can cause leukoplakia or that it is anything more than a secondary infection. By contrast, in the case of syphilitic leukoplakia where nothing is known of the mechanism of the production of the oral lesion, it would be thought to be perverse in the extreme to describe a case as one of "oral leukoplakia with superimposed syphilitic infection". Further, in those cases of so called "superimposed candidiasis", there has been nothing to show that there was in fact a pre-existing plaque which became infected.

In fact, unlike most other types of leukoplakia there is a good deal of evidence indicating the causative role of the infection in candidal leukoplakia. Leukoplakia is for instance common and is sometimes the main feature of mucocutaneous candidiasis in children, an age group which can hardly be said to be one prone to leukoplakia in general. In addition, the dermal lesions of mucocutaneous candidiasis show the same characteristic epithelial proliferation. Secondly, unlike other leukoplakias, the proliferative epithelial plaque of candidiasis can be reproduced experimentally either in rats or in chick chorioallantoic membrane (Cawson, 1973). Thirdly, the fact that Candida albicans can be shown by electron microscopy (Cawson and Rajasingham, 1972) to be an intracellular parasite of epithelial cells indicates a means by which the behaviour of these cells could be profoundly affected (figs. 12, 13 and 14).

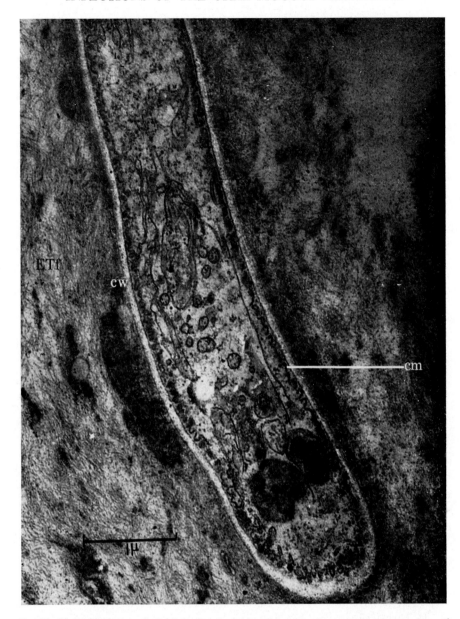

FIG. 12. Electron micrograph showing part of a hypha of *Candida albicans* within the cytoplasm of a human epithelial cell and surrounded by tonofilaments (ETf). The fungal cell wall (CW) and cytoplasm membrane (CM) are well defined as are the organisms' various organelles. (Reproduced from the *British Journal of Dermatology* by kind permission of the Editor.)

Under these conditions, the invading hyphae can be seen within the cytoplasm of the epithelial cells which appear otherwise to be undamaged and in no way disorganized. The hyphae are highly developed and show clearly a complete range of the organelles expected in a eukaryotic cell. By contrast, hyphae grown in artificial culture, though identical by light microscopy with those from human lesions (fig. 15), show a strikingly different intracellular organization by electron microscopy. These differences may perhaps reflect adaptive changes in the invading organism related to its intracellular environment.

Finally there may also be some relationship between iron deficiency—a common association with chronic candidiasis—and leukoplakia. Although atrophic changes in oral epithelia are the expected result of anaemia, leukoplakia can develop and has been described in the Paterson-Kelly syndrome.

There seem, therefore, to be adequate reasons for believing that invasion of epithelia by *Candida albicans* results in epithelial proliferation. While it would be unreasonable to state categorically that candidiasis is not a superimposed infection of leukoplakia it would not be possible to prove such a chain of events unless it could be established that a pre-existing, uninfected leukoplakia had been present. Until this is done there seems to be little basis for trying to distinguish candidal leukoplakia (in any of the variants of mucocutaneous candidiasis) from so called "superimposed candidiasis."

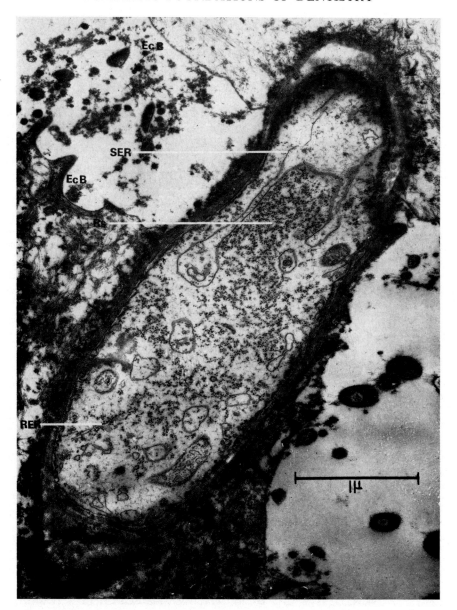

FIG. 13. Electron micrograph of an oblique section of a hypha (also from a human lesion) passing across the boundaries (EcB) of two epithelial cells. In this section the smooth and rough endoplasmic reticulum (SER, RER) and ribosomes (Rs) of the organism are clearly seen. (Reproduced from the *British Journal of Dermatology* by kind permission of the Editor.)

Diagnosis and Investigation

The clinical features of the different forms of candidiasis are now well known, and once the possibility is suspected confirmation of the diagnosis is usually straightforward.

Though admittedly uncommon, mucocutaneous candidiasis is the most probable diagnosis in a child with persistent white lesions of the tongue and buccal mucosa with angular stomatitis, and especially if there are also skin lesions. The oral plaques may vary from whitish flecks or thin whitish film to thick irregular plaque according to the severity of the case and age of the patient.

The first step in making a diagnosis is to make a direct smear by firmly scraping the lesions, and staining by Gram's method or PAS. In candidal leukoplakia, hyphae will be seen often in great numbers and embedded in epithelial cells or fragments of detached epithelium. Hyphae are always found in abundance in thrush, and this diagnosis should not be made if they do not appear in such numbers in a smear. In smears from denture stomatitis, however, hyphae may sometimes be difficult to find. The presence of a few yeast cells alone is probably of little significance.

In the case of thrush the clinical features and the presence of enormous numbers of hyphae in the smear should be sufficient to make the diagnosis, but in adults especially, some precipitating cause should be looked for if the patient is known not to have been having immunosuppressive or prolonged antibiotic therapy. A full blood

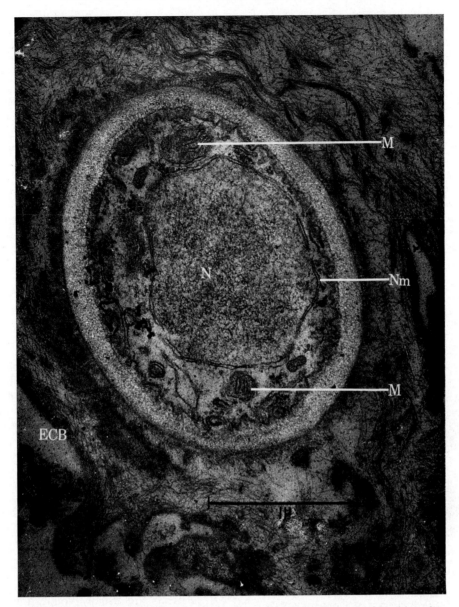

FIG. 14. Transverse section of a hypha within a human epithelial cell close to the cell boundary (ECB) and showing more detail of the epithelial tonofilaments. In this part of the hypha there are well defined but small cristate mitochondria (M) and the nucleus with its characteristic unit membrane (Nm) interrupted by pores can be seen. (Reproduced from the *British Journal of Dermatology* by kind permission of the Editor.)

picture and serum iron levels should be looked at, and the patient investigated for the presence of any latent disease.

In the case of candidal leukoplakia, biopsy (as in the case of any other chronic epithelial plaque) should be carried out to confirm the diagnosis and also to determine whether the epithelium shows any significant degree of atypia. The sections should, of course, be stained by haematoxylin and eosin and PAS. A full blood picture and serum iron levels (repeated if necessary) should be investigated. The report on the blood film may also indicate the presence of other deficiencies.

Though it is only occasionally positive in the older patients, the family history should be enquired into to ascertain the existence of other affected siblings and also

parental consanguinity. In the case of the candida endocrinopathy syndrome the appearance of the endocrine defect may occasionally be delayed until early adult life so that this possibility should also be remembered.

Therapeutic Considerations

In spite of the introduction of several specific antifungal agents, treatment of chronic candidiasis in particular remains difficult. Treatment of underlying disease, especially iron deficiency, is of primary importance, but even this is not easy and parenteral iron usually has to be given. The safest method of providing antifungal therapy is by mouth and 500,000 unit tablets of nystatin, or its equivalent, three times a day allowed to dissolve in the mouth represents an adequate regime. In the case of uncomplicated candidiasis secondary to antibiotic therapy the latter should be stopped if feasible, but if not, can be continued concurrently with oral nystatin or amphotericin B. In cases of severe chronic mucocutaneous candidiasis with immune defects the latter have been shown in some cases to recover once iron deficiency has been made good and the excessive antigenic load has been reduced by antifungal therapy. The clinical response also appears to be good. The alternative approach is to attempt repair of the immune defect by such means as the administration of transfer factor; this too may lead to clinical improvement but there are difficulties inherent in this type of treatment and it has been tried on only a small scale so far.

The usefulness of newer agents such as 5-fluorocytosine and clotrimazole has not yet been established for the management of this type of candidiasis though they have important applications for other forms of the infection.

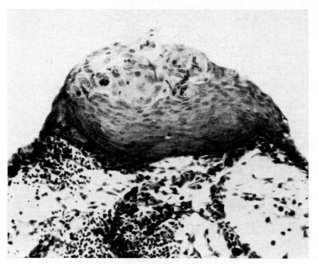

Fig. 15. Experimental candida infection of chick chorioallantoic membrane showing gross proliferation and formation of a thick epithelial plaque. There is an inflammatory cellular infiltration of the mesoderm but only a few hyphae can be seen in the superficial layers of the plaque in this section. (PAS × 220.) (Reproduced from the *British Journal of Dermatology* by kind permission of the Editor.)

ACUTE ULCERATIVE GINGIVITIS

(Syn. Acute Necrotizing, Ulcerative, Vincent's Gingivitis.)

This condition is a true gingivitis in that it appears to be dependent on the gingival anatomy and local biological environment for its development. The ulcerative process starts at, extends along, and (in the vast majority of cases) is restricted to the gingival margins. Occasionally contact ulceration develops on the adjacent mucosa but never (in so far as so absolute a term can be applied in medicine) originates there. Vincent's angina, characterized by pharyngeal ulceration, appears to be a separate entity which is not necessarily associated with gingival ulceration.

Aetiology

The predominant organisms found in acute ulcerative gingivitis are the anaerobic *Borrelia vincenti* and *Fusiformis*

fusiformis which are present in large numbers in the depths of the sloughs and in immediate proximity to the tissues. These organisms can be found in relatively small numbers in many if not most normal mouths, though this in itself should not provoke doubt about their aetiological role. Attempts to establish experimental infections by inoculation of these organisms have not, however, produced convincing evidence that the disease can be reliably reproduced, though in such circumstances it must be doubted whether the precise ecological conditions that exist in the human infection, have been reproduced (see also Chapter 15). More recently, the introduction of metronidazole and its demonstrable effectiveness in the treatment of acute ulcerative gingivitis has cast new light on the aetiology. Metronidazole has an unusual spectrum of activity (see also Chapter 17) being highly effective against *Trichomonas vaginalis*, moderately effective against *Treponema pallidum*, but inactive against Candida and the majority of bacteria. Metronidazole is also highly active against Vincent's organisms (being at least as effective as penicillin) and in view of its limited spectrum of activity this suggests that these organisms are likely to be the causative agents. The role of *Bacteroides melaninogenicus* is not clear.

Whatever the causative organism, acute ulcerative gingivitis appears to be an opportunistic infection which is unlikely to develop until environmental conditions are favourable. Most affected subjects have poorly cared-for mouths, many with malposed teeth, are often heavy smokers and in many cases have had a recent upper respiratory tract infection, either the common cold or influenza. During war-time conditions, ulcerative gingivitis was considerably more common than it is at present and though it does not appear that the disease is infectious, minor epidemics in barracks or the trenches were common. By contrast, ulcerative gingivitis is seen relatively infrequently in general practice in Britain today.

Clinical and Pathological Features

Patients are usually young adults; children are not affected in this country. The onset is usually rapid with soreness of the gingivae as the main symptom. Bleeding and increased salivation may also be noted. In most mouths there is evidence of neglect with accumulations of bacterial plaque and calculus. The ulceration characteristically starts at the tip of an interdental papilla, is crater-shaped, covered with greyish slough, and has an inflamed margin. Ulceration spreads laterally along the gingival margins or may penetrate deeply, rapidly destroying the papilla and crestal bone. In severe cases the regional lymph nodes may be enlarged and a little tender and there may be mild malaise.

Biopsies of these lesions show superficial ulceration with a slough of necrotic debris crowded with bacteria; in the deepest parts *B. vincenti* and *F. fusiformis* can be discerned but are difficult to demonstrate clearly against the background of other organisms and debris. The underlying tissue shows an intense inflammatory reaction but no specific features are obvious.

Investigation and Diagnosis

In most cases diagnosis is based on clinical grounds alone and since the clinical picture is usually so well defined and and there are no absolute criteria of diagnosis, this is inevitable. If, however, a swab is taken from the deep part of the superficial slough and stained by Gram's or (better) by Becker's method a heavy predominance of spirochaetes and fusiform bacilli will be seen, *i.e.* the picture is unlike that seen in simple marginal gingivitis or more advanced periodontal disease.

With regard to differential diagnosis, two conditions in particular must be taken into account. Occasionally the ulcers of herpes simplex are concentrated in the region of the gingival margins, and a few of these ulcers may fortuitously be situated at the tip of an interdental papilla. Cases of so-called Vincent's gingivitis in children usually prove to be herpetic infections. Careful examination is likely to show at least a few intact vesicles and that the individual ulcers are circular and spread away from the gingival margin. Characteristically, but not invariably, lymphadenopathy and malaise are also more severe than in Vincent's infection and may be disproportionately severe in relation to the extent of the oral lesions. If there is any doubt a direct smear, together with further virological examinations if needed (as outlined earlier), should clinch the diagnosis.

Another but less common problem is that of acute leukaemia. In acute monocytic leukaemia in particular the gingival margins are swollen as a result of infiltration by leukaemic cells, and may ultimately ulcerate. Gingival swelling is however the early and predominant feature while ulceration, when it develops, is much less precisely localized or defined than in Vincentiform gingivitis. In addition, anaemia is well advanced in those cases of leukaemia where oral ulceration has developed. Haematological examination will clarify this problem.

Management

Having confirmed the diagnosis the essential measure is to clean the mouth by removing the heavy mat of micro-organisms, slough, and calculus. The process is helped by frequent use of a hot mouthwash. In some cases if these measures are carried out meticulously and quickly and the patient maintains an adequate standard of oral hygiene (though this last item is the least likely to be implemented) chemotherapy may prove unnecessary. Metronidazole (200 mg. tablets twice daily on the first day then three times a day for two more days) is the drug of choice (see also Chapter 17) since it is effective, has minimal side effects, and avoids the problems associated with the use of penicillin. Recurrences are not uncommon and are made more likely by the poor standard of oral care of many patients with this disease.

REFERENCES

Cawson, R. A. (1973), "Induction of Epithelial Hyperplasia by *Candida Albicans*," *Brit. J. Derm.*, **89**, 497.

Cawson, R. A. and McSwiggan, D. A. (1969), "An Outbreak of Hand-foot-and-mouth Disease in a Dental Hospital," *Oral Surg.*, **27**, 451.

Cawson, R. A. and Rajasingham, K. C. (1972), "Ultrastructural Features of the Invasive Phase of *Candida Albicans*," *Brit. J. Derm.*, **87**, 435.

Dudgeon, J. A. (1970), *Modern Trends in Medical Virology*, 2nd edition (R. B. Heath and A. P. Waterson, Eds.). London: Butterworths.

Evans, A. D. and Waddington, E. (1967), "Hand, Foot and Mouth Disease in South Wales, 1964," *Brit. J. Derm.*, **79**, 6.

Higgs, J. M. and Wells, R. S. (1973), "Chronic Mucocutaneous Candidiasis: New Approaches to Treatment," *Brit. J. Derm.*, **89**, 179.

Joynson, D. H. M., Murray Walker, D., Jacobs, A. and Dolby, A. E. (1972), "Defect of Cell-mediated Immunity in Patients with Iron-deficiency Anaemia," *Lancet*, **ii**, 1058.

Valdimarsson, H., Higgs, J. M., Wells, R. S., Yamamura, M., Hobbs, J. R. and Holt, P. J. L. (1973), "Immune Abnormalities Associated with Chronic Mucocutaneous Candidiasis," *Cellular Immunology*, **6**, 348.

Watts, J. McK. (1961), "The Importance of the Plummer-Vinson Syndrome in the Aetiology of Carcinoma of the Upper Gastro-Intestinal Tract," *Postgrad. med. J.*, **37**, 523.

SECTION X

SALIVARY GLANDS

SECTION X

42. STRUCTURE AND INNERVATION OF SALIVARY GLANDS

J. R. GARRETT

STRUCTURE OF SALIVARY GLANDS

"Morphology alone is not enough"

Salivary glands are those glands whose secretions enter directly into the oral cavity. In most species there are three main paired glands, parotid, submandibular and sublingual, plus innumerable small mucosal glands distributed around the mouth. The glands show enormous structural and histochemical differences, not only between different species but also between different glands in the same individual and sometimes between similar glands in different individuals of the same species. Such complexities make unified concepts impossible and preclude simple classification according to cell type or function.

Problems of Nomenclature

The glands are composed of acini and ducts and it is commonly believed that the acini form a primary secretion which is secondarily modified in respect to ionic constituents by passage through the ducts, especially the striated ducts. The architectural arrangements of the acini and ducts are variable and most textbooks of histology give indications of the various patterns that occur. The acini which are considered the main secretory elements often have distinctive histological features and most classifications of the glands are based on the appearances of their acini. There have been numerous classifications with subsequent modifications over the years and those not versed in the subject tend to adhere slavishly to a current classification and are unaware that at best it is a poor representation of the truth.

The earliest classifications depended on the morphological appearances of the cells and soon the adjectives "serous" and "mucous" were being applied to the cells. "Serous" was used for parotid acinar cells because they resembled pancreatic cells and their secretions were thin and zymogen-containing. "Mucous" was applied to cells with appearances like the classical mucus-secreting, goblet cells. "Serous" is often rigidly applied to parotid glands but it was known before the turn of the century that many parotid glands contain mucous-like cells (see Langley, 1898). In addition, Bermann had described in 1878 special mucous glands associated with the parotid of man, rabbit, dog, cat, fox and bat, which subsequently have sometimes been spoken of as "Bermann's tubular glands".

The "serous" and "mucous" classification has the charm of simplicity but with the introduction of newer staining techniques it was found that many cells did not conveniently fit into either extreme group. It is now known that mucosubstances vary widely in chemical composition, consisting of protein and carbohydrate components. It is therefore not surprising that mucosubstance staining of similar-looking cells may be very different. Furthermore, staining is affected by fixation and preparation of the tissues and also by the maturity of the mucosubstance contained in individual cells. The history of the subject is well described by Yarington (1972) and the reader seeking more detail is referred to this article.

Salivary cells thus often appear similar unless stained for mucosubstances or for carbohydrate content, as with the periodic acid-Schiff (PAS) reaction. An additional intermediate term "seromucous" has been proposed for cells containing an appreciable amount of neutral and acidic carbohydrate; "mucous" cells being those containing large amounts of acidic carbohydrate and "serous" cells those which contain almost no acidic carbohydrate. This classification was based on alcian blue and colloidal iron staining. By this classification, the parotid glands of carnivores become seromucous as do the submandibular glands of rodents, and the demilunes of feline submandibular glands become "mucous". Later an additional term

enormous variations that are possible (see fig. 3) the mind boggles.

Perhaps the foregoing really means that, as each cell-type in each gland of each species has its own separate identity, only anatomically descriptive terms should be used and always qualified by species. Thus reference would be made

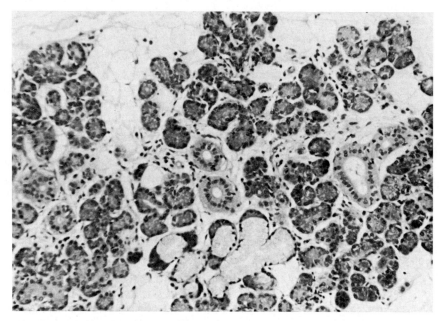

FIG. 1. Human submandibular gland from female of 75, showing acini interspersed with fat cells. A few mixed acini are present but most are of single cell type. Three striated ducts are also seen. Haematoxylin and eosin. × 135.

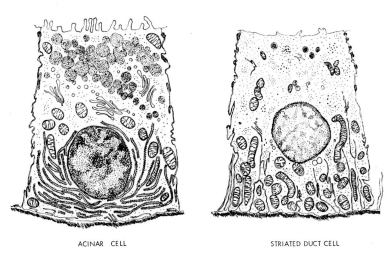

ACINAR CELL   STRIATED DUCT CELL

FIG. 2. Diagrammatic representation of acinar cell and striated duct cell; basal surfaces are associated with basement membrane, below, and luminal surfaces are above. The organelles are described in the text. The secretory granules in the acinar cell may be very variable.

"special serous" was introduced for cells which have little or no detectable mucosubstance, yet differ structurally from other serous cells. And so it will go on, no doubt.

It has been suggested that a classification based on the fine structural appearances of the secretory granules would be more satisfactory than one based on the histochemical affinity for mucosubstance; but when one considers the

to parotid acinar cells of the rat or submandibular central acinar and demilune cells of the cat. Terminology, however, becomes complex in glands such as human labial glands where not only "mixed" acini are found but also "non-mixed" acini not containing mucous cells.

It would seem that at one extreme are the obviously "serous" cells, containing zymogen granules, and at the other extreme are undoubted "mucous" cells, but in between a wide spectrum of possibilities exists.

Despite the problems of nomenclature and classification, an attempt will be made to describe the structure and innervation of the glands in broad general principles and relate them where possible to function.

features common to most salivary glands and will only point to differences where these may assist our understanding.

A recent review by Tandler (1972) provides a valuable basis for this topic.

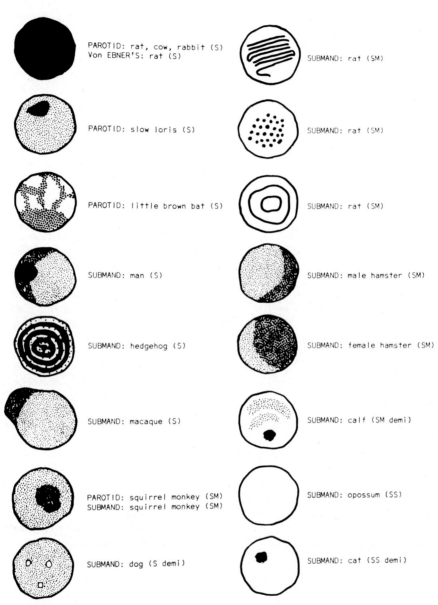

FIG. 3. Diagrammatic representation of a variety of secretory granules. (From Tandler, *Proceedings of Symposium on Salivary Glands and Their Secretions*, 1972, p. 11, University of Michigan, Ann Arbor.) Key (S) = "Serous" Cell, (SM) = "Seromucous" cell, (SS) = "Special Serous" cell, (demi) = demilune.

Epithelial Elements of the Glands

In simple terms the glands are composed of acini, intercalary ducts, striated ducts, collecting and main ducts, and parts of the tubulo-acinar complexes are usually associated with myoepithelial cells. As indicated previously, the detailed arrangement and extent of each element varies between glands. The ensuing account will concentrate on

Acinar Cells

Acinar cells (see fig. 2) are arranged around a lumen and are pyramidal in shape. The luminal surface usually exhibits microvilli. The stromal surface varies from straight in some glands to invaginated in others. The contiguous surfaces between acinar cells also show variable complexities. One or more intercellular canaliculi may be present between adjacent cells as prolongations from the main lumen. Desmosomes and other junctional complexes are found between the cells. These are often considered to create an impermeable barrier between the interstitial extracellular space and the saliva in the lumen, but this view may be too rigid. The possibility that there is a variable leakiness in epithelial junctional complexes, including those containing so-called "tight" junctions, is receiving increasing attention (see later under permeability).

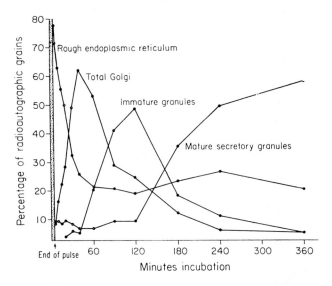

FIG. 4. Incorporation of leucine ³H into parotid acinar secretory protein. *In vitro* preparations of parotid lobules from rabbits, showing wave-like movement of the labelled secretory protein through intracellular compartments. (From Castle, Jamieson, and Palade (1972), *J. Cell. Biol.*, **53**, 308.)

The cytoplasm of the cells contains variable amounts of organelles and, in any one cell, these change with the functional state of the cell. In the basal parts of cells, rough endoplasmic reticulum is arranged in flattened cisterns bounded by a unit membrane which is studded with ribosomes on its cytoplasmic aspect. This is the system by which exportable protein is synthesized. The endoplasmic reticulum is most conspicuous at the stage when the cells are undergoing a phase of resynthesis after secretion and in mucosubstance-secreting cells the cisterns become widely dilated. A Golgi apparatus composed of flattened saccules or vesicles lined by smooth unit membrane is present, often in a supranuclear position. In truly "serous" cells part of this system contains condensing vacuoles for packaging the protein prior to its passage into secretory granules. In mucosubstance-secreting cells the Golgi apparatus becomes prominent at the intermediate stages of resynthesis and is believed to be responsible for processing carbohydrate moieties into the forming secretory material. In the resting cell the apical cytoplasm contains numerous secretory granules, each bounded by a unit membrane. These granules show an amazing variety of ultrastructural appearances (see fig. 3). Presumably some of the sub-structures relate to chemical constituents, possibly enzymes in a sequestered position, and to chemical reactions induced by

fixation. The secretory granules in "mucous" cells are often relatively large, have a tendency to coalesce, and frequently exhibit great variability in their electron density, even within the same cell. In resting cells the secretory granules tend to fill most of the cell, bulging the apical membrane and displacing the nucleus basally.

The cytoplasm of the cells also contains mitochondria in which respiratory enzymes for the cell are situated. A few or more lysosomes are present depending on the cell type and the need for lysosomes at the time the tissue was taken. These membrane-bounded organelles contain arrays of hydrolytic enzymes and are capable of digesting redundant cytoplasmic material; in so doing they help to ensure the continuing viability of the cells rather than the converse, as is popularly believed. In certain circumstances, they may have a role in secretory processes. Lipid droplets are frequently found. They are present in man and have been shown to increase in the parotid of the rat with starvation.

Functional studies have helped our understanding of the synthetic and secretory processes of the acinar cells. Castle, Jamieson and Palade (1972) studied the transport of leucine-³H through the cell and its incorporation into the secretory proteins of parotid acinar cells in rabbits and their results are shown graphically in fig. 4. These findings, in conjunction with similar extensive studies on the pancreas, are taken as evidence for a sequence of events beginning with synthesis of the exportable protein at the attached ribosomes of the rough endoplasmic reticulum. The protein is subsequently passed into a cisternal cavity of the reticulum and then moves to a transitional zone, where it is thought that elements bud-off to become Golgi vesicles. These vesicles ferry their enclosed contents to the next compartment, known as condensing vacuoles, which progressively fill and concentrate their content. In addition, the Golgi complex processes the polysaccharide moieties into the forming secretory granules. Gradually the immature granules become mature granules and reach a position in the apical region of the cell.

Numerous studies have been made on the morphological changes accompanying secretion but large pharmacological doses of secretory drugs have been used to induce secretion and thus some of the findings may represent changes at the extreme limits. Reflexly induced physiological secretion is likely to be a more gentle process. The changes induced by isoprenaline treatment in the parotid of the rat have been summed up diagrammatically by Amsterdam, Ohad and Schramm (1969), as is reproduced here in fig. 5. Secretion was accompanied by a depletion of zymogen granules through fusion of the granule membrane with the lumen membrane and discharge of the contents. The membrane of the zymogen granule once connected with the lumen acted as lumen membrane and this resulted in progressive increase in lumen space. Apposition between cells remained close at the luminal end. It is, however, often found that during secretion the basal part of the intercellular gap increases. After zymogen depletion the luminal size was rapidly reduced; this was believed to occur by withdrawal of luminal membrane, in the form of small, smooth vesicles, into the cytoplasm of the cells. It was considered by these authors that the amount of membrane lost in the lumen

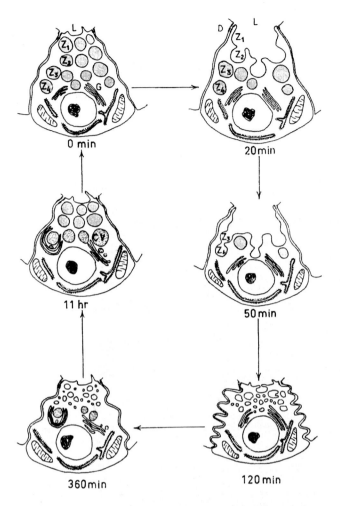

FIG. 5. Diagrammatic representation of sequential changes during secretory cycle induced by isoprenaline in parotid acinar cell of rat. Z_1–Z_4 = Zymogen granules secreted in that order. (From Amsterdam, Ohad and Schramm (1969), *J. Cell Biol.*, **41**, 771.)

was insignificant. However, following simple reflex secretion by this gland, membrane structures lying free in the lumina are a most conspicuous feature and it seems likely that much of the redundant membrane material is lost in the secretion.

In "mucous" cells the process is somewhat different. Sublingual glands of rats treated with pilocarpine and isoproteronol (Kim, Nasjleti and Han, 1972) showed that masses of fused granules and mucus discharged into the lumen through breaks in the apical membrane. Tandler (1970) found that in human labial glands, taken routinely, the contents of the cells were liberated into the lumen by an apocrine process which was sometimes so extensive that the cell failed to reconstruct its apical surface and the whole contents spilled into the lumen.

It should be pointed out that the major fluid production of saliva, water and ions, also occurs at the acini and this may continue after severe depletion of the exportable protein content of the cell. The mechanisms by which the fluid secretion occurs remain obscure.

Enzyme histochemistry of the glands shows great differences between the species (for example, see fig. 6) and between glands in the same species. Such studies do not help in the classification of the glands but it is anticipated that they will be of help for our understanding of secretory processes by individual glands.

Duct Cells

The first duct beyond the acinus is the intercalary duct, which ranges from a few to many cells in length, depending on the species. The cells are usually low cuboidal but may be columnar and they are unspecialized with only a few organelles present; however, they often contain some structures like secretory granules. The intercalary ducts are thought to act principally as conduits without causing much change in the saliva. It is sometimes considered that these

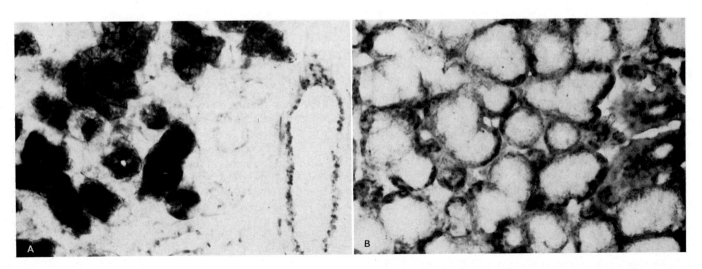

FIG. 6. Sections from submandibular glands showing great differences in histochemical staining for acid-phosphatase (lead method) in different species. × 270. A = Cat in which most of reaction product is diffusely arranged in central acinar cells with little or no staining in demilune cells. Interlobular duct on right shows lysosome-like staining but little is seen in striated ducts between it and acini. B = Dog in which reaction product is in granular lysosome-like staining, most marked in demilune cells; mucous parts of central cells show virtually no staining.

cells are pluripotential and can differentiate into acinar or other parenchymal cells should the need arise.

The striated ducts are next in line (see figs. 2 and 7). These also vary in their length and complexity between glands and species. The cells have complex foldings of their basal membranes with vertically orientated mitochondria within the folds. These features are responsible for the striated appearances seen by light microscopy and hence the name given to the cells. Cells with these characteristics are known to be associated with active transport of electrolytes and micropuncture studies have confirmed this to be so in the

cells may be revealed in some animals, such as the cat, by staining for alkaline phosphatase activity as the reaction product outlines the cells. Basal cells tend to be more common in the collecting ducts. Their function is obscure.

The main ducts receive attention from physiologists because they modify the ionic contents of fluid passing through the lumen, which makes them an interesting model system for studying such phenomena. The morphology of the main ducts has not been studied extensively to date. "Basal", "dark" and "light" cells have been observed in the submandibular duct of the rat; but in the case of the

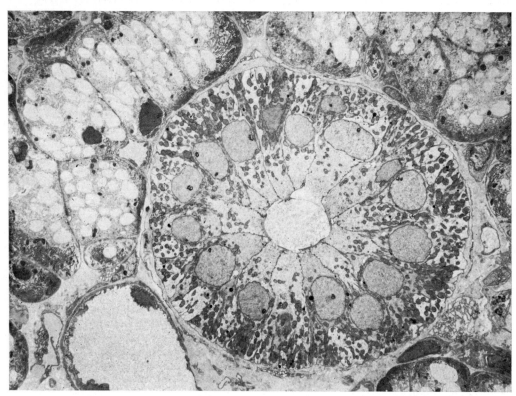

Fig. 7. Electron micrograph of submandibular gland of rabbit showing striated duct surrounded by acini and some capillaries. Note blebbing of one striated duct cell. × 1,700.

case of striated ducts (see Schneyer, Young and Schneyer, 1972). Sodium is resorbed from saliva, and potassium is passed into the saliva. The cells of striated ducts have variable numbers of desmosomes on their adjoining surfaces. Lysosomes are common in striated duct cells and lipofuscin granules are often present in older animals (see fig. 8). In a number of species some granules, looking like secretory granules, are seen in the apical cytoplasm and they tend to stain with PAS. Variable numbers of microvilli are present on the luminal surface and it is not uncommon to find apical blebbing of cytoplasm, which balloons into the lumen (see fig. 7). These blebs are thought to enter the saliva by an apocrine process. In some species the cells are not all of one type and may be described according to electron microscopical appearance as "light" and "dark" cells. The significance of the differences is not understood. In addition, it is not uncommon to find basal duct cells, which are small rounded cells in a basal position. These

rabbit it has been reported that besides the basal cells there is only one population of columnar cells, corresponding to the "light" cells of the rat.

As they approach the oral opening ducts tend to be lined by stratified squamous cells for a short distance. In many ducts, especially in man, scattered goblet cells are found in the main duct and they tend to increase under conditions of chronic inflammation, such as may result from the presence of a calculus. It should be appreciated that in man the luminal diameter of the parotid duct is much narrower than that of the submandibular duct, as is shown by sialography. With age, increasing numbers of oncocytes, special cells loaded with mitochondria, tend to be found in the ducts, particularly in the ducts of mucosal glands in man.

Myoepithelial Cells

Myoepithelial cells (figs. 9 and 10) are muscle-like cells with long tapering processes, which used to be called basket

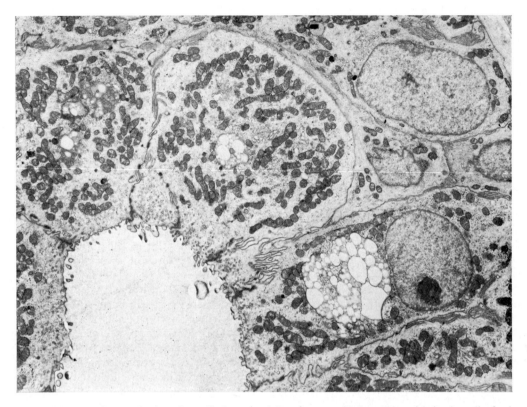

FIG. 8. Electron micrograph of a submandibular striated duct from an elderly male cat showing large lipofuscin granule on luminal side of nucleus in one cell. Parts of lipofuscin granules seen in other cells. × 4,800.

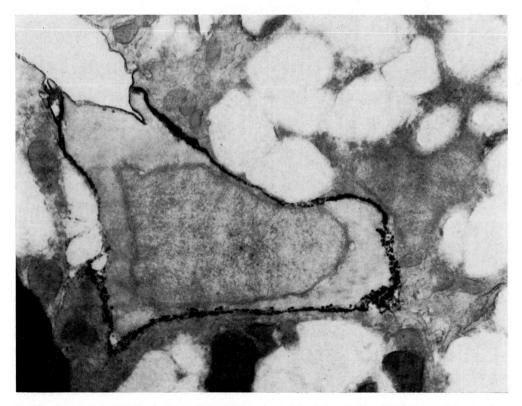

FIG. 9. Electron micrograph of submandibular gland of cat stained for alkaline phosphatase activity showing reaction product outlining surface of myoepithelial cell. × 17,500.

cells. They lie beneath the basement membrane on the outer aspects of parenchymal cells and embrace the under-lying parenchymal structures.

Their existence has been known for a long time but their prominence has only been realized in recent years as a result of modern techniques. The reason for this is that they are not readily identified by conventional microscopy. In many species, these cells contain histochemically detect-able alkaline phosphatase on their plasma membrane which enables them to be seen microscopically. This is not an invariable finding and in the glands of dog and man they show no reaction for alkaline phosphatase; however, in man, but not in the dog, they can be stained histo-chemically by an adenosine triphosphatase reaction. The cells are readily identifiable by conventional electron mi-croscopy and this may be enhanced in appropriate species by pre-staining for alkaline phosphatase (see fig. 9).

The frequency and distribution of myoepithelial cells is variable. In many species they are found around acini, along intercalary ducts, and in some species, such as the cat (see fig. 10), their processes may pass onto the beginnings of the striated ducts. In the parotid glands of rats (see fig. 10) their distribution is unusual and, although they are very dense along the intercalary ducts, the acini only receive processes from myoepithelial cells passing on to the base of the acinus but not embracing its outer surface.

bodies. Lipid droplets are sometimes seen. The myo-epithelial cells are hardy and withstand the atrophy induced by ligation, but end up with a bizarre architecture because of the underlying loss of parenchymal tissue, and thereafter they often contain increased lipid and also lipofuscin granules.

The cells are generally considered to be contractile. Pressure changes induced in the main duct by single-impulse nerve stimulation support this belief (Emmelin, Garrett and Ohlin, 1968, 1969) and these studies indicate that myoepithelial cells may remain contracted during secretion. Very high pressures can be induced without secre-tion by bradykinin in the dog. In the dog, it is possible to dissociate sympathetic myoepithelial activity from secre-tion, by the use of appropriate blocking agents. Such manoeuvres show that when myoepithelial cells are in-hibited the onset of salivary flow is delayed and, despite continuing secretion, only a low pressure is induced in the pressure system (Emmelin and Gjörstrup, 1973). This last feature must mean that myoepithelial activity helps to pre-vent back permeation of saliva into the gland if any obstruction to flow occurs.

The physiological role of the myoepithelial cells is not known exactly. They are not found in the pancreas, and thus are not essential for all exocrine secretory processes. Contraction of the myoepithelial cells may help to expel

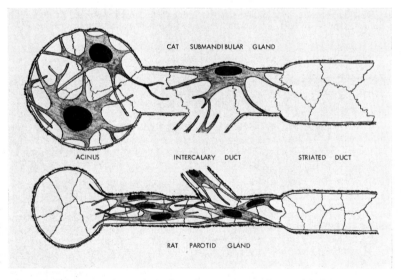

FIG. 10. Diagrammatic representation of arrangement of myoepithelial cells in cat submandibular gland (above) and rat parotid gland (below). Myoepithelial cells are shaded.

Ultrastructurally, their cytoplasm is similar in appearance to smooth muscle and immunofluorescent studies have shown that they contain a smooth-muscle actomyosin. Myofilaments are present particularly in the basal parts of their cytoplasm. Numerous vesicles and caveolae are present along the basal surface; they are somewhat less frequent on surfaces adjacent to secretory cells but some desmosomes are present here. The non-filamentous parts of the cell contain mitochondria, scattered elements of endoplasmic reticulum, Golgi complexes and lysosome-like

pre-existing saliva; it will also shorten luminal distance and thereby help secretory efficiency. They may have a role in supporting underlying structures against undue disten-sion which the secretion might otherwise induce. In addi-tion their contraction may help to express apocrine-type secretion from underlying cells. The unusual arrangement in the parotid of the rat may impart rigidity to the inter-calary ducts and also bring the acinar lumen over that of the intercalary duct, thereby aiding the passage of saliva.

Sexual Dimorphism of Glandular Structure

In the submandibular glands of adult mice there is a pronounced difference between males and females; the former have a greater preponderance of granular tubules, and their cells are more heavily loaded with granules. Since this was first described many other examples of sexual dimorphism in the structure of salivary glands have been identified, mainly in lower mammals and none as dramatic as in the mouse. A report has recently been published of sexual dimorphism to mucosubstance staining in the submandibular glands of miniature pigs, despite similar morphological appearances; unlike previously described examples, these differences occur before puberty. It is possible that sexual differences exist in the mucosubstance content of glands in higher mammals, but objective studies have yet to be done on this interesting possibility.

Stromal Elements in the Glands

The epithelial structures in the glands are separated and supported by connective tissue which contains blood vessels, lymphatics and numerous cells, all of which contribute to the functional integrity of the gland. Nerves are another important component and will be considered in a later section.

Blood Vessels

The glands are richly vascular. Secretion is dependent on a good blood supply; the flow of blood is greatly increased during secretory activity and secretion rapidly ceases if the blood circulation is obstructed. One or more arteries enter the gland and give rise to numerous arterioles which tend to follow the ducts in a counter-current direction and finally break up into numerous thin-walled capillaries. The distribution of capillaries is dense around the striated ducts and somewhat less dense around the acini. Collecting veins tend to follow the ducts and often more than one vein takes the effluent blood from the gland. In some glands, arterio-venous shunts are thought to exist but the subject is debated and their function is ill understood.

Lymphatics

Lymphatics are known to accompany the main vessels of the glands but little is known about their existence within the glands. There have been few studies on factors influencing their activity since the classical studies of Bainbridge who showed that there was an increased lymph flow accompanying secretion and also when the veins were obstructed. In human glands removed for inflammatory conditions, it is not uncommon to see dilated lymphatics around larger ducts within the glands. It is often difficult to identify the lymphatic vessels with certainty; but this is facilitated when per-arterial fixation is used, for, by this procedure, the blood vessels are washed out and the lymphatics remain full of coagulated lymph (see fig. 11). Using this technique it appears that the lymphatics within the gland are more prominent during secretion. It has been found in dogs that the marker protein, horseradish peroxidase, when injected via Wharton's duct, quickly appears within lymphatic channels.

Plasma Cells

Plasma cells (fig. 12) are a regular component of the interstitial tissues of salivary glands. The number present varies with the species and the gland. They are conspicuous in many of the mucosal glands of man. In the cat they are readily demonstrable by histochemical staining for non-specific esterase which shows that they are most abundant in the sublingual gland, somewhat less numerous in the parotid gland and least plentiful in the submandibular gland. Immunocytochemical staining shows that most salivary plasma cells contain IgA-type immunoglobulin. The IgA of

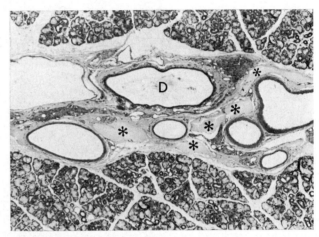

FIG. 11. Submandibular gland of cat after perfusion fixation during secretory activity, showing prominent lymphatics (*), containing coagulated lymph, adjacent to the main intraglandular duct (D). Blood vessels are empty. × 39.

the saliva is derived essentially from locally situated plasma cells. Factors inducing specific antibody secretion by these cells and the mechanisms whereby they localize in the glands are not yet understood. In its passage to the mouth, IgA becomes coupled with "secretory component" which is formed and secreted by certain cells in the glands. It is generally considered that an IgA pool exists in the interstitium of the glands and IgA molecules are selectively taken up and passed through secretory cells where they are coupled to "secretory component" before final passage into saliva. However, in view of the fact that, under certain circumstances, a permeability between glandular epithelial cells to proteins can occur (see later) it is wondered whether this may be a route of passage for IgA into saliva. The secretory IgA has a role in immunological protective mechanisms for the mucosa and presumably it also has a role in the defensive mechanisms of the gland itself.

Other Inflammatory Cells

It is not uncommon to find occasional small lymphocytic foci in the glands of man and experimental animals. They probably have a role in the normal protective mechanisms of the gland. Whether they are involved in induction of IgA-secreting plasma cells is not known. Under certain circumstances the number of lymphocytic foci becomes greatly increased and the condition is then described as focal lymphadenitis.

Occasional macrophages and polymorphonuclear leucocytes are often found in the glands and it is thought that they are involved in protective mechanisms aiding the maintenance of a normal *milieu*. They are found in very increased numbers after intra-glandular mucus extravasation caused by duct ligation and it is thought that they aid the removal of this extraneous material. Under physiological conditions it is possible that muscular obstruction may sometimes cause back permeation of saliva and at such times influxes of these inflammatory cells would play a protective role.

Morphological Studies on Glandular Permeability

It is generally considered that junctional complexes between adjoining epithelial cells in salivary glands create impermeable barriers to the passage of water and solutes. However, an increased permeability to certain sugars was found to occur in some glands during adrenergic stimulation which could only be explained by postulating diffusion through intercellular gaps.

The movement of a marker protein, horseradish peroxidase, is being used to pursue this problem. By harnessing

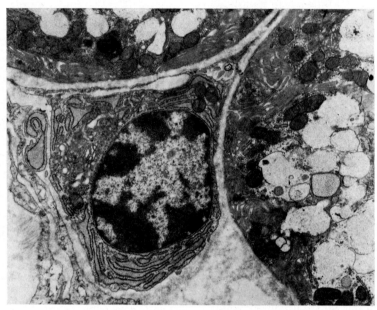

Fig. 12. Electron micrograph of submandibular gland from cat showing plasma cell lying between demilunar cells. Note cisterns of endoplasmic reticulum throughout cytoplasm of plasma cell and prominent Golgi saccules to left of nucleus. × 8,700.

Fibroblasts and Fat Cells

A matrix of collagen fibres is found around and between the parenchymal elements of the gland. Interspersed throughout the stroma are fibroblasts, sometimes with very long thin extensions. These cells presumably maintain the healthy architecture of the collagenous scaffolding in normal glands. At times of inflammation the fibroblasts tend to take on a more reactive form; the organelles increase, the rough endoplasmic reticulum becomes more prominent and they start actively laying down collagen. This is particularly prevalent in infective inflammatory conditions of the glands. The amount of collagen also tends to become much increased as a consequence of irradiation.

Fat cells (see fig. 1) are a common feature in the stroma of salivary glands. There are species and glandular differences and they are often most evident in parotid glands, especially in the rabbit. Glandular fat cells tend to show an increase with age. In man they are regularly found to some extent in submandibular and parotid glands, even in children. It sometimes seems that mild slow atrophy of the parenchyma leads to a replacement by fat cells but more rapid atrophy ends up with replacement by collagen, and intermediate gradations are possible.

the peroxidatic activity of this protein histochemically it is possible to produce a reaction product that can be seen at light and electron microscopical levels, thereby giving fine details of the sites of passage of the protein. Preliminary results indicate that horseradish peroxidase, with a molecular weight of approximately 40,000, is capable of passing between striated duct cells from the interstitium to the saliva in submandibular glands of rabbits.

No doubt species and glandular differences will be found in intercellular permeabilities. Many factors, including molecular size, lipid solubility, electrostatic charge, and tendency to bind with membranes or other proteins, will all affect the ability of any solute to diffuse between the cells. Nevertheless, potential spaces permitting permeability do exist between some salivary cells and it seems likely that neural and other activities may be able to modify the junctional complexes, thus allowing a greater or lesser permeability.

INNERVATION OF SALIVARY GLANDS

The importance of nerves for salivary secretion first became evident when, in 1851, Ludwig showed that stimulation of the chordalingual nerve in dogs caused a copious secretion of saliva from the submandibular gland. He also showed that the pressure of secretion would exceed the blood pressure and thus the process could not be a simple ultra-filtration.

Claude Bernard, probably the greatest physiologist of the nineteenth century, soon became involved in investigating the role of nerves in salivary secretion. He developed his ideas at lecture demonstrations in front of students and subsequently the lectures were beautifully written into book form in the mid-nineteenth century. He was aware of the reflex nature of secretion and not only studied the effects of stimulating cut nerves but also the effects of nerve section on reflex secretion induced by placing sapid substances on the tongue. By these means, the efferent nerve pathways to submandibular and parotid glands were mapped out and the pathways taught today are largely as Bernard described them. He showed that the parasympathetic nerves for the submandibular gland originated in the facial nerve, passed in the chorda tympani to join the lingual nerve and finally passed back to the gland as a distinct nerve travelling with the duct. He described how the parasympathetic supply to the parotid came via the lesser superficial petrosal nerve to the otic ganglion and finally through the auriculo-temporal

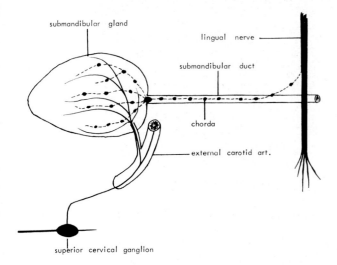

Fig. 13. Diagrammatic representation of autonomic nerve pathways to submandibular gland of cat. Sympathetic nerves = ———. Parasympathetic nerves = – – –●– – –, with swellings to represent ganglia within and without the gland. Distribution of nerves is similar in other animals if allowance be made for anatomical variations in position of the gland.

nerve, but he was in error in thinking that pre-ganglionic nerves came from the facial nerve for it is now known that they originate in the glossopharyngeal nerve. Bernard observed that stimulation of parasympathetic nerves caused a vasodilatation in the gland, but sympathetic stimulation caused a vasoconstriction; he also realized that normally there is sympathetic vasoconstrictor tone in the glands since section of these nerves caused a vasodilatation.

Many other workers became interested in the field and knowledge of the subject was amazingly extensive by the turn of the century, as was admirably recorded in a classical account by Langley in 1898.

Progress was less rapid during the next 50 years but attempts were made to generalize and simplify and to put salivary innervation on a simple conceptual basis. This was summed up in 1950 by Babkin who considered that in submandibular glands the parasympathetic nerves supply "mucous" cells and blood vessels, and sympathetic nerves supply blood vessels, "serous" cells and myoepithelial cells; a concept that is still often taught today. However, physiological studies had progressed beyond morphology, which had been stagnant for some time, and physiologists were beginning to challenge the Babkin concept (see Burgen and Emmelin, 1961). It was realized that parasympathetic nerves were largely responsible for the volume output of the glands and evidence indicated that all secretory cells had a cholinergic innervation while some, but not all cells, had an adrenergic innervation as well.

By the late 1950s the new techniques of histochemistry and electron microscopy were beginning to be used for morphological reassessment of the innervation of salivary glands, and a new era had started. As a consequence this subject has moved out of a period of simplicity into one of great complexity and it will require new thinking to establish where patterns of order lie.

Most of the glands depend on autonomic nerves to evoke secretion but some, such as the sublingual gland of the cat, can secrete "spontaneously" in the absence of nerve impulses; nevertheless, the greater part of salivary flow from these glands is still a nerve-mediated function. There is strong evidence that the parasympathetic neuro-transmitter in the glands is acetylcholine and the sympathetic transmitter is noradrenaline. No evidence exists for non-adrenergic non-cholinergic nerves in salivary secretory activity.

A general description of the present state of knowledge must suffice in this chapter; for greater detail the reader is referred to two recent reviews (Garrett, 1972, 1973).

Morphological Methods for Studying Autonomic Nerves

A. *NEUROHISTOLOGICAL TECHNIQUES*

(1) LIGHT MICROSCOPICAL HISTOCHEMISTRY—for the general distribution and relative density of the nerves.

(a) ACETYLCHOLINESTERASE (AChE)—to show principally, but not necessarily exclusively, cholinergic nerves (see fig. 14).

(b) CATECHOLAMINE FLUORESCENCE—to show adrenergic nerves (see fig. 14).

(2) ELECTRON MICROSCOPY—for details of innervation sites (figs. 15–18).

(a) CONVENTIONAL ELECTRON MICROSCOPY.

(b) CYTOCHEMICAL METHODS—to distinguish cholinergic and adrenergic axons.

B. *TISSUES EXAMINED*

(1) NORMAL CONTROLS.

(2) DENERVATED PREPARATIONS.

(a) For early degenerative changes (see fig. 18).

(b) For nerves remaining after denervation.

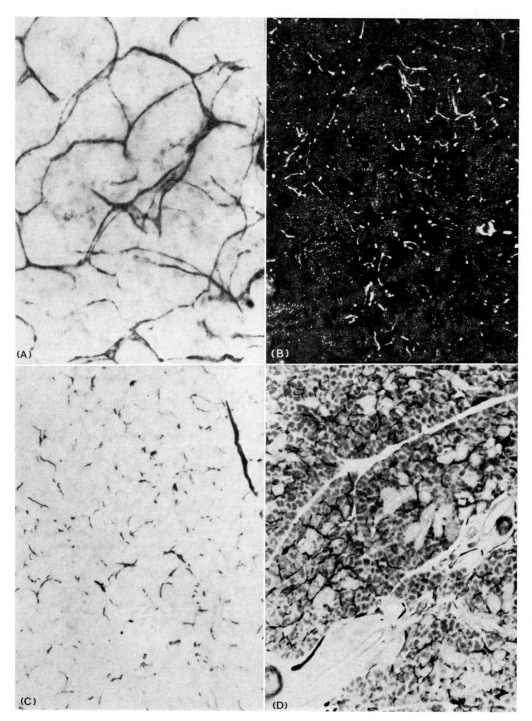

FIG. 14. Light microscopical histochemistry of nerves in salivary glands. (A) Submandibular gland of cat showing dense arborizations of AChE-positive nerve around acini. × 300. (B) Submandibular gland of cat showing formaldehyde induced fluorescence of adrenergic nerves which are most dense around blood vessels; also alongside acini and striated ducts. Ducts also contain non-specific fluorescent granules, possibly caused by lysosomes and lipofuscin granules. × 120. (C) Parotid gland of cat showing less dense innervation by AChE-positive nerves. × 120. (D) Submandibular gland from man showing AChE-positive nerves; density of nerves between that of submandibular and parotid glands of cat. Few positive nerves along collecting ducts. × 48.

General Findings

(1) Light Microscopy (fig. 14). As far as they have been tested the parasympathetic ganglia for the glands appear to be pure cholinergic ganglia in the old-fashioned sense, composed of cells with uniformly strong AChE activity and devoid of adrenergic elements. It should be mentioned that in many other systems the parasympathetic ganglia are now known to be much more mixed and complex.

AChE-positive nerves show very variable distributions in the glands. They tend to be more prolific than the adrenergic nerves. Usually they course back with the ducts and break down into complex arborizations around the acini. The overall density of AChE-positive nerves varies from gland to gland and species to species. Thus, vast numbers are found in the submandibular gland of the cat whereas relatively few are present in its parotid gland. In man the number is similar for both the submandibular and parotid glands, being somewhat between the extremes found in the cat.

Adrenergic nerves tend to enter the gland with the artery and course with the vessels. They also show a very variable distribution in different glands; for example, many adrenergic nerves are present in the submandibular gland of the rat but there are very few in its sublingual gland. In man the number in the parotid and submandibular glands is relatively similar.

(2) Electron Microscopy (figs. 15–18). Electron microscopy shows that the main nerve trunks entering the glands are composed predominantly of non-myelinated axons but some myelinated axons are also present; the latter are either pre-ganglionic nerves or afferent nerves. The non-myelinated axons are associated with Schwann cells. One or more axons lie in invaginations of the Schwann cell surface, thereby forming a Schwann–axon bundle which is surrounded by its own basement membrane. Although the cholinergic axons and adrenergic axons tend to reach the glands by separate routes, once inside the gland they cross and intermingle and it is common to find mixed axons in any one Schwann–axon bundle (see fig. 17). The Schwann cells are in end-to-end contact and are best thought of as a sort of scaffolding on which the axons can run in the interstices of the gland until they reach their ultimate destination.

Two types of neuro-effector site are found in salivary glands:

*(i) **"Interstitial"**, where an axon containing vesicles and running with a Schwann cell has a free surface adjacent to a salivary cell but lies outside its basement membrane and is separated by a gap of approximately 100 nm. (see figs. 15 and 17).

*(ii) **"Epithelial"**, where an axon containing vesicles lies beneath the basement membrane in intimate contact with

---

* Since writing this chapter the author's attention has been drawn to an article by Arnstein (1895, *Anat. Anz.* **10**, 410–419) in which neuro-effector relationships in salivary glands were classified as:

  EPILEMMAL if the axon remained outside the epithelial basement membrane,
  HYPOLEMMAL if the axon penetrated beneath the epithelial basement membrane.

These terms are now preferred to "Interstitial" and "Epithelial" used in the text or other terms in current use.

---

the adjacent salivary cells, and is separated by a gap of 20 nm. or less. This type of neuro-effector site has sometimes been called "intra-acinar" but it is now known that they can sometimes occur in "intra-ductal" sites as well; for this reason, the general term "epithelial" is preferred (see figs. 16 and 17).

The axonal vesicles vary depending on whether they are in cholinergic or adrenergic nerves. In cholinergic axons, most vesicles are clear agranular vesicles of about 40 nm. diameter and are thought to contain acetylcholine, but a few larger vesicles of about 80 nm. diameter and containing a dense core are also found. In adrenergic axons the small vesicles of about 40 nm. diameter contain a dense core which may be intensified for electron microscopical detection by pretreatment with the false transmitter 5-hydroxydopamine (5-0HDA). Adrenergic axons also contain some larger granular vesicles of about 80 nm. diameter. At innervation sites, it is not uncommon to find mitochondria in the axons as well. It is usually considered that when an impulse passes down the axon neuro-transmitter is released from the vesicles by a process of exocytosis. The activation of the adjacent effector cell will depend on the quantum of neuro-transmitter released, the closeness between the axon and effector site and the sensitivity of the effector cell membrane. No ultrastructural specialization has been found on the parenchymal side of neuro-effector sites in salivary glands.

It is unlikely that a single axon gives rise to a single neuro-effector site but probably any one axon can activate a number of cells on route before it physically terminates. Convergence of more than one axon on the same effector cell is not rare.

Some degree of electrotonic spread of activation may pass from cell to cell but there is little information on this possibility.

Beading is often associated with axons at sites that contain the most vesicles, both in "epithelial" or "interstitial" situations. It is not known whether the beading is static or, as seems highly possible, constantly moving in a peristaltic manner. If this be the case, then, it would seem that the activation site of salivary effector cells may also be constantly moving to some degree.

The type of effector site found, "interstitial", "epithelial" or mixed, varies widely between species, glands, cell types and nerve types. No self-evident pattern of order seems to exist with respect to the cell type or nerve type but presumably each gland has the right innervation for its own requirements.

Acinar Innervation

In most glands the density of nerves is greatest around the acini. The extent of the innervation of acinar cells differs enormously between glands and species. The age of the animal may also affect the picture since the number of "epithelial" axons decreases with age in some glands.

In the submandibular gland of the cat cholinergic "epithelial" axons occur adjacent to and between central acinar cells, but "epithelial" axons have not been found in association with demilune cells; these appear to receive their innervation by "interstitial" axons and in the cat parotid

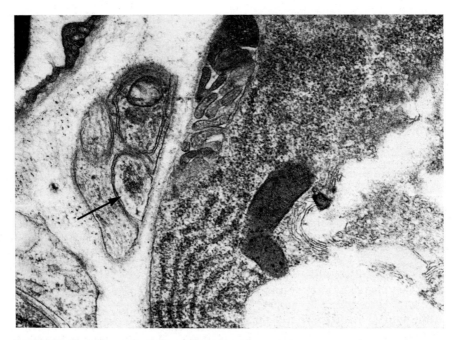

FIG. 15. Electron micrograph of submandibular gland from rabbit showing "interstitial" innervation site. Schwann-axon bundle shows one cholinergic axon (↑), containing agranular small vesicles, with free surface in relatively close proximity to adjacent acinar cell. "Interstitial" axons appear to be only type of innervation for acinar cells in the rabbit. × 33,300.

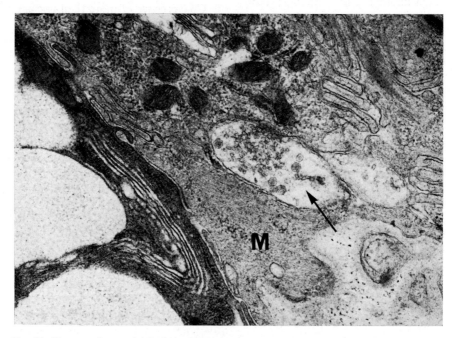

FIG. 16. Electron micrograph of submandibular gland from rabbit showing "epithelial" innervation site. Cholinergic axon (↑) containing agranular vesicles lies between granular tubule cell and myoepithelial cell (M). Acinar cell adjacent to other side of myoepithelial cell. × 33,300.

only "interstitial" axons have been observed. Contrasting with this, in rats only "interstitial" axons have been detected in submandibular glands whereas their parotid acini abound with "epithelial" axons.

"Epithelial" axons are mostly cholinergic but in the parotid gland of the rat and the rabbit many of the intra-acinar axons are adrenergic, and it is not rare to find a parotid acinar cell intimately associated with both an adrenergic and a cholinergic axon. Thus it is reasonable to assume that these cells receive a truly double innervation.

produce sympathetic saliva rich in amylase and parasympathetic saliva poor in amylase. Since the individual cells appear to have a dual innervation, it is likely that the neurotransmitter from the different nerves evokes different reactions from the same cells. Although something is known about the membrane changes accompanying neuroactivation virtually nothing is known about how these changes in the membrane bring about the complex chain of events in the cell from which secretion results, let alone how differences can occur in the same cell.

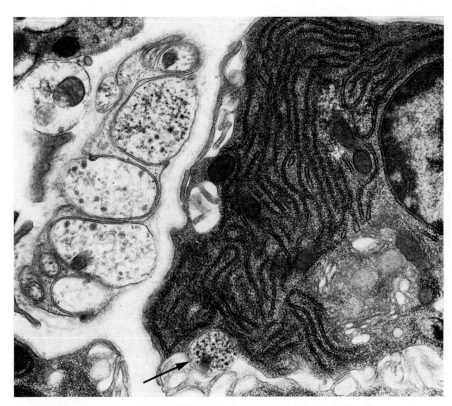

FIG. 17. Electron micrograph of parotid gland from rat showing both types of innervation site. Animal pretreated with 5-OHDA to enhance granular vesicles of adrenergic nerves. Adrenergic and cholinergic axon are in "interstitial" relationship with acinar cell; "epithelial" adrenergic axon (↑) also present beneath basement membrane. Cholinergic "epithelial" axons also exist in this gland. × 20,800.

Most workers have been unable to find "epithelial" axons in the major glands of man, but it is possible that this may reflect an age effect for tissue has usually been taken from older subjects. However, many "epithelial" axons have been found in human labial glands.

The relative roles of parasympathetic and sympathetic nerves in salivary secretory processes is still debated. It is usually found that parasympathetic stimulation causes a voluminous output of saliva. On the other hand, sympathetic stimulation may cause no overt secretion or, if it does, it is usually less voluminous than parasympathetic saliva but may contain a much higher organic content. Where documented, sympathetic and parasympathetic salivas have always shown qualitative differences. In mixed glands the possibility must always be considered that the different nerves are causing different cell populations to secrete. However, the monomorphic acini in parotid glands of rats

Nerve stimulation studies are extremely informative, albeit somewhat artificial; ultimately it is desirable to understand the respective roles of the different nerves in normal reflex secretory processes. Sometimes it is questioned whether sympathetic nerves have any role in reflex secretion. Recent experiments by Hodgson and Speirs (1974) give strong evidence for participation by sympathetic nerves in normal reflex secretion by parotid glands in rats. After unilateral section of the pre-ganglionic cervical sympathetic trunk, although reflex secretion was not inhibited, eating a solid diet caused little or no fall in glandular amylase, whereas on the side with intact innervation the usual big reduction in amylase content occurred.

In many glands, including those in which sympathetic stimulation does not cause saliva to flow, it is possible that the sympathetic impulses may modify the contents of the saliva being produced by parasympathetic activity. Thereby salivary constituents may be altered in relation to the type of food being eaten through reflex activity.

There are no obvious reasons for the wide differences in innervation patterns of different salivary glands. More needs to be known about normal flow rates, the contents of the saliva and the normal physiological requirements put upon the various glands.

Ductal Innervation

Innervation of the intralobular ducts is variable and tends to be less abundant than that of the acini. In most species, cholinergic axons are seen alongside striated ducts and occasionally are found beneath their basement membrane, as in the rabbit. "Epithelial" cholinergic axons tend to be found more often in intercalary ducts but this again is variable.

Adrenergic innervation of the intralobular ducts tends to be less extensive and in some species, such as the rat, adrenergic nerves have not been found alongside the striated

Extralobular ducts often have a variable loose association with cholinergic nerves but their role is not known. No adrenergic nerves have ever been detected along extra-lobular ducts.

Myoepithelial Innervation

Axons of either type are frequently found adjacent to myoepithelial cells, in an "interstitial" location, and convergence of more than one axon on the same cell is not rare. Where "epithelial" axons occur in acini they are often found lying between a myoepithelial cell and an adjacent acinar cell (see fig. 16). Thus, their innervation may be of the intimate or less intimate type depending on the gland or cells with which the myoepithelial cell is associated. Nevertheless, where tested they usually show a single impulse response, whether the innervation be "interstitial" or "epithelial", which would suggest that these cells have a high sensitivity for the neuro-transmitter. It is generally believed that myoepithelial cells are stimulated to contract by

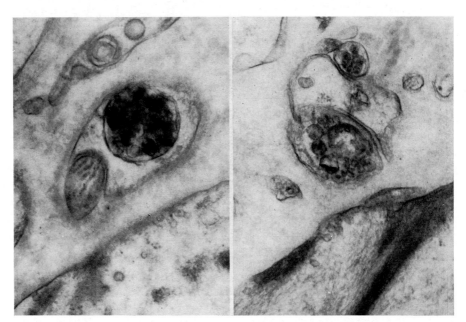

FIG. 18. Electron micrograph of parotid gland from dog, 48 hours after section of auriculo-temporal nerve, showing characteristic osmiophilic degenerative changes in axons adjacent to arteriolar smooth muscle cells thus confirming existence of parasympathetic vascular nerves. Illustrations are of different parts of same Schwann-axon bundle in adjacent sections and show that the degenerative changes are not uniform along the axons. × 43,300. (Garrett and Holmberg, previously unpublished observation.)

ducts. However, in a number of species, man included, adrenergic axons lie adjacent to striated ducts and in the rabbit they have even been found beneath the basement membrane of striated ducts.

Little is known about the role of nerves in striated duct function but the morphological evidence indicates that, if they can be influenced by neuro-transmitters, then nerves are present that can affect the cells. However, the nerves are rarely as frequent as to suggest that every cell has an innervation and, thus, electrotonic spread of activation may have a role.

adrenergic nerves and this is certainly the case in the dog, but in the cat the evidence for such is at best equivocal. Pressure studies support the belief that the myoepithelial cells are contracted by cholinergic axons in both species.

Vascular Innervation

Normally impulses in sympathetic nerves keep the glandular blood vessels in a state of vasoconstrictor tone; blockage of the sympathetic impulses causes a vasodilatation in the gland and stimulation of the nerves induces a vasoconstriction.

Bernard found that parasympathetic stimulation caused vasodilatation in the glands. However, the concept that this vasodilatation is caused by direct nerve mediation has been challenged and some workers consider that the vasodilatation is produced by a kallikrein release of bradykinin.

Morphological evidence, be it from denervation degeneration (see fig. 18), nerves persisting after denervation, or selective marking of adrenergic nerves by 5-OHDA, indicates that the muscular blood vessels in the glands receive an "interstitial" type of innervation of their outer muscle cells by both cholinergic and adrenergic axons, although the latter are usually present in greater numbers. Recent work shows that there is in fact a rapid nerve-mediated vasodilatation and this may be followed by a more sustained bradykinin vasodilation.

Axons of either sort are often seen in close proximity to capillary endothelial cells. Their role is not understood but it seems likely that if these cells can be activated by neurotransmitters then they are influenced by these nerves.

Revised Views on Nerve Pathways to Parotid Glands

Doubts have been cast over the years about the source and course of parasympathetic nerves for the parotid glands (see Babkin, 1950). Recently the subject has been reassessed in dogs by Holmberg (1972, a and b) using Bernard-like methods of cutting nerves and studying the effects of stimulating them for maximal secretory responses, and also by assessing changes induced by nerve section on maximal reflex secretion caused by citric acid on the tongue in animals coming round from light anaesthesia. He also studied the effects of nerve degeneration on the glandular content of choline acetyltransferase, which is the acetylcholine synthesizing enzyme in axons, and the denervation studies were backed up by light microscopical histochemical assessment of the nerves remaining in the gland. By these means Holmberg found that the vast majority, and sometimes perhaps all, of the pre-ganglionic nerves travel in the tympanic branch of the glosso-pharyngeal nerve and thereafter most nerves pass to, or are associated with, the main trunk of the mandibular nerve. After relay, presumably in the otic ganglion, which was too inaccessible for removal in recovery experiments, the nerves take a variable course. Some, but by no means all the post-ganglionic nerves, pass in the anatomically defined auriculo-temporal nerve. Other secretory fibres travel in branches which pass to the internal maxillary artery and then run with the artery in a direction counter-current to blood flow to reach the gland. A diagrammatic representation of these findings is shown in fig. 19. Interestingly, the secretory nerves passing with the internal maxillary artery were known to Bernard in 1879 but this information remained in obscurity until unearthed by Holmberg; these nerves should perhaps be called "Bernard's nerves". Besides the nerves passing with the artery and those in the auriculo-temporal nerve, Holmberg also found some secretory fibres in the facial nerve. However, despite extensive surgery involving sectioning of all these known secretory nerve pathways, a small number of nerves persisted; it seems therefore impossible to denervate completely the parotid gland of the dog and the source of the remaining nerves remains unknown.

Afferent Nerves

Glandular pain fibres undoubtedly exist and anyone who has suffered from obstructive episodes or even sialography is well aware of their presence. Little is known about the morphology of these nerves. Sensory endings have been described in association with the main ducts and they may also exist in the glands; their axons are thought to course in the main parasympathetic and sympathetic nerve trunks for the glands. It is also believed that sensory endings exist in the capsules of the glands and their nerves course with the somatic nerves supplying the area.

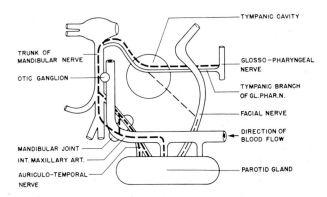

FIG. 19. Diagrammatic representation of parasympathetic nerve pathways to parotid gland of the dog. (From Holmberg, *M.D. Thesis*, 1972, Lund.)

Afferent impulses travelling from the submandibular gland in the chorda have been studied electrophysiologically in dogs. It has been shown that spontaneous activity is present and is greatly enhanced by increasing the pressure in the submandibular duct and this is thought to operate via baroreceptors in the gland.

CONCLUSION

Great strides have been made in recent years with structural studies of salivary glands and their innervation and, as a consequence, scientific understanding of the subject has improved. Aspects of recent advances have been discussed in this chapter but reference to the history of the subject has also been made as a reminder of the extent of knowledge long ago. Acquaintance with the history of a subject helps to prevent the repetition of mistakes. Recent work has answered some questions and posed many more to add to the long list of those unanswered. The field is wide open for further investigation.

REFERENCES

Amsterdam, A., Ohad, I. and Schramm, M. (1969), "Dynamic Changes in the Ultrastructure of the Acinar Cell of the Rat Parotid Gland During the Secretory Cycle," *J. Cell Biol.*, **41**, 753.
Babkin, B. P. (1950), *Secretory Mechanism of the Digestive Glands*, 2nd edition. New York: Hoeber.
Burgen, A. S. V. and Emmelin, N. G. (1961), *Physiology of the Salivary Glands*. Monographs of the Physiological Society, No. 8. London: Arnold.

Castle, J. D., Jamieson, J. D. and Palade, G. E. (1972), "Radio-autographic Analysis of the Secretory Process in the Parotid Acinar Cell of the Rabbit," *J. Cell Biol.*, **53**, 290.

Emmelin, N., Garrett, J. R. and Ohlin, P. (1968), "Neural Control of Salivary Myoepithelial Cells," *J. Physiol.*, **196**, 381.

Emmelin, N., Garrett, J. R. and Ohlin, P. (1969), "Motor Nerves of Salivary Myoepithelial Cells in Dogs," *J. Physiol.*, **200**, 539.

Emmelin, N. and Gjörstrup, P. (1973), "On the Function of Myo-epithelial Cells in Salivary Glands," *J. Physiol.*, **230**, 185.

Garrett, J. R. (1972), "Neuro-effector Sites in Salivary Glands," in *Oral Physiology*, p. 83 (N. Emmelin and Y. Zotterman, Eds.). Oxford: Pergamon.

Garrett, J. R. (1973), "Innervation of Salivary Glands. Morpho-logical Considerations," in *Secretory Mechanisms of Exocrine Glands*. Alfred Benzon Symposium, VII. (N. A. Thorn and O. H. Peterson, Eds.). Copenhagen: Munksgaard.

Hodgson, C. and Speirs, R. L. (1974), "The Effect of Preganglionic Cervical Sympathectomy on the Amylase Content of Parotid Glands in Fasted and Fed Rats," *J. Physiol.*, **237**, 56P.

Holmberg, J. (1972a), "On the Nerves to the Parotid Gland," in *Oral Physiology*, p. 17 (N. Emmelin and Y. Zotterman, Eds.). Oxford: Pergamon.

Holmberg, J. (1972b), "Secretory Innervation of the Dog's Parotid Gland," M.D. Thesis, Lund.

Kim, S. K., Nasjleti, C. E. and Han, S. S. (1972), "The Secretion Processes in Mucous and Serous Secretory Cells of the Rat Sub-lingual Gland," *J. Ultrastruct. Res.*, **38**, 371.

Langley, J. N. (1898), "The Salivary Glands," in *Textbook of Physi-ology*, Vol. 1, p. 475 (E. A. Schaefer, Ed.). Edinburgh: Young J. Pentland.

Schneyer, L. H., Young, J. A. and Schneyer, C. A. (1972), "Salivary Secretion of Electrolytes," *Physiol. Rev.*, **52**, 720.

Tandler, B. (1972), "Microstructure of Salivary Glands," in *Proceed-ings of Symposium on Salivary Glands and Their Secretions*, p. 8. (N. H. Rowe, Ed.) Ann Arbor: University of Michigan.

Yarington, C. T. (1972), "Diversity of Mucus Staining Characteristics of Human Salivary Glands," *Laryngoscope*, **82**, 2103.

43. SALIVARY SECRETION

C. DAWES

Types of salivary gland

Methods for collection of human saliva
   Whole saliva
   Parotid saliva
   Submandibular and sublingual saliva
   Minor glands
   Stimulated saliva

Factors influencing rate of flow

Secretory mechanisms
   Water and electrolytes
   Proteins and glycoproteins

Factors influencing salivary composition
   Inorganic constituents
   Organic constituents

Functions of saliva
   Protection
   Digestion
   Other functions

Saliva in diagnosis

THE DIFFERENT TYPES OF SALIVARY GLAND

In the human there are three pairs of major salivary glands, the parotid, submandibular and sublingual.

It has been found that adult parotid glands have a mean volume of 21·6 ml., as estimated by sialoangiography, with a range of 9·8–34·5 ml. and the submandibular glands a mean volume of 6·5 ml. with a range of 2·5–13·0 ml. The sublingual glands are of the order of 3–4 ml. in volume.

In addition to the major glands, minor glands are present in all areas of the oral cavity except for the anterior part of the hard palate and the gingivae. Figure 1 illustrates the secretion from minor mucous glands on the inner aspect of the lower lip. Recent studies have shown that although each individual gland is very small, the minor mucous glands as a whole contribute about 8 per cent of the total salivary flow.

The salivary glands in the human receive both para-sympathetic and sympathetic innervation but the former is the dominant as far as flow is concerned.

METHODS FOR COLLECTION OF HUMAN SALIVA

Whole Saliva

Unstimulated whole saliva can be collected by allowing saliva to drip from the lower lip into a funnel and thence into a graduated tube.

Stimulated whole saliva may be obtained if the subject is allowed to chew on some inert material such as paraffin wax (of melting point about 49°C) or on rubber bands. Soluble gustatory stimuli would, of course, contaminate the saliva.

Except during consumption of meals, unstimulated whole saliva forms the normal fluid milieu of the oral cavity. It has to be remembered, however, that whole saliva contains not only the combined secretions from the various salivary glands, but may also contain desquamated epithelial cells, leucocytes which enter from the gingival crevice or tonsils, bacteria from dental plaque or from microbial colonies on the soft tissues, food debris if a meal has recently been consumed, and gingival crevice fluid. Very little or none of the latter would be present in patients with healthy gingivae but in patients with gingival inflammation the flow of this fluid out of the gingival crevice is greatly increased.

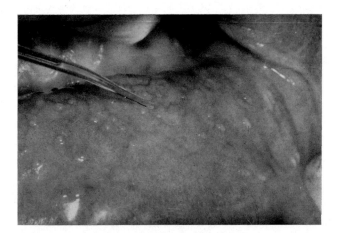

FIG. 1. A micropipette being used to collect minor mucous gland secretions from the inner aspect of the everted lower lip.

Whole saliva tends to be very viscous and heterogeneous because of cellular debris and precipitated mucin and on centrifugation yields material which has been termed salivary sediment. Sediment has a high bacterial content and in certain ways its metabolism resembles that of dental plaque. Many of the organic components of saliva are rapidly degraded by bacterial enzymes and enzymes released from leucocytes lysed in the hypotonic saliva. Thus, saliva should either be analyzed immediately after collection or stored frozen.

The proportional contributions from the different salivary glands do not remain constant but vary with flow rate and time of day. The restriction to inert stimuli ensures that only relatively low stimulated flow rates can be achieved.

Parotid Saliva

Of the major salivary gland secretions, parotid saliva is the most readily obtainable. In animals such as the sheep the parotid duct can be exteriorized but in the human the duct can either be cannulated directly with polyethylene tubing or covered with a Lashley cannula, illustrated in fig. 2. The inner ring is positioned over the parotid papilla on the inside of the cheek and saliva is allowed to flow down the shorter polyethylene tubing. The outer ring is connected to a suction bulb and negative pressure holds the cannula in place. With this device, parotid saliva can readily

be collected either without exogenous stimulation (unstimulated) or during masticatory or gustatory stimulation.

Submandibular and Sublingual Saliva

In some subjects the submandibular ducts can be cannulated directly, usually after a preliminary dilation of the duct, and in subjects with either a prominent lingual frenum or in whom the ducts enter the floor of the mouth close to the symphysis of the mandible, cannulation may be the only feasible approach. In many individuals a collection device made of silicone rubber can be positioned in the floor of the mouth and held securely in place with the tongue. Such a device is also illustrated in fig. 2 and may be custom-made for subjects with anatomical peculiarities. The centre well fits over the openings of both right and left submandibular

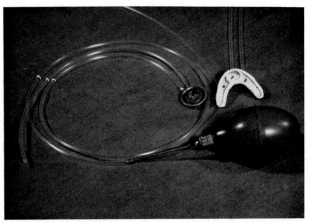

FIG. 2. Collection devices for parotid saliva and for submandibular and sublingual saliva.

ducts and thus collects saliva from both glands simultaneously. The side-arms cover the floor of the mouth at the sides of the tongue and sublingual saliva may be collected via the outer two tubes. The collection of sublingual saliva will rarely be complete because of the difficulty of locating the openings of the multiple ducts and because of the viscosity of the secretion.

Minor Mucous Gland Secretions

These secretions can be sampled directly by micropipette as shown in fig. 1.

Collection of Stimulated Saliva

There are two basically different methods of collecting stimulated saliva. One involves the use of a "constant" stimulus. For instance, for gustatory stimuli the subject may be instructed to suck on a sour lemon drop which is replaced every few minutes. However, flow rate may vary somewhat on different occasions. The second method uses a simple negative feedback approach to achieve a constant flow rate. Saliva is collected into a graduated centrifuge tube positioned in front of a mirror. The subject is able to calculate the flow rate with the aid of a stopwatch and regulate the intensity of sucking on a sour lemon drop to maintain a constant flow rate over extended periods of time.

FACTORS INFLUENCING SALIVARY FLOW RATE

(a) Control of salivary flow appears to be mainly nervous rather than hormonal. Even unstimulated flow ceases if the secreto-motor nerve is sectioned or anaesthesized, showing that the secreto-motor nerves are constantly active. Nervous control allows a very rapid reflex response to afferent stimulation (normally of the taste receptors).

depleted of about 8 per cent of its water content, salivary flow virtually ceases. On the other hand, hyperhydration by forced consumption of 1–2 l. of water has been shown to cause a significant increase in the flow rate of unstimulated parotid saliva.

(c) Recent studies have shown that biological rhythms can influence salivary flow rate. Circadian rhythms are those with a period of about 24 hr. and there is a circadian rhythm of fairly high amplitude in the unstimulated salivary flow rate, with peak flow rates in the afternoon. This is illustrated in fig. 3. The solid line is the cosine wave which fits best, by a least-squares method, to salivary flow rate data collected from eight subjects at several different times each day for many days in succession. The dashed line better represents the usual situation as it has been shown

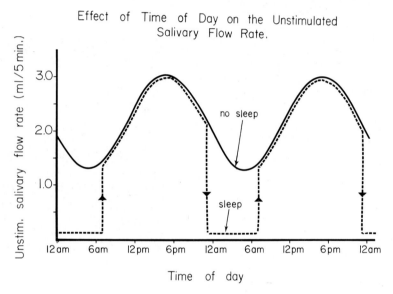

FIG. 3. Diagrammatic representation of the circadian rhythm in unstimulated salivary flow rate. Note that flow rate is virtually zero during sleep.

There is some evidence that catecholamines from the adrenal medulla reduce salivary flow rate in humans, probably by reducing the blood flow to the glands, which perhaps explains the dry mouth associated with fear.

During normal gustatory stimulation or when the motor nerves to a gland are stimulated directly, there is a great increase in blood flow to the gland. There is considerable controversy regarding the cause of increased blood flow but current evidence suggests that it is due both to activation of vasodilatory nerves and to release of vasoactive polypeptides. As saliva is ultimately derived from plasma, a high blood flow to the salivary gland is necessary if a high salivary flow rate is to be maintained.

Intravenous injections of substance P or physalaemin (from a South American toad) both stimulate salivation in some animals. These substances are small polypeptides and their secretagogue activity is not inhibited by prior administration of common inhibitors of known autonomic nervous system transmitters.

(b) The degree of cellular hydration is an important factor influencing salivary flow rate. When the body has been

that during sleep the salivary flow rate falls virtually to zero. This has great implications for preventive dentistry, as during sleep the saliva will be unable to wash away food debris or the products of bacterial metabolism. In addition, as will be discussed later, saliva at a low flow rate shows minimal buffering capacity and provides only small quantities of substances such as urea which promote base formation in the dental plaque. Thus perhaps the most important time of day to clean teeth, as far as reducing dental caries is concerned, is before going to bed.

Shannon and his colleagues have recently shown that the flow rate of unstimulated parotid saliva is reduced by as much as 75 per cent in blindfolded subjects. The flow rate is also affected by posture with highest flow rates in subjects in the standing position, somewhat lower flow rates in seated subjects and minimal flow rates in subjects who are recumbent. Whether the mechanisms involved are related to those which reduce salivary flow rate during sleep is not yet known.

Evidence has been produced of a circannual rhythm (having a period of about a year) in the flow rate of unstimulated parotid saliva collected from military personnel stationed in Texas. Minimum flow rates occurred during the summer months and may have been due to the fact that the subjects were slightly dehydrated, because of the hot weather. It would be of interest to reinvestigate this problem in a more temperate climate; but in any event, the findings have implications for salivary studies which extend over considerable lengths of time.

(d) The normal stimulus for salivation at rates of flow above the resting level is gustatory stimulation of the taste buds. Acid substances are the most potent gustatory stimuli and are widely used for experimental studies on stimulated saliva.

There is normally a negative-feedback system of the "proportional" type in that the salivary response is directly proportional to the intensity of stimulation. The saliva tends to dilute the stimulus (and also neutralize it if acid is the stimulus).

Ericson and his colleagues have shown that the maximum secretory capacity of the major glands is very strongly correlated with their size. This latter factor is the one which best explains differences between individuals in maximum secretory capacity. During intense experimental gustatory stimulation with acid there is essentially an "open" system in that the saliva produced in response to the stimulus is not allowed to dilute and neutralize the stimulus which is continously replaced. Hence it is not unreasonable that with maximum afferent stimulation the secretory response should be proportional to the size of the gland.

However, Ericson has also shown that the unstimulated salivary flow rate is rather poorly correlated with the size of the gland and with the maximum secretory capacity. During the collection of unstimulated saliva there is essentially a closed system as the saliva is still able to moisten the oral cavity but is allowed to drip out of the mouth instead of being swallowed. There would seem no reason why subjects with large salivary glands should require a higher unstimulated salivary flow rate. In fact, very little is known of the reasons for the large inter-individual differences in unstimulated salivary flow rate.

In a study on 661 healthy subjects, age 5–95, the mean unstimulated flow rate of whole saliva was 19 ± 14 ml./hr. (mean $\pm$ S.D.) with a wide range from 0·5–111 ml./hr. The saliva collections were carried out early in the morning before the subjects had had breakfast, and as this is the time of day when salivary flow rate is lowest, the above mean values must be considered as daily minima.

If a negligible salivary flow rate during sleep is assumed, an unstimulated flow rate of about 0·5 ml./min. during the waking hours and a flow rate of 2·5 ml./min. for 2 hr./day during meals, the total daily salivary flow rate may be calculated to be about 700–800 ml.

The contributions of the different glands to unstimulated whole saliva are probably about 65 per cent from the submandibular, 23 per cent from the parotid, 8 per cent from the minor mucous and 4 per cent from the sublingual. Since the submandibular gland is only about one-third of the size of the parotid gland and yet contributes three times as much to unstimulated saliva, it is apparent that size is unrelated to resting secretion rate. Even with maximal gustatory stimulation, the contribution of the parotid gland to the volume of whole saliva only rises to about 50 per cent.

(e) In the absence of gustatory stimuli the salivary flow rate can be increased by olfactory stimulation, by the smoking of tobacco, by irritation of the oesophagus and immediately prior to vomiting. As olfactory stimulation often precedes gustatory stimulation the increased salivary flow rate may be a useful anticipatory response. The increased flow rate in response to smoking may be a reflex response to substances in the smoke which dissolve in saliva and stimulate taste buds or it may be a reflex response to the general chemical irritation of the oral mucosa; it is possible, too, that ganglion cells may be stimulated.

A reflexly increased salivary flow rate will tend to reduce oesophageal irritation and, prior to vomiting, will tend to buffer the acid gastric juice and reduce the tendency for erosion of the teeth which occurs in patients who vomit frequently.

(f) A great number of studies have attempted to demonstrate psychic effects on unstimulated salivary flow rate. Although these effects may be present in certain individuals, they are of relatively small importance. It has been postulated that the sensation of mouthwatering prior to a meal is simply a sudden awareness of saliva already present in the floor of the mouth. There is some evidence that the secretory response to certain gustatory stimuli can be altered if the subject is given incorrect information about the nature of the stimulus.

(g) Although unilateral gustatory or mechanical stimulation elicits secretion from glands on both the right and left sides, the predominant response is unilateral. Receptors for mechanical stimuli are possibly in the periodontal membrane as anaesthesia of the lingual and inferior dental nerves reduces the response of the ipsilateral parotid gland to standardized mechanical stimulation.

SECRETORY MECHANISMS

For descriptive purposes, the secretion of water and electrolytes is described separately from that of protein although these normally occur together.

Secretion of Water and Electrolytes

The initial fluid secreted by the acinar cells is similar to that of an ultrafiltrate of plasma with respect to osmolarity and the concentrations of sodium, potassium and chloride. Typical values would be an osmolarity of 300 mOsm./kg. water; a sodium concentration of 146 mmol./l.; a potassium concentration of 4 mmol./l. and a chloride concentration of 100 mmol./l. The other types of anions present to balance the cations have not yet been determined. This initial secretion has the same composition whether parasympathetic or sympathetic stimulation is employed.

As the initial secretion travels down the salivary ducts its composition is modified, sodium and chloride being reabsorbed to a degree dependent on flow rate, and the potassium concentration is increased due to secretion of potassium into the saliva by the duct cells.

The acinar cells have a relatively low resting membrane potential of about -30 to -40 mV (inside of cell negative) which is typical of non-excitable cells and this is probably due to the cells having a relatively high permeability to sodium ions. In contrast, duct cells have a much higher resting membrane potential of about -80 mV.

As with most cells, the intracellular fluid of acinar cells is high in potassium and low in sodium, a ratio opposite to that in the primary secretion. Application of the Nernst equation suggests that chloride is probably passively distributed across the cell membrane whereas the distribution of sodium and potassium and also calcium is very far from equilibrium. There is always a tendency for potassium ions to leave the cell and for sodium and calcium ions to enter. The concentration gradients are normally maintained by an energy-requiring pump which pumps out sodium ions from

ion. The secretory potential also occurs in the presence of metabolic inhibitors such as dinitrophenol (DNP) showing that it is due to a passive permeability increase. However, the re-uptake of potassium after the secretory potential requires energy and is blocked by such inhibitors as DNP and ouabain.

Although the secretory potential always precedes secretion, it is possible to block secretion without affecting the secretory potential. Perfusion of a gland with a fluid of low calcium concentration, or in which sulphate is the main anion, will block secretion but not the secretory potential. Thus other events must follow the secretory potential before secretion is produced.

There is now evidence that two types of sodium pump are active in the acinar cell. Ouabain will block the activity of the pump which maintains the low sodium and high

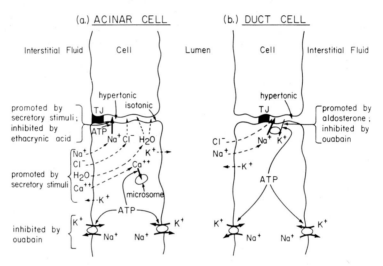

FIG. 4. Electrolyte transport by acinar and duct cells. T J, tight junction.
(From Diamond; Peterson; Schneyer *et al.*)

the cell and pumps in potassium ions. In a perfused gland the resting membrane potential is maintained after replacement of chloride by other ions and, as might be expected, is reduced if the external potassium concentration is increased.

When the gland is stimulated to secrete, the acinar cells develop a secretory potential. In most glands studied this secretory potential is a hyperpolarization of as much as 30 mV, but in certain glands it may be a slight depolarization. When this secretory potential was first described it was attributed to an influx of chloride ions. However, recent studies suggest that it is due to a passive increase in permeability to potassium and perhaps also to sodium. The loss of positively charged potassium ions accounts for the usual hyperpolarization and in those glands where depolarization occurs, this is presumably due to a proportionately greater uptake of sodium ions. The potassium is released from the acinar cells into both the venous blood and the saliva. In perfused glands the secretory potential can still be demonstrated after most of the ions in the perfusate have been replaced by sucrose to maintain osmolarity, after chloride has been replaced by sulphate or nitrate, and after sodium has been replaced by the tetramethylammonium

potassium concentrations intracellularly. This drug will prevent the re-uptake of potassium after a secretory potential but it will not affect secretion itself. On the other hand, a drug called ethacrynic acid has been shown to abolish secretion but not to affect potassium re-uptake after a secretory potential. Ethacrynic acid is thus believed to block the sodium pump which produces the primary isotonic secretion.

The mechanism thought to be involved in the secretion of isotonic fluid is illustrated in fig. 4a. In the presence of calcium ions, the initial cholinergic or adrenergic stimulus increases the permeability of the acinar cell membrane, allowing sodium, calcium and chloride ions, and water to enter and potassium ions to leave. It has been postulated that the pump affected by ethacrynic acid pumps primarily sodium ions from the cell into the intercellular canaliculi and that chloride ions follow passively. The initial secretion in the canaliculi is hypertonic; but since the lateral walls of the acinar cells are believed to be freely permeable to water, the fluid becomes isotonic by the time it reaches the acinar lumen. This mechanism is believed to be activated both by parasympathetic and sympathetic stimulation.

There has been recent interest in the possible role of cyclic adenosine 3′,5′-monophosphate (cAMP). Present evidence suggests that this substance is not involved in the secretory response to cholinergic stimuli but that it is involved in responses to adrenergic stimuli, as will be discussed later.

As the saliva travels down the salivary duct its composition is changed from one of isotonicity and by the time it enters the mouth the osmolarity may be only one-tenth of that of plasma, particularly at unstimulated flow rates. The mechanisms believed to be involved are illustrated in fig. 4b. There is believed to be a pump in the basal region of the lateral wall of the duct cells which pumps out sodium ions, partially in exchange for potassium ions, and chloride ions also leave passively into the intercellular space. It is believed that these lateral membranes, in contrast to the acinar cell membrane, are relatively impermeable to water. Thus, the fluid pumped out of the duct cells remains hypertonic. The short length of this region of the intercellular space will also reduce the area for water diffusion across the membrane.

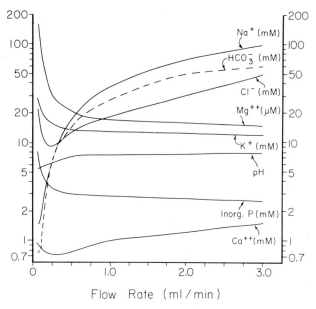

Fig. 5. The effect of flow rate on the concentrations of common electrolytes in parotid saliva. Note the logarithmic scale for the ordinate. Ideally, flow rate should be expressed as ml./g. gland/min.

Since potassium ions will tend to diffuse passively into the lumen from the duct cells, and sodium ions to move passively in the opposite direction prior to being pumped into the intercellular space, the net result is that the saliva becomes hypotonic, low in sodium and enriched in potassium. The effects of flow rate and other factors on these processes will be discussed in a later section.

Secretion of Proteins and Glycoproteins

Although certain salivary proteins such as immunoglobulin A (IgA) appear to be synthesized in plasma cells in the salivary glands and others, such as lysozyme, appear to be formed in the duct cells, most investigations have been concerned with protein synthesis and secretion from acinar cells.

The finding that over 98 per cent of the amylase from the rat parotid gland is secreted in response to injection of isoprenaline has facilitated a number of studies on the factors influencing protein synthesis and the secretory mechanisms in the acinar cells of salivary glands.

Protein Synthesis and Transport Within Acinar Cells

Studies using pulse labelling with radioactive amino acids have shown that the initial labelling occurs in the microsomal fraction of the cell. Proteins are synthesized on ribosomes attached to the rough-surfaced endoplasmic reticulum (RER). The proportion of ribosomes present as polysomes increases during active protein synthesis, as occurs 2–3 hr. after an injection of isoprenaline.

Autoradiographic studies, using the electron microscope, have shown that the newly synthesized protein is segregated within the cisternae of the RER and transported to condensing vacuoles of the Golgi complex by small smooth-surfaced vesicles located at the periphery of the Golgi complex. As the condensing vacuoles enlarge, they become zymogen granules and these leave the Golgi region and move towards the lumen of the cell. The whole process may take 2–6 hr. depending on the species.

The protein-backbones of glycoproteins are synthesized in the RER but the carbohydrate units are not attached until the protein has reached the Golgi region, which is very rich in glycosyl transferases. With the aid of inhibitors of protein synthesis, it has been shown that transport of newly synthesized protein from the RER is independent of continued protein synthesis and hence must be under separate control.

Studies, using the rat parotid gland, have shown a circadian rhythm in the rate of protein synthesis with maximum synthesis occurring at night during the time of feeding. In contrast, protein synthesis in the pancreas is not increased after stimulation of secretion. Mastication causes secretion of protein into the saliva and at the end of the feeding period the gland may have lost as much as 50 per cent of the total amylase content, far more than probably occurs with human salivary glands. Both synthesis and storage of protein are greatly reduced in rats maintained on a liquid diet to reduce mastication. Isoprenaline given to rats at 8 a.m., when protein synthesis is normally maximal, does not cause a further increase in synthesis but when given at 6 p.m. it causes both secretion and increased protein synthesis.

After isoprenaline injection, RNA and DNA synthesis reach a peak 24–28 hr. later. However, synthesis of secretory protein reaches a maximum after 8–12 hr. and occurs in the presence of drugs which inhibit nucleic acid synthesis. Thus the protein synthesis must be dependent on the existing messenger RNA.

Protein Secretion from the Acinar Cell

After administration of secretory stimuli, zymogen granules move towards the luminal border of the cell and the membrane of the zymogen granule fuses with that of the cell surface. Such contact is specific to the luminal membrane. The membrane then breaks down at the site of fusion and the contents of the granule are expelled into the acinar lumen, perhaps also with some membrane fragments. The lumen enlarges markedly due to incorporation of the membrane, and what was the inner aspect of the granule membrane then becomes external to the cell. After secretion, the lumen is reduced in diameter again by formation of intracellular vesicles from the lumen membrane. This process is illustrated in fig. 5, Chapter 42. The vesicle membrane is not reutilized as such to package more zymogen granules but is degraded, perhaps by lysosomes. Membrane to package the new zymogen granules is synthesized at the same time as the zymogen contents.

Secretory Stimuli

At present it is not certain whether parasympathetic or sympathetic nerves are primarily involved in protein secretion from human salivary glands although it has been reported that infusions of adrenaline or isoprenaline tend to increase salivary protein concentration by effects on β-adrenergic receptors.

It has recently been shown that adrenaline has both α- and β-adrenergic effects on the parotid acinar cells of rats. The α-adrenergic effect, which is blocked by phentolamine, results in vacuole formation within the acinar cell and release of potassium. There is no evidence that cAMP is involved in the α-adrenergic effect of adrenaline. The β-adrenergic effect of adrenaline, which can be blocked by propranolol, is the secretion of protein and this effect can be demonstrated at much lower doses than are necessary to elicit the α-adrenergic response. The response can be mimicked by injection of dibutyryl cAMP (which diffuses relatively easily into cells) and can be potentiated by theophylline (a drug which inhibits the phosphodiesterase which normally breaks down cAMP). Adrenaline activates adenyl cyclase, which forms cAMP from ATP and this stage is the one blocked by propranolol. The secretory response to both adrenaline and acetylcholine is energy-dependent.

GENERAL FACTORS INFLUENCING SALIVARY COMPOSITION

Type of Saliva

The composition of saliva varies according to whether it emanates from the parotid, submandibular, sublingual or minor mucous glands. For instance, the calcium content of parotid saliva is only about half that of secretions from the other glands. Minor mucous gland secretions show a virtual absence of bicarbonate and are also comparatively low in phosphate but high in magnesium. In addition, certain proteins or glycoproteins are secreted by particular glands; for instance, amylase is derived mainly from the parotid glands and blood-group substances from the sublingual and minor mucous glands.

Flow Rate

Flow rate influences the concentration of almost all components of saliva as will be discussed in more detail later.

Duration of Stimulation

The concentration of certain components of saliva such as protein, calcium, chloride and bicarbonate are dependent on the duration of stimulation. When the stimulated flow rate is held constant, the composition of saliva collected after 5 min. of stimulation may be quite different from that collected after 15 min. of stimulation. In addition, so-called "transient" changes in composition, such as an increase in potassium concentration associated with the secretory potential, occur at the very beginning of stimulation or when flow rate is suddenly changed.

Nature of the Stimulus

The concentrations of certain components of saliva depend on the type of secretory stimulation employed. In the human, both gustatory and pharmacological stimulation may be used whilst in animals, electrical stimulation of secretory nerves can be carried out. With similar flow rates, pilocarpine elicits a secretion containing higher protein and calcium concentrations than when gustatory stimulation is employed.

Serial Dependency of Sampling

Stimulation of secretion at one time may influence the composition of saliva collected on a subsequent occasion. This factor may be important when multiple collections are to be made on a given day. In general when gustatory stimuli are employed for 10–15 min. for a given collection, serial dependency of sampling can be avoided if a 2 hr. interval is maintained between successive collections.

Biological Rhythms

The concentrations of certain components of saliva are strongly influenced by the time of day at which collections are made. For instance, the sodium concentration in both unstimulated and stimulated parotid saliva shows a circadian rhythm of high amplitude with peak values in the early morning whereas potassium shows a rhythm of smaller amplitude with peak values in the afternoon. Appreciation of such rhythms is of importance if saliva composition is to be used as an index of systemic disease.

Plasma Composition

Salivary composition is dependent, to some extent, on the composition of the plasma. For instance, salivary urea and cortisol levels are strongly correlated with plasma levels of these substances. In addition, changes in the plasma concentrations of certain hormones many influence salivary composition. An increase in the plasma aldosterone concentration lowers the sodium and increases the potassium concentrations in saliva.

Diet

Although gross dietary deficiencies can influence the salivary composition there is little evidence that moderate changes in diet have much effect since the plasma concentrations of many components such as calcium or bicarbonate are very closely regulated. Diets high in protein increase blood urea levels which causes an increase in the urea concentration in saliva.

Genetic Effects

The best known genetic effects on salivary composition relate to the secretion of blood group substances in saliva.

About 80 per cent of the population possess the secretor gene and secrete blood-group substances of the appropriate ABO group in their saliva.

Inorganic Constituents of Saliva

Water

Water is always the main constituent of saliva and the saliva in humans is always hypotonic to plasma. At low flow rates the osmolarity of saliva may be only one-tenth that of plasma but at high flow rates it may be as high as three-quarters of the plasma osmolarity.

Sodium and Potassium

These two ions are the main cations in saliva, potassium predominating at low flow rates and sodium at high flow rates. The effects of flow rate on their concentrations in parotid saliva are shown in fig. 5. The saliva secreted in the region of the acinar cells may be assumed to have sodium and potassium concentrations of 146 and 4 mmol/l., respectively. Thus, at low flow rates almost all the sodium is reabsorbed as the saliva passes along the ducts whereas at high flow rates there is insufficient time for this to occur. In some subjects, it is possible to demonstrate a Tm value for sodium reabsorption (the maximum capacity for sodium reabsorption by the ducts). Because the saliva concentration of potassium at all flow rates is maintained above that in plasma, there must obviously be active secretion of potassium from plasma to saliva, as discussed in an earlier section. Furthermore, because the potassium concentration in stimulated saliva is relatively independent of flow rate, the secretion of potassium must be closely tied to the flow rate.

The effects of flow rate on the sodium and potassium levels in the other types of saliva are very similar.

Chloride and Bicarbonate

Although the minor mucous gland secretions contain virtually no bicarbonate, this ion is present in secretions from the major salivary glands, the concentration being extremely dependent on flow rate, as shown in fig. 5.

At low flow rates, chloride is the predominant anion and only a trace of bicarbonate is present. At low stimulated flow rates the chloride concentration falls below that in unstimulated saliva but at higher flow rates the concentration increases again. Figure 5 is misleading in that chloride and bicarbonate concentrations are also dependent on the duration of stimulation. For instance, at high flow rates the chloride concentration approaches plasma levels in the initial samples and then falls gradually to about half the plasma level with the bicarbonate showing a reciprocal rise. There appears to be an exchange of chloride for bicarbonate in the salivary duct and the efficiency of this exchange increases with duration of stimulation.

The pH of the saliva is related to the bicarbonate concentration by the Henderson-Hasselbalch equation:

$$pH = pK + \log \frac{[HCO_3^-]}{[H_2CO_3]}$$

The concentration of carbonic acid can be calculated from the partial pressure of CO_2 in the saliva ($[H_2CO_3] = 0.03 \times pCO_2$]) and as this is relatively constant and about equal to the pCO_2 in blood, the pH is dependent almost entirely on the bicarbonate concentration. At low flow rates the pH of parotid saliva may be as low as 5·3, rising to about 7·8 at high flow rates (fig. 5). The pH of saliva is particularly dependent on flow rate at flow rates just above the unstimulated.

Calcium, Inorganic Phosphate and Fluoride

The concentrations of these ions in saliva are important in any consideration of the processes of dental caries or dental calculus formation as the concentrations of calcium, phosphate and hydroxyl and fluoride ions determine whether saliva is undersaturated or supersaturated with respect to different salts of calcium phosphate such as hydroxyapatite or fluorapatite.

Saliva contains less calcium than does plasma (2·5 mM.) but more phosphate than plasma (1 mM.). Parotid saliva contains less calcium but more phosphate than do the other types of saliva and both calcium and phosphate concentrations are dependent on flow rate (fig. 5).

Since the second pK value for phosphoric acid is about 7·2, inorganic phosphate is present almost entirely as the mono and dihydrogen forms and the relative proportions are dependent on the pH of the saliva and thus on the flow rate. At all flow rates, the phosphate concentrations in parotid and submandibular saliva are above that in plasma and thus it is likely that the duct epithelium secretes phosphate into the saliva.

The critical pH of saliva is defined as the pH at which saliva becomes unsaturated with respect to hydroxyapatite or enamel mineral. Saliva is generally supersaturated with respect to hydroxyapatite; but if the pH is lowered by addition of acid and then the saliva is tested for its ability to dissolve hydroxyapatite, the critical pH is usually found to be between 5·5 and 6·5.

It is difficult to predict the critical pH for saliva for a number of reasons. Firstly, the calcium, phosphate and hydroxyl ion concentrations are flow rate-dependent and are different in different types of saliva. Secondly, the relative proportions of the different types of phosphate ions vary with pH and thus with flow rate. Thirdly, the concentrations of ionic calcium and phosphate vary because of variations in the concentrations of complexing agents such as proteins. Finally flow rate also affects the critical pH by changing the ionic strength (which tends to increase with flow rate) and the ionic strength influences the values of the apparent dissociation constants for phosphoric acid and the activities of the calcium, phosphate and hydroxyl ions.

Since dental caries occurs at the interface between enamel and the dental plaque and calculus is deposited within dental plaque, the critical pH for plaque fluid rather than for saliva is of more importance. Dental plaque has been shown to contain higher calcium and phosphate concentrations than an equivalent volume of saliva, so that the critical pH for plaque fluid is probably lower than that for saliva.

McCann (1968), in an important study on parotid saliva

collected at different flow rates from several individuals, has shown that with the exception of a few samples of unstimulated saliva, all other samples of saliva studied were supersaturated with respect to hydroxyapatite. Figure 6 illustrates his results regarding the degree of saturation of parotid saliva with respect to various calcium-containing minerals. All samples of unstimulated saliva were supersaturated with respect to fluorapatite and the difference from hydroxyapatite is because unstimulated saliva contains higher concentrations of fluoride ions than hydroxyl ions (about 10^{-6} M. fluoride ions and 2×10^{-9} M. hydroxyl ions).

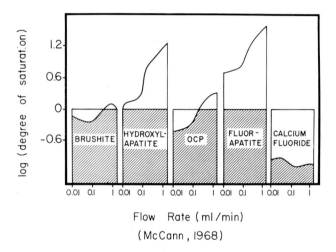

Flow Rate (ml/min)

(McCann, 1968)

FIG. 6. The effect of flow rate on the degree of saturation of parotid saliva with various calcium salts. Note that the scales for both ordinate and abscissa are logarithmic. Thus a value of 1·0 for the log (degree of saturation) indicates that the saliva is tenfold saturated with respect to the salt in question. Note that at all flow rates saliva is unsaturated with respect to calcium fluoride which can thus dissolve in saliva. Saliva is saturated with respect to both hydroxyapatite and fluorapatite but is only saturated with respect to brushite and octacalcium phosphate at higher flow rates.

It has been reported that the fluoride content of saliva is independent of flow rate and is about 10^{-6} M. (0·018 p.p.m.) in subjects drinking tap water containing a low fluoride concentration and is only slightly raised in subjects receiving dietary supplements of 10 mg. sodium fluoride per day. However, 1 hr. after a single dose of 10 mg. sodium fluoride, the salivary level of fluoride rose to about $1·6 \times 10^{-5}$ M. (0·3 p.p.m.).

Since plaque has also been shown to concentrate fluoride to levels much higher than those in saliva, it is necessary to know the fluoride level in plaque fluid in order to calculate whether the plaque fluid is or is not saturated with respect to various calcium salts. In general, it seems likely that under fasting conditions, plaque fluid will be supersaturated with respect to both hydroxyapatite and fluorapatite. Thus it is likely that inhibitors of crystal nucleation or crystal growth must normally be present in the plaque.

Iodide

Salivary glands of many species, including humans, are able to secrete iodide into saliva at concentrations greater than the plasma concentration. Studies with radioautographs have shown that this concentrating ability is located in the tubules rather than in the acini. Excessive intake of iodide, as may occur with consumption of certain cough medicines, may cause salivary gland enlargement and pain. In humans, salivary iodide is present almost entirely in the inorganic form and the concentration is inversely related to flow rate. The iodide-concentrating mechanism is independent of whether the patient is euthyroid, hyperthyroid or hypothyroid, but the salivary iodide concentration does depend on the plasma concentration. The resting gland accumulates iodide in the tubules and on stimulation an initial transient rise occurs in the iodide concentration in both saliva and venous blood.

Buffering Capacity

The three possible buffers of acid or alkali in saliva are bicarbonate, phosphate and protein. The proteins of saliva have negligible buffering capacity, as may be shown after dialysis of saliva to remove all small molecules. The concentration of phosphate may be 7–8 mM. at low flow rates but only 2–3 mM. at high flow rates (fig. 5). Since the pK_2 value for phosphate is about 7·2, and since the pH of unstimulated saliva is much lower than this, the phosphate in unstimulated saliva will be largely in the $H_2PO_4^-$ form rather than as $HPO_4^=$ and hence will be ineffective as a buffer. Since the phosphate concentration is low at higher flow rates, phosphate makes only a very weak contribution to the buffering capacity.

The bicarbonate concentration may be less than 1 mM. in unstimulated saliva (fig. 5) but may be as high as 60 mM. at high flow rates. Thus the buffering capacity of saliva is almost entirely due to its bicarbonate content and it is really only effective at high flow rates. The clinical importance of this is that if patients consume carbohydrate-containing foods prior to going to sleep, the saliva, because of the very low flow rate during sleep, will have not only a low pH but also a low buffering capacity against acid formed by the micro-organisms of the dental plaque.

Organic Components of Saliva

Proteins and Glycoproteins

There are a great number of organic constituents in saliva but the ones occurring in highest amounts are proteins and glycoproteins. These are mainly responsible for the physical properties of saliva such as its viscosity and spinnbarkeit, or ability to be drawn into long elastic threads. Sialic acid is a component of some of the glycoproteins and contributes to the viscosity of saliva. The glycoproteins consist of a polypeptide chain with short carbohydrate side chains and sialic acid, when present, is the terminal sugar residue. Its low pK value (2·6) ensures that it is fully ionized over the physiological pH range and the negative charges on adjacent terminal sialic acid residues repel each other. This repulsion prevents random coiling and the extended molecules cause the viscosity which is greatly reduced after cleavage of the sialic acid residues. The viscous secretions not only lubricate food particles but may also provide a diffusion barrier to protect the mucosal surfaces.

Over twenty different proteins have been separated from parotid and submandibular saliva by a variety of techniques such as electrophoresis and some have been identified by enzymatic and immunological techniques. Many plasma proteins appear in trace amounts in saliva but the majority of the proteins are synthesized by the salivary glands and are specific to saliva.

Certain proteins have been isolated in a relatively pure state and these include six isozymes of amylase, lysozyme, immunoglobulin A with its associated secretory component, and a group of proteins relatively rich in proline. Since the different salivary proteins are not all synthesized by the

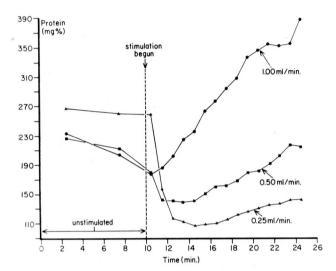

FIG. 7. The effects of flow rate and duration of stimulation on the concentration of total protein in parotid saliva. Fifteen subjects on three separate days collected two five-min samples of unstimulated saliva and then began sour lemon drop stimulation to maintain a constant flow rate of either 0·25, 0·50 or 1·0 ml./min. for the next fifteen min.

same type of cell, the relative concentrations vary with different saliva-collection conditions. Whereas amylase appears to be synthesized in acinar cells, lysozyme is produced by duct cells and immunoglobulin A by plasma cells located adjacent to the ducts. Secretory component, part of which is bound to dimers of IgA, is synthesized in the acinar cells. The relative amounts of those proteins believed to be derived from acinar cells increase with stimulation of salivary flow rate.

The protein concentration in human saliva varies from about 0·025 to as much as 1 g./100 ml. as compared with a plasma protein concentration of about 7 g./100 ml. The secretion of total protein is dependent both on salivary flow rate and on the duration of stimulation as may be seen in fig. 7. In addition, the salivary protein concentration in both unstimulated and stimulated parotid saliva shows a circadian rhythm of high amplitude as illustrated in fig. 8. These results contrast with what may have been expected from the rat experiments discussed earlier, in which maximum protein concentrations in the salivary glands of rats were found at the beginning of the feeding cycle. In humans though, minimum salivary protein concentrations were present in samples collected before breakfast.

The nature of the gustatory stimulus can also influence salivary protein concentration and marked variations with different stimuli and between individuals may be encountered as illustrated in fig. 9. It is possible that different gustatory stimuli can influence the ratio of cholinergic to β-adrenergic stimulation to the salivary gland.

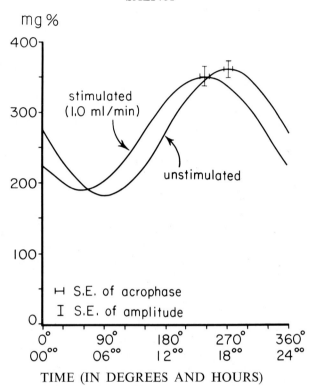

FIG. 8. Circadian rhythms in the protein concentration in unstimulated (7 subjects) and stimulated (8 subjects) parotid saliva. Subjects collected saliva about 5 times per day for about 11 successive days. Best-fitting cosine waves of period 24 h. were calculated by least-squares and the mean curves are shown.

Following prolonged stimulation of parotid secretion, there appears in the saliva the protein "core" of a glycoprotein present at the beginning of stimulation. Further study should facilitate understanding of the factors controlling glycosylation of the polypeptide chains of glycoproteins.

Many of the individual salivary proteins contain unusually large proportions of the basic amino acids, which accounts for their high isoelectric points, and their functions, if any, are largely unknown.

Non-protein Organic Components

Saliva also contains a large number of small-molecular-weight organic substances present in trace amounts. These include free amino acids, vitamins, hormones, products of intermediary metabolism and often drugs present in plasma. Most of these substances are present in saliva at concentrations far lower than in plasma and probably pass by diffusion through the epithelial cells of the salivary glands.

It is significant that glucose is present at a concentration of only about 0·05 mM. (1 mg./100 ml.) compared with a plasma concentration of about 5 mM. This means that for significant acid formation by the microorganisms of the dental plaque, an exogenous source of carbohydrate must be provided, although certain microorganisms can metabolize the carbohydrate components of salivary glycoproteins. However, because the urea concentration in saliva is usually just slightly below that in plasma, and because many plaque microorganisms can rapidly metabolize urea to form ammonia and carbon dioxide (a net production of base), the plaque pH in fasting subjects is usually maintained above neutrality.

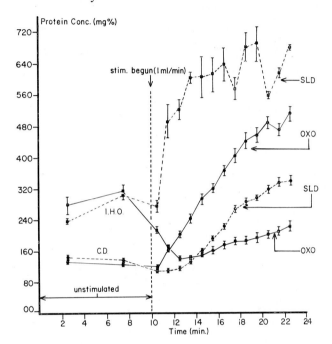

FIG. 9. The effects of duration of stimulation and the nature of the gustatory stimulus on the protein concentration in parotid saliva. On a given day, before breakfast, the subjects collected two 5-min. samples of unstimulated saliva and then thirteen 1-min. samples at a constant flow rate of 1 ml./min. using either sour lemon drops (SLD) or OXO, a beef bouillon cube with a predominantly salty taste, as gustatory stimuli. Subject IHO used each of the two stimuli 7 times and CD used each 13 times. The bars indicate SE for each individual point. The results for CD are fairly typical of the response of several other subjects and differ markedly from those for IHO.

THE FUNCTIONS OF SALIVA

Protection of the Entrance to the Alimentary Tract

Saliva tends to prevent the accumulation of bacteria in the oral cavity so that stomatitis is often associated with xerostomia. Anti-bacterial components, such as lysozyme and perhaps IgA, may either retard bacterial growth or act to repel invasion of the mouth by transient microorganisms. IgA may also play a role in the neutralization of viruses and limit the absorption of certain antigens.

Saliva is necessary for lubrication, dissolution and dispersion of hard food particles, and the glycoproteins facilitate the swallowing process. Certain salivary proteins readily adsorb to exposed crystals of hydroxyapatite so that the teeth are always covered by a layer of acquired pellicle. This process is the first stage of plaque formation.

Saliva acts as a solvent and thus is essential for taste. It is probably of great physiological significance that unstimulated saliva contains no bitter substances, virtually no sugar, very little sodium chloride and has a nearly neutral pH and low buffering capacity. These characteristics favour detection of low concentrations of bitter, sweet, salty and acid substances. Saliva acts as a good buffer at high flow rates. Not only will it buffer acid in the diet and that formed by the dental plaque but also acid gastric juice which enters the mouth during vomiting. Saliva also acts as a temperature buffer against hot or cold foods and drinks.

Digestive Functions

Saliva is necessary in order to taste substances not in solution. In addition, it serves to soften hard foods prior to formation of a bolus, and is necessary for swallowing. Although parotid saliva in particular contains a high concentration of amylase, this enzyme probably contributes very little to the digestion of starchy foods since saliva is in contact with food for only a short time before it is inactivated by the acid gastric juice. Amylase may help to dissolve starchy food particles retained on the teeth and oral mucous membranes.

Other Functions

Saliva is necessary for speech and also plays a role in water balance as reduced salivary secretion during dehydration is one of the signals of thirst.

Saliva also acts to form a peripheral seal, necessary for retention of full dentures, and an oral seal during suckling, for which purpose it is essential in the rat. When a rat is exposed to a hot environment, this stimulates the flow of saliva which the animal spreads on its fur in order to lose heat by evaporation of saliva rather than sweat, and a commoner example of the same principle is seen in panting in dogs and cats.

SALIVA AS A DIAGNOSTIC TOOL

Salivary secretion of blood-group substances has long been used in physical anthropology and the most common tested are the ABO and Lewis groups. About 70 per cent of the blood-group substances secreted in whole saliva are derived from the sublingual and minor mucous gland secretions, the remainder being derived from submandibular saliva. Because of the variable proportions derived from different glands, in different individuals, it would seem appropriate that family studies on the concentrations (rather than just the presence) of blood-group substances should be carried out on saliva from a single gland, preferably the submandibular. The recently reported genetical polymorphism of certain proline-rich salivary proteins should also be of value in physical anthropology.

In patients who have suffered trauma affecting the facial nerve, comparison of flow rates from the two submandibular glands is of value. Some authorities believe that, if the flow rate on the affected side is found to be less than 25 per cent of that on the uninjured side, the facial nerve should be surgically decompressed.

It has been shown that a fairly good correlation exists between the concentrations of mercury, urea and cortisol in plasma and the concentrations of the same substances in saliva. Thus, where repetitive sampling is required, as, for instance, to screen industrial workers for exposure to mercury, saliva sampling may be more acceptable than venepunctures.

The ability of the salivary glands to concentrate iodide may sometimes be useful in the diagnosis of certain thyroid disorders. After injection of radioactive iodide, the level of radioactivity in the saliva is usually much greater than in plasma. A reduction in the ratio may indicate a similar trapping defect for iodide by the thyroid gland. In patients where the plasma iodide level is too low for chemical analysis, such an analysis can be done on the saliva and if, after injection of radioactive iodide, the saliva/plasma ratio is measured, the plasma iodide concentration can then be calculated. (See also Chapter 44).

There has as yet been no corroboration of the report that the concentrations of calcium and potassium in stimulated whole saliva are significantly increased in patients with digitalis toxicity.

It has also been reported that the level of potassium in stimulated submandibular saliva is significantly higher in patients with primary aldosteronism than it is in normal subjects or those with pseudo-primary aldosteronism. Such a distinction is important as patients with pseudo-primary aldosteronism are not improved by adrenal surgery.

There is some evidence that patients with Addison's disease show high salivary sodium/potassium ratios whereas those with Cushing's disease show low ratios. It would seem important to control the time of saliva sampling in such tests because of the high amplitude of the normal circadian rhythm, particularly in the sodium concentration.

It has been suggested that the deposition of calculus is increased in patients with cystic fibrosis; this may be due to the higher levels of calcium, phosphate and protein present in submandibular saliva from such patients. In children with cystic fibrosis the submandibular saliva may be cloudy on collection and this is probably due to aggregation of a calcium precipitable glycoprotein. Even in normal subjects, submandibular saliva collected at high flow rates may appear cloudy and this is particularly likely to occur in subjects with high calcium concentrations in their submandibular saliva. It has been reported that the salivary sodium concentration, as measured by a sodium electrode at the opening of the parotid duct, is considerably elevated in infants with cystic fibrosis and that this may be a useful screening device.

REFERENCES

Dawes, C. (1972), "Circadian Rhythms in Human Salivary Flow Rate and Composition," *J. Physiol. (Lond.)*, **220**, 529.

Dawes, C. and Wood, C. M. (1973), "The Composition of Human Lip Mucous Gland Secretions," *Arch. Oral Biol.*, **18**, 343.

Ericson, S., Hedin, M. and Wiberg, A. (1972), "Variability of the Submandibular Flow Rate in Man with Special Reference to the Size of the Gland," *Odont. Revy*, **23**, 411.

May, M., Lucente, F. E., Harvey, J. E. and Marovitz, W. F. (1973), "Salivation Testing in Traumatic Facial Paralysis," *Ann. Otol. Rhinol., Lar.*, **82**, 17.

McCann, H. G. (1968), "Inorganic Components of Salivary Secretions," in *The Art and Science of Dental Caries Research*, p. 55 (R. S. Harris, Ed.). New York: Academic Press.

Petersen, O. H. (1973), "Acetylcholine-induced Ion Transports Involved in the Formation of Saliva," *Acta. physiol. Scand.*, supplementum 381.

Schneyer, L. H., Young, J. A. and Schneyer, C. A. (1972), "Salivary Secretion of Electrolytes," *Physiol. Rev.*, **52**, 720.

Shannon, I. L. (1972), "The Biochemistry of Human Saliva in Health and Disease," in *Salivary Glands and Their Secretion*, p. 94 (N. H. Rowe, Ed.). University of Michigan.

Shannon, I. L. and Edmonds, E. J. (1972), "Effect of Fluoride Dosage on Human Parotid Saliva Fluoride Levels," *Arch. Oral Biol.*, **17**, 1303.

44. DISEASES OF THE SALIVARY GLANDS

D. K. MASON AND D. M. CHISHOLM

Tests of salivary gland function
- Salivary flow rate
- Sialography
- Biopsy
- Scintiscanning

Developmental anomalies

Sialadenitis
- Bacterial
  - Acute
  - Chronic
  - Specific
- Allergic
- Viral
  - Mumps or epidemic parotitis
  - Salivary gland inclusion disease

Obstructive and traumatic lesions
- Fistula
- Sialolithiasis
- Mucoceles

Functional disorders
- Xerostomia
- Increased salivation
- Cystic fibrosis

Neoplasia

Sjögren's syndrome
- Xerostomia
- Glandular enlargement
  - Diagnostic methods
    - Salivary flow rate estimation
    - Labial salivary gland biopsy
- Hydrostatic sialography
- Salivary scintiscanning
- Other laboratory and experimental findings
- Treatment

Benign lymphoepithelial lesions

Sialosis

Changes with age

Disease of the salivary glands may occur either as a local condition or as part of a generalized disease process. In this chapter, diseases of the salivary glands will be considered from both local and general points of view. Special attention will be devoted to those areas of salivary gland pathology in which major advances have recently been made. Disease of the salivary glands interferes with gland function and may lead to profound intra-oral signs and symptoms. In addition to conventional techniques such as bacteriological and histopathological tests, special investigations of salivary gland function may be helpful in diagnosis. The broad outline of these tests will now be described.

TESTS OF SALIVARY GLAND FUNCTION

Salivary flow rate refers to the quantitative measurement of salivary secretion. For the major salivary glands the technique employs a modified Carlson Crittenden cup which is held in place over the main duct orifice by air suction (fig. 1). Collecting devices are available for both parotid and submandibular secretions. Saliva is collected into graduated measuring tubes and the most reliable results are obtained under conditions of maximal stimulation using a sialagogue such as 10 per cent citric acid solution. Many factors, however, including the time of day, age and sex of the subject, the effects of various commonly prescribed drugs and local or systemic disease, influence salivary flow rates; values obtained must be interpreted against this background.

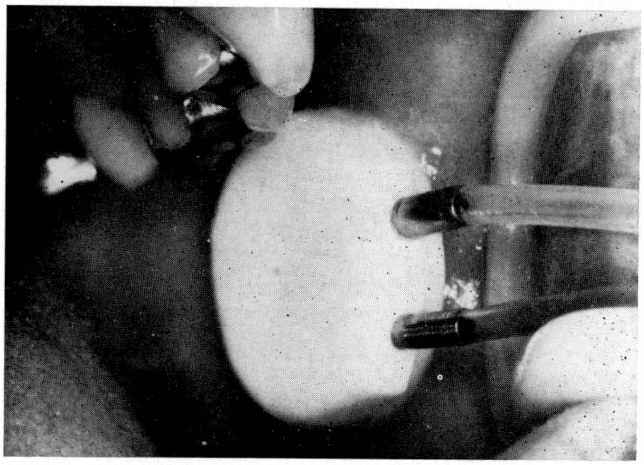

FIG. 1. Modified Carlson-Crittenden cup for collecting parotid saliva, placed in position over the duct orifice.

Hydrostatic Sialography refers to the introduction of a radio-opaque contrast medium into the salivary duct system. The method described by Park and Mason (1966) has some advantages over the conventional hand-injection techniques and allows a water-soluble contrast medium to flow into the duct system under constant pressure with minimal risk of damage to the gland. Simply, the medium such as "Hypaque" or "Triosil" is contained within a glass cylinder, placed approximately 90 cm. above the reclining subject's head, and is linked to a catheter which is inserted into the duct orifice of the gland to be examined. The medium is allowed to flow into the gland and a radiograph

—the filling phase film—is taken (fig. 2). The subject is then given a piece of lemon to suck in order to stimulate salivary secretion and thus rapidly expel the medium from the duct system. A second radiograph—the secretory phase film—is taken and normally no retention of medium will be observed.

Biopsy is a most valuable diagnostic procedure and is the only test which gives an indication of the nature of a disease process which may affect an organ or tissue. With regard to the major salivary glands care must be taken to avoid

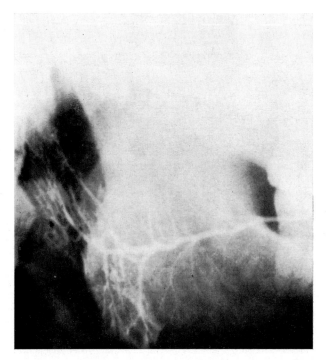

FIG. 2. Filling phase sialogram showing normal parotid duct structure.

damage to important neurovascular structures and minimize the risk of fistula formation. For these reasons, biopsy of the major glands is limited generally to the situation where neoplasia is suspected. However, in a number of disease processes where the salivary glands are affected generally, biopsy of the intra-oral minor salivary glands may be of great value.

Scintiscanning of the salivary glands is a most promising investigative technique. It is, however, a relatively new test and remains to be fully evaluated as a test of salivary gland function. It has the great advantage of examining all the major salivary glands at the same time. The technique takes advantage of the fact that the major and minor salivary glands, like the thyroid gland, concentrate iodide to many times the plasma level. An artificial isotope such as ^{99m}Tc pertechnetate, which is similar to iodide in ionic size, is injected intravenously. The detecting head of the scanner picks up the emissions from the head and neck region of the subject and translates them to a colour print-out thus giving an anatomical picture of the salivary glands.

DEVELOPMENTAL ANOMALIES

Aplasia or agenesis, the congenital absence of the major salivary glands, is uncommon. Any one of the glands or group of glands may be absent, unilaterally or bilaterally, and the condition gives rise to xerostomia and an increased caries rate (fig. 3).

Atresia is the congenital occlusion or absence of one or more major salivary gland ducts and is exceedingly rare. It may produce xerostomia and may lead to retention cyst formation.

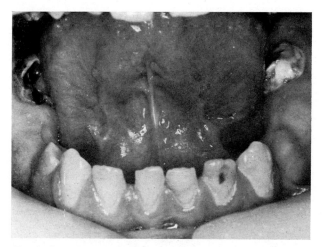

FIG. 3. Intra-oral view of the floor of the mouth of an 11-year-old boy with aplasia of the major salivary glands. Severe dental caries and profound xerostomia were present.

Aberrancy refers to the presence of salivary tissue at an abnormal site. An example is inclusion of salivary tissue within the ramus or body of the mandible. Usually, an anatomical communication exists with normally situated gland tissue and it may be considered an extreme example of developmental lingual mandibular salivary gland depression. Salivary gland tissue has also been reported in the base of the neck, middle ear, mastoid bone and within lymphoid tissue including the intra or paraparotid lymph nodes. It is important to note that such tissue may be the site of tumour formation.

SIALADENITIS

Inflammatory disorders of the major salivary glands are the result of bacterial or viral infection. Rarely an allergic reaction may result in sialadenitis. Infection is manifest by painful swelling of the affected gland with an alteration in salivary secretion rate and character, the saliva becoming cloudy and thick. Mixed infections usually ascend from the mouth, whereas specific infections tend to be blood-borne.

Bacterial

Acute Sialadenitis

Predisposing factors include reduction of salivary flow which is often a post-operative complication, especially of abdominal surgery when the patient is debilitated or dehydrated. Acute parotitis may follow the use of drugs which cause xerostomia, such as phenothiazine and its derivatives. The condition may also represent an acute exacerbation of a low-grade chronic non-specific sialadenitis. Clinically, acute sialadenitis presents as a painful swelling accompanied by low-grade fever, elevated erythrocyte sedimentation rate, leukocytosis, general malaise and headaches. In addition to these features, the overlying skin is reddened, trismus may be present, and oedema may involve the cheek, periorbital region and neck. A purulent discharge may be expressed from the affected duct by digital pressure. The micro-organisms involved include *Staphylococcus aureus*, *Streptococcus pyogenes*, *Streptococcus viridans* and pneumococci. The introduction of sulphonamides and antibiotics led to a marked reduction in the incidence of acute parotitis, but with the emergence of antibiotic-resistant *Staphylococcus aureus*, acute parotitis has become more prevalent again. The treatment includes rest, antibiotic therapy, and surgical drainage where necessary. The condition resolves or may become a low-grade chronic sialadenitis. Biopsy and sialography are contra-indicated in the acute stage.

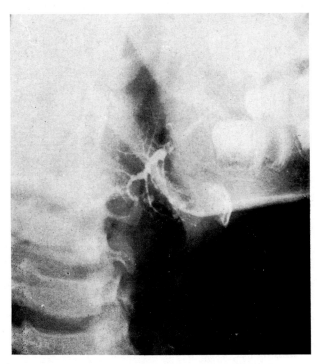

Fig. 4. Main duct dilatation as revealed by sialography. The patient was a 12-year-old girl with recurrent chronic parotitis.

Chronic Recurrent Sialadenitis

The aetiological factors are similar to those for acute sialadenitis. The condition usually is unilateral with pain and swelling in the preauricular, retromandibular or submandibular region. The duct orifice is reddened and a purulent discharge from the duct of the affected gland may be present, often described as having a salty taste. Salivary flow may be reduced and sialography (fig. 4) may show ductal dilatation. The histopathological features include

hyperplasia of duct epithelium, periductal lymphocytic infiltration, acinar atrophy and fibrosis leading to eventual disappearance of the acini.

Sialadenitis of Specific Origin

The salivary glands are seldom involved in specific inflammatory disorders. On rare occasions, however, they may be the site of granulomatous disorders such as tuberculosis, syphilis and sarcoidosis and are affected as part of these systemic disease processes. The term Mikulicz's syndrome is often applied to the condition of bilateral salivary gland and lacrimal gland enlargement due to a known cause, such as the specific granulomata as well as lymphoid neoplasia (see later). It is now known that uveoparotid fever or

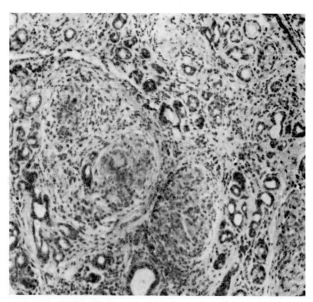

Fig. 5. Sarcoid granulomas in the minor salivary glands of a patient with Mikulicz's syndrome. × 75.

Heerfordt's syndrome is due to sarcoid involvement of the uveal tract, lacrimal and salivary glands. The minor salivary glands (fig. 5) may also be involved in this condition. Resolution is usually achieved by appropriate treatment of the systemic disorder.

Allergic Sialadenitis

Salivary gland enlargement as a localized allergic reaction is rare. Among the allergens reported are various foods, drugs such as chloramphenicol and oxytetracycline, various pollens and heavy metals. Allergic sialadenitis may be produced experimentally and the histopathological features include acute inflammation and parenchymal degeneration. Eosinophils in saliva may be helpful diagnostically, whilst sialography and blood eosinophil count may also be of value. In the treatment of allergic sialadenitis antihistamines are of limited value.

Viral Sialadenitis

Mumps or Epidemic Parotitis

Mumps is an acute, infectious, viral disease that affects primarily the salivary glands, especially the parotids. It occurs in all areas of the world and is the most common of all salivary gland diseases. It is endemic throughout the year in temperate climates but there is usually a seasonal increase in late winter and spring. The disease affects both sexes equally, and is usually contracted by children and young adults. Mumps virus, which has an incubation period of 2–3 weeks, is transmitted by direct contact or in droplets of saliva. The onset is sudden, with fever, headache, and painful swelling of one or more salivary glands, more commonly the parotids, which are involved bilaterally

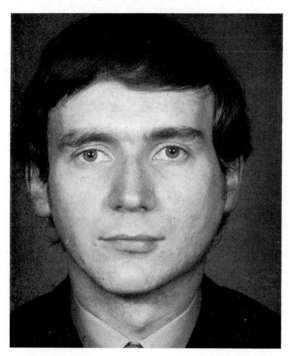

FIG. 6. Bilateral parotid salivary gland swelling in a male patient with mumps.

in 70 per cent of cases (fig. 6). Classically, one gland is affected at first. The swelling reaches a maximum within 2 days and diminishes over an additional week.

Adults who contract the disease may develop serious complications, such as orchitis and oophoritis, though sterility is rare. Other organs which may be affected are the pancreas, liver, kidney or nervous system.

A durable immunity results from mumps and in adults is detected by a positive reaction to skin-test antigen and by the presence of complement-fixing antibodies. In serum, a rise in antibody titre occurs within a week. The virus may be detected by complement fixation in saliva 2–3 days before the onset of sialadenitis and for about 6 days afterwards. Treatment is usually symptomatic with isolation for 6–10 days. Histologically a rather diffuse infiltration of the gland parenchyma by mononuclear cells and degeneration of acini is observed. It is important to note that parotitis may be caused by other viruses such as Coxsackie A, Echo virus, and the virus of lymphocytic choriomeningitis.

Salivary Gland Inclusion Disease

This rare condition usually affects infants in the first few days of life. Infection occurs transplacentally without evi-

dence of disease in the mother and debilitates the fetus, retards its development and gives rise to premature birth. There are no particular signs or symptoms. Hepatosplenomegaly, jaundice, thrombocytopenic purpura and involvement of the nervous system may be present. It has been reported that features of cytomegalic inclusion disease have been noted in 10–30 per cent of salivary glands of stillbirths, regardless of the cause of death. Adults are rarely affected, but in the known cases there is an association with severe debilitation such as occurs in terminal neoplastic disease. It is of interest that cytomegalovirus is associated with most cases of the postperfusion syndrome, an atypical mononucleosis-like illness. The most frequent clinical

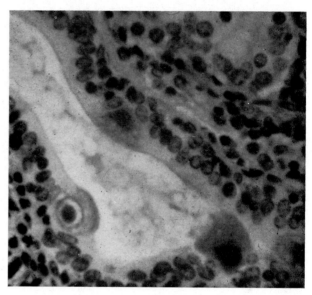

FIG. 7. Viral inclusion bodies within the cytoplasm of parotid duct cells. × 350.

manifestations are fever, hepatosplenomegaly and lymphocytosis and during the infection, immunological abnormalities may be induced. Diagnosis depends on the detection of characteristic cells in saliva, sputum or urine. Histologically, when the salivary glands are involved, numerous large doubly contoured inclusion bodies within the cytoplasm or nucleus of duct cells of affected glands are observed (fig. 7).

OBSTRUCTIVE AND TRAUMATIC LESIONS

In this category salivary duct fistula, sialolithiasis and mucocele formation will be discussed.

Salivary Duct Fistula

A salivary duct fistula is defined as a communication between the duct system and the skin which allows secretion of saliva externally. Though uncommon, salivary fistula is a troublesome and distressing condition. Internal fistulas may occur, but since they drain into the oral cavity they are asymptomatic and therefore of little consequence. A

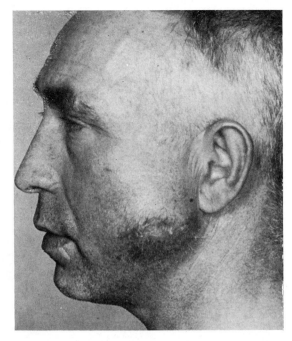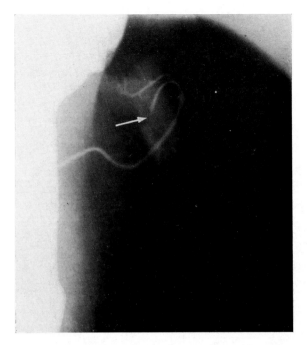

FIG. 8. Parotid salivary duct fistula formation arising as a complication of acute parotitis. (a) Facial swelling and fistula. (b) Confirmation of duct damage by sialography.

salivary duct fistula may be congenital though more commonly it follows trauma—for example, deep laceration of the cheek, as a complication of major gland surgery, or resulting from ulceration and infection associated with sialadenitis, large calculi or tumours.

In clinical practice wound infection is common in cases of duct fistula and granulation tissue and fibrous repair tissue may accumulate, leading to occlusion of the proximal duct and causing atrophy of the gland. More commonly, an external fistulous tract is established and the actual site of duct involvement may be determined by sialography (fig. 8). Treatment and management is primarily by surgical repair.

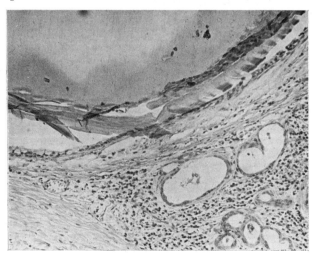

FIG. 9. Sialolith within the duct lumen of a minor salivary gland. Adjacent parenchymal tissue shows chronic inflammatory changes. × 95.

Sialolithiasis

Calcific masses within duct lumina leading to obstruction can be found in many organs of the human body, most often in the urinary tract, gall bladder and submandibular salivary gland. They may, however, also occur in the parotid and minor salivary glands, pancreas and lungs.

Salivary calculi are usually unilateral and round or oval, have a smooth or irregular surface, vary in size from 0·1–2·0 cm., and are usually yellowish. Calcium phosphates and carbonates comprise the major inorganic portion but iron oxide, sodium chloride, sodium or potassium thiocyanate and magnesium compounds may also be present. Mucopolysaccharides, cholesterol and uric acid are generally present.

The mechanism of formation and subsequent enlargement of sialoliths is complex. However, the concept of an initial organic nidus formation followed by the fairly uniform deposition of inorganic material appears to be supported by ultrastructural study.

Adults are more commonly affected, though sialolithiasis may occur in children, and the classical clinical signs and symptoms are those of pain and sudden enlargement of the affected gland, especially at mealtimes. Clinical diagnosis may be confirmed visually, by palpation and plain radiographs. Treatment, depending on the site and clinical features, is by surgical removal of the calculus though in some cases removal of the gland may be necessary. Histologically the affected gland will show the features of chronic sialadenitis whilst within the affected duct calcified material is observed (fig. 9).

Mucocele

Mucoceles may be superficial or deep and may vary in size from a few millimetres to 1 cm. in diameter. Those which are superficial are bluish, translucent, and rupture easily. Deeper-seated mucoceles have the same colour as surrounding oral mucosa. Recurrence is common, especially of the superficial type of lesion.

Histologically, mucoceles may be of two types, termed mucous extravasation cyst and mucous retention cyst.

The cause of the mucous extravasation cyst is considered to be mechanical trauma of minor excretory ducts leading to severance of the duct, with resultant spillage of mucous into the connective-tissue stroma. The mucous pool is localized or walled-off by a condensation of connective and granulation tissue (fig. 10). A mucous retention cyst refers

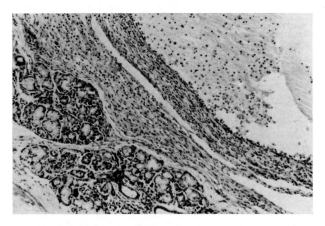

FIG. 10. Granulation tissue lining of a mucuous extravasation cyst (mucocele). × 30.

to a mucocele which results from a partial obstruction to the flow of saliva. As a consequence the duct dilates, resulting in a cystic lesion lined by simple columnar or pseudo-stratified squamous epithelium.

Mucoceles occur most commonly in the lower lip, followed by the buccal mucosa and floor of mouth. The palate and upper lip are rarely involved. A mucocele of anterior lingual salivary glands is often referred to as a cyst of Blandin-Nuhn. Ranula is the name given to a form of mucocele which occurs in the floor of the mouth and is associated with the ducts of the submandibular and the sublingual salivary glands. The ranula is usually a unilateral swelling, 2–3 cm. in diameter, which is soft, fluctuant and bluish-violet. Although generally painless it may interfere with speech, mastication and swallowing. Histologically it has a simple cuboidal epithelial lining and probably arises as a result of partial obstruction to the flow of saliva. A rather rare lesion, referred to as a deep ranula, is one which extends through and below the mylohyoid muscle and may extend as far back as the base of skull or into the neck. This lesion may take its origin from the cervical sinus, normally obliterated during embryonic life. The "true" cyst with a complete epithelial lining is usually about 1 cm. in diameter, and located within the affected salivary gland. The treatment for all lesions is by surgical removal or by marsupialization.

FUNCTIONAL DISORDERS

Xerostomia

Xerostomia, or dryness of the mouth, is a fairly common clinical complaint which can be extremely distressing to the patient. It is useful to distinguish between primary xerostomia, where a pathological lesion is present in the salivary glands as a manifestation of either localized or generalized disease, and secondary xerostomia where no detectable salivary lesion is present.

The causes of xerostomia are numerous and have recently been reviewed by Bertram (1967). Emotional and anxiety states and the effect of various drugs such as tranquillizers, hypotensive agents and atropine-containing medications are implicated in symptomatic xerostomia. Other causes include pernicious anaemia, iron deficiency anaemia, loss of fluid through haemorrhage, sweating, diarrhoea or vomiting, the polyuria of diabetes mellitus and diabetes insipidus and various vitamin and hormonal deficiencies. Primary xerostomia may be due to absence of salivary tissue, irradiation, glandular infection or obstruction and systemic disease in which the salivary glands are involved, such as Sjögren's syndrome.

In addition to dryness of the mouth, the patient may complain of a burning sensation, sore tongue, oral soreness and ulceration, and difficulty with denture retention. Xerostomia predisposes to infection of the pharynx and salivary glands and contributes to a marked increase in dental caries. The effects upon the oral mucosa include epithelial atrophy, inflammation, fissuring and ulceration.

Treatment is aimed at seeking and removing the cause. The use of a glycerine and lemon mouthwash is helpful in alleviating the symptoms in most cases. The use of sialogogues such as pilocarpine is of limited value and may be contra-indicated in some cases.

Increased Salivation

This condition is relatively uncommon, though it may be present during acute inflammatory conditions which lead to stomatitis, such as herpetic and aphthous ulceration, eruption of teeth, pregnancy and nausea. Mental retardation, epilepsy and cerebral injuries may give rise to a more permanent increased salivation. Attention to the cause together with bicarbonate mouthwashes are helpful for the temporary condition. The more permanent form may require the use of atropine-like drugs or extirpation of a gland.

Cystic Fibrosis

This serious, hereditary disorder of children and young adults may give rise to salivary gland dysfunction.

The disease affects the pancreas primarily, though exocrine glands are involved generally. The disorder in mucous glands leads to the production of a thick viscous secretion, stasis, duct dilatation, interstitial fibrosis and ultimately acinar atrophy. It is of interest that limited alterations are found in the composition of parotid saliva whereas significant elevations of various electrolytes, urea and uric acid and total protein are present in submandibular saliva. Two tests which reflect salivary gland dysfunction in cystic fibrosis have attracted attention in recent years. Firstly, the use of sodium-sensitive micro-electrodes has allowed easy and rapid detection of the increased sodium levels which are present in saliva in these patients. The convenience of this saliva test recommends its use as a less complicated screening test for cystic fibrosis than either the conventional sweat-test or duodenal aspiration. An important factor to note, however, is that the test must be carried out on unstimulated saliva since sodium is a salivary electrolyte which is flow rate-dependent. Secondly a minor labial salivary gland biopsy reflects the nature of the disease process in a majority of cases. The biopsy will show interstitial fibrosis, acinar atrophy and duct dilation together with the accumulation of eosinophilic plaque-like material within the duct lumina. At an ultrastructural level, apart from more mucus, the cells of the labial salivary glands show little difference from the normal.

NEOPLASIA

Salivary gland tumours are relatively uncommon, comprising fractionally more than 3 per cent of all tumours. In general, the incidence shows little variation between Europe and the United States where the major studies have been undertaken. However, slight exceptions include Eskimos who appear to be a high-risk group, and in the non-white populations of United States and Africa, females are affected more commonly than males. The parotid glands are by far the most commonly affected and tumours at this site are approximately ten times more common than those in either the submandibular glands or the minor glands taken as a group. Tumours of the sublingual salivary glands are even less common and therefore are extremely rare. It is of interest that certain racial groups show variation from this general situation. Amongst the Chinese in Malaya, for example, 30 per cent of salivary tumours occur in the submandibular glands, whilst in South Africa 29 per cent of tumours affect the palatal salivary glands. For intra-oral salivary gland tumours the palate is the commonest site, followed by the upper labial glands and buccal glands.

There is no evidence, either clinical or experimental, to suggest that in the salivary glands a pre-existing inflammatory, obstructive or traumatic condition predisposes to malignant change. There is evidence, however, that an association may exist between salivary gland carcinoma and breast cancer. The association with blood-group factors or secretors and non-secretors now appears unlikely. In experimental animals, salivary gland tumours may be induced by a variety of agents including carcinogenic hydrocarbons, ionizing radiation and polyoma virus. Almost without exception the lesions have been duct carcinomas of the squamous cell type, though tumours with adenomatous pattern have been produced on occasion.

Evidence has been provided, based on chromosome-marked cells, that tumours with predominant connective tissue features actually arise from epithelial cells and that mesenchymal cells do not contribute neoplastic cells to the tumour. A cell line having epithelial characteristics has been established from a human salivary gland pleomorphic adenoma.

It has been known for some time that both epithelial and mesenchymal mucins can be distinguished histochemically in the stroma of the pleomorphic adenoma. There are close morphological and functional similarities between smooth muscle cells and myoepithelial cells, and they have in common a closely related or identical protein which shows immunological cross-reactivity with actomyosin. Therefore, the concept of a myoepithelial cell having the ability to produce mixed stromal mucins in salivary tumours is an attractive one. Myoepithelial cells, however, present a problem of identification, especially at the light microscopic level, and histochemical stains cannot be relied upon to identify the cells. Myoepithelial cells have well defined ultrastructural characteristics (fig. 11) and electron microscopic studies have suggested that the myoepithelial cell plays an important role in the growth and development of pleomorphic adenoma, adenoid cystic carcinoma, adenolymphoma and oncocytoma. Quantitative ultrastructural comparison, however, of the cells of pleomorphic adenomas and of normal salivary glands, show that differences in percentage volumes of individual cell types are highly significant. A higher proportion by volume of cells of duct origin in pleomorphic adenoma (fig. 12) indicates that this cell, rather than the myoepithelial cell, is the principal cell of this tumour. However, more information is required in respect of the origin, ultrastructure and possible transformations of parenchymal cells in neoplasia before firm conclusions can be drawn as to the cells of origin of salivary gland tumours. The application to tumour material of an immunohistochemical method for identification of actomyosin in myoepithelium may be of considerable value.

In the past, some salivary gland tumours have been given not only a variety of names but also these terms have been applied to separate and different lesions. Recently, however, the World Health Organization has published a classification and concise description of salivary tumours, paying particular attention to the behavioural pattern of individual lesions (Thackray, 1972), and readers are referred to that manual as a starting-point for detailed study of individual salivary gland tumours.

SJÖGREN'S SYNDROME

Sjögren's syndrome, first described in 1933, consists of the triad of xerostomia, kerato-conjunctivitis sicca and, in one-half to two-thirds of patients, rheumatoid arthritis. Salivary gland and/or lacrimal gland enlargement may be present. In some cases, rheumatoid arthritis may be replaced by another connective tissue disease such as polyarteritis nodosa, systemic lupus erythematosus, progressive systemic sclerosis, polymyositis or dermatomyositis. The presence of two of these three main components is generally sufficient for the diagnosis of the syndrome. The term "sicca syndrome" is used when the connective tissue disorder is absent, i.e. only xerostomia and kerato-conjunctivitis are present.

Sjögren's syndrome is primarily a disorder which affects middle-aged females and is a common complication of

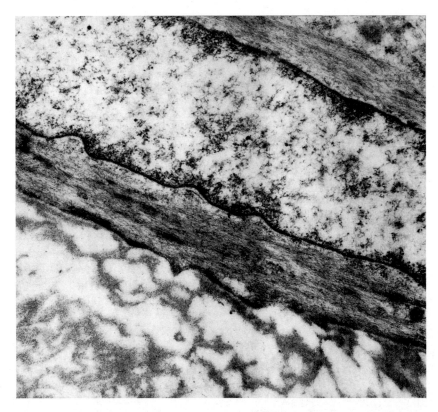

FIG. 11. Electronmicrograph showing the production of basement membrane-like material within the cyst-like space of an adenoid cystic carcinoma. A myoepithelial cell is present in relation to this material. × 9,100.

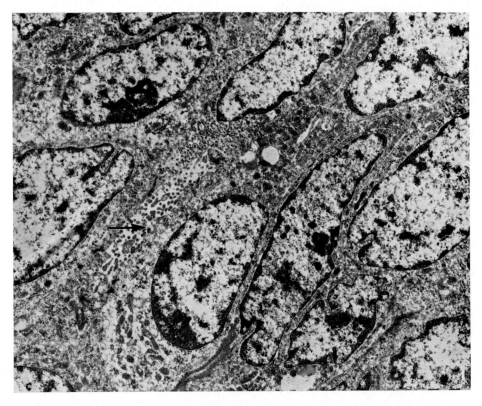

FIG. 12. Ultrastructural appearances of tumour cells from a cellular area of a pleomorphic adenoma. A duct lumen with short, stubby microvilli is indicated. × 4,750.

rheumatoid arthritis alone (Shearn, 1971). Though the cause of Sjögren's syndrome remains unknown, it seems likely that a combination of genetic, immunological, viral and/or environmental factors may play a role in the pathogenesis.

Xerostomia

Decreased salivation, difficulty in swallowing and mastication, increased fluid intake, abnormalities in taste sensation, oral mucosal soreness and ulceration are common symptoms. The oral mucous membranes appear dry, smooth and glazed, whilst lingual changes varying from slight reddening with mild fissuring to pronounced reddening with severe lobulation and deep fissuring are often present (fig. 13).

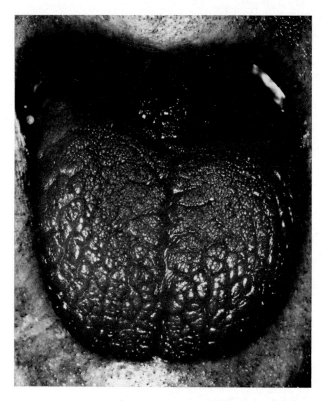

FIG. 13. Lobulated appearance of the tongue in a patient with Sjögren's syndrome.

The histopathological appearances of the oral epithelium in Sjögren's syndrome include basal-layer disruption, parakeratinization, lymphocytic infiltration and atrophy.

In patients with a natural dentition, rapidly progressive dental caries may be observed and patients with dentures have difficulty with retention and a high incidence of oral candidosis.

Salivary Gland Enlargement

Bloch et al. (1965) reported salivary gland enlargement in half of 62 patients studied, but our experience over a 10-year period has been that although a history of salivary gland enlargement may be elicited from approximately 30 per cent of patients, its presence is clinically apparent in only half that number. In the majority of cases, salivary swelling in Sjögren's syndrome occurs bilaterally and the parotid glands are more commonly affected. Patients with Sjögren's syndrome who develop lymphoid neoplasia are more likely to show salivary gland enlargement.

At present, there is no entirely satisfactory diagnostic test for the salivary gland component of Sjögren's syndrome. The diagnostic value of salivary function tests such as flow-rate estimation, labial salivary gland biopsy, hydrostatic sialography and ^{99m}Tc pertechnetate scintiscanning will now be considered.

Diagnostic Methods

Salivary Flow Rate Estimation. This method is a fairly reliable test of salivary gland function and 90 per cent of patients with Sjögren's syndrome, observed in the authors' clinic over a 10-year period had flow rate values below the normal range.

Labial Salivary Gland Biopsy. Although Sjögren himself reported labial gland involvement in a post-mortem study of one case, it was not until the histopathological features of groups of patients with various connective tissue disorders, including Sjögren's syndrome, were studied that the value of the labial biopsy was fully appreciated. Focal lymphocytic sialadenitis is present in approximately 70 per cent of patients with Sjögren's syndrome (fig. 14). The finding of local lymphocytic adenitis in the labial salivary glands in approximately 20 per cent of patients with rheumatoid arthritis alone is of interest, for this lesion may represent a sub-clinical form of Sjögren's syndrome in these patients. Conceptual support for the labial biopsy technique is provided by a post-mortem study in which focal lymphocytic sialadenitis could not be demonstrated in the labial glands.

Hydrostatic Sialography

Interpretation of sialographic abnormalities is based on criteria outlined by Bloch et al. (1965) and varying degrees of sialectasis are consistent findings in patients with Sjögren's syndrome.

Salivary Scintiscanning

Both qualitatively and quantitatively ^{99m}Tc pertechnetate uptake by the salivary glands is reduced in patients with Sjögren's syndrome. Approximately two-thirds of patient's with Sjögren's syndrome have uptake values below the lowest value for controls. Parotid gland involvement is more common than submandibular, and the parotid glands may be involved without the submandibular glands though the reverse does not hold and gland involvement is usually bilateral.

More recently, sequential salivary scintigraphy using the gamma camera has been shown to closely parallel reduction in flow rates and sialographic abnormalities in the syndrome.

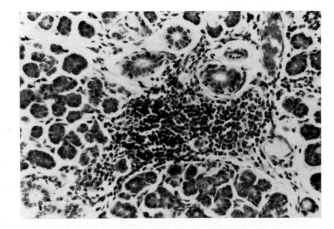

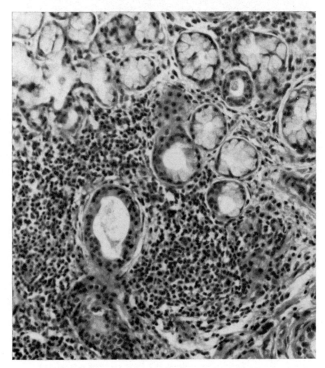

Fig. 14. Focal lymphocytic sialadenitis of the labial glands (above) and submandibular gland (below) of a patient with Sjögren's syndrome. Above × 30, below × 80.

Other Laboratory and Experimental Findings

An autoantibody to the cytoplasm of salivary duct cells has been demonstrated by indirect fluorescence. This antibody is considered to be a reflection of rheumatoid arthritis alone, rather than a manifestation of Sjögren's syndrome *per se*, and its pathogenic significance appears doubtful.

The histopathological features of the major salivary glands include acinar atrophy, focal lymphocytic sialadenitis and ductal hyperplasia leading to the formation of "epimyoepithelial" cell islands, though ultrastructural studies have failed to reveal the presence of myoepithelial cells in these cell islands. Virus-like particles, similar to murine C-type oncogenic virus have been reported within endothelial cells and lymphocytes in the parotid gland.

Although attempts to produce the salivary gland lesion of Sjögren's syndrome in experimental animals by immunization with salivary gland homogenates and Freund's adjuvant have met with limited success, a most interesting development has been the discovery that a series of abnormalities, resembling those of Sjögren's syndrome, occur spontaneously in NZB and NZWF mice. These abnormalities appear about the fourth month, together with other autoimmune phenomena, and increase in severity with age, particularly in females. In these animals, salivary amylase is reduced and the salivary protein concentration is elevated.

Malignant lymphoma may complicate Sjögren's syndrome in about 6–7 per cent of cases, and is more common in those with the sicca components only. Generally, such neoplastic change has an extra-salivary distribution, though malignant transformation may originate within the salivary glands. The prolonged state of immunological and lymphoid hyperactivity in patients with Sjögren's syndrome, especially those with the sicca syndrome, may be predisposing factors in the development of lymphoid neoplasia.

The role of cell-mediated immunity in the pathogenesis of Sjögren's syndrome has been demonstrated by the inhibition of macrophage migration *in vitro* by salivary gland extracts, whilst immunoglobulin synthesis by labial salivary gland lymphocytes has been shown.

Treatment and Management

A broad approach, directed both locally and systemically, is required in the treatment and management of the distressing symptoms of Sjögren's syndrome.

It is important that the oral mucous membranes be kept as moist as possible and, to this end, glycerine lozenges, methylcellulose (2 per cent solution) as a lubricant, and the salivary stimulant effect of boiled sweets may be of benefit to edentulous patients. A mouthwash containing citric acid (12·5 g.), essence of lemon (20 ml.) and glycerine (made up to 1 l.) has been used with success in our clinics. Patients should be encouraged to increase their fluid intake, and the importance of meticulous oral and dental hygiene should be stressed. Local infections such as candidosis should be detected and treated with appropriate antifungal agents. Salivary gland swelling usually subsides, but painful recalcitrant swellings may be treated with analgesics. Antibiotic therapy should be undertaken with care in view of the known tendency to drug allergies, especially to penicillin, in these patients.

Irradiation is contra-indicated for persistent salivary swelling in view of the known association of Sjögren's syndrome and lymphoid neoplasia. The use of corticosteroids does not appear to improve the sicca symptoms. Drugs which may cause or increase xerostomia, such as some tranquillizers and hypotensive agents, should be avoided or changed if possible. Parasympathomimetic drugs are contra-indicated in some cases. Immunosuppressive drugs, such as cyclophosphamide, have been tried recently and may cause an improvement of sicca symptoms in severe cases. However, this approach requires further study and cannot be recommended as a routine measure at the present time.

BENIGN LYMPHOEPITHELIAL LESIONS

In 1888 Mikulicz described a patient who had enlarged lacrimal and salivary glands. Histologically, the lacrimal gland showed a round cell infiltrate and acinar atrophy. The lesions recurred and were again excised but the patient died shortly thereafter from peritonitis. Retrospectively, it is impossible to know if this case represented a benign or malignant condition; but in the years since, cases of bilateral lacrimal and salivary gland swelling were labelled as Mikulicz's disease. A case of Mikulicz's disease is illustrated in fig. 15. In some patients, however, the cause of the

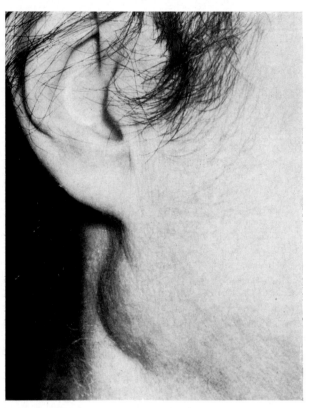

FIG. 15. Parotid swelling in a 54-year-old female patient with Mikulicz's disease (lymphoepithelial lesion).

glandular enlargement can be determined and it has been suggested that the term Mikulicz's syndrome be applied to such cases. Diseases which may give rise to lacrimal and salivary gland swelling include tuberculosis, syphilis, sarcoidosis, leukaemia and lymphoma. In 1953 Morgan and Castleman studied the clinical and pathological features of 18 cases of Mikulicz's disease and defined diagnostic histological criteria for the condition. Despite massive lymphocytic infiltration and acinar atrophy, the lobular architecture of the gland is retained. An additional characteristic feature is the intraductal proliferation of epithelial and myoepithelial cells giving rise to structures referred to as "epimyoepithelial cell islands" (fig. 16).

One year earlier (Godwin, 1952) in reviewing the histopathological features of Mikulicz's disease, suggested that the term benign lymphoepithelial lesion be applied to the condition. The term rapidly gained acceptance since it was aetiologically noncommittal and included the concept of non-malignancy. However, this concept has been disproved recently by evidence that a number of initially benign lesions undergo malignant transformation, usually in the direction of malignant lymphoma but occasionally also to undifferentiated carcinoma. A further area of confusion is the relationship between Mikulicz's disease or benign lymphoepithelial lesion and Sjögren's syndrome. Though the histopathological features are similar, if not identical, there is not enough clinical or investigative evidence to link the two conditions further. Clinical and laboratory studies have

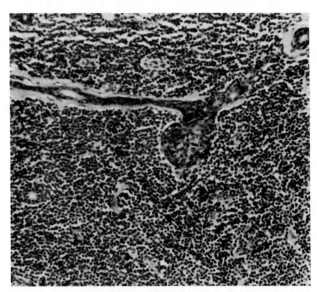

FIG. 16. Histopathological appearance of the parotid gland from a patient with Mikulicz's disease. Dense lymphocytic infiltration and an "epimyoepithelial cell island" are present. × 66.

been reported of patients with lymphoepithelial lesions in which none had the systemic manifestations associated with Sjögren's syndrome, nor developed any of the stigmata after a 10-year follow-up period. For the moment, it would appear that there is a case for considering the two conditions as separate entities. Further clinical and laboratory studies are required to be made before an association beyond the histopathological features can be made.

SIALOSIS

This is the term which has been used to describe a noninflammatory, non-neoplastic recurrent bilateral swelling of the salivary glands. The parotid glands are much more commonly affected than the submandibular glands. Histologically, the condition is characterized by serous acinarcell hypertrophy, oedema of the interstitial supporting tissue and atrophy of the striated ducts. The cytoplasm of the hypertrophic serous cells is more mucoid and less granular than normal. The lesion may progress to a lipomatosis of the affected glands. The majority of cases reported have been related to hormonal disturbances, chiefly ovarian, thyroid and pancreatic dysfunction, and to malnutrition, liver cirrhosis and chronic alcoholism. Drug-induced sialosis in experimental animals may follow the administration of various adrenergic and cholinergic drugs. In humans, parotid enlargement has been noted in patients taking medications such as phenylbutazone, iodide-containing compounds, thiouracil and catecholamines.

CHANGES WITH AGE

With increasing age individual cells or groups of cells in various glands undergo a striking change, becoming larger with an eosinophilic, granular cytoplasm. These cells have been called oncocytes, and neoplasms composed of similar

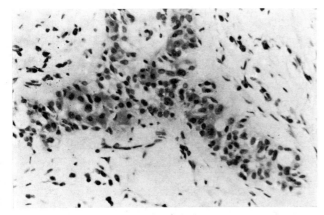

FIG. 17. Focal oncocytic hyperplasia affecting an epithelial cell island at the periphery of a pleomorphic adenoma. × 30.

cells sometimes occur. However, a non-neoplastic increase in number of oncocytes in the salivary glands may be termed oncocytosis. Oncocytosis would appear to be an age-related phenomenon, though in some instances inflammation or duct obstruction may provide the stimulus for oncocytic hyperplasia (fig. 17).

The ratio of functional acinar and duct cells to intracapsular fat and connective tissue in human salivary glands is seen microscopically to differ from subject to subject. A recent autopsy study has shown that when the values for the volume of functional mass of acinar and duct cells relative to that of fat and connective tissue in human submandibular glands were analysed in relation to age, a gradual significant reduction throughout adult life was found. Furthermore, the values reported were not related to the adiposity of the subject, no trend for change with age was found in the fresh net weights of the glands, and the results indicated a loss on average of a quarter of the relative secretory cell volume between childhood and old age, by which time the more severely affected glands had lost one-half.

This loss of functional reserve tissue may be association with the reported reduction with senescence of salivary flow rate and amylase activity. It is of interest that salivary gland enlargement has been noted to occur with greater frequency in older individuals, though whether or not this is due to fat accumulation remains speculative. Fatty replacement of salivary parenchymal tissue may occur, of course, as part of a pathological process or response such as malnutrition, following irradiation, sialadenitis and lipomatosis.

REFERENCES

Bertram, U. (1967), "Xerostomia. Clinical Aspects, Pathology and Pathogenesis," *Acta odont. scand.*, **25**, 1.

Bloch, K. J., Buchanan, W. W., Wohl, M. J. and Bunim, J. J. (1965), "Sjögren's Syndrome. A Clinical Pathological and Serological Study of Sixty-two Cases," *Medicine (Baltimore)*, **44**, 187.

Godwin, J. T. (1952), "Benign Lymphoepithelial Lesion of the Parotid Gland (Adenolymphoma, Chronic Inflammation, Lymphoepithelioma, Lymphocytic Tumour, Mikulicz Disease, Report of 11 Cases)," *Cancer*, **5**, 1089.

Morgan, W. S. and Castleman, B. (1953), "A Clinicopathologic Study of Mikulicz's Disease," *Amer. J. Path.*, **29**, 471.

Park, W. M. and Mason, D. K. (1966), "Hydrostatic Sialography," *Radiology*, **86**, 116.

Shearn, M. A. (1971), *Sjögren's Syndrome*, Vol. II, in the series "Major Problems in Internal Medicine," Philadelphia: W. B. Saunders Company.

45. THE STRUCTURE AND DEVELOPMENT OF BONE

J. J. PRITCHARD

Bone (that is to say, bony tissues), dentine, cementum and calcified cartilage are classified as mineralized, or calcified, connective tissues because their intercellular collagen-mucopolysaccharide matrices are in part hardened with an inorganic mineral rich in calcium. The matrices of bone, dentine and cementum are similar, but in calcified cartilage the matrix is distinguished by its high mucopolysaccharide/collagen ratio.

Bony tissues have in common a framework of hard material (mineralized bone matrix), a specialized cell population, and a special type of vasculature. Adult bone is readily divided into compact, and coarse cancellous, types: compact bone (fig. 1) appears to the naked eye to be composed of solid mineralized matrix, because the vascular channels are too fine to be seen, while in coarse cancellous bone the spongy character of the matrix framework is obvious. During its development bone (figs. 2 and 3) is not so readily classified. When first formed in fetal life, or in fracture repair, it is cancellous, but with so fine a texture that the cancellous structure cannot be distinguished macroscopically; as the bone matures this fine cancellous bone is gradually remodelled into either compact or coarse cancellous bone, or else it is removed altogether in the formation of a marrow cavity.

BONE MATRIX

Bone matrix has an organic component making up about one-third of its dry weight, and consisting of collagen fibrils aggregated into fibres and fibre bundles within a ground substance, or cement, containing mucopolysaccharides;

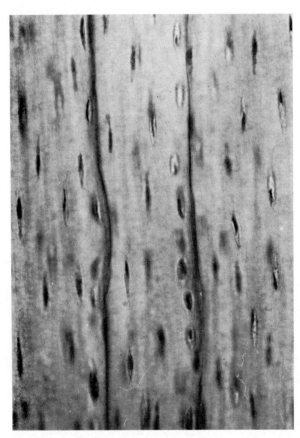

FIG. 1. Compact lamellar bone showing two cement lines. Adult rat tibia. Haematoxylin and eosin. ×234.

and an inorganic component making up some two-thirds of the dry weight, and chiefly consisting of calcium phosphate $(Ca_{10}(PO_4)_6(OH)_2)$ in micro-crystalline form.

Bone matrix is classified as lamellar or non-lamellar depending on whether or not it exhibits a laminated appearance in sections, especially when viewed with polarized light (fig. 5). In lamellar bone the fibre bundles are thin and uniform in size, and are arranged in sheets (lamellae).

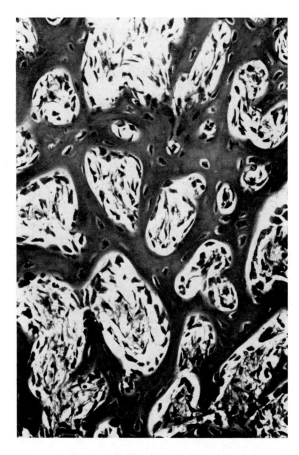

FIG. 2. Fine cancellous membrane bone. Newborn rat tibia. Weigert's haematoxylin and van Gieson. ×234.

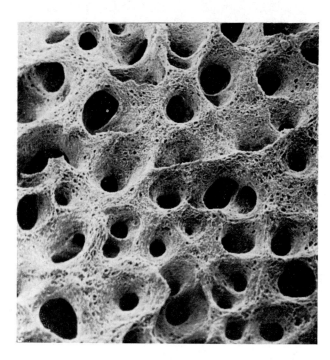

FIG. 3. Fine cancellous membrane bone. 5-month-fetal horse. Scanning EM. (Courtesy of Dr. A. Boyde.) × 60.

Lamellation is particularly clear when either the direction, or the density, of the fibre bundles differs significantly in alternate sheets (fig. 4).

In non-lamellar bone (often called woven bone) coarse and fine fibre bundles are mixed and a laminated arrangement is not seen. Coarse bundles are particularly numerous at sites accommodating attachment fibres from soft tissues, in which case the term bundle (or Sharpey-bundle) bone is often used.

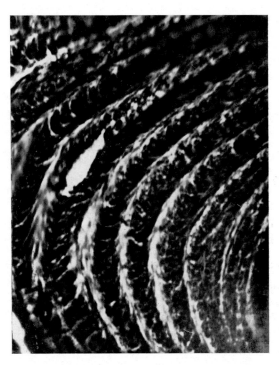

FIG. 4. Lamellar bone. Adult human parietal. Wilder. × 850.

In adult bone, whether of the compact or the coarse cancellous type, the matrix is mostly of the lamellar variety. In compact bone matrix the lamellae are arranged (fig. 5) either as concentric cylinders around blood vessels (concentric lamellar systems, osteons, Haversian systems), or in extensive stacks where the grain is parallel to the periosteal or medullary surface (circumferential lamellar systems, ground lamellae, surface bone), or else as fragments of osteons inserted between complete ones (interstitial lamellar systems). In adult cancellous bone matrix, interstitial lamellar systems predominate. In fine cancellous "fetal" bone the matrix is initially non-lamellar, but as it is remodelled it is consolidated and replaced and overlaid with lamellar bone.

BONE CELLS

The bone cells are a closely related group which include **osteocytes, osteoblasts, osteoclasts** and **osteoprogenitor cells**. The basic type is the **osteoprogenitor** cell, which can be in a dormant state, or it can be undergoing mitotic division, or it can be transforming into an osteoblast, or an osteoclast (or even into a chondroblast under certain circumstances).

Osteoblasts, which are heavily engaged in the manufacture of bone matrix, do not divide. Many of them become trapped in the matrix and change into osteocytes, while others probably revert to the osteoprogenitor state when their work is done. Osteoclasts are actively involved in bone matrix resorption: they are believed to arise by fusion of osteoprogenitor cells, but other modes of recruitment are also possible. When their work is done they may revert to being osteoprogenitor cells, but the evidence is not definite.

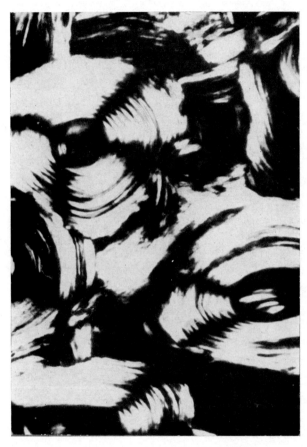

FIG. 5. Osteons (Haversian systems). Human femur. Polarized light. × 200.

Osteocytes are believed to "maintain" the bone matrix around them in some way, and they possibly regulate the flow of minerals and nutrients between bone and blood It is not known if they are capable of reverting to the progenitor state when released from their prisons as a result of resorption of the matrix around them. In regions of very active growth, especially if tissues are under compression, osteoprogenitor cells may transform into cartilage cells instead of osteoblasts, and cartilage rather than bone matrix is deposited.

Osteoblasts

These are large cells with an ovoid body about three times as long as it is broad (say, 8 × 25μm.) and a great many fine branching processes, mostly too fine to be seen with the light microscope. The nucleus lies at one end and occupies about one-third of the cell, an enormous Golgi complex occupies most of the middle third of the cell, while the other third shows an extensive granular endoplasmic reticulum, a fair number of mitochondria, some lipid granules and dense bodies, and areas with microfilaments and microtubules (fig. 6). In ordinary histological preparations an osteoblast is recognized by its situation on a bone matrix perimeter, by its large size, eccentric nucleus, and clear, eosinophilic Golgi area, and by its intensely basophilic cytoplasm outside the Golgi area (fig. 7). Histochemically, osteoblasts are characterized by intense alkaline phosphatase activity. *In toto*, osteoblast cytology indicates that the cell is heavily engaged in the manufacture of some secretion for export, and both circumstantial evidence, and evidence from autoradiographic studies using labelled proline and sulphate, indicate that collagen and mucopolysaccharides are being made. It is widely believed that the intense alkaline phosphatase activity of osteoblasts is associated in some way with the deposition of the inorganic, mineral component of bone matrix, but the details remain elusive. For greater detail refer to Pritchard, 1972.

Osteoclasts

These are large cells with many nuclei; it is possible that cells with similar functions, but with only one or two nuclei, have been overlooked. Cytologically, in addition to its numerous nuclei, an osteoclast is noted for its very large complement of mitochondria (fig. 8), its numerous lysosomes, and its complexly-folded "ruffled border" and cytoplasm laden with vacuoles where it is in contact with crumbling bone matrix. Histochemically, osteoclasts show marked acid phosphatase activity. These features are hallmarks of a highly energetic resorptive cell; and there is little doubt that osteoclasts are responsible for dissolving the inorganic part and digesting the organic part of bone matrix, but once again, the precise mechanisms are not known. For greater detail refer to Hancox, 1972.

Osteocytes

When recently buried in bone matrix these are similar to osteoblasts in their cytology, but as they mature they lose much of their complement of organelles, and shrink (fig. 9). The body of the mature osteocyte in lamellar bone is shaped like a melon seed, and neighbouring cells are well-spaced and orientated to conform with the grain of the bone. The body lies in a cavity called a **lacuna,** and its fifty or so major processes lie in minute tunnels called **canaliculi.** In non-lamellar bone the osteocytes are plumper, more crowded and more randomly arranged than in lamellar bone. There is little doubt that osteocytes, when young, can secrete a little more matrix around themselves, but the view, strenuously held in some quarters, that older osteocytes are effective in resorbing the bone matrix round them, receives little support from their cytological characteristics, which do not resemble those of a resorptive cell.

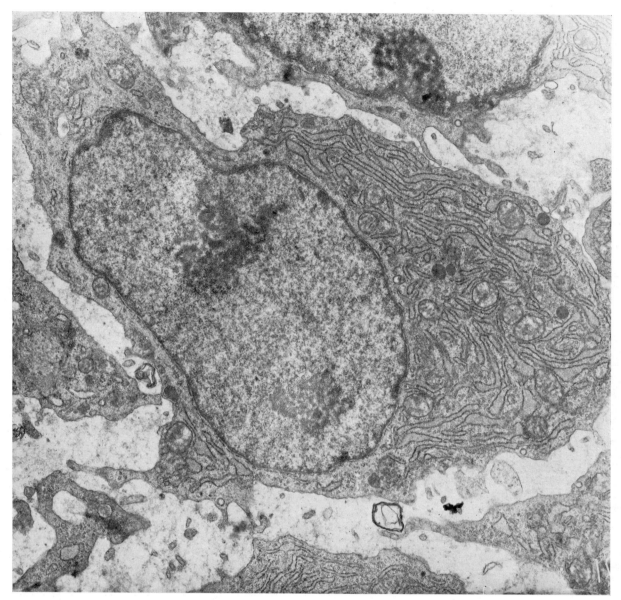

Fig. 6. Osteoblast. Newborn rat tibia. E.M. × 10,000.

Osteoprogenitor Cells

These were formerly known as osteogenic cells, cambial cells and pre-osteoblasts. In their dormant state they cannot be identified with certainty, but the inconspicuous flat cells lying next to inactive bone matrix surfaces are assumed to belong to their number. Near active bone surfaces, the cells showing mitotic figures, or which can be flash-labelled with tritiated thymidine, are regarded as osteoprogenitor cells, as are their immediate non-dividing neighbours in the same zone at the same distance from the bone surface. In active periosteum the cells between the fibroblasts of the fibrous periosteum and the osteoblasts on the bone surface are taken to be osteoprogenitor cells. However, the osteoprogenitor cells in the middle zone of the periosteum are not homogeneous in their cytology: those near the fibrous periosteum are more like fibroblasts, while those near the

osteoblasts are more like osteoblasts. Osteoprogenitor cells, in fact, form a graded series in which the osteoblast condition is approached from a fibroblast-like condition as a result of hypertrophy of cytoplasmic organelles, particularly the Golgi complex, but also of the granular endoplasmic reticulum and the mitochondrial complement. As a result, the cell gets much plumper and its nucleus gets pushed to one end so that the enormous Golgi complex comes to occupy the centre of the cell. Metabolically and chemically there is evidence of increasing activity also, as shown by histochemical reactions for enzymes, especially alkaline phosphatase, and by rates of uptake of isotope-labelled raw materials.

The conversion of osteoprogenitor cells into osteoblasts is fairly well documented, but the alternate pathways to osteoclasts and chondroblasts are less well known; in particular, there is little in the way of direct evidence of osteoclast formation through fusion of osteoprogenitor cells, while the complexities of cartilage cell maturation have not been satisfactorily unravelled, partly because cartilage cells can exist in so many forms. On the whole, the type of cartilage cell which is derived from an osteoprogenitor cell has more in common with an osteoblast, cytologically and histochemically, than the type of cartilage cell derived from ordinary perichondrium. For greater detail refer to Young, 1964.

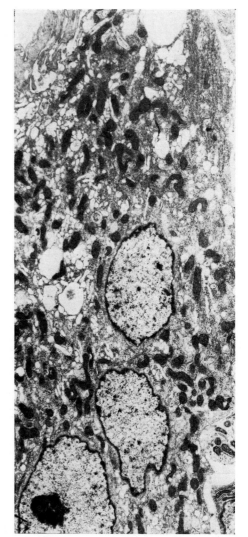

FIG. 8. Part of an osteoclast. Newborn rat tibia. E.M. × 4,000.

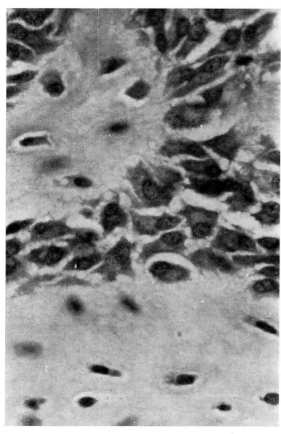

FIG. 7. Osteoblasts. Chick radius. Haematoxylin and eosin. × 730.

Finally, the point should be made that while, normally, osteoprogenitor cells are confined to the vicinity of bone surfaces, under abnormal circumstances they may appear in almost any connective tissue, and initiate **heterotopic** bone formation.

THE BLOOD VESSELS OF BONY TISSUES

Bony tissues are richly vascular. Between the arteries which enter, and the veins which leave a bone, there is a complex network of fine vessels. Where the bone is compact, the small vessels run in narrow canals, and are like capillaries, but longer and wider than usual (fig. 10). Where the bone is spongy the vessels tend to be in the form of dilated thin-walled venous channels, or sinusoids. It is probable that the direction of flow in the small vessels is mostly centrifugal, that is, towards the periosteum.

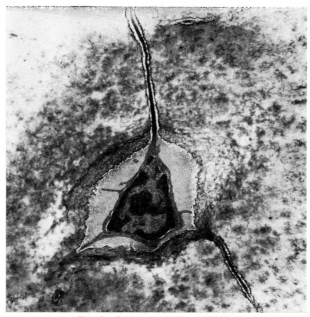

FIG. 9. Osteocyte. E.M. × 6,800.

PERIOSTEUM

The periosteum is a fibrous membrane which ensheathes a bone everywhere except at cartilage-covered surfaces and where tendons and ligaments are attached. It serves for muscle attachment, as a bed for blood vessels, and as a major agent in bone growth and repair. An important function of periosteum in the growth period is to form a strong bond between the shaft and epiphysis of a long bone. Its structure

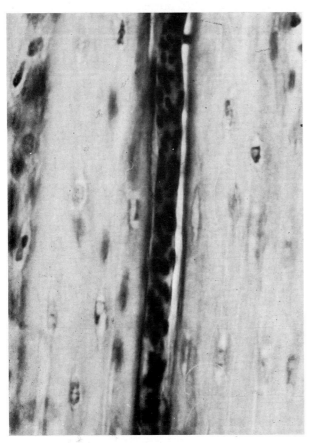

Fig. 10. Vascular canal in compact bone. Radius of chicken. Haematoxylin and eosin. ×350.

varies considerably. Around fetal bones the periosteum is clearly in two layers (fig. 11), an outer densely fibrous containing long thin fibroblasts, and an inner much less fibrous, containing plump osteoprogenitor cells, osteoblasts and osteoclasts. The outer layer becomes increasingly thick as it approaches the ends of the bone, where it is firmly attached. The inner layer continues into the interstices of the underlying fine cancellous bone without sharp demarcation. The inner layer is evidently actively engaged in bone formation and bone resorption at this stage. Around adult bones the periosteum is generally in the form of layers of dense fibrous tissue, firmly attached to the ends of the bone and to ligaments and tendons passing to the bone, but only loosely attached elsewhere by fibrous threads around the small vessels entering and leaving the bone surface. Osteoblasts and osteoclasts are rarely seen on the bone surface in adult life, and osteoprogenitor cells are almost

impossible to make out. However, if the bone is fractured, or damaged in any way, the periosteum locally returns to the fetal condition and within a few days osteoprogenitor cells are multiplying and osteoblasts and osteoclasts are active once again in the deeper layers of the membrane (Pritchard, 1964). Presumably, adult periosteum contains dormant osteoprogenitor cells which respond rapidly to a variety of stimuli by enlargement, multiplication and conversion into bone-forming or bone-destroying cells, or in some circumstances, into cartilage-forming cells. Indeed, cartilage formation by periosteum is not only a common event after injuries to bone (fig. 12), but is a normal event in the development of many bones. Thus the cartilage in the condyle of the mandible is originally periosteal.

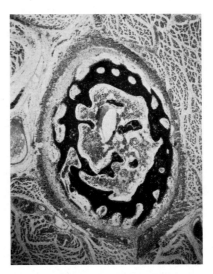

Fig. 11. Fibula, showing outer and inner layers of periosteum, periosteal bone and marrow cavity. Six-month-human fetus. Mallory. × 15.

BONE MARROW

The term "bone marrow" is usually restricted to the soft red or yellow tissue occupying the macroscopically visible cavities in a fresh bone. There is no agreed term, unfortunately, for the soft-tissue contents of the fine canals and spaces in the more solid parts of a bone: "endosteum" would have been a useful word if it had not been pre-empted for the cell layer of the marrow next to the bone. Bone marrow is essentially a framework of reticular tissue (reticulum cells and fibres) supporting blood vessels, especially venous sinusoids, and either colonies of developing blood cells, or large fat cells.

Reticulum cells readily turn into osteoprogenitor cells, and indeed could well be classed with them. The endosteum, and the contents of the finer canals and spaces in bone, are essentially marrow without blood-cell-forming colonies. The deeper layer of the periosteum, the tissues within the fine canals of compact bone, the tissue between the trabeculae of cancellous bone, and the bone marrow, are, in fact, anatomically continuous and functionally equipotential, at least so far as bone formation and destruction are concerned; they all readily generate osteoblasts and osteo-clasts from their osteoprogenitor reserves when suitably stimulated.

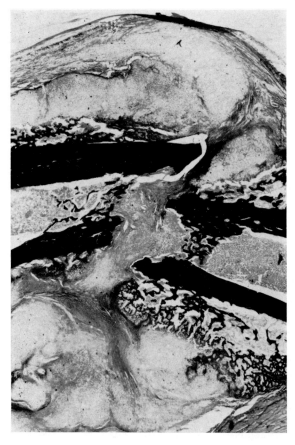

FIG. 12. Ten-day tibial fracture callus showing new bone and cartilage. Young rat. Weigert's haematoxylin and van Gieson.

OSSIFICATION

(bone formation, osteogenesis)

This section will be concerned first of all with the events accompanying the production of fine cancellous bone from precursor fibrous and cartilaginous tissues—that is to say, with the events of primary intramembranous and primary endochondral ossification (fig. 13).

Primary Intramembranous Ossification is characteristic of beginning ossification in the face and skull vault, and in early periosteal, tendinous and ligamentous ossification generally. In all cases, a fibrous framework with vascular interstices is first generated, and then the framework is converted into bone matrix through the agency of osteoblasts evolving from the local connective tissue cell population. The conversion of fibrous tissue into bone matrix involves the addition of more collagenous fibres, of cement, and of hydroxyapatite. The matrix before it is calcified is called "osteoid", which may thus be thought of as collagen plus cement. It is not the same as decalcified bone—rather it is uncalcified bone!

The **primary membrane bone** which results is in the form of a fine cancellous framework of non-lamellar bone matrix whose interstices are occupied by osteoblasts, osteo-progenitor cells and wide capillaries or sinusoids (fig. 2). Here and there plump osteocytes are buried in the matrix. Many of the fibre bundles in the matrix were present before ossification, and were passively incorporated in the osteoid and bone matrix later on. Where a great many coarse fibre bundles have been inherited from a tendon or ligament, the result is bundle bone; in it the osteocytes tend to lie in long columns between the coarse bundles. Where the fibre bundles have been taken over from the deeper layer of the

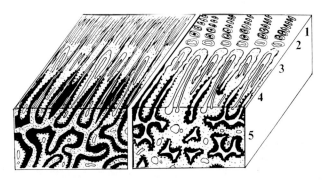

FIG. 13. Diagram comparing intramembranous and endochondral ossification in longitudinal and transverse section 1. Zone of growing fibrous tissue (left): zone of growing cartilage (right). 2. Zone of dead chondrocytes and calcified matrix (right). 3. Zone of vascular loops and progenitor cells. 4. Zone of bone formation on fibrous strands (left) and on calcified cartilage (right). 5. Network of fine cancellous membrane bone (left) and fine cancellous cartilage bone (right).

periosteum they tend to be variable in size and arrangement, and the osteocytes are more randomly arranged (ordinary woven bone).

Periosteum in which primary membrane bone formation (intramembranous ossification) is active, therefore ideally shows from outside in, first a layer of dense fibrous tissue containing elongated fibroblasts, then a zone of actively multiplying osteoprogenitor cells and new fibrous tissue, then a zone in which the new fibrous tissue has been converted into a network of osteoid, crusted with osteoblasts, and housing in its interstices wide, thin-walled blood vessels and osteoprogenitor cells, and finally a network of calcified osteoid, that is to say, bone matrix, with imprisoned osteo-cytes (fig. 13).

The network sometimes has its grain more or less perpendicular to the long axis of a bone, but more often the grain is oblique, and may be almost parallel to the long axis in some places, so that appearances are different in different planes of section, with the matrix sometimes resembling "chicken-wire" and sometimes parallel strips (fig. 13). A tendon or ligament into which bone is extending shows much the same general features except for greater fibre density in the precursor tissue, and greater regimentation of cells, fibres and blood vessels at the ossification front. Passing along the tendon or ligament towards the bone, normal tendon or ligament is followed by a zone in which the cells are enlarging and becoming more like osteoblasts, and then a zone in which groups of bundles encrusted with osteoblasts alternate with loose vascular and cellular tissue. These grouped bundles then become transformed to osteoid, and finally calcified, forming trabeculae of bundle bone matrix. It is possible in suitable sections to see long columns of cells passing from tendon to bone in which tendon cells, osteoprogenitor cells, osteoblasts and osteocytes follow one another in the same column, and are in register with the cells of neighbouring columns right across the tendon. In cross-section the appearances are totally different, the new bone having a frankly cancellous appearance. Not all tendons and ligaments ossify in this manner, however. In many situations the cells become chondroblasts instead of osteoblasts, and the tendon is converted into fibro-cartilage before undergoing endochondral ossification.

Primary Endochondral Ossification takes place at centres of ossification in cartilage models, and at the cartilaginous ends of growing bones. First of all, cartilage cells multiply and new cartilage matrix is manufactured; then the cells become greatly enlarged, they calcify the matrix around them, and then die, leaving a honeycomb of calcified cartilage matrix. This is immediately invaded by osteoprogenitor cells and blood vessels which resorb some of the partitions in the calcified cartilage network, so opening it up, and deposit bone matrix on the residual calcified cartilage partitions. Part of the resorption is undoubtedly carried out by multinuclear cells resembling osteoclasts, which in this context are called chondroclasts; but there is a body of opinion that other cells, including vascular endothelium, are also involved. Bone matrix deposition is carried out by osteoblasts which form from some of the osteoprogenitor cells. The first matrix contains fine uniform bundles of fibres, but is not obviously lamellated.

In sections across areas where endochondral ossification is active we see first of all a cartilage zone in which the cells are flat and multiplying, and piling up in parallel columns like so many stacks of coins. Then comes a zone in which the cells of the columns are less thin, and then a zone in which they are grossly swollen and spherical. The matrix around the last few cells in the columns of swollen cells is calcified, and the last cell of all is dead. Beyond this, one sees a zone where the residual calcified cartilage honeycomb, having lost its cartilage cells, has been colonized by blood vessels and marrow cells, and beyond this again, a more open network of calcified cartilage matrix coated with new bone matrix and osteoblasts (fig. 13). These successive zones are referred to usually as the proliferative, prehypertrophic, hypertrophic and calcified cartilage zones, the primary spongiosa (of vascularized calcified cartilage) and the secondary spongiosa (of fine cancellous bone).

The fine cancellous "cartilage" bone formed in this way differs from the fine cancellous "membrane" bone previously described in that it has calcified cartilage remnants in its matrix, and its fibre bundles are fine, uniform and regularly arranged.

Neither form of fine cancellous bone lasts long. The network is opened up through osteoclastic resorption in some places, and consolidated through osteoblastic accretionary action in others, so that both its general texture, and the fine structure of its matrix, change rapidly. Grossly it becomes compact, or coarsely cancellous, or else it disappears to make a marrow cavity, while in its fine structure it shows an increasing content of lamellar bone.

THE FORMATION OF LAMELLAR SYSTEMS

Fine cancellous bone may be thought of as a bundle of thin-walled hollow cylinders traversed by fine blood vessels, and with osteoprogenitor cells and osteoblasts lying between the vessels and the cylinder walls. Concentric centripetal deposition of new lamellar bone matrix within each thin-walled cylinder converts it into a thick-walled cylinder with only a narrow central vascular canal. Such a cylinder is termed a primary osteon—or primary concentric lamellar system.

Surface bone (circumferential or ground lamellar system) is formed by slow addition of lamellae parallel to the periosteal and medullary surfaces of existing bone.

The classical, or secondary, osteon (Haversian system) has usually a much wider diameter than the primary osteon, and is formed in a different way. First of all, a narrow vascular channel in a primary osteon or surface bone widens markedly, as a result of osteoclastic action which pays little or no heed to osteonal boundaries; and then osteoblasts appear and fill in the dilated channel with concentric lamellae. Secondary and primary osteons are easily differentiated because the former begin their filling-in with a thin layer of fibre-free cement, which remains as a readily-seen cement line around the completed osteon, whereas the primary osteons are not bounded externally by cement lines. Such lines are common in bone and indicate where the steady deposition of lamellae has been temporarily arrested (arrest lines, fig. 1), or where deposition has begun again after a period of resorption (reversal lines). Bone does not usually remain at the secondary osteon stage; such osteons in their turn are resorbed (or partly resorbed) and tertiary osteons take their place, and so on, the complement of fragmentary osteons (interstitial lamellar systems) steadily increasing, and the pattern of reversal lines becoming ever more intricate. Coarse cancellous bone is a conglomerate of interstitial lamellar systems separated by a jig-saw pattern of reversal lines, as betokens a tissue which has been remodelled many times in the course of its life.

It should not be supposed, however, that all compact bone in the adult skeleton is riddled with remodelled secondary osteons; much of it remains at the primary osteon stage, and in the bones of some small mammals, secondary osteons do not form at all.

BONE MATRIX FORMATION

So far little has been said about the way bone matrix is manufactured—about the chemistry of the process (described in detail in the next chapter), and the way this is controlled. The position is far from clear, but in a general way it is envisaged that osteoblasts secrete collagen molecules (tropocollagen), muco-polysaccharides and glycoproteins, and then, outside the cells, the collagen molecules aggregate into fibrils which can be seen with the electron microscope, and these in turn aggregate into fibres (visible with the light microscope), and fibre-bundles.

Fibre orientation and registration over a wide area is difficult to explain, but it is believed that the osteoblast is able to exert a decisive influence over the alignment of fibres in its immediate neighbourhood.

Some facts about mineralization are clearly established, however. Once begun, mineral deposition in lamellar osteoid proceeds rapidly until some 70 per cent of full mineralization is achieved in a day or two, but thereafter the completion of mineralization takes weeks or months. Non-lamellar bone, however, seems to complete its mineralization much more quickly, and so in a growing bone the lamellar parts, on average, are less well mineralized than the non-lamellar parts. It is also known that cement lines are heavily calcified, even though they are devoid of fibres. However, it would seem that where lamellae have a high cement–collagen ratio the collagen bundles calcify before the cement.

DEVELOPMENT AND GROWTH OF BONES

The general pattern of development and growth of a bone can be summed up as:

(a) The formation and growth of a fibrous, or a cartilage and fibrous model (*i.e.* a cartilage model wrapped in fibrous tissue);

(b) the formation and growth of a primary bony model within and at the expense of the fibrous, or cartilage and fibrous model;

(c) the emergence of the definitive adult bone through remodelling of the primary bone model; and

(d) maintenance, adaptation and repair of the adult bone through further remodelling.

Ossification begins in most bones in fetal life at points called primary centres of ossification, and most of the bony tissue of the adult skeleton is formed as a result of growth of these centres. However, outside the skull, and usually after birth, secondary centres of ossification appear in the extremities and projections of the cartilage models, and grow into bony epiphyses: for some time these are separated from the parts of the bones developed from primary centres by bands of cartilage, but eventually the cartilage disappears and the epiphyses fuse with the main body, or shaft, of the bone. In the skull, some bones are composite, in that parts developing from separate primary centres of ossification eventually fuse through disappearance of the intervening fibrous tissue or cartilage. Thus, there are many more centres of ossification than there are adult bones: the humerus, for example, develops from one primary and seven secondary centres, while the sphenoid develops from as many as fourteen primary centres.

The bone laid down at centres of ossification, and at the rapidly growing periphery of a mass of bone, is of the fine cancellous variety, but deeper in the bony mass remodelling of the bony tissue takes place through removal of some trabeculae, and thickening of others, so that the mass becomes either more compact or more openly (coarsely) cancellous. The fine cancellous bone, and especially the fine cancellous membrane bone, is typically non-lamellar, but the bone which thickens the trabeculae in the course of

remodelling is typically lamellar. Gradually, therefore, in the course of development non-lamellar bone is replaced by lamellar bone.

Development and Growth of a Typical Membrane Bone (*e.g.* the Parietal)

Before ossification begins there is a fibrous model for the whole skull vault termed the brain capsule. Centres of ossification for the parietals, left and right halves of the frontal, squamous temporals and supraoccipital, appear as islands of dilated blood vessels within the brain capsule, associated with which the capsule cells differentiate into osteoprogenitor cells and osteoblasts, the latter depositing a network of bony trabeculae interdigitating with the blood vessels. These events take place in the middle stratum of the

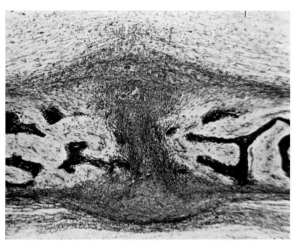

Fig. 14. Developing sagittal suture. Fetal sheep. Weigert's haematoxylin and van Gieson. ×50.

capsule (fibrous model): the outer and inner strata of the capsule remain fibrous, the former becoming a fibrous periosteal layer termed the pericranium, the latter delaminating into the periosteal layer (endocranium) and the meningeal layer of the dura mater. Between the centres of ossification, where the brain capsule is three-layered (fibrous, bony, fibrous) the capsule remains as a single fibrous layer. Through proliferation of osteoprogenitor cells, and differentiation of osteoblasts around the first-formed bony network at the centre of ossification, the network expands both in thickness and in area, but particularly in area, and more and more of the capsule becomes three-layered. It is as if the growing bone were splitting the capsule and insinuating itself between outer and inner fibrous layers. The unsplit capsule is of course growing at the same time, but the bones for a while grow faster, until eventually the bone edges advancing from the separate centres of ossification approach closely in many places, and begin to establish sutural relationships (fig. 14): in other places the edges remain relatively far apart leaving unossified areas of the capsule between them, known as fontanelles. At the sutures the ossification fronts of proliferating osteoprogenitor cells belonging to the adjacent bone surfaces are separated by a zone of loose fibrous tissue which becomes the sutural membrane

(Pritchard, Scott and Girgis, 1956). Bone growth at the sutural edges of the bone is not inhibited, because the pericranial and endocranial fibrous tissue bridging the bony gap continues to expand under the stretching stimulus provided by the growing brain, and so room is constantly being created for bone expansion. In addition, in most sutures, the growing bone edges pass each other and overlap to an increasing extent, the loose fibro-cellular tissue of the immature sutural membrane offering little hindrance. Later the sutural membrane becomes increasingly fibrous, and sutural bone growth slows down and stops. Further growth of the skull can then only take place by remodelling, that is to say, by adding new bone on the outer surface of the skull and removing old bone from the inner surface. Meanwhile, the main body of the bone is being remodelled from an initial fine cancellous state to a condition in which the bone consists of outer and inner tables of compact bone with a middle stratum of coarse cancellous bone (diplöe), in the interstices of which haemopoietic marrow finds a home, and blood-cell manufacture continues throughout life, except where paranasal air sinuses develop instead.

In adult life sutural membranes gradually disappear, and the separate cranial bones fuse, but unlike birds and most mammals which show this synostosis as soon as maturity is reached, some sutures in Man remain partially or completely unclosed even into extreme old age.

Development and Growth of a Long Bone (*e.g.* the Tibia)

Development begins with the rapid multiplication of mesenchymal cells and the formation of a "model" of closely packed cells. Most of these cells then become cartilage cells and secrete cartilage matrix around themselves, forming the primary cartilage model, but the more superficially placed cells form a fibrous membrane (perichondrium) around the cartilage model. The cartilage model grows partly by cell multiplication and new matrix production within the model (interstitial growth) and partly by addition of new cartilage on the outside as a result of the conversion of the cells of the deeper layer of the perichondrium into cartilage cells (appositional growth). Where cartilage models meet, an interzone of unchondrified fibrous tissue is left between them. This tissue for a while contributes to appositional cartilage growth on the adjoining ends of the models, but later it either breaks down to give a synovial cavity, or else forms a plate of fibro-cartilage, according to whether a synovial or a secondary cartilaginous joint is being formed.

The initial cartilage model is a miniature approximate replica of the adult bone. The onset of bone formation to give a primary centre of ossification is heralded by profound changes in the middle segment of the cartilage model. The cells become greatly enlarged (hypertrophied) at the expense of the matrix, which is reduced to thin septa between the cells. These septa then undergo mineralization, while the cells themselves die, leaving spaces termed primary areolae. These spaces do not remain empty but are soon colonized by blood vessels and progenitor cells derived from the perichondrium locally.

Before the cartilage cells die, however, the perichondrium around the hypertrophic segment of the cartilage model becomes increasingly vascular, and the deeper cells of the perichondrium transform into osteoprogenitor cells, some of which become osteoblasts and deposit a layer of bone matrix on the surface of the hypertrophic cartilage, to form a primary centre of ossification. Some of the progenitor cells then differentiate into chondroclasts, and these invade the underlying calcified cartilage ahead of blood vessels and undifferentiated progenitor cells. The chondroclasts remove some of the calcified cartilage partitions between the primary areolae, converting them into larger secondary

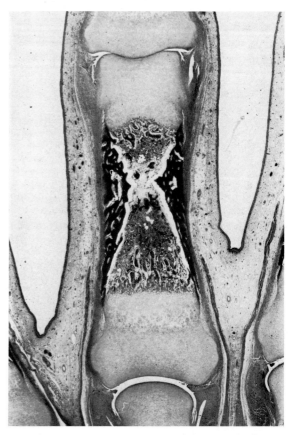

Fig. 15. Early development of a "long" bone (first phalanx of finger). Six-month human fetus. Mallory. × 15.

areolae. Those invading progenitor cells which follow the chondroclasts, and which lie against the calcified cartilage, become osteoblasts and deposit bone matrix on the surface of the cartilage. Ossification thus begins perichondrally and becomes endochondral a little later.

The cartilage model as a whole tends to be dumb-bell shaped, with a cylindrical shaft (cartilaginous diaphysis) and expanded globular ends (cartilaginous epiphyses: fig. 15). At each end, next to the epiphysis, the cartilage cells of the shaft multiply rapidly and pile up in columns to form a proliferative zone; next, in the direction of the middle segment of the shaft, the cells become greatly enlarged to form a hypertrophic zone which passes into a zone of calcified cartilage matrix and dying cells, and then into zones of primary areolae, and secondary areolae with endochondral bone formation. This general sequence is characteristic of the growing shaft until the end of adolescence. The shaft elongates at each end through the activity of the cartilage cells of the proliferative zone, while the bony portion of the shaft elongates at each end through endochondral formation at the expense of the zones of calcified hypertrophic cartilage. In addition the perichondral bone, which formed around the middle of the shaft, grows in length *pari passu* with the endochondral bone, always keeping in register with the hypertrophic zones at each end of the shaft (fig. 16). As this perichondral bone forms, the perichondrium over it becomes the periosteum. Perichondral bone is a type of membrane bone, and so the bony shaft consists of cartilage bone internally and membrane bone externally. The membrane bone thickens by centrifugal growth under the fibrous periosteum. The shaft, therefore, grows in length mainly by endochondral ossification at the expense of the growing cartilage model, and in breadth mainly by intramembranous ossification under the fibrous periosteum.

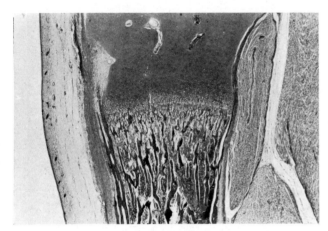

FIG. 16. Endochondral and perichondral ossification. Six-month human tibia. Haematoxylin and eosin. ×11.

The bone at the ossification "front" under the fibrous periosteum, and in the newly calcified cartilage, is of the fine cancellous variety (fig. 16), but it is soon remodelled. The earlier-formed endochondral, perichondral and periosteal bone is almost entirely removed by osteoclasts to produce a marrow cavity, which becomes colonized by haemopoietic cells. The outer portion of the shaft, on the other hand, gradually consolidates into compact bone with primary osteons. At the ends of the marrow cavity the newly-formed endochondral bone networks constitute the metaphyses. The zones of cartilage at the extreme ends of the shaft are termed growth cartilages, or epiphyseal plates (although strictly speaking, they are diaphyseal).

At the time of birth, long bones in general exhibit a largely ossified shaft (a hollow cylinder of compact membrane bone plugged at either end with fine cancellous cartilage bone) surmounted at each end by an expanded cartilaginous epiphysis. Between the epiphyses and the bony shaft there are plates of growth cartilage.

After birth, at times specific for each epiphysis, secondary centres of ossification appear, independently of the shaft ossification, in the cartilaginous epiphyses. In many cases, there is more than one secondary centre in an epiphysis.

Ossification extends radially at the expense of the epiphyseal cartilage, to produce a bony epiphysis (fig. 17). Where there are two or more secondary centres at the end of a bone, the bony epiphyses derived from them generally fuse into a compound bony epiphysis. Now all that remains of the cartilage model are the articular cartilages at the joint surfaces, and the growth cartilages. Sometime towards the end of adolescence the growth cartilages disappear, and the shaft fuses with the bone epiphyses. However, the bone is not now static, for remodelling continues throughout life, consolidating the bony framework here, and making it more cancellous there, partly as an adaptation to changing gravitational and muscular stresses, partly to make good "wear

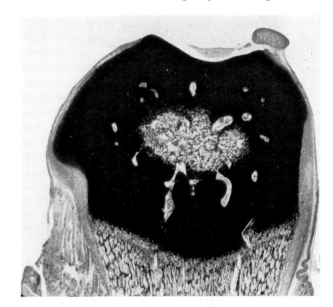

FIG. 17. Secondary centre of ossification, tibia. One-week-old rat. Haematoxylin, eosin, and toluidine blue.

and tear", and partly to maintain a certain amount of recently-formed bone whose minerals can readily exchange with those of the blood stream in the interests of general mineral homeostasis. In addition, dramatic changes in bone architecture take place after fractures and in most pathological conditions of the skeleton. Although the growth cartilages form but a small proportion of the whole bone, anatomically speaking, their functional integrity is in fact vital for efficient growth of the skeleton. The growth cartilages are the target for many influences, hormonal, mechanical, nutritional and infective, and their formative activities are rather readily depressed or disturbed. Fortunately they have considerable powers of recovery, so that temporary upsets can be made good later, and even if the growth cartilage at one end of a bone is severely damaged. compensatory overgrowth at the other end is probable.

SKELETAL GROWTH HARMONY

Although individual bones possess a considerable degree of autonomy in their development and growth, cartilage bones in particular developing surprisingly well *in vitro*, or when transplanted to soft tissues; nevertheless the skeleton is not just an assembly of bones, but an integrated structural and functional unit which serves the total unified needs of the organism. The same is true, of course, of subunits of the skeleton, like the skull, thorax and pelvis. In other words, the adult bones harmonize, and the growing bones must also harmonize, because the skeleton evidently maintains functional efficiency throughout the growing period. Such harmony is largely the result of genetic programming, but it is perfected by the mutual influences bones exert upon each other's development, and by the subordination of bone growth to higher authority. Thus in the skull, if a centre of ossification fails to appear, or if a developing bone is damaged so that it does not grow to the expected size, neighbouring bones overgrow to make up the deficiency, and the skull as a whole develops its normal shape and size, even if the sutural patterns are bizarre (Girgis and Pritchard, 1958).

On the other hand, if part of the brain is removed in a young animal, the skull vault fails to grow to its normal size, and accommodates itself to the smaller contents. By a similar token, in hydrocephalus the skull is much bigger than normal. By and large, the centres of ossification in the skull vault are rigidly programmed, but bone growth thereafter is negotiable within fairly wide limits—the bones growing at their edges wherever space is made available in the expanding fibrous brain capsule, which in turn grows in response to brain expansion. The brain is thus the prime mover, or pacemaker. However, premature synostosis of sutures in early childhood may prevent brain expansion and lead to blindness, idiocy and death unless bone is extensively removed.

The maintenance of skeletal harmony in the growing pelvis requires bodily migration of the ilium relative to the sacrum, because the iliac crest grows many times faster than the acetabular end of the bone. It has been shown that such migration is brought about through the pull of a strong sacro-iliac ligament, which lengthens only at about half the rate at which new bone is added at the crest.

The fine adjustment between the articulating cartilages in synovial joints is apparently regulated by mutual influences on each other's growth. Thus, if the femoral head is dislocated from the acetabulum in a young animal the head fails to achieve its expected size, while the acetabular cartilage flattens and atrophies, its matrix losing much of its mucopolysaccharide component. However, experiments have also shown that if the limb is amputated leaving the femoral head in its socket, acetabular development proceeds comparatively normally.

An interesting example of harmony in skeletal development is provided by the ends of bones (like the upper end of the tibia) where a strong tendon is attached to a tuberosity on the epiphysis (Badi, 1972). In such cases, while the rest of the epiphysis is attached to the shaft by means of the cartilaginous growth plate, the tuberosity is attached to the shaft by means of a stout, ligament-like, fibrous band (fig. 18). This ligament grows at its epiphyseal end, and is replaced by bone at its diaphyseal end, in harmony with cartilage growth and bone replacement in the cartilaginous growth plate, and the two processes have much in common, except that bone replaces the ligament by intramembranous ossification, while the cartilage is replaced by endochondral ossification. The situation is basically similar, however, at the ends of any long bone, whether there is a strong tendon attachment or not, for the fibrous periosteum is almost ligamentous as it crosses the plane of the growth cartilage to be inserted into the epiphysis, and the intramembranous ossification beneath it likewise keeps pace with the endochondral ossification at the junction of metaphysis and growth cartilage. Crilly (1972) has recently carried out experiments on the young chicken radius, from the results of which he postulates that the growth cartilages at each end

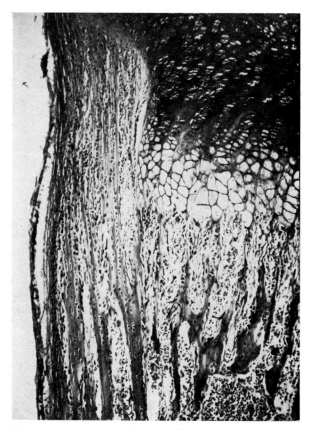

FIG. 18. Upper end of tibia showing both endochondral and intramembranous ossification. One-week-old rat. H. and E. × 95.

of the bone, as they move apart during development, produce tension in the periosteum and stimulate it to lengthen, and, at the same time, extension of intramembranous ossification in the deeper layer of the periosteum is induced in the direction of the extremities of the bone. Tension in the periosteum, on the other hand, holds back cartilage growth, for if the periosteum is cut circumferentially, the growth cartilages grow more rapidly than is normal, and the bone as a whole, in consequence, overgrows until periosteal continuity is restored. Thereafter, the growth cartilage furthest from the plane of periosteal section continues to grow faster than normal, while the nearer growth cartilage grows at a slower rate than normal. This kind of reciprocal influence between periosteum and growth cartilage is probably the means by which a great deal of skeletal harmony is achieved during growth, not only within a given bone, but also between neighbouring bones, so that the interaction between sacrum and ilium experimentally demonstrated in the developing pelvis is probably only a rather dramatic example of a widespread co-ordinating mechanism in skeletal development.

REFERENCES

Badi, M. H. (1972), "Ossification in the Fibrous Growth Plate at the Proximal End of the Tibia in the Rat," *J. Anat.*, **111**, 201.

Crilly, R. G. (1972), "Longitudinal Overgrowth of Chicken Radius," *J. Anat.*, **112**, 11.

Girgis, F. G. and Pritchard, J. J. (1958), "Effects of Skull Damage on the Development of Sutural Patterns in the Rat," *J. Anat.*, **92**, 39.

Hancox, N. M. (1972), "The Osteoclast," in *The Biochemistry and Physiology of Bone*, 2nd edition, Vol. 1, p. 45 (G. H. Bourne, Ed.). New York and London: Academic Press.

Pritchard, J. J. (1964), "Histology of Fracture Repair," in *Modern Trends in Orthopaedics. 4. Science of Fractures*, p. 67 (J. M. P. Clark, Ed.). London: Butterworths.

Pritchard, J. J. (1972), "The Osteoblast," in *The Biochemistry and Physiology of Bone*, 2nd edition, Vol. 1, p. 21. (G. H. Bourne, Ed.). New York and London: Academic Press.

Pritchard, J. J., Scott, J. H. and Girgis, F. G. (1956), "The Structure and Development of Cranial and Facial Sutures," *J. Anat.*, **90**, 73.

Young, R. W. (1964), "Specialization of Bone Cells," in *Bone Biodynamics*, p. 117 (H. M. Frost, Ed.). Boston: Little & Brown.

46. THE COMPOSITION AND CHEMICAL DYNAMICS OF BONE

J. E. EASTOE

Chemical composition

Inorganic constituents
Organic constituents
Collagen
Sialoprotein
Proteoglycans
Lipids
Peptides

Chemical dynamics

Hydroxyapatite and ion concentrations in plasma
Deposition and resorption of bone
Parathyroid hormone
Calcitonin
Vitamin D
Vitamin A
Vitamin C
Nucleation of the inorganic phase
The impossibility of homogeneous nucleation
Epitaxy
Solid phase transition
Cellular involvement in nucleation
The role of phosphatases in mineralization
Dynamics of the inorganic phase—a provisional analysis

INTRODUCTION

Bone is the hard mineralized **tissue** the presence of which characterizes the **organs** known as bones, the variously shaped components making up the vertebrate skeleton. Other tissues such as marrow, cartilage, periosteum and blood also occur in bones and together account for nearly half the weight of the skeleton, the overall composition of which is therefore different from that of its constituent tissue bone. This chapter will attempt an explanation in chemical terms of both the constitution of bone and the normal changes which this tissue undergoes.

The domain and scope of the tissue chemistry of bone is clarified by consideration of some histological and ultrastructural concepts. **Bone cells** (osteocytes) are usually distributed throughout bone, separated from each other by mineralized **extracellular material**. Neighbouring bone cells are more widely spaced than the cells of soft tissues, so that intercellular material occupies much of the total volume. Thus, in the overall chemical composition of bone the contribution from the extracellular material, which is highly characteristic of the hard tissue, predominates, whereas cells make only a small contribution.

The ultrastructure of the extracellular material shows two distinct phases, an **organic phase** and an **inorganic phase**. The inorganic phase is discontinuous and consists of very small discrete **crystals** and **amorphous material**. These are surrounded by a continuous organic phase consisting ultrastructurally of **collagen fibrils** and relatively structureless **interfibrillar material**. The material of the organic phase of bone has long been referred to as the "organic matrix", a term derived from the Latin word *matrix*, meaning womb or uterus. This derivation supplies the two main ideas implied by the term:

(a) a substance or medium enclosing other bodies; and
(b) a place or medium in which something is bred or developed.

The generalized histological use of the term organic matrix refers to any sort of extracellular continuum surrounding cells. This satisfies the first idea but not the second one, because the cells give rise to the extracellular continuum not *vice versa*. Both ideas are, however, satisfied by defining the matrix with respect to the inorganic crystals. The organic matrix of bone is thus more specifically the intricate fibrillar network which encloses the minute inorganic crystals in its interstices, the mineralization of bone involving deposition or development of mineral crystallites within the pre-existing matrix. The characteristics of a true matrix are that it should:

    (a) be in existence before whatever is bred;
    (b) participate in its development; and
    (c) enclose it spatially,

and the organic matrices of the vertebrate mineralized tissues, bone, dentine, cementum and enamel show all these features with respect to the inorganic crystallites.

The ultrastructure of the extracellular material of bone thus reveals the major chemical constituents, namely inorganic matter and collagen. Smaller amounts of high molecular weight substances occur in the interfibrillar organic material.

THE OVERALL CHEMICAL COMPOSITION OF BONE

Bone presents difficulties with regard to making precise quantitative statements concerning its chemical composition. These arise partly because bone occurs in close association with other tissues from which it must be separated, before it can be analysed, and partly because of continuous variation within the bone itself. In particular the degree of mineralization varies with the species, the site within the skeleton and the age of the individual. Mean values of 26·5, 21·1 and 15·8 per cent have been found for the total nitrogenous organic matter in dry, defatted femur shaft bone of man, ox and rabbit, respectively. These figures reflect substantial species differences in degree of mineralization. The content of organic matter in human femur diaphysis falls from 27·4 per cent at 7 years to 25·8 per cent at 65 years corresponding to a slow but steady increase in mineralization.

The main basis of these variations is that every piece of bone tissue becomes more heavily mineralized with time after it has been deposited. However, if it is resorbed and replaced by new bone, this will at first be comparatively lightly mineralized, resulting in local variations in composition of the remodelled bone. Thus, microradiography of a transverse section of cortical bone shows that while the newly laid-down Haversian systems (osteons) are comparatively radiolucent, older ones are more opaque to X-rays, because of their higher inorganic content. It is therefore difficult to suggest meaningful standard values for bone composition. The extent of total variation in the mineralization of osteoid tissue and osteons at the lowest and highest degree of calcification is summarized in Table 1.

Bone suitable for chemical studies is most easily prepared, if the starting material is carefully selected. Whereas cancellous and spongy bone require tedious work to remove associated soft tissues, compact bone is more easily prepared. Femoral diaphyses are a particularly convenient source of compact bone. Powdered bovine cortical bone has been used as a standard preparation to obtain an analytical "balance sheet" for bone (Table 2).

Two different experimental approaches have given results in reasonably good agreement. The values in the first column of figures were obtained by exhaustive extraction

TABLE 1

COMPOSITION OF OSTEOID TISSUE AND HAVERSIAN SYSTEMS AT DIFFERENT DEGREES OF CALCIFICATION
(Values other than density are given as μg./μl.)

Material	Density (g./ml.)	Hydroxy-apatite	Collagen	Non-collagenous Protein	Mucopoly-saccharide
Osteoid tissue	1·460	162	468	188	23
Osteons at the lowest degree of calcification	2·005	787	518	227	17
Osteons at the highest degree of calcification	2·211	1,207	523	34	17

Recalculated from the data of Pugliarello *et al.* (1970). Hydroxyapatite calculated from phosphorus × 5·4, collagen from hydroxyproline × 7·14, non-collagenous protein from non-collagenous nitrogen × 6·25 and mucopolysaccharide from hexosamines × 2·69.

of bone powder with hot water to convert the collagen to (soluble) gelatin. The weight of the insoluble residue (after correction for the residual "resistant protein") and 1·36 per cent of water-soluble inorganic salts have been used to calculate the percentage of inorganic matter. The approach used to obtain the values in the last column was to demineralize the bone powder by dialysis against ethylenediaminetetra-acetate (EDTA) and, after dialysing-away the excess of this salt, to evaporate the contents of the dialysis tube to give the dry weight of organic matter.

TABLE 2

COMPOSITION OF BOVINE CORTICAL BONE
(From Herring 1972)

	Per cent by Weight of Whole Dry Bone	
Inorganic matter	77·23*	76·04†
Organic matter	22·77	23·96
	Per cent by Weight of Organic Matrix	
Collagen	89·15*	88·48†
"Resistant protein"	4·87	0·98
"Osseomucoid"	1·14	
Chondroitin sulphate		0·81
Sialoprotein (bone)		0·80–1·15
CP–S glycoprotein		0·31–0·44
Lipids‡	0·42	
Peptides¶	0·54	
Other glycoproteins, proteins and matter not accounted for	3·88	7·18–7·66

* Figures in this column calculated from Eastoe and Eastoe (1954).
† Figures in this column from Herring (1972).
‡ From Leach (1958).
¶ From Leaver and Shuttleworth (1968).

The Inorganic Constituents

Possession of a separate extracellular phase, which is predominantly inorganic, distinguishes bone, dentine, cementum and enamel from the soft tissues. Fully formed bone contains enormous numbers of minute and tightly packed inorganic crystals (or crystallites), revealed by the electron microscope, and conspicuous because of their high density. Some amorphous calcium phosphate is also present. Agreement has not been reached concerning the shape and size of bone crystallites. Some investigators consider they consist of flat tablets, 35–40 nm. long in two directions and 2·5–5·0 nm. in the third. The crystals have also been interpreted as being rod- or needle-shaped, ranging from 15–150 nm. in length and from 1·5–7·5 nm. in the other two dimensions. The long (c) axes of the crystallites are almost certainly oriented parallel to collagen fibres. It has

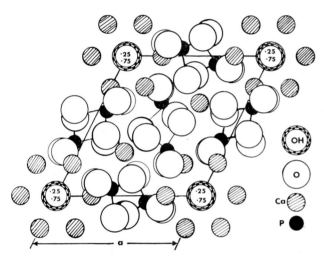

FIG. 1. Space lattice of hydroxyapatite projected on to the basal plane. For simplicity the distances of the atoms from the basal plane are omitted, except for the columnar hydroxy groups. Each phosphorus atom is surrounded by four equidistant oxygen atoms to form an orthophosphate (PO_4) group.

been suggested that inorganic crystals occur at regular intervals in relation to the 64 nm. axial repeat of the collagen fibrils, however, the exact location in relation to the fine structure of the spacing is uncertain.

Bone was first analysed in 1771 by Scheele, who showed that it contains calcium and phosphate. "Bone salt" is one of the rather large family of calcium phosphates, many of which occur as minerals. Attempts to fit a precise chemical formula to bone salt based on analysis were only partly successful owing to the complexity of the inorganic phase in bone. The analyses suggested that the inorganic portion of bone is a basic calcium phosphate. Other examples of basic calcium phosphates were found in the apatite group of minerals of which fluorapatite $3\,Ca_3(PO_4)_2 . CaF_2$ is the most abundant. On the basis of its chemical composition, it was suggested as long ago as 1862 that the inorganic component of dental enamel has a structure of the apatite type and the substance hydroxyapatite $3\,Ca_3(PO_4)_2 . Ca(OH)_2$ has since become accepted as the best approximate

representation of the crystallites in bone. The apatites are not only the most basic but also the most stable and least soluble of the calcium phosphates. The word apatite is derived from the Greek απαταω (I deceive) since the refractile mineral was sometimes mistaken for aquamarine. This derivation proved appropriately prophetic in respect of the part played by hydroxyapatite in living bone, which sometimes verges upon the paradoxical.

Half a century ago, the technique of X-ray diffraction analysis was first applied to determine crystal structures. The space lattice of hydroxyapatite worked out from the X-ray diffraction data is shown in fig. 1. It forms a rather complex pattern with a unit cell in the hexagonal system containing 18 ions and 44 atoms. The unit cell has two equal edges, a, inclined at 120° to each other and a third edge, c, perpendicular to these. The unit cell dimensions of bone crystallites and apatites are summarized in Table 3 The X-ray diffraction pattern of the inorganic portion of bone is closely similar to but more diffuse than that given by the mineral apatites because of the very small size of the bone crystallites and the presence of amorphous calcium phosphate. If bone is heated to 900°, its diffraction pattern becomes sharper because the crystals grow in size though the dimensions of the unit cell do not alter.

TABLE 3

UNIT CELL DIMENSION OF VARIOUS APATITES
(Lengths given in nm.)

	a	c
Fluorapatite	0·9371	0·6884
Hydroxyapatite	0·9421	0·6882
Bone	0·942	0·688
Bone (after heating at 900° for 2 hr.)	0·9421	0·6882

The composition of the inorganic portion of a standard preparation of bovine cortical bone is summarized in Table 4. In addition to the calcium and phosphate ions, already considered as major constituents of the inorganic phase, a substantial proportion of carbonate is present. Sodium, magnesium, potassium strontium, chloride and fluoride ions occur at levels below 1 per cent.

Although hydroxyapatite represents the most well defined constituent of the inorganic material in bone, it is not present in a pure state, nor is it the only inorganic phase present. The hydroxyapatite of bone corresponds to the mineral crystallites and its departure from purity is partly the result of their small size, which necessarily results in their having a very large surface area, calculated as 100 square metres per gram of apatite. This results in a significant proportion of the ions in the crystallites being either in or near the surface. Since the reactive crystal surface is in contact with tissue fluid within the extracellular region of bone, various ionic interactions can take place there including adsorption, ion-exchange and isomorphous replacement. These changes result in the composition of the

Table 4

INORGANIC CONSTITUENTS OF DRY, FAT-FREE
BOVINE CORTICAL BONE
(From Armstrong and Singer, 1965)

	%	Mequiv/gm
Cations		
Calcium	26·70	13·32
Magnesium	0·436	0·358
Sodium	0·731	0·318
Potassium	0·055	0·014
Strontium	0·035	
Anions		
Phosphorus	12·47	
as PO_4^{3-}		12·06
Carbon dioxide	3·48	
as CO_3^{2-}		1·58
Citrate	0·863	
as Cit^{3-}		0·138
Chloride	0·077	0·022
Fluoride	0·072	0·038

surface layer differing from that within the crystal and cause departures from ideal stoichiometry and the theoretical calcium/phosphate ratio of 1·67 for apatite. Adsorption probably accounts for the presence of sodium, potassium and chloride.

The status of the carbonate ion in bone is still largely unsolved. The amount present is substantial and although study of mineral and synthetic carbonate-containing apatites indicates that carbonate can enter the apatite lattice in minerals, all present data for bone suggest that most of the carbonate must be present in a second phase and not in the apatite structure.

Another inorganic phase, consistently observed, is amorphous calcium phosphate. This is especially characteristic of active calcification sites where new bone is being laid down and mineralization is beginning. However, most regions in bone show a continuous background scatter of X-rays attributable to amorphous calcium phosphate. The ash content of whole rat tibia has been found to progress from 22·9 per cent at 3 days of age to 54·0 per cent at 80 days. Over the same period, the content of amorphous calcium phosphate falls steadily from 67 to 37 per cent of the total mineral, while the crystalline apatite content rises reciprocally. Amorphous calcium phosphate has a calcium/phosphate ratio of 1·50, probably corresponding to a hydrated tri-calcium phosphate $Ca_3(PO_4)_2 \cdot xH_2O$. It is transformed both *in vitro* and in bone to extremely small crystallites of hydroxyapatite which subsequently grow in size and crystal perfection.

Bone contains up to 1 per cent of citrate, which is probably associated with the inorganic rather than the organic phase because it dissolves completely when bone is demineralized. The specific function of citrate in mineralized tissue has not been established. It is produced by metabolic activity in cells generally, including bone cells, and is probably co-precipitated with the inorganic phase. Similar co-precipitation occurs *in vitro* and the citrate of bone may be

purely adventitious in origin. The skeleton nevertheless contains a substantial part of the total citrate of the organism and contributes citrate to the tissue fluids during bone resorption. Lactate is also present in bone but at a level of only 0·1–0·3 per cent.

The Organic Constituents

Bone Collagen

The collagen of bone tissue accounts for nearly 90 per cent of the organic constituents (Table 2). When bone is demineralized, the inorganic crystallites are dissolved and the collagen remains forming a soft elastic model of the original hard tissue. Strong acids may cause some breakdown of collagen and demineralization with ethylenediaminetetra-acetate (EDTA) is preferable when preparing bone collagen for chemical investigation.

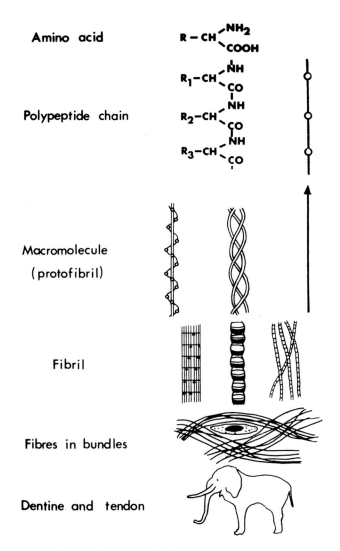

Fig. 2. Structural features of collagen at increasing orders of size represented at different levels. The method of representation is changed in order to relate the feature shown to both the next smaller and larger orders of size. Thus macromolecules are considered as stiff rods (arrows) which are oriented parallel to one another in the fibrils (Eastoe, 1967b).

The collagens occur widely as major extracellular structural constituents of connective tissues of mesodermal origin. These include not only the mineralized tissues—bone, calcified cartilage, dentine and cementum—but soft tissues also. The collagens share a common hierarchy of structural organization over many orders of size from the constituent amino acids of their polypeptide chains, to the macroscopic form of anatomical structures (fig. 2). This pattern, while showing minor variations between species and tissues, is remarkably uniform throughout the vertebrate sub-phylum. It is based on the collagen **macromolecule** which consists of three intertwining protein chains wound around each other, to form a triple helical structure (fig. 3). Whereas the individual protein chains of

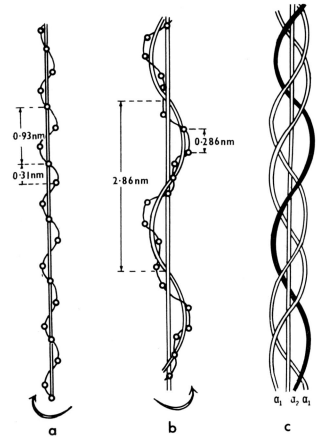

FIG. 3. The triple helix of collagen. (a) Single polypeptide chain wound in a left-handed helix of pitch 0·93 nm. with three amino acids per turn. (b) Here the axis of the simple helix in (a) is wound in a right-handed helix of pitch 2·86 nm. so that the polypeptide chain itself forms a compound helix. (c) Three units of the type shown in (b) arranged to form a triple helix. For simplicity only the three axes are shown.

collagen are highly flexible, the macromolecules are comparatively rigid structures like long thin rods with a length (280 nm.) greatly exceeding their diameter (1·4 nm.) and a molecular weight of approximately 300,000. Macromolecules are secreted by the fibroblasts (including osteoblasts) into the extracellular space where they function as pre-fabricated units for building a second much larger structural unit, the collagen **fibril.**

Fibrils are revealed by the electron microscope as long

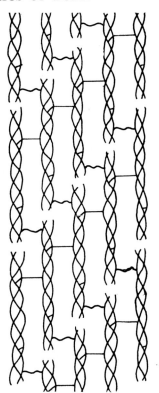

FIG. 4. Diagrammatic representation of intra- and inter-molecular cross-linking of collagen macromolecules within a fibril of insoluble collagen.

narrow curving structures with a regularly repeating pattern of cross striations having a periodicity of 64 nm. Bundles of parallel fibrils form the fibres of collagen, seen in histological sections with the optical microscope (fig. 2). Collagen fibrils are formed by **aggregation** of macromolecules, a process which involves the molecules becoming oriented parallel and in close proximity to each other and then drawing even more closely together by mutually attractive forces. These forces consist of large numbers of individually weak (non-covalent) bonds, such as hydrogen and electrostatic bonds. At this stage, the aggregation process can be reversed by the extraction of the young tissue with mild reagents such as neutral salt solutions or weak acids which break the weak bonds and release the collagen macromolecules, as **soluble collagen.**

Soon after it is formed, the collagen fibril begins to undergo a process known as **maturation** whereby it becomes decreasingly soluble in the mild reagents which extract soluble collagen from immature tissues. Maturation consists of the gradual formation of a few strong **covalent cross-linkages** between adjacent polypeptide chains in the fibril. They are formed at specific points determined by the chemical structure and may be either **intramolecular** cross links joining chains in the same macromolecule or **intermolecular** ones connecting chains in different but neighbouring macromolecules within the fibril. The entire fibril is thereby welded together by covalent bonds into what could be called a "giant molecule" (fig. 4). Lathyrism is a disease characterized by the formation of brittle collagen and caused by the ingestion of organic nitriles. These substances interfere with the formation of covalent cross linkages in collagen and so prevent its maturation.

Collagens have a distinctive composition characterized by the possession of two unusual amino acids, hydroxyproline and hydroxylysine, which do not occur in other proteins. One-third of all the amino acid residues in collagen consist of glycine, which has no side chain and occupies sequentially every third position along the collagen chains. One-ninth of the residues is alanine, with methyl side-chain groups, while the two imino acids proline and hydroxyproline together account for two-ninths of the residues (Table 5). Two features of the composition of collagen are essential for its triple helical structure. Firstly, by occupying every third position along the chain, the small glycine residue can be accommodated in the middle of the collagen macromolecule, near its axis, where there is insufficient space for any other kind of amino acid (fig. 3). Secondly, the imino acids, proline and hydroxyproline, impose an obligatory bend in the direction of the protein chain wherever they occur. This rigid bend fits the compound helical form taken up by each chain in the macromolecule and so helps to stabilize it. Although mammalian collagens conform rather closely to a common pattern of amino acid composition, there are minor differences between tissues and species (Eastoe, 1967a). However, there do not appear to be any consistent features which distinguish the composition of collagen of mineralized tissues from that of soft tissue collagens (Table 5).

TABLE 5

AMINO ACID COMPOSITION OF BONE AND SKIN COLLAGEN
FROM BOVINE AND HUMAN TISSUES
(Values are given as residues/1,000 amino acid residues)

	Bovine		Human	
	Skin*	Bone*	Skin†	Bone‡
Hydroxyproline	92	98	94	100
Aspartic acid	48	45	45	47
Threonine	17	16	17	18
Serine	38	34	36	36
Glutamic acid	72	74	73	72
Proline	129	123	128	123
Glycine	334	337	330	319
Alanine	105	109	110	113
Valine	19	20	24	24
Methionine	6·6	5·0	6·2	5·3
Isoleucine	11	11	10	13
Leucine	25	25	24	25
Tyrosine	4·7	4·3	2·8	4.5
Phenylalanine	13	13	12	14
Hydroxylysine	6·8	5·7	5·8	3·5
Lysine	25	26	27	28
Histidine	4·6	4·1	4·8	5·8
Arginine	48	50	51	47
Amide	(41)	(38)	(37)	(37)

* Data from Piez and Likins (1960)
† Data from Bornstein and Piez (1964).
‡ Data from Eastoe (1967a).

The main feature which distinguishes bone collagen from that of soft tissues is its insolubility in the neutral salt solutions and weakly acid solutions used to extract soluble collagens. Thus, less than 0·5 per cent of demineralized bone collagen is soluble in neutral salt solution and less than 1 per cent in dilute acid solution compared with approximately ten times these amounts from young skin and tendon. Two opposing explanations have been put forward to account for the high stability of bone collagen.

Glimcher, Katz and Travis (1965) consider that bone collagen is not highly cross-linked but that its stability results from strong non-covalent intermolecular forces, resulting from the particular mode of aggregation of collagen macromolecules within the fibrils in bone. This idea is based upon their findings that when they succeeded in dissolving an appreciable proportion of decalcified powdered bone in 3 per cent acetic acid after sequentially freezing at $-70°$ and thawing at $2°C$ or after denaturation in hydrogen-bond breaking reagents, a substantial proportion of the soluble collagen so formed was found to consist of α components (i.e. the individual protein chains, three of which intertwine to make up the macromolecule).

Miller, Martin, Piez and Powers (1967), however, consider that bone collagen is unusually highly cross-linked, which accounts for its low solubility. Thus they found that while 17 per cent of bone collagen is extracted by 5 M. guanidine hydrochloride, which breaks hydrogen and electrostatic bonds, only about 30 per cent of this (5 per cent of the total collagen) consists of α or β (i.e. a pair of α chains joined by a covalent cross-linkage) components. The remainder of the soluble material consists of aggregates of very high molecular weight (made up of many chains joined to each other by cross-linkages) together with degraded fragments from other chains.

Most of the available evidence appears to support this second view that bone collagen is more highly cross-linked than soft-tissue collagens. A much higher proportion of single chain (α) components can be separated from the bone collagen of animals which have been given β-aminoproprionitrile, so that they become lathyritic, than for normal bone collagen. Since lathyrism inhibits formation of cross-linkages, these would appear to be responsible for holding together the α chains of normal bone collagen. The composition of the separated α components of bone collagen are summarized in Table 6, it being disputed whether there are three or, as in most soft-tissue collagens, only two types of α chains. Identification of the peptides resulting from breaking the chains with cyanogen bromide at the widely spaced methionine units supports the view that there are two identical α_1 chains and one α_2 chain in chick bone collagen.

Further evidence for the highly cross-linked nature of bone collagen comes from the isolation of a reduced aldol, probably formed by condensation of the δ-semialdehydes of lysine and hydroxylysine. Sufficient is found in bone collagen to account for one cross-link for every two collagen macromolecules, a much higher proportion than in soft-tissue collagen. It is considered to represent an intermolecular cross-link which would account for the low acid solubility of bone collagen.

TABLE 6

AMINO ACID COMPOSITION OF THE α CHAINS OF BONE COLLAGEN
(Values are given as residues per 1,000 total residues)

	Francois and Glimcher (1967)			Miller et al. (1967)	
	α₁	α₂	α₃	α₁	α₂
Hydroxyproline	109	88	98	102	101
Aspartic acid	43·2	48·9	43·5	42	48
Threonine	20·0	19·8	19·1	19	18
Serine	26·8	30·3	26·4	28	28
Glutamic acid	79	67	78	78	65
Proline	114	112	114	118	120
Glycine	325	330	326	332	330
Alanine	126	105	125	128	104
Valine	13·0	30·0	15·7	14	26
Methionine	9·6	5·5	9·6	8·6	5·4
Isoleucine	6·6	19·0	8·2	6·3	18
Leucine	19·4	31·0	20·4	20	31
Tyrosine	4·6	4·5	4·1	2·4	2·5
Phenylalanine	14·1	14·8	14·6	14	14
Hydroxylysine	5·6	7·8	5·2	5·5	8·2
Lysine	31·0	24·9	29·9	29·0	24·0
Histidine	3·4	7·3	3·2	2·8	7·0
Arginine	49	54	57	49	50

Bone Sialoprotein

Bone sialoprotein, a substance apparently specific for bone tissue, was first isolated from bovine cortical bone in 1961. It is a typical **mucosubstance**, because its molecules contain both protein and carbohydrate moieties, and it probably occurs in association with interfibrillar material. Bone sialoprotein conforms more closely to the definition of a **glycoprotein** than to that of a **proteoglycan**, these representing the currently convenient terms for the subdivision of

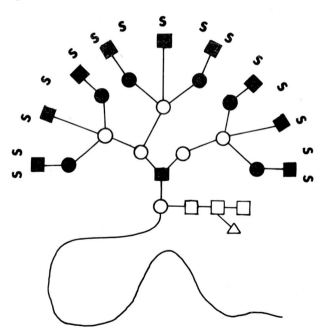

FIG. 5. Suggested possible structure for bone sialoprotein (Herring, 1972). S indicates sialic acid; ○ glucosamine; ● galactosamine; ■ galactose; □ mannose and △ fucose.

mucosubstances. Thus, proteoglycans have very long polysaccharide chains with only two alternating types of sugar residue, except at their junction with the protein part of the molecule. The polysaccharide chains of glycoproteins are shorter, do not have an alternation of types of sugar and have a wider variety of sugar residues, including (in addition to hexosamines, which occur also in proteoglycans) galactose, mannose, glucose, fucose and especially sialic acids.

TABLE 7

COMPOSITION OF SIALOPROTEIN FROM BOVINE CORTICAL BONE
(Data from Herring, 1972)

	% by Weight	moles/mole of BSP
Sialic acid	20·5	15·3
Galactose	8·2	10·5
Mannose	2·5	3·1
Fucose	0·7	1·0
Galactosamine	4·6	5·9
Glucosamine	4·6	5·9
Phosphate	1·4	3·4
Total of amino-acid residues	47·9	87·6
Lysine	1·59	2·52
Histidine	0·74	1·07
Arginine	0·76	1·04
Aspartic acid	8·80	15·20
Threonine	5·02	9·70
Serine	3·20	7·00
Glutamic acid	12·80	20·09
Proline	2·15	4·27
Glycine	3·49	10·71
Alanine	1·36	3·51
Valine	1·38	2·71
Methionine	—	—
Isoleucine	1·25	2·19
Leucine	1·43	2·53
Tyrosine	1·54	1·95
Phenylalanine	0·72	1·00
Tryptophan	0·87	0·98
Cysteic acid	0·81	1·10

The chemical composition of bone sialoprotein is summarized in Table 7 and its possible structure, is shown diagrammatically in fig. 5. Bone sialoprotein is characterized by its possession of sialic-acid groupings. Both N-acetyl- and N-glycollylneuraminic acids are present as terminal groups of the carbohydrate chains. These sialic acids are related to mannosamine and differ only in the type of substituent attached to the nitrogen atom.

Values ranging from 14·3–20·5 per cent of sialic acid in bone glycoprotein have been obtained and since the organic portion of bone contains 0·166 per cent of sialic acid, probably present as sialoprotein, the content of sialoprotein in bovine bone is in the region of 0·81–1·15 per cent of the matrix, which corresponds to 0·34–0·48 per cent of whole bone.

Compared with other glycoproteins, bone sialoprotein is unusual in having a very high content of sialic acid, which, together with the unusually large amounts of glutamic and aspartic acids with free side-chain carboxyl groups, in the protein chain, render bone sialoprotein very acidic. The single very highly branched carbohydrate moiety (fig. 5) with a high molecular weight of 9,220 is also unusual for a glycoprotein. It is attached to the protein at a single point.

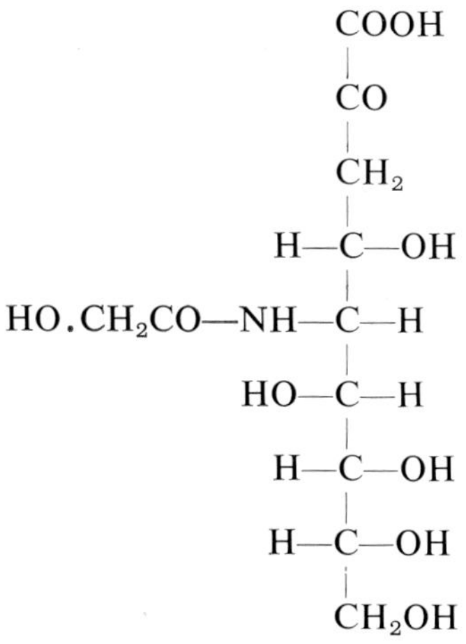

$$
\begin{array}{c}
\text{COOH} \\
| \\
\text{CO} \\
| \\
\text{CH}_2 \\
| \\
\text{H—C—OH} \\
| \\
\text{HO.CH}_2\text{CO—NH—C—H} \\
| \\
\text{HO—C—H} \\
| \\
\text{H—C—OH} \\
| \\
\text{H—C—OH} \\
| \\
\text{CH}_2\text{OH}
\end{array}
$$

FIG. 6. Structure of *N*-glycollyl-neuraminic acid.

The strongly acidic nature of bone sialoprotein gives it marked binding properties for cations. The trivalent yttrium ion is bound several hundred times more strongly than divalent calcium. The binding sites probably each consist of three carboxyl groups situated on the protein part of the molecule. A solution of bone sialoprotein at a concentration of 0·2 mg./ml. causes a 50 per cent inhibition of calcium phosphate precipitation.

Proteoglycans of Bone

The **proteoglycans** form a second group of muco-substances, associated with the interfibrillar material of connective tissues. Their molecules consist of a protein core to which are attached a number of carbohydrate chains of the **glycosaminoglycan** type. Glycosaminoglycans, also known as acid mucopolysaccharides, have very long chains of alternating hexosamine and uronic-acid units. The hexo-samine is derived from glucose, galactose or mannose by the substitution of an amino group (usually acetylated) for the hydroxy group on C2. The uronic acid is derived from either glucose or galactose by changing C6 from a primary alcohol to a carboxyl group, which makes the glycosamino-glycan a weak poly-acid. Sometimes ester sulphate groups are attached to the hexosamine residues and these render the mucopolysaccharide strongly acidic, so that it stains with Alcian blue dye in the presence of high concentrations of magnesium ions.

Chrondroitin 4-sulphate, which has alternating *N*-acetyl-galactosamine (sulphated on C4) and glucuronic-acid units, has been isolated from bovine cortical bone, in amounts representing 0·25 per cent of the organic fraction. It is the major glycosaminoglycan of bone. Chondroitin 4-sulphate from bone has a molecular weight of 56,000, indicating that the chains are at least twice as long as those found in other tissues. In fracture callus chondroitin sulphate rises initially to 2 per cent and then falls to 0·5 per cent after 3

weeks, in line with the general observation that muco-substances are abundant in the first extracellular substances to be formed in young tissues and subsequently decrease as collagen fibres form within the extracellular ground substance.

Three native proteoglycan components D1, D2 and D3 are present in bone, each of which can be separated in a form which is homogeneous on electrophoresis and centrifugation. The composition of these fractions is shown in Table 8. Components D1 and D2 are closely similar as

TABLE 8

COMPOSITION OF THREE PROTEOGLYCANS FROM
BOVINE CORTICAL BONE
(Data from Herring, 1972)

	D1	*D2*	*D3*
	(% of dry weight)		
Nitrogen	6·2	5·5	2·7
Amino acids	27·46	21·76	1·27
Uronic acid	17·1	22·1	30·1
Galactosamine	13·9	17·9	25·1
Glucosamine	1·7	1·2	<0·1
Hexose	5·2	4·2	0·9
Sialic acid	12·1	6·9	<0·05
Sulphate	8·5	10·9	16·9
	(residues per 1,000 total residues)		
Lysine	33	34	30
Histidine	24	20	49
Arginine	48	42	19
Aspartic acid	162	162	138
Threonine	75	87	81
Serine	111	97	111
Glutamic acid	200	194	131
Proline	61	63	83
Glycine	127	140	127
Alanine	40	38	73
Valine	29	31	26
Methionine	3	2	3
Isoleucine	15	19	33
Leucine	40	34	68
Tyrosine	15	19	12
Phenylalanine	15	16	20

regards the amino acid composition of the protein moiety, which is quite different from that of the "core protein" of the chondroitin sulphate-containing proteoglycan from cartilage but resembles bone sialoprotein (Table 7). The sugars galactose, mannose, fucose and xylose are present in D1; the first three of these are present in bone sialoprotein while xylose is known to form the link between the chondroitin sulphate chains of cartilage proteoglycan and serine residues on the core protein.

D1 has been shown to have one chondroitin 4-sulphate chain of molecular weight 22,000–27,000 attached to a bone sialoprotein chain, D2 to have two such chondroitin sulphate chains and one sialoprotein chain and D3 to consist of unattached chondroitin sulphate only. According to the strict definition complexes D1 and D2 have structural characteristics of both proteoglycans and glycoprotein. Nature ever confounds the folly of man in attempting to classify these complex extracellular structures by means of too rigid definitions.

Lipids

Adult bovine cortical bone contains a small amount of lipids amounting altogether to 0·067 per cent of the dry weight. Of these lipids 79·2 per cent are triglycerides, 13·3 per cent free cholesterol, 1·7 per cent cholesterol esters and 2·2 per cent phospholipids. The phospholipids of bone account for 0·08 per cent of the organic matrix of bovine cortical bone. Before demineralization sphingomyelin (28·3 per cent of total phospholipid), lecithin (24·5 per cent) and phosphatidylethanolamine (13·2 per cent) are extractable. Further quantities of these substances (9·4, 5·5 and 5·8 per cent respectively) can be extracted after demineralization together with phosphatidylserine (4·4 per cent) phosphatidylinositol (1·4 per cent) and phosphatidic acid (1·4 per cent). A supposed specific phospholipid of bone named calciolipin has proved to be an artefact.

Peptides from Bone

A wide range of peptides is extractable from bone by N-hydrochloric acid. Altogether, the "acid soluble nitrogen" of these peptides accounts for 0·134 per cent of the weight and 3·7 per cent of the total nitrogen of bovine cortical bone. The peptides have been separated by gel filtration on various grades of Sephadex into three fractions with molecular weights above 5,000, between 5,000 and 750 and below 750.

When citrate is extracted from dentine with dilute acid, it is associated with an arginine-rich peptide. The citrate is not firmly bound to the peptide, however, and the association may only occur during extraction. The overall significance of peptides in bone is not at present clear; some may be detached from high molecular weight material by hydrolysis with the cold acid.

THE CHEMICAL DYNAMICS OF BONE

The chemical changes which occur in bone can be arbitrarily but conveniently considered as falling into three categories which differ as regards the sites where they occur and the largest structural levels involved. Some consideration of both histology and ultrastructure is relevant to all three types of dynamic change, which, since they occur simultaneously side-by-side, necessarily overlap. They are distinguished here to simplify the many complex processes involved in bone metabolism by attempting to emphasize the basic principles which operate.

(1) The first kind of dynamic change involves the relationship between dissolved calcium and phosphate ions, in the blood plasma and tissue fluids, and existing hydroxyapatite crystals in bone. This is concerned with the tendency towards deposition of ions on the crystal surface under physiological conditions, thereby resulting in growth of the crystal. Such processes take place in the **extracellular** regions of bone.

(2) The second kind of change operating in bone is much more complex and concerns both the laying down of new bone and resorption of the old as a direct result of the cellular activity of osteoblasts and osteoclasts, respectively. Combination and co-ordination of these processes of bone construction and destruction result not only in the growth of bone but the continuous remodelling of the contour of the bone surface, which continues throughout life. They are also responsible not only for the complete turnover of the whole substance of bone, over a long time scale; but also for short- and long-term regulation of the concentrations of calcium, phosphate and, perhaps, citrate ions in the blood. The bone cells are enabled to control blood homeostasis by removing ions from blood to new bone or returning them from old bone to the plasma as occasion demands. These changes are controlled by the effects of various hormones and vitamins on the bone cells. The investigation of the effects of these substances has been largely responsible for our detailed knowledge of this second level of bone dynamics, which is essentially cellular, but results in the synthesis or destruction of the extracellular material.

(3) The final type of process to be considered has presented great experimental difficulties and a variety of theories. This is the mechanism by which the mineralization of bone is initiated. Possession of this mechanism presumably distinguishes bone from non-mineralizing mesodermal tissues. The basis of this vexed question is to decide how solid calcium phosphate first arises in bone in the absence of any pre-existing inorganic phase. This process is sometimes referred to as **nucleation**. It is not yet entirely clear where the process of nucleation takes place, since it is disputed whether it occurs simultaneously with secretion of the organic phase or somewhat later in the secreted matrix. While this process may occur at or near cell surfaces, the apatite crystallites, which are the final product of nucleation, are clearly extracellular. The apparent simplicity of the nucleation process is deceptive and it is still far from being completely understood.

Hydroxyapatite and Ion Concentrations in Plasma

The **total** concentration of calcium in plasma is normally approximately 10 mg./100 ml. and the concentration of inorganic phosphate 3·5 mg./100 ml. The normal product of calcium and phosphate is thus 35 (mg./100 ml.)^2; but under exceptional circumstances this product can vary widely from, for example, a low value of approximately 20, where vitamin D is deficient, up to 50 where there is an excess of this vitamin.

It is, however, the concentration of **ionized** calcium which is significant in relation to the solubility of slightly soluble calcium phosphates. The normal value for the concentration of **free** calcium ions in plasma is difficult to establish because rather less than half of the calcium is in the form of ions, reversibly bound to protein while some 5 per cent of the total calcium is complexed with citrate. The amounts and degree of ionization of both protein and citrate therefore affect the proportion of bound calcium and hence the concentration of free calcium ions. The values shown in

TABLE 9
SOLUBLE CALCIUM AND PHOSPHATE IN NORMAL
HUMAN PLASMA

	Concentration (mg./100 ml.)
Total plasma calcium	10
Protein-bound calcium (non-diffusible)	4
Calcium complexed with citrate (diffusible)	0·5
Free calcium ions	5·5
Inorganic phosphate ions	3·5
Ionic producs of plasma = 5·5 × 3·5 =	19·25 (mg./100 ml.)^2

Table 9, however, are generally accepted as representative of the ionic status of normal human serum. The ionic product for free calcium and phosphate ions in plasma is approximately 19 (mg./100 ml.)^2.

The solubility product of hydroxyapatite is a little indefinite because of the large number of ions in the lattice and that of the inorganic matter in bone rather more so, on account of the presence of carbonate and adsorbed cations. The solubility product is also affected by temperature, pH and the concentrations of foreign ions in solution. Despite these variables, it has proved possible to determine the solubility product experimentally in the region above pH7. At physiological pH and with concentrations of sodium, magnesium and chloride equal to those in plasma the solubility product of "biological" hydroxyapatite at 37°C is 9±1 (mg./100 ml.)^2.

The apatite crystals in bone are in contact with the extracellular fluid of the tissue and will approach equilibrium with it in respect of the concentrations of calcium and phosphate ions. Since bone crystallites are so small and have a relatively enormous surface area, equilibrium will be rapidly attained and then maintained by ions being either deposited on or leaving the crystal surface. The ionic calcium and phosphate concentrations in the extracellular fluid of bone cannot easily be measured. However, the hydroxyapatite crystals will tend to maintain the ionic product of this fluid at their solubility product of 9 (mg./100 ml.)^2. The ionic product for plasma [19 (mg./100 ml.)^2] considerably exceeds this value. Calcium and phosphate ions therefore diffuse from the plasma into the extracellular fluid, down the concentration gradient. The increased concentration of calcium and phosphate disturb the equilibrium at the crystal surface of the apatite, which is re-established by the crystal growing in size at the expense of ions from solution. The result is a net transfer of calcium and phosphate ions from the plasma to the inorganic crystals of bone.

This process will tend to take place wherever bone which contains apatite crystals has been deposited. It will be most rapid in young bone where the crystals are smaller and there is more space for diffusion of ions and growth of crystal surfaces. In principle, the process will continue even in old bone but at a greatly reduced rate since the apatite crystals eventually fill almost all the space available to them, greatly slowing down the rate of ionic diffusion. Since bone is continually being resorbed and deposited anew, a proportion of relatively young bone is always present. The degree of mineralization of the bone as a whole will thus be somewhat lower than that found in the oldest parts, where it approaches a maximum value similar to that reached in the bulk of dentine, which is not resorbed.

Considering a piece of bone tissue at any given time, quite independently of any deposition or resorption as a result of cellular activity, there will be continuous growth of apatite crystallites at the expense of plasma calcium and phosphate. This continuous drain of ions from blood to bone is a physico-chemical process not requiring participation of cells and is simply a consequence of the plasma levels exceeding the solubility product of apatite.

Deposition and Resorption of Bone

Long-term changes involving growth and remodelling of bone and shorter-term responses to counteract undesirable changes in blood-calcium and phosphate levels, both require the intervention of bone cells. Two types of cell are involved, osteoblasts, the primary function of which is to produce extracellular organic compounds and osteoclasts which destroy bone. Both types of cell operate at the edge of existing bone. Osteoblasts synthesize and secrete collagen and the various other organic constituents of the extracellular material as the "osteoid" layer, which is either unmineralized or very sparsely mineralized, compared with mature bone. In contrast, destruction of bone by osteoclasts is virtually a single-stage process in which the inorganic and organic constituents are removed completely, almost at the same place and time. Thus, intact bone remains almost up to the edge of Howship's lacunae. Much of the information required concerning the patterns of bone growth is stored genetically in the osteoblasts as shown by their behaviour in tissue culture. Osteoblasts and osteoclasts also have a marked response to certain substances, especially hormones and vitamins, which reach them through the circulation.

Parathyroid Hormone

The parathyroid glands have an important effect in controlling calcium metabolism. They secrete a hormone, parathormone (PTH), a polypeptide of molecular weight 10,000, which is the main regulator of calcium homeostasis. Parathyroid hormone maintains the concentration of total calcium in plasma at its normal level of 10 mg./100 ml. In the absence of PTH, the level falls to 6–7 mg./100 ml. where it is also controlled, perhaps by the effect of the solubility product of hydroxyapatite, already discussed. At this lower level, muscle excitability is increased with tetany as the main symptom.

Parathyroid hormone provides a feedback mechanism to raise the plasma calcium concentration above this lower level and to maintain it constant at its higher controlled level. Its chief mode of action is to stimulate osteoclasts to destroy bone, so releasing both calcium and phosphate ions into the blood and thereby augmenting the calcium concentration. The stimulus to secretion of PTH by the parathyroids is the calcium ion level of the blood flowing through these glands. Thus, if the blood calcium level begins to fall, parathormone secretion increases, resulting in an increase of bone resorption and restoration of the calcium status of the blood. By continuously monitoring the blood in this way, the parathyroids not only keep the calcium concentration up to the normal level but provide a means of taking calcium and phosphate out of bone and putting them back into blood. Thus, the continuous drain of calcium and phosphate from the plasma to the surface of growing hydroxyapatite crystals is balanced.

Parathyroid hormone may have another kind of action which affects kidney cells causing them to transfer phosphate from blood into the urine. The effect of the hormone in transferring phosphate from bone to blood would thus tend to be offset and the level of phosphate in the blood to remain constant. Although it stimulates phosphate transport, parathormone can thus be regarded as being primarily a regulator for plasma calcium concentration.

Calcitonin

The existence of a second hormone which affects bone in the opposite way to parathyroid hormone was long unsuspected and calcitonin has only recently been isolated and thoroughly investigated. It is a peptide hormone produced in the thyroid gland and has a straight chain containing 32 amino-acid residues.

Calcitonin is a highly potent inhibitor of bone resorption. Not only does it prevent existing osteoclasts from resorbing bone but it appears to inhibit the differentiation of new bone-resorbing cells. It may increase bone formation as a result of a gradual shift in the progenitor cells towards becoming osteoblasts by preventing their differentiation to osteoclasts. Calcitonin has a direct effect on osteoclasts blocking destructive action and resulting in a 20–50 per cent fall in the plasma concentrations of calcium and phosphate within 0·5–2 hr. Although the effect of calcitonin is in a direction contrary to that of parathormone it does not operate by inhibiting the action of parathormone since calcitonin is effective in parathyroidectomized animals. The mechanism of action of calcitonin appears to be to prevent synthesis or release of a specific collagenase produced by the osteoclasts, but the hormone affects neither the synthesis nor the maturation of collagen. It seems likely that, whereas parathormone can be regarded as the primary homeostatic agent in relation to blood, calcitonin is concerned with the balance between the formation of bone and its resorption. Calcitonin has recently been synthesized and has been used with some success in treating hyperparathyroidism and Paget's disease.

Vitamin D

Several vitamins have important effects on the chemistry of bone, perhaps the most striking being that of vitamin D. A severe deficiency of vitamin D in the diet of growing children results in the bone disease known as rickets, characterized by soft, twisted, misshapen bones, particularly bowed long bones. This is the result of the concentrations of calcium and phosphate ions in the plasma being too low for full mineralization of the extracellular organic material ("osteoid") of bone to keep pace with its synthesis by osteoblasts. Sometimes osteoid builds up as under-calcified seams in the diaphyses of long bones. The parathormone and calcitonin regulators are unable to ameliorate this condition because the body as a whole has insufficient calcium and phosphate from which to mineralize its skeleton. The most common ultimate cause is not deficiency of these ions in the diet but deficiency of vitamin D. The vitamin is necessary for the active absorption of dietary calcium, and thereby indirectly of phosphate, from the lumen, across the wall of the small intestine into the blood stream. The mechanism by which the vitamin stimulates absorption is complex and not yet altogether clear. It probably involves an active transport mechanism with adenosine triphosphate as an energy source. If vitamin D is deficient in the diet, calcium and phosphate absorption are reduced, the plasma levels fall and bone mineralization is incomplete. The rachitic condition can be relieved by giving the vitamin or alternatively by exposure of the skin to ultraviolet radiation (in sunlight) which converts the inactive precursor, 7-dehydrocholesterol, into vitamin D which eventually is converted to the active form, probably 1,25 dihydroxycholecalciferol. Osteomalacia is a disease of adults corresponding to rickets in which mineralization is incomplete but with the difference that little new bone growth occurs.

Vitamin D also has a direct effect on bone, similar to that of parathyroid hormone, in stimulating osteoclastic activity thereby resulting in the transfer of calcium and phosphate from bone mineral to the blood plasma. This effect occurs with physiological levels of vitamin D and it has recently been found that the action of parathormone requires the presence of vitamin D, thus establishing that the vitamin plays an essential part in bone resorption in the normal individual.

Vitamin A

In tissue culture, vitamin A causes the intercellular substance of long bones to lose its capacity to stain metachromatically with toluidine blue. This is followed by rapid resorption of bone, with effects similar to those produced by parathormone involving an increase in the number of osteoclasts and rapid breakdown of bone. It is known that, in cartilage, vitamin A releases cathepsin D from lysosomes. The released enzyme then degrades the core protein of cartilage proteoglycan, resulting in solubilization of the attached chondroitin sulphate chains. Possibly, an analogous change may occur in bone proteoglycan, resulting in loss of metachromasia.

Deficiency of vitamin A has been studied in dogs where it results in abnormal remodelling of the bones of the skull. The vitamin appears to act as a specific chemical controller of the functions of osteoblasts and osteoclasts at a level which involves liaison between their activities. Excess of vitamin A causes bone lesions in the living animal probably also because of imbalance of osteogenic and resorptive changes.

Vitamin C

Ascorbic acid is essential for the development of bone, as it is for all connective tissues. Collagen synthesis depends upon the presence of vitamin C (together with molecular oxygen, ferrous ions, pyruvate and the enzyme, collagen proline oxidase) for the hydroxylation of proline residues, in the intact collagen chains, to hydroxyproline. In the absence of ascorbic acid, this step does not take place and the unhydroxylated "protocollagen" remains within the osteoblast so that secretion of extracellular material ceases. Ascorbic acid is also necessary for the synthesis of galactosamine, which is essential for chondroitin sulphate formation. When ascorbic acid is given to a scorbutic animal, deposition of extracellular substance soon begins once more.

Nucleation of the Inorganic Phase

Mineralized mammalian tissues, including bone, are distinguished by possessing an extracellular inorganic phase of calcium phosphate. This substance does not occur in normal soft tissues and therefore fundamental knowledge of the mechanisms for the formation of apatite crystals in bone would help to establish the essential differences between mesodermal tissues which normally mineralize and those which do not. Though knowledge of nucleation mechanisms is still incomplete, a brief consideration of the main ideas involved concludes this chapter.

The Impossibility of Homogeneous Nucleation

Since the ion product of calcium and phosphate in blood plasma, 19 (mg./100 ml.)^2, considerably exceeds the solubility product of hydroxyapatite, 9 (mg./100 ml.)^2 (see p. 562), it would, at first sight, appear to be necessary to explain not so much why bone becomes mineralized but why all other tissues, including blood, do not. There are many factors preventing such ubiquitous and dangerous mineralization but the most basic one can be demonstrated by a simple experiment. If an artificial solution is prepared containing calcium and phosphate ions at the same concentration as in plasma, namely 19 (mg./100 ml.)^2, and placed in a clean sealed container, it can be kept indefinitely without separation of solid crystals. However, if hydroxyapatite crystals are introduced into this solution, they grow at the expense of ions from solution until the ionic product falls to 9 (mg./100 ml.)^2, when crystal growth stops, the system having reached equilibrium.

Suppose further, that a series of similar solutions is prepared with gradually increasing concentrations of calcium and phosphate from 19 (mg./100 ml.)^2 upwards. No solid separates from these solutions until an ionic product of approximately 35 (mg./100 ml.)^2 is reached, above which level precipitation occurs. However, the solid which separates is not hydroxyapatite but the less stable and more soluble calcium hydrogen phosphate, $CaHPO_4.2H_2O$, which has a solubility product of 35 (mg./100 ml.)^2.

From the first experiment, it is clear that the **homogeneous nucleation** of a substance (*i.e.* the initial production of crystals in the absence of any solid phase) must be carefully distinguished from the growth of existing crystals. Thus nucleation appears more difficult than **crystal growth**. The second experiment shows that homogeneous nucleation is particularly difficult to achieve, for substances such as

hydroxyapatite, having a complex ionic lattice. This is shown by the fact that homogeneous nucleation of another more soluble calcium phosphate takes place preferentially. It is now clear, in principle, why nucleation of hydroxyapatite does not occur in tissues generally and in plasma.

How then are hydroxyapatite crystals produced in bone and other mineralized tissues? Two alternative answers would seem to be "by epitaxy" or "by solid phase transition".

Epitaxy

The basic reason for the difficulty in bringing about homogeneous nucleation of apatite is probably the instability of clusters of ions in the hydroxyapatite lattice below a certain size. Below this critical size, ion clusters occurring by chance collision of dissolved ions fly apart almost as soon as they are formed, because of their thermal energy. Mineralization in bone does not take place in simple solution but in the presence of pre-existing solid, namely the organic matrix. Thus nucleation of apatite may be **heterogeneous**, some structure in the organic matrix helping to stabilize ion clusters below the critical size for homogeneous nucleation. Such a structure might be a pattern of charged groups which bears a spatial relationship to the apatite lattice. In this concept of *epitaxy* (Greek = on-arrangement), the inorganic ions are considered to build up on a pre-existing organic template of charged groups which holds the inorganic ions by electrostatic forces in suitable relationship to form the apatite lattice. The cluster of ions would thus be stabilized until it reached the critical size, when the crystal would grow spontaneously, provided that the ion product of the surrounding solution exceeded the solubility product for apatite.

While epitaxy is a feasible explanation of the mechanism of mineral nucleation in bone, the difficulty remains that none of its organic constituents has been convincingly shown to have epitactic properties.

Considerable evidence for collagen acting as an epitactic agent was assembled by Glimcher (1959). Certainly it is the most abundant organic constituent and the numerous crystallites occur between fibrils and on their surfaces. Although in recent years, doubt has been cast on both the deposition of the first formed mineral on specific sub-bandings of the fibril and on the location of mineral crystallites within fibrils, recent determinations of the intermolecular volume of collagen fibrils from demineralized bone by Katz and Li (1973) prove that at least 56 per cent of the inorganic matter of compact bone from ox femur shafts is present within the collagen fibrils.

Some investigators consider that chondroitin sulphate, with its large number of acid sulphate groups, which can bind calcium ions, acts in conjunction with collagen as a "local-factor" initiating mineralization. Others consider that chondroitin sulphate reduces the concentration of free calcium ions in solution, and behaves as an inhibitor of mineralization. Bone sialoprotein is also highly acidic and binds calcium ions, however it inhibits precipitation of hydroxyapatite *in vitro*. In living bone it may behave differently as PAS positive staining, characteristic of bone sialoprotein, is a feature of sites undergoing rapid mineralization.

Mineralizing zones in bone also stain with Sudan black, after treatment with pyridine. This suggests that a lipidic substance may act as an epitactic agent; but despite extensive searches for lipids specific to bone, only ones which also occur in soft tissues have been found.

Solid Phase Transition

Recently, the idea that hydroxyapatite may not be the first inorganic solid to be formed in bone has gained ground. A strong case for the occurrence of amorphous calcium phosphate $(Ca_3(PO_4)_2.xH_2O)$ in substantial amounts in bone has recently been made (Termine, 1972). Conditions which favour and inhibit its *de novo* formation from solution as well as those enhancing its stability or conversion to hydroxyapatite have also been established. Since amorphous calcium phosphate is abundant in very young bone and the proportion of hydroxyapatite subsequently increases, it seems reasonable to suppose that the relatively labile amorphous calcium phosphate may be the first inorganic solid to be formed in bone. It then presumably undergoes a solution-mediated phase transition, to give small imperfect crystals of apatite, which finally grow in size and perfection. If this is so, then amorphous calcium phosphate plays a central role in mineralization and the direct epitactic formation of apatite from solution assumes less importance. However, each of the three steps in the formation of apatite via amorphous calcium phosphate is quite sensitive to its molecular environment and nothing definite is yet known about the specific effects of macromolecular substances. It therefore seems wise to reserve judgment upon the possible role of the bone matrix.

Cellular Involvement in Nucleation

During the last few years, attention has been turned from the extracellular collagen fibrils to the more immediate vicinity of bone cells as the site where the first inorganic material is laid down. Thus, substantial amounts of calcium and phosphate have been demonstrated chemically within bone cells. Electron opaque granules, considered to be calcium phosphate, are laid down within the mitochondria of osteoblasts and osteocytes by expending energy derived from oxidative phosphorylation. These mitochondrial granules may be transported to the extracellular matrix during calcification but it seems more likely that they are a metabolic reserve to keep intracellular concentrations of calcium and phosphate constant. Studies of the participation of cells in the mineralization process are, however, only beginning.

The earliest calcification detectable in cartilage and bone may occur either in relation to cell surfaces, possibly in association with lipoprotein membranes, or in extracellular loci sometimes described as "vesicles". Such vesicles have pronounced phosphatase activity and contain amorphous calcium phosphate but little protein and polysaccharide. They may be formed from the Golgi apparatus or perhaps the plasma membrane. Vesicles are presumably extruded from the cell, either complete with calcium phosphate granules or with sufficient supplies of calcium and phosphate ions for deposition of mineral subsequently to occur within the vesicles but extracellularly. However, this is purely speculative as very little is yet known about these structures.

The Role of Phosphatases in Mineralization

In tissues undergoing mineralization there are increased amounts of enzymes of the phosphatase group, particularly alkaline phosphatases. These enzymes release inorganic phosphate ions by hydrolysis of organic phosphate esters. It was once considered that they are directly responsible for mineralization of hard tissues by a process involving precipitation of calcium phosphate as a result of the increased phosphate ion concentration.

This "alkaline phosphatase theory" was gradually abandoned, partly because of the realization that concentrations of organic phosphate substrates were too low for the mechanism to account for the precipitation of large amounts of bone mineral and partly because other organs, especially the kidney, have large amounts of alkaline phosphatase but do not normally calcify. Later it was realized that the deposition of hydroxyapatite crystals in bone is a more "organized" phenomenon than a simple precipitation of calcium phosphate and further that, as described on p. 562, the plasma concentrations of calcium and phosphate in any case exceed the solubility product of hydroxyapatite.

However, it still appears necessary to explain the presence of phosphatases in mineralizing tissues. In recent years there have been a number of suggestions concerning their role in calcification of which three are particularly interesting. The first concerns possible epitactic agents in so far as they may require to be phosphorylated by adenosine triphosphate (ATP) or possibly alkaline phosphatase as a necessary prerequisite to the formation of a seeding site.

Secondly, it has recently been shown that alkaline phosphatases are capable of splitting pyrophosphate ions into inorganic phosphate. Plasma, urine and probably tissue fluids in general contain an inhibitor of mineralization, identified as the inorganic pyrophosphate ion. This presumably operates by a mechanism whereby it occupies sites into which the phosphate ion normally fits and thereby disrupts the building-up of a stable apatite lattice. The presence of pyrophosphate in tissue fluids generally is another line of defence against the deposition of hydroxyapatite in non-calcifying tissues. Deposition of calcium phosphates in calcifying tissues would be made possible by the pyrophosphatase activity of the localized alkaline phosphatase there, which breaks down the inhibiting pyrophosphate ions.

$$OH^- + (HP_2O_7)^{3-} \rightarrow 2\,(HPO_4)^{2-}$$

Thirdly, phosphatases may be responsible for locally raising the phosphate ion concentration at cell membranes or within vesicles.

Dynamics of the Inorganic Phase—a Provisional Analysis

Many ideas have been put forward regarding the formation and significance of bone mineral but few are capable of unequivocal experimental proof. They have been considered individually in some detail to give an overall impression of current views on mineralization. There follows an attempt to select ideas which are reasonably well established and which appear at present to be converging towards a coherent picture.

The stable structural core of mineral metabolism in bone is undoubtedly the hydroxyapatite crystallites. Their mass is continuously added to by ions, ultimately derived from the blood which, in health, is supersaturated with respect to hydroxyapatite. This constant drift of ions from solution to solid phase appears potentially dangerous to the organism, but the impossibility of homogeneous nucleation of hydroxyapatite prevents its formation in sites other than the specialized hard tissues. In addition, the widespread occurrence of pyrophosphate as an inhibitor of mineralization in soft tissues provides a further check to uncontrolled mineralization.

Epitaxy of hydroxyapatite from ions in solution by the organic matrix has been widely explored but remains unproven. It seems more likely that creation of new hydroxyapatite crystals involves more direct cellular involvement just as does the destruction of existing crystals. The first formed mineral is probably amorphous calcium phosphate produced as a result of oxidative phosphorylation within cells raising the local ionic product above the level found in the tissue fluids. Amorphous calcium phosphate may then be produced intracellularly but more probably extracellularly on cell membranes or within vesicles invading the extracellular space, phosphatases perhaps being involved in raising the phosphate ion concentration. The transformation of amorphous calcium phosphate into hydroxyapatite and the recrystallization of the latter occur via solution in the extracellular tissue fluid. It is at this level involving the orderly re-organization of the more random amorphous calcium phosphate, produced under cellular influence, to the regular, oriented crystals of hydroxyapatite, that the extracellular matrix probably participates in the development of the stable mineral phase.

Increase or decrease in the potential total pool of hydroxyapatite only occurs as a result of osteoblastic and osteoclastic activity respectively. This permits not only bone remodelling but also mineral homeostasis of the entire organism. Although there is a constant ionic drain from blood to bone, the volume of bone resorbed in a given period only needs to equal that laid down in order to offset this drain, because the resorbed bone is more heavily mineralized than the new bone. Thus, in the healthy adult skeleton, release of calcium and phosphate ions from apatite by osteoclastic resorption is sufficient to maintain the blood ionic product above the apatite solubility product by an amount controlled by the feedback system of parathyroid hormone. Additional but reversed control of osteoclasts by the thyroid, acting through calcitonin, regulates the delicate balance of resorption and deposition and provides a further safeguard against extremes of cellular activity upsetting the far-from-simple process of mineralization in living bone.

REFERENCES

Armstrong, W. D. and Singer, L. (1965), "Composition and Constitution of the Mineral Phase of Bone," *Clinical Orthopaedics*, **38**, 179.

Bailey, A. J., Fowler, L. J. and Peach, C. M. (1969), "Identification of Two Interchain Crosslinks of Bone and Dentine Collagen," *Biochemical and Biophysical Research Communications*, **34**, 663.

Bornstein, P. and Piez, K. A. (1964), "A Biochemical Study of Human Skin Collagen and the Relation Between Intra- and Intermolecular Cross-linking," *J. clin. Invest.*, **43**, 1813.

Eastoe, J. E. (1956), "The Organic Matrix of Bone," in *The Biochemistry and Physiology of Bone*, 1st edition, p. 81 (G. H. Bourne, Ed.). New York: Academic Press.

Eastoe, J. E. (1967a), "Composition of Collagen and Allied Proteins," in *Treatise on Collagen*, Vol. 1, p. 1 (G. N. Ramachandran, Ed.). London: Academic Press.

Eastoe, J. E. (1967b), "Chemical Organization of the Organic Matrix of Dentine," in *Structural and Chemical Organization of Teeth*, Vol. 2, p. 279 (A. E. W. Miles, Ed.). London: Academic Press.

Eastoe, J. E. and Eastoe, B. (1954), "The Organic Constituents of Mammalian Compact Bone," *Biochem. J.*, **57**, 453.

Francois, C. J. and Glimcher, M. J. (1967), "The Isolation and Amino Acid Composition of the α Chains of Chicken-bone Collagen," *Biochim. biophys. Acta*, **133**, 91.

Glimcher, M. J. (1959), "Molecular Biology of Mineralized Tissues with Particular Reference to Bone," *Reviews of Modern Physics*, **31**, 359.

Glimcher, M. J., Katz, E. P. and Travis, D. F. (1965), "The Solubilization and Reconstitution of Bone Collagen," *J. Ultrastruc. Res.*, **13**, 163.

Hartles, R. L. (1960), "Chemistry of Bone and Tooth Minerals," *Annual Report of the Chemical Society for* 1959, p. 322.

Herring, G. M. (1972), "The Organic Matrix of Bone," in *The Biochemistry and Physiology of Bone*, 2nd edition, Vol. 1, p. 127 (G. H. Bourne, Ed.). New York: Academic Press.

Katz, E. P. and Li, S.-T. (1973), "Structure and Function of Bone Collagen Fibrils," *J. molec. Biol.*, **80**, 1.

Leach, A. A. (1958), "The Lipids of Ox Compact Bone," *Biochem. J.*, **69**, 429.

Leaver, A. G. and Shuttleworth, C. A. (1968), "Studies on the Peptides, Free Amino Acids and Certain Related Compounds Isolated from Ox Bone," *Arch. Oral Biol.*, **13**, 509.

Miller, E. J., Martin, G. R., Piez, K. A. and Powers, M. J. (1967), "Characterization of Chick Bone Collagen and Compositional Changes Associated with Maturation," *J. biol. Chem.*, **242**, 5481.

Neuman, W. F. and Neuman, M. W. (1958), *The Chemical Dynamics of Bone Mineral*, p. 173. Chicago: The University of Chicago Press.

Piez, K. A. and Likins, R. C. (1960), "The Nature of Collagen—II, Vertebrate Collagens," in *Calcification in Biological Systems*, p. 411 (R. F. Sognnaes, Ed.). Washington, D.C.: American Association for the Advancement of Science.

Posner, A. S. (1957), "The Structure of Bone Mineral," *Clin. Orthopaed.*, **9**, 5.

Pugliarello, M. C., Vittur, F., de Bernard, B., Bonucci, E. and Ascenzi, A. (1970), "Chemical Modifications in Osteones During Calcification," *Calcified Tiss. Res.*, **5**, 108.

Termine, J. D. (1972), "Mineral Chemistry and Skeletal Biology," *Clinical Orthopaedics*, **85**, 207.

Weidmann, S. M. (1963), "Mechanism of Calcification. Biological Aspects," *Proceedings of the 9th ORCA Congress on Dental Caries, Paris 1962*, p. 79. Oxford: Pergamon Press.

47. THE REACTION OF BONE TO TRAUMA AND INFECTION

M. S. ISRAEL

THE REACTION TO TRAUMA

Bone is frequently subjected to increased strain, and when this is of a high order a fracture may occur. The reaction of bone to severance provides excellent testimony to its healing qualities. The healing of a fracture can be described arbitrarily in three phases. Figure 1 illustrates these in greater detail.

Demolition and Formation of Granulation Tissue

Immediately after the fracture the bone ends are surrounded by a considerable haematoma which, by the rupture of the encompassing periosteum, spreads into the neighbouring muscles and fascia. The periosteum is itself distended by the blood clot. There is an immediate acute traumatic inflammatory response and the polymorphonuclear leucocytes, and more especially the macrophages, scavenge the blood clot and the necrotic debris. Prominent in this early phase of demolition is the appearance of osteoclasts which resorb bone spicules and fragments of jagged bone forming fringes at the broken ends. These osteoclasts are believed to form from the fusion of macrophages, and are classical giant cells with many nuclei. Within a few days the bone ends will have been rendered smooth, and much debris removed. There then follows the ingrowth of undifferentiated fibroblastic cells and vascular endothelial elements. These form granulation tissue, an early reparative tissue consisting of fibroblasts, thin vascular channels, and a variable number of inflammatory cells (mostly macrophages in uninfected fractures). Soon the fibroblastic cells lay down collagen fibres, so that the bone-ends become united by a young, vascular type of fibrous tissue. This should be well established within a week.

Formation of Provisional Callus

It is at this stage that the fibroblastic cells show their differentiated potential. Most of them secrete a characteristic ground substance called osseomucin, which is deposited between interwoven collagen fibres. This complex of ground substance and coarse collagen fibres forms the matrix called osteoid tissue into which there is a progressive precipitation of mineral salts to form woven bone. The term, woven, is derived from the random and intertwining pattern of the fibre bundles; they have no intimate association with blood vessels nor are they aligned to sites of stress. A few of the fibroblastic cells, instead of differentiating into osteoblasts as above described, show a chondral differentiation and lay down islets of hyaline cartilage which rapidly undergo calcification. Thus the provisional callus (of hard tissues) that unites the bone ends consists of a mixture of woven bone and calcified cartilage. The poorer the immobilization of the bone-ends the greater the amount of cartilage laid down. A considerable amount of cartilage will therefore be found in the provisional callus of a fractured rib and in experimental fractures in animals. The role of the periosteum in healing is essentially similar to that described in Chapter 45.

The mechanism of the calcification at this stage is not well understood, but the high content of alkaline phosphatase present in osteoblasts may be a factor. In the inflammatory phase of healing, the local pH is acid (the acid tide) and this helps to bring calcium into solution after osteoclastic resorption of bone fragments. In the later phase of healing the pH rises (the alkaline tide), and the alkaline phosphatase produced locally may be able to react more easily with plasma hexose monophosphate to produce a local supersaturation of phosphate. It might be that the calcium and phosphate precipitate in high saturation on the osteoid and cartilage matrix. Provisional callus should be abundant by two weeks, and easily visible radiologically.

It is found that bone is formed in electronegative regions and destruction occurs in regions of electropositivity. This is consistent with the enzymes produced by the osteoblasts and osteoclasts; the former cells are active at the cathode where alkaline conditions exist, whereas the latter are active at the anode where acid conditions are present. In this respect, the alkaline phosphatase of osteoblasts plays a part, as has already been noted, in osteogenesis, whereas the acid phosphatase and other lysosomal enzymes of osteoclasts act in an acid pH and aid in autolysis. (See also Chapter 35).

Formation of Definitive Callus

This is the final stage of fracture healing. There is active osteoclastic resorption of woven bone and calcified cartilage, and the ingrowth of blood vessels and osteoblasts into areas of resorption. In this way the hiatus produced by resorption is replaced by well-formed blood vessels surrounded by laminae of osteoblasts, which lay down bone fibres in concentric lamellae around the centrally disposed blood vessels. This is the basic Haversian system, and the bone arranged thus is described as lamellar bone (or adult bone). It forms thick trabeculae, and is laid down in lines of stress. It is therefore much more useful in bearing strain than the more primitive woven bone that it replaces. This process of lamellar bone replacement of woven bone and

nant of the fusiform bulging of the initial haematoma, is removed entirely to leave a smooth outer surface. The lamellar bone is the definitive callus and although it takes a long time for perfect bony regeneration to occur, in practice the limb (or jaw) is considered healed for regional use within a period of one to three months depending on the site of fracture. In many instances fracture union is expedited by internal fixation, especially in sites where delayed healing is to be expected, *e.g.* the neck of the femur.

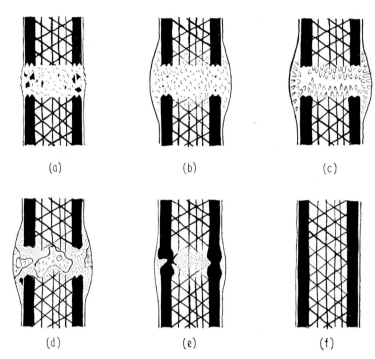

FIG. 1. Stages in the healing of a fracture: (a) Haematoma formation. (b) Stages 2 and 3. Acute inflammation followed by demolition. Loose fragments of bone are removed, and the bone ends show osteoporosis. (c) Stage 4. Granulation tissue formation. (d) Stage 5. The bone ends are now united by woven bone, cartilage or a mixture of the two. This hard material is often called callus and can be divided into three parts—internal, intermediate, and external. The intermediate callus is that part which lies in line with the cortex of the bone. The internal callus occupies the original marrow cavity, while the external callus produces the fusiform swelling visible on the outside of the bone. (e) Stage 6. Lamellar bone is laid down; calcified cartilage and woven bone are progressively removed. (f) Stage 7. Final remodelling.

calcified cartilage is the traumatic counterpart of intramembranous and endochondral ossification noted developmentally. It takes months, even years, to be completed and there is constant remodelling of lamellar bone in accordance with the local stress to which the area is subjected.

In this way regeneration of compact cortical bone results in the replacement of the irregularly laid down woven bone by massive seams of concentrically disposed lamellae. Near the surface, these assume a plate-like contour. The inner portions of the woven bone, if removed entirely, are replaced by thin trabeculae of cancellous bone. Thus, the "internal callus" is replaced by thin strands of lamellar bone around which there is a cavity containing fat cells or haemopoietic bone-marrow elements (depending on the bone involved), the "intermediate callus" becomes dense lamellar bone, and the "external callus", which is the rem-

Healing of the Post-extraction Tooth Socket

This follows the usual course of fracture healing except that periosteum plays little or no part in the healing process. The socket fills with clotted blood, and in a few days this is organized to granulation tissue and fibrous tissue. Woven bone is laid down, and this is gradually replaced by lamellar bone. There is a covering of compact bone, but as the alveolar bone is no longer needed to support the tooth, there is extensive remodelling with a reduced ridge in that area. At the same time as these osseous changes are occurring, there is epithelialization of the raw surface of the wound.

If the clot disintegrates too early, infection can involve the underlying bone and produce a localized osteomyelitis. This is called a "dry socket", and is extremely painful. The exposed bone undergoes necrosis and is sequestrated. Healing is slow.

Factors Influencing Healing of Fractures

Under certain circumstances fracture healing may be considerably delayed. Sometimes healing is never properly achieved and a fibrous union is all that results. In the worst cases, there may be no union at all, and a pseudarthrosis due to synovial differentiation of the fibroblastic tissue between the bone-ends develops. The main causes of delayed or impaired union are:

(a) **Inadequate immobilization of the fracture site,** which results in repeated damage to the granulation tissue and the provisional callus.

(b) **Infection** of the site as occurs in compound injuries. Not only is the reparative tissue destroyed, but the tension engendered by the purulent exudate leads to necrosis of the surrounding bone and the development of chronic osteomyelitis.

(c) **Ischaemia** leading to inadequate granulation tissue formation. This is typical of fractures of the neck of the femur, the shaft of the tibia, and the carpal scaphoid.

(d) **Deficiencies in dietary protein and vitamin C,** both of which are essential for collagen formation.

(e) **Inadequate apposition of the bone-ends** or the inter-position of non-osteogenic tissues, such as muscle or fat, or foreign bodies.

(f) **Pathological conditions of the bone** that may have predisposed to fracture, *e.g.* simple or aneurysmal bone cysts, hyperparathyroidism (osteitis fibrosa cystica) with its "brown tumours", giant-cell tumour of bone, and especially metastases from carcinoma elsewhere in the body. This is the commonest cause of a pathological fracture, and the usual primary sites of the tumour are the breast, lung, prostate, kidney, and thyroid.

Bone-grafting

Bone-grafting is an established means of expediting heal-ing at fracture sites notorious for slow regeneration. The graft may be autogenous, but homografts (from other indi-viduals) or even heterografts (from other species of animals) have been successfully used. In all cases, the osteocytic elements are destroyed. This is due to ischaemia in the instance of autografts, and also to the graft rejection reaction with homografts and heterografts. Nevertheless, the inert bone acts as an efficient framework through which new granulation tissue can grow, as well as providing a good support for the fracture ends. Sometimes it may effect excellent internal fixation. The operation itself stimulates an inflammatory reaction that sets in motion the formation of granulation tissue. The local source of bone salts pro-vided by the graft assists the repair process. The bone is removed by osteoclastic resorption, and is gradually replaced by the bone-forming granulation tissue in which woven and then lamellar bone are laid down.

Grafts of compact bone provide mechanical strength as soon as they are firmly united to the original bone-ends, but revascularization and remodelling of such a compact graft is relatively slow.

Grafts composed of fragments of cancellous bone, or small bone chips, take longer to become firm; but the greater amount of internal surface in such grafts allows for more rapid ingrowth of new soft tissues, and more rapid remodelling.

Other Traumatic Lesions of Bone

Whenever bone is subjected to severe trauma, there is a hypertrophy of the endosteal cells of the vascular spaces and the bone marrow and the cambial periosteal cells. They enlarge and assume osteoblastic morphology. There is also a proliferation, and in long-standing stress new bone is laid down, especially beneath the periosteum. This sub-periosteal new bone leads to the characteristic adventitious ridges seen on the shafts and processes of bones of those engaged in heavy physical or athletic labour. Expanding intraosseous lesions such as cysts and tumours lead in the same way to a marked periosteal reaction—the onion-like layers of new bone that form over an expanding Ewing's tumour is a classical example, and a somewhat similar appearance may sometimes be seen over a giant-cell tumour or an osteosarcoma (irrespective of its intrinsic osteogenic potentiality).

Severe injury may lead to **ischaemic necrosis.** Its relation-ship to certain anatomical types of fractures has already been noted, but a quieter, less obvious ischaemic necrosis may follow repeated traumatic episodes in growing bones. The necrosis that is the basis of the epiphyseal lesions in such childhood conditions as **Legg-Perthes disease** of the head of the femur is believed to follow the ischaemia of trauma. Ischaemic necrosis of bone is an important compli-cation of **decompression sickness** (caisson disease), which is traditionally attributed to bubbles of nitrogen gas blocking the lumina of small blood vessels, especially in the central nervous system and in bone. Masses of sickled red blood cells in **sickle-cell disease** are another cause of widespread bony infarction.

Ionizing radiation may also cause bone destruction. Adult bone is fairly resistant to the effect of ionizing irradiation, but the endochondral bone laid down during childhood is vulnerable to even moderate exposures. The damage affects the proliferating cartilage cells more than the newly-formed osteoblasts, and ossification may be greatly retarded.

In adult bone, only massive exposures lead to focal necrosis of bone—erroneously called "radiation osteitis", for there is little inflammatory reaction. The necrotic bone forms a sequestrum, and there may be a degree of periosteal reaction to produce a mild involucrum over the dead bone. Some areas of necrosis are liable to become secondarily infected, especially when the mandible is involved, and then an intractable, painful osteomyelitis develops.

An occasional complication of massive external exposure to ionizing radiation is the development of osteosarcoma. This is a much greater hazard of the deposition of radio-active elements in the bone itself. The classical example occurred in women engaged in painting dials of watches with a luminous paint containing mesothorium. By sucking the tips of the brushes they were using, they imbibed quantities of this radioactive element which produced not only radiation necrosis of bone but also multiple osteosarcomata.

The administration of strontium 90 to rabbits has been shown to lead to osteosarcomata related to the apices of the teeth, where the radioactive element became incorporated in the developing dental tissues. However, massive doses were involved, and there is no evidence of the development of jaw sarcomata in man from this cause.

THE REACTION TO INFECTION

The reaction of bone to infection is a combination of acute inflammatory destruction and attempts at repair by the laying down of new bone under the periosteum.

Acute Pyogenic Infections

By far the commonest type of pyogenic osteomyelitis is caused by *Staphylococcus pyogenes* (*aureus*). This is typically a disease of growing children, and the organism lodges in the metaphysis of a long bone. It reaches this final site as part of a bacteraemia; presumably the staphylococcus enters the blood stream during an insignificant skin infection. Less commonly the organism involved is the pneumococcus or a *Salmonella* species, usually *S. typhi*. Acute pyogenic osteomyelitis can also follow the local contamination of a bone, *e.g.* in a compound fracture or during open surgery. Again the infection is usually staphylococcal.

In the early phase of acute pyogenic osteomyelitis there is suppurative destruction locally, and the tension engendered by the inflammatory exudate in a rigid confined space soon occludes the regional blood vessels. This leads to extensive ischaemic necrosis of bone. The pus also tends to track beneath the periosteum, thus cutting off the periosteal blood supply to the bone and augmenting the necrosis. In the worst cases the whole shaft may become necrotic, but usually only a part is affected. This necrotic remnant cannot be cast off spontaneously, and it acts as a nidus for organismal growth in addition to preventing proper drainage of the pus. It is for this reason that inadequately treated osteomyelitis always becomes chronic—should the patient survive the acute phase and not die of septicaemia or pyaemia.

In chronic osteomyelitis the regenerative response of bone to infection becomes conspicuous. While the pus ruptures through the periosteum to the surrounding soft tissues and drains through the skin by multiple sinuses, the vascular periosteum lays down a sheath of new bone that surrounds the dead shaft, which is now merely a sequestrum. This sheath of new bone is called an **involucrum** (fig. 2), and the pus which bathes the surface of the sequestrum escapes through holes, or **cloacae**, in the involucrum. There is an attempt at separation of the sequestrum by osteoclasts which loosen it from its point of attachment to the living remnant of bone, but even if this detachment is completed the loose sequestrum cannot be shed from the area because of the poor drainage of the part. Only a radical surgical

excision can effect a cure of this form of chronic osteomyelitis, and in many cases this entails such a great removal of bone that the limb would be rendered useless. Amputation is therefore the usual end of chronic osteomyelitis. The right treatment is never to allow it to develop, by the expeditious use of antibiotics and (if necessary) surgical drainage in the acute stage.

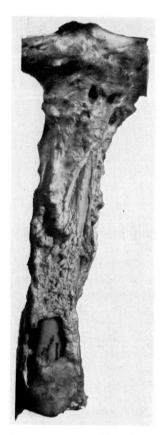

Fig. 2. Osteomyelitis of the tibia. The extensive central sequestrum is largely concealed by an exuberant involucrum formed from the detached periosteum. At the base of the shaft there is a cloaca through which the pitted sequestrum is visible. (Specimen HS44.1 from the Wellcome Museum of Pathology reproduced by permission of the President and Council of the Royal College of Surgeons of England.)

Another more localized type of chronic osteomyelitis is the classical **Brodie's abscess**, found at the metaphysis of a long bone—often the lower end of the tibia or fibula—in young people. In this instance the organism is of low-grade virulence in relation to the host's immune response (once more it is usually a staphylococcus), and the local suppuration is contained in an abscess cavity surrounded by thickened new bone laid down by surrounding osteoblasts. In due course the pus may become sterile. Radiologically there is a central area of radiolucency surrounded by dense bone. Drainage is curative.

When an organism of low-grade virulence infects the periosteum there may be a predominant laying-down of new subperiosteal bone, so that the whole area becomes thickened and sclerotic. This type of chronic pyogenic periostitis is unusual.

Acute pyogenic osteomyelitis is not uncommon in the jaw. An unusual, but well-recognized type affects the maxilla of newborn infants. The source of infection is sometimes undecided; it may follow birth trauma to the oral mucosa with subsequent contamination by the nurse or mother or by the teat of a feeding bottle, or else it may be haematogenous from an umbilical or skin lesion. The organism is *Staph. pyogenes*, and the infection starts around the crypt of the first molar tooth and the adjacent area of the anterior part of the maxilla. From here there is rapid spread to the orbit, palate, and paranasal sinuses. If penicillin therapy (with possible draining) is not started at once, there will be necrosis and sequestration of much of the maxilla, and a loss of much of both the deciduous and the permanent dentition on that side.

Osteomyelitis of the jaw in older children and adults usually follows a local injury with contamination of the deeper tissues. Haematogenous infections may occur, but are not common.

Tuberculosis

Osseous tuberculosis, like pyogenic osteomyelitis, is a haematogenous infection. Nowadays, the primary tuberculous lesion is almost invariable pulmonary, and the bone condition arises as part of a bacteraemia that occurs during the course of the infection. The organisms may lie dormant in the bone (and other organs) for years, and then become reactivated, often for no apparent reason. Often the pulmonary focus is scarred and healed when the bony lesion makes its appearance.

As in pyogenic osteomyelitis, tuberculous disease usually starts in the metaphysis. The classical tubercle follicle develops: a central zone of caseous necrosis surrounded by a layer of epithelioid cells (which are altered macrophages) and Langhans giant cells (fused macrophages with peripherally disposed nuclei), which is in turn encompassed by a dense diffuse envelope of lymphocytes in which there are also proliferating fibroblasts. As the disease spreads, neighbouring follicles expand and fuse, and bony trabeculae are replaced by advancing caseation and tuberculous granulation tissue. Soon, the caseous material undergoes liquefaction to form the **cold abscess** so typical of osseous tuberculosis. This extends beneath the periosteum, penetrates it, drains through the soft tissues, and eventually discharges through the skin by one or more sinuses. The abscess may extend over a considerable area of tissue, and drain at a site remote from the bony lesion. A good example is tuberculosis of the lumbar vertebral bodies draining via the psoas sheath into the groin.

Tuberculosis produces extensive bony destruction without any significant regenerative ossification such as is seen in chronic pyogenic osteomyelitis. The condition used to be called "tuberculous caries" and was encountered most often in the spinal column where, by destroying the

vertebral bodies, it led to an angular deformity of the spine called a "gibbus" (fig. 3).

Another distinctive feature of skeletal tuberculous is its destructive effect on cartilage. Whereas the epiphyseal plate holds up the progress of a pyogenic osteomyelitis, and suppurative arthritis is an unusual complication in most cases of this condition, in skeletal tuberculous disease early joint involvement is the rule. In some cases, this is due to an initial synovial infection from the bloodstream, but more often it is due to metaphyseal spread from a neighbouring

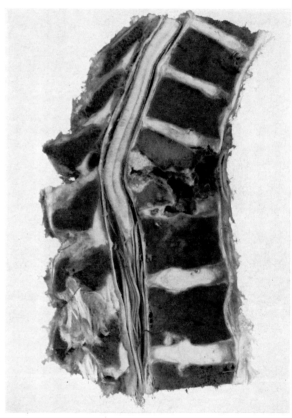

Fig. 3. Tuberculosis of the spinal column. Two adjacent vertebral bodies have been destroyed by progressive caseous necrosis, and the intervening intervertebral disc has disintegrated amid the debris. The result has been collapse of the two vertebrae with acute angulation of the spine. (Specimen S490.4 from the Wellcome Museum of Pathology reproduced by permission of the President and Council of the Royal College of Surgeons of England.)

bone. The angular gibbus of spinal tuberculosis is augmented by the destruction of the intervertebral discs adjacent to the diseased vertebral bodies. The hip and knee joints are the most commonly affected after the vertebral ones.

Syphilis

A mild periostitis is not uncommon in the secondary stage of syphilis, but like most of the other secondary-stage manifestations it is reversible and leaves no permanent trace.

It is in tertiary syphilis that the characteristic gummatous lesions of the bone develop, and these cause great destruction. A gumma consists of an irregular area of necrosis surrounded by reparative fibrous tissue containing many lymphocytes and plasma cells with rather fewer macrophages and only occasional giant cells. Obliterative endarteritis is a characteristic change in the neighbouring arteries and arterioles, and this adds to the necrosis by the ischaemia it causes. The result is a focal destruction of bone with cavitation. But in most cases of tertiary bone syphilis there is also a marked periostitis that leads to the production of new subperiosteal bone. The whole condition is called **syphilitic osteo-periostitis.**

The bones most commonly affected in syphilis are the tibia, ulna and clavicle, where the proliferative periostitis usually exceeds the gummatous destruction—the sabre tibia is a good example of this proliferative tendency that

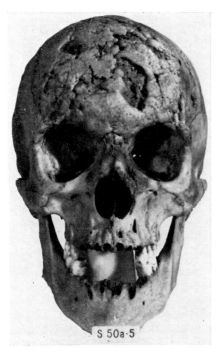

Fig. 4. Gummatous osteo-periostitis of the skull. The calvaria shows multiple areas of destruction, many of which are overhung by extensive layers of new bone. Thus there is focal destruction with generalized thickening. (Specimen S50a.5 from the Wellcome Museum of Pathology reproduced by permission of the President and Council of the Royal College of Surgeons of England.)

mimics the bowed tibia of rickets and Paget's disease—and the calvaria of the skull and the facial bones, where destruction is usually predominant. Well-known effects of tertiary syphilis are the perforated palate and the saddle-back nasal depression due to destruction of the nasal bones. In the worst cases there may be great focal destruction of the skull with reparative bony overgrowth around the hiatuses left behind (fig. 4).

The bony lesions of congenital syphilis resemble those of the tertiary stage: perforated palate and sabre tibia may occur. A more characteristic manifestation is the syphilitic epiphysitis, particularly around the elbow, seen in young infants. Here, as elsewhere, there is an infiltration of lymphocytes and plasma cells together with focal destruction

of the bone. The condition is painful, and the infant does not move the affected limb. The result is a pseudo-paralysis.

Yaws

Yaws is a treponematosis caused by *Treponema pertenue*, and it has many features in common with syphilis. The primary lesion is cutaneous, but unlike the chancre of syphilis, is extragenital and not venereally acquired. In the secondary stage, in addition to widespread skin eruption (with little mucosal involvement), there is often a considerable periostitis, so that bone pains are a common complaint. As in syphilis, this periostitis resolves spontaneously.

Tertiary yaws is almost completely confined to the skin and bones. Cardiovascular and central nervous system involvement is unusual. The gummatous lesions described in syphilis are frequently found in the bones in yaws. The lesions may result in a sabre tibia and roughened thickened radius and ulna. A more characteristic lesion is a destructive inflammation of the bones and soft tissues of the palate, nose and pharynx. This is called **gangosa** and it leaves in its wake great deformity. A localized periosteal overgrowth of new bone in the maxillary bone produces an exostosis-like lesion called **goundou** which may interfere with vision.

Other Infections

Actinomycosis sometimes affects the mandible and the base of the skull in the course of cervico-facial disease, and the result is a destruction of bone without fresh ossification. The related condition **maduromycosis**, which is the result of either nocardial or a frankly fungous infection of the soft tissues, usually of the foot or hand, leads to a similar tissue reaction. The bone is replaced by loculated abscesses, separated by fibrous septa in which colonies of the causative organisms are easily visible on microscopy. Their coloured "granules" can be isolated from the pus.

Cryptococcosis is a fungous disease that may cause destructive bony lesions when it becomes generalized, as may other fungous diseases, *e.g.* **blastomycosis** and **paracoccidioidomycosis**. In none of these is there new bone formation.

Hydatid disease of bone is associated with the production of confluent cysts that lead to gross osseous destruction with no attempt at bony regeneration. The pelvis is most often affected, and the disease is intractable. The causative agent is the cestode parasite *Echinococcus granulosus*.

CONCLUSION

The reaction of bone to uncomplicated injury is a rapid regenerative process that ends in perfect replacement by lamellar bone. Only where the local or general conditions are unfavourable is there delayed union, fibrous union, or non-union. Ionizing radiation may lead to osteosarcoma formation. Infective agents act predominantly to destroy bone; only in pyogenic and treponemal infections is the laying down of new bone a conspicuous feature.

48. METABOLIC DISEASES OF THE JAWS

L. WATSON AND J. M. FACCINI

Abnormalities of the jaws and teeth may result from many endocrine and metabolic disorders. This chapter will be devoted to manifestations of metabolic bone disease and no attempt will be made to give a systematic account of numerous rare diseases.

The three commonly occurring forms of generalized metabolic bone disease are osteoporosis, osteomalacia and osteitis fibrosa (the specific bone disease of hyperparathyroidism). Osteoporosis may be due to endocrine abnormalities such as Cushing's syndrome, hypogonadism and thyrotoxicosis. The jaws are affected by idiopathic osteoporosis in common with the other bones of the body whereas abnormalities of the jaws and teeth are surprisingly uncommon in osteomalacia. Osteitis fibrosa is less common but is important because it may exhibit dental manifestations. Abnormalities of growth hormone production may also produce striking changes in the jaw.

Other rarer disorders will be described because they have obvious dental features or are important in differential diagnosis. These include osteogenesis imperfecta, osteopetrosis, fibrous dysplasia and Paget's disease of bone.

OSTEOPOROSIS

Albright and his associates (see Albright and Reifenstein, 1948) clearly characterized osteoporosis as a disorder of too little bone of normal composition, a definition which has never been seriously challenged. It is not a single disease entity but constitutes a non-specific reaction of the skeleton to a number of different stimuli. Osteoporosis is by far the commonest form of metabolic bone disease and among the commonest of all disorders.

Pathogenesis

The classic speculations of Albright focused attention on the endocrine nature of the disease and led for a time to some rigidity of thought about pathogenesis. It has since become clear that osteoporosis is a normal ageing process in the skeleton of all adults and that it increases slowly in degree beginning soon after the age of 20 years.

Nevertheless, this view of osteoporosis cannot explain all the features of the disease for it may become clinically apparent at any age and other aetiological factors have been implicated. These may be well defined causes of accelerated bone loss, such as immobilization. Disuse osteoporosis is a major problem in orthopaedic surgery and potentially in space exploration. Endocrine abnormalities such as Cushing's syndrome, hypogonadism and thyrotoxicosis are other good examples of well defined pathological processes which may result in bone loss. Usually, however, the nature of the accelerating factor cannot be defined (idiopathic osteoporosis).

Calcium Dynamics and Biochemical Findings

There are important biochemical differences between the three major forms of metabolic bone disease as shown in Table 1.

In most cases of osteoporosis the plasma levels of calcium, phosphorus and alkaline phosphatase are normal. Hypercalcaemia is uncommon though it may occur in acute osteoporosis following immobilization, especially in children. The urinary calcium excretion may be normal, increased or decreased depending on the stage of the disease.

The level of faecal calcium is usually raised and in immobilization it may be very high, even exceeding intake. Since the urinary calcium may also be considerably raised

TABLE 1

BIOCHEMICAL FINDINGS IN METABOLIC BONE DISEASE

	Plasma				Urine
	Calcium	Phosphorus	Alkaline Phosphatase	Urea	24-hour Calcium
Osteoporosis	N	N	N	N	N or ↑
Osteomalacia due to vitamin D deficiency or malabsorption	N or ↓	↓	↑	N	↓
Osteitis fibrosa: Primary or tertiary hyperparathyroidism	↑	↓ or N or ↑	↑	N or ↑	↑ or N or ↓
Secondary hyperparathyroidism due to renal-glomerular failure	N or ↓	N or ↑	↑	↑	↓
Secondary hyperparathyroidism due to vitamin D deficiency or malabsorption	N or ↓	↓	↑	N	↓

↑ = above normal
↓ = below normal
N = normal

in these circumstances, such subjects may have a large negative calcium balance, sometimes as great as 500 or 600 mg./day. However, in most idiopathic osteoporotics and in some of known origin the overall external calcium balance is not strikingly negative. Thus, the calcium balance picture in osteoporosis varies in degree, depending probably on the stage and activity of the disease, the nature and intensity of aetiological factors and perhaps the response to treatment. Many published balances are clearly from patients in an inactive phase.

Some workers believe that decreased intestinal absorption of calcium is the cardinal factor in the production of osteoporosis, which may also result from simple dietary deficiency of calcium. However, high faecal calcium is more likely to be the result of bony dissolution than its cause. This view is supported by quantitative microradiographic studies which show bone formation rates to be normal in most cases of osteoporosis, while bone resorption rates are increased.

Histology

There are also important histological differences between the three major forms of metabolic bone disease. In osteoporosis the bone appears qualitatively normal but there are fewer trabeculae in a given area than would be expected. It can readily be distinguished from osteomalacia where failure of mineralization of bone matrix results in a characteristic histological appearance due to abnormally large amounts of osteoid. Osteoporosis is also distinct from

osteitis fibrosa in which osteoclastic resorption of trabeculae is associated with fibrous replacement of lacunae.

Clinical Features

Osteoporosis is often asymptomatic, the diagnosis being made from an X-ray film taken for some other purpose. Bone pain is not uncommon, however, especially in the back and osteoporosis is probably the commonest cause of backache in the elderly. Pain may occur in other situations such as long bones, pelvis, sternum, hands and feet. Pathological fractures of the femoral neck are a well-recognized feature of osteoporosis in the elderly. Localized osteoporosis may also occur at sites of immobilization such as healing fractures or arthritic joints.

The jaw is involved in this generalized ageing process in common with the other bones, hence the need for greater care with dental procedures in old people. Nonetheless, spontaneous jaw fractures are unusual in osteoporosis. The process is more pronounced and obvious in the alveolar bone where it is accelerated by the removal of teeth. In the rare cases of juvenile osteoporosis there is no abnormality of dentition despite the severity of the disease.

Treatment

From the very nature of the condition, it is not surprising that treatment is difficult and often unrewarding. Some general points are of importance:

(a) any obvious aetiological factor should be removed, such as Cushing's syndrome, steroid administration, thyrotoxicosis or immobilization;

(b) in adults, the realistic aim of treatment is to arrest the course of the disease and relieve symptoms;

(c) in children, where growth potential still exists in the skeleton, good improvement may occur if aetiological factors can be removed; and

(d) patients should be advised to be as active as possible—thus preventing further osteoporosis due to immobilization.

Apart from analgesics, the sex hormones are the mainstay of drug treatment in adults. It is wise to ensure that the intake of calcium and vitamin D is generous, but there is no evidence that large doses of vitamin D or calcium have further beneficial effect.

RICKETS AND OSTEOMALACIA

These conditions result from deficiency of vitamin D or resistance to its actions. In childhood the effects are most striking at the epiphyses of long bones producing characteristic rickety changes. In adults, in whom the epiphyses are fused, the long bones are softened, producing bone pain, tenderness, deformity or pathological fractures. Radiologically the characteristic lesion in adults is the pseudofracture, or Looser's zone. As already noted the histological picture is striking and usually diagnostic. Biochemical findings are characteristic with low (or normal) plasma calcium, low plasma phosphorus and raised alkaline phosphatase levels (Table 1).

Most of the published work on the effect of vitamin D on the dental tissues has been derived from experimental animals in which severe rachitogenic diets have interfered with calcification and matrix formation of both enamel and dentine. Changes described in the alveolar bone of rachitic dogs show that this is affected in the same fashion as spongy and cortical bone elsewhere in the skeleton—failure of the matrix to calcify producing large amounts of uncalcified or poorly calcified osteoid.

Clinical Features

Surprisingly, quite severe or prolonged vitamin D deficiency in childhood producing the typical symptoms of rickets is not necessarily associated with disturbances in the dentition. Studies on children with rickets have not revealed enamel or dentinal hypoplasia, and skeletal development assessed by cephalometry has not shown gross abnormalities; nor has delayed eruption been noticeable. It may be that in these instances the deficiency is not sufficiently severe to damage developing teeth, but experience suggests that the incidence of dental lesions in rickets is very low in this country. The published accounts of hypoplasia of the teeth in rachitic children are of some antiquity. A question of great interest is why patients with extensive changes in their skeleton do not have corresponding changes in the dentition. No ready answer comes to mind.

HYPERPARATHYROIDISM

Primary hyperparathyroidism was established as a clinical entity about 45 years ago when the first parathyroid tumours were removed at operation. The early diagnoses were made in hypercalcaemic patients with severe and extensive osteitis fibrosa and parathyroid tumours were then thought to be very rare. Albright's group soon realized that parathyroid tumours were common and produced more varied clinical manifestations than had at first appeared. Their experience has been confirmed in many centres and there is now good evidence that the prevalence of parathyroid tumours is greater than one case per thousand of the adult population.*

Albright and Reifenstein (1948) defined **secondary hyperparathyroidism** as a condition in which more parathyroid hormone is manufactured than is normal, but where the hormone is needed for some compensatory purpose. This is found most commonly in prolonged renal-glomerular failure and in osteomalacia in which there is reactive hypertrophy and hyperplasia involving all four parathyroid glands.

The term **tertiary hyperparathyroidism** was later introduced to describe cases in which parathyroid tumours had apparently developed after prolonged secondary hyperparathyroidism due to renal-glomerular failure or mal-

absorption syndromes with osteomalacia. These cases would formerly have been classified as primary hyperparathyroidism (Davies, Dent and Watson, 1968). The term tertiary hyperparathyroidism implies the importance of aetiological factors in parathyroid tumour formation.

Pluriglandular Syndromes

Genetic factors may be important in the production of parathyroid tumours. When found in families, hyperparathyroidism is usually associated with tumours of other endocrine glands. There are two genetically distinct pluriglandular syndromes (Steiner, Goodman and Powers, 1968); parathyroid tumours are associated in the one with adenomas of the pituitary (producing acromegaly) and the pancreas (producing the Zollinger-Ellison syndrome or hyperinsulinism) and in the other with phaeochromocytomas, medullary thyroid carcinoma or, less commonly, with Cushing's syndrome. This latter group may rarely be associated with multiple oral mucosal neuromas—an important early diagnostic sign.

Calcium Dynamics and Parathyroid Hormone Action

The plasma calcium level is an important bodily constant which is normally maintained within a narrow range despite large daily exchange of calcium between the intestine, the bloodstream, the kidneys and the bones. Even minor deviations of the plasma calcium from the normal range may cause severe symptoms and extensive disease.

It is generally agreed that the principal function of parathyroid hormone (PTH) is to maintain a normal plasma calcium level, that hypocalcaemia is the best stimulus to the secretion of PTH, and that the reciprocal relationship between plasma calcium and PTH levels is a good example of a feed-back mechanism. The many actions of PTH have been reviewed in Chapter 46.

There is debate about the relative importance of peripheral sites of action of PTH in regulating plasma calcium. The view most commonly held is that the prime action of PTH is to control the dynamic exchange of calcium between bone and bloodstream. Others consider that renal excretion and perhaps gastrointestinal absorption of calcium are more important sites of physiological regulation in the maintenance of normal plasma calcium levels.

There is also clear evidence that PTH has at least three direct actions on bone:

    (a) it promotes osteoclastic resorption;
    (b) it promotes osteocytic osteolysis; and
    (c) it may inhibit or stimulate osteoblastic activity.

These actions account for the varied histological appearances which may be seen in hyperparathyroidism with osteitis fibrosa, whether primary, secondary or tertiary.

The mechanism whereby PTH produces its actions at the cellular level is uncertain and appears to be complex. There is evidence that it causes release of adenyl cyclase on the inside of cell membranes with resulting increase in cyclic 3'5'-AMP. This, in turn, results in increased RNA synthesis, followed by increased production of enzymes and

---

* For some time, primary hyperparathyroidism was considered synonymous with the presence of a parathyroid tumour, usually a single adenoma, and less commonly multiple adenomas, parathyroid carcinoma or primary water-clear cell hyperplasia. Later, the occurrence of primary chief-cell hyperplasia of all four parathyroid glands was recognized as a pathological entity. The histological distinction between these entities may be difficult (Faccini, 1970).

organic acids in some target cells with decreased production in others. There may also be changes in membrane permeability, both in cell organelles and in the cell membrane itself. The end results include increased osteoclastic bone resorption and other actions reviewed elsewhere, such as phosphaturia and enhanced renal tubular reabsorption of calcium.

A most interesting unsolved question is why so many patients with parathyroid tumours and excess PTH secretion have little or no evidence of osteitis fibrosa. It has been demonstrated that circulating PTH levels are significantly higher in patients with osteitis fibrosa than in those without clinical or radiological evidence of bone involvement. The former also have much larger tumours and there is good correlation between serum PTH levels and tumour size (O'Riordan, Watson and Woodhead, 1972). It appears therefore, that the development of overt osteitis fibrosa may be a quantitative expression of these increased levels. Why parathyroid tumours should behave in these different ways remains undecided. Current theories include differences in calcium absorption, vitamin-D intake and PTH release; none is completely satisfactory.

Histology

The characteristic histological features of osteitis fibrosa are osteoclastic resorption of bony trabeculae with fibrous replacement of the resulting Howship's lacunae and the adjacent marrow. There is an increase of newly formed trabeculae of bone and in the number of bone surfaces covered by osteoid (fig. 1). In decalcified sections especially, similar changes may be seen in fibrous dysplasia, Paget's disease, at the periphery of an aneurysmal bone cyst or at a fracture site within a solitary bone cyst.

More advanced cases may lead to the production of localized areas of resorption and fibrosis large enough to give a cystic appearance on radiological examination. In other cases, solid masses of soft tissue known as brown tumours may occur. Histologically these are composed of large numbers of osteoclasts in a loose vascular fibrous stroma; another prominent feature is the predilection for the periosteum which is often involved first and most prominently.

All these features are well seen in the jaw where cyst formation, giant-cell lesions, generalized loss of bone substance with fractures, and subperiosteal erosion involving the lamina dura have all led to an eventual diagnosis of primary hyperparathyroidism. The giant-cell lesion of hyperparathyroidism is indistinguishable histologically from the giant-cell granuloma whether central or peripheral. It is therefore imperative in all cases of oral giant-cell lesions in adults to exclude hyperparathyroidism.

Radiology

Subperiosteal erosions of the phalanges and of the terminal digital tufts (fig. 2) are the most characteristic radiological signs. In more advanced cases the same process is seen at the outer end of the clavicle, the medial surface of

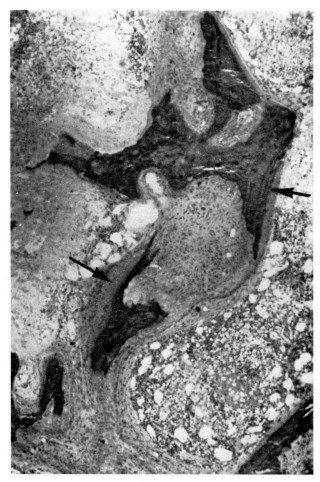

FIG. 1. Osteitis Fibrosa of Hyperparathyroidism. Irregular resorption of calcified trabeculae with fibrous replacement of bone and marrow and osteoid lining bone surfaces (arrows). Haematoxylin and Eosin. × 48.

the neck of the femur, the lower end of the femur and the inner surface of the upper end of the tibia.

Areas of gross loss of bone with fibrosis or brown tumour formation produce a cystic appearance on radiological examination. These cyst-like areas appear most commonly in the jaw and at the ends of long bones and they are usually associated with signs of generalized osteitis fibrosa. Sometimes they occur alone and a radiolucent lesion in the jaw may be the first and only sign of a parathyroid tumour.

Early workers stressed the importance of loss of the lamina dura as a diagnostic sign in primary hyperparathyroidism. More recently, its diagnostic limitations have become apparent. Many patients with hyperparathyroidism are edentulous for the disease is much more common in older people. Even when teeth are present the loss of lamina dura is a non-specific sign for it may disappear in periodontal disease, in osteomalacia and in secondary hyperparathyroidism.

Clinical Features

In all large series of parathyroid tumours renal stones are the commonest manifestation, and overt osteitis fibrosa occurs less frequently. Among the first 300 patients with parathyroid tumours diagnosed and treated at University College Hospital, London, 162 (54·0 per cent) first sought treatment for symptoms of renal stones whereas only 67 (22·3 per cent) had overt osteitis fibrosa. Other patients exhibited mental symptoms, gastrointestinal manifestations, hypertension, pluriglandular syndromes, myopathy or joint pain (see Table 2). It is therefore a mistake to think of obvious bone disease as an essential part of hyperparathyroidism.

TABLE 2

PRIMARY MANIFESTATION OF THE DISEASE IN THE FIRST 300 PATIENTS WITH PARATHYROID TUMOURS DIAGNOSED AND TREATED AT UNIVERSITY COLLEGE HOSPITAL, LONDON

	No. of Patients	%
Renal stones and nephrocalcinosis	162	54
Osteitis fibrosa	67	22·3
Gastrointestinal manifestations	16	5·3
Psychiatric disorders	10	3·3
Symptoms of hypercalcaemia *per se*	9	3
Hypertension	4	1·3
Associated with other endocrine disease	4	1·3
Neonatal hypocalcaemia in the patient's baby	1	0·3
Relative of affected patient	1	0·3
Myopathy	1	0·3
Accidental	25	8·3
	300	

On the other hand, the first manifestation of many parathyroid tumours is still osteitis fibrosa which remains a major feature of hyperparathyroidism, whether primary, secondary or tertiary. It has a predilection for several sites, notably the fingers, ends of long bones, and the jaws.

All degrees of osteitis fibrosa are seen. In the early stages it causes vague aches and pains which may be widespread and are often diagnosed wrongly as rheumatism, myositis, fibrositis, arthritis, neuritis or lumbago. Later, severe bone pain and tenderness occur with gross loss of bone substance leading to fractures and deformities which may have a fatal outcome from mechanical respiratory failure. Bone tenderness is a common finding which often disappears within a day or so after the parathyroid tumour is removed, although many months are required for complete bone healing.

In a series of 67 patients with osteitis fibrosa, 10 had obvious lesions in jaws which was the first feature of the disease to be recognized in many cases. Details of this series are shown in Table 3. It is noteworthy that cyst-like lesions and epulides were about equally common and that evidence of osteitis fibrosa elsewhere in the skeleton was found in only half the cases. Osteitis fibrosa may be localized entirely to the jaw.

Diagnosis

The characteristic clinical, radiological and histological features will usually ensure an accurate diagnosis of osteitis

TABLE 3

INVOLVEMENT OF THE JAW IN PRIMARY HYPERPARATHYROIDISM— 10 CASES TREATED AT UNIVERSITY COLLEGE HOSPITAL, LONDON

Case	Sex	Age	Jaw Lesion	Rest of Skeleton Involved	Plasma Levels Pre-operatively		
					Ca mg./100 ml.	P mg./100 ml.	Alk. Phos. K.A. Units
1	M	43	Cyst-like	—	17·1	2·0	21
2	M	28	Cyst-like	+	15·8	2·4	86
3	F	59	Cyst-like	+	13·0	2·5	30
4	M	67	Epulis	—	10·9	2·4	13
5	M	22	Epulis	+	14·8	2·3	13
6	F	51	Epulis	—	11·3	1·9	6
7	M	60	Epulis	—	11·6	2·2	13
8	F	19	Cyst-like	+	14·8	1·9	19
9	F	52	Epulis	+	12·3	1·5	19
10	F	56	Epulis	—	12·4	2·0	12

fibrosa. Biochemical findings are then essential for distinction between primary, secondary and tertiary hyperparathyroidism. In the diagnosis of hyperparathyroidism without osteitis fibrosa, biochemical findings are of cardinal importance. Patients with parathyroid tumours (primary and tertiary hyperparathyroidism) almost always have hypercalcaemia and the typical biochemical findings (see Table 1) are in contrast to those of secondary hyperparathyroidism, osteomalacia and osteoporosis. Parathyroid hormone assay (now available by a technique of radioimmunoassay) is a valuable further diagnostic aid and the plasma level is almost always raised in patients with parathyroid tumours and osteitis fibrosa. Confident diagnoses can still be made without this assay for the radiological changes of osteitis fibrosa when taken with the other biochemical features are characteristic.

Differential Diagnosis of Hypercalcaemia

The diagnosis of hyperparathyroidism is more difficult when osteitis fibrosa is absent. In such cases, the demonstration of significant hypercalcaemia is a cardinal feature. The other causes of hypercalcaemia are then considered (see Table 4) and there is no substitute at this stage for careful clinical and radiological assessment. Other laboratory procedures then become of value in differential diagnosis (Watson, 1972a, b, c).

Treatment

In primary and tertiary hyperparathyroidism, any medical treatment is a poor substitute for surgical removal of the abnormal parathyroid tissue which will cure the hypercalcaemia and most other effects of the disease. The prognosis is usually good in these cases once the tumours have been removed. Osteitis fibrosa resolves completely and there is usually marked improvement in the other features.

In secondary hyperparathyroidism oral administration of the correct dose of vitamin D will raise the plasma calcium by enhancing calcium absorption and so remove the stimulus to parathyroid hyperplasia. The alkaline phosphatase level falls coincidentally with healing of the osteitis fibrosa.

TABLE 4

CAUSES OF HYPERCALCAEMIA

1. Excessive parathyroid secretion:
   primary and tertiary hyperparathyroidism
2. Excessive administration of vitamin D, or calcium, or both:
   (a) self-medication with vitamin preparations;
   (b) accidental overdosage in treatment of hypocalcaemia or other conditions; and
   (c) milk-alkali syndrome
3. Increased sensitivity to small doses of vitamin D:
   (a) sarcoidosis; and
   (b) perhaps some cases of "idiopathic" hypercalcaemia of infancy
4. Bone diseases:
   (a) secondary carcinoma involving bone;
   (b) multiple myeloma, leukaemia, Hodgkin's disease and other reticuloses involving bone;
   (c) Paget's disease (in periods of increased activity or after immobilization); and
   (d) rarely in osteoporosis due to
       (i) immobilization especially in childhood; and
       (ii) thyrotoxicosis
5. Other causes:
   (a) carcinoma, sarcoma, and reticuloses without bony involvement;
   (b) adrenal insufficiency
       (i) acute following adrenalectomy; and
       (ii) Addison's disease (rarely);
   (c) hypercalcaemic periostitis

DISORDERS OF THE PITUITARY

Pituitary growth hormone affects bone directly by acting on endochondral and periosteal new-bone formation and, indirectly, by its effects on calcium and phosphate transport in the kidney and gut. Studies on pituitary dwarfs and acromegalics have shown that growth hormone increases the absorption of calcium from the gut and its excretion by the kidney; while, in contrast, the renal excretion of phosphate is reduced. The overall effect depends on skeletal maturity.

Hypopituitarism

In children pituitary deficiency leads to dwarfism. It is very rare and in many cases the cause is unknown. The condition is usually not recognized until the second or third year as the body proportions are normal. Bone growth is retarded along with body development and, despite the fact that the epiphyses remain open, bone formation remains defective at the growth cartilage. The effects on the teeth are less severe than those in the bony skeleton and this results in the crowding of normal sized teeth in small jaws. The deciduous teeth are not resorbed and their consequent retention aggravates the crowding. Severe malocclusion develops through a failure of the condylar growth cartilage to contribute to mandibular development.

Hypopituitarism is more common in adults but there are no specific effects on the jaws from pituitary deficiency after skeletal maturation.

Hyperpituitarism

This is due to excessive secretion of growth hormone by pituitary acidophil adenomas. The effects are determined by the age at which the adenoma occurs: in young individuals the result is gigantism; if the epiphyses have closed acromegaly ensues.

Gigantism

The condition is usually diagnosed with the approach of puberty. Initially, growth is symmetrical but subsequently becomes more exaggerated in the peripheral skeleton; acromegalic features, including mandibular prognathism, begin to appear at puberty. The teeth are of normal size and mineralization and consequently are spaced.

Acromegaly

After closure of the epiphyses growth hormone can no longer influence longitudinal growth; it continues to stimulate cell division of chondrocytes in articular cartilage, however, and this may result in arthrosis. Induction of soft-tissue growth and periosteal new bone formation continues and this has an effect on the acral skeleton—the phenomenon which prompted Marie to coin the term acromegaly.

The soft tissues of the face are coarsened and the hands and feet are large. The cranium is thickened and the facial bones expanded. The maxillary and ethmoidal sinuses are dilated and the sella turcica is widened. These are important radiological signs in the diagnosis of acromegaly. Another useful radiological sign is a significant increase in heel-pad thickness. However convincing the clinical and radiological signs may be, the diagnosis is finally established by radioimmunoassay of growth hormone levels in the plasma.

The effects on the jaws are profound and the excessive growth in length and width of the mandible results in characteristic prognathism. The lips and tongue are also hypertrophied and the pressure of the latter on the alveolar ridges enhances the spacing of the teeth.

FIBROUS DYSPLASIA

Fibrous dysplasia is a disease entity affecting one or several bones. It may be associated with metabolic disturbances and, in the past, it was confused with hyperparathyroidism; there is no evidence, however, to connect the two conditions aetiologically although histological features may be similar. It occurs in monostotic or polyostotic forms—the latter when associated with cutaneous pigmentation, endocrine dysfunction and precocious puberty being known as the Albright syndrome.

Clinical Features

In most cases of fibrous dysplasia with jaw involvement the disease is monostotic, the maxilla being affected more often than the mandible. Of 14 cases studied recently, 11 were monostotic and only 2 of these occurred in the mandible.

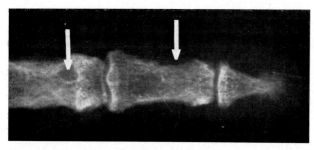

FIG. 2. Radiograph of the phalanges in a patient with osteitis fibrosa. Note the subperiosteal erosions in the phalanges (arrow) and in the terminal tuft of the distal phalanx. There is also a small cyst-like lesion (arrow).

Widespread polyostotic fibrous dysplasia nearly always appears in childhood. In such circumstances, it may lead to unsightly deformities which are usually the first feature recognized. Involvement of the jaws may prevent teeth from erupting.

The radiological appearances range from a distinct radiolucency that has to be differentiated from a cyst to a more typical dense ground-glass appearance (fig. 3). This depends on the amount of osseous tissue present. The margin of the lesion is often ill-defined and, in the maxilla, suture lines may be expanded. The biochemical findings are usually within normal limits.

Pathology

The essential lesion consists of fibrous tissue containing islands and trabeculae of woven bone (fig. 4) and, occasionally, more amorphous calcified material. The cellularity of the fibrous stroma varies.

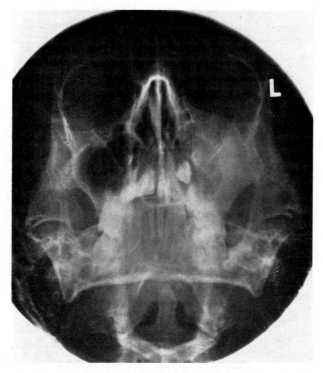

FIG. 3. Radiograph showing fibrous dysplasia of the left maxilla in an eight-year-old boy.

In biopsy material, particularly if the tissue is sparse, the lesion may be difficult to distinguish from early Paget's disease, especially as an increase in cement lines, frequently thought to be pathognomonic of Paget's disease, can be present in fibrous dysplasia. Osteitis fibrosa can be confused histologically with fibrous dysplasia but the biochemical findings are distinctive.

Confusion also arises over the use of the term ossifying fibroma to describe a circumscribed lesion which may not be distinguishable histologically from monostotic fibrous dysplasia. Whether or not an ossifying fibroma is regarded as a focus of fibrous dysplasia, such lesions are usually rapidly growing and require different treatment.

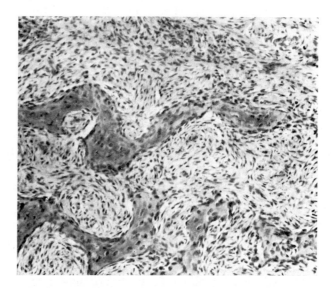

FIG. 4. Fibrous dysplasia. Ramifying trabeculae of newly formed bone in a cellular fibrous matrix. Haematoxylin and Eosin. × 116.

Treatment

Surgery is needed for correcting the deformity caused by fibrous dysplasia, either for aesthetic reasons or to restore function. Because fibrous dysplasia in children tends to slow down or to be arrested with the cessation of skeletal growth, it is usually recommended that surgery be delayed when possible. In the case of localized, rapidly growing lesions of young people, however, operation is frequently called for early in the course of the disease and this can often effect a cure (Williams and Faccini, 1973).

PAGET'S DISEASE

Paget's disease of bone is a common disorder in people over the age of 40 years. Manifestations in the jaws, however, are relatively uncommon and usually occur in association with involvement of the skull.

Clinical Features

Paget's disease occurs most commonly in the vertebral column, particularly the lumbo-sacral region, and in the skull. Progressive involvement of the skull leads to deafness and to changes in the shape and size of the head. Lesions in the jaws can occasionally be the first symptom, especially when maxillary involvement interferes with the function of an upper denture. Pain is often an early symptom and this may occasion a dental consultation. The cardinal biochemical finding is a raised level of plasma alkaline phosphatase. The plasma calcium may also be raised during periods of increased activity or after immobilization (Table 4).

Radiology

The teeth characteristically exhibit hypercementosis; initially there may be rarefaction around the roots sometimes associated with root resorption. This is followed by the more distinctive feature of mottled radiopacity (fig. 5). Eventually, the bone and cementum may become too dense for even high penetration intra- or extra-oral radiographs.

Pathology

Initially, there is an increase in bone turnover with an increased number of osteoclasts and trabeculae lined by plump osteoblasts. Fibrous tissue can replace the marrow and the appearance may be similar to that of hyperparathyroidism. Later the cement lines become more prominent, and the quantity of bone increases producing the special mosaic pattern of Paget's disease of the bone.

Treatment

Until recently there was no effective form of treatment; but during the last few years, enthusiastic claims have been made for the value of calcitonin, mithramycin, glucagon and even the phosphonates. Evidence is accumulating that long-term treatment with calcitonin may relieve the pain, lower the alkaline phosphatase level and even produce radiological improvement. At present this is the treatment of choice.

OSTEOGENESIS IMPERFECTA

Osteogenesis imperfecta constitutes a spectrum of disorders, ranging from the lethal form of the disease—frequently associated with death *in utero* or stillbirth and marked by extreme fragility of bones—to a condition in which cortical bone is simply thinner and more fragile. Blue sclerae, and impaired hearing resulting from otosclerosis, often accompany the disease but are not invariable features. The involvement of the teeth is equally variable, as is exemplified by the paradox of severe disturbances in bone associated with normal teeth and vice versa.

The disorder, which is inherited through an autosomal dominant gene of variable penetrance, is basically due to abnormal collagen resulting in an inadequate bone matrix. There is currently no effective treatment.

Clinical Features

In the form manifested from birth, the survivors are dwarfed and, frequently, have crippling skeletal deformities. In the later onset form, the individual may give a history of having suffered fractures on many occasions. Fractures heal at a normal rate in both forms of the disease but may be associated with exuberant callus formation, especially in the more severe forms.

The oral manifestations consist of thinning of cortical bone in the jaws and defective formation of enamel and dentine. In affected teeth the crown is small, tends to suffer fractures of enamel and to be lost early; the roots are reduced in length and breadth, while the pulp cavities are frequently obliterated (fig. 6).

Few reported cases of osteogenesis imperfecta even mention the teeth but it would appear that there is no clear-cut relationship between the forms of osteogenesis imperfecta and dentinogenesis imperfecta.

Pathology

The structural disturbance in dentine is indistinguishable from the opalescent dentine seen in dentinogenesis imperfecta without bone disease. A puzzling feature is that so severe a mesenchymal disorder, sufficiently generalized to cause excessive joint mobility and a skin translucency as well as the skeletal defects, can sometimes be associated with normal dentine.

In the severe, lethal forms of the disease there is a failure of formation of cortical bone. Biochemical and electron microscopic studies have shown an abnormality of crosslinkage of collagen (Francis, Smith and Macmillan, 1973). In the late-onset type of disease the histological features are normal.

OSTEOPETROSIS

This condition contrasts strikingly with osteogenesis imperfecta, the basic defect being a failure in resorption of the primary spongiosa which, in the lethal variant, eventually occludes the medullary cavity, producing marrow failure. The genetic basis is complicated, but a severe autosomal recessive type and a benign autosomal dominant type can be distinguished.

Clinical Features

Severe Type. Due to the inexorable growth of spongy bone the marrow is gradually obliterated; symptoms are, therefore, mostly related to marrow failure and to compensatory extra-medullary haematopoiesis. If the child survives the effects of marrow failure—a possibility with repeated transfusions—it will suffer pressure effects on cranial nerves and blood vessels with resultant blindness and facial palsy. The bone, furthermore, is subject to osteomyelitis. Radiology reveals dense bone due to a failure in remodelling, there is a gradually increasing diameter of the shaft of long bones, initially in the metaphysis and, eventually, in the diaphysis. The head is usually mis-shapen and radiologically the skull and jaws are dense. There are profound effects on the dentition: the teeth are slow to erupt and are then shed prematurely. Osteomyelitis is a well recognized complication of dental extraction.

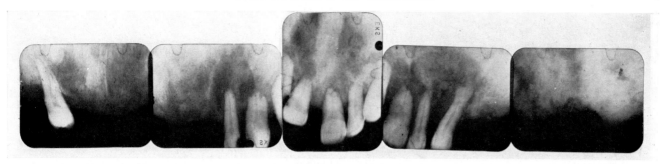

FIG. 5. Intraoral radiographs of maxilla in a case of Paget's disease, showing periapical resorption of roots and bone, as well as hypercementosis and dense opacities in the left molar region.

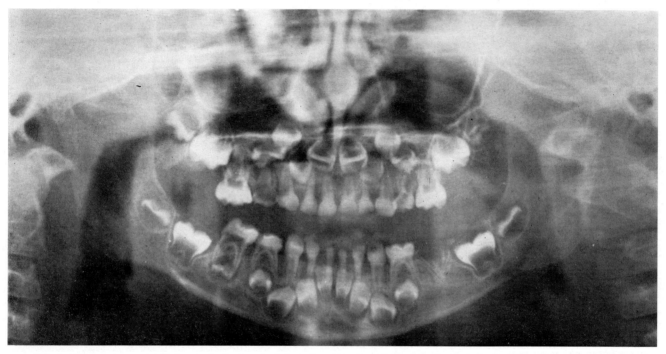

FIG. 6. Orthopantomograph from a case of osteogenesis imperfecta showing thin cortical bone and associated dentinogenesis imperfecta.

Benign Type. This form of osteopetrosis is less common than the recessive severe type. It may be discovered only accidentally on routine radiography as an increased density of the diaphyses of long bones which may also show a lack of remodelling. There is no attendant anaemia and the dental effects consist simply of a delay in eruption.

Pathology

In the severe form of the disease, the defect lies in a failure of the normal resorptive process to keep the shaft hollow and trim the metaphysis into a narrow diaphysis. The medullary cavity consequently becomes filled with a mass of unresorbed bone.

REFERENCES

Albright, F. and Reifenstein, E. C. (1948), *The Parathyroid Glands and Metabolic Bone Disease.* Baltimore: Williams and Wilkins.

Davies, D. R., Dent, C. E. and Watson, L. (1968), "Tertiary Hyperparathyroidism," *Brit. med. J.,* **3,** 395.

Faccini, J. M. (1970), "The Ultrastructure of Parathyroid Glands Removed from Patients with Primary Hyperparathyroidism: a Report of 40 Cases, Including 4 Carcinomata," *J. Path.,* **102,** 189.

Francis, M. J. O., Smith, R. and Macmillan, D. C. (1973), Polymeric Collagen of Skin in Normal Subjects and in Patients with Inherited Connective Tissue Disorders," *Clin. Sci.,* **44,** 429.

O'Riordan, J. H., Watson, L. and Woodhead, J. S. (1972), "Secretion of Parathyroid Hormone in Primary Hyperparathyroidism," *Clin. Endocr.,* **1,** 149.

Steiner, A. L., Goodman, A. D. and Powers, S. R. (1968), "Study of a Kindred with Phaeochromocytomas, Medullary Thyroid Carcinoma, Hyperparathyroidism and Cushing's Disease: Multiple Endocrine Neoplasms, Type 2," *Medicine,* **47,** 371.

Watson, L. (1972a), "Diagnosis and Treatment of Hypercalcaemia," *Brit. med. J.,* **1,** 150.

Watson, L. (1972b), "Hyperparathyroidism—Primary, Secondary and Tertiary," in *Modern Trends in Endocrinology,* **4,** 353 (F. T. G. Prunty and J. Gardiner-Hill, Eds.). London: Butterworths.

Watson, L. (1972c), "Diseases of the Parathyroid Glands," in *Medicine (Endocrine Disease),* p. 148 (R. I. Bayliss and R. Hall, Eds.). London: Medical Education (International) Ltd.

Watson, L. (1973), "Endocrine Bone Disease," *Practitioner,* **210** 376.

Williams, J. Ll. and Faccini, J. M. (1973), "Fibrous Dysplastic Lesions of the Jaws in Nigerians," *Brit. J. Oral Surg.,* **11,** 118.

49. MUSCLE FUNCTION AND THE OCCLUSION OF THE TEETH

D. C. BERRY and R. YEMM

Mandibular rest position

What is "overclosure"?

Some aspects of oral function

MANDIBULAR REST POSITION

Although Magnus was writing in general terms when he stated in 1925 that "every movement starts from and finishes in some posture", the conclusion would have been as apt if he had been discussing jaw movements and mandibular posture. It is but a small step to state that in the understanding of any movement it is fundamental to understand the starting and finishing position. For the lower jaw this is frequently the mandibular rest position. Indeed, one widely used method for clinical assessment of this position is to make measurements on completion of a movement.

The mandibular rest position has been defined as "the postural position of the mandible determined by the resting length of the muscles which elevate or depress the mandible when the person is sitting or standing in an upright position" and also as the position when "the mandibular musculature is in a state of minimal tonic contraction to maintain posture and overcome gravity" (Ramfjord and Ash, 1971). This much has become generally accepted since the time of the first descriptions of the position. However, more consideration is justified, since it is probably the start-line and the finishing-post for mandibular movements. Is mandibular resting posture a constant fixed position as first reported? If not, how and when does it vary and under what influences? If it does change is anything else affected, how much, and does it matter?

It has become clear that, far from being a fixed position, the mandibular resting posture is variable both over short periods and in the long term.

Short-term changes in resting posture can be detected by examination of the relationships between the teeth of the upper and lower jaws. The most obvious and easily demonstrated of these variations occurs with postural changes of the head and body. For instance if, with the trunk erect, the head is tilted forward, the separation of the teeth (freeway space, interocclusal clearance) reduces, and also the mandible moves forward relative to the maxilla. The converse occurs if the head is tilted backwards. This simple observation has some interesting implications for dental prosthetic and oral rehabilitation clinics.

Although it has not been confirmed objectively, the reduced ("negative") air pressure in the oral cavity following a swallow, due to anterior and posterior seals, appears to raise the mandible and reduce the freeway space compared with the state when the intraoral air pressure has equilibrated with the surroundings. The subjective observation that the mouth drops open during sleep could be related, although head posture changes or a reduction of lip activity are other factors. ("Habitual" lip activity to maintain an anterior oral seal might be expected to lift the mandible).

An apparently rapid change in resting-posture accompanies removal of an appliance (*e.g.* a full denture) from the lower jaw in many people. Perhaps related is a similar change occurring when the lower natural dentition is removed.

Longer-term studies of jaw position are obviously difficult to perform, and the teeth cannot be used as fixed reference points. There is evidence, from a study of face heights of a population subdivided into age groups (Tallgren 1957), that systematic changes in mandibular rest position occur with ageing. Tallgren reported an increase in face height and thus presumably an increase in the separation of the mandible and maxilla, of the order of 4 mm. during adult life; this in individuals who retain the natural dentition. Different changes are reported in edentulous patients. The most obvious, and undisputed, change in the resting relationship between mandible and maxilla is that which accompanies skeletal growth. No doubt there are other circumstances in which resting posture changes, but these examples serve to illustrate the type of posture with which we have to deal.

It will be apparent from the preceding paragraphs that, although the mandibular rest position is recognized as being variable, the extent and circumstances of its variability are by no means perfectly understood. Uncertainty also exists with respect to the underlying mechanisms responsible for the position. As a starting-point for consideration of present knowledge, it is worthwhile to discuss the current hypothesis for maintenance of relaxed posture elsewhere in the body. It was held for many years that skeletal or voluntary muscles were active at all times, even when a muscle or muscle group was resting. Thus, even when the arm was hanging freely beside the body, a small but significant number of fibres was thought to be contracting. This state was termed "tonus", and was considered responsible for resting or relaxed posture. The hypothesis was derived initially from the study of decerebrate animals in which, at least in muscles having a supporting or anti-gravity role, this state of affairs exists.

More recently, it has been recognized that skeletal muscles can and do switch-off completely. This applies even to some important "anti-gravity" muscles in the human standing erect, and it has been shown that the mechanical properties of the skeleton, muscles and ligaments are appropriate to permit this. Indeed, it might be a worthwhile feature to incorporate at the design stage, since it would be inefficient to expend muscle energy doing nothing. A mechanical aspect which has been shown to be of importance is elasticity, particularly of muscle, but also of ligaments of which the elastic ligament of the neck is an example.

It has become accepted, therefore, that for many if not all parts of the body complete relaxation can occur, and in these circumstances posture depends on an equilibrium between external forces, such as gravity, and non-active internal forces such as elasticity of related tissues.

It is generally considered that human mandibular resting posture is governed by muscle tone, supporting the jaw against gravity and maintaining the position within close limits. This hypothesis arises first from analogy with that formerly advanced for other parts of the body, and second from studies of the activity of human jaw muscles using electromyographic techniques. However, since the muscle tone theory has been virtually abandoned as far as other parts of the body are concerned, it is reasonable to reappraise its application to the mouth. In this reappraisal there are two questions to be answered.

First, is continuous activity of all or any of the muscles associated with the jaw characteristic of mandibular rest position and, second, what part if any do tissue physical properties such as elasticity play in determining posture?

Many electromyographic (EMG) studies of human jaw muscles have included observations of their electrical activity when the mandible is in the rest position. In general the conclusion has been that, at this position, the muscles exhibit their least activity. However, various findings have been reported, including complete absence of activity, intermittent activity, and continuous low-level activity. None of these findings can be regarded as fully objective because of the inherent limitations of EMG techniques.

Various types of electrode are employed to sample extracellular voltage charges accompanying the action potentials of skeletal muscle fibres. None gives a reliable sample of the activity of a whole muscle. For instance, needle electrodes only sample relatively small volumes, in which probably all activity is detected. Surface and subdermal electrodes sample more widely, often too widely, but it has yet to be proved that they are capable of detecting voltage changes of all the fibres of a muscle.

Whatever the electrode type, the signals available are small. Despite advances in recent years, the amplification required contributes "noise" to the EMG before it can be examined. The noise contains similar frequency components to those of the EMG itself, and this imposes limitations on the ability to distinguish biological components. "Noise" could mask activity, or activity could be interpreted as noise. Either way, the decision becomes essentially subjective.

In addition, some muscle fibres do not produce action potentials in the usual way. These are so-called "slow" fibres which, though common in lower orders, have only been located in a few specialized eye and ear muscles in mammals. If such fibres were present, active muscle tension could exist without detection by EMG techniques. However, the limited evidence available suggests that this type of fibre is not present in the jaw muscles.

Further uncertainties arise from the use of human subjects. Recorded activity may not be essential for maintaining resting posture. Naive subjects should be used, but may be unable to relax fully, because they are unfamiliar with, and slightly worried by, the experimental situation. Environmental stresses have been shown to initiate muscle activity in mandibular elevator muscles. Knowledgeable subjects who understand the objectives of the study may hold the mandible in what they assess to be their rest position; their assessment may be wrong, or activity of both elevator and depressor muscles may be employed unnecessarily to fix the position of the mandible.

It is clear, therefore, that EMG techniques cannot provide an objective answer to the question of involvement of continuous activity of jaw muscles in maintaining the rest position of the mandible, beyond the observation that the activity is minimal. In any case, as a preceding section shows, the mandible is not stabilized in a precisely controlled position by muscle tone.

The role of tissue elastic forces is also uncertain, primarily through lack of investigation. Indirect evidence of the importance of elasticity was obtained in an EMG study in which it was shown that slow closure of the mouth is associated with a reduction of depressor muscle activity until about the rest position, after which elevator muscle activity is necessary to complete the movement. This observation is consistent with the first part of the movement depending upon elastic recoil of the elevator muscles, and the second phase occurring against elastic extension of depressor muscles (fig. 1). More recently, it has been shown that in the rat, elastic properties of the soft tissues of the jaws can produce by themselves a jaw position which corresponds very closely with the rest position.

Perhaps the best working hypothesis for the mechanism underlying mandibular posture is that tissue elastic properties are the primary governing factor, a state of equilibrium between these being the basic rest position of the mandible, and that other factors influence that position from time to time. For instance, changes in head posture, as well as causing changes in the direction of gravitational forces, would result in changes in the length of the depressor muscles and hence in the resultant equilibrium length of the elevator muscles. Removal of teeth, or an appliance, from the lower jaw results in a change in the effect of gravity as well as changes in posture of lips and tongue; either or both of these could influence the equilibrium. It is reasonable also to postulate that gradual changes in tissue elastic properties occur with age or with varying use and function, causing a gradual change in rest position. For instance, it is generally thought that elasticity of tissue diminishes with age. Similarly, muscle utilization may increase or decrease with resultant parallel effects on the muscle tissue, such as hypertrophy with increased usage, which may influence the passive properties of the muscles concerned. The establishment of a rest position at an early age and its subsequent maintenance during growth would, on the tissue elasticity hypothesis, be dependent upon there being a relationship

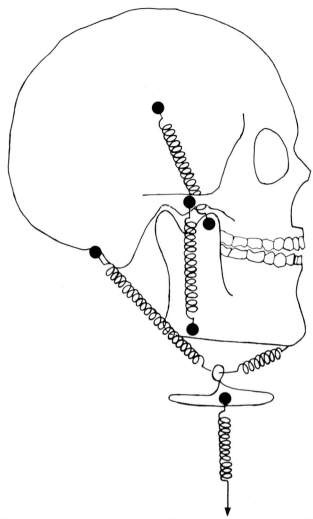

FIG. 1. A diagram to show the mandibular rest position as an equilibrium position depending upon the elastic properties of muscles. The diagram does not represent all the jaw muscles, but demonstrates that a change in tension in any muscle, or any change in an outside influence, such as gravity, will necessitate an adjustment of the equilibrium.

between growth rates of skeletal and soft tissues. Such a relationship clearly exists.

This concept of mandibular rest position as being an inbuilt property of the system of bone and soft tissues suggests that the rest position may be the keystone for occlusion. The teeth may fit themselves into the available vertical space, rather than the vertical space be adjusted by continuous muscle activity to suit the teeth.

WHAT IS "OVERCLOSURE"?

This question commonly arises in one of two possible situations:

(a) the full denture wearer;
(b) the fully or partially dentate subject who is considered to need some form of "occlusal rehabilitation".

In both situations, it is necessary to compare the difference in total face height between the rest position of the mandible and its position when the teeth occlude. This difference, the freeway space or inter-occlusal clearance,

is itself subject to variation: first, because of the several factors which can cause changes in the rest position of the mandible itself, and second, because it is apparent that differences of the order of 0·5 cm. in the size of the freeway space are common between individuals. It has been suggested that there is a relationship between the size of the free-way space and the type of occlusion present, but this has not yet been proved.

The clinical problem, in both (a) and (b) above, is therefore one of estimating the size of the freeway space in any individual, and comparing this estimation with another, which is a guess based on experience, at the size of the free-way space considered to be correct for that individual. It is not surprising that the answer is sometimes wrong.

Before looking at the difficulties of the clinical problem in greater detail, it is necessary to consider how the constancy of facial heights is maintained—if indeed it is.

The important facts can be found mainly in two publications—Tallgren (1957), Murphy (1959)—and they are these:

(a) on a natural diet, attrition occurs rapidly;
(b) compensatory mechanisms exist to reduce resulting changes in occluding facial height. These are eruption, and alveolar bone growth. These compensatory mechanisms are built-in to the individual and as far as is known are not controllable by external factors; and
(c) it would seem that the two dynamic processes, the attrition and the compensatory mechanisms, should be in balance. However, the rate of attrition is mainly controlled by diet. Thus, any process, such as civilization, which renders the diet less abrasive or more refined, reduces attrition. Very abrasive diets, such as in some Aborigines and Eskimos, increase attrition. In either case the balance is upset.

Other factors which are important in varying the rate of attrition, although probably not as important as diet, are the muscle activity used in chewing, and the presence of bruxism or clenching.

The muscle activity used in normal chewing is a variable factor, but in general can be expected to follow the general physique and is also affected by age: a secondary result is the limitation of diet as age increases because of the inability to chew it. Clearly, the presence of "stress-induced" muscle activity can not only be a factor in directly opposing eruption and alveolar growth, but can cause loss of tooth substance by attrition. It can therefore be postulated, on theoretical grounds, that in Man the masticatory system has a built-in mechanism for maintaining the occluding height at a constant level, and at the same time protecting the teeth from the harmful effects of wear, as long as the food eaten and the use made of teeth ensure that the rate of attrition is precisely correct. It is, of course, a characteristic of biological systems that constant stability is unlikely. Usually such systems tend to function by means of sensitive feedback mechanisms, around rather than exactly on a mean level. This characteristic need not upset the concept that, under ideal conditions, wear and tear on the masticatory system does not reduce its efficiency. Indeed, wear may be essential to provide this efficiency.

Under circumstances where the diet is abrasive, and muscle activity high, attrition may be increased so that the rate of loss of tooth substance is greater than the increase in facial height provided by the factors of eruption and alveolar growth. As Murphy (1959) has shown, this situation can obtain in Aborigines, and the result is that the total occluding face height decreases with age, rather more so in males than in females. It can therefore be said that in this situation overclosure exists. The assessment of the extent of the overclosure must, for the present, remain as before, a matter of hopeful guesswork.

In civilized countries, it is not usual to find that the diet is abrasive. Certainly it is possible to find individuals with gross attrition, but these have either adopted an abrasive diet because they are vegans, or have a dietary predilection for one type of abrasive food, such as nuts, or have very high levels of stress-induced muscle activity. They may request treatment because their "teeth are wearing away". Although no work can be found which gives any guide to the comparability of these people to the Aborigines with respect to the balance of the equation, it is unlikely that they could have such a high rate of attrition, in spite of their peculiar dietary habits or level of stress. The supposition that overclosure must exist simply because of considerable loss of tooth substance must therefore be

any permanent form of restoration of lost tooth substance be attempted.

The opposite situation with respect to occlusal wear is more commonly found in Western civilization. The diet is one in which refined foods predominate, and attrition is minimal. The teeth usually have long clinical crowns and steep cusps. According to what has been said, it should therefore be expected that eruption and alveolar growth should combine to produce an increase in total occluding face height with age as long as the natural teeth are present. This theory is supported by the findings of many investigators. It is curious that, in spite of this, it is not usually taught that occluding face height increases with age, and the probable reason for this is that the rate of increase is slow, amounting to about 4 mm. over the whole of adult life, and that today the average individual loses his teeth in middle age before the normal increase in occluding face height becomes of any great clinical significance. As Tallgren has pointed out, an interesting point in connection with this steady increase in occluding face height is that the freeway space remains extraordinarily constant at between 2–3 mm. (fig. 2). It might be concluded that, if the freeway space remains constant although the total occluding facial height increases, no degree of "open-bite" can exist.

There are, of course, several factors to consider. As well

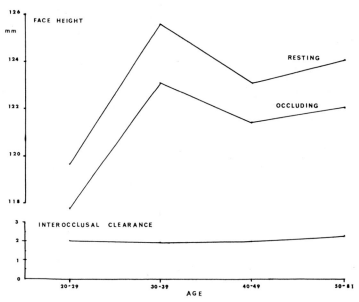

Fig. 2. Re-drawn from Tallgren (1957). It will be noted that during adult life the increase in both resting and occluding facial heights is of the order of 4·0 mm., while the interocclusal clearance remains remarkably constant at about 2·0 mm.

resisted. It should certainly be tested by the short-term use of a simple acrylic overlay appliance. If no overclosure exists, it is unlikely that the appliance will be tolerated. From what has been said previously about muscle activity it is clear that tooth loading may be excessive because the freeway space can be reduced by the appliance. If vanity overcomes discomfort, the risk is that the appliance will cause intrusion of the natural teeth until the former freeway space is restored. Only if the appliance is easily tolerated, with no muscle discomfort after several weeks of use, should

as attrition being reduced by the refined diet, muscle activity is also low—chewing is largely unnecessary. It could be suggested that the occlusal load might increase because the teeth have increased in height by eruption and alveolar growth, and in such circumstances the freeway space could be reduced. That this does not occur to any significant extent may be due to balancing changes in both the factors involved in increasing occluding facial height and in those tending to decrease it.

The clinical problem can now be examined in the light of

the foregoing considerations. Although these are somewhat theoretical, there is little scientific work on this subject other than that already mentioned.

In the full denture wearer overclosure may arise in three ways:

(a) the estimation of the correct vertical dimension may be wrong when the dentures are made and an excessive freeway space provided;

(b) alveolar resorption, particularly if the dentures are some years old, will reduce the vertical dimension; and

(c) attrition of the teeth, particularly if these are the comparatively soft acrylic variety, will also cause loss of occluding facial height.

In all these cases the freeway space will be increased, for there are no compensatory mechanisms to maintain it at a fairly constant level, and overclosure is therefore present. An additional check can be obtained by inspecting the occlusion of the dentures. It is usually possible to relate the dentures to each other, out of the mouth, in the position in which they were set up. If, when the dentures are returned to the mouth, this position is more retruded than any that can be achieved, then overclosure is probably present. The reason for this is that, as alveolar resorption and wear of the teeth proceed, the mandible must rotate further upwards in order to bring the teeth together. In doing so, because the axis of rotation is near the condyles, an inevitable forward component of the upward movement is necessary. In the case where the teeth are porcelain, this attempt to produce occlusion may involve "jumping-the-bite" because the teeth are too hard to allow the incisal wear necesary for gradual accommodation to overclosure. If this does happen, there may also be some degree of real rather than apparent forward movement of the mandible.

Even though there may be little doubt that overclosure is present, it is not usually wise to correct this in every case. Old people who have become accustomed to an overclosed occluding position are often happier as they are. Only if the overclosure is causing dissatisfaction with appearance—and even here caution should be exercised—or mandibular dysfunction pain, should correction be attempted. In spite of the former view that overclosure is commonly associated with facial pain (the so-called Costen's syndrome), this association will be found rarely in full denture wearers. It is more common to find that muscle pain is related to a long period of wearing dentures of too great a vertical dimension. But it is certainly true that muscle pain is much less common in full denture wearers than in dentate subjects. It might be thought that the diagnosis of overclosure is more simple in denture wearers than in patients with natural dentitions: this is not so. The average human is an adaptable creature, and the masticatory system can tolerate variations in total face height to a surprising degree. There are certainly some individuals whose masticatory systems are much less tolerant and in these the occluding height must be correct to within 2–3 mm. whether wearing full dentures or possessed of a natural dentition. Such people are fortunately not common. If they were, many of the restorative procedures which involve increasing the occluding face height would fail at the outset. That they do succeed at all is more usually

due to the gradual re-establishment of the original occluding face height by the intrusion of the natural teeth. This cannot occur in full denture wearers, but it is surprising how rapidly accelerated resorption beneath a lower denture can occur if the vertical dimension is too great. A further factor which is relevant to full denture wearers is appearance. Much discomfort due to an excessive vertical dimension will be tolerated if the appearance is approved of.

It is indeed this very quality of tolerance which makes the diagnosis of overclosure in full denture wearers often difficult. Rarely does overclosure, unless gross, noticeably reduce the efficiency of dentures, for on modern diets a high level of efficiency is not required. It also seems that the masticatory system can adjust itself to maintain some degree of constancy of the freeway space, for in many cases of gross overclosure it is clinically obvious that, in function, a freeway space of usual dimensions exists. In such a case, it is possible that two basic mandibular positions are used; the true resting position, and an habitual resting position from which chewing movements begin and at which they end. If this is indeed so, then a re-programming of the muscle activity concerned must be continually taking place. "The rest face height adapts itself to alterations in the morphologic face height" (Tallgren 1966).

The remaining situation in which overclosure may occur is in the partially edentulous who do not wear dentures. In some cases, although a few teeth may be retained, there may be no remaining occlusal contact or stop. The situation here is similar to that seen in the completely edentulous subject who does not wear dentures. When no occlusal stop remains, there is usually a slight but gradual reduction in total face height. To consider whether overclosure exists seems irrelevant, for anything resembling a functional dental occlusal level is impossible.

However, if in the hypothetical case of the partially edentulous but non-denture wearing subject occlusal stops do exist, as may happen if the upper and lower anterior teeth are retained, much depends on the stability of the remaining occlusion. If the load on the teeth is such that because they are few in number they are moved, either by intrusion or by proclination, then the occluding face height will change, the freeway space will theoretically increase, and of course overclosure will be present. But, and this is important, Tallgren has shown that the rest face height may adapt to this re-arrangement. The total face height is reduced but the freeway space remains the same. At this stage, the insertion of dentures made to the correct occluding height will initiate a change in the total face height back to its original value, the freeway space still remaining the same. Perhaps this confusing state of affairs has been best summed-up by Tallgren (1966): "The rest position of the mandible, due to its inconstancy . . . constitutes an unreliable reference for assessment of the occlusal vertical dimension." Unfortunately there is no other reference, as yet, which can be used quickly and easily at the chair-side.

SOME ASPECTS OF ORAL FUNCTION

Of the many functions of the mouth, chewing has received the most attention, probably because it is in this activity that the teeth as specialized structures are most involved. In swallowing and speech, the teeth play a secondary role to functions which primarily concern the muscles of the region. (See also Chapter 50.)

In chewing, co-ordination of muscle activity results in movements of the jaws to use the teeth to cut, grind and crush food placed in the mouth. The movements are complex. Cinephotography has shown that even in a single subject successive chewing cycles are different, varying both in the amount of opening and also in the path taken by the mandible (Ahlgren 1966). Some of this variation is probably due to the changing nature of the food as it is reduced. However, even with a material of fairly constant properties such as chewing gum, the chewing strokes differ. In addition, most subjects periodically change the side of chewing. Even greater differences in the pattern of jaw movement are seen when different subjects are compared.

The relationship between the upper and lower teeth during a chewing stroke is uncertain. For incision, with an unworn occlusion used for modern diets, the lower jaw is protruded to enable the incisors to function as cutting edges, and when tooth contact is approached the lower incisors are positioned to slide up the palatal surface of the upper incisors so providing a shearing action similar to the action of scissors. When incising some foods, it seems unlikely that this last phase is necessary or indeed that it occurs.

In chewing between premolar and molar teeth it has been shown that the lower teeth approach the opposing teeth eccentrically, the closing phase generally taking place with the mandible deviated towards the working side. This is achieved by a forward movement of the condyle of the temporomandibular joint on the side opposite to that occupied by the food bolus. The last part of the chewing stroke involves not only the final closure, but also a sliding movement between the upper and lower teeth, brought about by a return of the contralateral condyle to a more retruded position. This produces a grinding motion between the opposed occlusal surfaces. The occurrence of tooth contact in this process is difficult to study because contact may take place anywhere on the occlusal surfaces, which makes tooth contact monitoring difficult or impossible. Indeed, this final phase of closing may be directed by anterior tooth contact, for instance between upper and lower canines. While some reports contend that tooth contact rarely if ever occurs, others state that contact is the usual termination of the chewing stroke. Until more perfect methods of testing are devised, the truth must remain in doubt, but it seems fairly clear that centric occlusion, with maximum interdigitation of the cusps of upper and lower teeth, does not occur in each chewing cycle. In any case, the recorded observations of tooth contact were of modern dentitions, relatively unworn by present-day diets. The effects of more "natural" diets on wear of teeth, and hence upon their occlusal shapes must be considered as well. Tooth contact at the end of a chewing stroke, between single or only a few cusps, may be in a sense unphysiological.

The muscle activity involved in chewing is complex. Not only are there many muscles which participate, but also the distribution of activity varies between the different muscles.

Using EMG techniques to study muscle activity, the picture which emerges is essentially one of co-ordinated reciprocal activity of the elevator or jaw-closing muscles and the depressor or jaw-opening muscles. Careful study of the individual muscles has revealed some characteristic patterns. For instance, activity in the medial pterygoid muscle during the closing phase usually starts before that in the masseter or temporal muscles. As might be expected from the cinephotographic results, differences are seen between successive cycles. An important muscle is the lateral pterygoid, which contributes to opening of the mouth, to protrusion, and to the lateral movement of the mandible during chewing between the molar teeth. Activity is not limited to the muscles of the working side; the contralateral muscles are also active, though sometimes to differing extents.

The jaw-closing muscles are capable of exerting extremely large forces, and under some circumstances such forces arise in chewing and could cause damage unless applied in a controlled manner. At times, sudden changes occur during the closing phase of a chewing cycle. For example, the teeth may suddenly encounter a resistant object in otherwise soft material, or conversely a hard object may suddenly fracture. In the first instance, the sudden arrest of movement could cause a rapid and damaging rise in local force; in the second, sudden movement might result in harmfully forceful tooth-to-tooth contact. The fact that damage rarely occurs under circumstances such as these may be due to reflex changes in the activity of the muscles. Two distinct reflexes have been demonstrated in human subjects which may provide a measure of protection. It has been shown that when a hard object is encountered, the closing movement is very rapidly arrested, and is followed by opening of the mouth. The response may be initiated by a sudden increase in the firing rate of mechanoreceptors in the periodontal ligament. A reflex opening response has been demonstrated in decerebrate and lightly anaesthetized animals which has been attributed to these receptors. In the animal response there is an active participation of the depressor muscles, which has not so far been demonstrated in the conscious human, either to tooth stimulation or to stimulation of mucous membrane. In the latter case, noxious stimuli appear only to result in a brief inhibition of the elevator muscles.

In the second situation, where sudden fracture of brittle food material occurs while under pressure between the teeth, there is a reflex response which will at least contribute to the arrest of movement. Very rapidly after release of the load, inhibition of the jaw-closing muscles takes place, followed by an increase in the activity of a jaw-opening muscle, the digastric. It seems likely that this response is due to the muscle spindles of the closing muscles. The rate of firing of these receptors would be expected to decrease as soon as the jaw started to close as unloading takes place, which would reduce the drive to the elevator muscles and perhaps also reduce inhibition of the depressors.

Control of the chewing process itself is much more complex. For some years it has been generally held that the cyclic movements arise from reflexes. Jaw closing was said to occur because the mouth-open position stretches and stimulates muscle spindles in elevator muscles. The impulses from the spindle receptors then initiate elevator muscle activity; this is the so-called stretch reflex. Activity thus stimulated continues until tooth contact occurs. At this point stimulation of periodontal mechanoreceptors inhibits closing activity and initiates opening. According to the reflex hypothesis, the cycle then repeats. Such a mechanism may account for oscillations of the mandible seen in decerebrate preparations, where reflexes are much more sensitive because of the loss of controlling influences from higher centres, but it seems unlikely that it can account for the complexity of movement seen in the conscious human, or indeed in any other animal.

Partly as a result of this reflex-based hypothesis, much interest has centred upon muscle response to tooth stimulation in the human. The foregoing hypothesis would predict that a jaw-opening reflex would result. However, even forceful mechanical stimulation does not activate depressor muscles. The only response reported is a brief inactivation of elevator muscles, lasting about 15 msec., seen as a silent period on the EMG if the stimulus is applied during a period of elevator muscle activity. Furthermore, there is a possibility that this response is at least partly due to receptors other than those of the periodontal ligament.

The existence of nervous pathways implicated in the chewing process by the reflex hypothesis has been amply demonstrated by animal experiments. However, it must be concluded that, even though the reflex pathways exist, they are not capable of maintaining a cyclic movement without a major input from elsewhere in the nervous system.

The objections to the simple reflex hypothesis may be summarized:

(a) inability to initiate appropriate movements by experimental stimulation in the intact conscious animal;

(b) the complexity of the natural movements is difficult to explain by such a simple system of automatic responses;

(c) the jaw-closing muscles are active for an appreciable time after forces build up between the teeth, when reflex excitation from muscle-spindle stretch is reduced, and when reflex inhibition from periodontal receptors should be high; and

(d) the natural chewing cycle is too slow to be accounted for by the rapid reflex responses demonstrated in animal experiments.

A more recent alternative to the reflex hypothesis is the proposal that movements depend upon a central oscillator. Such a mechanism is proposed also for other cyclic or rhythmic body movements.

According to this hypothesis the basic open and close sequence is governed from the central nervous system. Sensory inputs, from teeth, oral mucous membrane, muscles and joints influence the precise form of the movement by feeding back through the reflex pathways. In support of the central oscillator hypothesis, it has been shown that stimulation of some regions of the brain initiates cyclic jaw movements even when many, if not all, the sensory pathways from the mouth have been destroyed and hence the supposed reflex system for maintained cycling disabled.

A mechanism of this type for chewing provides a more acceptable explanation for the observed complexity and overall voluntary nature of the process. The role of sensory input and reflex arcs becomes that of one means of modifying basic movements to changing local conditions, and perhaps providing safety mechanisms or overload protection. For instance, information from periodontal ligament receptors during initial chewing of hard, resistant material may limit the build-up of force or initiate opening earlier than is normal. Some of the deficiencies of chewing by wearers of full dentures may be due to the abnormality of a part of the normal sensory information, despite the fact that the chewing process is basically unchanged.

Although bruxism and subconscious clenching are not usually regarded as normal functions, in both cases the teeth are involved in forceful contact through muscle activity. Bruxism, or nocturnal tooth grinding, does not appear to be a consequence of activity limited to the oral muscles, since it occurs during periods of light sleep in association with movements of the whole body. It may also be associated with periods of dreaming. It has often been stated that a trigger to bruxism is the presence of premature or irregular tooth contacts. While this may be so, it is at least as reasonable to consider that the discovery of these contacts, through pain or attrition of the affected teeth, or through muscle pain when the contact is made, is a consequence of bruxism. If forceful, unconscious jaw movements take place, unusual tooth contacts may arise. Although treatment applied to the affected teeth, to diminish loading or to remove restrictions on jaw movement, may be successful in alleviating the symptoms, this does not prove that tooth contacts are the initiating factor.

The association of bruxism with other body activity suggests a central rather than local origin. Certainly there is no evidence that stimulation of periodontal mechanoreceptors can cause prolonged activity of elevator muscles to produce the protracted and forceful closing forces associated with bruxism. Stress in everyday life has been suggested as an aetiological factor in bruxism, and this is in general agreement with the observation that at times of stress, sleep may be difficult to achieve.

Stress may also be a factor in relation to protracted clenching of the teeth. Experiments have shown that stress can cause increased activity in many muscles, including the jaw-closing muscles. Equivalent and compensating activity is unlikely to occur in depressor muscles, if only because of the size difference. Prolonged muscle activity and clenching of the teeth, arising in this manner, may be a factor in initiating some clinical conditions such as disorders of the muscles themselves. It has been shown that voluntary clenching can lead to muscle pains and that some patients with muscle pain exhibit an exaggerated muscle response to experimental stress. In addition, the opinion is sometimes expressed that clenching contributes to periodontal breakdown in some patients and there is experimental evidence that some denture patients suffering from protracted soreness under their dentures may be abnormally susceptible to clenching when under stress.

REFERENCES

Ahlgren, J. (1966), "The Mechanism of Mastication," *Acta odont. scand.*, **24**, suppl. 44, 1.

Beyron, H. (1964), "Occlusal Relations and Mastication in Australian Aborigines," *Acta odont. scand.*, **22**, 597.

Magnus, R. (1925), "Animal Posture," *Proc. roy. Soc., B.,* **98**, 339.

Murphy, T. (1959), "Compensatory Mechanisms in Facial Height Adjustments to Functional Tooth Attrition," *Aust. Dent. J.,* **4**, 312.

Ramfjord, S. P. and Ash, M. M. (1971), *Occlusion*, 2nd edition, p. 12. Philadelphia: W. B. Saunders.

Tallgren, A. (1957), "Changes in Adult Face Height Due to Ageing, Wear and Loss of Teeth and Prosthetic Treatment," *Acta. odont. scand.*, **15**, suppl. 24.

Tallgren, A. (1966), "The Reduction in Face Height of Edentulous and Partially Edentulous Subjects During Long-term Denture Wear," *Acta. odont. scand.,* **24**, 195–239.

50. THE MANDIBULAR JOINT:

DEVELOPMENT, STRUCTURE AND FUNCTION

H. J. J. BLACKWOOD

Development

Postnatal growth

Structure of the adult joint

  The mandibular condyle
  Temporal bone
  Articular disc
  Joint capsule and ligaments
  Blood supply
  Innervation
  Articular remodelling

Function

INTRODUCTION

In man and in mammals the mandibular joints comprise the articulation between the condyles of the mandible and the squamous portion of the temporal bones. From an evolutional standpoint, this articulation is regarded as the secondary jaw joint having developed in the mammal-like reptiles to replace the primary or reptilian type of joint which existed between the posterior end of Meckel's cartilage (articulare) and the quadrate. With the emergence of the mammals the primary joint became incorporated in the middle ear and persists as the malleoincal joint thus serving the function of hearing. Reflecting this evolutional change, the mandibular or secondary jaw joints develop somewhat later in embryonic life than the joints of the primary skeleton. In the mammalian embryo, however, these phylogenetic events are recapitulated in the development of this region.

DEVELOPMENT

The mandibular joint develops in the condensation of mesenchyme cells separating the developing squamous portion of the temporal bone from the condylar cartilage which forms on the dorsal surface of the developing mandibular ramus. In man, intra-membranous ossification commences in the squama of the temporal bones in the 30 mm. CR embryo and differentiation of the cartilage of the mandibular condyle takes place about the 50 mm. CR stage of development. Growth of the condylar cartilage brings the mandible into close relationship with the temporal bone and in the 55–65 mm. CR fetus the upper and lower joint cavities make their appearance as two slit-like spaces in the intervening mesenchyme. The development of the joint cavities serves to delineate the future articular disc which at this stage is seen to be continuous ventrally with the developing lateral pterygoid muscle and dorsally with the perichondrium covering Meckel's cartilage. The relationship of the disc to the lateral pterygoid muscle and Meckel's cartilage at this stage of development has prompted the view that the medial portion of the disc may be developed from the tendon of the lateral pterygoid muscle.

From this stage onwards there is rapid growth of the condylar cartilage which forms a cone-shaped mass tapering anteriorly where it is surrounded by the developing membrane bone of the mandibular ramus (fig. 1). The anterior extremity of the cartilage extends as far as the crypt of the second deciduous molar, and posteriorly (where it forms the articular surface of the condyle) it is covered by a cellular perichondrium. This perichondrium is in continuity with the adjacent periosteum. Subsequently, the anterior portion of the cartilage is invaded by vascular mesenchyme and replaced by endochondral bone formation, but the posterior part persists in cartilage forming the mandibular condyle. Growth of the cartilage continues by apposition from the covering perichondrium and replacement of the deep surface by endochondral bone formation. In the 130 mm. CR human fetus vascular canals can be seen to form within the cartilage and constitute a regular feature of the growing cartilage up to the second or third year of life. The blood vessels within the canals originate in the medullary cavity of the condyle and form a fine vascular plexus close to the articular surface of the cartilage. Vascularization of the cartilage at this stage may facilitate its rapid growth.

Posteriorly, the developing mandibular joint is in open

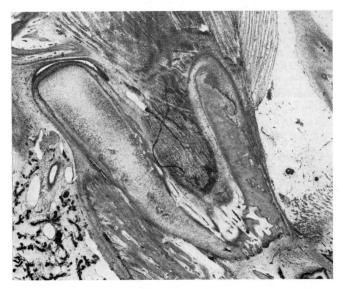

FIG. 1. Section of the condylar cartilage and developing mandibular joint in a human fetus at approximately 12 weeks intra-uterine life. Haematoxylin and eosin × 19.

continuity with Meckel's cartilage and the structures of the middle ear. This communication between the joint and the middle ear persists until the 270–300 mm. CR stage when the growth of the squamo-tympanic fissure effectively separates the two structures. The joint capsule develops by condensation of the surrounding mesenchyme and is usually well demarcated in the 180 mm. CR fetus.

POSTNATAL GROWTH

After birth, there is very rapid growth of all components of the joint. The mandibular condyle grows by endo-chondral ossification and within the cartilage three distinct cell zones can be distinguished, namely the articular, proliferative and hypertrophic zones (fig. 2). As its name implies, the surface articular zone provides the articular covering of the condyle and consists of dense fibrous tissue in which the collagen fibres are arranged mainly parallel to the articular surface. Beneath this the cells of the proliferative zone are small and closely packed and by their mitotic activity provide the main growth centre of the condyle. The cells of this zone differentiate to become the chondroblasts and chondrocytes of the hypertrophic zone. Within the hypertrophic zone, the cells first secrete the cartilage matrix and then undergo hypertrophy; the cartilage matrix mineralizes and is ultimately resorbed and replaced by endochondral bone formation.

The process of cell renewal and growth within the cartilage has been studied by many investigators in a variety of animals using tritium labelled thymidine (Blackwood, 1966a). These studies indicate that the main growth activity of the cartilage is confined to the proliferative zone and renewal of the cells of the articular zone would appear to take place independently probably in response to wear o the articular surface. The histochemical reactions of the cartilage (Greenspan and Blackwood, 1966) and the metabolic activity as measured by uptake of S^{35}-sulphate and

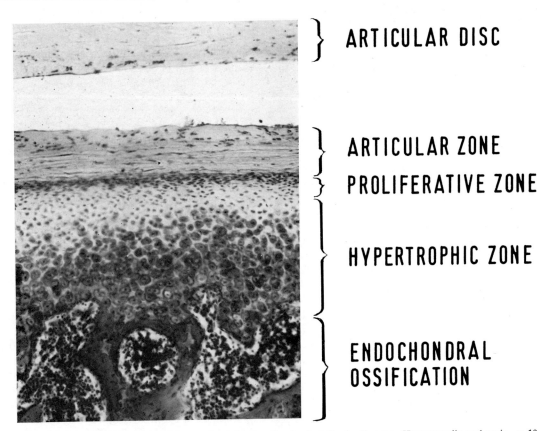

} ARTICULAR DISC

} ARTICULAR ZONE
} PROLIFERATIVE ZONE

} HYPERTROPHIC ZONE

} ENDOCHONDRAL OSSIFICATION

FIG. 2. Section of the growing condylar cartilage showing the clearly defined cell zones. Haematoxylin and eosin × 100.

H³-glycine have tended to confirm the functional aspects of the component zones of the cartilage.

Controversy exists as to whether the condylar cartilage acts as a primary growth centre, somewhat similar in function to the epiphyseal plate of a long bone, in promoting the downward and forward growth of the mandible, or whether growth of the cartilage is purely adaptive to maintaining the relationship of the condyle to the articular fossa and temporal bone. It may well be that within this controversy the two elements of mandibular growth are being confused, namely the contribution by the cartilage to growth in height of the mandibular ramus and growth of the body of the mandible which is entirely in membrane bone. The facial deformity resulting from unilateral hyperplasia of the

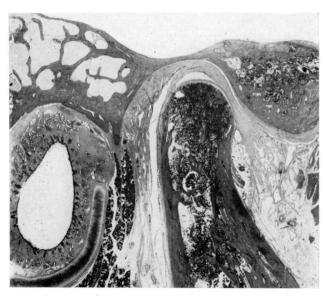

FIG. 3. Sagittal section through the mandibular joint of a young adult showing the relationship of the joint to the external auditory meatus and parotid gland posteriorly and to the middle cranial fossa superiorly. Haematoxylin and eosin. × 3

mandibular condyle is evidence of considerable growth-potential in the condylar cartilage and where agenesis of the condyles occurs the body of the mandible can still be seen to develop to a considerable extent. However, it must be acknowledged that an element of adaptive growth is essential and this property is inherent in the human mandibular condyle throughout life (Blackwood, 1966b).

At birth the articular surface of the temporal component of the mandibular joint is flat and angulated slightly laterally. The articular disc is closely adapted to both surfaces of the joint and maintains the congruity between this flattened surface and the convexity of the condylar cartilage. The adult contour of the temporal surface of the joint, that is the marked convexity of the articular eminence and concavity of the articular fossa, is not fully achieved until the permanent dentition has erupted. This is brought about mainly by apposition of bone in the region of the articular eminence and some resorption of bone in the area of the articular fossa. During this stage of growth, the articular disc also assumes its characteristic biconcave form and the fibres within the disc become more definitely orientated.

STRUCTURE OF THE ADULT JOINT

The Mandibular Condyle

The adult mandibular condyle is roughly elliptical, the largest diameter being medio-lateral and the shortest antero-posterior (fig. 3). The articular surface, as in the growing condyle, is covered by fibrous tissue. On the posterior aspect of the condyle this covering is thin and is applied directly to the sub-articular bone. Over the convexity of the condyle, the articular covering is much thicker and here there is a layer of fibro-cartilage between the surface fibrous articular layer and the sub-articular bone (fig. 4). The proliferative zone appears as a thin line of cells along the line of junction between the fibro-cartilage and the articular layer. In older joints the proliferative zone may not be very distinct but the cells of this zone are capable of proliferative activity at any time throughout life and play an important part in the remodelling and repair of the articular surfaces (Blackwood, 1966b). In microradiographic examination of the articular surface of the mandibular condyle mineralization can be seen to extend from the sub-articular bone to a varying depth into the adjacent fibro-cartilage. In the normal joint the mineralization front is smooth (fig. 5) but it may become irregular in the aged or osteoarthritic joint.

Temporal Bone

The articular surface of the temporal bone comprises the concavity of the articular (glenoid) fossa posteriorly and anteriorly the convexity of the articular eminence. The articular surface extends from the anterior margin of the squamo-tympanic fissure to the tubercle of the articular eminence, and is bounded medially by the suture between the squamous portion of the temporal bone and the great wing of the sphenoid. The bone of the articular fossa is normally very thin and this part of the joint surface is lined by a thin layer of fibrous tissue (fig. 6). Anteriorly, the covering of the articular eminence is much thicker, and there is a layer of fibro-cartilage between the surface fibrous articular zone and the bone; as in the condyle a less well-defined proliferative zone of cells can be distinguished between these two layers (fig. 7). The slope of the articular eminence shows wide individual variation and is subject to change during life especially in association with disease of the joint.

Articular Disc

The articular disc or meniscus consists of dense fibrous tissue and is roughly elliptical with a thin central area and thickened anterior and posterior margins. Posteriorly the disc splits into an upper lamina, which is attached to the margin of the squamo-tympanic tissue, and a lower lamina which blends with the periosteum of the posterior surface of the neck of the condyle. This posterior attachment of the disc is sometimes referred to as the retro-discal pad and it contains elastic and fatty tissues and numerous large vascular spaces. Anteriorly the disc is attached to the anterior

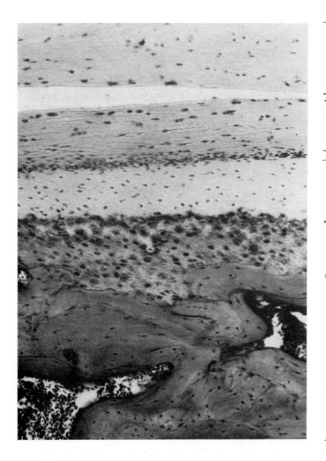

ARTICULAR DISC

ARTICULAR ZONE
PROLIFERATIVE ZONE
FIBRO-CARTILAGINOUS ZONE

CALCIFIED CARTILAGE

SUB-ARTICULAR BONE

FIG. 4. Section of the articular covering of the adult mandibular condyle showing the arrangement of the cell layers. Haematoxylin and eosin. × 100.

edge of the articular eminence above and to the articular margin of the condyle below. Some fibres of the lateral pterygoid muscle are inserted into the anterior and medial edges of the disc and during movement the disc tends to follow the mandibular condyle.

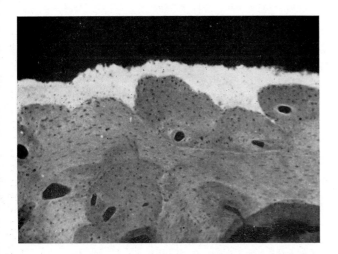

FIG. 5. Microradiograph showing the subarticular bone and minerali-zation of the adjacent fibrocartilaginous layer. (Blackwood, *J. dent. Res.* **45**, 1966.)

Joint Capsule and Ligaments

Anteriorly and posteriorly the joint capsule is thin, but medially and laterally it is strengthened by the capsular ligaments. The lateral ligament is especially strong and is termed the temporo-mandibular ligament. The spheno-mandibular and stylo-mandibular ligaments are sometimes referred to as accessory ligaments of the mandibular joint, but it is doubtful whether they have much influence on mandibular movement. The synovial lining of the joint may form synovial folds or villi in the fornices of the joint and these are probably responsible for the control of synovial fluid.

Blood Supply

The main arterial supply to the joint is the internal max-illary artery through its deep auricular branch. The ptery-goid plexus of veins is in close relationship to the medial aspect of the joint. There is a rich vascular plexus in the capsule and particularly in the posterior attachment of the articular disc but the central part of the disc is avascular.

Innervation

The nerve supply to the mandibular joint is from the mandibular division of the trigeminal nerve through its auriculo-temporal branch. Only free nerve endings have

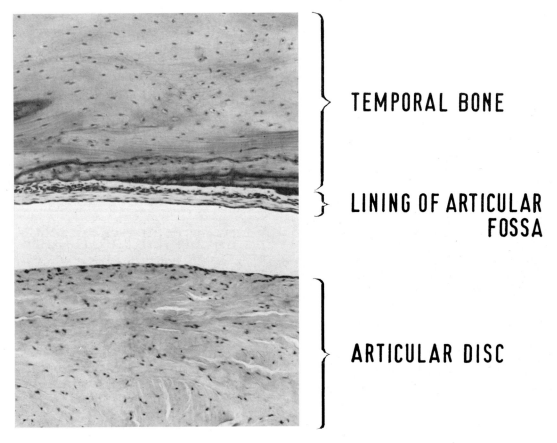

FIG. 6. Section through the temporal bone showing the very thin lining of the articular surface of the glenoid (articular) fossa. Haematoxylin and eosin. × 100.

been described in the joint capsule and periphery of the articular disc but the central part of the disc is not innervated.

Articular Remodelling

Remodelling of articular surfaces of joints takes place continuously throughout life and such remodelling activity has been described in the human mandibular joints (Blackwood, 1966b). Three types of remodelling take place; progressive remodelling in which there is addition of tissue to the joint surface thereby increasing the vertical dimension of the articular surface; regressive remodelling in which tissue is removed resulting in decrease in the vertical dimension of the articular surface; and peripheral remodelling which results in the addition of tissue to the margins of the articular surface such as may be found in lipping or osteophyte formation. The changes are thought to compensate for the changing relationship of the jaws which may result from occlusal wear or through loss of teeth; in fact, the extent of remodelling has been shown to have a direct correlation with the number of missing teeth. Remodelling of the articular surfaces has also been demonstrated in experimental animals in response to alteration of the vertical and antero-posterior relationships of the jaws.

FUNCTION

The movements of the mandible comprise depression and elevation (as in opening and closing movements of the jaw), side to side (or lateral) movements, and protrusion and retrusion. (See also Chapter 49).

Jaw opening from the position of centric occlusion is initiated by contraction of the lateral pterygoid muscles which cause rotation and a slight translatory movement of the condyles forward in the lower joint compartment. With further opening, movement is transferred to the upper joint compartment and the condyles together with the disc slide downward and forward on the articular eminence. This movement is effected by the continued contraction of the lateral pterygoids, mainly the superior fibres of the muscle, and the co-ordinated relaxation of the masseter, temporalis and medial pterygoid muscles, and contraction of the anterior belly of the digastric and supra-hyoid muscles. In extended opening the condyle and disc move on to the convexity of the articular eminence but there is considerable individual variation in the extent to which this forward translation of the condyle takes place. On closing the jaw, the condyles and disc are returned to the articular fossa by the contraction of the masseter, temporalis and medial pterygoid muscles with relaxation of the lateral pterygoids.

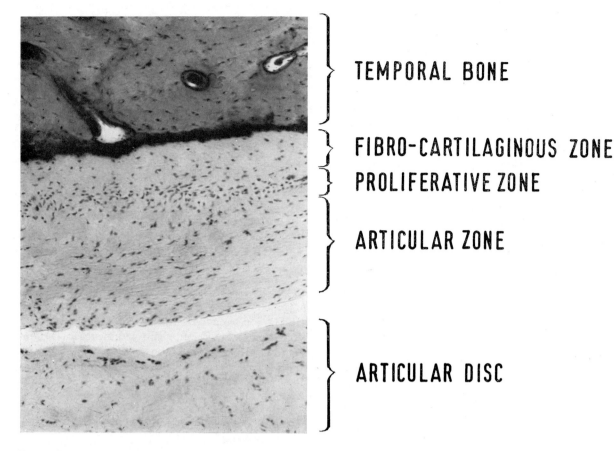

TEMPORAL BONE

FIBRO-CARTILAGINOUS ZONE
PROLIFERATIVE ZONE

ARTICULAR ZONE

ARTICULAR DISC

FIG. 7. Section through the articular eminence in the adult mandibular joint showing the relatively thick articular covering of this area of the joint. H. and E. × 100.

The disc at all times follows the movement of the condyle and its return path with the condyle may be aided by the elastic tissue present in the loose posterior or retro-discal attachment.

During rotational or side-to-side movements the condyle on the side to which the jaw is moving is held in the articular fossa by the contraction of the muscles on that side, while on the other side the condyle is drawn forward on to the articular eminence by contraction of the lateral and medial pterygoids of that side. If the jaw is moved in the opposite direction the position of the condyles within the joint is reversed.

The mandible may also be protruded and retruded. For protrusion, both condyles are moved forward on the articular eminence by contraction of the medial and lateral pterygoids while the mandible is supported by the tonic contraction of the masseter and temporalis muscles. In the retruded position the condyle is drawn backward in the

articular fossa by the contraction of the horizontal fibres of the temporalis muscle.

The movements of the condyle of the mandible within the joint during mastication, deglutition and speech are a complex of those outlined above. It is doubtful if the ligaments associated with the joint, namely the capsular ligaments, sphenomandibular and stylomandibular ligaments have much influence other than in the extreme limits of movement of the joint.

REFERENCES

Blackwood, H. J. J. (1966a), "Growth of the Mandibular Condyle of the Rat Studied with Tritiated Thymidine", *Arch. Oral Biol.*, **11**, 493.

Blackwood, H. J. J. (1966b), "Cellular Remodelling in Articular Tissue", *J. dent. Res.*, suppl. 3, **45**, 480.

Greenspan, J. S. and Blackwood, H. J. J. (1966), "Histochemical Studies of Chondrocyte Function in the Cartilage of the Mandibular Condyle of the Rat", *J. Anat. (Lond.)*, **100**, 615.

51. THE MANDIBULAR PAIN-DYSFUNCTION SYNDROME

P. A. TOLLER

Clinical features

Investigations
  Opaque arthrography
  Ultramicroscopy of the condyle
    Normal
    Abnormal

Treatment

Lubrication of the joint

Hypothesis
  Clicking
  Locking
  Resolution
  Degeneration

The commonest complaint affecting the temporo-mandibular joint involves a set of symptoms which include clicking of the joint, periodic inability to open the jaw (locking), and pain associated with the joint or its musculature. Schwartz (1959) summarized current observations on the condition and applied the descriptive term pain-dysfunction syndrome (PDS) and this has gained wide acceptance, although Laskin's term myofascial pain-dysfunction (MPD) is also frequently used. There is little agreement as to the precise cause of all the symptoms and in these circumstances a variety of empirical treatments has grown up, based upon what is found to benefit the patients and ameliorate their symptoms. Greene's (1973) nationwide questionnaire revealed wide divergency of opinion as to cause and treatment throughout the United States by practitioners, specialists and teachers.

A scientific approach to the problem should preferably include a study of all relevant facts and a search for new facts, an hypothesis to account for the observations, and a treatment policy the success of which would tend to confirm the correctness or not of the assumed underlying principles.

CLINICAL FEATURES

PDS is a world-wide problem encountered more frequently in countries and communities with advanced social systems, which may in itself suggest a relationship with neurotic tension. Boering (1966) contributed an excellent clinical analysis of the occurrence of PDS and his findings are generally supported by a study of 1,435 cases by the present author. The syndrome is predominantly experienced by women: reports from 10 different authors in various parts of the world revealed remarkable consistency in the sex ratio of those afflicted by PDS, a mean ratio from these reports being very nearly F:M = 3:1.

In patients with PDS little or no abnormality is to be seen on radiographs of the joint; earlier reports of backward displacement of the condyle in centric occlusion have been discounted by many clinicians, and the use of radiography in the diagnosis of this condition is tending to lapse as its results are rarely of much use. PDS is not statistically related to other rheumatic diseases. It is rarely related to a history of direct extrinsic trauma, neither is it related to a history of juvenile dental irregularities nor their correction by orthodontic procedures. Studies have shown that a sudden condylar displacement due to surgery or trauma does not alone lead to PDS, and this has been confirmed in many patients following partial resection of the mandible for malignancies; the contralateral joint which remained did not develop the symptoms of pain-dysfunction syndrome or arthritis.

Many experienced clinicians have the impression that the syndrome has a relationship with neurosis, discontent, or tension-producing situations. A wide survey of professional opinions in the U.S.A. with regard to the nature and causes of PDS revealed that a large majority had concluded that emotional stress was the main contributing cause of the condition. Bruxism is not uncommon, and it is likely that about 40 per cent of all sufferers are given to nocturnal bite-grinding habits.

It has frequently been stated that a freeway space of 4 mm. is too large and can be productive of joint symptoms. In fact, a freeway space of as much as 4 mm. is uncommon in PDS cases, neither is the symptom particularly common in full denture patients where the freeway spaces have become larger than 4 mm. With advancing age there is a tendency towards loss of teeth, increased dental irregularity and increased freeway space, but after the age of about 30 years there are fewer complaints about the temporomandibular joint.

Boering found that unilateral tooth loss seems to be significant in the production of temporomandibular joint symptoms, and that joint disturbances are most common on the side with the better dental articulation, which is the side of preference in chewing. However, Franks (1967) reached the opposite conclusion; namely, that the dysfunction occurred more frequently on the side with the greater tooth loss, and consequently on the side opposite to that of preferential chewing. But in spite of such seemingly conflicting evidence there is no doubt that unilateral dental irregularity (63 per cent) is common, and unilateral tooth loss (66 per cent) still more common in cases of PDS. The largest group of all PDS patients have 3–4 missing dental units, but as the number of missing teeth increases beyond six so the incidence of pain-dysfunction syndrome decreases, and it is difficult to establish a tight statistical relationship between tooth loss and prevalence of PDS.

It has commonly been stated that PDS is most frequently seen in young unmarried females, but this is not supported by the facts. The mean age of presentation is about 30 years, and although the ratio is F:M = 3:1, a recent analysis of 1,000 consecutive cases revealed that there was a ratio of married to unmarried women of nearly 2:1.

Although PDS is not of rheumatic character the sex ratio is very similar to that of most rheumatic diseases. It is also similar to the sex ratio of patients attending psychiatric clinics for the treatment of neurosis.

The prevalence of symptoms of clicking, locking and pain have been studied in a group of 1,000 cases with the following results:

Age at First Manifestation	Predominant Joint Symptoms		
	Clicking	Locking	Pain
15–25 years	75%	40%	31%
26–39 years	49%	48%	51%
40–65 years	27%	50%	90%

This revealed that in the younger age group, the predominant symptom was clicking; in the middle age group, symptoms of clicking, locking and pain were equally distributed; and in the age group of over 40 years the predominant symptom was pain. This may suggest a difference in the character of the condition relative to age.

Boering has found that at least one of the main symptoms of clicking, locking, or pain in the temporomandibular joint has been experienced by approximately one-fifth of the general population by the age of 30 years.

Joint stiffness, locking and pain are much more frequent in the morning; patients often report having awoken one morning with a stiff jaw and with pain related to the joint. Often by mid-morning the range of movement has become more normal, and then clicking may recur.

Prolonged histories of clicking joint are more likely to be followed by an acute episode of locking and pain; the locking takes place at the point in the range of movement where clicking used to occur. Patients often tolerate clicking, but they are intolerant of locking and pain which causes them to seek advice.

RESULTS OF SPECIAL INVESTIGATIONS

The technique of electromyography has been used experimentally by a number of workers; but the practical contributions of these studies to the clinical aspects of PDS are strangely deficient, and electromyography has never developed into a widely-used diagnostic tool. However, the results certainly confirm that there is neuro-muscular involvement in this syndrome, and the technique has sometimes been able to show which muscles exhibit abnormality of activity during periods of discomfort in the joint. It is, of course, possible that the main muscle hyperactivities occur during periods other than those during which the symptoms are experienced by the patient, namely hyperactivity during sleep or during eating or grinding habits. However, it is to be hoped that further investigations along this line will soon be productive of data that are of clinical value.

Opaque Arthrography

Locking, intermittent or continuous inability to open the jaw fully, is often associated with failure of full forward sliding of the meniscus in the upper joint compartment, and substantial demonstration of the failure of free forward sliding of the meniscus is given by opaque arthrographic examinations. An arthrogram from a case of periodic locking is demonstrated in fig. 1 where the absence of the

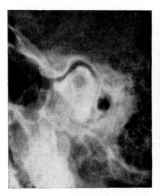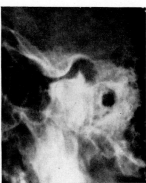

FIG. 1. Opaque arthrogram of lower joint cavity in a case of periodic locking of left temporomandibular joint. From the normal closed position (L) the condyle cannot move in front of the eminentia on attempted jaw opening (R), and a sharp tension deformity develops at the meniscal reflexion of the posterior synovial sulcus.

normal change in the shapes of the opaque-filled lower synovial sulci demonstrates a small early shift forward of the disc coincident with rotation movement of the condyle on the under-surface of the disc, but failure of that disc to slide fully down and forward over the eminentia articularis, with tension deformity of the posterior synovial attachment. The contralateral side shows the typical normal forward glide of the disc (fig. 2).

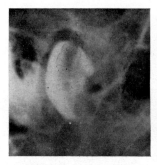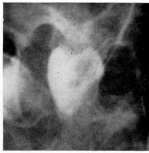

FIG. 2. Normal lower cavity opaque arthrograms. Closed position (L) and with the jaw open (R) showing typical change in shape of the lower synovial cavity.

In another case in which the lower compartment was filled with radio-opaque medium the strong forward pressure produced tenting of both margins of the lower synovial edges in the attempt to urge the disc forward (fig. 3).

In other cases of simple clicking the upper cavity arthrograms taken first in the closed position, then just at the point of click, and then after the click had taken place all demonstrate the hesitation of the meniscal glide at a similar point in its excursion (fig. 4).

Strong forward pressure in another case at this point of locking produced distortion of the meniscal shadow in the upper joint cavity (fig. 5), but this forward pressure failed to unlock the condition.

Application of local analgesia to the nerve supply of the joint, in the course of arthrographies, often relieved the condition of locking and allowed patients temporarily to open widely. This strongly supports the assumption that a neuromuscular mechanism is concerned with the condition.

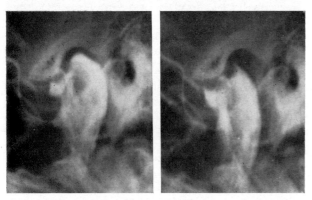

FIG. 3. Opaque arthrogram of lower joint cavity in a case of prolonged locking of the jaw. Fairly normal in closed position (L), but both anterior and posterior synovial edges drawn into tents as the meniscus fails to slide forward (R), as the condyle endeavours to come forward.

When an aqueous radio-opaque solution was introduced into either the upper or lower joint cavities in the absence of local analgesia, it was unusual for the symptoms of locking or clicking immediately to be influenced. This suggested that the lubricating effect of the synovial fluid, which must be diluted and its volume increased by such an action, plays little or no part in the condition. It is known that the efficiency of lubrication of a hyaline-surfaced joint is strangely independent of the viscosity of the lubricating (synovial) fluid, but that the sliding efficiency rests more in the integrity of the cartilaginous surface itself, and this is likely to be true also of the fibrous-surface temporomandibular joint.

Ultra-microscopy of Normal Human Condyle Surfaces

Operations for conservative surgical procedures on the joints of patients who failed to respond to all previous treatments (Toller 1974a) have provided opportunities for taking fresh specimens for examination by transmission electron micrography. A number of normal specimens from fresh cadavers provided a background against which biopsies from the PDS cases could be compared.

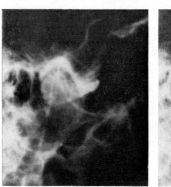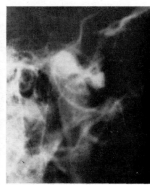

FIG. 5. Upper cavity arthrograms in a patient with intermittent locking at the point of clicking. (L) Normal sigmoid shape of upper cavity arthrogram in the jaw-closed position. (R) The slightly distorted meniscal shadow in this attempted open position corresponds with sticking of the disc and its failure to advance along the eminentia to eliminate the anterior synovial sulcus.

Ultra-microscopy reveals the basic structure of the articular surface of the condyle to be composed of a dense meshwork of bundles of collagen fibrils interspersed with fibrocytes. The wavy interlacing of collagen forms an extremely tough wear-resisting structure.

At the extreme articular surface the collagen structure ends rather abruptly (fig. 6). Between the collagen and the synovial cavity there is a narrow zone of a faintly fibrillar material which is more electron-dense than the underlying ground substance. This smooth-surfaced zone varies from between 1 and 3 microns in thickness and it probably corresponds with the lamina splendens as described in other

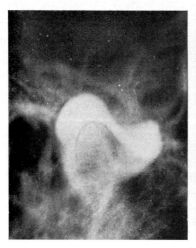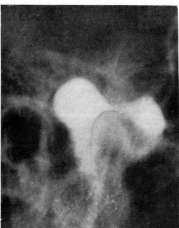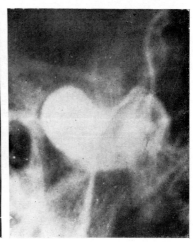

FIG. 4. Upper cavity arthrograms in a case of clicking joint. (a) Closed position appears normal. (b) Position of click with hesitation of condyle and meniscus. (c) Jaw-open position after clicking.

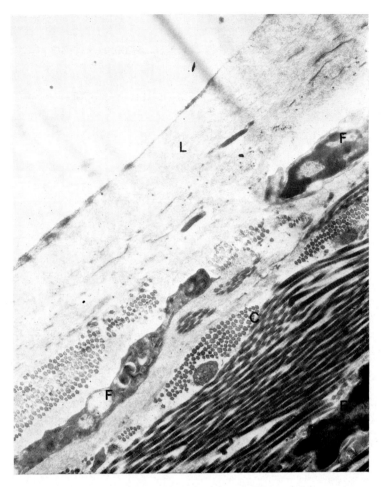

FIG. 6. Electron-micrograph of normal human mandibular condyle articular surface. The flat faintly fibrillar extreme surface (lamina splendens) zone of 3 μ thick (L) overlies interlacing bundles of collagen (C). Sections of three fibroblasts (F) may be seen. × 12,000.

joints (Weiss and Mirow, 1972). The articular surface of this zone is smooth, while its undersurface follows the undulations of the main collagen structure and seems to effect a smoothing-out of any irregularities of the main architecture which may correspond to the presence of large collagen bundles.

The fibrocytes near this articular surface have much reduced cytoplasm and few intracellular organelles, but their nuclei are large and intact, and the cells seem to retain their integrity right up to within a few microns of the articular surface. In the non-load-bearing surface of the condyles, the collagen structure is less dense, the amorphous layer broader, and the cells have more cytoplasm with correspondingly more intra-cellular organelles.

Abnormal Condyles

Departures from this normal pattern were seen in the specimens of condyles from patients with known histories of pain and dysfunction.

An early change was the irregular loss of the lamina splendens, and the development of unevenness of the extreme surface (fig. 7). Some underlying collagen bundles were exposed at the articular surface and there appeared to be some amorphous patches between the bundles.

The next stage was the total loss of all the amorphous layer (fig. 8), and at the same time the most superficial collagen masses consisted only of small-diameter fibrils. This layer of small-diameter collagen was about 2 microns thick and loss of the amorphous layer always corresponded with diminution in the diameter of the superficial collagen population. Total loss of the normal amorphous layer exposed a minutely irregular surface of fine collagen fibrils to the articulation, while directly beneath lay the collagen structure of normal composition.

In the non-load bearing areas of the "abnormal" condyles the amorphous zone was lost and the entire surface structure was loose (fig. 9), with diminution of collagen fibril size, loss of collagen itself, and many fibrocytes tenuously supported by surrounding matrix. The fibrocytes near the first stage abnormal surface showed a great increase of cytoplasmic vacuoles and intracellular inclusions of unnatural variety. There was loss of density and quantity of nuclear chromatin in the most superficial fibrocytes and massive vacuolization of their cytoplasm, distortion of

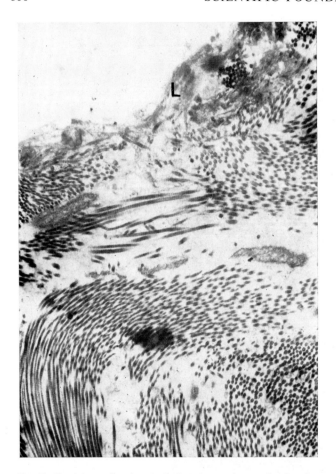

FIG. 7. Condylar surface in pain-dysfunction syndrome, showing disruption of surface lamina splendens zone (L) over a normal collagenous architecture. × 6,500.

their mitochondria and gross enlargement of the cisternae of their cytoplasmic reticulum. These features suggest abnormal activity followed by cell death.

Specimens from patients with severe and prolonged histories of joint disability displayed more obvious disorganization at the articular surface (fig. 10). The surfaces were irregular with accumulations of structureless material interspersed with haphazard orientation of fine collagen fibrils (which lay in a manner suggestive of denaturation and dissolution of their ground substance). The superficial cells had lost their cytoplasm, their position represented by degenerate nuclei, which were the last cytological features to lose integrity. In the surrounding disorganized mass were many remnants of cytoplasmic disintegration. This altered articular layer could extend deeply into the collagen matrix, recognizable elements of normal collagen being almost obliterated by structureless material.

The agency responsible for the alteration of the interfibrillar ground substance and the collagen seems to act from the direction of the synovial cavity; this suggests either mechanical stress at the articular surface or a chemically mediated factor acting via the synovial fluid. Excessive cell death might liberate lysosomal enzymes sufficient to bring about such changes.

RESPONSE TO VARIOUS FORMS OF TREATMENT

An unselected group of 100 patients of all ages presenting with PDS, were given no active treatment other than reassurance and advice with regard to relaxed jaw movements, and three months afterwards could be classified as:

	Cured	Improved	Not Improved or Worse
A similar group of patients was treated by reassurance and advice and this group also received some alteration of their natural occlusion by cuspal adjustment, and similar procedures. At the end of three months they were assessed as follows:	59%	23% (82%)	18%
	39%	37% (76%)	24%
Cobin (1969) published the results of his own conservative treatments as follows:	71%	12% (83%)	17%

Since the criteria of individual clinical assessors vary, and quantification of clinical impressions is notoriously difficult, it may be better to combine those who show improvement or cure (i.e. those who are satisfied and need no further clinical attention). The patients who fail to show improvement are clearly distinguishable from the rest. When recorded in this way, it is noticeable that in all three groups the percentages of patients showing cure or improvement are rather similar, and that there seems to be a failure of primary conservative treatment in nearly one-fifth of all cases.

When considering this rather crude assessment it should be remembered that the cases showing only improvement, and those failing to improve at all, receive further active treatment by different physical methods such as biting splints. A satisfactory method of showing results of different types of treatment and which allows for successive types of treatment according to various previous diagnoses is that displayed by Thomson (1971) where the results of simple conservative treatments are first shown, successively followed by results of more elaborate therapies applied to those in the original groups whose response to earlier treatments had been inadequate.

Conservative and reversible treatment should be employed before irreversible treatments, which include permanent alterations to the occlusion. Primary reversible treatments include reassurance, training in relaxed jaw movements, thermotherapy, anti-anxiety drugs and biting appliances. Failure to respond adequately or permanently to such conservative methods may necessitate adjustment of the natural occlusion.

It is likely that sub-clinical abnormalities in the joint

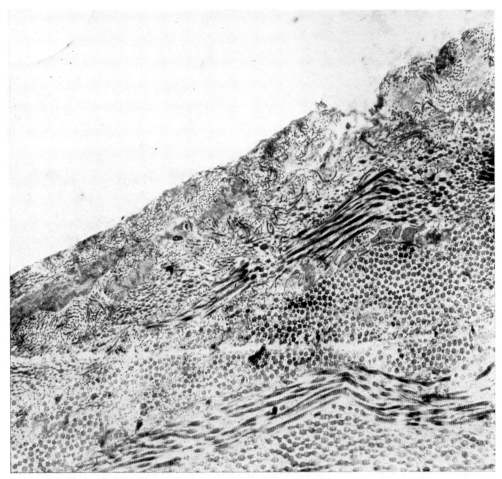

FIG. 8 Articular surface in pain-dysfunction syndrome showing loss of normal surface layer and the appearance of small diameter collagen at the surface, intermixed with some amorphous matter. × 12,000.

might be brought to a clinical level of awareness by alterations of neurotic threshold due to anxieties. In such cases it is not easy, and may not be possible, to submerge the symptoms to their previous level by symptomatic treatment and it becomes important to treat the anxiety or neurotic element as well as the symptoms (concurrently with any physical factors which may be discovered), in order to reduce the likelihood of relapse.

After preliminary consultations and reassurances it is often wise to apply a removable upper biting appliance, as it assists in revealing abnormal cuspal contacts when the act of occlusion is inspected after wearing the appliance. Soft wax, slightly adhesive on one side so that it sticks to one set of teeth, can be used with soft tapping closures of the teeth to reveal premature dental contacts and allow them to be adjusted by grinding and polishing. In this manner the patient's own jaw is used in place of any external articulating mechanism.

The upper acrylic biting splint is usually retained by Adam's cribs to the first molar teeth, and is made so that all the lower teeth can contact its bite plane (total occlusive splint), the thickness of this plane being made less than the freeway space. The wearing of such a splint during day-time is inconvenient and socially unacceptable for most persons, but when worn at night it is usually readily tolerated.

Greene (1973) has shown interesting results from the use of three types of splints in the treatment of patients with PDS. One group (71 cases) was treated with the application of an entirely non-occlusive splint fitting only over the soft tissues of the palate having no direct effect on the dental occlusion, and 40 per cent of these cases showed a positive response to the wearing of such an appliance. In another group treated with splints which only covered the anterior teeth and which disoccluded the posteriors, there was a positive response in 50 per cent of the cases. The third type of splint provided full occlusal coverage for the upper teeth, and the response in these cases was positive in 80 per cent.

It is difficult to know how the bite splint works but a number of conjectures are possible; for instance, the bite plane may simply free interlocking cusps and remove the effects of simple reflex nerve impulses derived from isolated premature contacts. Many clinicians find it wise progressively to thin down the posterior bite plane of the appliance after it has been worn for a few weeks, the effect being to depress the anterior lower teeth away from the hard bite on the back of the upper front teeth. This enables the mandible to adjust very slightly forward in occlusion, and allows natural easement of the intra-articular relationship and pressures.

Since it is generally observed that PDS symptoms are

more severe in the morning, it may be that damaging muscle activity takes place during the preceding night during sleep. In such cases, a bite splint worn at night may not only prevent injurious proprioceptive impulses due to certain interlocking cusps or premature cuspal contacts, but the plate may in fact be so gross an intrusion into the natural condition that it has the effect of simply preventing the working of a subconscious muscular habit, possibly by the establishment of an absurdly different one.

that the full occlusal biting splint is a valuable means of treatment for resistant cases of PDS, particularly for those who have not shown early response to reassurance and to the correction of more obvious irregularities of the occlusion.

LUBRICATION OF THE JOINT

Consideration of these clinical and experimental observations has prompted questions concerning factors that may cause the apparent intermittent failure of sliding movement

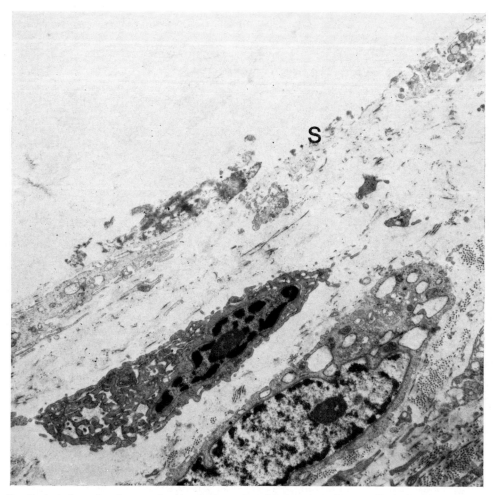

FIG. 9. Articular surface from non-load bearing area of condyle from case of severe pain-dysfunction syndrome showing loose architecture with loss of fibroblast integrity toward surface (S). × 7,500.

Certainly the early-morning locking syndrome is common, and the locking tends to disappear by mid-morning, only to reappear on waking the following day. It is possible that during sleep the condyle establishes a close-packed position in the glenoid fossa which would not favour the circulation of synovial fluid required for normal metabolism of articular tissue, and the factors which encourage or allow free sliding movement of the articular components might thus be diminished. An occlusive biting appliance may prevent the final establishment of centric occlusion during sleep and so prevent the condylar and meniscal articular surfaces from becoming so congruent and pressed together that free sliding is impaired (Toller, 1961).

Whatever the precise means of action, there is no doubt

of the meniscus. It seems natural to ponder over whether there can be a significant rise in articular friction.

It has been suggested that the change in shape of the flexible meniscus from the closed to the open positions of the jaw may alter the properties which govern the low-friction qualities of the joint, especially during the early phases of movement in the upper joint cavity. It seems likely that under certain conditions of loading the upper joint surfaces could become too congruous at some point, as, for example, if the flexibility of the disc allows its initial upper convexity to be transformed into a concavity during normal sliding motion over the eminentia articularis, at which point the cohesion between the surfaces could rise sharply.

The low-friction properties of joints are largely a function of the chemico-physical nature of the sliding surfaces and the interposed fluid film (boundary lubrication), and hydrodynamic lubrication by the fluid film probably plays only a secondary role. The physical condition related to this phenomenon might be likened to the difficulty of sliding two plane glass surfaces over one another even in the presence of abundant lubrication between them; if loads across them are excessive they begin to stick. The prevention of sticking of such congruous surfaces can be achieved by altering the

ties in the nature of the sliding articular surfaces of condyles observed by electronmicroscopy have been mentioned, and have been interpreted as alterations of both the collagen matrix and the interfibrillar ground substance. These ultramicroscopically altered articular surfaces are extremely likely to exhibit marked departures from normal low-friction qualities. It is not difficult to visualize intermittent or prolonged sticking between two such surfaces in sliding contact, especially under conditions of abnormal muscular

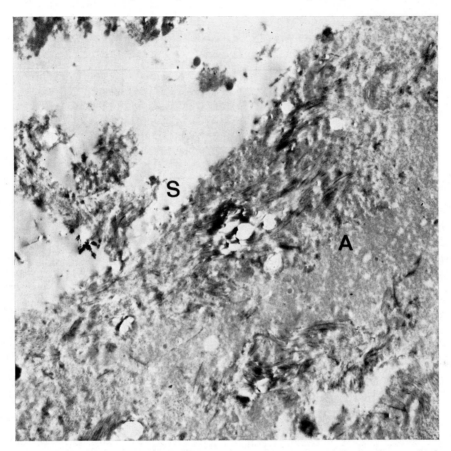

FIG. 10. Condylar articular surface (S) from a patient with a prolonged history (five years) of painful dysfunction. The collagen matrix is being replaced by a mass of amorphous material (A) and appears to be breaking up. × 7,500.

nature of the fluid between them, not merely by increasing its viscosity but by altering its chemical nature so that one part of the molecule of the lubricating fluid has an affinity for each sliding surface. By virtue of such an affinity, a monomolecular film adheres to the surface and so absorbs any free molecular activity of the surface which would otherwise be available to attract molecules on the opposite sliding surface, and so sliding takes place within this interface. Such a boundary lubricant is specific for the particular substances comprising the sliding planes. Thus water or even glycerine is a bad lubricant for two glass surfaces but a watery solution of oleic acid is a good one.

Should repeated excessive loading of the temporomandibular joint give rise to changes in the physical nature of the sliding surfaces, any resultant variations in frictional qualities would become clinically important. Abnormali-

loading. Indeed, persistent movement under such conditions would be likely to bring about their disintegration, unless the excessive loading were relieved. It would seem possible that articular erosion and signs of osteoarthrosis could arise in severe and unrelieved cases of pain-dysfunction syndrome.

HYPOTHESIS

From these findings, the following hypothesis can be constructed of a possible sequence of events leading to pain-dysfunction syndrome:

Clicking Joint

Repetitive muscular overloading of the joint surfaces occurs. (This may be due to dental inadequacies or irregularities, or to neuro-muscular habits, or to a combination of such factors leading to lack of harmonious muscle action in jaw movements).

Frictional hesitations of movement of the meniscus arise.

The meniscus sticks early in the range of movement, but as jaw opening continues the meniscus suddenly recommences its forward movement to completion, with a release of energy, audible as a click (comparable with the sudden ejection of an apple pip from between pressed finger-tips).

Locked Joint

The muscle load may increase, and alterations in the articular surface (identifiable at an ultrastructural level) may interfere with the free sliding of the upper joint components.

The disc fails to slide forward to complete its excursion and remains stuck. (This will produce continuous "locking of the jaw" in the position where it used to click).

Resolution

The muscular overload may spontaneously cease, in which case full movement may recommence in the upper joint compartment.

Joint overload may not cease, but subarticular remodelling of the bony elements of articulation may so modify the shapes of articular surfaces as to allow free sliding movements, and indeed to relieve the overload itself.

Degeneration

If resolution fails to take place a far worse condition may supervene with break-up of articular surface tissue and subsequent bony erosion. This is termed "Temporomandibular Arthropathy" (Toller, 1974b), which is a special form of osteoarthrosis peculiar to the temporomandibular joint.

If the above hypothesis were correct, then it would be logical to direct treatments towards a reduction of muscular disharmony and overload. It would be wise to adjust cuspal contacts which interfere with normal occlusal movements. Restoration of lost functional dental units would be indicated, either with fillings, bridgework or dentures. It is difficult to determine the extent to which the strict restoration of "height of bite" is necessary and this is usually a subjective assessment. A lost height of bite would hardly seem to contribute to muscular overload, but such loss may well be associated with repetitive impulse actions which could be traumatic, and which could initiate changes at an ultra-structural level in the sliding articular surfaces.

Since so many of the complaints of clicking, locking, or pain occur in the morning, and often on waking, it may be presumed that inharmonious muscle actions during sleeping hours produce a traumatic effect in the joint itself. The wearing of a full occlusal-coverage acrylic biting splint at night may relieve the effect of dental irregularities. Indeed, it may be so gross an intrusion into the mechanism that unconscious muscular habits become broken, possibly with the establishment of other patterns of muscular movement which may not in themselves be traumatic.

An important aspect of treatment is to reassure the patient. The use of relaxant or tranquillizing drugs may have a place in some instances. It is always necessary to encourage the development of jaw movements which are quietly controlled and relaxed.

REFERENCES

Boering, G. (1966), *Arthrosis Deformans van het Kaakgewicht*. Groningen: Drukkerij Van Denderen.
Cobin, H. P. (1969), "Treatment of the Temporomandibular Pain-dysfunction Syndrome," *N.Y. St. dent. J.*, **35**, 552.
Franks, A. S. T. (1967), "The Dental Health of Patients Presenting with T.M.J. Dysfunction," *Brit. J. Oral Surg.*, **5**, 157.
Greene, C. S. (1973), "Survey of Current Professional Concepts and Opinions about the Myofascial Pain Dysfunction Syndrome," *J. Amer dent. Ass.*, **86**, 128.
Schwartz, L. L. (1959), *Disorders of the Temporomandibular Joint*. Philadelphia: W. B. Saunders & Co.
Thomson, H. (1971), "Mandibular Dysfunction Syndrome," *Brit. dent. J.*, **130**, 187.
Toller, P. A. (1961), "The Synovial Apparatus and Temporomandibular Joint Function," *Brit. dent. J.*, **111**, 355.
Toller, P. A. (1974a), "Temporomandibular Capsular Rearrangement," *Brit. J. Oral Surg.*, **11**, 187.
Toller, P. A. (1974b), "Temporomandibular Arthropathy," *Proc. Roy. Soc. Med.*, **67**, 153.
Weiss, C. and Mirow, S. (1972), "Ultrastructural Study of Osteoarthritic Changes in the Articular Cartilage of Human Knees," *J. Bone J. Surg.*, **54A**, 954.

52. DEGENERATIVE DISEASE OF THE MANDIBULAR JOINT

P. A. TOLLER AND L. E. GLYNN

Characteristics of mandibular osteoarthrosis

    Incidence
    Dental state
    Radiographic features
    Dental history

Correlation of clinical, radiological and histological
    observations

    Fibrillation
    Denudation and eburnation
    Perforation
    Sub-articular collapse
    Erosion
    Repair

Response to treatment

    Intra-articular corticosteroids
    Condylectomy

Pathogenesis of osteoarthrosis

While rheumatoid arthritis is primarily a disease of synovial tissue, osteoarthrosis is considered to be a disease of articular cartilage. In recent years it has generally been agreed that the disease is of a degenerative nature, but dispute continues with regard to the precise cause. A diagnostically important and scientifically perplexing feature of degenerative disease of the mandibular condyle is that both its clinical and its histopathological characteristics differ from those seen in other diarthrodial joints.

CHARACTERISTICS OF MANDIBULAR OSTEOARTHROSIS

A recent clinical survey (Toller, 1973) was based on a series of 150 cases derived from a study of about 2,000 cases of temporomandibular joint lesions seen over the past 20 years, and this suggested that osteoarthrotic cases constitute about 8 per cent of all the temporomandibular joint lesions which have been studied in one clinic during this period. Salient clinical findings from this study are summarized in Tables 1 and 2 and fig. 1. None of these patients had an abnormally raised sedimentation rate, and none was seropositive for rheumatoid factor. Nineteen cases of confirmed rheumatoid arthritis affecting the temporomandibular joints were found among the whole series of joint cases during this period, that is, a 1 per cent incidence of rheumatoid arthritis in this clinic compared with 8 per cent incidence of degenerative joint disease over the whole period. This is reasonably similar to a series of 400 temporomandibular joint cases which included 14 per cent arthrosis deformans from all causes, in Holland.

No case of bilateral active disease was seen, but in six cases the painful and degenerative disease subsequently started in the condyle opposite to the one in which the disease process had been seen to resolve and become symptomless. Ten other cases were noted where healed lesions were apparently present in the opposite condyle. Clinical polyarthritis was not manifest in any of this series, but complete clinical examinations were not carried out on all patients, and data regarding the occurrence of osteoarthrotic lesions in other joints were not recorded.

TABLE 1

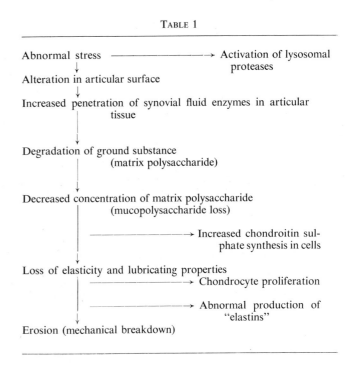

Dental State

Dental state was recorded only as good, fair, or badly kept teeth, in addition to adequately or inadequately supported occlusion, the latter when three or more functional molars were missing or improperly restored, or where the freeway space in full denture cases exceeded 5 mm. The general standard of dental health and care among these patients was fairly high and only about one in three was judged to have inadequately restored dentitions. Although impaired dental efficiency has been said to bear a relationship to the occurrence of the pain-dysfunction syndrome, no such relationship was obvious in this series of osteoarthrosis patients. Striking clinical improvement did not follow appropriate attention to the dental state. However, about one-half had a history of pain-dysfunction systems at some previous time in the affected joint and this suggests a relationship between the occurrence of untreated pain-dysfunction syndrome and the later onset of degenerative joint disease.

Radiographic Features

One of the reasons why osteoarthrosis of the temporomandibular joints has not been more frequently recognized is that the most important sign, that of erosion of the mandibular condyle, is not easy to detect on the transcranial radiographic projection which is commonly used to

(Toller, 1969) whereby it is usually, but not always, possible to achieve a sharply defined image of the articular surface with minimal distortion and no overlying bony shadows.

The onset of symptoms in mandibular osteoarthrosis may be sudden or gradual, and probably does not correspond closely with radiographic appearances. In some instances radiographic changes are recognizable before symptoms arise and there is evidence to show that the erosive disease can run its full course without the patient having been aware

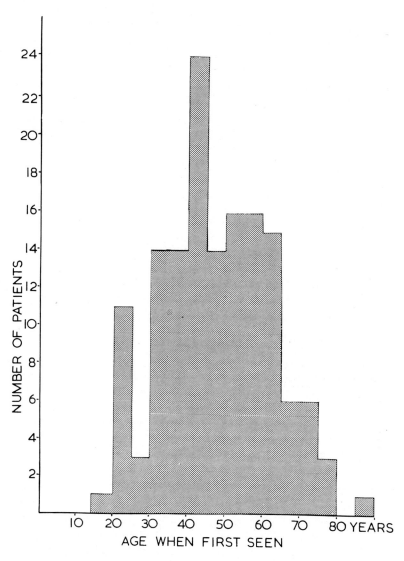

Fig. 1. Histogram showing ages at first attendance of patients diagnosed as mandibular osteoarthrosis.

study this joint. With this projection, the central ray must pass through several overlying anatomical features so that fine detail of the bony surface of the condyle is reduced. Radiographic techniques such as tomography are more revealing of the state of the articular surface, but inherently are never really sharp and their technical complexity makes them unsuitable for routine examination. The simplest radiographic technique for showing the state of the bony surface of the condyle is the transpharyngeal projection

of it. In other cases, the joint can become acutely painful before radiographic changes are detectable. Whatever the clinical form taken, radiographic changes are essential to a definitive diagnosis of this condition.

The first radiographic appearance of mandibular osteoarthrosis is a loss of integrity of the articular bony end-plate, at or near the point of articular contact on the anterior or superior aspect of the condyle; rarely, if ever, are bony changes encountered on the posterior aspect. This early

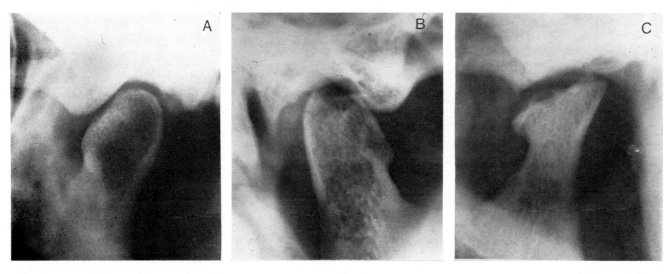

FIG. 2. Transpharyngeal radiographs of three patients with degenerative joint disease, each in a different stage of the development of erosion of the condylar surface.

change may be diffuse or punctate (fig. 2a). Histological examinations of resected condyles, which will be mentioned later, suggest that thickening and sclerosis of the bony end-plate precedes this rarefaction, but this has not often been detected radiographically. The next stage, after one or two months, is the appearance of a shallow conchoidal excavation in the articular surface corresponding with considerable pain, tenderness, stiffness and obvious crepitus (fig. 2b). Soon rarefaction expands into a fully developed erosive

TABLE 2

Signs and Symptoms	% of Total Cases
Pain on movement	96
Radiographic changes at first attendance	86
Crepitus	67
Some limitation of jaw movement	64
Deviation of jaw on opening	45
Tenderness over condyle	41
Aching in joint or side of face	21

TABLE 3

FURTHER CLINICAL FINDINGS

	% of Total Cases
Sudden onset symptoms	52
Gradual onset symptoms	48
Good dentition, adequately supported bite	70
Poor dentition or inadequately restored bite	30
Relevant history of trauma	5
Previous history of pain-dysfunction syndrome	34
Previous lesion on contra-lateral side	8
Females	85
Males	15

lesion as the total bony size of the condyle is reduced. This lesion shows as a shallow saucer-shaped erosion with a fairly sharp periphery (fig. 2c).

Osteophytes, rarely present, are usually found at the anterior edge of the lesion (fig. 3a) but some radiographs suggest that they occur occasionally at the lateral margin of the lesion (fig. 3b), and radiographs taken in another plane suggest that these osteophytes are calcifications in the region of the temporomandibular ligament. The osteophytic lipping at the anterior edge of the condyle near the insertion of the external pterygoid muscle is probably a late state in the disease and may be clinically unimportant.

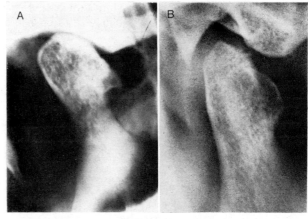

FIG. 3. Radiographs of mandibular condyles showing two types of osteophyte: (A) Anterior osteophytic lipping. (B) Osteophytes in lateral capsular reflection which appear in this radiographic projection as on superior condylar surface.

Although radiographic changes are usually to be seen at first attendance, it is important to note that severe erosions may develop more obviously two or three months after the first symptoms (fig. 4). As the severity of the symptoms increases or persists, osteoporosis of the condyles may become more extensive. In a few cases that respond to early

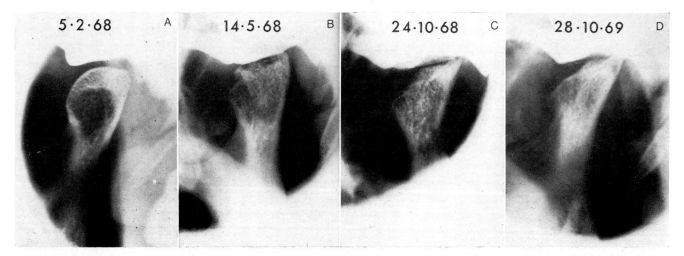

FIG. 4. Serial transpharyngeal radiographs showing development and course of mandibular O.A. Male aged 48, treated conservatively. (A) Sudden onset of acute pain and crepitus on movement with limitation of jaw opening. (B) Less pain, still tender, crepitus but increased opening. (C) No pain, no tenderness, increased range of movement, but still deviation on opening. (D) No pain at all, no crepitus, and full range of movement.

conservative treatment with the subsidence of symptoms, radiographic irregularities disappear within a few months. In other cases symptoms may disappear completely in spite of severe condylar erosion, and there is by no means a close correlation between radiographic appearances and clinical symptoms.

The last state in nearly every case is for the reduced condyle to form a new mineralized articular surface (fig. 5), and this reduced condyle appears radiographically as having a shorn-off appearance; it can, however, function with surprising efficiency and freedom from symptoms, although the dental occlusion is by no means always altered.

Radiographic involvement of the eminentia articularis was detected in 14 per cent of the series reported here. In each of these cases the associated erosion of the condyle was severe, and the mean age of the patients with upper joint cavity involvement was 62 years, which was higher than the mean age of the whole series. The clinical course of the disease with wider joint involvement did not differ markedly from that of patients whose condyles only were affected.

It is difficult to assess the extent of the involvement of the meniscus in mandibular osteoarthrosis, owing to its radiolucency. In 20 cases which were treated by minimal condylectomy, and where it was possible to inspect the joint as a whole, the meniscus appeared generally to be intact in 16 of them. When the upper joint cavity was opened, the articular surfaces generally appeared little affected.

Dental History

Clinical follow-up studies have been carried out on a fairly large group of patients who had received no active treatment for long periods, whose chief complaint had been pain, and all of whom showed radiographic changes. The majority suffered from marked joint pain, crepitus and discomfort for about nine months, followed by a gradual burning-out of the condition over the next two or three years with a little residual, but painless disability. The end-result of extensive bony remodelling is usually an alteration

in shape and reduction in size of the condyle. The reduced and altered condyle can be seen to be functional and free from pain many years after an arthrotic episode. It seems possible that about 5 per cent of all cases never become spontaneously free from pain and disability.

Ankylosis of the joint has not been observed to follow erosive arthrosis, and cannot be regarded as a complication of this disease. If a policy of watching is adopted, there is an even chance that the main symptom of pain will have completely disappeared at the end of one year after clinical presentation, but it is not possible to anticipate which cases will naturally resolve and primary conservative treatment should be instituted in all cases to relieve pain and to give encouragement.

CORRELATION OF CLINICAL, RADIOLOGICAL AND HISTOLOGICAL OBSERVATIONS

The structure of the mandibular joint differs in one important aspect from other diarthrodial joints (except the sterno-clavicular joint) in that the condylar articular surface is not covered with hyaline cartilage but with a layer of mature fibrous tissue; this lies above a stratum of cartilage which surmounts the convexity of the bone (fig. 6). Osteoarthrosis of diarthrodial joints is usually described as a primary disease or degeneration of hyaline cartilage, but there is no hyaline cartilage on the surface of the temporomandibular joint, and it is possible that this essential structural difference may account for the unusual clinical manifestations of pathological changes.

Clinical manifestations differ from those seen in other joints in age of onset, sex differential, infrequency of osteophytes, early spreading subarticular osteoporosis (erosion), and in the relatively rapid clinical course with tendency to natural repair.

Owing to the focal nature of the articular lesions, and the frequent juxtaposition of degenerative and reparative processes occurring in a single joint at any particular time, a confusion of interpretation can easily arise. The histological

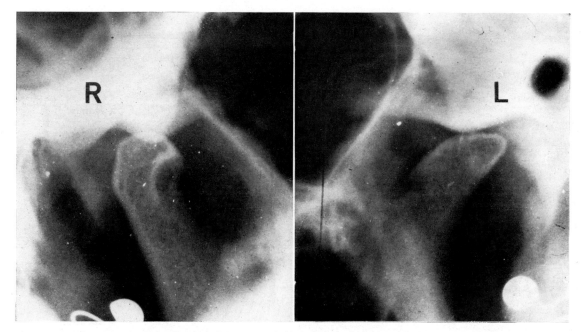

FIG. 5. Woman aged 35 who had suffered a painful osteoarthritic episode in the left condyle 14 years previously which had lasted for 3 years. Since then no pain, mandibular movements free, and function normal. The left condyle shows typical size and shape of spontaneously healed osteoarthritic lesion.

appearance of a particular focus cannot be judged as typical of the whole joint, but by studying serial sections of pathological material from well documented cases it has been possible to relate histological appearances to the pattern of observed symptoms and radiographic changes.

Stage 1 (Fibrillation)

Commencing in the area of articular contact (through which pass the greatest loads) there is a loosening of peripheral fibres in the articular surface. There appears to be a progressive lack of cohesion between the collagen bundles allowing fluid to collect between them (fig. 7), after which they fray off into the synovial cavity. This probably corresponds with "fibrillation" in other diarthrodial joints.

Immediately beneath the fibrous articular layer an organized hypertrophy and mineralization of the cartilaginous zone results in consolidation of the articular end-plate. In the sub-articular zone bony trabeculae may undergo some remodelling, but the bone marrow itself remains intact.

At an early stage another phenomenon may sometimes be encountered, possibly pathognomonic of the condition, namely clusters of cells in the surface zone (fig. 8). Large clusters of chondrocytes seen in osteoarthrosis are probably derived by repeated cell division which is not typical of normal articular cartilage, and there is evidence that the same is true of a fibrous articular surface.

Denudation and Eburnation

The articular surface becomes progressively denuded as all fibrous tissue is lost. Deposition of bone within the cartilaginous layers results in an eburnated, highly mineralized bony articular surface (fig. 9) apparently often articu-

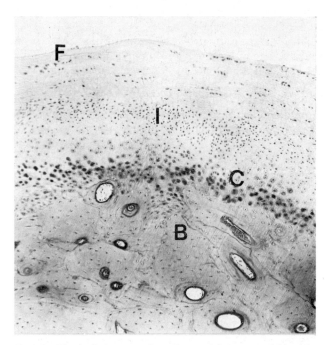

FIG. 6. Histological preparation of normal human condyle, male aged 27, showing fibrous articular surface (F), intermediate cellular zone (I), cartilage zone (C), bony end-plate (B). × 66.

lating successfully with the under-surface of the intact joint meniscus. The bony surface can become non-vital in parts, and yet remain mechanically intact (fig. 10).

From the clinical standpoint this stage may be akin to healing without appreciable deformation, and resembles eburnation seen in other joints. It is likely that a new fibrous surface can grow in from the synovial edges to re-cover the exposed bone. Preservation of the intra-articular meniscus

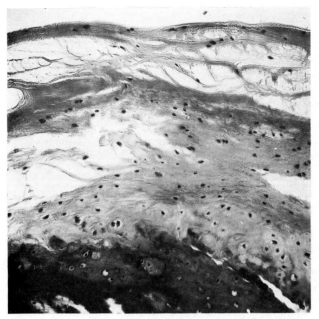

FIG. 7. Articular surface of condyle showing early interfibrillar fibrous degeneration over normal cartilage and bone. × 100.

would appear to be of the utmost importance for the successful and painless functioning of the joint following this stage of apparent repair.

At this stage radiographs may show little change in the shape or size of the condyle, although some diminution of the apparent joint space (distance between the main bony surfaces) would be expected, even if not easily detectable. The shadow of the lamina dura might be seen to become more dense. Pain on movement, tenderness, stiffness and crepitus are clinical features expected at this stage.

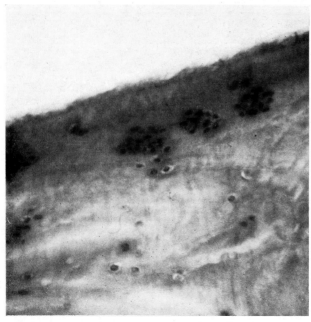

FIG. 8. Abnormal cloning of cells at the articular surface in a mandibular condyle, other parts of which had displayed both surface fibrillation and an erosive defect. × 100.

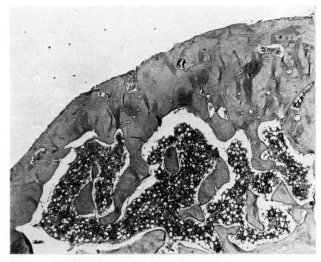

FIG. 9. Condyle showing complete loss of all fibrous articular zones, presenting a thickened bony articular surface beneath which there is a normal bone marrow. × 33.

Stage II (Perforation)

The bony end-plate may next become thinned and defective and be insufficient to separate the articular cavity from trabecular bone (fig. 11), in which case fibrosis occurs within the marrow spaces. This reaction extends upwards into the defects in the bony end-plate, in which attempts at bony repair can cometimes be seen and may be successful.

This stage could be seen on radiographs as a small break in the articular surface. Although it is likely that perforation of the bony end-plate would be accompanied by pain, perhaps of sudden onset, case histories suggest that it can almost certainly be painless in some instances.

Sub-articular Collapse

The apparently successfully repaired articular surface following Stage 1 can later fail in a way typical of conventional osteoarthrosis in other joints, namely, subarticular collapse. Punctate failures can take place through the bony

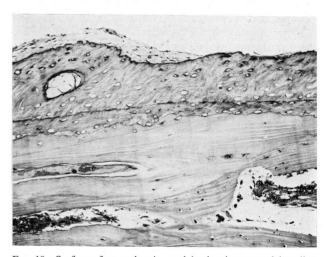

FIG. 10. Surface of an arthrosic condyle showing normal lamellar bone surmounted by a narrow zone of dead bone with empty lacunae, over part of which a fibrous surface extends. × 60.

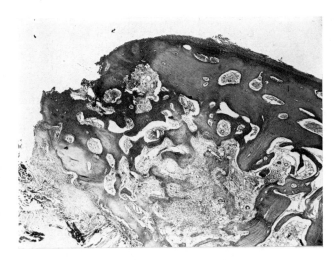

FIG. 11. Osteoarthrosic condyle showing loss of fibrous articular surface with perforation of bony end-plate and underlying fibrosis of the bone marrow. × 18.

end-plate possibly in association with sub-articular micro-fractures. The intra-articular pressures of normal movement may induce the formation of a small cyst-like space which gradually enlarges in size, in a fashion similar to that described in osteoarthrosis in other diarthrodial joints. The space may at first be lined with a fibrous layer, often richly vascular (fig. 12), but the walls may later give way to generalized trabecular bone destruction indistinguishable from

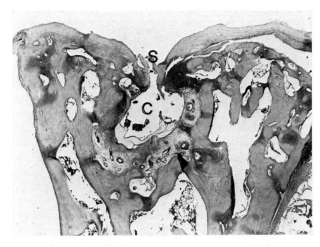

FIG. 12. The flattened surface of this condyle is broken by a small stoma (S) communicating with a synovial "pressure cyst" (C) beneath the articular surface. × 18.

Stage III. Such massive erosion of the articular surface, spreading from a single point (not necessarily that of articular contact) has been seen radiographically in some cases. It is worth noting that sub-articular collapse has appeared on radiographs as a bony erosion even though the overlying articular fibrous covering was found to be unbroken after subsequent condylectomy. Such cases (fig. 13) may not be uncommon.

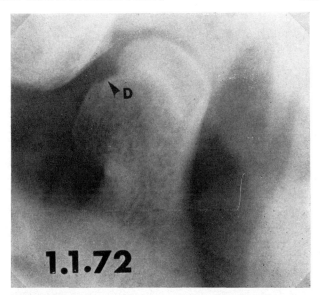

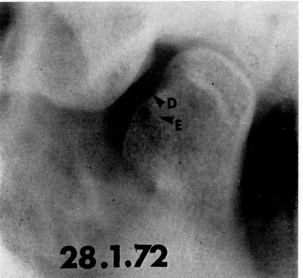

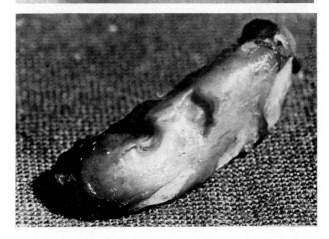

FIG. 13. Two radiographs showing the rapid development of a small "erosive" lesion (E) adjacent to a previous articular defect (D). Male aged 29 with pain, stiffness and crepitus for 6 months. Surgical specimen of condylar surface from the same patient (condylectomy 9.2.72) showing that each bony defect was still covered by a fibrous articular surface, suggesting subarticular collapse at these two places.

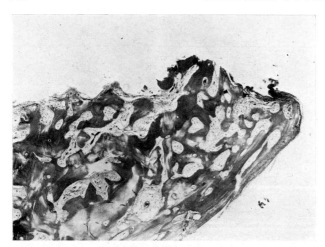

FIG. 14. Eroded condylar surface from a typical advanced case of O.A. Much trabecular remodelling is taking place; there is a complete absence of inflammatory reaction. × 15.

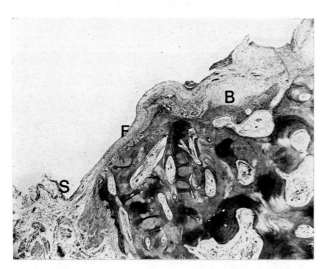

FIG. 15. Anterior margin of a grossly eroded condyle showing new bone formation at (B) and an overgrowth of fibrous tissue (F) originating at the synovial margin (S). The cancellous spaces are fibrosed. It seems likely that a process of repair is taking place giving rise to a new fibrous articular surface over a repaired bony end-plate. × 45.

Stage III (Erosion)

If repair is not successful the defect becomes larger, more trabecular bone is lost, and the lesion extends in depth (fig. 14). In the underlying cancellous spaces, fat and haemopoietic elements are replaced by fibrous tissue. At first, this fibrotic marrow is seen directly beneath the articular defect, but later fibrosis spreads throughout the marrow of the entire condylar head. Fibrotic reaction in the marrow spaces takes place whenever cancellous bone is in direct communication with the synovial cavity, as though the access of synovial fluid to cancellous spaces has a fibrosing affect.

While the erosive lesion spreads, pain may not be as severe as in the early stages of the disease, but crepitus is marked. Radiographic changes become most obvious at this comparatively late stage. Severe degrees of erosion may exist with no pain at all. Stiffness of the joint may also become less marked at this stage. As in so many other joints afflicted with osteoarthrosis clinical features often bear surprisingly little relationship to the severity of histological changes.

Stage IV (Repair)

No histological section has been seen in which the stage of massive erosion has been succeeded by complete repair with reformation of a satisfactory bony end-plate, but many radiographs show that this final and clinically satisfactory stage may be attained. Some condyles excised from cases with long histories of intractable pain and dysfunction, and which exhibited gross erosion of the bony end-plates with fibrosis of the marrow, showed evidence of repair, namely an ingrowth of new fibrous articular surface in continuity with the synovial edge (fig. 15), as well as underlying osteogenesis. It seems likely that a new fibrous articular surface re-forms from the synovial margins and a new cortical end-plate forms beneath it. Radiographs show that this re-formed articulation can be of abnormal shape, but clinical experience suggests that it can function with remarkable efficiency. This type of spontaneous repair would obviate the need for surgical interference, so that it is unlikely to be encountered in histological investigations.

It is likely that the presence of the intra-articular disc markedly influences the expression of this disease, enabling function to be maintained between an altered condylar surface and the upper part of the joint. Should the disc become damaged after the condyle has lost its fibrous articular surface, severe trouble will probably follow and it is unlikely that any form of repair will ensue without deformity and limitation of movement. There seems to be no justification for meniscectomy in the treatment of this condition.

RESPONSE TO TREATMENT

Active conservative treatment is directed first to the correction of any dental deficiency or inadequacy of masticatory function, the correct height of bite being especially important in denture wearers. Steps should also be taken to alleviate pain by general methods and anodynes, and massage over the joint and the masseter region with a minimal amount of counter-irritant unguent, containing methyl salicylate, is often of real comfort; this can be supported by infra-red therapy.

The pattern of pain and crepitus symptoms was observed after the instigation of simple conservative treatment outlined above. About one case in three was free of pain six months after the commencement of active treatment, but about 90 per cent still had crepitus. Crepitus remains in some cases for many years after pain has been eradicated and good movements have been established with adequate function. The symptom of crepitus seldom worries patients, and it does not readily respond to treatment by conservative methods.

In the majority of cases treatment is palliative to encourage the patient, to relieve pain, to preserve function and to prevent or minimize deformity. The disease still seems to run its course, although it is hoped that treatment will shorten the course or make it more tolerable.

Intra-articular Corticosteroid Therapy

The clinical results of treatment with single intra-articular injection of a corticosteroid drug in suitable cases are better than simple conservative procedures alone. Intra-articular hydrocortisone usually has a pain-relieving effect lasting on average about 10 weeks, and in cases of severe pain and limitation of movement this should be considered in the non-surgical approach to this disease, with a view to tiding the patient over into a naturally less painful phase. Its use as a sole treatment is to be deprecated, but it may be indicated when, after several months, the pain has shown insufficient response to conservative procedures. A well-practised and meticulous technique is required to introduce 0·5 ml. of an aqueous suspension containing 12 mg. of prednisolone trimethylacetate into the lower joint compartment below the meniscus, preferably after a simple auriculo-temporal nerve block with lignocaine.

The pain-relieving effect of intra-articular corticosteroid seems to encourage a reduction of the diseased articular surface in those cases where radiographic changes at the joint surfaces are already well advanced. The intra-articular application of catabolic steroids could be deprecated on the grounds that they promote further disruption and destruction of the joint tissues, but long-continued observation and experience justify its use in selected cases. Many patients are well satisfied and continue in comfort and adequate function after the degenerative disease has run its natural course, and it would seem that a single corticosteroid treatment shortens this course. Multiple injections are inadvisable.

It has been found that in about two-thirds of cases there is complete relief of pain, with improved function, and no further active treatment is necessary. The best responses are to be found in the age group over 35 years, and the results in younger age groups generally are poor.

In an important series of experiments the articular surfaces of mandibular condyles in healthy macaque monkeys showed histological damage after six injections of hydrocortisone in circumstances in which the changes most likely resulted from the use of the drug. It is not possible to say with certainty whether comparable damage to condylar surfaces can be attributed to the use of hydrocortisone in humans, since intra-articular corticosteroid therapy is customarily used on patients who have considerable radiographic erosions before treatment; certainly, however, some erosions tend to become more obvious after such therapy, although all symptoms are often permanently improved. Some regard such treatment as a safe and palliative procedure in the local treatment of arthritis, but others suggest caution because the steroid might interfere with a local protective mechanism and thus encourage a damaging level of physical activity. It is possible that this could account for the increased rate of condylar erosion in steroid-treated cases of mandibular osteoarthrosis, but this could serve to speed up the disease process towards its natural resolution—a sort of pharmacological arthroplasty. If insufficient improvement follows corticosteroid treatment, surgical treatment of the joint should be considered.

Mandibular Condylectomy

Both clinically and radiographically, the final condition of a "burnt-out" case of the more severe type resembles the results of a sub-total condylectomy. Cases which show little or no response to conservative lines of treatment and which have been inadequately relieved by intra-articular corticosteroid may be considered for surgical treatment. The advent of precise and fully sterilizable bone-cutting drills has enabled the operation of condylectomy via a small pre-auricular incision to be developed to a stage where there is now little trauma to the surrounding tissues; only the diseased portion of the condylar surface need be removed and the integrity of the upper joint cavity can be preserved. The absolute importance of unilateral operation at any one time is stressed; an anterior open bite can very easily result from a simultaneous bilateral condylar resection.

Post-operatively, the relief of pain and increase in range of movement of the affected joint is often dramatic for the patient, and the operation has much to recommend it in cases of severe intractable pain and disability where all conservative methods have failed.

PATHOGENESIS OF OSTEOARTHROSIS

The marked differences in clinical osteoarthrosis between the mandibular joint and other joints is interesting and merits discussion. The sex distribution (F: M = 6:1) does not correspond with that of osteoarthrosis found in other joints where there is usually an equal distribution of disease between the sexes. This sex ratio differs, also, from that which has been widely reported for the mandibular pain-dysfunction syndrome, where the ratio is F: M = 3:1. Nor does the ratio correspond to that observed for rheumatoid arthritis recently stated as F:M = 2·7:1 in a southern English county. There is no clear relationship between the occurrence of mandibular osteoarthrosis and impaired dental efficiency, and experimental reports tend to support this. The effect of unilateral dental function on the temporomandibular joints in rhesus monkeys has been carefully studied and no evidence has been found of a relationship between such unilateral function and either adaptive changes in either joint, or the incidence of degenerative joint disease. Neither did studies in the human suggest that asymmetrical dental function is directly related to the onset of osteoarthrosis in the temporomandibular joint. It thus seems that purely dental factors, at least in the young and middle-aged groups, may be of comparatively little importance in the aetiology of degenerative joint disease of the mandibular condyle. Certainly, it is difficult to believe or understand how so small an organic disability as dental inadequacy could initiate so severe a lesion as that to be seen in fig. 14, but it is significant that a majority of radiographically detected lesions occur at the area of articular contact and it is just possible that an alteration of load carriage of a less obvious neuromuscular nature cannot be excluded from the aetiology. The likelihood would seem to be that this disease is multifactorial in origin.

The disintegration of the articular surface in early lesions suggests fundamental tissue failure, and histological evidence points to dissolution of the ground substance which

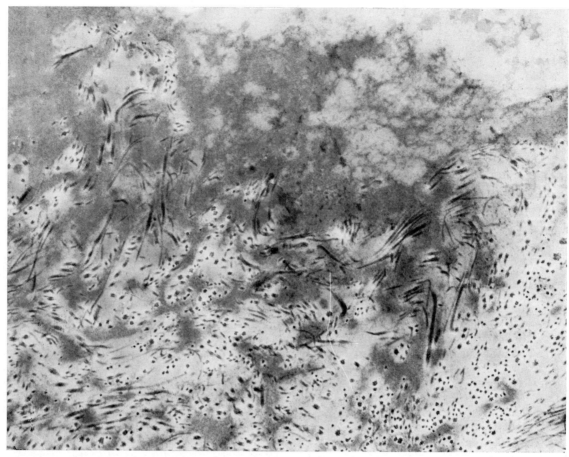

FIG. 16. Transmission electron-micrograph of articular surface of arthrosic mandibular condyle, showing disorganisation of the collagen arrangement, variation in size of collagen fibrils, and the apparent alteration of the interfibrillar ground substance. × 21,300.

binds collagen fibres together. An alteration of inter-fibrillar ground substance might be brought about by chemical, hormonal, or enzymatic effect via the synovia, while the physical destruction of fibres could be brought about by mechanical means such as intermittent impulse loading mediated via the musculature.

The predominant involvement of the condyle in temporo-mandibular osteoarthrosis merits further comment. Although the actual loads must pass across all four interfaces of the joint, it seems possible that the greater total bearing surfaces of the meniscus and upper joint cavity may spread the load in this region, and thereby diminish the possible damaging affects of excessive usage. Similar loads concentrated on the relatively smaller zone of articular contact on the condyles might more readily stress their articular tissues beyond their physical limits of tolerance.

Ultra-microscopic studies of the surfaces of human mandibular condyles affected by early osteoarthrosis suggest an alteration of the surface inter-fibrillar ground substance together with a denaturation of surface collagen (fig. 16). Electron-micrographic studies have also revealed in the deeper layers of the fibrous articular surfaces aggregations of convoluted elastic-like structures which have provisionally been termed "vermiform bodies". It is thus possible that one of the responses of mandibular articular tissues to stress is a kind of reactionary elastosis, which further contributes to structural weakness. These studies are insufficiently advanced to make further commentary at this stage.

A schematic representation of the process of osteoarthrosis at the articular layer has been suggested as in Table 1 following Bollet (1969).

It has been almost universally held that osteoarthrosis is primarily a disease of articular cartilage and that its nature is degenerative, not inflammatory. Although this concept of the disease has stimulated extensive study of the chemistry of both normal and osteoarthrotic cartilage it has signally failed to reveal any underlying cause. The precedence of loss of proteoglycans over loss of collagen in the genesis of the osteoarthrotic lesion does, however, point to some local action of hydrolytic enzymes, and cartilage cells themselves have been regarded as the main site of enzyme production. Since it is the most superficial layers of cartilage, however, that show the first signs of the disease, it is difficult to accept that cells situated within the cartilage are the primary source of the enzymes responsible.

An alternative source is the cells lining the synovial membrane. Electron microscopy has clearly distinguished two main types of lining cell: type A, characterized by a multiplicity of cytoplasmic processes, large numbers of lyso-

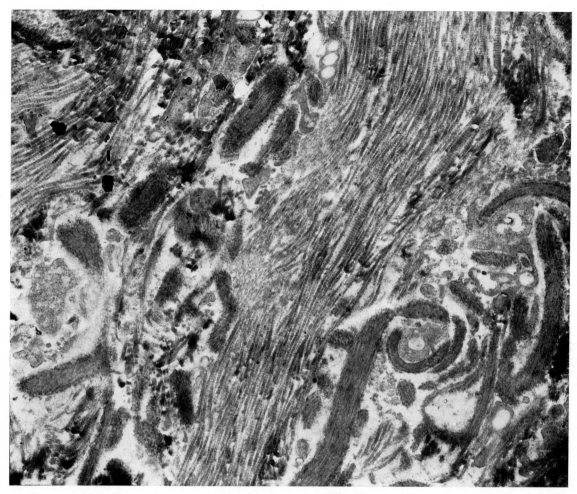

FIG. 17. Electron-micrograph from deeper layers of the fibrous articular surface of an arthrosic condyle showing the dense bundles of normal collagen interspersed with aggregation of "vermiform bodies". These are abnormal collections of elastic-like structures. × 12,000.

somes and considerable phagocytic activity; and type B, in contrast, relatively lacking in cytoplasmic processes, with few lysosomes, but richly endowed with rough endoplasmic reticulum. On the basis of structure, it would appear that the A cells are phagocytic scavengers and that the B cells are active secretors of protein.

Apart from a relatively small number of intermediate cells, the A and B cells each contribute about half the total cell composition of the synovial lining. It is evident, therefore, that the synovial lining of normal diarthrodial joints is capable of phagocytic and digestive activities of a high order, and since function determines structure it may be presumed that normal joint activity results in a significant production of wear-and-tear material whose removal from the joint space is essential for the maintenance of normal function. This clearing function of the A cells involves phagocytosis with subsequent fusion of phagosome and lysosome in order to bring enzyme and substrate particle into mutual contact within the environment of the A cell itself. Whenever such activity occurs on a large scale it is reasonable to suppose that some leakage of enzymes occurs into the extra-cellular (i.e. synovial) space. If such released enzymes are not to lead to digestion of the surface layers of

the articular cartilage it is essential that inhibitors of the enzymes should be simultaneously available. The most potent of such natural inhibitors are found in the α_2 macroglobulin component of the serum proteins. This, however, as its name implies, is composed of large molecules (mol. wt. 900,000) and is probably incapable of passage through the capillary walls of an uninflamed synovium. For access of such a molecule to the extra-vascular space a process of active synthesis and secretion would be required such as could well be provided by the B type of lining cells. At present there is no clear evidence as to the nature of the material synthesized by these cells but similar cells in normal connective tissue have been shown by the fluorescent antibody method to contain significant quantities of α_2 macroglobulin.

Therefore the hypothesis proposed is that osteoarthrosis results from an imbalance between the two cell types in the synovial lining leading to an excess of leaking enzymes over secreted inhibitors, possibly in combination with predisposing factors.

A criticism of this hypothesis is that the presence of uninhibited proteolytic enzymes in the synovial fluid should lead to a uniform attack upon the whole surface of the articular cartilage and not be confined, as it is in the early stages, to the obvious areas of pressure. The enzymes themselves, however, are macromolecules and incapable of penetrating into normal cartilage because of the space-occupying character of its own macromolecules as recently shown for immunoglobulins in the *in vitro* studies of Fell and Barratt (1973). Some extra factor is therefore required to permit the intimate contact between enzyme and substrate needed for enzyme activity. The alternative pressure and relaxation of the weight-bearing areas may well provide this extra factor, especially if such muscle loading across the joint surfaces is excessive.

REFERENCES

Bollet, A. J. (1969), "An Essay on the Biology of Osteoarthritis," *Arth. and Rheum.*, **12**, 152.

Fell, H. B. and Barratt, M. E. J. (1973), "The Role of Soft Connective Tissue in the Breakdown of Pig Articular Cartilage Cultivated in the Presence of Complement-sufficient Antiserum to Pig Erythrocytes," *Int. Arch. Allergy*, **44**, 441.

Toller, P. A. (1969), "Transpharyngeal Radiography for Osteoarthritis of the Mandibular Condyle," *Brit. J. Oral Surg.*, **7**, 47.

Toller, P. A. (1973), "Osteoarthrosis of the Mandibular Condyle," *Brit. dent. J.*, **134**, 223.

53. RHEUMATOID ARTHRITIS

L. E. GLYNN

Diagnostic features

Effects on cartilage and bone

Extra-articular manifestations

Underlying causes

Experimental studies
    Interpretation

Rheumatoid arthritis may be defined as a subacute or chronic, non-suppurative inflammatory polyarthritis affecting mainly the peripheral joints, usually in a symmetrical fashion, running a prolonged course of exacerbation and remission and accompanied by signs of systemic disturbance such as anaemia, weight loss and raised erythrocyte sedimentation rate (Duthie, 1969). It is unfortunately an extremely common disease affecting in Britain 2·1 per cent of males and 5·2 per cent of females, with incidence rising with age to 6 per cent in males over 75 and 16 per cent in females between 65 and 74. No age is exempt, not even infants in the first few months of life. However, in the juvenile age-group, defined to include all individuals under 16 years old, the disease tends to run a more benign course and to show certain differentiating features which probably justify its separate designation as Still's disease.

DIAGNOSTIC FEATURES

For comparative studies of pathogenesis, aetiology, treatment and prognosis, it became evident about 20 years ago that some agreed definition of the disease was essential. This led to the now widely held criteria laid down by a committee of the American Rheumatism Association and revised in 1958 and again in 1963 These criteria have proved invaluable and are given here in outline as they provide not only the basis for diagnosis but also an excellent picture of the clinical state. They are:

(a) morning stiffness;

(b) pain on motion or tenderness in at least one joint;

(c) swelling in at least one joint due to the thickening of the soft tissues or effusion;

(d) swelling of at least one other joint with an interval of not less than 3 months between the two events;

(e) symmetrical joint swelling, *i.e.* simultaneous involvement of the same joint on both sides of the body;

(f) subcutaneous nodules over bony prominences or in the vicinity of joints;

(g) X-ray changes typical of the disease. These include increased radiolucency in the vicinity of the affected joints and erosions of the bone at the margins of the articular cartilages; and

(h) positive tests for the presence of rheumatoid factor (*v.i.*).

The disease is described as classical if it presents seven of these criteria, definite if it shows five and probable with only three. A large proportion of cases present no diagnostic difficulty and are characterized by morning stiffness and a progressive arthritis affecting particularly the metacarpo-phalangeal and proximal interphalangeal joints in a symmetrical fashion. It is, however, important to exclude the many other conditions that may first appear as a polyarthritis, including other diseases of the connective tissues such as systemic lupus erythematosus, dermatomyositis, and scleroderma as well as a host of other conditions, including rheumatic fever, gout, tuberculosis, psoriatic arthritis, ulcerative colitis, rubella, haemophilia, Sjögren's disease (keratoconjunctivitis sicca) and several rarer conditions.

Although the small peripheral joints of the hands and feet are by far the most frequently affected, no joints are exempt, not even the crico-arytenoids, and the temporo-mandibular joints are not infrequently affected although progressive damage is fortunately rare. The pathological changes in the affected joints are highly characteristic. The earliest changes are seen in the synovial membrane and include proliferation and hypertrophy of the lining cells together with infiltrations of lymphocytes and plasma cells, the former tending to concentrate around the small blood vessels. Occasionally, the aggregations of lymphocytes come to resemble closely the lymphoid follicles of anti-genically stimulated lymph nodes with their germinal centres of pale blast-type cells. Polymorphonuclear leuco-cytes, which predominate in the synovial fluid, contribute insignificantly to the cellular infiltrate of the membrane itself. Vascular changes are conspicuous; the membrane is hyperaemic with an apparent increase of small vessels, especially venules. Increased permeability of these vessels is presumably responsible for the exudation of fluid resulting in oedema of the soft tissues and distension of the synovial space. This increased permeability is also responsible for the considerable extra-vascular deposition of fibrin, both within and upon the synovial membrane, where it seems to resist the normal processes of digestion and/or organization by which accumulations of fibrin are normally removed.

EFFECTS ON CARTILAGE AND BONE

Although the pathological changes may remain confined to the synovial membrane for several months, the disease process eventually extends to cartilage and bone. The pro-liferating cells of the membrane extend across the articular cartilage forming the so-called pannus, which is followed by the death of underlying cartilage cells and progressive dissolution of its intercellular matrix. At the same time, similar extensions of the inflamed synovium extend deep to the cartilage and erode the adjacent bone, resulting in mar-ginal erosions which are a typical radiological feature at this stage. This destruction of bone and cartilage may extend to involve any or all of the other intra-articular structures, such as menisci, ligaments, and tendons, result-ing in loss of stability, whilst the associated fibrosis leads to contracture, deformity, and even to fibrous ankylosis. Dissolution of the various tissues is presumably accom-plished by the release of a variety of enzymes from the lyso-somal granules present in large numbers not only in the synovial cells but also in the polymorphonuclear and other inflammatory cells present. The access of these lysosomal enzymes to their appropriate substrates in the extracellular tissues is obviously a factor of importance in the patho-genesis of the rheumatoid joint and it is therefore of great interest that the normal ability of the lysosomal membrane to control this access is greatly impaired in rheumatoid tissue.

EXTRA-ARTICULAR MANIFESTATIONS

The lesions of rheumatoid arthritis are by no means con-fined to the joints. It is now well recognized that this is a systemic disease in which no single tissue appears to be entirely exempt. The systemic nature of the affection shows itself most obviously in anaemia, loss of weight, and the various changes in plasma proteins that are such a com-mon feature of the disease. These changes are responsible both for the raised erythrocyte sedimentation rate (attribut-able to increased fibrinogen and gamma globulin) and for the power of rheumatoid sera to potentiate the agglutination of a variety of particles when treated with subagglutinable doses of immune globulins. The observation that rheuma-toid sera could, for example, cause the agglutination of sheep red cells which had been previously treated with a sub-agglutinating dose of a rabbit anti-sheep red cell antiserum forms the basis of the Rose Waaler test for rheumatoid factor. This factor is now known to be itself an antibody, capable of reacting with the rabbit antibody on the sheep red cells used in the test. The complete understanding of the phenomenon had to await further studies in basic immunology which showed that human immunoglobulins fall into several classes, now designated as IgG, IgM, IgA, IgD and IgE. The classical rheumatoid factor is an IgM immunoglobulin which behaves as a specific antibody to certain chemical groups present on IgG molecules. These groups, however, are not present exclusively on human IgG molecules but are also found on similar immunoglobulins of other species, e.g. the rabbit. It may well be asked why the rheumatoid factor does not react in vivo with the IgG in the circulation. The most probable answer is that a reac-tion does indeed occur but is extremely weak because of the relatively inaccessible nature of the chemical groups involved when the IgG is in its native state. Deformation of the IgG molecules such as occurs when, for example, they react either specifically with an antigen such as a sheep red cell or non-specifically, as with a latex particle, exposes these groupings and allows them to form a firm bond with the rheumatoid factor, which becomes manifest by the clumping of the coated particles. Rheumatoid factor is therefore an auto-antibody, auto since it reacts with group-ings present in the individual producing it. Its appearance in some 85 per cent of all patients with rheumatoid arthritis supports the view that the basis of the chronic rheumatoid process is an auto-immune reaction against one or more constituents of the connective tissues, either in their native state or more probably in a state of deformation as a result of wear and tear or of some inflammatory process.

The extent to which other organs are involved varies widely, but in general the more severe the disease the more probable are the extra-articular manifestations. These in-clude vasculitis, which probably plays a part in most of the lesions, subcutaneous nodules, a granulomatous endo-carditis in which lesions resembling the subcutaneous nodules may occur, peripheral neuropathy, myopathy, pul-monary interstitial fibrosis with or without intra-pulmonary nodules (Caplan's syndrome), and amyloid degeneration. With the decline in the incidence of tuberculosis and chronic bacterial infections, such as osteomyelitis, rheumatoid arthritis has become the commonest condition in Britain predisposing to amyloid degeneration.

UNDERLYING CAUSES

Views as to the nature and cause of rheumatoid arthritis have changed with the fashions of disease aetiology. During the great bacteriological era at the turn of the century it was natural to assume that a specific micro-organism was the root cause. No single organism has withstood critical appraisal and the last to be dismissed in this way are the mycoplasmas and the diphtheroids. Nevertheless, it would be premature to disregard any participation of micro-organisms in the pathogenesis of this disease. With the demonstration that symptoms could be dramatically allevi-ated by administration of corticosteroids such as cortisone, it was naturally assumed that some endocrine imbalance involving these and related steroids was the underlying cause and, more particularly, that this imbalance was attributable to faulty adaptation to stress which normally led to an increased secretion of cortisone-like steroids. When adaptation to stress was inadequate, an excess of the so-called mineralo-corticoids was postulated and to this excess the various lesions were attributed. Unfortunately for the acceptance of this hypothesis, nothing resembling a rheumatoid lesion could be produced experimentally by induced imbalance of the kind postulated, and further-more no evidence of arthritis appeared in human subjects in whom such imbalance was present as a result of aldo-sterone-secreting tumours.

The current view ascribes all the lesions of rheumatoid arthritis to the interaction within the affected tissues of one or more antigens with cells of the immunological system, especially lymphocytes and plasma cells. The evidence in favour of such an interaction is now reaching compelling proportions. The main facts are as follows. Reference has already been made to rheumatoid factor and its immuno-logical significance, and to the histological features that are indicative of a local immunological reaction, namely the concentrations of plasma cells, lymphocytes, and lymphoid follicles. The immunological role of plasma cells has, more-over, been confirmed by the demonstration within them of immunoglobulins of both IgG and IgM classes; and by the use of fluorescein-labelled heat-aggregated IgG it has been clearly shown that a proportion of the plasma cells contain and presumably secrete rheumatoid factor. The plasma cells at the periphery of subcutaneous nodules have simi-larly been shown to contain immunoglobulins and rheuma-toid factors. The capacity of cells in the rheumatoid synovium to secrete immunoglobulins has been confirmed by more direct methods. It has been found that fragments of synovial membrane removed by therapeutic synovectomy will, in tissue culture, secrete newly synthesized immuno-globulins into the culture medium with an efficiency com-parable, weight for weight, to that of explants of spleen. The immunoglobulin-synthesizing cells of the synovium are, however, screened from extra-synovial antigens since syn-ovial explants from subjects recently immunized with tetanus toxoid showed no specific antibody in the immuno-globulins released into the culture medium. This important finding was interpreted by Herman et al. (1971) as evidence that the immunocytes of the rheumatoid synovial membrane are already committed in their response to some other antigens, presumably already present in the membrane itself.

Immunoglobulins are a constituent part of the plasma proteins and their appearance in inflammatory exudates is not itself evidence that the inflammation is immunologically induced. The simultaneous presence of complement com-ponents, e.g. C3, strengthens the hypothesis but in the absence of any known and demonstrable antigen the key evidence is lacking. Nevertheless, the presence of complexes of IgG and βIc (a complement component) and of IgM and IgG in the synovial tissue of rheumatoid individuals sug-gests that some, at least, of the inflammation is mediated by these complexes. The importance of such complexes in a variety of inflammatory states is now well established. The activation of complement by the immune complexes leads to the local release of several agents responsible both for changes in vascular permeability and for the local accumulation of inflammatory cells. The phagocytosis of these complexes by the inflammatory cells results in labiliz-ation of their lysosomes with release of enzymes into the tissue resulting in further damage and inflammation.

EXPERIMENTAL STUDIES

The evidence pointing to an underlying immunological pathogenesis of rheumatoid arthritis is thus far both histo-logical and serological. Further strong support is also available from attempts to induce a rheumatoid type of lesion in experimental animals. A comprehensive review of these attempts up to 1960 was published in that year by Gardner who concluded, somewhat pessimistically, that the disease was essentially one of humans, or perhaps pri-mates, and therefore not reproducible in animals of a lower order. However, Banerjee and Glynn (1960) and Dumonde and Glynn (1962) were able to show that two of the most characteristic lesions of the disease, namely the nodules and the chronic apparently self-perpetuating arthritis could be produced in rabbits by essentially immunological methods. Thus Banerjee and Glynn (1960) found that although a subcutaneous implant of rabbit fibrin into a rabbit was rapidly removed and replaced by a small fibrous scar, a similar implant of foreign fibrin resists the normal processes of removal and can readily be identified several weeks later. Particularly striking, however, was the resemblance between the retained implant with its local inflammatory response and a typical subcutaneous rheumatoid nodule. So close is this resemblance that it strongly suggests the probability of the nodule itself being the expression of a reaction to local antigenic material.

Even more striking were the results of Dumonde and Glynn in their attempt to reproduce a rheumatoid type of arthritis. With the results of Banerjee and Glynn in mind they studied the reaction of the rabbit knee joint to injec-tions of fibrin, particularly when the animal had been previ-ously immunized in various ways to the injected material. It soon became apparent that when immunization was ob-tained with the use of Freund's complete adjuvant, in which the antigen was incorporated, inflammatory arthritis fol-lowed joint challenge; this arthritis resembled in all its pathological minutiae the joint lesion of rheumatoid arthritis. These include villous hyperplasia of the synovial membrane, proliferation of its lining cells, oedema, lymphocyte and plasma cell infiltration, lymphoid follicle formation with germinal centres, pannus formation, cartilage destruction and marginal erosion. Of even greater significance however, is the tendency of the experimental lesion to become chronic, so that active inflammation with progressive joint destruction is still evident after intervals approaching three years without any further manipulation of the experimental animals subsequent to the single joint challenge.

It is perhaps important to emphasize that although the early experiments of Glynn and his colleagues made use of fibrin as the stimulating antigen, their subsequent experiments have clearly shown that virtually any good protein antigen can take its place.

INTERPRETATION

The major question arising from this experimental arthritis is why the inflammation remains active, apparently indefinitely. The relevance of this question to the problem of rheumatoid arthritis is self-evident. Three possibilities have been considered. In any chronic inflammatory condition however primarily induced, there is always the possibility of secondary infection, either exogenous or the result of lighting-up some latent infection. No evidence of infection has thus far been obtained to account for the continuing nature of the experimental lesion. The second and perhaps more probable explanation is the persistence in the inflamed tissue of sufficient antigen to maintain both the immunological stimulus and the inflammatory reaction resulting from the interaction of antigen and antibody. Attempts to monitor the persistence of the antigen by labelling it with ^{125}I have not entirely resolved the question, although it seems extremely unlikely that the amount retained after six months would be adequate for this purpose. It is, moreover, doubtful whether the deposit of immune complexes within the articular cartilage and other avascular structures of the joint can play a significant role. The quantities involved and their rate of release would seem to be quantitatively inadequate.

This leaves a third alternative: namely, that the immunological reaction and the inflammation are maintained not by residues of the initiating antigen but by the acquisition of antigenicity by one or more of the components of the inflamed joint itself; in other words, an autoantigen. As mentioned previously, some 85 per cent of all rheumatoid arthritics show evidence of a capacity for this type of reaction in the presence within their serum of rheumatoid factor. This is not to say that interaction between this factor and its antigen (denatured IgG) is actually responsible for the chronicity of the lesion. There are many potential autoantigens in joint tissue and there is evidence that at least some of these are involved. Thus, antibodies to collagen have been found and, more recently, evidence of cell-mediated immunity to synovial antigen(s). Attention directed towards potential auto- and other antigens in the affected tissues of rheumatoid arthritis is comparatively recent and it is highly probable that several others will soon be found. Any complex macromolecule is potentially auto-antigenic, especially if it tends to undergo gross configurational changes during normal or pathological metabolism. Such molecules include the immunoglobulins, fibrinogen, collagen and various structural proteoglycans of the connective tissue.

The study of experimental arthritis has thus distinguished two phases in the evolution of the chronically inflamed joint. The first is the direct result of the interaction within the joint of a foreign antigen with antibody or sensitized cells reacting specifically with this antigen. This reaction only persists as long as sufficient antigen remains, a period which, judged by experimental studies in the rabbit, is unlikely to exceed 6–12 months. Any duration of active inflammation beyond this implies the advent of a second phase, attributable to the appearance within the affected tissues of a new antigen presumably derived from the affected tissues themselves.

REFERENCES

Banerjee, S. K. and Glynn, L. E. (1960), "Reactions to Homologous and Heterologous Fibrin Implants in Experimental Animals," *Ann. N.Y. Acad. Sci.*, **86**, 104.

Dumonde, D. C. and Glynn, L. E. (1962), "The Production of Arthritis in Rabbits by an Immunological Reaction to Fibrin," *Brit. J. exp. Path.*, **43**, 373.

Duthie, J. J. R. (1969), *Textbook of the Rheumatic Diseases*, p. 259 (W. S. Copeman, Ed.). Edinburgh: E. S. Livingstone.

Gardner, D. L. (1960), "The Experimental Production of Arthritis. A Review," *Ann. rheum. Dis.*, **19**, 297.

Herman, J. H., Bradley, J., Ziff, M. and Smiley, J. D. (1971), "Responses of the Rheumatoid Synovial Membrane to Exogenous Immunisation," *J. clin. Invest.*, **50**, 266.

SECTION XIII

54. DIAGNOSTIC AND THERAPEUTIC RADIATION

R. W. STANFORD

Sources of Radiation
  Ionizing radiation
    Electromagnetic
    Sub-atomic particles
  Non-ionizing radiation
    Ultrasound
    Lasers
    Infra-red
    Microwaves

Physical properties of radiation
  Ionizing
  Non-ionizing

Detection and measurement of radiation
  Ionizing
  Non-ionizing

Hazards associated with radiation
  Ionizing
    Somatic effects
    Genetic effects
  Non-ionizing

Applications of radiation
  Ionizing
  Non-ionizing

For many years ionizing radiations have been used as an aid to diagnosis and for therapeutic purposes. Used wisely and with discretion these radiations have made major contributions both to preventive dentistry and medicine and to the treatment of certain diseases. That they will continue to make these contributions is beyond doubt; nevertheless increasing sophistication and discrimination in their use is to be striven for. Concomitant with this is the need for careful appraisal of the possible uses of non-ionizing radiations where these provide an acceptable substitute for ionizing radiations or a new approach to diagnostic or therapeutic procedures.

The kinds of ionizing radiations most commonly employed are:

(a) sub-atomic particles such as electrons and neutrons; and

(b) electromagnetic radiations such as X-rays and gamma rays. Sources of these radiations range widely from simple X-ray tubes, such as are used in dental radiography, to highly sophisticated accelerators, and include both natural and artificial radioactive isotopes.

Development of the conventional X-ray tube during the past two decades has been aimed largely at providing smaller sources of X-rays at higher intensities, improved shielding, and better control of the size and quality of the smaller source (that is, the focal spot) diminishing geometrical unsharpness, whilst the high intensity beam reduces the exposure time and thus unsharpness due to voluntary and involuntary patient movement. Unnecessary radiation to both patient and operator is diminished by the better shielding. More accurate control of the size of the beam enables smaller areas of the patient to be irradiated whilst filtration diminishes the relative intensity of soft X-rays which are too heavily absorbed by tissue to contribute useful information on the radiograph. These steps also reduce substantially the dose to the patient.

The availability of the image intensifier, whereby lower intensity X-ray beams may be used to obtain smaller but much brighter images than are available on the simple fluorescent screen, enables dynamic studies to be undertaken, and a variety of aids are used to exploit these techniques. The reduced image may be photographed on 35, 70, or 100 mm. film or may be viewed remotely through a closed circuit television chain and recorded on videotape. Such facilities enable pre-programmed investigations to be carried out, ranging from single exposures through high speed radiography and cinematography. X-ray tubes and control equipment used in such procedures are frequently designed to provide pulses of X-rays of time length and frequency that need not be synchronized to the mains frequency, as is normally the case.

Of far-reaching importance is the recent introduction of a diagnostic X-ray technique which may well become the greatest advance made in the last 50 years. A beam of X-rays a few millimetres in width is passed transversely through the head and caused to scan linearly across the head. The emergent beam is detected electronically and the intensity of the beam expressed as a function of the path length and the absorption coefficient of the various body tissues traversed by the beam. The X-ray beam and detector are together moved through one deg. in the selected transverse plane and the procedure repeated. This process is continued until the system has rotated through 180 deg. in this plane. Some thirty thousand simultaneous equations are obtained for each rotation and solved using a computer. The solutions are expressed as varying degrees of brightness of a matrix on a television monitor. The resulting picture is a radiograph of the transverse slice of the body under investigation. The results so far obtained

621

in the sub-speciality of neuroradiology, to which, at present, this technique is applied, are undoubtedly superior to any other existing form of investigation.

Ionizing radiations used for therapeutic purposes must be chosen so as to provide high doses of radiation in prescribed volumes of tissue which are usually deep seated. It is therefore necessary that such radiations shall be of high energy and capable of deep penetration. These high energies are obtained by accelerating electrons to high speed and then allowing the electron beam to impinge directly on to tissue or on to a suitable metal target from which X-rays emerge and then impinge on to tissue. The energies required range up to tens of millions of electron volts. Alternatively gamma rays obtained from a disintegrating radioactive source may be used.

It is impracticable to accelerate an electron to the required energy by using a conventional X-ray tube and applying to it an electrical voltage of tens of millions of volts. Two alternative approaches are normally employed. In the linear accelerator a radio wave of frequency some thousands of megahertz* is produced and caused to travel inside a hollow metal tube of precise dimensions. This tube is known as a wave guide and the radiation travels inside it much as water travels inside a pipe. The speed at which the wave travels is caused to increase by varying the dimensions of the guide. Electrons are injected into the guide at the same velocity as the wave and travel on the crest of the wave much as a surfer travels on a water wave. As the velocity of the wave increases the electron is accelerated thus increasing in velocity and energy. Although the initial velocity of the electron requires a voltage of only some tens of thousands of volts the final velocity after acceleration is that which would be acquired had it been accelerated by a steady voltage of some millions of volts.

Circular acceleration as is produced in the cyclotron and betatron makes use of different physical principles. A moving electrical charge which is subjected to a steady magnetic field in a direction perpendicular to the line of motion experiences a force in the mutually perpendicular direction. The combined effect of the original velocity and the perpendicular force causes the charge to move in a circular path. In the cyclotron a powerful electromagnet produces an intense magnetic field, circular in cross section and many tens of centimetres in diameter. The charged particle such as a deuteron moves in a circular path transverse to the magnetic field. It is caused to increase in velocity twice in each revolution by means of an electric field alternating at the appropriate frequency and directed along the path of the particle. The cyclotron is not normally used to accelerate electrons but is more frequently employed to accelerate particles such as deuterons, which are then allowed to fall upon a target and produce radioactive substances. For clinical work the electron is required, and this is accelerated by a betatron. In this instrument the electron moves in a circular path round an axial magnetic field which varies in strength in a cyclical fashion. This variation induces an accelerating voltage along the path of the electron thus causing the electron

velocity to increase rapidly. In later instruments the actual voltages employed are of the order of tens of thousands whereas the final energy of the particle is that corresponding to acceleration through a steady voltage of tens of millions of volts.

High energy gamma rays are produced during the nuclear disintegration of certain radioactive substances, the most commonly employed being Cobalt 60. A fundamental property of all radioactive substances is that the atoms undergo disintegration at a rate proportional to the number of atoms present. In consequence of this the time required for one half the number of atoms in a given sample to disintegrate is fixed and is known as the half life. The intensity and energy of the gamma rays emitted are unique to the element concerned. Radioactive cobalt emits gamma rays having energies in the range 1·17 to 1·33 MeV. and of sufficient intensity to provide a high dose of radiation. Sources used for therapeutic purposes range in activity from tens of millicuries up to thousands of curies.* Since the radiation is emitted continuously in all directions it is necessary to shield the sources when not in use and to provide means whereby the size of the gamma ray beam can be controlled when used for treatment purposes. Shielding is achieved by surrounding the source with dense material such as lead or tungsten which, for intense sources, has a mass of several thousands of kilograms. An aperture in the shielding, from which a beam of gamma rays can emerge, is controlled in size by means of articulated "jaws" also constructed from dense material. These jaws provide the means of controlling the dimensions of the gamma ray beam.

The development of compact high output neutron tubes similar to conventional X-ray tubes has opened up the possibility of using neutrons for therapeutic treatment. Within the tube, neutrons are produced by bombarding a tritium target with deuterium ions producing an output of more than 10^{12} neutrons per second with energies of about 14·3 MeV. The neutron source is approximately 40 mm. in diameter and emits the neutrons almost isotropically. Shielding is essential to reduce the intensity to acceptable levels outside the area of the beam used for treatment. For this purpose a mutilayer protective shield comprising an inner core of iron and an outer layer of polythene and oil surrounds the tube save for the area from which the neutron beam is required to emerge. The dimensions of the emergent beam are determined by collimators constructed from suitable materials such as boron-loaded polythene.

Non-ionizing radiations include ultrasound, laser light beams, infra-red radiation and microwaves. Ultrasonic radiation is normally produced from the oscillations of crystals. Quartz was used originally for this purpose but increasingly a wide range of synthetic crystals is being introduced. Laser light beams most commonly originate from electrical discharges through gases. Infra-red radiation is emitted by any heat sources including the body.

---

* The Hertz is a unit of frequency corresponding to 1 cycle per second.

* The curie unit is a unit of radioactivity and is defined in terms of the number of disintegrations taking place in a given time. A substance undergoing $3·7 \times 10^{10}$ disintegrations per second is said to have an activity of 1 curie.

Sound waves are a longitudinal wave motion, that is to say the particles of the medium through which the sound is propagated vibrate about a mean position in the direction of propagation of the wave. Thus a series of compressions and rarefactions is produced. Any source of sound, whether it be in the audible range of frequencies up to 14 kHz. or in the ultrasonic range of frequencies from 20 kHz. to several megahertz, produces mechanical oscillations. In the case of ultrasound these oscillations are produced by a crystal exhibiting the piezo electric effect. This property is possessed by certain anisotropic crystals the effect being that, when the crystal is compressed along a particular direction, the faces of the crystal perpendicular to this direction acquire an electric charge. The reverse effect is also true, that is to say the crystal will expand or contract in this direction if an electric field is applied to these faces. An ultrasound transducer consists of a suitable crystal rigidly attached by one such face to a metal electrode. A second electrode, usually in the form of a thin conductive layer, is attached to the opposite face. Across the electrode an oscillating voltage is applied thus causing this opposite face to vibrate. To obtain maximum movement of this face it is necessary that the frequency of the applied oscillations match the natural frequency of oscillation of the crystal. Under these circumstances resonance occurs and a significant amount of power is dissipated from the moving face in the form of ultrasound.

For diagnostic purposes ultrasound is used in much the same way as radar. Short pulses of electrical oscillations are applied to the crystal thus providing pulses of ultrasound. If such a pulse is reflected back to the crystal face, arriving at an instant in time between the application of the electrical pulses, the reverse process takes place. In this instance the ultrasound compresses and extends this crystal face and produces electrical charges on the opposite faces of the crystal. The time interval elapsing between the emission of a pulse of ultrasound by the crystal and the return of this pulse by reflection back to the crystal, is related to the distance travelled by the pulse in the medium before reaching a reflective surface. Thus the distance of the reflecting surface from the crystal may be determined. The results of this are generally viewed in one of two ways known as "A" scope and "B" scope presentations. In "A" scope presentation the transmitted pulse is caused to start the electron beam of a cathode ray tube moving horizontally across the tube at a constant rate, thus producing a horizontal trace known as the time base. The return pulse causes a vertical deflection of the electron beam thus showing a spike on the time base. The distance of this spike from the origin of the trace is a measure of the distance traversed in the medium by the pulse of ultrasound. In "B" scope presentation the electron beam is caused to move radially from the centre of the cathode ray tube but the beam is suppressed so that no trace appears on the tube face. The return pulse is caused to remove this suppression and thus brighten the trace at the appropriate point. With this method of presentation the transducer is mounted in such a manner that it can be moved in one selected plane only and any such movement causes a similar movement of the radius

along which the electron beam moves in the cathode ray tube. Thus a cross-sectional plan of all reflected pulses in this plane is shown on the tube.

Sources of ultrasound designed for therapeutic use are fundamentally the same as those already described. Important differences are firstly the need for power output which is some thousands of times greater, and secondly the need for continuous as opposed to pulsed output. Since there is no interest in the reflected waves such equipment does not require to present data as in "A" scope or "B" scope techniques. However it may be necessary to bring the sound waves to a focus at some point within the irradiated material. For this purpose lenses are employed and these, unlike those used in optics, are normally constructed from metal. Because of the relative velocity of sound in metal and liquids the shape of these lenses is opposite to those used for light. Thus a converging lens has a concave face whereas for light it would have a convex face. It is also necessary that there should be controlled variation of the power output and this is normally obtained by variation in amplitude of the electrical oscillation applied to the crystal.

The theory underlying the production of laser light is referred to later. The apparatus required for this consists of a gas-filled tube through which an electrical discharge takes place. A suitable high voltage power supply of conventional design is coupled to the tube. Of the gases known to be suitable, a mixture of helium and neon or carbon dioxide is most commonly used. The construction of the discharge tube is characterized by two features, namely, a narrow tube of dimension millimeters or less to concentrate the discharge, and optically flat inclined windows at the ends of the tube. At either end of the tube mirrors are mounted to cause the light to be reflected back into the discharge tube. One of these mirrors is partially silvered to permit the controlled escape of light rays. Both mirrors are aligned with great precision since any maladjustment will prevent the production of the laser beam. The size of this apparatus is related to the power output required. At low power both tube and power supply may be contained in a cover some few centimetres square and some tens of centimetres in length which is comfortably held in the hand. High power laser may be some hundreds of centimetres in length, correspondingly large in cross-section, and will require specially designed mountings to handle the mass involved.

Sources of microwave radiation are essentially circuits in which electric currents oscillate at the required frequency. The circuit is designed to resonate at this frequency and frequently comprises a cavity resonator. Power is fed into the resonator from a thermionic valve. Output power is taken from the resonator by cable to a suitable antenna from which it is radiated into space as a radio wave.

THE PHYSICAL PROPERTIES OF RADIATION

Ionizing Radiation

Although sub-atomic particles tend to be thought of as discrete but minute particles of "solid" matter and electromagnetic radiations as waves, in fact this distinction is neither real nor, on occasions, does it assist in understanding the various processes involved when these radiations interact with matter. Particles have certain wave characteristics associated with them as is well shown by diffraction of electrons. Waves have certain particulate characteristics as is demonstrated by photographic and photoelectric effects. It is more appropriate to recognize that waves and particles have associated with them an amount of energy normally expressed in a unit known as the electron volt.* In the case of particles this energy may be equated to the kinetic energy, whence is derived the concept of the particle moving at a velocity which may be extremely large. By comparison the wave may, for most purposes, be regarded as moving at a fixed velocity and the concept of energy is here related to the wave consisting of a series of discrete packets of energy or quanta.

Of fundamental importance are the interactions that take place when these radiations pass through matter. Whatever the nature of these interactions the radiation loses energy and whilst there may be primary, secondary, or tertiary processes involved, the ultimate effect is for the lost energy to be dispersed as thermal energy. For the most part the energy of the radiation is vastly in excess of the binding energy of molecules and of orbital electrons. Thus the probability exists that these bonds can be broken by energy absorbed from the radiation. Accompanying this process is the release of electrons of varying energy and a trail of ionized atoms and molecules. Thus the track of an ionizing particle is characterized by a transfer of energy along the track to the matter through which the particle is passing. This energy transfer is most usefully measured in terms of keV. per micron track length. It is to be noted that transfer is not the same for all particles and depends, in a complicated way, upon the energy and charge of the particles, even when the primary beam is mono-energetic. Almost invariably there is a spread of energy in the primary beam thus further complicating the process. These interactions are complex but in general result in

(a) the production of electrons of varying energy; and
(b) the production of X and gamma rays of varying energy.

In consequence of this the linear energy transfer also varies within the absorbing material. Thus for electrons having energies in the range 1 keV. to 1 MeV. in water the energy transfer varies from 12–0·25 keV. per μm., the greatest transfer taking place with the least energetic particles. A similar situation obtains for X and gamma rays. X-rays having a nominal energy of 200 keV. transfer energy at a rate varying from 0·4–36 keV. per μm. in water whereas gamma rays from Cobalt 60 having energies of 1·17 and 1·33 MeV. in the same absorber transfer energy at from 0·2–2 keV. per μm. Neutrons lose energy by collision with atomic nuclei, somewhat after the manner of two billiard balls colliding. Neutrons may have a wide range of energy and at the lower end of this range the energy loss can occur by absorption into the

nucleus producing nuclear changes. The new nucleus may be unstable and lose energy by the emission of particles or electromagnetic radiation. These emissions subsequently transfer energy to the absorbing material.

As a consequence of these energy losses the primary beam of radiation is attenuated when passing through an absorbing substance. The attenuation varies with

(a) the energy of the radiation; and
(b) the atomic number of the absorbing material;

and thus coefficients of absorption are not fixed quantities.

Non-ionizing Radiation

Unlike electromagnetic radiation ultrasound is totally dependent upon a material medium for transmission and as the medium varies so does the velocity of the ultrasound. It is in fact a mechanical wave motion consisting of a series of compressions and rarefactions of the medium moving in the direction of propagation of the wave motion. The frequency is much in excess of those to which the ear can respond and may be as much as several megahertz. The particles of the medium vibrate about a mean position at this frequency with an amplitude depending upon the intensity of the wave. For a given intensity the kinetic energy of these particles depends upon the square of the frequency. Similarly the accelerating force giving rise to this kinetic energy depends upon the square of the frequency. It is these large velocities and accelerating forces which give rise to internal frictional forces in the medium through which the ultrasound passes. Ultimately the mechanical work done against these frictional forces results in the production of heat. This heat represents a loss of energy from the wave motion thus attenuating the intensity of the ultrasound beam. Other mechanical effects such as cavitation may occur to a degree dependent upon the intensity of the radiation. It is usual to express the attenuation in decibels per cm.* This varies with the medium but for a given medium increases logarithmically with frequency.

Ultrasound can be reflected and refracted in a manner somewhat similar to audible sound. Reflection takes place at interfaces between media where there is a change in their specific acoustic impedance. This impedance depends upon the density of the medium and the velocity of ultrasound in that medium. In practice this implies that at a solid-gas interface there is total internal reflection. For this reason an ultrasonic generator cannot transfer energy through air and must be coupled to a medium by a substance, usually an air-free liquid, which has a suitable matching impedance. Refraction of ultrasound arises from the same cause as refraction of light, that is variation of velocity in different media and so it is possible to construct and use lenses. Sources of ultrasound can be constructed to produce a highly directional beam by using a single source of dimensions at least ten times greater than the

---

* The electron volt is that amount of energy acquired by an electron in moving through a potential difference of 1 V. The numerical value is $1·602 \times 10^{-10}$ J., and the symbol eV.

* The decibel is a simple number expressing the ratio of two powers. Thus if the powers are p^1 and p^2 their relative levels in decibels are $10 \log_{10}(p^1/p^2)$.

wavelength of the radiation. This is in contrast to visible light where the source is an atom or molecule having dimensions which are many times smaller than the wavelength of the light which is emitted equally in all directions.

Radiation in the form of laser light has ultimately the same characteristics as ordinary light, that is to say it can be reflected, refracted and attenuated when incident upon an absorbing material. However, there are certain limitations attaching to conventional light sources which do not apply to laser beams and thereby confer upon the laser beam those features which render it especially useful. These limitations are:

(a) a spread of wavelength in the radiated energy;
(b) collimation can only be achieved with mirrors and lenses resulting in loss of intensity;
(c) sources of great brightness can in general operate only for a short period of time;
(d) it is impossible to increase the brightness of an image over that of a source; and
(e) lack of coherency.

By definition, a laser is a device that amplifies light by means of the stimulated emissions of radiation. The most commonly used light generator is an electric discharge through a gas, with a feed-back mechanism in the form of mirrors. In general, energy is supplied to the laser medium, that is the gas, to ensure that more atoms in the medium are in an excited state than are in the normal unexcited state. Under these circumstances one excited atom may stimulate another so that both produce light output which is identical. As the light beam progresses through the medium this process is repeated. Mirrors at either end of the discharge path reflect the beam back and forth thus giving the opportunity in each traverse for further light to be produced and creating a resonant cavity. Partial silvering of one mirror permits the escape of some of the beam. The inherent properties of light produced in this manner are:

(a) spatial and temporal coherence;
(b) very small divergence of the light beam;
(c) high intensity; and
(d) monochromaticity.

Light from a conventional source derives from the individual atoms or molecules comprising that source. These emit the light in a random and unco-ordinated fashion so that the light waves from each source bear no fixed relationship to one another. The reverse situation obtains with laser light for which there is a constant phase relationship between two points on a series of equal amplitude wavefronts, and a correlation in time between the same points on different wave fronts. Light having these characteristics is described as coherent. The temporal coherence of the laser beam derives from the fact that the light emitted is close to being monochromatic whilst the spatial coherence is largely responsible for the fact that the angular divergence of the beam is of the order of milli-radians.

Perhaps the most important characteristic of the laser beam is its enormous intensity which is normally expressed as watts per cm². In many cases the laser output is not delivered continuously but in pulses. Thus the peak pulse power as well as the mean power is a relevant parameter. The power delivered at any point may be still further increased by focusing the beam to remove or diminish the beam divergence. Under these circumstances peak powers of the order of hundreds of megawatts may be produced providing a brightness vastly in excess of sunlight. In passing through matter energy absorbed from the laser beam is manifested as heat. The absorbed energy depends upon the wavelength of the light and upon the optical absorption spectrum of the medium as in the case of conventional optical absorption. In consequence of this the greatest thermal stress will arise in regions of maximum absorption. Additionally with high intensity beams pressure waves may be set up, giving rise to a transient sonic wave. This wave can cause simple mechanical disruption of the absorbing material due to shear stresses. Associated with the laser beam is an electrical field, the magnitude of which is estimated to be comparable with the inter-atomic binding forces. The effects resulting from the interaction of these fields have yet to be fully assessed but may result in the release of high energy particles or X and gamma rays.

Infra-red radiation extends from the red end of the visible spectrum over a wide range of longer wavelengths. All objects at a temperature above absolute zero emit infra-red with an intensity and range of wavelengths dependent upon the temperature of the source and the nature of the emitter. A surface emitting all the wavelengths appropriate to the temperature of the surface is a perfect emitter, described as a black body. Similarly such a surface will also absorb all radiation incident upon it. A black body in no way relates to the colour of the surface; thus, for example, human skin, whatever the colour, is almost a perfect black body. Since all objects commonly encountered are at a temperature above absolute zero, all objects emit infra-red. Equally all such objects receive radiation from their surroundings. Whether the temperature of the object rises or falls depends upon whether the rate at which heat is received is greater or smaller than the rate of loss. Ultimately any such object will reach the temperature of the environment. Radiation emission and absorption do not then cease but the exchange continues under conditions of dynamic equilibrium. Change of temperature of the object or the surroundings, or the introduction of another object at a different temperature, will disturb the equilibrium. Unequal emission and absorption will take place until the equilibrium is re-established.

The absorption characteristics of infra-red arise primarily from interactions with molecules. They are, therefore, dependent both upon the nature of the absorbing material and the energy or wavelength of the radiation. Absorbed energy is manifested as heat which may be conducted and convected away from the region of absorption. The effects of the release of heat are, therefore, dependent upon the thermal properties of the absorbing material. If the rate of delivery of heat is greater than the rate of loss of heat from the region of interest a local rise in temperature will occur. Thus the effect of short pulses of high intensity radiation are likely to be entirely different from the effects of the same amount of radiation delivered at a steady rate.

The interaction of microwave radiation with biological tissues is far from being fully understood. Disruption of chemical bonds or of the electronic structure of atoms appears unlikely and it is more probable that either the electric or magnetic field associated with the waves is responsible. The distribution of electric charge on a water molecule is known to be asymmetrical so that in an electrical field these molecules will tend to align themselves parallel to the field. In a high frequency field the orientation of the molecules will tend to follow the changes in direction of the field. Physical work done against internal frictional forces is then dissipated in the form of heat. Thus the heating effect of microwaves in tissue is likely to be affected by the water content. However in the human body water content varies in the different layers of skin, fat, and muscle and the microwaves are reflected at the various interfaces. The mechanism of absorption of energy in the body is complicated and as yet not fully understood.

DETECTION AND MEASUREMENT OF RADIATION

Although quantitative measurement is frequently difficult, effective use of radiation requires exact measurement if the biological effects are to be understood. Early recognition of this principle by those concerned with the use of ionizing radiations for therapeutic treatment of malignant disease led to the definition of units of dose. The use of physical units to measure doses delivered by the non-ionizing radiation in the biological sciences is, however, comparatively rare.

Ionizing Radiation

The classical unit is the roentgen which is based upon the quantity of electric charge produced in air by the radiation. Defined in this manner the roentgen is essentially a physical unit capable of realization under laboratory conditions by allowing a precise mass of air to be irradiated and measuring the charge produced. The practical instrument derived from this laboratory procedure is the ionization chamber. In this the ions produced in a small air-filled container are collected by electrodes and measured and recorded by suitable electronic circuits.

As a clinical unit the roentgen is of limited value; accordingly a second unit of absorbed dose, the rad, is now in common use. This unit is defined simply in terms of the absorbed energy, in J per kg. of absorbing material. The biological effect of an absorbed dose of radiation depends upon a number of factors such as the system irradiated, the rate of absorption of energy, the kind of ionizing radiation used, and the degree of oxygenation of the tissues. Thus the dose in rads must be further modified by a factor known as the relative biological effectiveness (RBE) or quality factor (QF). The resulting biological dose is expressed in terms of a unit known as the rem.

The quantity capable of direct measurement is the exposure in roentgens, the numerical value of which must be converted by these factors to absorbed dose in rads and biological dose in rems. For low energy X-rays absorbed in soft tissue these conversion factors are approximately unity. In this particular case the exposure in roentgens is numerically the same as the biological dose in rems. However there are marked differences in these values when, for example, electrons are used and when the target tissue is bone.

Non-ionizing Radiation

The introduction of ultrasound as a radiation for use in diagnosis and therapy entails a need for establishing dosage. Since the ultimate form of energy derived from the absorption of ultrasound is heat, a calorimetric method of determining dose would seem to be appropriate. However this technique is essentially a laboratory procedure and unsuited for the purpose of clinical measurement. Instead a direct measurement of temperature rise in biological material may be determined by the insertion of fine thermocouples into the material under investigation, provided the presence of these does not distort the structure or affect the rate of absorption of energy.

A further accepted method of determining the power output of a transducer is by pressure measurement. Since ultrasound is conveyed by particles of the medium moving in the direction of propagation of the wave, changes in momentum must occur if these particles impinge upon a solid medium. This medium experiences a force due to these changes and this force is simply related to the rate of change of momentum and, hence, is related directly to the power of the ultrasound beam.

As with ultrasound, so with the laser any attempt to quantify the interaction effects of its radiation requires a knowledge of the magnitude of output levels. Essentially such knowledge must take into account both the total energy in the beam and the area of cross section of the beam, so that the unit employed is joules per square centimetre. There are, however, other factors of significance, notably the beam divergence and the pulse duration. Combination of these factors enables a statement of the rate of delivery of energy or power in watts per square centimetre to be made. If this power is related solely to the time during which the laser pulse is delivered then the figure obtained reflects the peak power output, but if averaged over a number of pulses it becomes mean power. In general terms statements of power output require to be qualified with a clear reference both to the measurement technique and to the various beam parameters taken into account.

Commonly the method of measurement requires that the total pulse energy shall be absorbed with a suitable device and the resulting rise in temperature determined. Suitable absorbing devices are a hollow cone or a loosely but randomly packed ball of insulated copper wire. Multiple reflections take place inside the cone, with a percentage of beam energy being absorbed at each reflection and the resulting temperature rise measured with thermistors or thermocouples. In the case of the copper wire the temperature rise is determined from the change in electrical resistance.

Measurement of infra-red radiation also poses problems which are essentially calorimetric. Because the therapeutic use of this radiation has for many years been conducted on a subjective basis little effort has been devoted to the development of suitable detectors. In contradistinction to this the diagnostic use of infra-red emitted by the human body has been subject to more scientific and objective analysis, and detectors for measurement of long wavelength infra-red are much better developed.

Such instruments as are available for measuring high intensity sources of infra-red are based upon the total absorption of the radiation by a black body. The temperature of the black body is measured using thermocouples or thermistors. It is necessary to ensure that the black body is in a constant temperature environment and this may be achieved by surrounding all but the surface exposed to the radiation with a water cooled enclosure.

Long wave-length infra-red, such as is emitted by the human body, is detected by using semi-conducting substances such as indium antimonide and mercury cadium telluride. The absorption of the infra-red radiation releases electrical charge carriers in proportion to the total energy absorbed. Since such release can also be produced due to the energy of electrons at ambient temperature the required sensitivity can be obtained only if the detector is cooled to liquid nitrogen temperature.

True dosimetric measurements on biological systems exposed to microwave radiation cannot as yet be made. Direct measurement of radiation intensity is made using suitably calibrated radio receivers. The insertion into the radiation field of heterogeneous absorbing material modifies the intensity distribution of the radiation. Frequently temperature measurements at various sites in the absorber are the only meaningful observations that can be made.

HAZARDS ASSOCIATED WITH RADIATION
Ionizing Radiations

The consequences of the interaction of ionizing radiation with tissue are assumed to arise from the production of ion pairs along the track of the radiation. Oxidation and reduction reactions are known to be initiated when certain chemical solutions are exposed to ionizing radiations. It is reasonable to suppose that similar reactions take place in the aqueous solutions occurring within the cellular organization of living tissue. Nevertheless despite extensive researches no comprehensive theory of radiation effects at the sub-cellular level is as yet extant. There is an "accidental" flavour associated with radiation damage which is unlikely to be explained solely on the basis of the energy being delivered as quanta and hence the concept of probability that a quantum of radiation will achieve a damaging "hit". Moreover, the subsequent history of any cellular or micro-cellular damage is likely to be affected by metabolic repair processes. Thus, although dose-effect relationships may be postulated many factors may inter-

vene to modify the effect of a given dose. It is clear that knowledge in this field is far from exact; nevertheless, there is a general consensus of thought that, whatever the magnitude of the dose, damage will occur.

Such data as are available concerning biological damage are derived from animal experiments and from observations on humans exposed to radiation occupationally or as a result of accident. Much of the evidence so gained is related, more especially in the case of humans, to the effects observed in individuals exposed to relatively high doses. Of much greater concern are the likely consequences of low dose, chronic irradiation in relatively small groups such as radiation workers, or low dose irradiation of large numbers of persons such as arises from the diagnostic use of X-rays and gamma rays. Extrapolation of data from animal experiments and from the relatively small groups of humans referred to earlier is difficult and uncertain, involving assumptions of dubious validity concerning dose-effect relationships. It is from this state of informed ignorance that judgments must be made concerning acceptable levels of exposure. Although in many countries statute law imposes no limitation on the amount and kind of radiation that may be used for diagnostic or therapeutic purposes, there are strong ethical considerations to be borne in mind by all who use this tool. None would deny its great value but there is a deep and serious obligation upon all users to weigh the cost against the benefit and to proceed with proper caution.

The detectable somatic effects of radiation in the person exposed to radiation are well documented. Inhibition of cellular mitosis is one of the earliest effects and can readily be demonstrated in tissue cultures. Cellular death, and clumping and fragmentation of chromosomes are recognized effects. Production of free radicals in aqueous solution and their probable reaction with nucleoproteins may be assumed to play a part in the process. There remains a wide gulf between these partial explanations and the known effects of skin damage, late induction of carcinoma, haemolytic effects, and the possible effect of premature aging. The correlation between damage and single doses from high intensity sources, more especially when the whole body is irradiated, is reasonably established. There is no such correlation between damage and the same dose delivered over a much longer period of time. At low levels comparison is sometimes made with the background radiation arising from naturally occurring radioactive substances and cosmic rays. However, this radiation varies widely throughout the world as do also the social, economic, ethnic and environmental backgrounds of the persons exposed to it. Nevertheless, in default of better standards, it is sometimes assumed that, as a rough yardstick, a dose of radiation of the same order as background delivered at the same rate is unlikely to cause damage which may be specifically attributed to the radiation.

Still less well documented and even less well explained is genetic damage. By extrapolation from animal experiments it is assumed that irradiation of the gonads can increase the spontaneous gene mutation rate. It is further presumed that such mutations will introduce into a population unwanted or deleterious genetic changes. Such changes are frequently, but almost certainly incorrectly, assumed to be gross. It seems more probable that, in fact, there would be an increase over the whole range of genetic abnormalities, many of which might be regarded as little more than social handicaps. Even if this is the case it in no way diminishes the undesirable nature of such changes. Nor indeed does it in any way modify the likelihood that changes, once induced, may endure for many generations before they disappear.

The mechanism responsible for these changes is inadequately understood. Equally obscure is the dose of radiation to produce a given change in the spontaneous gene mutation rate. Data from individual cases are of little help and indeed it is possible to select published data to support almost any level of dose giving rise to damage. It is in fact unlikely that any study which is not based upon careful observation of large numbers of persons over several generations will produce conclusive evidence.

It follows from the foregoing that there is no safe dose of radiation and that all levels of radiation are likely to cause a degree of damage. Difficult though it is, an attempt to define levels of dose which, in the light of present knowledge, produce an acceptably low level of damage is essential. Levels of dose which confer an acceptable degree of risk, compatible with that arising from everyday life, have been established by the International Commission on Radiological Protection and are maintained under continuous review. These levels are regarded as maximum doses and in practice many users of ionizing radiations can proceed with their work and receive substantially less than these maximum levels. There is, however, more concern and greater difficulty in establishing similar levels for the general public who may well be exposed to increasing doses arising from the clinical use of radiation and the increasing number of peaceful uses of atomic energy.

Non-ionizing Radiation

Since the introduction of ultrasound into biological sciences studies have been made and are continuing in an attempt to define levels of power at which cellular damage occurs. Experimental work with animals suggests that there exists a threshold dose for cellular damage which is immediately visible. This threshold dose is likely to be dependent upon the intensity of the source and the duration of the irradiation. It is also possible that sub-threshold damage of a different nature may occur and that the effects of this damage may not become manifest until some later time. The power output utilized in this type of experimentation is at least an order of magnitude greater than that used for diagnostic purposes. It might be expected that if cellular damage is to occur with these low powers then such damage would most likely be detected in the fetus subjected to ultrasonic examination. Whilst the possibility of damage demands constant vigilance, nevertheless present evidence suggests that the use of low intensity ultrasound confers no detectable cellular damage.

A complete laser safety programme is essential if these sources are to be used without hazard. The areas of the body at risk are:

(a) the eye;
(b) the skin; and
(c) the respiratory tract.

The portion of the eye most at risk depends upon the wavelength of the light. Thus the eye is relatively transparent to radiation over the wavelength range 400–1,400 nm. and, therefore, can be affected not only by the visible light (400–700 nm.) but also by short wavelength infrared. Laser light emitted in the visible range is focussed by the eye on to the retina and since the brightness of the beam may be thousands of times greater than that of the sun retinal burns are readily produced. At longer wavelengths greater absorption may take place in the cornea, the lens, and the aqueous and vitreous humour and damage to these regions of the eye is more likely. Research into eye damage continues and values for maximum safe levels of irradiation are still subjects for debate.

Damage to the skin may arise from acute or chronic exposures. The former is most likely to result from the direct exposure of the skin to the laser beam and is, therefore, confined to a small area. Chronic exposure arises from scattering of the beam and may involve all or part of the normally exposed skin. Acute exposure gives rise to skin burns which result from the absorption of the heat energy in skin pigmentation. The extent and depth of the burn depends upon the rate of dissipation of power at the site of irradiation and may, because of the relative transparency of the skin to various wavelengths, even involve underlying organs. Little is known concerning the total effect of chronic irradiation which, therefore, remains as an area to be assessed.

Respiratory tract damage may arise from air pollution as a result of the release at the site of irradiation of particles such as bacteria, tumour fragments, or metal fragments. The possibility of biological harm to the operator clearly depends upon the nature of the particles, the extent to which they are explosively erupted from the site, and the extent to which they are assimilated into the body. Safety measures to guard against each of the hazards are necessary and are relatively simple to implement.

The hazards arising from infra-red radiation are significantly less than those from the laser beam because of the much reduced intensity from sources in common use. Accordingly such precautions as may be required are minimal and amount in general to much scaled down versions of those applicable to laser beams.

Reported pathological effects of microwave radiation relate primarily to haematological changes, production of defects in the lens of the eye, and damage to the testes. The bulk of evidence for these effects stems from animal experiments and is thought to arise from thermal damage. There is, however, concern over possible non-thermal damage which may affect the central nervous system. Much remains to be done before these effects are substantiated and before permissible exposure levels for humans are the subject of international agreement as is the case for ionizing radiations.

APPLICATIONS OF RADIATION

Ionizing Radiation

The conventional uses of X-rays for diagnostic purposes are sufficiently well known to require no further discussion. However, the methods normally adopted to extract information from the modulated beam of X-rays emerging from a patient are inefficient and result in loss of data. Thus further progress may be expected in the analysis of these data by computer techniques. Extending and modifying the conventional image intensifier, solid state amplifiers, smaller in physical size and more efficient in data capture, may well add greater scope to diagnostic X-ray techniques. The photographic emulsion has for long been regarded as the method of choice for recording the X-ray beam. Despite this, electrostatic techniques making use of xerographic and triboelectric effects provide methods of recording in which control of contrast and detail are as good as, if not superior to, those obtained with film.

Techniques that employ radioactive substances now constitute an important element in the diagnostic armamentarium. Apart from their use as laboratory tools, their application to *in vivo* measurements and observations on patients is expanding rapidly. A suitable compound, labelled with a gamma emitting radioactive element, which is selectively absorbed by normal or abnormal tissue or is incorporated in a physiological process, is adminstered. An external detector measures the emission of rays from a large volume of body tissue or from many small adjacent areas of the body. The former detectors are described as probes and the latter as gamma cameras or rectilinear scanners. Probes have long been used to investigate metabolic and cellular processes whilst cameras and scanners provide elegant methods of directly imaging the size, shape and normality of body organs. Computer processing of the data obtained provides objective assessment of the information content of images and physiological parameters. As they develop, these techniques, more especially parametric analysis, under dynamic conditions, may be expected to become powerful diagnostic tools.

The dosimetry, planning and apparatus for the delivery of X and gamma rays for orthodox treatment of cancer now have a precision far exceeding the prediction of biological results. To conventional radiations have now been added the high Linear Energy Transfer radiations of electrons and fast neutrons. Penetration of electrons is related to their energy which, in turn, affects the size and complexity of the generator. Selectively, electrons of energy about 12 MeV. are used for treatment of superficial lesions. Following early unsuccessful attempts, radio-biological research has pointed the way for the use of fast neutrons. Clinical trials are now in progress to evaluate the efficacy of this radiation in treating suitable tumours such as squamous cell carcinoma of the bladder, cervix, brain and pharyngeal tract.

Non-ionizing Radiation

Microwave radiation at 433 MHz. is the most recent radiation to be used for both detection and treatment of cancer. Using a cylindrical antenna system the patient is partially enveloped in a bath of radiation. Little data of a scientific, cytological, or histopathological nature are available to support or disprove claims made for this treatment. Controlled trials may justify the use of this technique alone or in combination with other established methods.

Ultrasound provides a recognized, if as yet relatively undeveloped, means of investigating soft tissues and certain dynamic processes. The shift of mid-line structures of the brain using A scope presentation, and examination of the pregnant uterus and the abdomen with B scope presentation, are established uses. Using Doppler techniques measurement of fetal heart rate and peripheral blood flow are equally well established. Much remains to be done in the biological and physical aspects of ultrasound if this facility is to be fully exploited.

The diagnostic uses of thermographic techniques are necessarily restricted to the examination of factors affecting skin temperature. When the uncovered skin is in dynamic thermal equilibrium with constant temperature surroundings, the factor of prime importance is peripheral blood supply. By scanning the infra-red emitted from the area of interest the skin temperature is used to modulate the brightness of a television monitor thus producing a "temperature picture". Any pathological, traumatic, or surgical factor affecting peripheral blood supply may be seen. Tumours of the breast, peripheral vascular insufficiency, placental site and blood supply to skin flaps have been investigated with this technique.

The potentialities of the laser beam in diagnostic and therapeutic medicine have yet to be fully realized. Apart from some experimental applications in surgery the most frequent use is for the treatment of detached retina. The inherent properties of laser light render it suitable for microscopic transmission and thus for micro-surgery, even on a cellular basis. As holographic techniques are developed for study of motion lasers will be the light source of choice.

55. ELECTROSURGERY AND CRYOSURGERY

D. E. POSWILLO

INTRODUCTION

The biological effects of such physical factors as heat, cold and ionizing radiation have been used for centuries in the course of medical and dental practice. Both heat and cold behave like ionizing radiation in one particular respect; the maximal lethal effect is obtained when they are applied to cells undergoing mitosis. For this reason, the first attempts to employ heat and cold for tissue destruction were directed to the local removal of tumours. Limitations in the original equipment prevented the most effective application of these physical agents in the therapeutic field. Nevertheless, interest in such methods of treatment has persisted over the intervening years, and today both electrosurgery and cryosurgery have defined roles in the management of dental and surgical disease.

ELECTROSURGERY

The use of heat as a surgical tool was known to the Egyptians about 3,000 B.C.; Hippocrates *circa* 400 B.C. used heat for opening abscesses, and Celsus employed the cautery to control haemorrhage. Soon after the discovery of electricity, surgeons developed an electrocautery which coagulated tissues by heat. The invention of the spark-gap generator made high-frequency electrosurgery possible, and soon after this, in 1891, d'Arsonval discovered that an electric current oscillating 10,000 times or more per second could be passed through living tissue without causing painful muscular contractions. This finding made possible the development of electrosurgical apparatus capable of incorporating the patient as part of an electrical circuit, and using an active electrode at a chosen place for the selective destruction of living tissues. Thus the electrosurgical instrument differs from the electrocautery. The former heats the tissues between two electrodes which do not become hot themselves, whereas the latter utilizes an element with a high resistance which becomes "burning" hot when the current is passed through it. Most modern electrosurgical equipment involves the use of two electrodes. In machines with a high power output, one element is an earth-plate attached to the patient. This is the principle employed in most large diathermy machines in operating theatres. In dental surgical practice, however, the machines have a lower output, less than 400 W., and the electrodes can be made less cumbersome, thus avoiding the necessity for an "indifferent", or earth-plate. The two terminals in the popular Birtcher Hyfrecator are separated by insulating material, and together they form an integral diathermy unit.

When electrodes of about equal size are employed, warmth but no tissue destruction is obtained because the current is evenly dispersed. When electrodes grossly unequal in size are used, and the small electrode is applied to the tissues, all the heat energy potentiated by the current radiates towards the small electrode and produces an intense destructive effect.

Instrumentation

Most modern electrosurgical apparatus used in dental and oral surgery is compact, portable, and simple to use. A large selection of interchangeable active electrodes can be fitted into the insulated handle. The intensity of the current can be controlled, and variations made according to the thickness of the selected electrode, the density of the tissues, viscosity of the saliva, presence of blood, and fluctuations in the electric supply. The electrode may be a needle, a ball, or a loop in basic design. It is operated by a foot-switch and applied to the tissues with precision and absence of pressure. Rapid and accurate movements should be used to guide the electrode to perform the tissue destruction, using brush-like strokes. Adhesion of charred tissues to the electrode is indicative of faulty technique. The active electrode should not be held in contact with bone; soft tissues over bone can be cut or coagulated adequately without substantial damage to the underlying hard tissues, provided that the electrode is kept moving. When performing cutting procedures a high current intensity is desirable. The reverse is true for electrocoagulation procedures, where a low current output is more desirable.

Variations in construction of the high-frequency generator produce differences in oscillation patterns which are reputed to be of clinical significance. The three principal types of oscillation found in equipment in current use are:

(a) Damped oscillations from "spark-gap" equipment;
(b) undamped periodically-interrupted oscillations from "tube current" machines; and
(c) high-frequency current from "fully-rectified tube" machines.

"Spark-gap" equipment produces more charring and damage to underlying structures than the high-frequency currents produced by tube generators. Bearing in mind that the cutting properties of the "tube generators" are better than the "spark-gap" appliances, the variations which arise from operative technique are at least as likely to affect the result as differences in the basic equipment. For this reason, the expenditure of large sums of money on expensive apparatus would seem to be contraindicated.

A recent investigation of the technical aspects of electrosurgery has revealed that the electrode tip configuration, the power level, and the operative technique can account for many of the clinical similarities observed when appliances are switched from "cut" to "coagulate". To achieve the maximum desired effect, be it coagulation or cutting, great attention must be given to electrode shape. A small change in electrode dimension can cause a great change in electrode surface area and wide variations in both current density and local heat dispersion.

The Biological Effects of Surgical Diathermy

Electrosurgical currents act on all tissues in a similar fashion, first to produce cellular dehydration and disintegration, and subsequently coagulation necrosis. These effects may be varied in three ways, namely coagulation, fulguration and cutting.

Coagulation is the simple direct application of heat by local contact of the electrode. There is a consequent drying-out of the cells when the current is applied. It is especially useful to seal off bleeding vessels or arrest general vascular oozing in cut tissues, or to coagulate ulcerated surfaces, or destroy granulation tissue.

Fulguration occurs where the electrode is held at a short distance from the tissues, with the creation of a "spark-gap". This induces destructive coagulation of tissues with charring of the surface. It is useful for the destruction of papilliferous and granulomatous growths, tissue tags, and sinus openings.

Cutting involves the use of the diathermy as a scalpel. The electrode is moved through the tissues to produce tissue disintegration and cleavage with minimal coagulation of adjacent tissues. It is useful in many ways in the practice of conservative dentistry and periodontology.

The general morphology of coagulated tissues is preserved but cellular and fibrillar detail are lost. The degree of injury diminishes as the distance from the point of wounding increases (fig. 1). After 24 hr. the wound is covered with a fibrin layer in which polymorphonuclear leucocytes are enmeshed. The leucocyte invasion increases in the following 48 hr. and the wound becomes covered with necrotic debris. After four days the necrotic surface has been replaced by inflammatory cells and fibrin. Fibroblasts appear in the depths of the wound, and by eight days organization of the covering clot is almost complete. By 18 days dense bundles of collagen fibres appear in the depths of the wound, which is covered by a thin, pale, epithelial cover. At four weeks little evidence of any wound (fig. 2) remains except slight erythema, or a poorly defined depression on the skin surface. It has been shown in non-human primates that electrosurgery retarded healing of oral mucosa by 10–14 days when compared with scalpel excision. The degree of scar tissue

formation following electrosurgery was less than that which followed repair of the surgically excised wound (fig. 3). Similar results have been observed in the gingival region in dogs and the degree of bone injury following gingival electrosurgery was seen to be much greater than that which followed sharp excision.

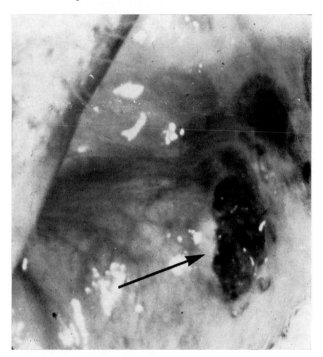

FIG. 1. Electrosurgical wound on the oral mucosa of the buccal sulcus; the tissues in the treated area are coagulated and charred.

The Specific Uses of Electrosurgery in Dental Surgery

In the field of restorative dentistry, electrosurgery has been used for desensitizing hypersensitive cervical erosions, and for sterilizing root canals. Gingival and granulation tissues overgrowing the margins of deep cavities can be "wiped" away with the cutting current, providing clear bloodless access for cavity preparation. In the preparation of crowns and bridges, electrosurgery is used to elongate the clinical crown, for exposing and reclaiming retained roots, for post preparations, and for preparing a pre-impression trench around the base of a crown preparation.

In periodontal practice, electrosurgery is used for gingivectomy, frenectomy, removal of granulations from infrabony pockets, and re-contouring the gingivae.

In the field of prosthetic dentistry electrosurgery is frequently used for the elimination of hyperplastic tissues in the sulcus area, and for extending the ridge available for prosthetic retention. Hypertrophic mucosa may be removed by cutting or coagulating currents; bloodless submucous resection can be carried out with the cutting electrode.

In the sphere of orthodontics electrosurgical apparatus may be used to expose buried teeth prior to banding for traction into the arch; for the resection of labial and lingual frena, for exposing the clinical crown of partly erupted teeth, and for controlling hyperplastic gingivitis associated with orthodontic bands.

Oral surgeons have used electrosurgery for the resection of peri-coronal flaps, for the destruction of benign lesions of the gingival and oral mucosa, for the removal of mucous retention cysts, and fibrous hyperplasias commonly seen in denture wearers, and for biopsy and palliation of malignant

As with most other aids to dental practice, good results depend upon a thorough understanding of the limitations of the technique. To assist in an appreciation of the merits and defects of electrosurgery these will be annotated briefly, with the shortcomings and dangers listed first.

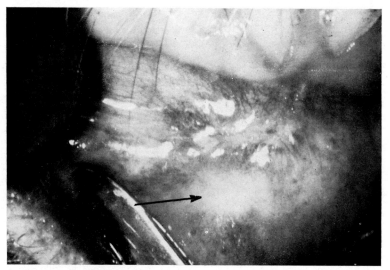

Fig. 2. Appearance of healed wound shown in fig. 1. There remains only a slight indentation of the tissues with some colour change.

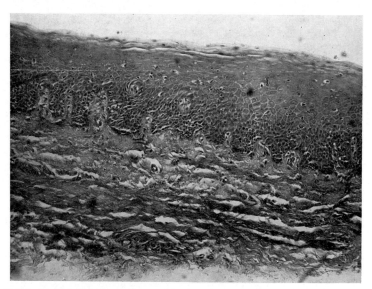

Fig. 3. Healed electrosurgical wound in the palate stained to show collagen fibres in the submucosa. Observe the loose yet regular arrangement of the tissues in the base of the wounded area, and the absence of scarring.

neoplasms. It is useful for the control of haemorrhage, for the coagulation of adherent tags of soft tissue, and the "sparking" of margins of cystic cavities where residual remnants may be difficult to remove by other mechanical means.

For almost all procedures in which electrosurgical apparatus is used the pain evoked by the procedure warrants the use of local analgesia. The exceptions are the use of the electrosurgical machine for pulp vitality tests and for the treatment of hypersensitive dentine and sterilizing root canals.

Disadvantages

(1) The most severe hazard is the rare danger of electrocution. Regular maintenance of the equipment should prevent this occurrence, but such accidents have occurred in the past.

(2) The danger of fire and explosion must be appreciated, and the machine must never be used in situations where inflammable agents such as ether, ethyl chloride, or cyclopropane are even standing exposed in the same room, let alone in use on the patient.

Care should also be taken to avoid using spirit-based skin preparations immediately prior to use of the electrosurgical machine. Sparks from electrosurgical equipment have been known to ignite such inflammable skin lotions, causing local burns.

(3) When an "indifferent" or earth electrode is used great care must be taken to avoid burns from this electrode. Burns may occur from a multitude of causes, and all who use such equipment must be thoroughly familiar with these risks. Regular inspection of apparatus should be carried out to prevent serious complications from arising. In this respect, it is timely to mention that contact between the active electrode and a metal retractor may cause damage to tissues which the operator is aiming to protect. For this reason, wooden or plastic retractors should be used in the vicinity of the electrocautery.

(4) The odour of scorching tissue associated with electro-coagulation is frequently objectionable to the patient.

(5) The technique of electrosurgery is exacting, and the equipment easily misused by an inexpert operator.

(6) The procedures are painful, and can only be carried out with adequate local or general anaesthesia.

(7) Patients often complain of excessive pain in the healing stage, which is frequently prolonged.

(8) The effect of the electrosurgical instrument on underlying structures, notably bone, emphasizes the disadvantage of this technique where deep structures, in the floor of the mouth for example, may be damaged or destroyed because of the low self-limiting effect of the coagulating current.

Advantages

(1) Small operations can be completed with the minimum of fuss in a bloodless field.

(2) The apparatus is simple to use, and to set up; it is not unduly expensive.

(3) The techniques of electrosurgery are readily learned.

(4) A variety of electrodes may occasionally provide access to otherwise difficult sites for the destruction of tissues.

(5) Some additional advantages and disadvantages of electrosurgery have been revealed by animal experiments. The reduction in scar tissue formation which follows electrosurgery supports its value in the treatment of hyperplastic lesions of the buccal and lingual sulci where the preservation of a scar-free deep sulcus is imperative for prosthetic rehabilitation. It has been suggested that results obtained by electrosurgery with partially rectified current are less satisfactory than those from equipment with fully rectified current, properly employed. The difference is attributed to the reduced heat dispersion and greater self-limiting capacity of fully rectified currents.

CRYOSURGERY

The effects of low temperature on living cells and tissues have been the subject of fascinating studies since Robert Boyle reported almost 300 years ago that cells were killed by freezing. A great deal of research has been done in the field of cryobiology to investigate the effects of freezing and thawing on microorganisms, red blood cells, embryos, and various organs and tissues. It was not until the basic cryobiological research and the capacity for improved instrumentation were combined that the clinical application of cryosurgery became a practical proposition. Today local freezing can be achieved in many parts of the body for destruction of both benign and malignant lesions.

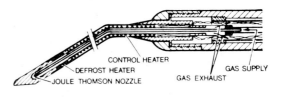

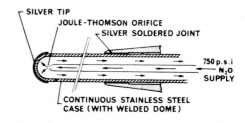

Fig. 4. Diagrammatic design of the Nitrous Oxide cryo-probe operated on the Joule–Thomson principle of the rapid expansion of gas.

Instrumentation

Cryosurgical equipment for use in dental and oral surgery is of two principal types. One is the Amoils-type unit in which expanding gas, by the Joule-Thomson effect (fig. 4), produces rapid freezing at the probe nozzle. This machine produces a temperature of about $-70°C$ at the probe tip. The other form of apparatus in common use is the liquid nitrogen apparatus which has a probe-tip temperature of about $-170°C$. Both forms of apparatus are controlled by a footswitch, leaving the hands free for manipulating the probe and tissues. Various shapes and sizes of applicators, or cryoprobes, are available. Those most useful in dental surgery are the tonsillar probes, and the general purpose probe. Each applicator produces an iceball of specific size and configuration which should be related to the geometrical design of the lesion to be treated. Sophisticated equipment with electrically operated defrosting systems is available at the upper end of the price range; non-electric systems occupy an intermediate position, and simple canisters of liquid nitrogen, used either as local sprays or with interchangeable probe-like nozzles are available in the cheaper range of appliances. The Amoils systems, electric or non-electric, operated by compressed nitrous-oxide gas, have been found to be of great value in dental and oral surgery.

The Biological Effects of Cryosurgery

Most tissues freeze at about $-2.2°C$, and lethal damage may be done to cells by a combination of factors induced by the freezing process. The object of cryosurgery is to freeze tissues and cells in order to kill them. But not all cells react in the same way to the same low temperature. Epithelial cells, for example, are particularly susceptible to low temperatures. Fibroblasts, on the other hand, are remarkably resistant. Individual cells respond in different ways to freezing depending on such external variables as the freezing rate, the rate of thawing, and the effect, if any, of local protective agents that may be present. Cell death, in an iceball induced by a local source of cold, may occur because of a number of factors. Intracellular ice formation and shifts in the concentration of cell or tissue electrolytes have all been implicated in the process of cryodestruction. The rate at which the tissues are frozen has an important effect on the extent of cell death. At rapid cooling rates, both intracellular and extracellular ice crystals form rapidly. If the rate of cooling is slow, cellular shrinkage keeps pace with loss of water to the external environment and the rate of intracellular ice crystal formation is reduced. At slow

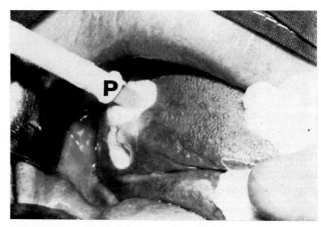

FIG. 5. Iceball formation in lesion of the tongue being treated by freezing probe (P).

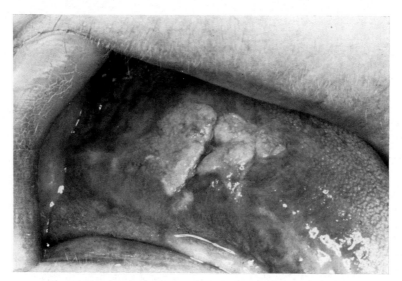

FIG. 6a. Premalignant lesion of tongue prior to treatment by cryosurgery.

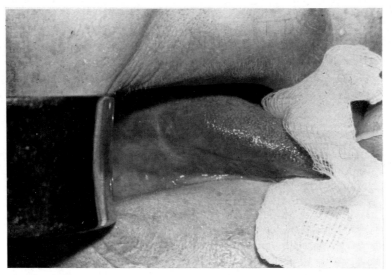

FIG. 6b. Area of tongue one year after removal of lesion by cryosurgery. Note the absence of indentation and scarring.

cooling rates, the concentration of salts which interacts with the lipids of the cell membrane to cause cell death is at a maximum. In fast cooling rates the time for salt injury to occur is greatly reduced. There is obviously a cooling rate at which these two extremes balance out. Among the many factors which may account for cases of individual susceptibility or resistance to freezing among cells of different types will obviously be the permeability of the cell to water. Cells that have survived the initial effects of cold, dehydration and ice-crystal formation may fail to survive the effects of thawing. Minimum tissue damage occurs if thawing is quickly accomplished and the crystal growth

Clinical Changes Following Cryosurgery

The gross clinical changes which follow the application of the cryoprobe pursue a predictable pattern. The warm point of the cryoprobe should be placed on moist tissues before freezing commences. Highly keratinized surfaces should be treated with an application of a water-soluble jelly before the probe is applied. During freezing an iceball forms (fig. 5) and continues to enlarge for about one minute, when equilibrium between the heat source and the cold source is reached and the iceball remains stationary in size. Freezing is sustained for a variable period of minutes

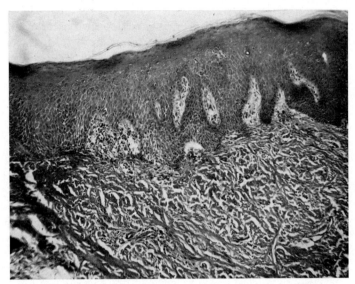

Fig. 7. Section of palatal mucosa one month after cryosurgery. Compare the very loose arrangement of the collagen bundles in the submucosa with those seen following electrosurgery (fig. 3).

phase by-passed. The cycle of a rapid freeze, followed by slow thaw produces the maximum lethal effect.

Freeze-thaw rates can be further modified by factors which reduce the heat input. Digital compression of feeder arteries, or the use of local or general vasoconstrictors all reduce the heat source of neighbouring tissues in the vicinity of the iceball, and promote the lethal effects of cryosurgery.

In some way not as yet understood, cells which have been subjected to one freeze-thaw cycle are stressed, and succumb more readily to repeated freeze-thaw interventions. Thus repeated cycles enhance the thermal conductivity of the tissues and allow the formation of a larger iceball.

Regardless of these physical effects of freezing, cells throughout the cryolesion are affected by the process of ischaemic infarction. Within 20 min. of the disappearance of an ice-ball there is a near-complete shutdown in the vascular supply to the affected part. It has been shown by carbon labelling techniques that the endothelial cells lining the capillaries and venules are swollen, with damage apparent in the organelles. Microthrombi form, leading to areas of infarction within and around the cryolesion. These vascular changes enhance the total destructive effect and probably play a part in the total volume of necrosis induced beyond the immediate area of contact of the cryoprobe.

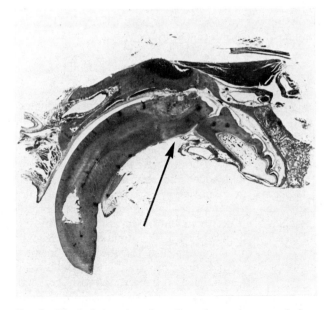

Fig. 8. Histological section of continuously growing upper incisor tooth of a Wistar rat subjected to freezing to −20°C for one minute at point of development indicated by arrow. Observe subsequent local damage to developing hard tissues, but eventual partial recovery.

depending on the nature of the lesion being treated; the source of refrigerant is then cut off. Soon after the onset of thawing the probe becomes detached and is withdrawn. The iceball thaws slowly, spontaneously for 2–3 min. and this is followed by redness, swelling, and sometimes vesiculation over 2–4 hr. The swelling may increase in the next 24 hr. Superficial necrosis appears after 2–3 days. On the skin, a dry eschar forms on the wound; in the mouth it is covered with a yellow-grey slough. Repair and re-epithelialization takes place deep to the slough, which separates off after 10 days in the mouth and up to 20 days on the skin. After separation there is a clean surface to the wound. Cryowounds rarely become infected, even in dirty conditions. Oral lesions heal without evidence of scarring (figs. 6a and b). On the skin, scarring is minimal, but the epidermis may remain thin and depigmented for many months. Animal experiments have confirmed the clinical impression that the amount of mature collagen found in the cryoscar is appreciably less than that which follows excision or electrosurgery (fig. 7).

Where bone or cartilage are included in the iceball the cellular elements are temporarily destroyed, but the skeletal architecture remains. Subsequently the osseous or cartilaginous framework is repopulated by new cells, with the return of vitality.

Nerves are affected by the cryoprobe, and both the Schwann cells and nerve axon undergo early degenerative changes. This produces a degree of paraesthesia which disappears remarkably rapidly. Because of the preservation of the integrity of the nerve sheath, the effects of Wallerian degeneration are rapidly reversed, with accurate restoration of function within a month or two.

Freezing to −30°C in the vicinity of the apex of the continuously growing incisor of the rat produces disorganization and death of a proportion of the ameloblasts and odontoblasts, and vacuolation of the pulp tissues. Within 14 days the cellular elements are replaced, but visible defects of varying degree remain in the hard tissues developing at the time of the insult (fig. 8).

The Specific Uses of Cryosurgery in Dental and Oral Surgery

Cryodestruction may be carried out with or without local anaesthesia. The treatment and healing periods are uncomplicated by infection, pain or odour. Hyperplastic and granulomatous lesions, polyps, epulides, and papillomas all respond well to cryosurgical intervention with complete healing and no tendency to recurrence. Where fibrous hyperplasias are removed by cryosurgery loss of sulcus depth is minimal, and scarring is absent. Dramatic results are achieved in the treatment by cryosurgery of vascular and pigmented naevi. No other treatment to date has proved as simple and effective for the management of haemangiomas. Cryosurgery is rarely, if ever, followed by troublesome haemorrhage. It is often used with great effect to control epistaxis, and haemorrhage following dental extractions in haemophiliacs.

Where chronic pain from long-standing erosive lesions such as lichen planus is revere, and the lesion fails to respond

to conventional measures, cryosurgery has proved to be completely effective. Such lesions may recur, however, and cryosurgery should be combined with biopsy and used with reservation in chronic ulcerative states.

Mucosal white patches, both hyperkeratotic and ulcerative, respond with remarkable speed to treatment with the cryoprobe. These lesions frequently involve areas such as the cheeks, palate, floor of mouth and lip commissure where excision and grafting are extremely difficult and painful. Cryosurgery is now the treatment of choice for such lesions, especially where there may be premalignant or early malignant changes in the condition (fig. 9a and b).

Many successful cases of eradication of malignant oral disease by cryosurgery have been reported in the literature. The cryoprobe has the distinct advantage over other surgical methods in that, theoretically, all malignant cells are trapped in the iceball until killed; spread of the tumour should therefore be greatly reduced. There is an added possibility that cryodestruction of a malignant lesion may provoke antigen formation through the liberation of lipoprotein complexes from cell membranes. The rise in circulating antibodies found following cryosurgery, combined with an increase in lymphocyte activity, may have a profound influence on the prognosis of a case. Much research remains to be done in this field of cryotherapy for malignant disease. At present, the role of cryosurgery in the treatment of malignant disease can be delineated as follows:

(a) it may be used for the control and palliation of recurrence when all conventional treatment has failed;
(b) it may be used as the primary treatment:

    (i) for accessible early lesions without lymphadenopathy;
    (ii) where age or debilitation mitigate against major surgery and/or intensive radiotherapy or chemotherapy.
    (iii) for multiple skin lesions, *e.g.* basal cell carcinomas; and
    (iv) in developing countries where the incidence of oral malignancy exceeds the provision of facilities for treatment, and where high standards of ablative and reconstructive surgery and radiotherapy are difficult to achieve.

Advantages and Disadvantages of Cryosurgery

Cryotherapy represents a major advance in the management of oral disease. However, like other new methods of treatment introduced to control oral or dental disease, it is not a universal panacea.

The most serious disadvantage of cryosurgery, particularly in the management of premalignant and malignant lesions, is the lack of opportunity to examine and sample an excised specimen microscopically. This disadvantage is countered, to some extent, by the fact that frozen tissues may be biopsied simply, without pain or subsequent haemorrhage, while in the frozen state and then immersed in fixative and treated as a routine specimen for biopsy purposes. The quality of the tissues thus available for diagnostic pathology is adequate for most purposes.

A further disadvantage of cryosurgery is the lack of cer-

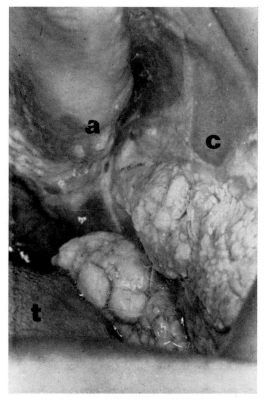

FIG. 9a. Verrucous carcinoma of lower alveolus and cheek (C) which had recurred twice in 15 months following surgical stripping of the mucosal lesion. (a = upper alveolus, t = tongue.)

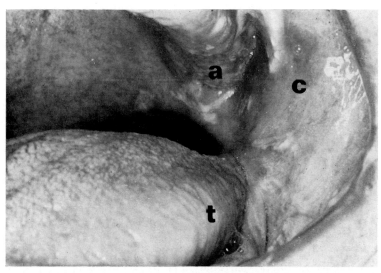

FIG. 9b. Same patient shown in fig. 9a two years after treatment of lesion with cryosurgery. There is no local recurrence in the treated area, and some reduction in size of the hyperkeratotic areas which were not treated.

tainty that the boundaries of the iceball coincide with the area of total cell death, or even that each and every cell within the iceball has been effectively destroyed. The depth of penetration of the iceball is difficult to estimate, but it coincides exactly with the dimensions of the iceball formed on the freezing probe immersed in a glass of water at body temperature. In practice these disadvantages are nullified in part by the increasing ability of the operator to assess the "area of kill" associated with a particular probe design, and the facility of multiple coverage of a lesion. This latter provides overlapping zones of destruction, designed to destroy any cells left alive in the "escape zone".

The cryoprobe is less effective on skin and dry, crusted lesions. In such conditions, the area under treatment must first be thoroughly moistened with a water-soluble jelly to enhance probe contact.

The over-extension of a cryolesion to adjacent normal structures is of less concern than a similar incident with the electrocautery or scalpel. Structures such as nerves, cartilage, bone and blood vessels on the periphery of the lesion are less severely affected by cryosurgery than by other methods of destruction, and the capacity of the frozen tissues for repair is greater. Thus, in the management of malignant lesions, over-treatment rather than under-treatment should be the aim of the operator, all other factors being equal. There are occasions in clinical cryosurgery around the face and jaws when it is difficult to apply the cryoprobe to the precise areas under treatment; the equipment is relatively inflexible and is not easily adapted to areas

difficult of access. It is anticipated that improved probe design will overcome this difficulty to some extent as technical innovations are made.

Cryosurgery has the potential advantages of being easily applicable, by repeated interventions with or without anaesthesia, and over long intervals with the minimum of unpleasant side-effects or terminal sequelae. It can prevent or control haemorrhage, even in the most vascular situations. It controls dissemination of tumour cells by immobilizing them within the cryolesion until destroyed. It is not accompanied or followed by unpleasant odour or infection, and it is followed by relatively painless healing without scar formation. Clinical experience has already shown that cryosurgery has great advantages over conventional methods in the treatment of multiple small lesions, and in the palliation (or even cure) of lesions that have failed to respond to all other conventional methods of treatment.

It seems certain, now, with increased clinical use and extended understanding of basic cryobiology, that cryosurgery will become an effective and essential tool in the management of oral lesions. By continued careful selection, and postoperative follow-up, the role of cryosurgery in the management of benign oral lesions may well be expanded. It is even possible to envisage the cure of oral malignancy without the radical destruction so often associated with current forms of therapy. Improved instrument design and tissue-freezing by local physical means or other related procedures should further enhance the application and value of cryosurgery.

56. THE HAEMOSTATIC MECHANISM AND ITS DEFECTS

R. G. MACFARLANE AND ROSEMARY BIGGS

Components of the Haemostatic Mechanism
> The blood clotting mechanism
> Thrombin generation
> Additional plasma factors
> Interaction of clotting factors
> Platelets in haemostasis
> Changes in vessels

Defects and their correction
> Congenital defects
> > Diagnosis
> > Treatment
> > Complications
> Acquired defects
> > Platelet deficiency
> > Other abnormalities

The evolution of the circulatory system of the higher animals has entailed a corresponding evolution of automatic safeguards to prevent disastrous loss of blood in the event of vascular damage. In lower animals primitive haemostatic mechanisms can be discerned, such as the agglutination of corpuscles, and the formation of precipitates in the vicinity of tissue damage, and it is tempting to view these as the evolutionary precedents of the complex platelet and plasma reactions to injury which characterize the mammalian haemostatic mechanism.

The importance of this mechanism to survival should not be underestimated. Though injuries to large vessels may cause fatal bleeding unless something is done to promote artificial haemostasis by such things as tourniquets, ligatures, sutures, or dressings, the natural mechanism does cope, with great efficiency, with bleeding from the smaller vessels and, since these are far more numerous and are far more liable to damage in ordinary life than the major vessels, this efficiency is literally of vital importance. The fact that the bleeding from minor injuries ceases spontaneously is so familiar that it is accepted without thought of the hydrostatic forces which have been overcome to achieve this effect. Even experienced surgeons often seem to be unaware of what they owe to nature when their patients do not bleed to death; they make their incisions, clamp, cauterize or ligate a few dozen of the larger vessels they have cut, and feel that they have made the major contribution towards haemostasis, whereas in reality thousands of small cut vessels have been sealed by a natural process the failure of which would be catastrophic. Artificial hæmostatic measures which are effective in supplementing the normal mechanism are relatively useless without it, and many patients with haemostatic defects have bled to death from apparently trivial injuries despite every effort to stop the bleeding by conventional surgical means. During the past two decades considerable advances have been made in the understanding of the normal haemostatic mechanism and its defects, and in the development of effective methods for the treatment of the latter.

THE COMPONENTS OF THE HAEMOSTATIC MECHANISM

Normal haemostasis in a wound area is achieved by the interlocking operation of three different mechanisms, which, as will be seen, are to some extent dependent on each other. The first is coagulation of the blood; the second is adhesion and aggregation of platelets, and the third is the reaction of damaged vessels. The effect of clotting and platelet adhesion is to produce an obstructive mass in the wound area, and the effect of the vascular reactions is to reduce or divert blood flow in the vessels supplying it. Haemostasis normally only operates where and when it is needed. If it fails when required, the patient may bleed to death, and if it operates in the wrong place, he may die of thrombosis.

The Blood Clotting Mechanism

Few biological phenomena have been so intensively studied as the coagulation of blood. For two centuries it has led to experiment, speculation and argument. Much of the discord has been resolved by an internationally agreed numerical nomenclature for the different clotting factors (see Table 1) which has shown that most disagreements were about words and not facts, so that a reasonably coherent and acceptable account can be given in less space than would have been possible 10 years ago.

The solidity of the clot is due to **fibrin**, a polymer which, though it forms only about 0·2 per cent of the weight of the clot achieves remarkable strength by its interlacing, adhesive fibres. The precursor of fibrin is **fibrinogen**, a plasma protein of high molecular weight. Its molecule is split by the enzyme **thrombin**, into one major and several minor (peptide) fragments. The major fragments, having lost negative charges, tend to polymerize by electrostatic attraction followed by hydrogen bonding, becoming aligned end-to-end and side-to-side to form the typical fibrin strands. A later change associated with a specific plasma factor **(Factor XIII)** results in a strong linkage, probably due to a transamidation reaction.

Thrombin Generation

Thrombin does not exist in the circulating blood in amounts sufficient to cause detectable coagulation. It is generated from an inert precursor, **prothrombin**, an α-globulin present in a concentration of about 10–15 mg./100 ml. plasma. The mechanism by which prothrombin is activated to thrombin has been a source of controversy during the past 30 years. It is agreed that there are two

TABLE 1

THE PLASMA CLOTTING FACTORS AND SOME OF THEIR PROPERTIES

Roman numeral	Common synonyms	Molecular weight	Isoelectric point	Ppt by $(NH_4)_2SO_4$	Cohn fractionation	Electrophoresis	Stability at 56°C	Adsorption by inorganic gels
I	Fibrinogen	3.4×10^5	5.5	25%	I	Fibrinogen	Labile	0
II	Prothrombin	6.9×10^4	4.2	—	III-2	α Globulin	Stable	+
III	Thromboplastin	—	—	—	—	—	—	—
IV	Calcium catalyst	—	—	—	—	—	—	—
V	Ac-globulin labile factor	2.9×10^5	5.3	45%	III	—	Labile	0
VII	Proconvertin S.P.C.A.	5.0×10^4	—	—	III-2	β Globulin	Stable	+
VIII	Antihaemophilic globulin	3×10^5 to 5×10^6	—	33%	I	β_2 Globulin	Labile	0
IX	Christmas factor PTC	5×10^4	4.0–5.0	33–50%	IV	β Globulin	Labile	+
X	Stuart Prower factor	8.6×10^4 (bovine)	5.5	—	—	α Globulin	Labile	+
XI	P.T.A.	—	4.0–5.2	33–50%	III, IV-1	Between β and γ globulins	Labile	+
XII	Hageman factor	8.0×10^4		33–50%	III, IV-1		—	—
XIII	Fibrin stabilizing factor	1.3×10^5	5.4	33%	III	γ Globulin	Stable	—

main stimuli, both relevant to normal haemostasis, which cause prothrombin activation through a chain of intermediate reactions. The first is the action of some factor released from damaged tissue, and the second is contact of the blood with any one of a variety of surfaces other than the surface of normal vascular endothelium.

Thromboplastin. During the first half of this century the tissue-activated system was the most intensively investigated. It was supposed that a specific factor known as "thromboplastin" or "thrombokinase" released by damaged cells or platelets activated prothrombin directly. Since calcium ions were also required, 4 clotting factors were therefore recognized, thromboplastin, calcium, prothrombin and fibrinogen, and the reaction was set out as follows:

$$\text{Tissue Thromboplastin} + \text{Ca}^{++}$$
$$\text{Prothrombin} \xrightarrow{} \text{Thrombin}$$
$$\text{Fibrinogen} \xrightarrow{} \text{Fibrin}$$

Additional Plasma Factors

The wide use of the "prothrombin time" test, introduced by Quick in 1935, soon revealed the fact that other factors must be involved. This test consists of adding tissue thromboplastin and calcium to citrated blood or plasma, and recording the clotting time. According to the above theory this time is determined by the prothrombin concentration only, provided that fibrinogen is adequate, but cases were soon discovered in which clotting was delayed despite normal prothrombin and fibrinogen concentrations.

Factors V, VII, and X. These factors were postulated to explain the haemostatic defects in patients whose plasma

samples had long prothrombin times; these factors are required for the normal activation of prothrombin by thromboplastin; a deficiency of any one of these would lengthen the prothrombin time. The first was called Factor V, by Owren (1947), the next was called Factor VII by Koller et al. (1951) (the term Factor VI was used in another context and this term is not now used). Some time later, another factor found to be required for the action of thromboplastin was called Factor X (Koller, 1955). Thus, the activation of prothrombin by this extrinsic system requires the factors set out on the left-hand side of Fig. 1.

During the elucidation of this extrinsic system it became apparent that there must be other factors concerned with normal clotting. For example, it was obvious that there

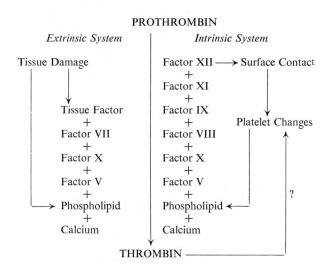

FIG. 1. The factors concerned with the activation of prothrombin following surface contact, and by tissue damage.

was something wrong with the clotting mechanism in haemophilia, since haemophilic blood might have a grossly prolonged clotting time in glass, though it clotted normally with added tissue thromboplastin. Investigation of the normal mechanism of clotting without such added thromboplastin revealed a whole system activated by contact with foreign surfaces. This recalled the pioneer work of Lister (1863) whose demonstration of the effect of surface contact was overshadowed by later preoccupation with thromboplastin.

Factors VIII, IX, XI and XII. Investigation of this "intrinsic system" which proceeded in different centres over a number of years showed that at least four other plasma factors were involved. One of these is deficient in haemophilia and was called "anti-haemophilic globulin" (AHG), now Factor VIII. Another, deficiency of which causes Christmas disease, is called Factor IX, a third is Factor XI, and the last to be defined is Factor XII (Hageman factor) a protein with a special affinity for glass or similar surfaces. In addition, Factors X and V, being also required, are common to both the intrinsic and extrinsic systems. These factors are set out on the right-hand side of Fig. 1. They have been defined and identified by a variety of fractionation techniques including differential precipitation and adsorption, chromatography, electrophoresis and the use of specific antibodies. The identification of specific factor activities has depended on the natural occurrence of deficiency states in which the patient's plasma forms a test system. Some of the properties of the different factors are set out in Table 1. The most important outcome of this study of the properties of coagulation factors lies in its application to the preparation of therapeutic concentrates.

Interaction of Clotting Factors

Most physiologists would not be content with a list of components of a biological mechanism and a fragmentary knowledge of their physical or chemical properties; they would want to know how they work together. Countless experiments have provided a mass of data on reactions between practically every combination of clotting factors. Out of all this has come a consensus of opinion that they react, probably in pairs, and in a preferential sequence.* On the intrinsic side, the first reaction is between a surface and Factor XII, followed by reactions involving Factors XI, IX, VIII, X, V, and prothrombin in that order. Phospholipid is also required, and is derived from platelets. The extrinsic system involves tissue factor, Factors VII, X, V, and prothrombin so that Factor X is the meeting point of these two systems.

Factor X appears to be activated enzymatically in both systems to yield an active product, itself an enzyme, which then activates prothrombin in the presence of Factor V, phospholipid and calcium. It later appears that most of the other factors are activated in a similar way, and are probably proenzymes like prothrombin, each yielding an enzyme capable of activating the next proenzyme in the sequence. The evidence for this view

*Some authorities do not agree with this view; see Seegers 1965.

is not complete but is sufficiently strong to support it as a working hypothesis (Macfarlane 1964, 1965) which provides a rational picture of the clotting process and its evolution. In this view the clotting factors form an enzyme "cascade" resembling the electronic cascade of a photomultiplier or amplifier. Each enzyme activates a larger amount of the next proenzyme so that there is a "gain" of production rate, stage to stage, and the minute stimulus of surface contact is transmitted as a rising wave of activity culminating in an almost explosive generation of thrombin.

Critics of coagulation theory have complained of, or ridiculed the idea that so many factors are required to produce a clot, but they accept the fact that a radio set with 9 transistors gives better reception than one with 4. This idea of the clotting mechanism is set out in Fig. 2,

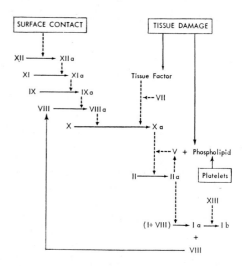

Fig. 2. A comprehensive scheme of the clotting mechanism based on existing evidence. Factor X is activated both by the intrinsic (surface contact) system and the extrinsic (tissue) system. Thrombin (IIa) acts, not only on fibrinogen to form fibrin (Ia) but also on the platelets to release phospholipid and on Factor VIII first to mobilize it and then destroy it. Factor XIII (or fibrin-stabilizing factor) acts on fibrin to produce stable fibrin (Ib).

each activated product being designated by the letter "a". There are certain complications; thrombin has "feed-back" effects on earlier reactions, so that once it begins to appear it greatly accelerates its own production. These effects are on Factor VIII, and also on the platelets, causing their aggregation and the release of phospholipids (Platelet Factor 3). Phospholipid itself seems to act as a surface catalyst, adsorbing clotting factors which are normally present in minute concentrations and thus potentiating their interaction. Another, and most important feature of the clotting mechanism is the rapid destruction of all the active products, including thrombin, so that within a few minutes of the completion of clotting these activities have virtually disappeared. It is this effect which is probably the most important safeguard against thrombosis, yet its mechanism is still largely unknown.

Platelets in Haemostasis

Morphological studies of the solid masses which form spontaneously at the site of vascular injuries show that, particularly in the case of smaller vessels, fibrin is not the only or even the main component. As long ago as 1882 Hayem recognized that such hæmostatic plugs were mostly composed of aggregated "hematoblasts" (platelets) and he predicted that a shortage of platelets would result in persistent bleeding. These observations have been repeatedly confirmed but it is only within the past decade that an understanding of the mechanism underlying this platelet aggregation has begun to emerge.

At first it was supposed that fibrin formed a cement which held the platelets together, but more detailed studies, in particular electron microscopy, showed that platelet aggregation was not dependent on fibrin formation, and could, in fact, occur in its absence. It became clear that platelets are not merely passive globules of protoplasm, but are packed with active substances relevant to the haemostatic mechanism and also, incidentally, to the processes of inflammation and repair. These substances include enzymes, such as acid phosphatase, glycolytic enzymes, cathepsin, and, perhaps most important in the haemostatic mechanism, ATP-ase. Platelets contain a high concentration of ATP, (adenosine triphosphate), and the pharmacologically-active amines 5-hydroxytryptamine (serotonin), adrenalin, nor-adrenalin, and (particularly in the rabbit) histamine. They also contain a contractile protein (thrombosthenin) which is probably responsible for clot retraction and the consolidation of platelet clumps, and various other factors concerned with clotting.

Platelet Behaviour

The physical behaviour of platelets during their aggregation is related to biochemical changes which have been intensively studied (Born 1965, Marcus and Zucker 1965). Following contact with certain surfaces or activation substances, the platelets undergo what was termed "viscous metamorphosis" by earlier workers, though this term is now in disrepute. Essentially this process consists of the appearance of pseudopodia-like protrusions, an increased stickiness, and the clumping of adjacent platelets into masses with a loss of visible granules, and finally, by light microscopy, a loss of cell outlines so that the mass appears to be amorphous.

These changes can be analysed into 3 separate stages which can be reproduced experimentally *in vitro*, and which may be termed adhesion, cohesion, and fusion.

Adhesion. This refers to the adhesion of individual platelets to any solid surface. Their lack of adhesion to the vascular endothelium, or to the circulating blood cells is a striking and essential fact of normal blood flow, but they at once adhere to any damaged vascular surface. In shed blood, they adhere to almost any surface with which they come in contact, in particular the glass which forms most laboratory apparatus. Platelets also adhere actively to collagen fibres or particles. A few substances such as some silicones, plastics, waxes, and oils do not promote adhesion, nor are they so effective as glass in activating the clotting system.

The mechanism of adhesion is still unexplained. The fact that it occurs almost instantly, and as actively at 0° as at 37°C, suggests that it does not depend on time-consuming biochemical reactions. It would therefore seem to be a physical process involving some special properties of the surfaces of the platelet and the substance to which it adheres, which have not yet been defined. Most adhesive surfaces are water-wettable, but some are not, and some water-wettable surfaces, notably living vascular endothelium, are non-adhesive. Measurements of surface electrical charge and zeta potential have not provided a general explanation. Though it has been shown that normal, negatively charged platelets will adhere to a positively charged surface, not all adhesive surfaces have such a charge and the observation that a degree of impact is necessary for platelet adhesion suggests that long-range forces of repulsion have to be overcome by the momentum of the platelet moving towards a surface, and that subsequent adhesion is due to short-range forces at present undefined.

Once adhesion has occurred, the platelet undergoes biochemical changes which have an effect on the behaviour of other platelets in the vicinity. The most important of these is the so-called **release reaction**. This entails the breakdown of ATP, the release of ADP, serotonin and other amines into the surrounding medium, and the release of Platelet Factor 3, as well as other activities which promote contact activation and intrinsic coagulant activity. These activities are mainly released at the platelet surface.

Cohesion. The next stage is platelet cohesion, that is the adhesion of one platelet to another so that solid masses of aggregated platelets are built up. These can form at the site of already adherent platelets at a surface so that the masses are anchored, or they can form in a suspension of platelets to produce visible clumps or floccules, a reaction which has provided the indicator for a great deal of recent experimental work. Platelet cohesion can be produced by many agents, but the most important is ADP (adenosine diphosphate). This substance, in a concentration of 0·04 μg./ml. will cause visible clumping *in vitro* in 60 seconds, and it will greatly enhance platelet aggregation *in vivo*. Other agents will also cause cohesion, in particular thrombin, serotonin, adrenalin and nor-adrenalin, but it is significant that all these cause the release of ADP from platelets. In addition, inhibitors which block the cohesive action of ADP also prevent the action of these other agents, and it therefore seems likely that ADP is the final common factor in platelet cohesion.

The mechanism by which ADP produces this effect is at present unknown, but it appears to be quantitatively involved, with calcium, in the formation of an inter-platelet binding compound. It is a feature of such ADP induced platelet clumping that the process is reversible, the platelets becoming re-dispersed, apparently intact, on the destruction of ADP, or the removal of calcium ions. Electron microscopy of platelets clumped by ADP, or which have formed an intravascular mass by contact with a small area of minor endothelial damage, shows similar pictures in each case. The platelets form a compact mass in which the outline of individual platelets is distinct, with granules and other structures well preserved.

Fusion. In the next stage of aggregation, fusion occurs and the picture changes. This change is seen particularly in the so-called haemostatic plug at the site of gross vascular disruption with haemorrhage. The platelets, particularly at the periphery, lose their granules, and appear as swollen, empty envelopes. Next, their membranes become indistinct, so that actual fusion appears to be taking place, often accompanied by the appearance of fibrin in the vicinity. *In vitro*, these changes can be brought about by the action of thrombin. It would seem, therefore, that thrombin may have two actions on the platelet, first, the release of ADP causing platelet cohesion, and second, a possibly enzymic action on some constituent of the envelope (possibly resembling fibrinogen) which leads to fusion. The end result is a tough, adherent, irreversibly compacted mass of platelets reinforced with the fibrin also produced by the action of thrombin on the plasma.

Changes in the Vessels

The third component of the haemostatic mechanism is the reaction of the vessels themselves. Active constriction of arteries and veins at the site of injury is often seen, and is probably an important haemostatic factor where larger vessels are concerned. There are many instances in which individuals have survived the accidental amputation of limbs despite considerable delay in the application of a tourniquet or other surgical aid to haemostasis, and it is difficult to believe that any natural process other than vascular constriction could stop the bleeding from a major severed artery. In the case of smaller vessels the importance of constriction is less obvious, though it can be seen in damaged arterioles and venules and also in undamaged vessels in their vicinity. It is sometimes seen in experimental preparations, such as the hamster cheek pouch, that a damaged area may be virtually by-passed by the blood supply as the result of the opening up of vascular shunts and alternative anastomotic pathways.

The reaction of the smallest vessels, the capillaries, is probably important. They often disappear from view after injury in experimental preparations. It is probable that the disappearance of these vessels is due in part to active contraction of myofibrils in the endothelium. Their endothelium becomes sticky, and outside pressure may then cause their walls to adhere together in such a way that the lumen is obliterated. Another factor is the increase in vascular permeability which occurs in these smaller vessels following trauma. This results in a leakage of plasma into the tissue spaces, raising the extravascular pressure, and also a packing of the red cells retained in the vessels with a consequent rise in viscosity, both processes causing a reduction in flow.

The mechanism of these reactions is obscure. The constriction of large muscular vessels is presumably mediated through their nerve supply, and results from the stimulus of trauma. The reactions of the smaller vessels may be due to the vaso-active substances released in the area of injury, particularly by the platelets. Such substances are found in fresh serum, or in blood escaping from a wound, and they probably include **serotonin** and the **catecholamines**. Other substances produced under these conditions are derived from activation of the kinin system, including **bradykinin** which causes local pain and increases vascular permeability. This sytem is linked to the clotting mechanism since it is activated by Factor XII (Hageman factor).

The Haemostatic Mechanism as a Whole

The three components of the haemostatic mechanism described are closely integrated and interdependent. Clotting is dependent on the platelets for the phospholipid essential for its normal operation, and platelet aggregation is dependent on the action of thrombin. Fibrin formation is required to consolidate platelet masses, and vascular reactions are probably dependent on the vaso-active substances released by the platelets, which are also, perhaps, activated by the clotting mechanism.

The timing of the different events in this complex operation, and the relative importance of its component parts depends largely on the nature and extent of the injury. The smallest vessels are probably sealed effectively by platelet plugs alone, formed as the result of their contact with exposed collagen, and without the co-operation of the clotting mechanism. But without the co-operation of clotting such platelet plugs will not be consolidated, and they will not have sufficient permanence or mechanical strength to be effective in vessels larger than arterioles and venules. Conversely, clotting without adequate platelet or vascular function seems to be incapable of arresting bleeding from even the smallest vessels.

In larger injuries, the clotting mechanism is an essential addition to platelet aggregation for effective hæmostasis, generating the thrombin which causes platelet fusion, and fibrin which is required for their reinforcement. In still larger vessels the formation of a hæmostatic plug is mechanically difficult in the face of the rapid flow and high pressure of the escaping blood, and in such cases vascular constriction, a profound fall in blood pressure, or artificial aids are required to prevent exsanguination. A general scheme of the interactions of these various components is shown in Fig. 3.

DEFECTS IN THE HAEMOSTATIC MECHANISM AND THEIR CORRECTION

Defective haemostasis may result from a quantitative or functional deficiency of one or more components of the normal mechanism. These defects may occur in the clotting mechanism, the platelets, or the vessels. In many cases they are life-long and hereditary, with a well marked genetic pattern; they may be acquired, sometimes manifesting as acute emergencies, or they may be the result of treatment, with, for example, anticoagulants.

The correlation of quantitative studies of haemostatic factors with clinical experience in cases of abnormal bleeding has made it possible to predict the results of any particular defect. This knowledge, together with the increas-

TABLE 2

Haemostatic Defect by Clinical History and Examination

Platelet and Vascular Disorders	Coagulation Defects	
	Extrinsic Defect	*Intrinsic Defect*
Platelet count Bleeding time Prothrombin consumption index Platelet function tests	One-stage prothrombin time Two-stage prothrombin test Assays of factors II, V, VII and X	Thromboplastin generation test Assay of factors XII, XI, IX, VIII.
	Final stage and clotting	
	Tests for fibrinogen (factor I) and fibrin stabilizing factor (factor XIII)	

ing availability of effective therapeutic materials, has revolutionized the treatment of patients with haemostatic defects. These relatively recent advances have permitted the development of a logical approach to treatment based on accurate laboratory diagnosis and reliable assays of specific coagulation factors.

The laboratory methods are not simple techniques that can be relied upon to give good results in any routine laboratory and must include specific assays of coagulation factors, in addition to the more familiar general tests of coagulation function. Moreover the administration of therapeutic materials is not all that is necessary to ensure the patient's safety. Much skill and experience are required for the safe use of these materials in all circumstances. For these reasons the treatment of patients who have serious haemostatic defects should, wherever possible, be carried out at special centres. In all instances treatment in nonspecialist hospitals should be carried out with friendly advice from a special centre and should be restricted to emergency diagnosis and treatment wherever possible.

Congenital Defects in the Clotting Mechanism

Table 1 lists 12 coagulation factors all of which are thought to be involved in the normal clotting mechanism. Of these, Factors I, II, V, VII, VIII, IX, X, XI, and XIII may be deficient (or defective) and deficiency of any one of them causes a haemorrhagic state. Factors III and IV (tissue factor and calcium) are never defective and lack of Factor XII, which causes a severe *in vitro* coagulation defect, never causes any disturbance of the haemostatic mechanism. The failure of Factor XII deficiency to cause any haemostatic defect has always been rather difficult to explain but recent work has suggested that Factor XII is mainly concerned with coagulation systems in glass tubes and that, in the presence of platelets and the absence of glass, this factor may contribute little to normal clotting.

The diagnosis of patients having defects in the haemostatic mechanism

The distinction between the various components of the haemostatic mechanism depends very much on the taking

of a careful clinical history and making a clinical examination which should include enquiry about the sites most commonly affected by bleeding (joints and muscles in haemophilia and Christmas disease, and epistaxis and gastro-intestinal tract in platelet-vascular disorders). The time of onset of bleeding after injury is important (immediate and profuse in platelet-vascular disorders; delayed and persistent in coagulation defects). An enquiry about other members of the family may give a clue to the mode of inheritance. The degree of trauma required to cause bleeding will also give a good idea of the severity of the defect.

Having taken a history it is possible then to proceed to a systematic laboratory study along the lines indicated in Table 2 and following approximately the scheme of Fig. 3. In fact this systematic approach is often a waste of time since the clinical history may give a very good idea of the diagnosis. For example, a baby boy presenting with a massive lumpy haematoma on the head, with no underlying fracture, with no sufficient traumatic cause and whose maternal uncle has haemophilia, will be found to have haemophilia.

The treatment of patients with coagulation defects presents many special problems, both in laboratory testing for diagnosis and control of treatment and in clinical management. Since such patients are so rarely encountered, treatment in the United Kingdom is coordinated by Special Haemophilia Centres designated by the Area Health Authorities, from whom a list may be obtained. The discussion which follows provides a brief guide to the general principles that underlie the treatment of patients having coagulation defects.

Treatment of Patients with Coagulation Defects

Haemophilia (Factor VIII deficiency) is the commonest coagulation defect and the general principle of treatment for patients with coagulation defects will be illustrated by reference to this condition. The circumstances which influence effective treatment for all patients with coagulation defects are:

(1) The half-life of the infused material. A short half-life will clearly necessitate frequent dosage.

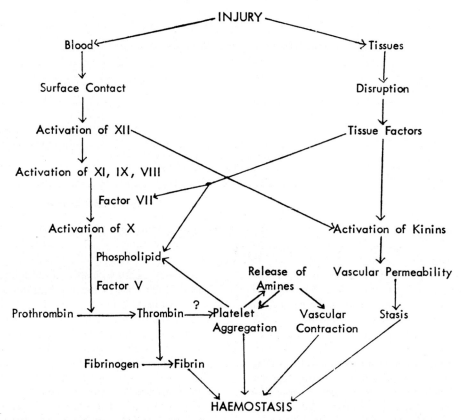

FIG. 3. A diagram illustrating the factors concerned with haemostasis, and their inter-relation.

(2) The availability of therapeutic materials.

(3) The plasma concentration of the particular factor required for effective hæmostasis related to the patient's lesion.

Table 3 refers to these different aspects in respect of the recognized coagulation defects. It should be noted that all these defects are rare, some extremely so.

Haemophilia. This is the commonest and most important of the hereditary clotting defects, with an incidence of about 5–6 per 100,000. It is inherited as a sex-linked recessive character, heterozygous females being carriers but usually haemostatically normal, and the very rare homozygous female being affected like the hemizygous male. Different grades of severity occur, and breed true. The relationship of blood levels of Factor VIII to clinical severity is shown in Table 4. In the severely affected patient, bleeding can occur from or into any part of the body subjected to even slight trauma, but superficial scratches and needle pricks usually do not bleed abnormally, probably because of normal platelet function, and the bleeding time test is therefore normal. Bleeding from external wounds cannot be controlled by any of the usual haemostatic measures, and tight dressings, plugs, cauteries, sutures or ligatures are usually worse than useless since they create further tissue damage. Haemorrhage into the deep tissues may be widely infiltrating and cause damage to muscles, nerves, or other organs, and in the mouth, throat or neck it can cause asphyxia. Repeated haemorrhage into the joints is a most charac-

teristic feature, leading to joint destruction and permanent crippling.

The haemophilic defect can be corrected by intravenous infusion of materials having Factor VIII activity. The half-life after infusion of all materials is short and thus daily or twice daily infusions may be required. The preparations available for treatment are listed in Table 5. It will be seen that neither whole blood nor plasma contains a sufficient concentration of Factor VIII to raise the patient's plasma concentration of Factor VIII to high levels. Whole blood should in fact only be used to replace blood lost and should never be relied on as a haemostatic agent.

Plasma is relatively ineffective when compared to concentrates and may sometimes cause dangerous reactions in multiple transfused patients. Plasma should now never be used to treat patients in the United Kingdom since there is now no shortage of effective concentrates if the commercial preparations of human factor VIII are taken into account. The concentrates of factor VIII at present available include cryoprecipitate and a small amount of freeze-dried concentrate made by the National Health Service. It is planned to increase supplies of this concentrate and ultimately to have all the concentrate required made within the NHS in freeze-dried form. Until this time several commercial firms are selling a high quality freeze-dried human concentrate which is available through Haemophilia Centres.

The animal material is more concentrated than most

TABLE 3

REPLACEMENT THERAPY REQUIRED BY PATIENTS WITH VARIOUS COAGULATION DEFECTS

Deficient factor	Half-life of infused activity (hours)	Blood concentration required for effective haemostasis	Materials for effective replacement therapy		
			Plasma	Concentrate	Source of concentrate
I	120	50–100 mg.%	Effective	Effective	Fibrinogen
II	80–120	40% of normal	—	Effective	"Prothrombin complex" (II, VII, IX, X)
V	15–24	10–15% of normal	Effective	Not needed	—
VII	5	10% of normal	Probably ineffective	Short duration of effect	"Prothrombin complex" (II, VII, IX, X)
VIII	10–18	15–20% Controls spontaneous bleeding 50% Controls traumatic bleeding	Effective for spontaneous bleeding	Required for traumatic bleeding	Human AHG Animal AHG
IX	15–30	As for Factor VIII	Probably effective for spontaneous bleeding	Required for traumatic bleeding	"Prothrombin complex" (II, VII, IX, X)
X	60–70	15–20%	?	Effective	"Prothrombin complex" (II, VII, IX, X)
XI	60–70	?	Effective	Not needed	—
XII	50–70	0	Not needed	Not needed	—
XIII	80–120	1–5%	Effective	Not needed	—

of the present human preparations, it is available commercially in England, and it is clinically effective. However, being derived from animals (porcine and bovine) it may give rise to non-specific sensitization reactions if administered often. The animal preparations are particularly useful in the treatment of patients who have antibodies to Factor VIII (see below).

The amounts of therapeutic material required to treat a particular patient on a particular occasion will depend very much on the lesion from which he is suffering. From Table 4 it is clear that the most serious and most frequent bleeding episodes occur in patients with no detectable plasma Factor VIII and these patients are in fact the most numerous. Table 6 gives the post-infusion plasma Factor VIII concentrations required in these severely affected patients for different types of lesion. Haemarthroses, seen before marked swelling has occurred, will respond to modest treatment and plasma may be an adequate thera-

TABLE 4

THE RELATIONSHIP BETWEEN OBSERVED NATURAL BLOOD LEVELS OF FACTOR VIII AND THE OCCURRENCE OF HAEMORRHAGIC SYMPTOMS

Blood level of Factor VIII %	Haemostatic efficiency in the untreated patient
50–100	Normal
25–50	May experience excessive secondary haemorrhage after major surgery
10–25	Bleeding after major surgery, dental extraction and accidents is usual but usually not lethal
0–10	Severe bleeding after surgery. Haemarthroses and deep haematomata follow minor trauma
0	Severe and frequent spontaneous bleeding with crippling and residual deformity in the untreated patient. Surgical bleeding disastrous in the untreated patient

TABLE 5

THE FACTOR VIII CONTENT OF AVAILABLE THERAPEUTIC MATERIALS AND THE BLOOD LEVELS OF FACTOR VIII THAT MAY BE ACHIEVED FOLLOWING INFUSION. 1 UNIT IS THE AVERAGE FACTOR VIII ACTIVITY OF 1 ML. OF NORMAL PLASMA

Therapeutic material	Factor VIII units/ml.	Dosage units/kg.	Post infusion Factor VIII % of normal
Fresh whole blood	0·3	4·5*	5–7*
Fresh or frozen plasma	0·6	12*	15–20*
Cryoprecipitate	2·8	20–80	30–100+
Freeze dried human concentrate	2·8	20–80	30–100+
Animal freeze dried concentrate	10–15	100–200	100+

* In the case of whole blood and plasma the dose to be given is limited by the infusion volume that can safely be administered to the patient.

peutic material. One dose in these cases may be curative and most haemophilic centres treat such cases as outpatients. The more traumatic the lesion clearly the more treatment will be required and it is here that judgment and experience are important. For major surgery the general rule is that treatment should continue until healing is complete. Dental extraction may be an exception to this rule. It has been found that one dose of Factor VIII sufficient to raise the patient's plasma level of Factor VIII to 50 per cent of normal at the time of operation may be sufficient if epsilon amino caproic acid (EACA) is given by mouth for ten days post-operatively. Presumably the antifibrinolytic action of EACA preserves the clots formed at operation and thus promotes haemostasis. EACA could well have a beneficial effect in other surgical operations.

TABLE 6

THE RELATIONSHIP BETWEEN THE TYPE OF LESION IN SEVERELY
AFFECTED HAEMOPHILIC PATIENTS AND THE PLASMA CONCENTRATIONS
OF FACTOR VIII REQUIRED FOR HAEMOSTASIS

Lesion	Post treatment haemostatic level	Dose of Factor VIII required units/kg.	Duration of treatment
Early haemarthroses, early haematomata	15–25	10–16	One dose may suffice
Serious haemarthroses and haematomata	25–50	16–35	1–3 daily doses
Dental extraction	50	35	1 dose with EACA may suffice (see text)
Major surgery	50–100+	35–70	Daily or twice daily infusions until healing is complete

These considerations apply to severely affected patients. Mildly affected patients with 10 to 25 per cent of Factor VIII in their plasma should never be forgotten. They may bleed badly after surgery and require almost as much therapeutic material as the severely affected patient to ensure safe haemostasis. The normal general appearance of many of these patients at clinical pre-operative assessment may lead to a too optimistic view of haemostatic function in the patient.

Complications of Treatment

There are two serious complications of treatment: one is the development of serum hepatitis and the other is the development of specific antibodies to Factor VIII.

Severely affected hæmophilic patients receive very many infusions and the concentrated material is made from pools of normal plasma donations. A single patient may thus receive material derived from several thousand donors in a year. The risk of hepatitis is therefore high and many patients do at some time give positive tests for hepatitis associated antigen or antibody. Fortunately only about 3 per cent of patients develop clinical illness.

The second serious complication is the production of specific antibodies which destroy infused Factor VIII. At present about 5 per cent of treated patients develop these antibodies. Patients who have antibodies are difficult to treat and for them the animal concentrates may be useful since the antibody is usually less potent towards animal Factor VIII than towards human material.

Factor IX deficiency (Christmas Disease), is the next commonest hereditary clotting defect, with an incidence in this country of about 2–3 per million. Its symptoms and inheritance are similar to those of haemophilia. Its specific treatment consists in the infusion of concentrates of human Factor IX, or, in milder cases or those with minor injuries or operations, infusions of plasma.

Factor XI deficiency. This deficiency is inherited through an autosomal gene with partial dominance. The deficiency is strongly linked to Jewish ancestry and its frequency varies from one region of the world to another. Treatment with plasma is usually effective.

Afibrinogenaemia. Fibrinogen deficiency may occur as total afibrinogenaemia inherited as a recessive character. Bleeding is not usually as severe as that of severe haemophilia, despite the complete incoagulability of the blood. Normal thrombin generation occurs in this condition but not in haemophilia, and it is supposed that the lack of the thrombin action on platelet function is an additional haemostatic defect in haemophilia. Temporary treatment of afibrinogenaemia consists in the infusion of sufficient fibrinogen to bring the blood level to 100 mgm. per cent, or more. The half life of fibrinogen is 2–5 days.

Other hereditary coagulation defects. Deficiencies of Factors II, V, VII, X, and XIII are exceedingly rare. The inheritance is autosomal and recessive in most cases. Treatment consists of replacement of the appropriate missing factor (see Table 3).

Von Willebrand's disease is a haemorrhagic state inherited as a simple dominant, in which all three components of the mechanism appear to be involved. Clinically it manifests as repeated episodes of bleeding, particularly from the mucous membranes, gastrointestinal and uterine tracts. Trauma, particularly to the nose, mouth or throat, such as tooth extraction or tonsillectomy may lead to persistent bleeding. The laboratory findings are complex. The bleeding time is prolonged, and, though the clotting time may be normal, there is a deficiency of Factor VIII in many cases, down to levels of 0 to 10 per cent of normal. The platelets are normal in number, and most estimates of platelet function are also normal, but there is evidence of impaired adhesion of platelets to glass and some evidence of impaired adhesion to damaged tissues in vivo. There is also evidence of a capillary abnormality in the form of dilated and tortuous vessels seen by skin microscopy. Temporary improvement of the general haemostatic mechanisms can be obtained by plasma transfusions which raise the blood level of Factor VIII, both by reason of the Factor VIII infused and also because the normal plasma stimulates the production of Factor VIII by the patient; which effect, apparently unique to this condition, is still unexplained. It is found that infusions of Factor VIII or plasma to these patients may also temporarily reduce the bleeding time and improve the ability of the platelets to adhere to glass.

From the point of view of surgical intervention, the raising of the plasma concentration of Factor VIII is as important as in haemophilia. If the operation site is accessible, local pressure to secure a dry field at the time of operation together with Factor VIII treatment may give post-operative haemostasis.

Acquired Coagulation Defects

Acquired coagulation defects are much more commonly encountered than congenital defects but are mercifully usually of short duration.

Defibrination syndrome. This syndrome is associated with gross reduction in clottable fibrinogen, reduction in platelets and in blood clotting Factors V, VIII, and XIII. The blood also usually contains fibrin degradation products derived from lysis of fibrinogen or fibrin, and there is reduction in plasminogen concentration. The condition complicates some cases of abruptio placentae, intrauterine fetal death, and severe surgical procedures, particularly pulmonary operations and open heart surgery. It may also occur in patients with leukaemia or disseminated carcinoma. The patient usually suffers profound shock and severe bleeding occurs from the uterus, operation site or venepuncture holes, or the patient may bleed spontaneously.

The condition is in most cases associated with diffuse intravascular clotting and in fact some experts refer to the condition as "DIC." The presence of products of lysis of fibrinogen or fibrin and the reduction in plasminogen (presumably due to consumption of this factor in producing lysis) has, in the past, led to the belief that lysis is the primary cause of the syndrome, but now it is usually accepted that the lysis follows and perhaps compensates for the prior clotting of blood.

Treatment obviously depends on the cause. If intravascular clotting is primary, anticoagulants such as heparin may be indicated. In fact dramatic improvement has been brought about by heparin infusion in some cases. To give heparin to a seriously ill patient whose blood is escaping rapidly from the surface and into the tissues is, however, a difficult decision, and discretion must be used in selecting patients for such treatment. If lysis were the cause then anti-fibrinolytic agents should be preferred but in fact anti-fibrinolytic treatment has led to dangerous and widespread thrombosis in some patients. In any event it seems logical (and is practically effective) to replace the fibrinogen and other factors by whole blood or plasma infusions.

Factors II, VII and X, deficiencies. Acquired deficiencies of Factors II, VII and X are often combined because these factors are all produced in the liver, and are dependent on Vitamin K for their synthesis. In some cases of liver disease, Factor II (prothrombin) deficiency may be the main defect and, though insufficient to cause an overt hæmorrhagic state, or even a gross prolongation of the one-stage "prothrombin time" test, may be severe enough to cause abnormal haemorrhage following surgical operation. A specific assay of Factor II is therefore advisable in such cases before any operation. Vitamin K deficiency as a result of obstructive jaundice or steatorrhoea is usually revealed by a prolongation of the prothrombin time test, and it too may result in serious bleeding at operation unless corrected.

Treatment of these conditions is, firstly, the administration of Vitamin K, which may have to be in the form of Vitamin K$_1$ by injection; in cases where the liver cannot utilize the vitamin or synthesize prothrombin for other reasons, a "prothrombin complex" concentrate containing Factors II, VII, IX and X can be infused.

Factors VIII and IX. Acquired deficiencies of Factors VIII and IX are rare, and are usually due to the development of antibodies opposing their normal function.

Platelet Deficiency

Platelet deficiency may be quantitative or qualitative, inherited or acquired. The clinical picture in such conditions is usually different from that of defective coagulation. Bleeding tends to be spontaneous, in the form of persistent oozing of blood, particularly from mucous membranes, and of petechial haemorrhages, or ecchymoses in the skin. The bleeding time test is prolonged, but the blood clotting time is usually normal since the deficiency of Platelet Factor 3 is seldom absolute, and a fraction of the normal amount is sufficient to cause clotting in the normal time, though the quantitative conversion of prothrombin is reduced. Deep tissue haemorrhages are rare, and bleeding into joints very rare, but serious gastrointestinal or uterine bleeding may occur, and the risk of cerebral haemorrhage is appreciable.

Secondary thrombocytopenic purpura. The commonest form of platelet deficiency is secondary thrombocytopenic purpura, due to the action of chemical poisons, ionizing radiations, drugs and toxins on the bone marrow, to invasion of the marrow by malignant tissue or leukaemia, and to the various forms of aplastic anæmia. In such conditions the onset of haemorrhagic thrombocytopenia is often terminal, but successful treatment or remission of the underlying condition may be possible in some cases and in these the use of platelet transfusions, steroids, and if the defibrination syndrome is a factor, heparin treatment may be indicated.

Idiopathic thrombocytopenic purpura has similar symptoms, but without obvious cause or marrow involvement. Occasionally platelet antibodies can be demonstrated, and the good response to steroid therapy, or splenectomy, suggests that an auto-immune state may be involved in a proportion of cases. Again, acute bleeding episodes may sometimes be controlled by platelet transfusions, perhaps allowing an emergency splenectomy to be carried out safely. In such cases the platelets from 5 to 10 pints of freshly collected blood should be given as a concentrated suspension in plasma and this amount repeated daily until the patient shows signs of improved platelet production or haemostasis.

Hereditary thrombocytopenia is rare; **congenital thrombocytopenia** may occur in babies born of thrombocytopenic mothers, but is usually of short duration.

Thrombocythaemia and **thrombocytosis,** conditions in which there is a pathological increase in platelets, may be associated not only with thrombotic tendencies, but particularly with abnormal bleeding. This seems to be due, in some cases, to abnormal platelet function.

Thrombasthenia or Glanzmann's disease. Qualitative platelet abnormalities are rare and the underlying defect is often obscure. Different workers use a great variety of tests to detect the abnormalities and no well established and generally agreed classification exists. The commonest features include dominant autosomal inheritance, failure of platelets to agglutinate on the addition of ADP, and reduced coagulant activity. Treatment by infusing normal platelet concentrates may be helpful if surgery is required.

Other Abnormalities Causing Haemorrhage

Purely vascular abnormalities causing haemorrhage are rare, apart from the degenerative vascular diseases. **Haemorrhagic telangiectasia,** inherited as a simple dominant, can lead to profuse bleeding from the dilated capillaries forming the lesions, which may be in the nose, gastro-intestinal or pulmonary tracts. General treatment is usually ineffective. Accessible bleeding can be stopped by temporary local pressure, which allows time for the formation of a haemostatic plug. **The Ehlers Danlos syndrome** is often associated with abnormal bleeding. Such cases present diagnostic difficulties, since most laboratory tests are normal, and the characteristic hyperextensibility of the joints, particularly of the fingers and elbows, and the lax skin and stretched scars may be missed unless specifically looked for. Various oral abnormalities, such as notched incisors, microdontia, and friable gingivae have been reported in association with this syndrome, but none is diagnostically specific. In this condition the friability of the vessels and their supporting tissues seems to be the cause of the bleeding.

Abnormal Intra-vascular Thrombosis

Finally, there must be mentioned excessive haemostasis, in the sense of its occurrence in functional intact vessels causing thrombosis. The pathogenesis of this condition is now the centre of much attention and experiment and there are continuing efforts to detect the occurrence of a *pre-thrombotic state* of the blood which would favour thrombosis. Increase in stickiness or in numbers of platelets, increase in the concentration or activity of various clotting factors, decrease of normal inhibitory factors and of fibrinolytic activity have been demonstrated in a proportion of cases of established thrombosis, and in conditions such as the post-operative period in which thrombosis is apt to occur. But no overriding abnormality has been found to be consistently associated with thrombosis. One is left with the impression that a thrombus is the result of a concatenation of the predisposing circumstances recognized for many years: a local abnormality in the vessel wall, disturbances in the blood flow, and an increased coagulability of the blood (and platelet activity) which may occur from time to time as the result of a variety of extraneous factors. In combination these may tip the scale towards thrombosis, though separately they might not disturb the natural balance of the haemostatic mechanism.

FURTHER READING

Biggs, R. and Macfarlane, R. G. (1962), *Human Blood Coagulation and its Disorders*, 3rd Ed. Oxford: Blackwell.

Biggs, R. and Macfarlane, R. G. (1966), *The Treatment of Hæmophilia and other Coagulation Defects*. Oxford: Blackwell.

Born, G. V. R. (1965), "Platelets in Thrombogenesis. Mechanism and Inhibition of Platelet Aggregation", *Ann. Roy. Coll. Surg. Eng.*, **36**, 200.

Duthie, R. B., Matthews, J. M., Rizza, C. R., and Steel, W. M. (1973), *The Management of Musculo-skeletal Problems in the Hæmophilias*. Oxford: Blackwell Scientific Publications.

Esnouf, M. P. and Macfarlane, R. G. (1968), "Enzymology and the Blood Clotting Mechanism", in *Advances in Enzymology*, Vol. 30 (Ed. F. F. Nord). Interscience Publishers.

Hardisty, R. M. and Ingram, G. I. C. (1965), *Bleeding Disorders, Investigation and Management*. Oxford: Blackwell.

Hayem, G. (1882), "Sur le méchanisme de l'arret des hémorrhagies", *C.R. Acad. Sci. (Paris)*, **95**, 18.

Koller, F., Loeliger, A. and Duckert, F. (1951), "Experiments on a new Clotting Factor (Factor VII)", *Acta. Haemat.*, **6**, 1.

Koller, F. (1955), "Le facteur X", *Rev. Hemat*, **10**, 362.

Lister, J. (1863), "Croonian Lecture on the Coagulation of the Blood", *Proc. Roy. Soc.*, **12**, 580.

Macfarlane, R. G. (1964), "An Enzyme Cascade in the Blood Clotting Mechanism; its Function as a Biochemical Amplifier", *Nature*, **202**, 498.

Macfarlane, R. G. (1965), *A Clotting Scheme for 1964 in Genetics and the Interaction of Clotting Factors*, p. 45. Stuttgart: Schattatteuer-Verlag.

Macfarlane, R. G. (Ed.) (1970), "The Hæmostatic Mechanism in Man and Other Animals", in *Proceedings of a Symposium held at the Zoological Society of London*, December 1969. Academic Press.

Marcus, A. J. and Zucker, M. B. (1965), *The Physiology of Blood Platelets*. New York and London: Grune and Stratton.

Owren, P. A. (1947), "The Coagulation of Blood, Investigation of a new Clotting Factor", *Acta. Med. Scand.*, Suppl., 194.

Quick, A. J. (1935), "The Prothrombin in Hemophilia and in Obstructive Jaundice", *J. Biol. Chem.*, **73**, 109.

Rizza, C. R. and Biggs, R. (1971a), "Hæmostasis and Blood Coagulation", in *General Anæsthesia*, 3rd ed. (Eds. T. Cecil Gray and J. F. Nunn), Vol. I. London: Butterworths.

Rizza, C. R. and Biggs, R. (1971b), "Hæmophilia Today", *Brit. J. Hosp. Med.*, **6**, 343.

57. RESUSCITATION

J. P. PAYNE

Collapse in the dental surgery

Emergency measures

Methods of resuscitation

Post-resuscitation considerations

Moral and ethical considerations

INTRODUCTION

In some respects, the practice of dentistry carries the same risks as that of surgery: for example, when local anaesthetic drugs are used to infiltrate the tissues, when intravenous agents are given to induce sleep, or when inhalation agents are administered to provide general anaesthesia, the risks do not differ significantly whether the patient is about to undergo major surgery or a simple tooth extraction. These risks, which are not negligible, include drug sensitivity, severe respiratory depression and even cardiac arrest; thus it is important for the dentist to be completely familiar with the management of such conditions. Moreover, it should not be forgotten that certain conditions dangerous to life can develop anywhere, at any time, and the dental surgery is no exception. Indeed, the anxiety associated with a visit to the dentist could well provoke a severe heart attack or a cerebro-vascular accident in a susceptible patient; under these circumstances, immediate and major resuscitative measures may be required. Furthermore, sudden severe haemorrhage from a peptic ulcer, or as a complication of pregnancy, may give rise to circulatory collapse sufficiently severe to need prompt treatment, including blood transfusion. And even bleeding from the nose or from a tooth-extraction socket has been known to need massive blood replacement. Rarely, a sudden severe and sometimes fatal anaphylactic shock has followed exposure to an antigen to which the victim has been sensitized. Formerly this condition, which is manifested by acute respiratory obstruction and hypotension, usually resulted from the venom of wasps and other stinging insects; but recently, the introduction of drugs capable of combining with body proteins, together with the more frequent use of parenteral routes of administration, has made drug treatment an increasingly important cause of anaphylactic shock. In this respect, the parenteral use of certain forms of penicillin, often given prophylactically, has given rise to anxiety.

A further general point on resuscitation deserves mention. At a time when road casualties have reached epidemic proportions in the western world, and when much thought has been given to the management of mass casualties, the need for experts trained in life-saving emergency procedures has never been greater. Theoretically, the dentist, with his background and training, and particularly with his experience of airway maintenance, is better qualified than most to provide such assistance. In practice however, the story is somewhat different; like the medical practitioner, the dentist often feels incapable of rendering assistance to patients in need of emergency resuscitation and, possibly justifiably in view of his ignorance, is reluctant to become involved in emergency situations. He is thus reduced to the status of an ineffective bystander. The explanation for this apparent paradox lies in the fact that no formal instruction in resuscitation techniques or even in elementary first-aid is provided during medical or dental training at undergraduate level. It is indeed a sad commentary on the priorities in our medical and dental schools that students interested in first-aid have to enrol in the St. John Ambulance or similar organizations to obtain the necessary training.

COLLAPSE IN THE DENTAL SURGERY

As emphasized, the need for resuscitative measures may arise from many causes but in the dental surgery it is most likely to be due to some mishap related either to the surgery or to the anaesthetic technique. Surgical mishaps, with the exception of excessive bleeding, are often mechanical in nature and usually give rise to airway obstruction. A badly placed or dislodged pack, for example, may allow blood, mucus and other debris to reach the larynx and on occasion the pack itself may become impacted. The consequent laryngeal spasm may be sufficiently severe to endanger life. Likewise the inhalation of such debris or, more rarely, of an extracted tooth, may lead to bronchospasm, respiratory obstruction and pulmonary oedema.

Mishaps due to the anaesthetic technique are most commonly related to the drugs employed. In the case of local anaesthetic drugs frank overdosage is rare and toxic effects are usually confined to young children, and then only when the drug has been injected intravenously. Occasionally, however, allergic reactions which occur in all age-groups follow their use and are associated with rashes and swellings. When toxicity is marked, oedema of the larynx may occur and in extreme situations generalized convulsions have been reported. However, the main source of danger with injections of local anaesthetic agent is not the drug itself but the associated vasopressor used to curtail uptake and to reduce bleeding. In most instances, this is either adrenaline or noradrenaline, and both drugs are capable of producing serious side-effects including ventricular fibrillation and cardiac arrest, but more often the side-effects observed are confined to sweating, palpitations and fainting. Fortunately such reactions are well-known and the pattern of management once they have occurred is clearly defined. Less well-known are the consequences of the inter-action of these vasopressors with many of the compounds now prescribed for the treatment of depression. The availability of specific therapeutic substances for such treatment is a relatively new phenomenon but it has important implications for dentists which extend far beyond the management of depression.

The chance discovery that isoniazid, introduced for the treatment of tuberculosis, could inhibit amine oxidase led to a deliberate search for related drugs with a more specific inhibitory action for use in the treatment of certain psychiatric disorders. These new compounds fell into three groups: (a) those related to the amphetamines; (b) the hydrazines, the primary action of which is a powerful inhibition of amine oxidase; and (c) those like imipramine with only a mild amine oxidase effect but yet effective antidepressants. The significance of amine oxidase is that it is a naturally occurring enzyme which destroys adrenaline and noradrenaline in the body, thereby limiting their actions. It was soon discovered that the amine-oxidase inhibitors interacted with amines in food, leading to severe hypertensive crises. It is now known that this occurs because amines such as tyramine, phenylethylamine and tryptamine are found in certain foods such as cheese, meat extracts and beans; the harmful effects that could follow the ingestion of these substances are normally avoided because they are rapidly broken down by amine oxidase, but they are preserved by amine oxidase inhibition. In addition, interaction occurs with other drugs; morphine and pethidine are potentiated and this can result in excitement, coma and hyperthermia; the actions of adrenaline, noradrenaline and ephedrine are enhanced and prolonged; the effects of hypotensive drugs may be distorted and those of the barbiturates potentiated. It is clear, therefore, that before the dentist administers any drug in his surgery he would be wise to question the patient about current drug therapy; it is infinitely easier to avoid the occurrence of a drug interaction crisis than to treat it once it has developed.

As far as general anaesthetics in dentistry are concerned the traditional methods involve the use of nitrous oxide. Originally a single-dose method was employed; the gas was inhaled from a bag through a face-mask until unconsciousness was reached, whereupon the mask was removed and the dentist has approximately thirty seconds in which to complete the extractions before consciousness returned. The addition of oxygen to the nitrous oxide to provide a nitrous oxide-oxygen mixture increased the operating time, and this was further extended at the beginning of the present century by the introduction of the nasal mask which allowed the administration of the anaesthetic to continue throughout the operative procedure.

Paradoxically, the addition of oxygen increased the dangers of nitrous oxide anaesthesia because, for most administrators, the mere presence of oxygen was assumed to guarantee safety and little thought was given to the amount needed. Today it is generally accepted that an inspired concentration of less than 20 per cent oxygen is potentially dangerous, and when it is considered that some degree of respiratory obstruction is virtually inevitable while the dentist works in the mouth the recommendation by some authorities that the inspired concentration of oxygen should never be less than 50 per cent makes sound clinical sense. For satisfactory anaesthesia under these circumstances,

either heavy premedication is required or the anaesthetic needs to be supplemented by an intravenous agent, such as pethidine, or by an inhalation agent like halothane. The greatest single danger during general anaesthesia is a deficiency in the oxygen supply to the tissues which may result from respiratory obstruction, from central respiratory depression, or from an inspired breathing mixture deficient in oxygen. But whatever the cause, the end result is the same if the hypoxia is severe and prolonged; irreversible cerebral damage and cardiac arrest are inevitable if severe hypoxia is not relieved. The most obvious sign of danger is cyanosis, and it should never be allowed to persist. It indicates the presence of a substantial amount of desaturated haemoglobin in the circulating blood and as such represents a deficiency in the amount of oxygen available in the blood. Unfortunately, the absence of cyanosis is no guarantee of safety. If, for example, the red blood cells have a low haemoglobin content as in certain types of anaemia, severe hypoxaemia may exist without cyanosis. For cyanosis to be obvious a minimum of 5 g. per cent unsaturated haemoglobin must be present in the blood; the amount of saturated or oxyhaemoglobin present is relatively unimportant. Furthermore, in negroes and other dark-skinned patients pigmentation may prevent the detection of cyanosis until the degree of hypoxaemia is sufficiently severe to be determined by other means.

The advent of intravenous anaesthesia has made little substantial difference to the risk of hypoxia. Indeed, the technique of administering small repeated doses of barbiturates by the intravenous route for conservative dentistry has proved to be just as controversial as some of the earlier methods, and certainly the evidence presented to support the claims of superiority is far from convincing. Undoubtedly the technique has advantages in skilled hands, but the danger to the patient when intermittent injections of barbiturate are given by a single-handed operator-anaesthetist, whose attention is distracted by a delicate or complicated manoeuvre, needs no further emphasis.

The dangers are not lessened by the usual position of the patient undergoing dental treatment. When a general anaesthetic is administered for major surgery the supine position is most commonly adopted, but when a general anaesthetic is given for a dental procedure the patient is more likely to be sitting upright in a dental chair. The additional risk, especially in the elderly, of prolonged hypotension during anaesthesia in this position, particularly if the intravenous route has been employed, has yet to be fully evaluated. Moreover, there is evidence to suggest that episodes of fainting are not uncommon in this position and frequently go unnoticed by the anaesthetist. If this is the case then undoubtedly the inadequate circulation, together with the effects of the anaesthetic, could lead to cerebral damage. It remains to be seen how many such cases can be identified, but on general physiological principles it can be argued that the upright position during general anaesthesia is difficult to justify.

EMERGENCY MEASURES

When collapse occurs, resuscitation procedures fall naturally into two categories. Firstly, emergency measures are effected to protect the victim and to restore vital functions when necessary. Secondly, more specific therapy is needed to deal with individual problems such as pain, blood or fluid loss, hypoxia, tissue damage and bone injuries. In many instances, the emergency treatment of laying the victim flat and maintaining a clear airway is sufficient, and this must always include a check for the presence of foreign material causing obstruction. If the victim is conscious,

METHODS OF RESUSCITATION

The techniques of cardiopulmonary resuscitation are simple and easily learned. They have the further advantages that no detailed knowledge is necessary and that no special equipment is required; the rescuer needs only his hands to compress the victim's heart and a sufficient vital capacity and reserve of energy to inflate his lungs rhythmically.

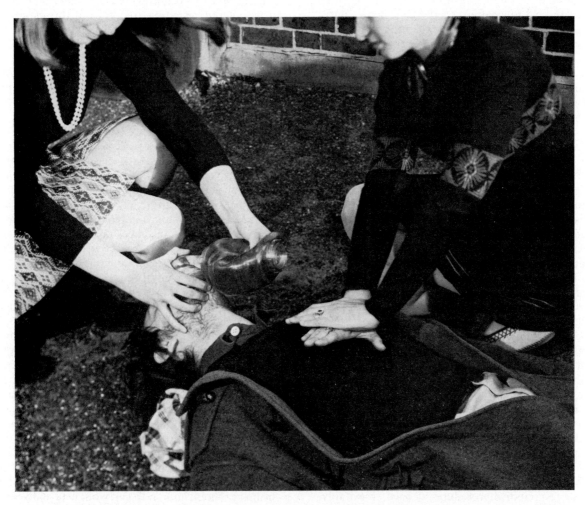

FIG. 1. Application of external cardiac compression combined with positive pressure ventilation.

reassurance will be required and persistent bleeding should be stopped or at least reduced by packing the wound which, in any case, should be shielded from contamination.

In patients moribund or apparently dead the full cardiopulmonary resuscitation procedure should be started at once without waiting for the arrival of specialist help or equipment. If not delayed, the use of mouth-to-mouth ventilation combined with external cardiac compression significantly reduces the loss of life when sudden respiratory or cardiac arrest occurs as a result of trauma or drugs in otherwise healthy individuals and, even when cardiovascular or other disease is the cause, some reduction in mortality has been achieved by prompt measures.

When cardiac compression is started (see fig. 1) it is important to avoid damage to the ribs and to such underlying structures as the liver and spleen. Accordingly, it is suggested that only the heel of the hand should be used to exert pressure on the chest wall and this is best done with the long axis of the hand laid against the lower end of the sternum. The other hand is then placed at right-angles over the first, and with the arms held rigid sufficient pressure is applied at 1 sec. intervals to move the sternum approximately 4–5 cm. with each stroke. This compresses the heart against the spinal column and produces an appreciable pulsation palpable in the carotid and femoral arteries. As each compression movement is withdrawn, the hands should be lifted momentarily just clear of the chest, to allow full expansion. A firm background is essential for effective cardiac compression and the hospital ward or dental surgery floor is excellent for this purpose, but if the victim is on a bed or on soft ground some form of rigid support such as a board or a tray should be placed under his back at the first opportunity. If the rescuer is alone, the cardiac compression should be interrupted at 15 sec. intervals to allow two rapid and full lung inflations by mouth-to-mouth or mouth-to-nose ventilation, and this pattern should be followed until help arrives. If assistance is available the lungs should be inflated once every 5 sec. without disturbing the rhythm of the cardiac compression.

Sometimes the victim starts to breathe spontaneously as soon as the hypoxia has been relieved, and this is always associated with a prompt return of the heart beat. Occasionally, however, prolonged resuscitative efforts may be needed and these may have to be continued until the victim is admitted to hospital unless the evidence of death is incontrovertible. In hospital, the decision to discontinue resuscitation in the absence of signs of life is the responsibility of the receiving clinician, preferably in consultation with an experienced specialist.

The decision to start resuscitative measures is sometimes equally difficult. Time is the most important single factor in all successful resuscitative procedures and no elaborate time-consuming system of diagnosis can be tolerated. If the victim has stopped breathing, and if the carotid and femoral pulses are absent, external cardiac compression should be started forthwith. Fixed dilated pupils support the accuracy of the diagnosis and their prompt reduction in size once resuscitation has been started provides confirmation that the circulation to the brain is at least adequate. But if it is known that the victim is suffering from a terminal illness, or that he has been apnoeic and pulseless for longer than 10 min., no attempt at resuscitation should be made. Almost certainly, if the heart has been stopped for longer than 5 min., irreversible brain damage will have occurred and under these circumstances resuscitative efforts are unjustified. Unfortunately, the rescuer faced with an apnoeic and pulseless victim is rarely presented with precise information, and he has little alternative but to initiate resuscitative procedures at once. Inevitably such decisions raise serious medico-legal and ethical questions, some of which have been discussed in detail in the *Proceedings of the Second International Symposium on Emergency Resuscitation* (Lund and Lind, 1968).

Recently, a possible alternative to external cardiac compression has been proposed. It is claimed that, in some instances, a sharp blow will depolarize the ventricles of the heart and produce a systolic contraction. It is further claimed that rhythmical chest pounding with the fist will restore normal cardiac contractions in cases of cardiac asystole, although apparently it is ineffective if ventricular fibrillation is present. It is difficult to understand why a heart that is fibrillating does not respond to such treatment when an arrested heart does so, and it may be that the technique has not been fully investigated; certainly it has not been fully documented. Indeed, the method itself remains to be proved, but as the time needed to carry out

the manoeuvre is so short it is probably worth attempting in every instance of cardiac arrest.

Occasionally the heart will not respond to any external method of stimulation and the rescuer is left with no choice: he must open the chest, preferably by an incision in the fourth left intercostal space, separate the adjacent ribs and apply direct manual compression to the heart. For this purpose it may be necessary to use both hands inside the pleural cavity to compress the heart antero-posteriorly but it is sometimes possible to carry out this manoeuvre with one hand by direct rhythmical compression of the heart against the inner surface of the sternum and the adjoining ribs. Obviously it would be preferable to carry out such heroic measures with the proper instruments and under sterile conditions in the operating room, but in practice it may have to be done with a pen-knife on the floor of a dental surgery or even by the roadside.

Once the immediate problem of maintaining the circulation has been resolved the next step is to establish the type of cardiac arrest. If the chest is open this can be done by direct inspection, but when external cardiac compression is used an electrocardiograph will be needed. In particular, a distinction needs to be made between circulatory failure due to cardiac asystole and that due to ventricular fibrillation; in the latter instance, normal rhythm may not be restored until the heart has been defibrillated electrically and this demands specialized equipment.

Since the fundamental defect caused by cardiac arrest is a failure of oxygen transport to the tissues, the provision of oxygen to the lungs must be an essential component of the overall management of resuscitation. Thus external cardiac compression by itself is useless; it must always be accompanied by some form of artificial ventilation except perhaps in the case of infants in whom the cardiac compression may also serve to establish some degree of respiratory gas exchange. Over the years, different methods of artificial ventilation have been introduced, but except in special circumstances such as mutilating injuries to the mouth and nose they have all been replaced by mouth-to-mouth or mouth-to-nose resuscitation. The main reason for this change is that the method is both easy to learn and easy to apply, as witnessed by the success of the Norwegians in training their primary schoolchildren to carry out artificial ventilation in this way.

Perhaps at this stage it should be emphasized that, even today, respiratory obstruction and failure are among the commonest causes of preventable accidental death and that cardiac arrest is usually secondary to respiratory arrest, yet simple manoeuvres such as removing vomitus or other debris from the throat, providing a clear airway by supporting the chin or by placing the victim in the semi-prone position or establishing mouth-to-mouth or mouth-to-nose ventilation could save more lives than any other emergency procedure. The greatest single cause of unsuccessful resuscitation is unnecessary delay in initiating the resuscitation procedure, which should be undertaken the moment that the respiratory arrest is recognized.

Once the decision to start artificial respiration has been taken, the first task of the rescuer is to make sure that the mouth and the throat are free from blood, vomitus, dislodged teeth, dentures or other foreign bodies. In the absence of suitable suction apparatus, this is best done by sweeping round the mouth with two fingers wrapped in a gauze swab or in a handkerchief. Thereafter the victim's head is extended on the neck and the mouth held slightly open. Then, having taken a deep breath, the rescuer presses his mouth against that of the victim and exhales gently but steadily until the patient's chest is seen to expand. The whole procedure, which is repeated at intervals of 4 sec. until such time as spontaneous breathing returns, is facilitated if the victim's nostrils are pinched firmly during each inflation.

It can scarcely be denied that many potential rescuers find direct mouth-to-mouth ventilation aesthetically distasteful, particularly when the victim's mouth has been full of blood, broken teeth or vomit or when the breath is saturated with tobacco or alcohol. Accordingly, various refinements of the mouth-to-mouth technique have been devised to avoid direct contact with the victim. These include the use of simple or double airways and others which incorporate a one-way valve system.

In patients with severe face, neck or chest injuries, tracheal intubation provides the best method of ensuring a clear airway, but unfortunately many doctors and dentists are not competent to carry out intubation and in the small minority of patients who need to be intubated tracheotomy or laryngotomy is the only alternative. But except in skilled hands tracheotomy is a relatively complicated procedure and laryngotomy is probably to be preferred. For this purpose the crico-thyroid membrane, the soft relatively avascular tissue between the thyroid and cricoid cartilages, must be identified and incised. This is most easily done by extending the neck to throw the thyroid cartilage into prominence; immediately below it the membrane can be palpated with ease (see figs. 2a and b). A single transverse incision is then made through skin, fascia and membrane into the larynx with whatever instrument is available. Ideally a scalpel should be used, but a penknife is equally effective and even a razor blade and a pair of scissors have been employed successfully. Once the incision had been made, it is a relatively simple task to insert a tube into the trachea.

When artificial ventilation has to be maintained over a longer period, some form of hand-operated and preferably self-inflating bag should be substituted for mouth-to-mouth ventilation; several such bags have been specifically designed for emergency use. Two of the most widely used in the United Kingdom are the Ambu Resuscitator and the Laerdal Resusci-bag. The Ambu-bag is made of neoprene rubber which is very resistant to heat, light and damp. The Laerdal bag, which shares these properties, is composed of a transparent plastic material. They are both self-inflating, and each incorporates a one-way valve to prevent rebreathing and carbon dioxide accumulation; in addition, a simple attachment on the inlet valve allows oxygen to be used instead of air for inflation of the lungs.

POST-RESUSCITATION CONSIDERATIONS

In this connection it should be stressed that, except in cases of transient cardiac arrest, the need for oxygen is virtu-

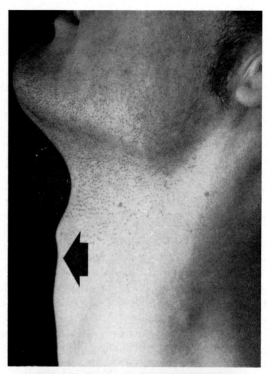

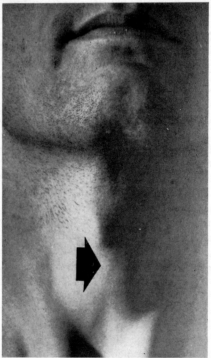

FIG. 2. (a) and (b). Landmarks for laryngotomy. Position for incision (arrowed).

ally universal in the immediate post-arrest period even in those patients in whom the return of spontaneous breathing appears to be both prompt and adequate; oxygen should therefore be provided at the earliest opportunity. This is because, almost invariably, after an arrested heart has begun to beat spontaneously its output is only slowly restored to normal. Since tissue oxygenation is dependent on blood flow as well as on the oxygen-carrying capacity of the blood, any deficiency in these variables reduces the oxygen availability at tissue level, sometimes substantially in those patients in whom blood loss has contributed to the cardiac arrest. The provision of an oxygen-enriched mixture, therefore, can ensure that the oxygen requirements of the tissues are met by increasing the amount carried per unit volume of blood. The oxygen availability in blood is a function of the concentration of oxygen present in the air reaching the lungs, of the efficiency of the respiratory gas exchange mechanisms in the lungs, and of the haemoglobin content of the blood.

One further aspect of cardio-pulmonary resuscitation needs discussion. Every patient who has sustained respiratory or cardiac arrest should be admitted to hospital for further observation and treatment, not only because of the risk of further pulmonary and cardiac damage, but also because a period of cardiac arrest is frequently followed by the development of cerebral oedema which, if not properly treated, can lead to serious and permanent brain damage. Unfortunately, many such patients tolerate movement badly and their transfer to hospital raises additional problems. Firstly, in some victims of cardiac arrest the state of the circulation remains so precarious for many hours after the restoration of a normal heart beat that even the postural changes induced by stretcher manipulation may be sufficient to cause a further cardiac arrest. Secondly, the patient tends to be highly vulnerable during the ambulance journey, partly because many ambulances are inadequately equipped to deal with emergency situations and partly because not all ambulance crews are suitably trained to deal with these emergencies. Thirdly, the frequent braking and acceleration necessitated by modern traffic conditions impose additional strains on the victims, particularly those who have suffered head injuries or fractures of the lower limb.

Accordingly, wherever possible, specialist advice should be sought before a decision is taken to move a patient who has been resuscitated after cardiac arrest. Unfortunately, it is still true that many victims who respond initially to cardio-pulmonary resuscitation fail to survive because continued management is inadequate. Consequently, although it has been argued that successful cardio-pulmonary resuscitation can be achieved without any special equipment, this does not relieve the clinician of the responsibility to ensure that in situations of high risk every possible means of supporting life is available if required. Thus, in the dental surgery, which must be included in the category of high risk, the dental surgeon has a moral if not a legal obligation to provide the basic equipment needed.

Among other requirements a supply of oxygen, together with a method of administration, takes high priority. Oxygen is normally provided in cylinders of different sizes; but small self-generating chemical packs, such as those used for mine-rescue work, have certain advantages. The methods of oxygen administration may vary; in most dental surgeries the substitution of a facemask for the nasal attachment on the standard anaesthetic machine is both convenient and effective, especially when supplemented by suitable airways; but some dentists prefer to have separate resuscitation equipment and a self-inflating hand-operated face-mask and reservoir bag is a useful safeguard should the oxygen supply become exhausted. In addition, a selection of cuffed endotracheal tubes together with a battery-operated laryngoscope of the type commonly used in anaesthetic practice are useful adjuvants on the rare occasions when intubation becomes necessary. Possibly of greater use in emergency situations is a powerful suction apparatus, but this is usually standard equipment in the dental surgery.

Although drugs have little part to play in the initial resuscitation procedures, once the heart is beating regularly and consciousness is restored a strong analgesic drug such as morphine does much to allay anxiety and relieve pain. In this respect, it is perhaps worth noting that the regulations concerning the control of dangerous drugs (1971) have recently been strengthened, and dentists may have to consider whether their system of storage and record-keeping is still within the law.

MORAL AND ETHICAL CONSIDERATIONS

The availability of sterile packs containing certain basic necessities such as airways, endotracheal tubes, gauze swabs and dressings as well as a few essential instruments in high-risk areas is becoming increasingly common and is both opportune and time-saving. In this connection some doctors now carry such emergency packs in their own cars and, indeed, in some countries all doctors are compelled by law to do so. Such laws obviously reflect the deep anxiety felt over the steadily increasing morbidity and mortality produced by accidents of all kinds. In particular, the high incidence of multiple casualties in air and train disasters and motor-way crashes, together with a greater recognition of the need for properly organized resuscitation procedures, are matters of some public concern. Already anxiety is being expressed through the press and the broadcasting media about the unsatisfactory nature of resuscitation facilities and casualty evacuation in some areas. Moreover, it has not gone unnoticed that many doctors are incapable of applying their theoretical knowledge of resuscitation, and the position is not improved by the fact that medical and dental students still qualify without any formal instruction in resuscitation techniques or even in elementary first-aid.

It seems likely that the strong moral pressure exerted by public opinion, reinforced by the outspoken comments of those doctors most closely concerned with resuscitation, will force a much greater direct involvement of all doctors and dentists in the management of resuscitation. In the first instance, this means that medical and dental schools will need to provide formal training in first-aid and resuscitation techniques, and a strong case can be argued for making this part of the first-year curriculum with revision courses annually until graduation.

REFERENCES

Lund, I. and Lind, B. (1968), "Aspects of Resuscitation", *Acta anaesth. Scand.*, suppl. 29.
Misuse of Drugs Act (1971), London: H.M.S.O.

58. CLINICAL TRIALS

G. N. DAVIES

INTRODUCTION

In dentistry as in medicine no agent for the prevention, treatment or control of disease can be recommended for general use until its safety and efficacy have been evaluated and confirmed by thorough clinical testing in humans. Following the thalidomide disaster, the regulatory authority of governments has been greatly strengthened in many countries. In the United States, for example, the Federal Food, Drug and Cosmetic Act has been amended to ensure that a new drug cannot be distributed for use in man without approval by the Food and Drug Administration. Special permission is required before a clinical trial can be undertaken, and is granted only when the rigidly prescribed requirements are met.

In the United Kingdom a Committee has been set up to ensure that an adequate investigation is made of the possible harmful effects of drugs before administration to man. This Committee has no legal powers of enforcement but it has successfully executed strong moral pressure to ensure that clinical trials are properly controlled. In the Netherlands the approval of a Government Commission is required before any product claiming to have therapeutic or preventive effect can be sold on the open market. In 1966 the National Health and Medical Research Council of Australia endorsed a comprehensive statement setting out the circumstances in which clinical experimentation is permissible and stressing the scientific and moral standards that must be adhered to. The Council emphasized the desirability of consultation, the continuing duty of the investigator towards the subject, the need for provision of full facilities, and the obligation to ensure comprehension by the subject before accepting his consent.

Statement of the Aim

The first step in planning a clinical trial is to define succinctly and precisely what it is hoped to prove and to consider whether these aims can be ethically fulfilled (Hill, 1962). As a general principle, the aim should be to answer a few specific questions. The research should be designed to avoid introducing a large number of variables into a trial in the hope that the relative effect of each on the efficacy of the agent can be assessed by statistical subtleties at the conclusion of the trial. As Hill (1962) says: "Too often an attempt to answer many questions at one time results in answering none wholly or none clearly".

The scientific sophistication of modern dentistry has greatly increased the demand for proper assessment of preventive and therapeutic measures. Clinical trials can thus have a wide range of objectives such as the evaluation of diagnostic procedures, or therapeutic and preventive measures, and of techniques and equipment. The variety is such that all clinical trials cannot be conducted in exactly the same way. The objectives determine the details of the design. Nevertheless there are some features common to all and it is with these features that this chapter is concerned.

Conditions That Must be Satisfied Before a Clinical Trial is Undertaken

Clinical trials on humans should not be contemplated until there is substantial evidence that the agent or procedure to be tested is potentially efficacious and safe. The rationale for its use must be scientifically acceptable and, wherever possible, there should be evidence from *in vitro* and/or animal studies to establish its potential usefulness. This may not always be feasible. In a few cases such as an assessment of various methods of toothbrushing there can be no scientific or moral objection to beginning with a pilot study on humans. In either case a preliminary test or pilot study is highly desirable. Clinical trials are expensive in terms of time, personnel and materials. A properly designed pilot study will permit a preliminary cost-benefit analysis of the proposal. Such an analysis will enable the investigator to determine whether or not the potential benefits are commensurate with the cost of mounting a full-scale clinical trial. Another advantage of a pilot study is that it will enable the investigator to facilitate the conduct of the main clinical trial by evaluating such factors as patient acceptance, familiarity of the personnel with the criteria and methods, cooperation of resource personnel such as health and education authorities, and the general adequacy of the protocol to meet unexpected contingencies.

An important feature of both *in vitro* and animal studies is that the conditions should simulate as closely as possible the conditions that apply in man. The very poor correlation between the results of *in vitro* tests and those of clinical trials of agents for the prevention of caries may be attributed to the use of unrealistic test procedures with saliva instead of plaque, powdered enamel instead of intact enamel and higher concentrations of the agent and longer reaction times than those used clinically (American Dental Association, 1972).

The results of tests of potential agents for the prevention of caries in animals and man have also given contradictory results in many cases, *e.g.* ammoniated dentifrices, phosphates, antibiotics and trace elements. On the other hand, there has been a high positive correlation between the results of animal studies and clinical trials of agents like fluorides which affect the chemistry of enamel. Rats and hamsters are the most commonly used animals for testing potential agents for the prevention of dental caries even though there are considerable differences between rodents and man with respect to individual factors affecting caries such as tooth morphology, ultrastructure of enamel, physical and chemical properties of saliva, and the oral microflora. Because of the difficulty in making appropriate allowances for such differences, increasing attention is now being given to the use of monkeys for caries research. The chemical composition of their saliva is somewhat different from that of human saliva but the microbial ecology of the mouth is similar and monkeys can adapt themselves to dietary regimens which are known to promote caries in man. The main disadvantages of using non-human primates for this purpose are associated with cost and the stringent measures required for maintaining a colony in a healthy state. These animals, however, have obvious advantages for experimental studies of other oro-dental problems such as the factors influencing growth and development, diseases of oral soft tissues, biological reactions to filling materials, and endodontic and surgical procedures.

Suffice it to say as a generalization that if a particular agent is effective in preventing a disease in non-human primates it can more readily be expected to be effective in man than can an agent whose action has been tested only on rats or hamsters. Similar arguments apply to tests of toxicity. There are well-established differences between species in their reaction to drugs which is presumably why the Food and Drug Administration in the United States generally requires that, as a minimum, acute toxicity tests should be undertaken in two species of animals and that the route of administration be the same as that to be used in the proposed clinical trials in humans.

Under no circumstances should a clinical trial in humans be undertaken if animal studies indicate that acute toxicity is likely. Whether or not a clinical trial should proceed in the face of evidence of minor side effects is a matter of clinical judgment. A decision to proceed will only be made if the benefits greatly exceed the disadvantages of the side effects.

Before a clinical trial can be started it will be necessary to obtain the approval of appropriate government, professional and voluntary agencies as well as the permission of the participants. Government agencies include health departments and education departments; professional agencies include medical and dental societies; voluntary agencies include parent-teacher groups and service clubs. Time spent in explaining the objectives and general design of the study to key personnel in such groups will greatly facilitate the smooth running of the trial itself. If school children are to be used as participants it is essential to obtain the permission and co-operation of their teachers. Planning should ensure that there are minimal interruptions in school routine.

The co-operation and support of the participants is essential to the success of any clinical trial. This can best be achieved not only by ensuring that they understand what is required of them but also by providing evidence of relevant government, professional and voluntary agency approval and a clear description of the significance of the investigation. Permission to participate by adults or the parents or guardians of children should be obtained in writing. If any side-effects from the use of the test agent are anticipated these must be explained to the participants at the time their co-operation is solicited.

Once the objectives of the trial have been defined and the requisite co-operation assured, it is necessary to design the study in such a manner that answers can be obtained with the least expenditure of money, materials, personnel, labour and time. It is essential to obtain statistical advice at the initial planning stage. This will ensure that the most appropriate experimental design and method of statistical analysis of the results is adopted. This is a complex task. Ideally a statistician should participate actively in all aspects of planning. He must have a clear understanding of the aim of the investigation, the results of any pilot studies, the reliability of any measurements or techniques of examination, the variability of the data to be collected, the magnitude of the benefits which would be regarded as of practical significance, the level of statistical significance which the investigator regards as appropriate, and the possibility of any adverse effects and constraints upon the design of the trial imposed by time, cost, and the actions of the participants and co-operating agencies.

EXAMINER ERROR

The measurement of any human attribute is subject to error, first, because of inherent variability in the attribute itself. For example, the number of microorganisms per unit volume of saliva varies not only from day to day but also at different times during the same day.

Secondly, the ability of the investigator to count or measure to a consistent standard is dependent upon such obvious characteristics as his training, experience, tactile sense, visual acuity and physical fitness. It also depends upon technical factors. This is particularly important in the assessment of both dental caries and periodontal disease. Dental caries proceeds from an initial lesion which cannot be diagnosed clinically, to an advanced lesion which can be recognized by the simplest method of examination.

Between these two extremes is a stage that has been called the "Transition Zone". The probability of making a reliable and consistent diagnosis of caries at the level of the initial microscopic lesion is zero. The probability of making a consistent diagnosis at the level of the gross lesion (characterized by extensive cavitation) should be close to 1·0. Within the transition zone, however, diagnoses are likely to be unreliable and depend heavily upon the examiner's skill, judgment and physical characteristics already enumerated. Examiner error in the clinical assessment of dental caries is largely due to the inability of the examiner to make an unequivocal distinction between a doubtful lesion and a true lesion (or between a sound and a carious tooth). This diagnostic error poses singular difficulties because only one type of error is disclosed—namely the change from a positive diagnosis at the first examination to a negative diagnosis at the second. This is known as a reversal. Since it is uncommon for an overt lesion to heal itself, an examiner may think it is justifiable to correct an "obvious" diagnostic error, but if he does it will tend to bias the results by inflating the estimate of the true caries increment. Since the increment of caries is smaller when an effective agent is used the bias decreases the chance of detecting a real effect when testing a preventive agent. The inability of an examiner to maintain absolute reproducibility in his examinations can easily be demonstrated by having him perform duplicate examinations on the same group of subjects over a period of time which is short enough to exclude the possibility of real changes in the condition being examined. Under ideal conditions, if one subtracts the results of the first examination from the results of the second the discrepancies should be distributed symmetrically about zero and the mean discrepancy should be zero. In such a situation, there is a reasonable assurance that the methods of examination are satisfactorily standardized and that the diagnostic criteria are being applied consistently. At least the examination errors are occurring randomly and no systematic error is apparent.

Similar difficulties arise in the diagnosis of periodontal disease. Few people have any difficulty in recognizing advanced destructive periodontal disease but errors of considerable magnitude occur in the diagnosis of early gingivitis; moreover, the assumption that gingivitis can be equated with early periodontitis is unproven.

Calibration

In any clinical trial it is essential for the examiners to be trained to render consistent clinical judgments. Otherwise, each examiner will interpret and apply written instructions in his own way and this will result in excessive within-examiner and between-examiner variability. Between-examiner variability can, of course, be eliminated by having all the assessments or measurements done by one examiner. Even so, the problem of within-examiner variability remains.

When more than one examiner is used in a trial each should, as nearly as possible, participate to an equal extent in the examinations of each experimental and control group. Regardless of the number of examiners used, it is essential that they undergo a period of calibration training before the trial begins. This training is necessary to ensure uniform interpretation, understanding, and application of the diagnostic criteria for the conditions which are to be observed and recorded; to ensure that individual examiners can examine to a consistent standard; and to ensure that variations between examiners are minimized. During the training period each examiner should make a series of independent recordings on the same subjects on different days until "acceptable" reproducibility is attained. "Acceptable" is difficult to define but it has been suggested that it is reasonable to expect an agreement of 85 per cent or better for most measurement procedures or indices.

Calibration training should continue until satisfactory or "acceptable" reproducibility is attained. Any examiner who is unable to examine to a consistent standard should be dropped from the team. If all examiners are unable to be consistent the diagnostic criteria and methods should be re-examined and modified.

Duplicate examinations should be done before a trial begins and also on randomly selected subjects at intervals during the trial. The examiner should not know which subjects will be re-examined and sufficient time should be allowed to elapse between duplicate examinations so that original diagnostic decisions or measurements cannot be remembered. The results of the duplicate examinations should be published with the results of the trial so that the magnitude of the examiner error can be assessed by the reader of the report.

It is advantageous to combine the calibration trial with a pilot survey. If subjects chosen for the calibration trial are representative of the general population with respect to those factors which influence the condition being examined, the results will provide a tentative assessment of the range of conditions likely to be encountered in the main clinical trial. This will greatly facilitate planning.

Recorders as well as examiners should participate in a calibration trial since it is what is recorded on the examination form that determines the outcome of the study. At the 1972 Conference on Clinical Testing of the American Dental Association special attention was paid to the precautions which should be observed in order to obviate recording errors.

THE DESIGN OF A CLINICAL TRIAL

Detailed descriptions of the design and analysis of clinical trials of preventive or therapeutic agents will be found in American Dental Association (1972); Chilton (1967); Finney (1955); Fisher (1951); Grainger (1972); Hill (1960, 1962) and Horowitz et al. (1973).

Written Plan or Protocol

It is essential to have a written set of instructions (called a protocol) in which all procedures, criteria and terms are clearly defined. Full details of the manner in which the trial is to be conducted should be given. It should be drawn-up in consultation with a statistician and should include a hypothetical description of the results.

All the examiners and recorders taking part in the trial should discuss and approve the protocol and must then follow the instructions exactly. Once the trial has begun there should be no change in either the method of assessment or in the criteria. If exceptional circumstances demand a revision of the protocol, data accumulated before the change must be clearly differentiated from those obtained after the change.

Description of the Type of Clinical Trial

The essential feature of a clinical trial is that the effect of a new agent or procedure on one group of subjects is compared with the effect on another group of subjects of a standard procedure or a placebo. If everything, except the new procedure under test, has remained constant over a period of time it may be possible to plan a trial with past events and observations as the standard of comparison. Such occasions are rare. Hill (1962) cites the example of a disease for which the fatality rate was 100 per cent. If recovery is used as the criterion of success then if the administration of a drug leads to the recovery of any patients there is clear evidence that the drug concerned has some value.

Similar but less spectacular examples occur in dentistry, for example, in connection with clinical trials of fluoridation of public water supplies. A base-line survey is made to determine the prevalence of dental caries in a specified group of subjects in a particular community. The water supply is fluoridated and subsequent surveys are undertaken to find out whether or not the prevalence of the disease (or conversely the age specific proportion of subjects caries-free) changes over time. This type of trial is known as a **Prevalence** (or Cross-Sectional) Study. The major weakness of this type of investigation is that it is difficult to establish with certainty that factors other than fluoride have not influenced the observed changes in prevalence of the disease. On the other hand replication of the trials with results which consistently confirm the beneficial outcome of the original trials gives the requisite credibility to the effectiveness of fluoride.

The more common type of trial is one in which there are concurrent controls. The test agent or procedure is administered to one group of subjects while another group similar in their characteristics to the treated group is either given no treatment or is given a placebo. Examinations or measurements are made at the beginning of the trial and at periodic intervals of time to determine the appearance of new cases of the disease or condition (this is known as an **Incidence** Study) or to determine any changes in the severity of the disease or condition. Both of these sub-types are known as longitudinal studies.

In some clinical trials there are ethical reasons why the results should be subject to continuous analysis as they become available. This will permit the trial to be discontinued as soon as it can safely be concluded that one treatment is more effective than another. This is known as a **Sequential** Trial. In clinical dentistry the sequential approach might be used in a long-term investigation of an acute disease such as acute necrotizing ulcerative gingivitis where the recovery of a patient can occur in a few days but where the prevalence of the condition is so low that the trial

might take place over a period of months or years. Statistical tests are available for detecting significant differences between two proportions and differences between the means of paired observations. For each test the investigator must decide in advance the magnitude of the differences he wishes to be certain of detecting. The sequential analysis of the results can then be performed by simple graphical methods.

The ideal clinical trial is one in which all known variables except the one under test are held constant. This cannot always be achieved in clinical or biological research so that it is necessary to use some device designed to correct for the effect of other variables which may be changing in an unknown or uncontrollable way during the study. The usual way of doing this is to divide the group of subjects into an experimental group (the treated group) and a control group (the untreated group) by a random process which ensures that each subject has an equal chance of being allocated to either group. The experimental group is given the test treatment. The control group may be given no treatment; but this is not always satisfactory, because the psychological effect of getting some treatment can itself influence the course of some diseases. One alternative is to give the control group an "inert" treatment known as a **placebo**, but the weakness of this design is that the experiment can only show if the treatment is better than nothing. For this reason, it is often better to design a study to compare the new treatment with a standard treatment. This design is not used as often as it should be. Large numbers of new treatments are constantly being devised but there is insufficient information about which one is best. This type of experiment is known as a **controlled trial**. The simplest example is one in which an attempt is made to compare two agents under standardized conditions. But when an investigator seeks to compare several treatments or to compare different effects of a single agent it would be extravagant to set up a controlled trial for each pair. Furthermore, the results would often be far from satisfactory because comparisons were not all made under the same conditions or because an essential feature of the investigation was to examine the interactions of various combinations of treatments.

Refinements in the designs of experiments with the latter type of objectives owe much to agricultural research and especially to the work of Fisher (1951). In field experiments the ultimate experimental unit that receives a treatment such as a fertilizer, method of cultivation, seed or time of sowing is the **plot**. This term has been transferred to many other types of experiments although the plot may be entirely different from an area of agricultural land. The plot may be a tooth, a dental patient, or a sample of saliva. Whatever the units to which treatments are to be applied each treatment must be allocated to two or more plots so that the variation between units treated alike can be assessed.

When an investigator wishes to compare several treatments simultaneously he must plan to make comparisons with maximum precision in order to keep the total number of plots that can be used within the limit of his resources. For example, if the growth of four strains of bacteria were to be compared, the plot might be a single inoculated plate on which some assessment of growth (*e.g.* number of colonies) was to be made. If the total number of plates is limited they should be divided at random into four equal groups to which the strains will be allocated at random. For convenience, it is best to ensure that the number of plots is a multiple of the number of treatments.

Sometimes it is possible to group the plots which share a common characteristic (usually with equal numbers of plots per group). These groups are termed **blocks**. A block may be a single litter of animals, a set of blood or saliva samples obtained from one person, a series of determinations made on one day or by one man, or a set of inocula on one agar plate destined to receive doses of different antibiotic preparations. In short, any property of the plots that can be determined before an experiment begins can form the basis of grouping into blocks. The object of grouping plots into blocks is, of course, to reduce variation in the experiment as a whole. Blocks are formed in such a way that each contains as many plots as there are treatments to be tested, and one plot from each block is randomly selected for each treatment.

Randomized blocks are frequently valuable in tests of technique. Assume, for example, that it is desired to compare counts of lactobacilli made on five different plates from the same sample of saliva. Repeated tests by the same method would allow the possibility of differences peculiar to the technique of dilution. Instead one plate could be counted from each of five different dilutions. Here the blocks—the different dilutions—give a broader basis for any inferences that might be drawn and serve to supply information about errors due to differences in dilution.

RANDOMIZED BLOCK DESIGN TO DETERMINE NUMBERS OF LACTOBACILLI COUNTED ON FIVE DIFFERENT ALIQUOTS OF THE SAME SAMPLE BY THE SAME OPERATOR

Plate	Dilution				
	I	II	III	IV	V
A					
B					
C					
D					
E					

The statistical analysis of the experiment involves partitioning the variation between all observations into a component representing differences between dilutions, another representing differences between plates and a third from which the residual variance or error can be assessed.

An expansion of the Randomized Block Design is the **Latin Square Design**. Since bacteria tend to clump together, variations in the counts of lactobacilli from different aliquots of the same sample of saliva may be caused by variations in the length of time the samples are shaken before a dilution is made. An experiment using a Latin Square Design can be undertaken to determine the extent of technical variations (or sources of error) due to samples, dilu-

tions, shaking time and the residual experimental error. In the randomized block design, the sources of variation were partitioned into three categories: between plates, between dilutions, and the residual or other sources of variation not specifically accounted for. In the Latin Square Design the influence of a further source of variation (shaking time) is determined.

LATIN SQUARE DESIGN TO DETERMINE THE EXTENT OF TECHNICAL VARIATIONS IN COUNTING LACTOBACILLI

Aliquot	Dilution				
	I	II	III	IV	V
A	a	c	b	e	d
B	e	d	c	a	b
C	d	a	e	b	c
D	c	b	a	d	e
E	b	e	d	c	a

Five different aliquots of the same sample of saliva (A–E) are collected and each aliquot is subjected to five dilutions (I–V) and each dilution is shaken for a specified period of time (a–e). The shaking times (a–e) are allocated in such a way that each dilution is subjected to each shaking time.

Larger and more complex designs are possible but those mentioned serve to re-emphasize the important fact that a statistician should be consulted during the planning stage of an experiment.

The Null Hypothesis and Tests for Significance

All clinical trials are experiments in which an attempt is made to find out whether an expected event will happen or to find out which of two or more "treatments" is effective. In the first type of experiment, the result is compared with the probability that the event could have occurred by chance. In the second type of experiment, a determination is made of the probability that the difference between two or more "treatments" could have occurred by chance. Before the experiment is begun it is tentatively assumed that the outcome will be negative (viz. the expected event will not happen or there is no difference between the drugs). This tentative negative assumption is known as the **Null Hypothesis**.

The assumption is then put to the test by experiment. If it is proved wrong (the expected event does happen or Drug A is significantly better than B) the result is decisive. On the other hand, if the assumption is not proved to be wrong the result is said to be not proven under the conditions of the experiment. It is important to realize that the Null Hypothesis can never be proven by experiment. What can be done is to assess the probability that it is not true. Another way of describing this concept is to say that the outcome of an experiment is expressed as a probability that the result could or could not have occurred by chance.

Statistical Significance

When an appropriate statistical test has been applied to experimental data, it is customary to describe the results in terms of statistical significance. The selection of the appropriate level of significance depends upon the nature of the experiment and the importance of the outcome and this choice should be made at the planning stage. If the statistical test reveals that the probability of the observed result occurring by chance is more than 5 per cent it means that the same sort of result could have been obtained by chance five or more times in a hundred trials. The 5 per cent level is customarily accepted as the borderline between statistical significance and non-significance. On the other hand, if the probability of the observed result occurring by chance is 1 per cent or less the Null hypothesis can be rejected with considerable confidence and the alternative hypothesis embraced that the result is "real" or "significant". In dental research it is common to express a probability of 5 per cent as "significant" and a probability of 1 per cent or less as "highly significant".

In everyday usage the word "significant" means "noteworthy" as in the statement—"There is a significant improvement in his work". In statistics, however, "significant" means "beyond the likelihood of chance". Whenever a result has practical significance, it should be possible to demonstrate that the result is statistically significant. The reverse, however, does not necessarily apply. A result may be statistically significant but have no practical importance. For example, in a controlled clinical trial to determine the effect of a new dentifrice on dental caries, it was found that the control group developed an average of 0·67 newly decayed tooth surfaces in a year whereas the experimental group developed an average of 0·29 newly decayed tooth surfaces in a year. The percentage difference (57 per cent) is statistically significant (P is less than 1 per cent) but the absolute reduction of 0·38 decayed tooth surfaces per person per year is of no practical consequence. Clearly, the sound interpretation of the results of a clinical trial depends not only on technical methods of analysis but also on the application of common sense and the elementary rules of logic.

Selection of Groups to be Studied

In most cases, a clinical trial is designed to test a preventive or therapeutic agent in such a way that it will be possible to draw conclusions applicable to a much larger population than the group from which the data are actually collected. If such an objective is to be attained it is essential to ensure that the subjects selected for study are representative of the population to which the generalizations are intended to apply.

It is usually not practicable to include the whole population in a clinical trial, so it is customary to study a small number (or sample) of the parent group and by induction draw conclusions which apply to the whole of the parent group.

It is necessary to dispel the myth that a complete count is necessarily more accurate than a properly selected sample. On the contrary, accuracy may tend to decrease with increasing numbers especially when the counts or measurements are tedious and monotonous.

A sample can provide information within limits which can be calculated provided that every single individual in the parent group has an equal chance of being chosen in the sample. Such a sample is known as a **Random Sample**.

The word Random has a specific meaning. It does not mean haphazard. The best way to get a true random sample is to assign a number to each individual in the parent group and then select the requisite number of individuals by using a Table of Random Numbers. These tables have been derived by a computer so that although there is no pattern connecting the numbers each digit tends to occur with equal frequency when the table is viewed as a whole.

Generally speaking, the larger the sample the more accurately will it reflect the characteristics of the parent group. This accuracy increases with the square root of the sample size so that a sample must be increased 100-fold to get a 10-fold increase in accuracy. The other factor which affects the size of the sample is the amount of variability in the parent group.

Whenever there is a great deal of variation between individual members of a parent group, there is an appreciable risk that a small random sample will contain by chance a disproportionate number of some minority group. To minimize this risk, a sample would need to be relatively large and the cost of obtaining such a sample might be prohibitive. To overcome this disadvantage it may be better to use a **stratified random sample**. To do this the parent group is first divided into a number of groups or strata which are as homogeneous as possible in respect of the feature being studied and then a random sample is taken from each stratum. This technique is widely used in market research and opinion polls for it is fairly easy to classify people into occupational, economic, social, educational and religious groups and other strata.

The method of selecting the sample must not be correlated with the attribute under study. For example, the prevalence of dental caries in a city could not be estimated from the records of patients attending a Dental Hospital, nor could it be estimated from the records of private dentists. In either case, the economic status of the sample would not be representative of the whole population. Further, their dental status is unlikely to be similar to that of the whole population because not all or even most of the population seeks regular dental care.

Finally, the allocation of subjects to experimental and control groups in a clinical trial should be done in such a way that the subjects are not aware of the groups to which they belong (this is called a **Single Blind Trial**) or, preferably, in such a way that neither the investigator nor the subjects know the groups to which the subjects belong (this is called a **Double Blind Trial**).

Procedures in which randomization is abandoned completely in favour of matching or pairing techniques have a restricted application in dental research. They are not usually recommended for several reasons. Firstly, because it is rare for matching to account for all the variable factors which may influence the outcome of the experiment. Secondly, because it is very difficult to prevent subjective influences from biasing the allocation of subjects to groups. Thirdly, because the loss of one of a matched pair forces the rejection of both.

Before the clinical trial begins it is desirable to check the comparability of the control and experimental groups with respect to those factors, if any, which are known to exert an influence on the condition being observed. This is especially important when numbers in the groups are small.

Not even the random assignment of subjects to groups can ensure that the groups are exactly equal in all respects. However, randomization does ensure that they will differ by an extent that is predictable and can be allowed for in the analyses of the results. The great advantage of randomization or stratified randomization is that it removes the influence of the investigator's personal judgment.

Generally speaking it is easier to demonstrate the presence or absence of benefit from a therapeutic or preventive agent in a homogeneous group than in a heterogeneous group (for example, in twins or captive populations such as children and adults living in institutions). The disadvantage of such groups, however, is that they are not representative of the general population and this restricts the inferences that can be drawn from the experiment. As a general rule, there is a greater need for stratification with heterogeneous groups than with homogeneous groups.

Administration of the Agents to be Tested

It has already been suggested that bias in a clinical trial can be minimized by the use of Single Blind and Double Blind techniques. This is not always possible. For example, the use of a stannous fluoride solution for topical application may cause superficial staining of teeth and thus serve to identify the subjects receiving this treatment.

There are two precautions which, when possible, should be taken to ensure that neither the subjects nor the examiners recognize the group to which subjects are assigned. The first precaution is to ensure that the test agent and the placebo or control agent are similar in as many respects as possible, e.g. appearance, smell, colour, taste, packaging, and method of administration. The second precaution is to identify the treatment and control agents by a numerical, alphabetical or alphanumeric code. Several codes may be assigned to each agent but when a subject needs a new supply of agent he should be given the same coded package as he was given initially. Confidentiality of the code can be assured by asking the statistical consultant to arrange the random allocation of agents (and codes) to individual subjects and then by keeping the identification of the coded agents under strict security by an independent authority such as the Registrar of a University or a Bank until the trial is completed or until the principal investigator requests identification of a coded agent.

Special difficulties arise when the nature of the agent under test (e.g. local anaesthetic agent) necessitates the administration of graduated doses and when the actual dose is dependent upon such factors as age or body weight. As a general rule, a specific treatment schedule should be prescribed and adhered to strictly. If this is not done it will not be possible to determine the optimum dosage. Also,

if the clinician is free to vary the dosage according to his own judgement of the patient's needs it will not be possible to compare the effects of different treatments at the end of the trial. Hill (1962) makes this point colourfully in the following words: "The main danger of this free-for-all trial is the apparently almost overpowering attraction to some clinicians of circular motion".

Length of the Study and the Frequency of Examinations

Decisions on both these points depend upon the nature of the disease process and the rapidity with which a favourable response to the agent may be expected. A clinical trial of an agent which is expected to prevent or cure an acute disease such as acute necrotizing ulcerative gingivitis can be of shorter duration than one designed to test the effectiveness of an agent for the prevention of a chronic and relatively slowly progressing disease such as dental caries. One advantage of the sequential trial over the controlled trial is that the experiment can be terminated as soon as a definite result has been demonstrated.

An obvious problem in the conduct of a clinical trial of an agent for the prevention of caries is that no precise estimate is available of the average time for an initial lesion to reach a size that is clinically detectable. It would seem, however, that a clinical trial which is restricted to a duration of one year or less can neither provide valid evidence of the ability of an agent to prevent the initial attack on sound enamel nor permit an estimate of the duration of its effect.

In some studies, the length of the trial may be determined by the need to protect the control group. For example, it has been suggested that clinical trials of mouth rinses to inhibit dental plaque should last a minimum of eight days and a maximum of 21 days. Such a period of time serves to demonstrate potential effectiveness, but to ascertain sustained effectiveness a much longer trial is essential.

Sample Size

The number of persons needed for a clinical trial depends upon the anticipated magnitude of the differences between the experimental and control groups, the extent of the errors of measurement, the variability of the observations, and the level of significance which the investigator desires to achieve. When large differences between test and control groups are expected, samples can be smaller than when small differences are expected.

The methods of estimating sample sizes are fully described in appropriate statistical textbooks. When the minimal size of the groups has been calculated, it is customary to make additional allowances for the loss of subjects during the course of the trial. Estimates of expected differences between groups, the variance of the observations and the extent of examiner error can be made from a pilot study or from a similar study reported in the literature.

Loss of Subjects

No matter how carefully a clinical trial is planned, some loss of subjects from experimental and control groups is inevitable. It is essential to determine whether or not the loss of subjects occurred with equal frequency from each group. The success of the trial may very well be prejudiced if withdrawals occur with unequal frequency and for different reasons in different groups. An excessive loss of subjects from one group may occur because the treatment or agent is unacceptable. Results should be reported both for subjects who were present for some examinations and for those subjects who were present for all examinations. Baseline findings for the original sample and for the subjects remaining at the end of the study, should be compared so that the effect of loss of subjects on the balance of the original groups can be determined. In reporting the results, it is also necessary to account for all subjects who withdraw from the trial at different stages and to give the reason for their withdrawal.

Data Collection

Careless or improper recording and tabulation of data can be a significant source of error in a clinical trial. It is important to ensure that an examiner makes his diagnosis or measurement without any reference to the results of a previous examination. Failure to observe this precaution results in examiner bias.

The simplest way to avoid this type of error is to use a separate record form for each examination. Record forms should be designed to promote simplicity and ease in the transcription of data. The number of items to be recorded should be confined to those which are essential to the investigation. During the initial stages of a clinical trial, it is desirable to check transcription errors by recording the examiner's calls on a tape-recorder and cross-checking them against what was written on the form by the recorder.

Statistical Analysis of the Results

The plan of analysis is determined by the design of the trial and this should be incorporated in the written protocol in consultation with a statistician. The objectives of the analysis are to determine the extent of effectiveness of the experimental agent; to determine the overall effect and to elucidate, if possible, the mode of action of the agent.

Interpretation of the Results

It is important to assess not only the statistical significance of the results of the experiment but also to establish their practical importance.

The practice of presenting results as percentage reductions can be misleading. In the interpretation of percentages, it is essential to pay equal attention to the numerator and the denominator. When results are expressed in terms of percentage reductions it is appropriate to ask "Per cent of what?" It is also advantageous when results are expressed as a percentage change to give the confidence limits of that change. If the 95 per cent confidence limits are used the results will be expressed as a range. For example, a range of 12–46 means that, if the study were repeated, 95 times out of 100 trials one would expect the percentage reduction to lie within the range of 12–46 per cent.

Cost-benefit Analysis

Every report of a clinical trial should contain an analysis of the benefits to be obtained from the preventive or therapeutic agent in relation to the costs of implementation.

An important effect of a preventive measure is a reduction in the cost of treatment. Cost/Benefit Analysis may be defined as a systematic method for measuring the value of all the costs and benefits of a programme. Cost-effectiveness analysis is a simpler procedure in which the costs of achieving a given output are compared. Cost-effectiveness may be assessed in terms of the number of hours of professional time required to achieve a stated benefit. Savings in the cost of dental treatment may be assessed from fee-schedules of private practitioners and in a public health programme from data on the operating expenses of the service. There are other benefits to be derived from the prevention of disease but it is not possible to assess them in financial terms. Such benefits of course include less pain, discomfort and anxiety, and less time lost from school and industry.

Costs of implementation include the actual cost of the agent itself, the cost of any equipment and supplies necessary to apply the agent, and the salaries of personnel involved in the administration of the agent.

Properly done cost-benefit and cost-effectiveness analyses assist public health administrators and members of the practising profession to decide whether the cost of a certain procedure is justified by the results achieved.

Publication

The final step in the conduct of a clinical trial is the publication of the results. If the report is to be published in a scientific journal it will need to be reasonably brief and must be drafted according to the format of the journal concerned. The contents of the report should include some or all of the following:

(a) a succinct and clear statement of the aim of the trial;
(b) a description of the materials and methods including the subjects, the data collected and method of collection, the method of assessment and criteria, the sampling method, calibration of examiners and recorders and the reliability and reproducibility of the data, method of statistical analysis, and costing analysis;
(c) the results;
(d) a discussion in which results of particular interest are highlighted, the significance of the results is explained and suggestions are made for further work to elucidate some interesting results;
(e) a brief summary and statement of conclusions;
(f) acknowledgements;
(g) references; and
(h) appendices.

BIBLIOGRAPHY

American Dental Association (1972), *Principles for the Clinical Testing of Cariostatic Agents*. Chicago: American Dental Association.

Chilton, N. W. (1967), *Design and Analyses in Dental and Oral Research*. Philadelphia and Toronto: J. B. Lippincott.

Finney, D. J. (1955), *Experimental Design and its Statistical Basis*. London: Cambridge University Press.

Fisher, R. A. (1951), *The Design of Experiments*. 6th edition. Edinburgh and London: Oliver and Boyd.

Grainger, R. M. (1972), "Committee Consensus on Design and Analysis and Introduction to Analyses and Design of Clinical Trials", in *Proc. Conf. on Clinical Testing of Cariostatic Agents*, pp. 50 and 53. Chicago: American Dental Association.

Hill, A. B. (1960), *Controlled Clinical Trials*. Oxford: Blackwell Scientific Publications.

Hill, A. B. (1962), *Statistical Methods in Clinical and Preventive Medicine*. Edinburgh and London: E & S Livingstone Ltd.

Horowitz, H. S., Baume, L. J., Backer Dirks, O., Davies, G. N. and Slack, G. L. (1973), "Principal Requirements for Controlled Clinical Trials of Caries Preventive Agents and Procedures", Mimeographed Report, F.D.I., London.

59. DENTAL IMPLANTS

R. B. JOHNS

General considerations

  Implant-tissue interface
  Implant materials
    Metals
    Polymers
    Ceramics
    Vitreous carbon

Dental implants

  Classification
    Retentive
    Supportive
  Implant-tissue interface
    Epithelial attachment
    Infection

GENERAL CONSIDERATIONS

This chapter is concerned with man-made devices, the purpose of which is either the restoration of function or the replacement of deficient tissues, with particular reference to the specific problems of dental implants. Implants may be composed of any material or combination of materials which are not vital at the time of implantation, and they may be totally buried, partially buried, or buried but exteriorized (fig. 1). The relationship between the implant and the tissue may alter with time because the period over which an implant is to function can be indefinite. The term permanent or temporary prosthesis is arbitrary.

Examples of implants which are totally buried include cardiovascular prostheses, bone plates, joint replacements, some radiotherapy devices, and substances used to augment deficient soft tissues either for aesthetic or functional considerations.

Partially buried implants are normally used only on a temporary basis. Examples are hypodermic needles, sutures which are used to approximate soft tissues, drainage tubes to allow the passage of fluid from deep seated infection, and external splints for the direct fixation of sections of fractured bones. In each of these examples the underlying tissues are protected to some extent from the ingress of infective organisms by the close adaptation of epithelium to the implant. For those which are intended to remain *in situ* for longer periods the flow of exudate beside the implant provides an additional protection to tissues exposed by a surface discontinuity which cannot be repaired as long as the prosthesis is in place.

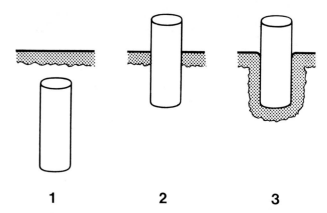

FIG. 1. Diagram to illustrate the three possible relationships an implant may have with the tissues: (1) Represents total implantation without epithelial involvement. (2) Represents partial implantation with discontinuity of the epithelium. (3) Represents partial implantation with exteriorization by the establishment of epithelial continuity.

Implants which are buried but exteriorized rely on the epithelium proliferating in such a way that the continuity of this tissue is re-established and with it the ability to prevent the ingress of bacteria to deeper structures. The desquamation of epithelial cells must not be impeded to the extent that there is an accumulation of necrotic material at sites remote from an external surface. Examples of this group include tympanic drains, some ocular prostheses, and one particular variety of dental prosthesis inserted through the alveolar ridges.

Implant-Tissue Interface

Any material which is implanted, whatever relationship it may have with the tissues, will evoke some reaction from the environment; this may be local or systemic. It is possible for both types of reaction to occur concurrently according to the tissues through which the implant passes. The implanted material itself will similarly be affected by the environment.

The extent of these interactions will depend not only on the material involved, its shape and surface finish, but also on the chemical and mechanical forces to which it is subjected. For example, in the presence of an inflammatory reaction there is a lowering of pH and an alteration in oxygen tension, both factors which are likely to accelerate corrosive degradation. Where orthopaedic endoprostheses are concerned, complex mechanical stresses arise at the bone/implant interface. These result from the distribution of the various forces involved, which are not in the general direction or of the same magnitude as those to which the bone is accustomed. The aim of those concerned with the design and use of total hip replacement is to reduce the extent of the transmitted load per unit area to an acceptable level. It is for this reason that a luting agent is used to provide a firm, intimate contact over as wide an area as possible and that the design of the prosthesis is such that the forces, which will act through it, will be orientated in a direction acceptable to the bone. The disparity between the moduli of elasticity of this, or any other type of load-bearing implant and that of the bone, is an additional complicating factor in these considerations. The capacity of the bone to adapt to such a variety of stresses depends on those factors which control its metabolism.

There is however concern over the reaction implant materials might evoke from some tissues. It has been noted that heterotopic bone has formed in synthetic sponges implanted in soft tissue. Such metaplasia, particularly in regions such as the breast in which malignant changes occur relatively frequently, would seem to contra-indicate their use. In recent years attention has been drawn to the fact that tumour formation can be induced by implanted material other than chemical carcinogens. Implanted films have been found to act in this manner, and since pore size has been shown to be a determining factor it is clear that in this instance it is the physical rather than chemical properties of the implant that constitute a hazard to the patient.

It is also clear that where articular surfaces are involved detached fragments of material can result from wear. These will pass into the tissue surrounding the implant. From this situation they may be removed and ultimately eliminated from the body; alternatively, they may remain in the vicinity of the implant and become encapsulated in such a way that they are less likely to cause irritation to the tissue.

Even if repair or maintenance of buried implants were possible, such procedures would constitute a hazard to the patient, as well as being both difficult and costly. Those implants which have to function mechanically often have to do so frequently and for long periods: it has been estimated, for example, that in the case of heart valve prostheses there are 40×10^6 functional movements a year, and in the case of artificial knee joints and total hip replacement each articular surface may have to withstand at least six times the body weight for each step taken. During the course of a year such a prosthesis may be loaded 1 to 2.5×10^6 times. It must be remembered, however, that the age and general health of a patient inevitably make such estimates extremely variable.

Implant Materials

Innumerable materials and combinations of materials have been implanted into the body. At present the two classes commonly used are metals and polymers. Each has specific applications although in combination with one another they may acquire additional usefulness. In addition ceramic materials are being used to a limited extent and vitreous carbon is being investigated as a possible implant material.

Metals

There are three types of alloy in common use; corrosion resistant steels, chrome cobalt molybdenum alloys and titanium and its alloys; for composition and physical properties see Tables 1–4 (British Standards, BS 3531, 1974). When considering metals as implant materials it is necessary to understand that their structure is crystalline and one in which the bonding between atoms is the result of a sharing of electrons. Both mechanical properties and chemical reactivity are extremely variable and may be altered by changes in crystalline structure due to heat, stress, or contact with electro-chemically reactive elements or compounds. Metals all have a tendency, to some extent, to return to a lower energy state, usually by reacting with oxygen. If stress is imposed on a metal which at the same time is in a corrosive environment there will be an accelerated degeneration in its physical properties.

TABLE 1

SPECIFICATION (BRITISH STANDARD 3531: 1974)
FOR WROUGHT AUSTENITIC STAINLESS STEEL

Stainless Steels

Element	Composition A	Composition B
Carbon	0·08% max.	0·03% max.
Silicon	1·00% max.	1·00% max.
Manganese	2·00% max.	2·00% max.
Nickel	11·0–16·0%	11·0–16·0%
Chromium	16·0–19·9%	16·0–19·9%
Molybdenum	2·0–3·5%	2·0–3·5%
Sulphur	0·030% max.	0·030% max.
Phosphorus	0·045% max.	0·045% max.
Iron	Balance	Balance

TABLE 2

SPECIFICATION (BRITISH STANDARD 3531: 1974)
FOR CAST AND WROUGHT COBALT–CHROMIUM ALLOYS FOR
SURGICAL IMPLANTS

Cobalt–Chromium Alloys

Element	Cast Alloy (percentage)	Wrought Alloy (percentage)
Chromium	26·5–30·0	19·0–21·0
Molybdenum	4·5–7·0	—
Iron	1·0 (max.)	3·0 (max.)
Nickel	2·5 (max.)	11·0 (max.)
Other metals (total)	1·0 (max.)	—
Carbon	0·35 (max.)	0·05–0·15
Silicon	1·0 (max.)	1·0 (max.)
Manganese	1·50 (max.)	2·0 (max.)
Tungsten	—	14·0–16·0
Cobalt	Balance	Balance

This phenomenon shows more than a purely cumulative effect of the individual corrosive and stress processes; metallic implants which behave in this manner not only lose some of their mechanical properties but may also release products which are cytotoxic.

Those metals and alloys which are suitable for use as implants resist corrosion by a protective oxide layer of limited thickness. For a metal to function satisfactorily in a hostile environment such as that provided by the tissues, it is necessary for this film to become re-established as quickly as possible should it become damaged. In some instances the oxide layer can be thickened electrolytically to increase the protection which it affords to the underlying metal. Stress within the implant, whether local or general, or variations in oxygen tension, can initiate a progressive breakdown in the protective oxide film. Changes in pH due to haemorrhage, tissue damage, or bacterial activity can similarly sustain or even initiate corrosion.

As distinct from corrosion, metals also exhibit the phenomenon of ion migration into the surrounding tissues, and in some cases this can give rise to local pigmentation. The migration of various ions from alloys is not necessarily in the same proportion as the individual metallic constituents of the alloy concerned or the reactivity of the component elements. One of the largest migrations of ions has been shown to take place from titanium, the least reactive of all metallic implant materials.

The possibility of malignant changes being induced either locally or at more distant sites, is extremely unlikely. The number of malignant neoplasms reported in patients

TABLE 3

MECHANICAL PROPERTIES OF METALLIC SURGICAL MATERIALS IN CURRENT USE,
FROM BRITISH STANDARD 3531 : 1974

Metal	Specific gravity	Young's modulus N/mm^2 (= MPa)	Tensile strength N/mm^2 (= MPa)	Fatigue limit (percentage of) tensile strength
Cold worked stainless steel	7·9	200,000	1,000	30
Cast cobalt-chromium alloy	7·8	200,000	700	43
Wrought titanium type T160 (bar products)	4·5	127,000	660	45

TABLE 4

SPECIFICATION (BRITISH STANDARD 3531: 1974) FOR TITANIUM*

Element	Wrought (For Machining)	Alloy TA 10–13	TA 28
Aluminium	—	5·5/6·75%	5·5/6·75%
Vanadium	—	3·5/4·5 %	3·5/4·5 %
Iron	0·20% max.	0·30% max.	0·30% max.
Carbon	0·10% max.	0·10% max.	—
Oxygen	0·50% max.	0·20% max.	0·20% max.
Nitrogen	0·05% max.	0·05% max.	0·05% max.
Hydrogen	0·01% max.	0·1025% max.	0·0125% max.
Titanium	Balance	Balance	Balance

* Provisional specification.

with implants is thought to be no more than might be expected in the normal course of events.

Polymers

Materials of this type are usually based on a low molecular weight molecule, containing a carbon or silicon atom, from which a macro-molecule is built up; this formation, described as a polymerization, is usually brought about by the action of heat or a chemical activator. If more than one basic molecule is involved the reaction is termed poly-condensation and may result in the production of a simple by-product molecule, the presence of which may be undesirable.

The lack of toxicity of macro-molecules is a measure of their stable unreactive state. However, their degradation or the alteration of their physical properties may be influenced by a number of factors. For instance, the presence of an oxidizing agent, or some wavelengths of electromagnetic radiation, are both factors capable of initiating a progressive breakdown of the macro-molecule or a molecular chain scission. Lipids in the blood have been shown to become absorbed by a silicon polymer when used as a heart valve replacement, resulting in the failure of the prosthesis due to distortion.

It has also been noted that further disadvantages of polymers, such as polymethylmethacrylate, are that polymerization is rarely complete and some residual monomer may leach out, causing tissue irritation. Other more reactive agents which can also pass into the tissues and give rise to adverse effects are traces of anti-oxidants, which are incorporated in order to delay spontaneous polymerization. Similarly stabilizers, intended to resist the break-up of the macromolecules, and plasticizers, included to modify the physical characteristics of the polymer, are also liable to leach out. Nevertheless in spite of both its potential irritation and its exothermic reaction, polymethylmethacrylate has been widely used clinically both as a luting medium in total hip prostheses and in the repair of cranial bone defects. As a dental implant material, however, its use has evoked conflicting reports of both success and failure.

Another polymer, polytetrafluorethylene (PTFE), is not only extremely well tolerated by the tissues but is capable of functioning as an articular surface in conjunction with a metallic alloy in joint prostheses. Not only does it provide minimal frictional resistance at the interface but the rate of wear is extremely low. Those wear fragments which are produced are well tolerated by the tissues.

Ceramics

This class of material is based on the regular structure of metallic and non-metallic elements whose bonding is ionic. Ceramic oxides are for the most part in their highest oxidation state and therefore they cannot corrode and are stable in an adverse environment. Although some ceramics have considerable strength, as a class they lack ductility and are brittle. The compatability of some ceramics with living bone and the ease with which tissue will grow into porosities has led to a renewal of interest and research into this class of material.

If current research is successful, direct bonding between an implant and the hydroxyapatite crystals in bone may lead to direct fixation of prostheses for the support of artificial limbs. Also it may prove possible to use certain biodegradable ceramics to fill bone defects on a temporary basis in place of graft material.

Vitreous Carbon

This material, which is similar to some ceramics, is processed from a polymer by pyrolysis. It is a glass-like substance with a variety of forms determined by the method of fabrication. It is said to have none of the disadvantages of polymers because there are no additives to leach out. In most circumstances it is inert in the tissue environment although one variety has been shown to undergo a physical change under the influence of an imposed EMF. The physical properties of vitreous carbon are similar to metallic implant materials except for a low modulus of elasticity and low impact strength. As it is black it may be aesthetically unacceptable in anterior regions of the mouth if implanted only just below the surface of the mucosa.

DENTAL IMPLANTS

Most dental implants fall within the classification "partially buried" (fig. 1). The exceptions are diodontic [*sic*] or endodontic endosseous implants, totally buried magnets, and those prostheses retained by rods placed in holes trepanned through the alveolar ridge.

Classification of Dental Implants

A classification of dental implants based primarily on function is set out in Table 5. The term "retentive" is used to denote an implant which has the sole purpose of providing additional retention for a prosthesis, all functional loads being transmitted through the mucous membrane with or without the involvement of teeth. A "supportive" implant not only provides retention but also relieves the mucous membrane or teeth of part or all of the transmission of functional loads to the jaws.

Retentive Implants

Retentive implants cover what might appear to be the major prosthetic problem. However there are many clinical situations, particularly those aggravated by senility, which make the mucous membrane less able to withstand a function for which it is not suited. Retentive implants include mucosal inserts; these are stud-like metallic projections processed on to the fitting surface of a denture. The studs are positioned above the more fibrous regions of the mucoperiosteum. Before the denture is inserted a small cruciate incision is made in the tissue beneath each stud, the intention being that healing around these extrusions will be sufficiently fibrous to provide additional retention.

TABLE 5

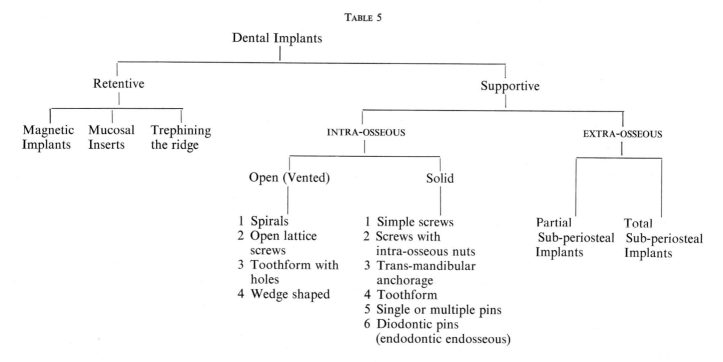

Magnetic implants are designed to be in two parts. One, made of a magnetized cobalt/platinum alloy, is inserted into an artificial bony crypt created within the alveolus. The magnet is covered with tantalum gauze, to promote the formation of a fibrous capsule above it. A second magnet, orientated to attract the one embedded within the bone, is processed into the denture.

The trepanning of a suitably shaped alveolar ridge can also provide absolute retention. A locking rod is designed to pass through two parts of a denture and the intervening epithelialized tunnel within the alveolus. It is therefore impossible to remove the denture so long as the rod is in place.

Supportive Implants

The two subsections of the supportive group are based on differences in the dissipation of functional loads.

The extra-osseous section is exemplified by subperiosteal implants which direct functional loads from small intraoral abutments to a framework constructed to fit either directly on to the alveolar bone or to shallow channels cut within it. The construction of these implants necessitates a preliminary operation at which the mucoperiosteum is reflected to allow for the surgical preparation of the bone and for an accurate impression to be taken. At a second operation the tissue is reflected again and the implant is inserted. This procedure allows the framework to be in close apposition to the bone and to be retained initially by the suturing of the fibrous mucoperiosteum over it and later by the proliferation of periosteum around the framework.

The other section of this group of implants is the intra-osseous category within which there are two sub-divisions. The first are solid implants inserted either directly into the socket of recently extracted teeth or into suitably shaped defects prepared in the bone. The retention of these implants relies on surface irregularities of the intrabony portion of the implant. The size of the irregularities will determine the type of tissue that will proliferate into these defects. Some solid implants are of a tooth form and on the grounds of simulating a physiological transfer of forces to the alveolus it would seem that they may have some advantages. However it is clear that sufficient alveolar bone must be present to make this type of implant practicable. Small diameter pins have been used; these are inserted divergent to one another so that the disparity in their paths of insertion or of withdrawal once they are securely attached to one another, is resisted by the bone. Although this type of implant may be stable initially, this stability does not persist and limited movement develops in a number of directions. It has been suggested that these pins should be sufficiently long to terminate in cortical bone. If this precept were followed, nerves and blood vessels would be put at risk and the nasal cavity and antra could be perforated.

Also in this sub-division are those implants which gain access to the deeper structures through standing teeth. These diodontic implants are indicated for those teeth which have inadequate periodontal support and are unable to withstand the functional demands to which they are subjected. There is little choice, with this type of implant, in selecting the direction in which it can be placed. Again, therefore, there is the concomitant risk of damage to related structures. It has been suggested that, by exposing the whole buccal aspect of the tooth, it may be possible to transfix a root by inserting an implant in a more favourable direction. Such an alteration in alignment would not only weaken the tooth itself but it would place a considerable strain on the cementing medium over a limited area of contact.

The second sub-division of the intra-osseous category covers those implants which have spaces within that portion of their structure designed to lie within the bone. This configuration allows not only fibrous tissue but also bone to form within the general outline of the implant. Various designs have been suggested, most of which are intended to give immediate retention of the implant within the bone. Fenestrated screw-shaped implants fulfil both the demand for retention and space for tissue ingrowth. Wedge-shaped implants which are thin in cross-section and which are forcibly driven into slots prepared in the cortical bone of the alveolus, have also been used. It appears that the wedging effect and stress induced within the bone may well stimulate rapid bone formation. This, therefore, shortens the transitional period from immediate stabilization due to wedging to stability derived from tissue ingrowth.

The retention and rigidity of a dental implant largely depends on the bone formation which takes place through or over the implant as well as on the surface irregularities which may be present. In the case of small surface defects or porosities the degree of mineralization will be influenced by the depth and diameter of the irregularities as well as the material of which the implant is made. As long as porosities are inter-connecting, mineralization of tissue will take place within some ceramic materials where the diameter of the porosities is 150 μm or more. Below 100 μm however, only fibrous tissue is found. It has been reported that using titanium fibres sintered on to a solid core, pore sizes of 170–350 μm have been formed, into which bone has proliferated. An intimate contact of bone with the metal fibres appears to have been effected with this method.

Using metal alloys, ceramics and polymers, various forms of porosity are being investigated to determine not only the type of tissue ingrowth induced but also the effect on the strength of the materials themselves.

The Tissue-Implant Interface in Function

The forces which act through the tissue/implant interface are the result of functional movements of the mandible and the oromusculature. In the natural dentition these forces act through the periodontal membrane, the function of which depends on the stretching or distortion of collagen, as well as the haemodynamic and visco-elastic components associated with the fibrous tissue elements. This complex mechanism meets the needs arising from the characteristic movement of teeth both at rest and under a variety of load conditions.

Whether an implant is resting on bone or is partially buried within it, the histological appearance of the soft tissue which separates it from the bone shows little resemblance to a periodontal membrane. The differences are first that the space between the implant and the bone is often extremely narrow. Secondly, those fibres which are present are orientated parallel to the implant surface and not in bundles at an angle to it. Thirdly, the tissue is much less vascular than that seen associated with a tooth. The

tissue which surrounds an implant therefore resembles an encapsulation of a foreign body rather than a specialized support mechanism such as the periodontal membrane. Nevertheless there is no reason why such a tissue should not be capable of transferring forces from an implant to bone provided that these are within the physiological limits of the bone.

Clearly these limits will vary, not only from person to person, but also with the total force to which the interface is subjected as well as the area of contact the implant has with the tissues. However, the direction of these forces may be altered to some extent by the use of narrow occlusal surfaces and minimal cuspal interferences of the intra-oral part of the prosthesis.

Epithelial Attachment

All those dental implants which gain access to deeper structures by passing through the epithelium must, at some point, have a region which is in intimate contact with that tissue. It would obviously be desirable if this contact were similar in structure and function to that which occurs adjacent to teeth. Depending on a number of factors, including the histological technique employed and the time over which experiments took place, the extent to which epithelium can be shown to proliferate beside an implant varies. Assessments of this proliferation have differed from total exteriorization, shown by the re-establishment of the continuity of the epithelium round the implant, to a downgrowth apparently limited to a few millimetres from the point where the epithelium was penetrated.

In those instances where only a limited proliferation beside an implant has occurred it has not been clear what mechanism has prevented the continued growth of the epithelium. It may have been the presence of inflammatory cells which interfered with this progression but there has not been any evidence that, as in the case of teeth, it has been due to the presence of fibres extending from the crestal bone to a cementum-like surface on an implant. Histologically the epithelium adjacent to an implant may appear to have some similarities to junctional epithelium but it has not yet been demonstrated that this tissue behaves in an analogous manner; neither is it clear to what extent the reaction of the epithelium is due to the chemical or physical surface characteristics of the implant.

Those implants which have been completely surrounded by epithelium as referred to above have been described as being completely exteriorized. It has been suggested that this is a stable physiological response to an implant. However, this stability must depend on the continued elimination of those epithelial cells which are desquamated at sites remote from their ultimate shedding into the oral cavity.

Infection

When totally enclosed orthopaedic implants are used either in bone plating or as total hip replacement a number of failures are due to supervening infections. In the oral cavity it is clear that all implants are inserted under conditions where bone is exposed to bacterial contamination and is, to a varying extent, damaged by their placement. Although a number of implants may fail initially for this reason there does not appear to be an inevitable failure due to infection.

In the assessment of success or failure of implants it is important that undue significance should not be attributed to apparent radiographic success. The evidence of such diagnostic aids is particularly susceptible to misinterpretation. Experimental work on animals has also shown that even apparent clinical success has not been supported by the histological findings. Radiographs are indicators only of the osseous response: therefore they will reveal failures due to osteolysis, but new bone formation does not necessarily indicate success because of the possibility that failure can also originate in the soft tissues.

There can be some justification for using this type of prosthesis if the implant can remain within the tissues without evoking a severe reaction. The use may still be acceptable even if the adjacent tissue does not resemble that which is normally found associated with a tooth. The design of both the implant and the superstructure should allow unimpeded examination of the tissues. It should also be possible to assess the stability of the implant free of any auxiliary support. A possible future design of dental implants may be on the basis of a composite structure. This would incorporate a solid core with a porous coating for that portion which would be within the supporting tissue. There would also be a region specifically designed to permit an epithelial attachment at the level where the implant would penetrate into the oral cavity.

60. FRAMING AND TESTING OF HYPOTHESES

SIR WILFRED FISH

This final chapter is concerned with framing and testing hypotheses—an appropriate subject for discussion in a book devoted to the scientific foundations of dentistry, for "hypothesis" is simply the Greek word for a foundation. Translated literally it means "that which is placed underneath". The chapter heading, therefore, goes straight to the heart of the matter and calls for a discussion of the method by which the science of dentistry has been and still is being built up.

The foundations of modern dentistry, or for that matter of modern medicine too, are scientific; but they are of comparatively recent development as will shortly appear. Using the word in a different sense, however, the foundation, or origins of dentistry as a practical art or craft were anything but either recent or scientific. Dentistry, like medicine or astronomy developed over the centuries as an empirical corpus of knowledge, which, so far as dentistry is concerned, was for the most part applied to the development of surgical or merely technical procedures related to the teeth.

Not surprisingly, mixed with much that was true and valuable in this heterogeneous collection of fact and inference were concepts which in many instances have proved to be false and have had to be abandoned. Inevitably much suffering must have been caused, but on the other hand we have inherited the outstanding contributions of such men as Hippocrates, Galen, Vesalius, Harvey, Hunter, Pasteur, Lister, and many more who could be added to the list.

Moving more directly into our own field, the scientific

foundations of dentistry are of very recent origin indeed, and with few exceptions hardly stretch back beyond the later years of the last century. The investigations of Sir John Tomes and of W. D. Miller spring to mind, but sixty years ago nothing was known of the histopathology of the periodontal tissues and very little of the physiology of the teeth themselves, and with the brilliant exception of Miller, human and comparative dental anatomy had absorbed most of the time of the few investigators who had concerned themselves with the scientific background of dentistry.

But to return for a moment to the actual word "hypothesis", the Oxford Dictionary definition is very helpful and quite adequate so far as medical practice is concerned in all its branches; though practitioners with a philosophical turn of mind will quite properly want to accept it only with certain reservations to which reference will be made later. The word hypothesis when used in science is defined by the Oxford Dictionary as a "provisional supposition which accounts for known facts, and serves as a starting-point for further investigation by which it may be proved or disproved".

It will be immediately seen that this is not the way the word is used when a youngster first meets it at school. On being introduced to Euclid, he finds that the word "hypothesis" is used to denote a statement of fact which must, for the purpose of the argument, be accepted as such. For instance, in seeking to prove that the two basic angles of an isosceles triangle are equal it is necessary to accept as a hypothesis that the two sides are equal. It is, then, common practice to say AB = AC by hypothesis; and the phrase "by hypothesis" is one which every school-boy learns to treat with respect as definitely excluding any contrary argument.

Unfortunately, in science generally, as appears from the dictionary definition, exactly the opposite is the case and could give rise to some confusion. A hypothesis may be nothing more than a mere suspicion, an informed guess, formulated in an attempt to account for observed phenomena. It is not a foundation on which one can build and must not be so regarded until it has been tested and as far as can be determined, found to be accurate. It is only after much evidence has accumulated to indicate that it is true, and provided that no circumstance has arisen to cast a doubt on its accuracy that it may be used as a foundation for further investigation or as a basis for clinical procedures. Even so, it must continue to be treated with reserve as is shown by another phrase often used by responsible scientific people. They will say "But of course that is only an hypothesis", and this phrase must be recognized as a warning that the matter referred to calls for further investigation before it is acted upon. It is not established fact.

A hypothesis must, therefore, have certain features. It must be precise and unambiguous and it must above all be susceptible of being tested; that is an absolute requirement if it is to have any value. It would be as useless to generate a hypothesis that could not be tested as it is dangerous to publish or to act upon one that has not been shown to be reliable. That statement does not, however, indicate that a hypothesis may not be discussed until some means has been found by which it may be tested. As will appear later, some of the most important discoveries in science have had to wait years for verification; and indeed it has been argued that a scientific statement can never be finally proved to be true.

Elaborating this argument, known as "Hume's problem", Sir Karl Popper says "Science is not a system of certain, or well-established, statements; nor is it a system which steadily advances towards a state of finality. Our science is not knowledge (*epistémé*); it can never claim to have attained truth or even a substitute for it such as probability".

He does not, however, despise science on that account but adds: ". . . the striving for knowledge and the search for truth are still the strongest motives of scientific discovery". What he does assert is that whatever experimental support a particular scientific theory may have it is always possible that some further discovery will undermine its acceptance. This is of course the inherent weakness of inductive reasoning, that is of the procedure by which it is sought to establish general laws by the production of isolated findings and particular instances. This is also the reason for taking exception to the word "proved" in the dictionary definition; perhaps "tested" would be more appropriate. Referring to those things we think we have discovered, Popper says: "Our method of research is not to defend them in order to prove how right we were. On the contrary, we try to overthrow them." Our purpose in doing this is not only to continue to test the accuracy of our findings, but to open up new fields of discovery as will later appear.

The procedure is generally referred to as 'The Scientific Method' which involves, first of all, a careful assessment of all the known facts related to a specific problem. Then if some inconsistency appears, or if an opportunity seems to present itself of providing some useful additional knowledge, the scientist must carefully estimate what the true facts are likely to be. In doing this he will have generated his hypothesis, and it remains for him to find a means of testing it. This is the way modern science has been built up; but the method itself did not spring into being ready-made; it had to evolve, and there can be no doubt that the great masters to whom I have referred, together with many others, made essential contributions also to this process of evolution.

For instance, Vesalius in his incomparably beautiful and inspiring masterpiece *De Humani Corporis Fabrica* (1543) established, as Doctors Saunders and O'Malley remind us, "with startling suddenness the beginning of modern observational science and research". I am sure that these authors would wish us not to fail to give due weight to the word "modern" in this statement, for observational research was the method assiduously followed by the old masters as will be seen in a moment; but the dark ages had intervened and right up to the middle of the sixteenth century the teaching of anatomy was based on garbled translations of their work, translations which had already passed through several languages, and the information thus obtained was supported by the very minimum of further practical investigation. In fact such dissections as were carried out were in the nature of ceremonial tributes to the great teachers of an earlier age, rather than being designed either to verify the accuracy of that teaching, or to discover new facts.

The importance of the observational approach, reintroduced so emphatically and in such magnificent detail by Vesalius is directly illustrated by him in the dental field; and particularly so by two items in plate 9 of the *Fabrica*. The first of these is a drawing of the meniscus from the temporomandibular joint, and the other is a section of a molar tooth displaying the pulp chamber and root canals. The latter drawing is a little out of proportion, but it is one generally attributed to Jan Stefan van Kalkar, one of the lesser lights of Titian's workshop in Venice, where most of the illustrations in Vesalius' masterpiece were produced.

The significance for us of the molar tooth illustration, however, lies in the fact that it does display a pulp chamber, and thus controverts Galen who said that teeth were solid. Science obviously was waking up from its long sleep. To controvert anything that Galen said was, in those days, nothing short of heresy. Even so, we may ask, why did not Galen look to see before he ventured on that pronouncement? All he needed was a hammer, a large stone, and an extracted tooth! But Galen had undertaken an enormous task and had far more exciting things on hand. He spent all his time experimenting on and dissecting all kinds of animals, including anthropoid apes. It is only necessary to recall that he described the anatomy of the submaxillary and sublingual salivary ducts, although he did not know their function, to excuse him for not smashing up a tooth; and anyhow, the scientific method was in its infancy.

It was this "first step", this habit of looking to see for

oneself that Vesalius reintroduced and adorned so magnificently, thereby establishing once again the importance of minute and scientifically accurate observation; for that kind of observation must inevitably lead to informed speculation and experiment. Informed speculation leads to the generation of a hypothesis, and to further observation and experiment, that are the means by which a hypothesis is tested.

It may sometimes appear that the generation of a hypothesis is nothing more than a flash of inspiration—a bright idea that suddenly occurs to one and which on mature reflection is seen to be either worth exploring or conversely may prove to be mistaken. There is an element of truth in this, inasmuch as a possible solution to a problem may occur suddenly to one when walking the dog or luxuriating in the bath; but it will only occur to someone who has spent many hours exploring the subject and has come to realize that there is a problem, that something is missing or that there is an apparent contradiction in the accepted facts.

It is not easy to classify hypotheses, nor would it be very useful to do so, but it is possible to enumerate several circumstances which give rise to the framing of them. In addition to the instances where there appears to be a contradiction between generally accepted facts or where there is an obvious gap in our knowledge, a scientist or a clinician, indeed anyone with an enquiring mind who has studied a subject deeply, may see an opportunity to extend the frontiers of knowledge in some new direction, and in order to seize this opportunity must formulate a hypothesis.

Such a situation arises when some natural phenomenon is seen to recur, for no obvious reason, but with persistent regularity, and the observer will generate a hypothesis in an attempt to discover some significant underlying cause. Then again, some unusual occurrence may be observed that appears to the observer to demand an explanation, which so far has not been forthcoming. In seeking it, the observer is trying to formulate a hypothesis. Perhaps it will meet the case most comprehensively to say that whenever there appears to be an opportunity of increasing human knowledge—a temptation which no true scientist can resist—the first step is to formulate a hypothesis.

In medicine generally, and therefore in our own specialized field, hypotheses are most frequently set up in an attempt to discover more about biological phenomena, or else to discover the cause of some abnormal or diseased state of the tissues with a view to the framing of a further hypothesis outlining a method of treatment which would appear to hold out a reasonable prospect of being beneficial.

Sometimes this process is observed to operate, as it were, in reverse, and a hypothesis is evolved to correct some procedure which having mistakenly been taken into practice is observed to have had unfortunate consequences. An example of this stems from the practice in the first world war of irrigating wounds. Seeking to explore the rationale of this treatment, Fleming discovered that the irrigation washed away the leucocytes more effectively than it removed the bacteria. Accordingly, in the Spanish civil war, wounds were plastered up after *debridement* and then left undisturbed for several weeks. When finally opened up and the mass of offensive pus washed away, the wounds were found to be far healthier than those that had been irrigated.

Up to this point, therefore, an attempt has been made to arrive at a definition of a hypothesis and to discuss its importance as an essential factor in building up scientific knowledge. Reference has also been made to some of the circumstances in which hypotheses are generated; but we have made little progress in discovering how one should set about generating one.

The fact of the matter is that a scientist cannot suddenly decide to frame a hypothesis out of thin air. What happens is that when he is studying his particular branch of knowledge from every aspect—as he must—he either gradually or suddenly becomes aware of an inconsistency or a problem of some kind and settles down to try to formulate his difficulty as precisely as possible and to put up an anticipated solution which is a hypothesis, or theory, to account for the discrepancy, or solve the problem; whereupon it remains for him to devise a means of testing the accuracy of his anticipated solution.

That is why the step forward that Vesalius took was so important when he made up his mind to look for himself in order to discover the true facts, instead of repeating the sometimes fallacious teachings of bygone days; for that is the first and most important step in the effort to build up a firm scientific foundation for any branch of science.

The next step is not so easily defined. Albert Einstein is quoted with approval by Sir Peter Medawar* as saying: "If you want to find out anything from the theoretical physicists about the methods they use, I advise you to stick closely to one principle: Don't listen to their words, fix your attention on their deeds."

I shall therefore confine myself, in trying to indicate how a hypothesis may be generated and tested, to recording several examples of methods that have been used in various scientific disciplines. They will perhaps indicate a few of the infinite variety of circumstances that call for the setting up of a hypothesis and some of the different means of testing them, that have been found appropriate. One example will in addition recall the appalling consequences of a false hypothesis in medicine being published and almost universally acted upon without having been adequately tested.

Before setting out these examples, however, one other matter calls for comment; it is a consideration of the kind of people who have formulated hypotheses which on becoming established have had far-reaching consequences on various aspects of civilized life. In the first place, they have all been people who were industrious, enthusiastic and capable of thinking logically; all these qualities are required if the necessary groundwork is to be accomplished to ensure that the problem to be solved is clearly set out and understood. It is sometimes said that genius is 90 per cent perspiration and only 10 per cent inspiration. There is much truth in the *cliché*, and thereby quite a large number of people are excluded from the enterprise, but a man who is likely to produce these new concepts—whether he be a clinician or a research worker in a laboratory—must have much more than a propensity for hard work; he must also have an enquiring mind coupled with a marked streak of originality and ingenuity. He must be one of those people, not always

* *Induction and Intuition in Scientific Thought* by P. B. Medawar. Methuen & Co. Ltd., London.

easy to get on with, who constantly ask "why?" when something is being explained to them. "How does it work?" "Could it not be better done some other way?" "Is there not some alternative explanation more likely to be correct?"

Karl Popper carries the eccentricities of original scientists to even greater lengths. "Bold ideas," he says, "unjustified anticipations, and speculative thought, are our only means for interpreting nature; our only organon, our only instrument, for grasping her. And we must hazard them to win the prize. Those amongst us who are unwilling to expose their ideas to the hazard of refutation do not take part in the scientific game."

A propensity for taking chances and even scientific curiosity are not perhaps such rare endowments, but the next requirement is one that reduces the number of candidates very drastically indeed. In seeking to satisfy his curiosity, a research man must have either inherited or acquired the habit of looking to see for himself. He must be a man who would not only be anxious to try the experiment, but would always prefer to do so rather than to look up what someone else said in a book.

William Harvey, who discovered the circulation of the blood early in the seventeenth century, puts the case for personal investigation very clearly in his introduction to his book The Generation of Animals. He is making the point that our intellectual knowledge is derived from, and is secondary to, sensory perception of events and of material objects. He continues:

"And hence it is that without the due admonition of the senses, without frequent observation and reiterated experiment, our mind goes astray after phantoms and appearances. Diligent observation is therefore requisite in every science, and the senses are to be frequently appealed to. We are, I say to strive after personal experience, not to rely on the experience of others; without which indeed no one can properly become a student of any branch of natural science."

He goes on to invite the "Gentle reader" not to take his (Harvey's) own word for what he tells him about the generation of animals but adds:

". . . I appeal to your own eyes as my witness and judge. For as all true science rests upon those principles which have their origin in the operation of the senses, particular care is to be taken that by repeated dissection the grounds of our present subject be fully established. . . . The method of investigating truth commonly pursued at this time therefore is to be held erroneous and almost foolish, in which so many enquire what others have said, and omit to ask whether the things themselves be actually so or not."*

In other words, "seeing is believing"; but apart from the importance of personal observation and experiment so clearly outlined some three and a-half centuries ago, there is the complementary danger in having too frequent re-

course to books. It is all too easy to become confused by reading masses of material often containing conflicting and accordingly unsubstantiated statements.

Even if the statements are not contradictory, there is a great danger of cramming the mind with masses of irrelevant detail. All one's mental energy is used up in sorting it out and storing it. A little knowledge may be a dangerous thing, but too much of it can suffocate originality. I think it was Sir James Jeans who said that the mark of a highly intelligent person was that he was able to select and remember the facts that were and would be of use to him and reject and forget the rest. In this very instance, is it not more important to have remembered what was said than to remember, for certain, who said it?

Professor David Hilbert of Gottingen University, perhaps the greatest mathematician of his time, is reported to have asked a group of mathematicians "Do you know why Einstein said the most original and profound things about space and time that have been said in our generation? Because he had learned nothing about all the philosophy and mathematics of time and space."*

There appears to be a remarkable consensus of opinion on this matter. In his fourth Fawley Lecture at Southampton University (October 17th, 1957) "The Strategy of Research", Sir George Thompson cites his father's views with approval. His father (J. J. Thompson of the Cavendish Laboratory, Cambridge) was accustomed to say that "the advice often given to students to start a problem by looking up the literature on it was wrong. They should start by thinking about it for some time for themselves; for once having read the ideas of others they would find it very difficult to produce original ones of their own. Afterwards read the literature."

One other important point should be made; it appears with great clarity in the discovery of penicillin. Discovery is often said to be a matter of luck. That is not so, unless it be agreed that luck is the ability to recognize the importance of a significant happening and take advantage of it at the moment when it occurs. Would we have discovered penicillin if we had picked up that Petri dish that Fleming found, unwashed, after a holiday weekend?†

But before moving on to consider in more detail other examples of hypotheses that have markedly influenced the course of one branch or another of science, a few general comments may be made on methods of testing hypotheses. Broadly speaking, there are two principal procedures. It may be possible to design an experiment that would appear to settle the matter or it may be necessary to extend one's observation of individual patients or of natural phenomena, as the case may be, in some particular direction.

As has been suggested, in neither case can final proof be attained, though this does not relieve the investigator of the requirement that his experiments must be as closely controlled as possible and his observations as frequent and

---

* From E. A. Parkyn's Introduction to Harvey's Motion of the Heart and Blood in Animals. Everyman's Library. J. M. Dent and Co., London.

* Bernstein, Jeremy. The New Yorker, March 17th, 1973, p. 45.
† As a matter of fact there was an element of luck in it too. Dr. Ian Maclean, who shared Fleming's laboratory with him at the time, promised to wash those dishes, but he could not resist the temptation to be happily carried off by the rugger team to attend a match in the West Country. "But for that," as Maclean used to say with a chuckle, "Fleming would never have discovered penicillin."

detailed as he can make them in order to exclude coincidence. Even so, the uncertainty inherent in inductive reasoning must always lead to caution in applying new "discoveries" in the treatment of human beings—if only because no scientific law can be conclusively verified however many experiments support it, whereas any scientific law could and might be conclusively falsified by a single experiment or observation.

As Bryan Magee puts it—however many white swans one may encounter, it is not certain that "All swans are white"; but the discovery of just one black swan falsifies the statement completely. It is not even true to say that repeated experiment increases the probability that the result consistently obtained is absolutely reliable. For instance, however often it is shown, at sea-level, that water boils at 100°C repetition of this demonstration will not alter the possibility or indeed the probability that someone else may try boiling it at the top of a mountain and get a different result.

An important responsibility, in fact the most important part of a scientist's duty in testing a hypothesis, takes its origin from this ever-present possibility that an exception may arise that falsifies his thesis. The requirement is that when he has reason to believe that he has discovered some new "fact" of science, he shall devote all this energies to trying—as Popper says—to overthrow his own discovery. If he succeeds in doing this he will admittedly have to modify his hypothesis, but he will also have discovered some new fact—as it were by chance—that may prove to be of greater value than his original discovery. If the water boiler climbs the mountain and finds that his 100°C rule no longer holds good, he will want to discover some new rule relating his altitude to the new boiling-point. Thus science grows—fertilized by its own integrity.

This approach as it applies to dentistry will be considered in some detail with instances illustrating how it has been used with advantage to explore problems with which the practitioner was faced; for it is in this field that the ultimate responsibility is brought to bear on the clinician. As Sir George Pickering points out ". . . it must always be remembered that so far as human disease is concerned, the first observation and the final proof, in so far as proof can ever be final, is made in man".*

The responsibility of the clinician is two-fold. It is he who has the best opportunity to find out in the first instance what additional knowledge is needed, and what further investigations should be embarked upon for the good of his patient. Sir Almroth Wright used to say that it was "the pain in the mind" induced by his inability to help his patient that drove him to devote most of his life to research.

At the other end of the investigation when a hypothesis has been formulated and tested in the laboratory, a further test must be carried out on the patient, once again by the clinician, and it is only when that proves successful that the hypothesis can be accepted for regular incorporation in clinical practice; even so, it must continue to be observed with a careful and critical eye for a long time.

The importance of recognizing this responsibility cannot be too strongly emphasized. Every operation and every

* *Medical Research. Priorities and Responsibilities*, W.H.O., 1970, p. 46.

course of treatment is, as Sir George reminds us, an experiment on a human being; and the result obtained should be recorded and so regarded. It forms the background of experience of the surgeon or physician and every clinician should remember that to take into general use a form of treatment that has not been subjected to the most stringent test is "amoral and antisocial". He adds that a good test a clinician should always apply is to ask himself whether he would carry out the procedure on a member of his own family or submit to it himself under corresponding circumstances.

At the same time a sense of proportion must be preserved, and the patient must not be deprived of the benefit of some valuable new discovery while philosophers argue the frailty of inductive reasoning. Scientific facts may not be absolutely verifiable, nor may we be able to say with certainty that they are even probably true, but if a particular procedure has always produced the desired result so far, we are so constituted that we shall place much confidence in the possibility that the luck will hold.

Perhaps by way of seeing how the procedure works out in practice, we may turn to one or two examples of the formulation and testing of hypotheses, and the first example, taken from the field of physics and astronomy, came about as the result of a most meticulous and prolonged observation of the four moons of Jupiter by the Danish astronomer Roemer in 1675.

It is an example of how a man who had made a very accurate and detailed study of a series of natural phenomena noticed a regularly recurring variation in the sequence of events for which there was at the time no adequate explanation.

If his observations had not been so precise or had not been pursued with so much diligence over so long a period, he would never have noted these variations and it would not have been possible for him to generate his hypothesis—a hypothesis which, having been tested, has been accepted as one of the most important laws of nature. The law is that light travels with a finite velocity, a velocity which (*in vacuo*) is now known to be constant.

Roemer's discovery came about in this way. He made out a time-table for the revolutions of Jupiter's four moons and found that in general they kept very accurately to schedule; but there was one important variation. When Jupiter was at a greater distance than average from the earth the moons appeared to run late; and correspondingly when Jupiter and Earth were nearer together than average the moons were early.

Roemer accordingly framed the hypothesis that this could be explained by assuming that the messenger which reached him—namely the light reflected from the moons—did not travel at an infinite velocity as had been assumed, but travelled at a finite speed and so took longer to reach us when Jupiter was further away from us and less time than average when it was nearer to us.

In support of this hypothesis, Roemer was able to calculate what this velocity was and arrived at a figure close to the value which is now generally agreed. His hypothesis was widely accepted because it fitted all the known facts so completely; and though Roemer did not live to see it, it was established beyond all reasonable doubt, 50 years later, when Bradley discovered the phenomena of aberration.

Our concern, however, is not with physics but with medicine and dentistry where biological problems are presented, and in this field the questions are not so clear-cut nor are the answers so precise and unambiguous. A page or two of dental history from the early part of this century may serve as an example to illustrate how and why hypotheses are sometimes developed but will also emphasize the danger of publishing or acting on a hypothesis that has not been adequately tested. It will in addition illustrate ways of testing hypotheses that have been devised, and the widely recognized fact that the solution of one problem often raised other, even more difficult ones.

In 1904 a paper was published in the Transactions of the Royal Society of Medicine suggesting that septic teeth and tonsils constituted a focus from which infection could spread throughout the body and cause disease in organs remote from the source of infection. No systematic attempt was made to prove the accuracy of this hypothesis but it was widely accepted on general principles, so widely in fact that twenty years later the Transactions published a paper containing a list, spreading over several pages, of diseases said to be caused or adversely influenced by focal infection; but once again still without any convincing evidence.

The application of this untested and as it was ultimately shown, fallacious, hypothesis was limited at first to cases where only obviously septic teeth were involved; cases in which pus could be expressed from the pockets or in the case of tonsils where there was a visible purulent discharge from their follicles. There was at that time, of course, no conservative treatment of periodontal disease—beyond scaling the teeth. At a later stage, as dental radiography developed, "dead teeth" were added to the black-list, showing, as they generally did, areas of apical rarefaction of the bone. On extraction the root canals and apices of most of these teeth were found to be infected. There was, therefore, evidence of infection related to the teeth but there was also a remarkable lack of any attempt to relate this infection experimentally or directly to the various diseases it was supposed to cause or influence. The list of these diseases included such diverse conditions as rheumatoid arthritis and diabetes (before insulin was made available).

It became the practice of many dentists to send extracted teeth to bacteriologists for culture, often at the request of the patient's doctor, whereupon a copious and mixed growth of organisms was obtained from the apices and sides of the root of practically all of them, irrespective of whether the pulp was alive or dead. This finding, though not perhaps very logically, provided additional ammunition for those who recommended the "clearance" of all teeth, and often of tonsils too, as a routine treatment for a very large number of diseases.

The final doom of teeth in general seemed to have been sealed when it was found that samples of blood taken from patients whose teeth had just been extracted were found to be infected with mouth organisms. The samples were taken for convenience while the patient was still anaesthetized or still in the dental chair, a circumstance that was subsequently shown to be of the greatest significance.

As to the damage that this untested hypothesis caused, it was responsible for the extraction of millions of sound teeth over a period of some 30 years. Soldiers were rendered unfit for front line service in the 1914–18 war because their sound natural teeth were extracted and their dentures broke or were lost or failed to cope with the "hard tack" that was often the only food available.

The most tragic result was that children (and adults too) suffering from rheumatic fever, involving the endocardium, which was not normally a threat to life, often had their teeth extracted; and the resulting bacteriaemia converted this rheumatic endocarditis into the infective variety from which they usually died. This was before antibiotics were available.

It will be clear from these notes that in a small percentage of cases patients were put at very serious risk, but it is unnecessary to emphasize to dental clinicians the widespread misery and disfigurement inflicted on so many other young patients by rendering them edentulous. The end results of these mutilations are still to be seen in the facial contours of older people today in whom bone resorption has emphasized the disfigurement caused by early extraction of the teeth.

From the medical angle the imaginary improvement that some doctors claimed to have observed in their patients' general condition was in many cases due to the fact that their misery was now concentrated on their dental problems and oral discomfort rather than on their rheumatism or whatever.

It is not surprising, therefore, that eventually the actual evidence that infection spread to other organs was subjected to more careful scrutiny. There could hardly have been a better reason for proceeding to test hypotheses that were leading to so much sickness and discomfort, and in some of these investigations the process of testing led to the need for new hypotheses to be generated.

For instance, the argument that swallowing pus must be harmful and especially liable to cause gastro-enteritis was one of the first to come under review. When an attempt was made to test this hypothesis, it was found that the bacteria on being swallowed were immediately killed and digested by the gastric juice; but this was not discovered until an enormous number of teeth had been sacrificed on that particular altar.

Then the hypothesis that rheumatoid arthritis was caused by oral sepsis was explored. It seemed reasonable at that time to suppose that if this were the case the organisms from the teeth would be found in and around the affected joints. They never were. They could not be demonstrated either histologically or bacteriologically. Thus, having found the original hypothesis to be false a new one had to be formulated. Accordingly, an alternative suggestion (that is an alternative hypothesis) was set up, to the effect that if not the organisms themselves, it was possibly some soluble toxic matter produced in relation to the septic teeth or tonsils that found its way to and affected these joints; but this lost support because of the presumption that if such toxic substances had been present collections of round cells should have been attracted to the site to deal with them, and nothing of the kind was ever found. Accordingly, a third hypothesis has since been formulated based on the phenomenon of auto-immunity (see Chapter 12).

There was a similar absence of bacteria when a corresponding investigation was made of the tissues surrounding the live teeth themselves *in situ*; yet when similar teeth were extracted they were all found to have bacteria on their roots. Cultures taken at biopsy under sterile conditions from the alveolar bone adjacent to these teeth were all negative; and at post-mortem it was found that the bone surrounding live teeth was consistently sterile and uninflamed.

The scientific foundation of this theory of focal infection was clearly turning out to be very shaky indeed; but up to this point the evidence against the theory was of a negative character. A positive hypothesis was therefore called for. It was that both the organisms on the roots of live teeth which were discovered after extraction of these teeth and also the bacteriaemia which followed immediately after extraction were due to the operation itself, and that the organisms were derived from the periodontal sulcus. This new hypothesis was suggested by the observation that the same strains of mouth bacteria were found in all three situations.

A method by which this hypothesis could be tested was worked out. It was decided to choose live teeth that for convenience were not too closely in contact with their neighbours but which displayed marked chronic marginal gingivitis. Under either general or local anaesthesia a cautery was passed rapidly but completely round the gingival sulcus of the selected tooth thereby effectively sterilizing it. The tooth was then immediately extracted before any saliva could reach it and re-infect the sulcus. Twelve teeth were extracted in this way and subjected to the usual bacteriological test. The apices, root canals and sides of the roots of all these teeth were found to be sterile except for an odd colony which the bacteriologist was satisfied to attribute to incidental atmospheric contamination.

The control comprised the innumerable live teeth extracted without sterilization of the sulcus, virtually all of which had shown severe contamination with precisely the same organisms as could be cultivated direct from the sulci before extraction. The experiment was further controlled by taking blood samples approximately one minute after extraction of these teeth. The samples were all found to be sterile whereas extraction without sterilization of the sulcus almost always produced a bacteriaemia as demonstrated in a blood sample similarly taken one minute after extraction.

An interesting corroboration of the accuracy of this hypothesis lay in the fact that close examination of the pulps of healthy live teeth, extracted without sterilization of the sulcus, occasionally disclosed bacteria actually in the lumen of the capillaries. These bacteria were obviously only in transit; they could not have been lodged even temporarily in such a situation.

In this way it was established that both the infection on the roots of live teeth and also the bacteriaemia observed after extraction originated from the gingival sulcus and that both were caused by the operation. It seemed reasonable to suppose, therefore, that the pumping effect of the movements of the tooth in its socket during extraction coupled with the wounds caused by the beaks of the forceps and the tearing of the tooth attachment introduced bacteria into the vessels of the pulp before the tooth attachment finally gave way. It also seemed likely that the bacteria entering the blood and lymphatic vessels of the periodontal membrane would either immediately or ultimately be destroyed as they passed through the lymphoid tissue of the cervical glands or the spleen or other lymphatic tissue of the body; in which case the bacteriaemia would be purely transient. In the event, this proved to be the case and samples of blood taken 10 min. or more after the extraction were invariably found to be sterile.

These findings, coupled with the facts that extraction of the teeth never seemed to cure any of the diseases they were alleged to have caused and that patients who had been edentulous for years seemed to get these same diseases just as often as those with oral sepsis, caused the focal infection theory to die a natural, albeit a lingering, death. It took almost 25 years and the theory lingered on in places until the Second World War; but of course work had been going on at the other end of the problem too, and the physicians had arrived at the same conclusion as the dental research workers.

Perhaps one other example of a hypothesis being generated to solve a clinical problem may be cited. It shows how the investigation of one hypothesis leads to the inception of another. In this further example a different kind of procedure had to be adopted in testing its accuracy.

Following on the demonstration of bacteria being forced into the blood stream by the operation of extraction of a tooth, other dental operations came under scrutiny. For example, where the pulp had become exposed under a carious lesion and an abscess had formed in the pulp, it was usual either to extract the tooth or to remove the pulp under local anaesthesia using a barbed broach. This latter procedure was not infrequently followed by the development of an acute apical abscess or conversely by a chronic granuloma. In either event, it was clear that the apical canals were infected.

In the case of those teeth that were extracted immediately on presentation in the casualty department, it was found on histological examination that in most instances the radicular portion of the pulp was alive and the abscess was confined to the pulp chamber at the point of exposure. Moreover, the living apical part of the pulp showed in most cases a normal structure, apparently free from both bacteria and inflammation.

Since the apical canals were so often infected after surgical removal of the pulp but not before, and in the light of experience of the cause of the bacteriaemia and infection of the apices following the extraction of live teeth, it seemed probable that the root canals of a tooth which were sterile before the operation of pulpectomy were also infected at the time of operation, but in this instance from the abscess in the pulp.

It is hardly necessary to use any imagination at all to realize that thrusting a barbed broach through the abscess and down into the canal would in itself infect the canal; but how much more would the next manoeuvre of pulling the pulp out of the pulp chamber suck the infected fluids down into the root canals? Not only so but the operation was almost certain to cause a general bacteriaemia, and since this was a simple matter to determine, it was checked and found to be the case. A bacteriaemia invariably followed the avulsion of an infected but still vital pulp by using a barbed broach, under nitrous oxide anaesthesia.

The hypothesis having therefore been framed, the following experiment was carried out using only single-rooted teeth. After full exposure of the necrotic pulp with as little disturbance of it as possible, nitrous oxide anaesthesia was induced and a fine cautery loop was used to burn out the pulp debris *in situ*. This probably destroyed all the bacteria in the pulp chamber; but to avoid the danger that some had remained alive the contents of the root canal were also burnt out with an electrically heated root-canal probe, and the accessible part of the canal, thus sterilized, was immediately filled and sealed-off. A blood sample was taken as soon as the operation was over and in no case had it caused a bacteriaemia. The final test of this hypothesis on the human subject was that, having cautiously taken this procedure into practice, subsequent radiological checks were carried out for many years on the teeth so treated and only in one case did the tooth show any evidence of apical infection—and in this case there had been an obvious fault in procedure.

These examples have been chosen to show the general approach that is employed in generating and testing a hypothesis in clinical dental practice. They illustrate more clearly than any mere affirmation could that research is primarily the responsibility of the clinician, not of the research worker in the laboratory. The laboratory research department is basically established to enable the clinician to obtain more easily and conveniently the scientific information he needs to treat his patients more efficiently. Of course, skills have become so complex and time-consuming in both fields that to be expert in both is more than one man could contrive.

Admittedly the laboratory research department must be staffed by extremely competent scientists; and inevitably they will wish to spend at least a proportion of their time seeking to assuage their thirst for an answer to some intriguing problem that has emerged, though the solution might not immediately be clinically useful; but their first responsibility is to increase the clinician's efficiency.

It is unfortunate that the men who are concerned with laboratory research should tend to become isolated from clinical experience; but they should certainly be invited to observe the results when their findings have been put into practice. It would be equally sad if clinicians were to feel themselves shut out of the laboratories or were to acquiesce with apparently contented resignation in leaving their microscopes and histological material behind them in dental school when they go out into practice.

It cannot be over-emphasized in teaching students that the careful basic instruction they receive in school in anatomy, histology and physiology is only a preparation for the study and treatment of dental disease in the living human patient. Dental pathology and especially histopathology must provide the background of every operation they perform, if they are to deserve and achieve the status of scientific professional people.

If it be agreed that every operation on a patient is an experiment, then it follows that these operations should not be performed except by surgeons who are thoroughly conversant with every anatomical detail of the tissues on which they are operating and of the changes that may take place when these tissues are disturbed or attacked by disease. If a student finds that he is unable to become interested in the scientific background of his professional activities, he would be well advised to seek other fields of employment before he becomes too committed.

Every clinician should himself also be carrying out some kind of investigation, making some effort to discover better clinical procedures based on a constantly growing understanding of the disease processes he daily observes. Unless he is prepared to regard his daily practice in this light he can hardly claim to be more than a technician carrying out such mechanical procedures as he has been taught.

It is all-important to realize that to frame hypotheses and put them to the test is not the prerogative of ancient astronomers or modern boffins. This method of seeking new knowledge (or satisfying curiosity, or assuaging Almroth Wright's "pain in the mind") is within the compass of the practising clinician providing that he has the will to work and the intellectual discipline to examine his results impartially and objectively.

INDEX